AF183421

Clinical Guide to Musculoskeletal Medicine

S. Ali Mostoufi • Tony K. George • Alfred J. Tria Jr.
Editors

Clinical Guide to Musculoskeletal Medicine

A Multidisciplinary Approach

Springer

Editors
S. Ali Mostoufi
Department of Orthopedics and Rehabilitation
Tufts University School of Medicine
Boston, MA, USA

New England Spine Care Associates & Boston
Regenerative Medicine
Cambridge, MA, USA

Tony K. George
Restorative Orthopaedics Spine &
Sports (ROSS) Institute
Somerset, NJ, USA

Alfred J. Tria Jr.
Department of Orthopedics
Rutgers-Robert Wood Johnson Medical School
New Brunswick, NJ, USA

ISBN 978-3-030-92041-8 ISBN 978-3-030-92042-5 (eBook)
https://doi.org/10.1007/978-3-030-92042-5

© The Editor(s) (if applicable) and The Author(s), under exclusive license to Springer Nature Switzerland AG 2022
This work is subject to copyright. All rights are solely and exclusively licensed by the Publisher, whether the whole or part of the material is concerned, specifically the rights of translation, reprinting, reuse of illustrations, recitation, broadcasting, reproduction on microfilms or in any other physical way, and transmission or information storage and retrieval, electronic adaptation, computer software, or by similar or dissimilar methodology now known or hereafter developed.
The use of general descriptive names, registered names, trademarks, service marks, etc. in this publication does not imply, even in the absence of a specific statement, that such names are exempt from the relevant protective laws and regulations and therefore free for general use.
The publisher, the authors and the editors are safe to assume that the advice and information in this book are believed to be true and accurate at the date of publication. Neither the publisher nor the authors or the editors give a warranty, expressed or implied, with respect to the material contained herein or for any errors or omissions that may have been made. The publisher remains neutral with regard to jurisdictional claims in published maps and institutional affiliations.

This Springer imprint is published by the registered company Springer Nature Switzerland AG
The registered company address is: Gewerbestrasse 11, 6330 Cham, Switzerland

To my father Dr. Kazem Mostoufi. My greatest teacher, role model, and the best physician I know.
To my mother Shokooh and sister Shiva for lifelong guidance, support, and love
To my children Cameron, Yasmine, and Ariana. You keep me on my toes and give me a purpose in life to be the best dad I can be.
To my wife, Eva. Your unconditional love and selfless support have been instrumental in my academic and professional journey. I love you.
—S. Ali Mostoufi

For Dr. John Neville Insall who taught me so much.
—Alfred J. Tria Jr.

To God, the giver of life abundant.
To Dad, for discipline and counsel.
To Mom, for prayer and unconditional love.
To Mridula, Aden, and Arielle for love and support.
To Dr. Mostoufi, for friendship and guidance.
To Dr. Tria, for vision and boldness.
—Tony K. George

Foreword

When Dr. Fred Tria called and invited me to write the foreword to *Clinical Guide to Musculoskeletal Medicine: A Multidisciplinary Approach,* I told him I would be delighted. For almost four decades, Fred and I have been friends and professional colleagues, collaborating and editing several textbooks. He has always been a driving force striving to enrich the medical community with contemporary and relevant publications on conditions of the musculoskeletal system. This current book, which he co-edited with Ali Mostoufi, MD, and Tony George, DO, is a comprehensive compendium of musculoskeletal disorders that all clinicians will find a valuable addition to their personal library.

This is a comprehensive text with chapters on the spine, and upper extremity and lower extremity injuries written by experts in orthopedic surgery, neurosurgery, physical medicine, neurology, radiology, and anesthesia. Adding to the contemporary nature of the book are sections on sport specific injuries and regenerative medicine. The format of each chapter provides an in-depth description of the etiology and clinical presentation of specific musculoskeletal disorders with instruction on the physical examination, diagnostic tests, and imaging, along with non-operative and operative treatments. All chapters are supported with descriptive illustrations, images, and figures, providing the foundation for the differential diagnosis for maladies of each anatomic site. This helps establish standards of practice, clinical guidelines, and an interdisciplinary approach, which the reader will find as a valuable clinical guide.

Both acute and chronic musculoskeletal maladies are common conditions. A wide spectrum of specialists require a working knowledge of these injuries, including but not limited to orthopedic surgeons, physiatrists, and primary care physicians. While this may be the anticipated target audience, it is my expectation and hope that this book will be a valuable resource for all healthcare providers.

Giles R. Scuderi, MD, FACS, FAAOS
Zucker School of Medicine at Hofstra/Northwell
Hempstead, NY, USA

Foreword

The *Clinical Guide to Musculoskeletal Medicine: An Interdisciplinary Approach* represents a long-overdue addition to the educational resources for medical students, residents, fellows, both early- and late-career practicing physicians, and other musculoskeletal clinicians.

Deficiencies in medical student knowledge in musculoskeletal medicine have been well documented in the literature. Musculoskeletal problems number among the most common seen by primary care providers, yet US medical school instruction in musculoskeletal medicine has been found to be practically absent or inadequate by many.

There is a need for an easily digestible and understandable resource that will be embraced by individuals that want to become proficient in the practice of musculoskeletal medicine. The authors/editors of the "*Clinical Guide*" have successfully achieved this goal. The editors, Drs. Mostoufi, George, and Tria are committed educators that put together a dedicated group of multidisciplinary physician authors to fill this need and focus on valuable clinical musculoskeletal information.

The "*Clinical Guide*" presents pertinent musculoskeletal pathologies and treatments in a well-organized and concise way. It addresses the more commonly challenging musculoskeletal pathologies that clinicians are faced with and potential treatment options when treating patients day to day. Each chapter dedicated to a particular pathology covers clinical presentation, physical examination, diagnostic workup, and treatment. In addition, there are chapters dedicated to innovative and established treatments such as regenerative medicine and spinal surgeries. This enables the clinician to learn in an organized way and use the book as a reference when working in the clinical realm. Also, illustrations, tables, and relevant imaging are embedded in the individual chapters and enhance this book as an educational tool.

Finally, the interdisciplinary approach of this book, inclusive of physical medicine and rehabilitation and orthopedics, gives the clinician multiple tools to work with when addressing musculoskeletal pathologies and challenges with their patients. This is essential when attempting to achieve optimal clinical outcomes.

In closing, as an educator and physical medicine and rehabilitation residency program director for over 25 years, I am grateful to this team of musculoskeletal clinicians for filling this much needed void. The editors have addressed an essential need in medical education, and they have done so in a concise, learner friendly, and effective way. Their efforts should be congratulated!

Thank you Drs. Mostoufi, George, and Tria!

Sara Cuccurullo, MD
Professor and Chairman, Department of Physical Medicine and Rehabilitation
Hackensack Meridian School of Medicine, Nutley, NJ, USA

Medical Director, Vice President, JFK Johnson Rehabilitation Institute, Edison, NJ, USA

Residency Program Director, Rutgers – Robert Wood Johnson Medical School
New Brunswick, NJ, USA

Physician in Chief, HMH Rehabilitation Care Transformation Services
Boston, MA, USA

Preface

Musculoskeletal conditions including spine disorders, tendinopathies, and joint disease are remarkably common, leading to disability and impairment. Subspecialty training in musculoskeletal conditions has always been popular among trainees; however, over the last two decades, there has been a renewed interest largely due to rapid expansion in the minimally invasive procedures in spine care and sports medicine using fluoroscopes, endoscopes, robotics, and ultrasound in addition to significant clinical interest in regenerative medicine. Minimally invasive spine, sports, and regenerative treatments have complemented advances in rehabilitation (PT/OT) and modern MIS surgical techniques available to patients suffering from degenerative or acquired skeletal conditions.

Clinical Guide to Musculoskeletal Medicine covers the most common MSK diagnoses that a seasoned clinician or a resident/fellow in training will encounter in an outpatient setting or at a sports sideline. We believe this book is valuable across many specialties, including physiatry, orthopedics, sports medicine, rheumatology, neurology, internal medicine, pain medicine, and physical therapy. The book is unique since many chapters are written as a collaboration between non-surgical and surgical providers such as physiatrist, orthopedist, and physical therapists. The contributing authors have been carefully selected based on their expertise in the topic, and they are members of highly respected academic institutions in the USA and across the world.

This book is divided into X parts. The first nine parts are based on body parts, including the head, spine, pelvic/trunk, and all major joints. Each joint is subdivided into four anatomical regions (anterior, lateral, medial, posterior), corresponding to the patient's chief complaint at the time of visit. Part X is dedicated to various conditions that intersect musculoskeletal conditions and other medical disciplines. Throughout the book, topics are presented in a uniform format so the reader can rapidly access needed information with ease. The format includes Synonyms, Current ICD-10 code, Description, Clinical Presentation, Physical Exam, Diagnostic Workup, and Treatments (medical, rehabilitation, procedures, surgery). Many chapters focus on the modern minimally invasive spine and sports medicine procedural and surgical techniques to enhance the book's utility. A portion of the book is dedicated to regenerative medicine, covering the basic science as well as its musculoskeletal applications based on the current body of evidence.

As editors, we are grateful to our contributing authors for lending their expertise and producing evidence-based information presented in this book. Without our authors' generosity, this book would not have been possible. We thank Kristopher Spring and his team at Springer, who were instrumental in bringing this book to publication. Finally, we are grateful to our patients who trust us with their lives and inspire us to explore the boundaries of science and produce educational material for the next generation of musculoskeletal physicians.

Boston, MA, USA S. Ali Mostoufi, Editor-in-chief, MD, FAAPMR, DABPM

Acknowledgments

We would especially like to recognize the contributions of our two associate editors: Dr. Jason Zaremski and Dr. Timothy Tiu. They both dedicated an extraordinary amount of time to help develop and finish this text.

Jason is an associate professor at the University of Florida and works as a non-operative musculoskeletal and sports medicine physician and as the university's NCAA collegial team physician. He has published more than 100 peer-reviewed articles, posters, and abstracts specific to all areas of sports medicine. His unique interest in upper extremity injuries and injuries specific to throwing was central in developing the sections on the upper extremity. He is an elected member in the board of directors of the American Medical Society for Sports Medicine (AMSSM) and a fellow of the American College of Sports Medicine (ACSM).

He is an elected member in the board of directors of the American Medical Society for Sports Medicine (AMSSM) and a fellow of the American College of Sports Medicine (ACSM).

Tim is Assistant Professor of PM&R/Sports Medicine at the University of Miami and the medical director of the Lynn Rehabilitation Center there. He has a strong interest in sports medicine and US-guided interventions in sports medicine and orthopedics. His publications on ultrasonography and biomechanical manipulation made him especially valuable in editing the chapters on the lower extremity. He is involved with the American Medical Society for Sports Medicine (AMSSM) as well as the American College of Sports Medicine (ACSM).

We thank them both and wish them even greater success in the future.

Contents

Contributors

Magda Aldousany, DPT Department of Kinesiology & Sport Sciences, University of Miami School of Education and Human Development, Miami, FL, USA

Swetha Ann Alexander, MBBS Department of Internal Medicine, University of Connecticut, Farmington, CT, USA

Kelly Alhooie, DPT OrthoPelvic Physical Therapy, Sterling, VA, USA

Todd Alter, MD Rutgers-Robert Wood Johnson Medical School, Department of Orthopedic Surgery, New Brunswick, NJ, USA

Armando Alvarez, MD, MPH Department of Physical Medicine & Rehabilitation, University of Miami Miller School of Medicine, Miami, FL, USA

Jomar Aryee, MD Department of Orthopaedics, Rutgers-Robert Wood Johnson Medical School, New Brunswick, NJ, USA

John Avila, PT Department of Physical Medicine and Rehabilitation, Northwestern University Feinberg School of Medicine, Chicago, IL, USA

Ogochukwu Azuh, MD Department of Physical Medicine and Rehabilitation, Memorial Healthcare, Owosso, MI, USA

Chandler Berke, MD Department of Orthopaedics, Rutgers-Robert Wood Johnson Medical School, New Brunswick, NJ, USA

William A. Berrigan, MD Clinical Sports Medicine Fellow, Department of Physical Medicine and Rehabilitation, Emory University School of Medicine, Atlanta, GA, USA

Joanne Borg-Stein, MD, FAAPMR Associate Professor, Department of Physical Medicine & Rehabilitation, Spaulding Rehabilitation Hospital, Massachusetts General Hospital, Harvard Medical School, Boston, MA, USA

Chief of Physical Medicine and Rehabilitation, Newton Wellesley Hospital, Medical Director: Spine Center at Newton Wellesley Hospital, Newton, MA, USA

Haylee Borgstrom, MD, MS, FAAPMR Clinical Instructor, Department of Physical Medicine & Rehabilitation, Spaulding Rehabilitation Hospital, Massachusetts General Hospital, Harvard Medical School, Boston, MA, USA

Robert Bowers, DO Assistant Professor and Director of the Emory Baseball Medicine Program, Department of Orthopaedics and Physical Medicine and Rehabilitation, Emory University School of Medicine, Atlanta, GA, USA

David P. Brown, DO Professor, Physical Medicine & Rehabilitation, Rutgers -Robert Wood Johnson Medical School, Medical Director Electrodiagnostics & Sports Medicine, JFK, Johnson Rehabilitation Institute, Edison, NJ, USA

Andrzej Brzezinski, MD Department of Orthopaedics, Rutgers-Robert Wood Johnson Medical School, New Brunswick, NJ, USA

Ryan Budwany, MD WVU Center for Integrative Pain Medicine, Morgantown, West Virginia, USA

Andrew J. Butler, MD Department of Orthopaedic Surgery, Robert Wood Johnson University School of Medicine, New Brunswick, NJ, USA

Department of Orthopaedic Surgery, Rutgers-Robert Wood Johnson Medical School, New Brunswick, NJ, USA

Charles Cassidy, MD Chairman and Professor, Department of Orthopedic & Rehabilitation Medicine, Tufts University School of Medicine, Tufts Medical Center, Boston, MA, USA

Department of Orthopedic Surgery, Tufts Medical Center, Boston, MA, USA

Department of Orthopedics, Tufts Medical Center, Boston, MA, USA

Ya-Ting Chen, MD Department of Physical Medicine and Rehabilitation, Harvard Medical School, Boston, MA, USA

Chu H. Chiang, MBBS, MSc Trauma and Orthopaedic Registrar, Kent Surrey and Sussex Deanery, NHS Foundation Trust, Canterbury, Kent, UK

Joseph Chin, MD Department of Physical Medicine and Rehabilitation, New York Presbyterian Weill Cornell Medical Center, Columbia University Irving Medical Center, New York, NY, USA

Nicholas J. Coccoluto, BS Tufts University School of Medicine, Boston, MA, USA

Eileen M. Colliton, MD Department of Orthopedic & Rehabilitation Medicine, Tufts Medical Center, Boston, MA, USA

Jeanie Cote, MD Department of Neurology/Neuroimmunology, Memorial Healthcare, Owosso, MI, USA

Ashley Cotter, PT MGH Brigham Rehabilitation Services, Harvard Medical School, Boston, MA, USA

Alexander M. Crawford, MD Harvard Combined Orthopaedic Residency Program, Harvard Medical School, Boston, MA, USA

Gerard D'Onofrio, DO Department of Rehabilitation Medicine, New York Presbyterian, New York, NY, USA

Abhijeet Danve, MD FACP Assistant Professor of Medicine (Rheumatology); Director of Yale Spondyloarthritis Program, Yale School of Medicine, New Haven, CT, USA

Timothy R. Deer, MD, DABPM Professor of Anesthesia, West Virginia School of Medicine, CEO of The Spine and Nerve Center of the Virginias, Charleston, WV, USA

Kevin De Jesus, MD Department of PM&R and Sports Medicine, University of Puerto Rico School of Medicine, San Juan, PR, USA

Arthur Jason De Luigi, DO, MHSA Chairman, Department of Physical Medicine & Rehabilitation, Mayo Clinic Arizona, Phoenix, AZ, USA

Director of Sports Medicine, Mayo Clinic Arizona, Mayo Clinic School of Medicine, Phenix, AZ, USA

Stephanie DeLuca, MD Clinical Fellow, Department of Physical Medicine & Rehabilitation, Spaulding Rehabilitation Hospital, Harvard Medical School, Charlestown, MA, USA

Abby Dillard, PT, DPT Department of Physical Therapy and Occupational Therapy, Duke University Health System, Durham, NC, USA

Cathy Duddy, PT, DPT, MS, CSCS Department of Physical Therapy, Mount Auburn Hospital, Harvard Medical School, Cambridge, MA, USA

Christopher Elmore, MD Department of Physical Medicine and Rehabilitation, Tufts Medical Center, Boston, MA, USA

Steven Falowski, MD Director, Functional Neurosurgery, Neurosurgical Associates of Lancaster, Lancaster, PA, USA

Jaleh Fatehi, MD Department of Neurology, University of Alberta, Edmonton, Canada

Abdolrahman Fazli, MD Orthopedic Department, Queen Elizabeth The Queen Mother Hospital, East Kent Hospitals University, NHS Foundation Trust, Margate, UK

Department of Orthopedics, Manipal Academy of Higher Education, Manipal, India

Luis Feigenbaum, PT, DPT Senior Associate Athletics Director for Performance, Health and Wellness, Miller School of Medicine, University of Miami, Miami, FL, USA

Andrew Felber, BA Tufts University School of Medicine, Boston, MA, USA

Gisela Figueroa, DPT Department of Rehabilitation Medicine, New York Presbyterian, New York, NY, USA

Richard Fontanez, MD Department PM&R and Sports Medicine, University of Puerto Rico, San Juan, PR, USA

Physical Medicine, Rehabilitation and Sports Medicine Department, University of Puerto Rico, School of Medicine, San Juan, PR, USA

Tony K. George, DO, FAAPMR Restorative Orthopaedics Spine & Sports (ROSS) Institute, Somerset, NJ, USA

Professor Emeritus, Department of Orthopaedics, Rutgers-Robert Wood Johnson Medical School, New Brunswick, NJ, USA

Ashleigh Gibula, BS Tufts University School of Medicine, Boston, MA, USA

Figueroa Gisela Department of Rehabilitation Medicine, New York Presbyterian, New York, NY, USA

Anna H. Green, MD Robert Wood Johnson University School of Medicine, Department of Orthopaedic Surgery, New Brunswick, NJ, USA

Laura Griffin, DO, FAAO Professor, Chair of the Osteopathic Principles and Practices Department, Kentucky College of Osteopathic Medicine, University of Pikeville, Pikeville, KY, USA

Padma Gulur, MD Professor of Anesthesiology and Population Health Sciences, Executive Vice Chair, Department of Anesthesiology, Duke University School of Medicine, Durham, NC, USA

Daniel Haddad, MD Department of Orthopaedics, Rutgers-Robert Wood Johnson Medical School, New Brunswick, NJ, USA

Jonathan M. Hagedorn, MD Department of Anesthesiology and Perioperative Medicine, Division of Pain Medicine, Mayo Clinic, Rochester, MN, USA

Mo Hamouda, MD, DABPM Assistant Professor, Department of Anesthesia, University of Colorado School of Medicine, Denver, CO, USA

Andrew Hecht, MD Professor, Orthopedics and Neurosurgery, Icahn School of Medicine at Mount Sinai, Chief of Spine Surgery for the Mount Sinai Health System, New York, NY, USA

Jennifer Hoffman, MD Assistant Professor, Department of Orthopaedics & Rehabilitation Medicine, Tufts University School of Medicine, Boston, MA, USA

Jennifer Soo Hoo, MD Assistant Professor, Department of Rehabilitation Medicine, Medical Director in Sports Medicine, Weill Cornell Medicine, New York, NY, USA

Associate Director of Sports Medicine Fellowship, New York Presbyterian, New York, NY, USA

Casey Imbergamo, MD Department of Orthopaedics, Rutgers-Robert Wood Johnson Medical School, New Brunswick, NJ, USA

Zacharia Isaac, MD Assistant Professor of Physical Medicine and Rehabilitation, Harvard Medical School, Medical Director of the Comprehensive Spine Care Center, Brigham and Woman's Hospital, Boston, MA, USA

Savion Johnson, MD Department of Anesthesiology, Duke University School of Medicine, Durham, NC, USA

David J. Kennedy, MD President, Spine Interventional Society, Professor and Chair, Department of Physical Medicine & Rehabilitation, Vanderbilt University, Nashville, TN, USA

Woo A. Kim Department of Orthopedics, Kent Surrey and Sussex Deanery, NHS Foundation Trust, Kent, UK

Augustine Lee, MD Department of Physical Medicine and Rehabilitation, Vanderbilt University Medical Center, Vanderbilt University School of Medicine, Nashville, TN, USA

Harry M. Lightsey IV, MD Harvard Combined Orthopaedic Residency Program, Harvard Medical School, Boston, MA, USA

Lei Lin, MD, PHD JFK, Johnson Rehabilitation Institute, Edison, NJ, USA

Garett Lui, MD Department of Orthopedics & Rehabilitation Medicine, Tufts University School of Medicine, Boston, MA, USA

Gerard Malanga, MD Founder, New Jersey Orthopaedic and Sports Medicine, Founder, New Jersey Regenerative Institute, Hanover, NJ, USA

Department of Physical Medicine & Rehabilitation, Rutgers School of Medicine, Newark, NJ, USA

George Ross Malik, MD Shirley Ryan Ability Lab & Department of Physical Medicine and Rehabilitation, Northwestern University Feinberg School of Medicine, Chicago, IL, USA

Jonathan S. Markowitz, MD Department of Orthopaedic Surgery, Icahn School of Medicine at Mount Sinai, New York, NY, USA

Julio A. Martinez-Silvestrini, MD Baystate Rehabilitation Care, University of Massachusetts Medical School – Baystate, Longmeadow, MA, USA

Adjunct Faculty, Tufts University School of Medicine, Boston, MA, USA

Associate Professor, University of Massachusetts Medical School – Baystate, Longmeadow, MA, USA

Baystate Physical Medicine and Rehabilitation, Baystate Medical Center, Springfield, MA, USA

Joshua Martin, MD New Jersey Regenerative Institute, Hanover, NJ, USA

Regenerative Orthopedics and Sports Medicine (ROSM), Reston, VA, USA

Kenneth Mautner, MD, FAAPMR Director of Primary Care Sports Medicine Fellowship, Emory University, Atlanta, GA, USA

Associate Professor, Department of Orthopaedics and Physical Medicine and Rehabilitation, Emory University School of Medicine, Atlanta, GA, USA

Kelly C. McInnis, DO, FAAPMR Program Director, Harvard–Spaulding PM&R Sports Medicine Fellowship, Assistant Professor of Physical Medicine and Rehabilitation, Harvard Medical School, Boston, MA, USA

Rojeh Melikian, MD DISC Spine and Sports, Marina Del Ray, CA, USA

Steven Mennona, MD Department of Orthopaedics, Rutgers-Robert Wood Johnson Medical School, New Brunswick, NJ, USA

William Micheo, MD Professor and Chairman, Department PM&R and Sports Medicine, University of Puerto Rico, San Juan, PR, USA

Derek Miles, PT, DPT Department of Physical Therapy, Barbell Medicine, Cincinnati, OH, USA

Emily Mostofi, MD Department of Neurology, University of Alberta, Edmonton, AB, Canada

Seyed Behrooz Mostofi, MBBS, FRCS (Tr &Orth) Consultant Orthopaedic Foot and Ankle surgeon, East Kent Hospitals University, NHS Foundation Trust, Canterbury, Kent, UK

Visiting Professor, Department of Orthopedics, Manipal Academy of Higher Education, Manipal, India

S. Ali Mostoufi, MD, FAAPMR, DABPM Assistant Professor, Department of Orthopedics and Rehabilitation, Tufts University School of Medicine, Boston, MA, USA

New England Spine Care Associates & Boston Regenerative Medicine, Cambridge, MA, USA

Department of Orthopaedics, Rutgers-Robert Wood Johnson Medical School, New Brunswick, NJ, USA

Ariana Mostoufi Medical Illustrator, Junior at Concord Carlisle High School, Concord, MA, USA

Behzad Mostoufi, DDS, MDS, FACDS Department of Oral and Maxillofacial Surgery, University of Maryland, Baltimore, MD, USA

Cameron Mostoufi Department of Mechanical Engineering, Purdue University, West Lafayette, IN, USA

Emanuel Mostoufi, MD Department of Neurology, University of Alberta School of Medicine, Calgary, CA, USA

Yasmine Mostoufi Medical Illustration and Image Optimization, Senior at Landmark High School, Beverly, MA, USA

Medical Illustration and Image Optimization, Senior at Landmark High Schoo, Beverly, MA, USA

Matthew H. Nasra, MD Robert Wood Johnson University School of Medicine, New Brunswick, NJ, USA

Department of Orthopaedic Surgery, Rutgers-Robert Wood Johnson Medical School, New Brunswick, NJ, USA

Giorgio Negron, MD Department of Orthopaedics and Physical Medicine and Rehabilitation, Emory University School of Medicine, Atlanta, GA, USA

Amanda Nelli, MD Duke Anesthesiology, Durham, NC, USA

Oluseun Olufade, MD Assistant Professor of Orthopaedics and Physical Medicine & Rehabilitation, Emory University School of Medicine, Atlanta, GA, USA

Bobby Oommen, MD Champlain Spine & Pain Management, Champlain Valley Physicians Hospital, The University of Vermont Health Network, Plattsburgh, NY, USA

Sagar S. Parikh, MD Assistant Professor, Hackensack Meridian School of Medicine, Nutley, NJ, USA

Gabriel S. Perrone, MS, MD Department of Orthopaedics, Tufts Medical Center, Boston, MA, USA

Eric W. Pettyjohn, MD Sports Medicine Fellow, UF Health, University of Florida, Gainesville, FL, USA

Carolyn Poston, PT The Spine and Nerve Center of the Virginias, Charleston, WV, USA

Tricia Prince, DO, MS Assistant Professor, Department of Physical Medicine & Rehabilitation, University of Miami Miller School of Medicine, Miami, FL, USA

Marina Protopapas, DO National Spine and Pain Centers, Fairfax, VA, USA

Paragi Rana, MD Assistant Professor of Anesthesiology, Yale School of Medicine, New Haven, CT, USA

Monica E. Rho, MD Chief of Musculoskeletal Medicine at Shirley Ryan Ability Lab, Associate Professor, Department of Physical Medicine and Rehabilitation, Northwestern University Feinberg School of Medicine, Chicago, IL, USA

Cara Rodriguez, OTR/L, CHT Department of Physical and Occupational Therapy, Tufts Medical Center, Boston, MA, USA

Department of Occupational Therapy, Tufts Medical Center, Boston, MA, USA

Darren C. Rosenberg, DO Assistant Professor of Physical Medicine and Rehabilitation, Harvard Medical School, Boston, MA, USA

Director, Osteopathic Manipulative Medicine, Spaulding Rehabilitation Network, Boston, MA, USA

Riley Rousakis, MS, OTR/L Boston Sports & Biologics PC, Private Practice, Wellesley, MA, USA

Department of Physical Medicine and Rehabilitation, Veterans Administration Medical Center, Boston, MA, USA

Tomas Salazar, MD JFK, Johnson Rehabilitation Institute, Edison, NJ, USA

John M. Sands, DDS, MD Department of Oral and Maxillofacial Surgery, University of Maryland, Baltimore, MD, USA

Michael F. Saulle, DO, FAAPMR, CAQSM Assistant Professor of Rehabilitation and Regenerative Medicine, New York Presbyterian Weill Cornell Medical Center, Columbia University Irving Medical Center, Tarrytown, NY, USA

Dawood Sayed, MD, DABPM Professor of Anesthesiology and Pain Medicine, The University of Kansas Health System, Vice Chairman of the Board, The American Society of Pain and Neuroscience (ASPN), Chief of Pain Medicine, The University of Kansas Health System, Kansas City, KS, USA

Sean Schowalter, MD Department of Physical Medicine & Rehabilitation, Spaulding Rehabilitation Hospital, Harvard Medical School, Charlestown, MA, USA

Charles Scott, MD Assistant Professor of Rehabilitation and Regenerative Medicine, Columbia University Medical Center, New Yourk, NY, USA

Shiv T. Sehra, MD Rheumatology Division Chief, Mount Auburn Hospital, Harvard University, Cambridge, MA, USA

Assistant Professor of Medicine, Harvard Medical School, Boston, MA, USA

Fernando Sepulveda, MD Professor, Department PM&R and Sports Medicine, University of Puerto Rico, San Juan, PR, USA

Physical Medicine, Rehabilitation and Sports Medicine Department, University of Puerto Rico, School of Medicine, San Juan, PR, USA

Margaret Shields, MD Department of Orthopaedics and Rehabilitation Medicine, Tufts Medical Center, Boston, MA, USA

Jeremy Silver, MD Department of Orthopaedics, Rutgers-Robert Wood Johnson Medical School, New Brunswick, NJ, USA

Andrew K. Simpson, MD, MBA, MHS Assistant Professor and Director of Minimally Invasive Spine Surgery, Department of Orthopaedic Surgery, Brigham and Women's Hospital, Harvard Medical School, Boston, MA, USA

Alexandra St Clair, MS, OTR/L Department of Occupational Therapy, Tufts Medical Center, Boston, MA, USA

John Stelmach, MD Department of Orthopaedics, Rutgers-Robert Wood Johnson Medical School, New Brunswick, NJ, USA

Kyungje Sung, MD Department of Orthopedics & Rehabilitation Medicine, Tufts University School of Medicine, Boston, MA, USA

Department of Orthopedic & Rehabilitation Medicine, Tufts Medical Center, Boston, MA, USA

Walter I. Sussman, DO, FAAPMR Department of Orthopedics & Rehabilitation Medicine, Tufts University School of Medicine, Boston, MA, USA

Boston Sports & Biologics PC, Wellesley, MA, USA

Roy Taborda, MD Department of Physical Medicine & Rehabilitation, JFK Johnson Rehabilitation Institute, Edison, NJ, USA

Adam Tenforde, MD Assistant Professor, Department of Physical Medicine and Rehabilitation, Harvard Medical School, Director of Running Medicine at Spaulding National Running Center, Spaulding Rehabilitation Hospital, Harvard Medical School, Charlestown, MA, USA

Timothy Tiu, MD, FAAPMR, CAQSM Assistant Professor, Department of Physical Medicine & Rehabilitation, University of Miami Miller School of Medicine, Miami, FL, USA

Medical Director, Christine E. Lynn Rehabilitation Center Outpatient Clinics, Miami, FL, USA

Alfred J. Tria Jr, MD Department of Orthopaedics, Rutgers-Robert Wood Johnson Medical School, New Brunswick, NJ, USA

Kristian Von Rickenbach, MD Department of Physical Medicine & Rehabilitation, Spaulding Rehabilitation Hospital, Harvard Medical School, Charlestown, MA, USA

Omar Walli, MD Department of Physical Medicine & Rehabilitation, University of Miami Miller School of Medicine, Miami, FL, USA

Martin Weaver, MD Department of Orthopaedics and Physical Medicine and Rehabilitation, Emory University School of Medicine, Atlanta, GA, USA

Kirkham B. Wood, MD Professor of Orthopedic Surgery, Stanford University School of Medicine, Palo Alto, CA, USA

Grace X. Xiong, MD Harvard Combined Orthopaedic Residency Program, Harvard Medical School, Boston, MA, USA

Peter K. Yi, MD Assistant Professor of Anesthesiology. Director of Pain Fellowship Program, Duke University School of Medicine, Durham, NC, USA

Nadia N. Zaman, DO Assistant Professor Department of Orthopedics & Rehabilitation Medicine, Tufts University School of Medicine, Boston, MA, USA

Jason L. Zaremski, MD, CAQSM, FAAPMR, FACSM Clinical Associate Professor, Divisions of PM&R, Sports Medicine, & Research, Department of Orthopaedics and Rehabilitation, UF Health, University of Florida, Gainesville, FL, USA

Kevin Zhang, MD Departments of Orthopedics & Rehabilitation Medicine, Tufts University School of Medicine, Boston, MA, USA

Peter A. Everts, PhD, FRSM Chief Scientific Officer, Research and Science Division, Gulf Coast Biologics, Fort Myers, FL, USA

Glenn Flanagan II, MD Naples Regenerative Institute, Naples, FL, USA

Luga Podesta, MD Director, Regenerative Orthopedics & Sports Medicine, Naples, FL, USA

Physical Medicine and Rehabilitation and Sports Medicine at Western University of Health Sciences, Pomona, CA, USA

Part I

Head and Face

Section Editor

Tony K. George

Sports-Related Facial Trauma

1

Behzad Mostoufi and John M. Sands

1.1 Description

Sports-related facial injuries are common at any age and will inevitably be encountered by the practicing physician [1]. With a systematic approach, maxillofacial trauma can be recognized and managed appropriately. Sideline primary survey followed by a detailed secondary survey should be performed to determine the setting in which the patient needs to be treated. Proper identification of injuries and a fundamental understanding of when to make referrals will lead to the cohesive multidisciplinary management of athletes.

While increased regulations and protective gears have reduced the number of sports-related trauma, facial injuries are still a frequent occurrence. Approximately 11–40% of all sports injuries involve the face [2, 3]. The anatomical location appears to be the same in pediatric and adult patients [4]. These injuries are often a sequela of a direct impact with a ball or player-to-player contact. Maxillofacial trauma and fracture patterns vary significantly depending on the mechanism of injury, age of the individual, and a variety of other factors [5]. However, most sports-related facial traumas translate into soft tissue injuries or fractures of nasal bones, zygomaticomaxillary complex (ZMC), mandible, and dentoalveolar process [6].

1.2 Facial Anatomy

The face is a complex functional unit containing many critical structures and managing facial trauma can become overwhelming. However, with a systematic approach, one can easily begin to unpack these individual units to create a thorough assessment and plan.

The soft tissue of the face can be described as multiple distinct facial esthetic components consisting of areas of uniform color, texture, thickness, and mobility. It is among the most vascular tissues of the body with extensive collateral flow making it resistant to ischemia and infection. Within the facial soft tissue, several critical components deserve special attention. These include the motor and sensory nerves, the lacrimal system, and the parotid gland/duct. The primary sensory innervation of the face is from the three branches of the trigeminal nerve. Paresthesia is a common finding due to nerve contusion at the site of injury. The muscles of facial expression are innervated by the five branches (facial, zygomatic, buccal, marginal mandibular, and cervical) of the facial nerve. Crossover communication between the frontal and marginal mandibular branch with adjacent branches is only about 15%, while crossover among the other branches is approximately 70%. Therefore, injury to these two nerves can cause prominent facial muscle weakness on clinical evaluation. The lacrimal system is located in the medial portion of the eyes and is particularly at risk in lacerations involving the inferior lid. The parotid gland primarily overlies the masseter in the posterior jaw. The parotid duct exits the parotid gland, travels over the masseter, and pierces through the buccinator muscle before entering the oral cavity at the level of the second maxillary molar. One can generally locate the position of the duct by drawing an imaginary line from the tragus to the lateral commissure of the mouth. Any lacerations to the cheek require identification and evaluation of the duct for injury.

The facial skeleton can be divided into thirds. The upper third extends from the hairline to the level of the supraorbital ridge. Fractures in this area involve the frontal bone, frontal sinus, and orbital bone. The middle third spans from the inferior of the supraorbital rims to the incisal edge of the maxillary teeth. This region is by far the most prominent and complex consisting of the orbits, nasal bones, zygoma, and maxillary bones. The lower third of the face is the mandible and the teeth it supports. The facial skeleton is composed of four horizontal and four vertical bony buttresses that act as strongholds during periods of applied external forces (photo). Spanning between these pillars are thin sections of cortical

B. Mostoufi (✉) · J. M. Sands
Department of Oral and Maxillofacial Surgery, University of Maryland, Baltimore, MD, USA
e-mail: BMostoufi@umaryland.edu

© The Author(s), under exclusive license to Springer Nature Switzerland AG 2022

S. A. Mostoufi et al. (eds.), *Clinical Guide to Musculoskeletal Medicine*, https://doi.org/10.1007/978-3-030-92042-5_1

bone that serve as functional airbags during the time of increased pressure. Management of midface fractures focuses on realignment and plating along these buttresses to restore the facial width and height. The mandible is a U-shaped bone with multiple vectors of pull from the masticatory and suprahyoid muscle groups. This results in zones of compression and zones of tension at the time of fracture. Management of fractures in the mandible is oriented around fixation at the zones of osteosynthesis. These lines correlate to strong, dense areas of the mandible that are capable of resisting functional stress and make ideal locations to place screws and plates.

1.3 Evaluation

1.3.1 Sideline Primary Evaluation

As with any trauma, initial evaluation of sports-related facial injuries begins with a primary survey (sideline), assessing the patient's airway, breathing, circulation, and mental status. While the majority of sports-related head trauma is managed conservatively, the provider should always be proactive in securing an airway in the setting of altered mental status and maxillofacial fractures. The clinical presentation of closed head injuries such as skull base fractures may not be obvious. If not recognized early, may have devastating consequences.

1. Airway Injuries

   Airway injury can be life threatening. Most contact sports are classified as low-impact mechanisms and are generally at low risk for having loss of airway. However, injuries resulting in mandibular fractures can quickly turn into airway emergencies if there is significant cervicofacial swelling in the setting of an unstable jaw, and/or pull of muscles in bilateral mandible fracture.
2. Bleeding
   - *Laceration*: The face is highly vascular; therefore, extensive hemorrhage from facial wounds can be encountered. The majority of these wounds can be managed primarily with firm pressure for initial hemostasis.
   - *Epistaxis* caused by a nasal injury can be a profuse source of bleeding as well. Epistaxis is classified as an anterior or posterior nasal bleed. Anterior nasal bleeds are most common and involve disruption of the Kiesselbach Plexus. These can be managed by direct pressure or a topical vasoconstrictor as an adjunct. Contrary to belief, the application of an ice pack to the posterior neck (cryotherapy) has not shown to have a significant difference in the reduction of microcirculatory nasal blood flow [7].
   - *Posterior nasal bleeds* secondary to disruption of the sphenopalatine artery are rare but can be catastrophic as nasopharyngeal bleeding can compromise the patient's airway. These are best managed with nasal packing and transfer to an emergency center.

1.3.2 Secondary Survey

Once all potentially life-threatening injuries are excluded, the secondary survey is performed. Each sports medicine provider should develop a systematic routine to provide a thorough examination. It is the author's preference to evaluate each component of the face through inspection, evaluation of sensory and motor nerve function, and palpation of bony prominences in a top to bottom fashion. Proper identification of injuries and a fundamental understanding of when to make referrals are imperative in the management of facial trauma.

The time, location, and nature of the incident are among the important information that clinicians should gather. To simplify, one can remember to inquire where, when, and how the patient sustained an injury.

1. *Scalp*: Examiner should thoroughly palpate the scalp as if you were "washing someone's hair with shampoo". This will allow the clinician to feel lacerations or indentations that might otherwise be covered by hair. Occasionally, blood on the gloves will indicate a laceration that would have otherwise gone unnoticed.
2. *Forehead/Bony Orbits:* Moving inferiorly, inspect the forehead for any abrasions or contusions. Palpate the superior and inferior orbital rims to complete a circumferential evaluation of the orbital rim.
3. *Ophthalmologic survey*: Attention is now brought back to the orbits. A thorough examination of the eyes is mandatory as injuries such as hyphema, ruptured globe, or retrobulbar hematoma are considered ophthalmologic emergencies [8]. First, inspect the orbits for any signs of injury including periorbital ecchymosis, hyphema, chemosis, subconjunctival hemorrhage, proptosis, or enophthalmos. The discrepancy of gross visual acuity is highly indicative of the presence of injury. Have the patient gaze in all directions in an "H" pattern to assess the extraocular muscular range of motion. Confirm that the pupils are equal in diameter, round, and reactive to light. Document any discrepancy.
4. *Zygomatic arch*: Continue to palpate the Zygoma and Zygomatic arch starting from lateral of the nose moving posteriorly to the tragus of the ear. Fractures of the ZMC will result in facial widening and loss of malar projection. This can best be observed by looking at the patient from the worm's eye view. Paresthesia of the infraorbital

region is a common finding. Evaluation for trismus is the only true functional indication for the repair of the zygomatic arch as an impingement on the coronoid process of the mandible can result in limited mouth opening.

5. *Nose*: Next, with a nondominant hand on the patient's forehead stabilize the head while evaluating the integrity of the nasal bones with the dominant hand. Examination of the nose includes the nasal bones, cartilage, and nasal septum. Swelling, crepitus, deviation of the dorsum, and epistaxis are frequently seen during times of injury. The intranasal examination includes evaluation for septal deviation and septal hematoma with good lighting and a nasal speculum.
6. *Maxilla*: Mobility of the maxilla is then assessed by placing the dominant hand on the maxillary incisors and alveolar process, attempting to move the maxilla in all directions. Throughout this time, document any pain, crepitus, or presence of step-offs which is suggestive of an underlying fracture.
7. *Midface evaluation*: Blunt trauma to the midface can result in a Le Fort fracture pattern which is defined by the separation of the pterygoid plates. This can best be assessed clinically by grasping the anterior maxillary teeth and firmly attempting to move the maxilla in all directions while stabilizing the forehead. The presence of Le Fort injury will present as midface mobility.
8. *Mandible*: Pain, asymmetry, malocclusion, occlusal step defects, sublingual ecchymosis, and paresthesia of the lower lip/chin area are all pathognomonic signs for mandibular fractures. Palpating the extraoral boundary of the mandible could be difficult due to swelling and edema. Careful intraoral examination for step deformity and any mobile segments should be performed by placing the index figure on the occlusal surface of the posterior teeth and thumb on the inferior border of the mandible extraorally. Place the other hand in the same manner on the anterior aspect of the mandible. While holding firmly, gently move the segments and observe for any movement and/or pain. Clinicians should inspect dentition for mobility, bleeding, and fracture fragments to prevent aspiration risk. Gingiva and oral mucosa should also be examined for lacerations.
9. *Lip/Tongue/Cheek*: The lips, tongues, and cheeks are susceptible to lacerations when compressed against the dentition. The oral cavity must be carefully examined for loose, missing, or fractured dentition. Be sure to carefully evaluate adjacent soft tissue for displaced tooth fragments.
10. *Cranial Nerves/Facial Nerve*: The cranial nerves are evaluated next. Using the back of your index finger, gently swipe the patient's forehead, cheek, and mental region bilaterally with a paintbrush-like motion. This will quickly evaluate any change in sensation of the three branches of the trigeminal nerve. To evaluate the five branches of the facial nerve, ask the patient to raise their eyebrows, shut their eyes tight, pucker their cheeks, and purse their lips. Note any muscle weakness or facial asymmetry.

1.4 Management of Soft Tissue Injuries

Sports-related soft tissue injuries often present as contusions (bruising), abrasions, lacerations, and hematomas.

A. *Contusions* are primarily managed with a cold compress to reduce swelling followed by moist heat to remove inflammatory mediators.
B. *Abrasions* require thorough irrigation as most wounds are contaminated with dirt, rocks, or particles from the field. After the wound is appropriately irrigated, topical antibiotic ointment and nonadherent dressing are applied.
C. *Lacerations* represent the most common type of facial injury encountered in the athletic setting. Management includes thorough irrigation of the wound, disinfection, and reapproximation of tissue (Fig. 1.1). Tetanus vaccination is also indicated if the patient is not up-to-date with the shot. Superficial lacerations without separation of the wound edges may be closed with Steri-strips, Dermabond, or simple interrupted sutures. A nonresorbable monofilament suture on a fine needle (i.e., 5–0 Prolene on RB needle) is ideal as it has good tensile strength and is the least reactive with tissue. Most sutures can be removed in 5–7 days to reduce the risk of scarring. For deeper lacerations with separated or jagged wound edges, consultation with a facial specialist such as Oral and Maxillofacial Surgeons or plastic surgery is indicated.
D. *Hematomas*: Management primarily involves cold compress for the first 48 hours and application of heat thereafter. However, complications associated with hematomas include expansion, overlying skin necrosis, or infection and warrant immediate intervention. Auricular and septal hematomas deserve special attention because of their potential associated complications. Auricular hematomas develop after compression or blunt trauma to the ear and subsequent shearing of the skin from the highly vascular perichondrium. Failure to adequately drain these hematomas can result in hardening and scarring leading to a permanent deformity of the auricle also known as "cauliflower ear". Treatment involves incision and drainage of the hematoma and application of a compressive bolster. Septal hematomas appear as purple, grape-like, swelling from the nasal septum. Treatment includes incision and drainage followed by anterior nasal packing. Failure to recognize and treat can result in septal necrosis and saddle nose deformity as a result of loss of septal support.

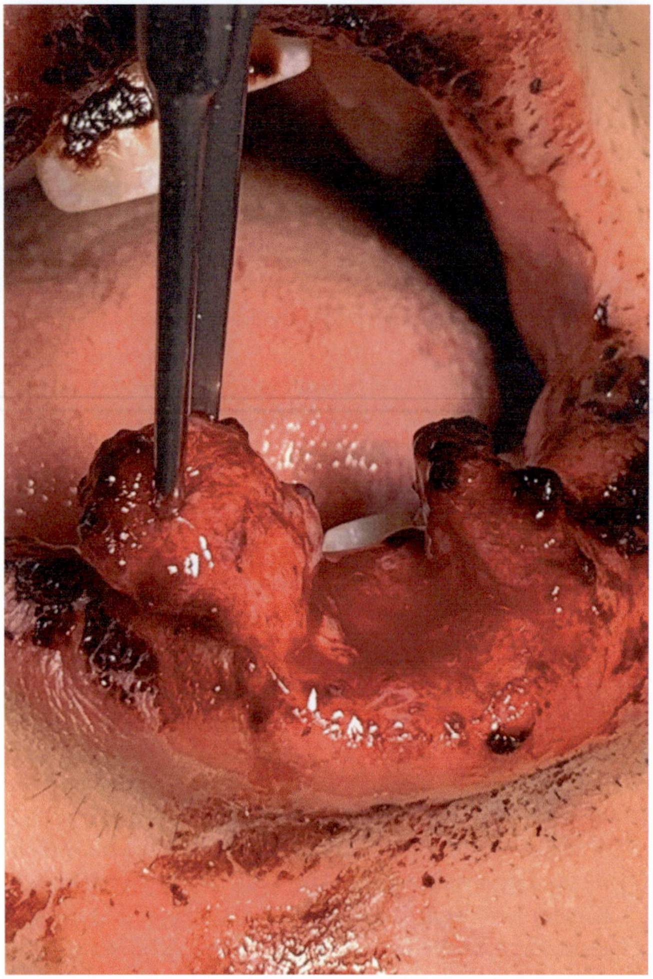

Fig. 1.1 Lip laceration following skateboard forward fall accident (X-games)

1.5 Orbital Fractures

One-third of all orbital fractures are secondary to sport injuries [9]. When an injury to the eye occurs, a thorough examination should be performed as previously described. Orbital fractures commonly present with periorbital ecchymosis, chemosis, and subconjunctival hemorrhage. The presence of enophthalmos, exophthalmos, hypoglobus, hyphema, and diminished visual acuity or other visual changes warrant immediate surgical consultation (Fig. 1.3). The medial orbital wall and inferior orbital floor are strategically designed to fracture during times of impact and increased pressure. This allows the contents of the orbit to expand into the adjacent paranasal sinuses, serving as an anatomic airbag to prevent globe injury. This fracture pattern is often referred to as orbital "blow out". Occasionally, the inferior rectus muscle will get trapped below the orbital floor bony segments resulting in impaired extraocular movement (Fig. 1.2). This is also a time-sensitive surgical emergency as failure to reposition the inferior rectus can result in necrosis and scar contracture of the muscle. Orbital entrapment can be ruled out by evaluating extraocular movement or a forced duction test. CT imaging may show herniation of the muscle without clinical signs, which may not require surgery. The majority of the orbital floor and orbital wall fractures are managed conservatively with surgical intervention only indicated in instances of enophthalmos, limited extraocular movement, and persistent diplopia. Conservative management includes protective eyewear, sinus precautions, and 4–6 weeks of reduced physical activity.

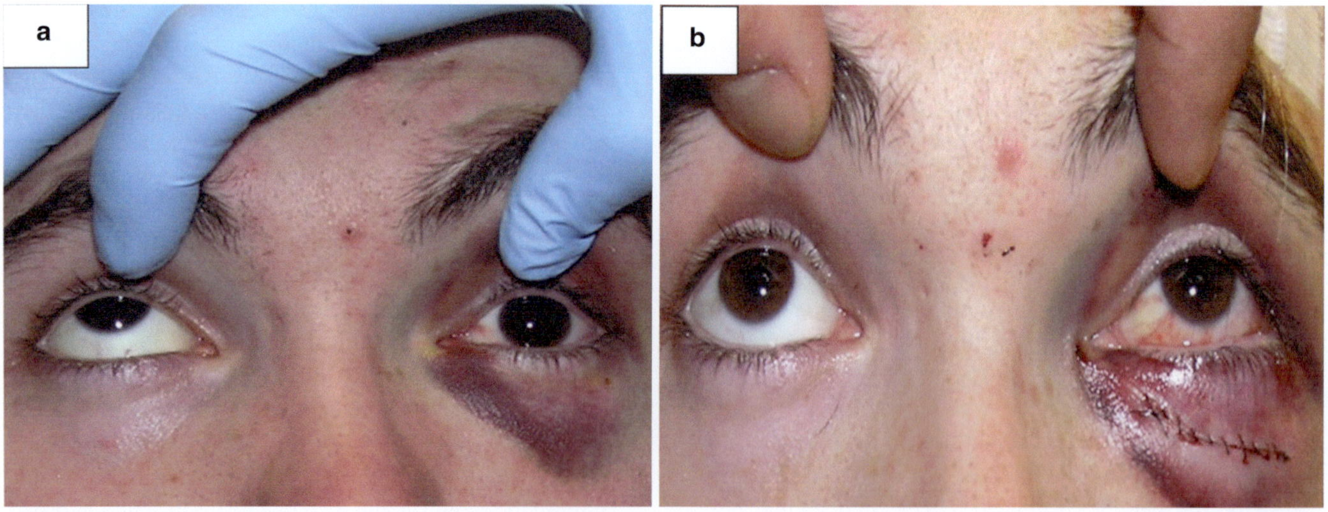

Fig. 1.2 (**a**) Left Orbital floor fracture. Note the restricted upward gaze in left eye due to inferior rectus entrapment, normal right side. (**b**) Normal movement after the Open Reduction Internal Fixation

1.6 Nasal Fractures

Because of its prominent location on the face, the nose is the most commonly fractured facial structure associated with sports-related facial injuries. Clinical findings associated with nasal fracture include epistaxis, swelling and tenderness of the nasal dorsum, periorbital ecchymosis, and deviation of the nasal bridge. Palpation can demonstrate mobility, bony irregularities, or crepitus. The intranasal examination should be conducted under proper lighting with a nasal speculum to evaluate for septal deviation and septal hematoma. Treatment ranges from simple closed reduction at the bedside under local anesthesia to open reduction of severely displaced fractures in the operating room. Swelling at the time of insult makes cosmetic evaluation and close reduction difficult. Whenever possible, it is best to wait 4 to 7 days for the swelling to subside before treating nasal fractures. Treatment focuses on realignment of the septum and nasal bones followed by external and internal splinting. Splints are maintained for 7–10 days, and players are cleared to return within 4–8 weeks following reduction.

1.6.1 Zygomaticomaxillary Complex Fractures (ZMC)

The ZMC and zygomatic arch make up the prominence of the face and sports-related fracture of this bony complex is not uncommon. Clinical findings commonly associated with ZMC fractures include periorbital ecchymosis, subconjunctival hemorrhage paresthesia in the infraorbital nerve distribution, and depression of the zygoma. Ophthalmic evaluation including visual acuity is also paramount in ZMC fractures as the majority of patients will report visual changes. One of the cardinal signs of ZMC fracture is that there is no posterior limit to the subconjunctival hemorrhage. Depression of the zygomatic arch can impede the coronoid process of the mandible during mouth opening, resulting in a limited range of motion. Therefore, documentation of maximum interincisal opening is standard during the evaluation of ZMC fractures. Treatment varies depending on the severity of the fracture and the degree of displacement. Indications for surgical intervention include cosmetic deformity and impaired function, most often in the form of trismus. The presence of either of these findings indicates surgical consultation.

1.6.2 Mandible Fractures

Clinical findings include malocclusion, limited mouth opening, mobility of segments, occlusal step defects, and floor of the mouth ecchymosis. As the mandible is a horseshoe-shaped structure, fractures rarely present as isolated fractures. They are almost always bilateral unless proven otherwise (Fig. 1.3). Simple, nondisplaced mandibular fractures can be managed conservatively with closed reduction, often in the form of maxillomandibular fixation (MMF) [10]. Comminuted, grossly displaced, or open fractures require anatomic reduction and internal fixation in the operating room. Athletes with jaw fractures should not return to play until healing has occurred or they are out of MMF, which generally takes 4–6 weeks.

1.6.3 Dentoalveolar Fractures/Tooth Avulsion

Dentoalveolar Trauma: Term Dentoalveolar consists of the alveolar bone and the associated teeth. Signs and symptoms of dentoalveolar trauma include intraoral bleeding, tooth malposition, malocclusion, and mobility of the affected segment. Inspection of the adjacent structures is critical as teeth may be lodged in the surrounding soft tissue (Fig. 1.4), lips,

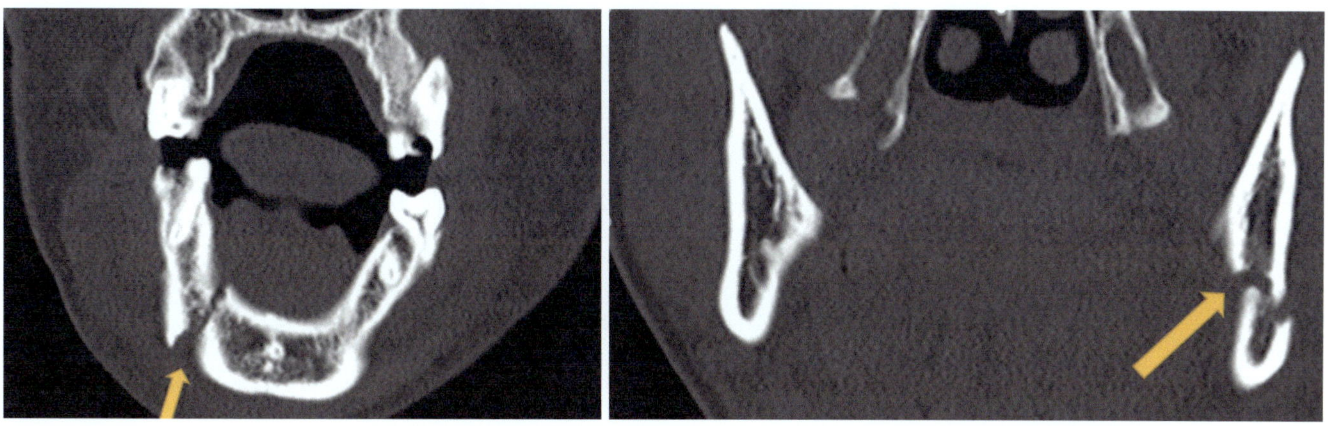

Fig. 1.3 Coronal view CT showing displaced fractures of Right Parasymphysis and Left Angle of the mandible following player to player contact in pick-up football game with no protective headgear used

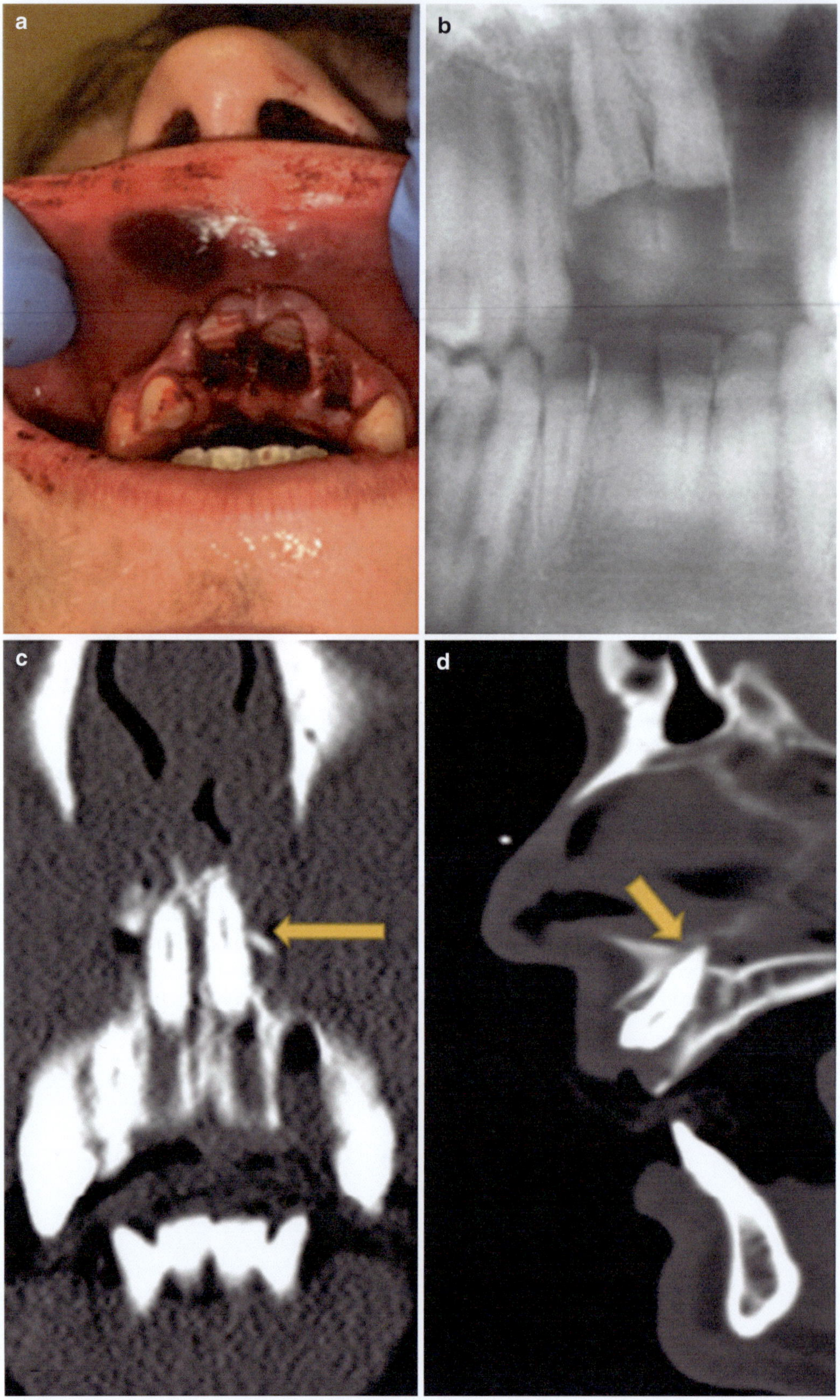

Fig. 1.4 Maxillary dentoalveolar fracture, cephalad displaced teeth violating the nasal floor (arrows) and avulsed left lateral incisor following Trampoline accident. Hematoma on the labial aspect of upper lip due to impact. Both Coronal and sagittal CT demonstrate nasal floor violation. (**a**) Oral photograph, (**b**) Pan Film, (**c**) Coronal CT view, (**d**) Sagittal CT view

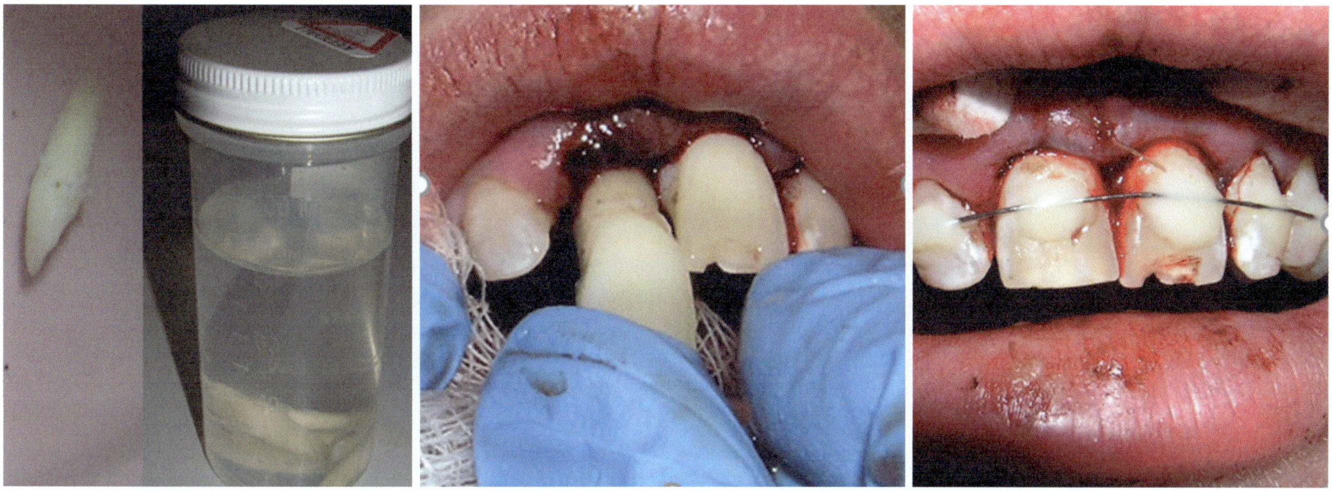

Fig. 1.5 Tooth avulsion due to unprotected backyard football injury. Patient brought avulsed teeth to the ED which was placed in normal saline followed by gentle irrigation. Middle image shows reimplantation followed by stabilization using 24-gage wire and light cure composite – Note that splint extended two teeth distal on either side

and tongue. Management involves reduction and fixation of the fracture with splints.

Tooth avulsion is the complete separation of the tooth from the alveolus which is an urgent situation (Fig. 1.5). The prognosis for the viability of the tooth and success replantation is inversely proportional to the length of time of tooth out of the socket. Reimplantation of the tooth within 30 minutes has >90% chance of tooth survival; after more than 2 hours, the chance of survival is 5% [11]. Continued nourishment and maintenance of the periodontal ligament are critical to tooth survival. This can be ensured with proper handling and transportation of the tooth. Do not scrub or brush the root of the avulsed tooth. Instead, gently handle the tooth by its crown. If the tooth cannot be immediately replanted into its socket, it should be gently irrigated with normal saline water and transported in the appropriate medium Photo. Hank's balanced solution can maintain the periodontal fibers for days; however, this may not be readily available on the field or in emergency rooms. Cold milk, followed by saliva, is a sufficient transport medium in an emergent situation. Once implanted, outpatient follow-up with a general dentist within 24 hours is indicated.

References

1. Rui P, Ashman JJ, Akinseye A. Emergency department visits for injuries sustained during sports and recreational activities by patients aged 5–24 years, 2010–2016. Natl Health Stat Report. 2019;2019(133):2010–6.
2. Carniol ET, Shaigany K, Svider PF, et al. "Beaned":A 5-year analysis of baseball-related injuries of the face. Otolaryngol Head Neck Surg (United States). 2015;153(6):957–61. https://doi.org/10.1177/0194599815602668.
3. Hwang K, You SH, Lee HS. Outcome analysis of sports-related multiple facial fractures. J Craniofac Surg. 2009;20(3):825–9. https://doi.org/10.1097/SCS.0b013e3181a14cda.
4. MacIsaac ZM, Berhane H, Cray JJ, Zuckerbraun NS, Losee JE, Grunwaldt LJ. Nonfatal sport-related craniofacial fractures: characteristics, mechanisms, and demographic data in the pediatric population. Plast Reconstr Surg. 2013;131(6):1339–47. https://doi.org/10.1097/PRS.0b013e31828bd191.
5. Liu C, Legocki AT, Mader NS, Scott AR. Nasal fractures in children and adolescents: mechanisms of injury and efficacy of closed reduction. Int J Pediatr Otorhinolaryngol. 2015;79(12):2238–42. https://doi.org/10.1016/j.ijporl.2015.10.011.
6. Echlin P, McKeag DB. Maxillofacial injuries in sport. Curr Sports Med Rep. 2004;3(1):25–32. https://doi.org/10.1007/s11932-004-0042-9.
7. Berry D, Carlson JN, Singletary E, Zideman DA, Ring J. Use of cryotherapy for managing epistaxis in the first aid setting: a scoping review. Cureus. 2021;13(5):e14832. https://doi.org/10.7759/cureus.14832.
8. Kaur J, Chopra R. Three dimensional CT reconstruction for the evaluation and surgical planning of mid face fractures: a 100 case study. J Maxillofac Oral Surg. 2010;9(4):323–8. https://doi.org/10.1007/s12663-010-0137-1.
9. Murphy C, O'Connell JE, Kearns G, Stassen L. Sports-related maxillofacial injuries. J Craniofac Surg. 2015;26(7):2120–3. https://doi.org/10.1097/SCS.0000000000002109.
10. Mostoufi B, Sands J, Patel M, Warburton G, Caccamese J. Fracture propagation associated with intermaxillary fixation screws in maxillofacial trauma. Int J Oral Maxillofac Surg. 2020;49(4):491–5. https://doi.org/10.1016/j.ijom.2019.09.006.
11. Reehal P. Facial injury in sport. Curr Sports Med Rep. 2010;9(1):27–34. https://doi.org/10.1249/JSR.0b013e3181cd2c04.

2 Concussion

Emily Mostofi, Jaleh Fatehi, and S. Ali Mostoufi

2.1 Synonyms

- Cerebral concussion
- Commotio cerebri
- Mild traumatic brain injury

2.2 ICD 10 Codes

S06.0X0 - S06.0X9

2.3 Description

Definition of Sport-Related Concussion based on the Fifth Consensus statement on concussion in sport is: "A traumatic brain injury induced by biomechanical forces" [1]. It may be caused either by a direct blow to the head, face, neck or elsewhere on the body with an impulsive force transmitted to the head [1]. It typically results in the rapid onset of short-lived impairment of neurological function that resolves spontaneously [1]. In some cases, signs and symptoms evolve over several minutes to hours. Sport-related concussion may result in neuropathological changes, but the acute clinical signs and symptoms largely reflect a functional disturbance rather than a structural injury and, therefore standard structural neuroimaging studies reveal no abnormality [1].

E. Mostofi · J. Fatehi
Department of Neurology, University of Alberta, Edmonton, AB, Canada

S. A. Mostoufi (✉)
Department of Orthopedics and Rehabilitation, Tufts University School of Medicine, Boston, MA, USA

New England Spine Care Associates & Boston Regenerative Medicine, Cambridge, NJ, USA
e-mail: ali.mostoufi@tufts.edu

Sport-Related Concussion results in several signs and symptoms that may or may not involve loss of consciousness [1]. Resolution of the clinical and cognitive features typically follows a sequential course however, in some cases, symptoms may be prolonged [1, 2]. The majority (80–90%) of concussions resolve in a short period (10–14 days), although the recovery timeframe may be longer in children and adolescents [1, 2].

Frequency of concussion is approximately 3.8 million/year in United States, half of which may be undiagnosed or unreported [2]. New information indicates that females may be more susceptible to concussion than males (in high school and collegiate levels) [5]. Concussion is more prevalent in certain positions in the field as well as certain sports including basketball, hockey, rugby, and soccer and American football, equestrian sports [1, 2, 4].

The biggest risk factor in developing first sports-related concussion is participating in contact sports that have a highest chance of collision resulting in head injury. Risk factor for prolongation of symptoms and/or recurrent concussion may include female athletes, younger age, previous history of concussion, and pre-existing conditions such as learning siblings, attention deficits, and migraine headaches [4]. Table 2.1 outlines differential diagnosis of concussion.

2.3.1 Mechanism of Injury

The exact mechanism of concussion is unknown. Concussion is due to rotational acceleration of the brain during the fall, motor vehicle accident or sports injury [3]. Although concussion is frequently associated with direct impact to the head (examples are helmet to helmet contact during tackle or head to turf during fall); there is no evidence that direct impact is

Table 2.1 Differential diagnosis of concussion

Differential diagnosis of concussion	
Intracranial hemorrhage	Headache disorders and Migraines
Skull fracture	Sleep dysfunction
Attention Deficit Disorder	Anxiety, depression, PTSD

© The Author(s), under exclusive license to Springer Nature Switzerland AG 2022
S. A. Mostoufi et al. (eds.), *Clinical Guide to Musculoskeletal Medicine*, https://doi.org/10.1007/978-3-030-92042-5_2

necessarily required to develop concussion [4]. Animal and human studies support the concept of postconcussive vulnerability. After the first concussion, there is greater susceptibility to sustaining another concussion and that subsequent concussions occur with less force and take longer to resolve [5]. Animal studies have shown poorer cognitive outcomes in the setting of repeated head injury [6].

2.4 Clinical Presentation

This condition is a diffuse injury and does not have a focal neurological deficit such as limb weakness, pupillary dilation. Symptoms may include headache, nausea and/or emesis, dizziness, photophobia, confusion, difficulty concentrating, poor sleep, and/or poor appetite, to name a few (Table 2.2). It should be noted loss of consciousness may present with a concussion rarely but does not indicate severity of concussion. Often the first concussion is mild and expected to recover 10 days [1]. These symptoms can sometimes persist as a postconcussive syndrome with continued memory and concentration difficulties, headache, personality changes, fatigue, and insomnia [7].

2.5 Physical Examination

2.5.1 Concussion Assessment at Sideline

Athletes are assessed for concussion and its severity at the time of injury. The *Sport Concussion Assessment Tool (SCAT)* is a standardized tool for evaluating injured athletes for concussion and can be used in athletes aged from 13 years and older. SCAT has been adopted by major sporting authorities including Olympic committee, NCAA, FEI, and FIFA [8]. The clinician should assess the concussed athlete, go through the sports concussion assessment tool, and make a clinical judgment regarding the concussion, ability to return to game, as well as red flags that require urgent care evaluation. Concussion signs and symptoms evolve over time, and it is important to consider repeat evaluation in the assessment of concussion [16]. Elemental SCAT testing includes the following:

Table 2.2 Symptoms of concussion based on sports concussion assessment tool [16]

Symptoms of concussion based on sports concussion assessment tool (SCAT 5) [16]		
Headache	Sensitivity to noise	Sensitivity to light
Pressure in the head	Balance problem	Difficulty concentration
Neck pain	Neck pain	Difficulty remembering
Dizziness	Feeling slowed down	Fatigue or low energy
Blurry vision	Feeling like "in a fog"	"Do not feel right"
Confusion	Drowsiness	Trouble falling asleep
More emotional/irritability	Sadness	Nervous and anxious

1. *Glasgow Coma Scale*: GCS evaluates athletes' ability to "eye-opening", "verbal response", and "motor response". A score of 13–15 is a mild concussion, a score of 9–12 is a moderate head injury, and the score of 3–8 is a severe head injury.
2. *Maddocks score*: It is a series of questions from the athlete, and he/she is asked to give the response they can. Questions include "what venue are you at", "which half it is now", "who score last in this match", "what did you play last week", "did you team when the last game". It has a low false-negative rate and false-positive of 29–68% [8].
3. *Cognitive assessment*: It includes questions such as what month it is, what date it is today, what day of the week it is today, what year it is, what time is it right now. Orientation score is given and documented.
4. *Concentration/Recall*: Immediate recall is tested by asking the athlete to recall a series of numbers in reverse order months in reverse. Delayed recall is a repetition of the recall testing 5 minutes after the end of the immediate recall testing.
5. *Cervical spine/neurologic examination*: Cervical spine and its cervical root are tested to evaluate for concomitant cervical injury.
6. *Balance or coordination exam*: SCAT testing uses a modified balance error scoring system which includes double-leg stance, single-leg stance with nondominant feet, tandem stance with nondominant foot at the back, and total error. Left and right are both tested. The surface in which balance is tested as well as shoe wear is documented [16].
7. *Memory testing*: At the sideline, memory is tested. Five words are given to the athlete, and he should recall as many as they can. It is trialed three times and the clinician would provide the same list to them and ask for recall. It could be done with five words or a 10-word list.
8. *Red flags* (Table 2.3) are symptoms that develop as a result of direct or indirect blow to the head of the athlete which would result to removal from participation and evaluation by licensed healthcare provider and possible transfer to urgent care for further evaluation.

2.5.1.1 Return to Play Guidelines

An athlete should not be returned to play on the same day of the injury. An athlete requires medical clearance with a stage rehabilitation program and would be progressed from initial no activity/sport and physical/cognitive testing into a light aerobic exercise program, followed by sport-specific exercise

Table 2.3 Red flags are symptoms in concussion, requiring immediate evaluation by licensed healthcare provider and possible transfer to urgent care

Red flag symptoms in concussion	
Neck tenderness or pain	Double vision
Weakness, tingling, burning in the arms/legs	Severe or increasing headaches
Seizure or convulsion	Loss of consciousness
Deterioration of conscious state	Vomiting
Inability to recognize people or places	Slurred speech
Increased in restlessness	Agitation or combative athlete

program. Once these stages are completed, an athlete may first enter a noncontact drill followed by a full contact practice, and eventually return to game. There should be no less than 24-hour in between each stage. If athletes have recurrence of symptoms, progression in the stages should be halted. The final determination regarding concussion diagnosis and fitness to play is a *medical decision* based on clinical judgment.

2.5.2 Evaluation at Concussion Clinic

For many healthcare providers, the first chance to assess a young athlete with a suspected concussion will not be on the sidelines, but an office. The clinician should collect detailed medical history, conduct a full neurological and musculoskeletal examination, and plan for care if the athlete remains symptomatic. Collecting detailed history is a very important step in evaluating concussed athletes which should include the history of previous head injuries, learning disabilities, attention deficit hyperactivity disorder (ADHD), mood disorders, previously vestibular disturbances, any previous neurological deficits, or conditions.

2.5.3 Physical Examination

- *Inspection*: Close examination of head and neck for any fractures or structural injuries. Inspection should include looking for any bruises and hematomas.
- *Musculoskeletal examination*: Full musculoskeletal examination should be conducted. In many cases with concussion, cervical spine injuries are missed. Clinicians are responsible for examination of the cervical spine and management of findings. Clinical examination may be combined with imaging and if there is a suspicion of cervical injury, return to play should be delayed.
- *Neurological examination*: Detailed neurological examination is conducted including cranial nerves and peripheral nerves an examination of the cervical spine roots, sensory testing, motor testing and reflect this. Specialized testing including vestibular ocular motor screening is conducted as part of neurological examination of concussed athlete.
- *Vestibular ocular motor screening*: This screening tool will test the following five domains. Abnormalities in these domains are present in up to 69% of adolescents after a minor traumatic brain injury [8].
  1. Smooth pursuits
  2. Horizontal and vertical saccades
  3. Near point of convergence distance
  4. Horizontal vestibulo-ocular reflex
  5. Visual motion sensitivity
- Gait/Balance: It includes tandem gait and Romberg examination to assess the patient's balance and motor coordination. Berg Balance testing is another tool to assess balance and may be used for prediction of rehabilitative outcome in acquired brain injury including concussion [15].
- The King–Devick: This test is based on measurement of the speed of rapid number naming (reading aloud single-digit numbers from three test cards), and captures impairment of eye movements, attention, language, and other correlates of suboptimal brain function. This test can be effectively administered by nonmedically trained laypersons as well (parents at sideline) [9].
- ASIA classification-based exam: If there is any finding compatible with spinal cord injury, examination based on The American Spinal Injury Association Impairment Scale (ASIA) should be conducted. This scale examines both the sensory and motor function of all the dermatomes and myotomes. It is a standardized and widely accepted method of evaluating spine trauma that is associated with spinal cord injury.

2.6 Diagnostic Workup

Concussion is largely a clinical diagnosis, but certain tests are ordered to assess for coexisting injuries.

2.6.1 CT Scan

Often performed at the emergency room to rule out intracranial bleed and/or fractures.

2.6.2 MR-Based Imaging

In general, there is a limited role for standard MRI in diagnosis of concussion. Structural or metabolic alteration in the brain after concussion may lead to utility of laboratory and advanced neuroimaging techniques to assist with managing patients with persistent symptoms. Advanced imaging includes functional magnetic resonance imaging, positron emission tomography, H magnetic resonance spectroscopy, and perfusion imaging [1]. At this time, such imaging modalities are primarily for concussion research and large prospective randomized studies are lacking in their clinical application.

2.6.3 Serum Biomarkers

A number of research studies have been conducted to identify biomarkers that could detect concussion, but most have been studied in severe concussion [10, 17]. These are serum biomarkers pointing toward neural injury including S100β, Glial Fibrillary Acidic Protein (GFAP), Neuron-Specific Enolase, Ubiquitin C-Terminal Hydrolase, Alpha-II Spectrin Breakdown Products, Tau Protein (tau), and Neurofilaments. Validity and utility of such biomarkers are still being studied but NIH funded research [18] noted two of the proteins were associated with the length of time needed by the athletes to return to play: tau and GFAP. Athletes who needed less than 2 weeks of recovery time had significantly higher tau within the first 48 hours after an injury. In contrast, GFAP was significantly lower for these athletes. Nf-L was not linked with the length of time needed for recovery [18].

2.6.4 Neuropsychological Testing

Neuropsychological assessment is a key component of the multidimensional approach recommended by international consensus guidelines for evaluation of athletes affected by sport-related concussion [11]. Neuropsychological tests are an objective measure of brain-behavior relationships and are more sensitive for subtle cognitive impairment than clinical exams. Although not all the concussions require neuropsychological testing, it should be considered as part of the comprehensive concussion management strategy rather than in isolation [2]. Neuropsychological testing is helpful in postconcussion management of athletes with persistent symptoms or complicated courses but is not a predictor of recurrent concussion or long-term complications. The exact timing and frequency of neuropsychic testing have not been conclusively determined yet [2].

2.7 Treatment

2.7.1 Medical Management

Treatment of a concussion is primarily supportive. This involves initial limitation of physical and cognitive activity, followed by a gradual return to previous activity levels. The Centre for Disease Control and Prevention (CDC) outlines a 6-step protocol for return to play to guide sports athletes, coaches, trainers, and medical staff [12]. An athlete should only move to the next step if they do not have any new symptoms at the current step. If an athlete's symptoms come back or if he or she gets new symptoms, this is a sign that the athlete is pushing too hard [12].

- *Step 1*: Back to regular activities (Such as School, Symptom permitting)
- *Step 2*: Light aerobic activity
- Begin with light aerobic exercise only to increase an athlete's heart rate. This means about 5–10 minutes on an exercise bike, walking, or light jogging. No weightlifting at this point.
- *Step 3*: Moderate activity
- Continue with activities to increase an athlete's heart rate with body or head movement. This includes moderate jogging, brief running, moderate-intensity stationary biking, and moderate-intensity weightlifting (less time and/or less weight from their typical routine).
- *Step 4*: Heavy, noncontact activity
- Add heavy noncontact physical activity, such as sprinting/running, high-intensity stationary biking, regular weightlifting routine, noncontact sport-specific drills (in three planes of movement).
- *Step 5*: Practice and full contact
- Young athlete may return to practice and full contact (if appropriate for the sport) in controlled practice.
- *Step 6*: Competition
- Young athlete may return to competition.

2.7.2 Rehabilitation

2.7.2.1 Cognitive Behavioral Therapy

Small-scale studies are done on cognitive behavioral therapy in management of postconcussive symptoms in children and adolescents. Such studies do not support the effectiveness of cognitive behavioral therapy for severity of symptoms of postconcussion syndrome; however, it might be an effective treatment option for improving depression, anxiety, and social integration in individuals with traumatic brain injury (21). Large-scale randomized studies are lacking in this area.

2.7.2.2 Aerobic Exercise

Emerging research supports the use of mild to moderate aerobic exercise for treating sport-related concussion and persistent postconcussive symptoms. The studies conclude subsymptomatic threshold aerobic exercise is safe, effective in sports-related concussions and in this group of postconcussive persistent symptoms [3].

The effect of exercise on baseline SCAT performance in male professional Rugby players was studied. Both rest-

SCAT and exercise-SCAT were tested and compared [13]. Symptom endorsement was greater when assessed after exercise than at rest. Orientation score was improved during SCAT5s performed after exercise-SCAT, but only when rest- and exercise-SCAT were conducted on the same day. Concentration score was impaired during exercise-SCAT. No other cognitive submodes were affected by exercise. Total errors during Modified Balance Error Scoring System increased during exercise-SCAT, as a result of increased errors made during single-leg balance, irrespective of testing sequence, with 42% of players making more errors in exercise-SCAT, compared to 28% making more errors in rest-SCAT.

2.7.2.3 Vestibular Rehabilitation

Concussion symptoms normally resolve within 10-14 days [1], but vertigo, dizziness, and balance dysfunction persist in 10-30% of cases requiring treatment [14]. Vestibular rehabilitation following concussion utilizes similar tools and techniques employed when treating those solely with peripheral pathology. Sport injury results in concussion, but also may result in peripheral and central injuries, leading to prolonged course of vestibular rehab. Comorbidities including cognitive and behavioral issues, visual-perceptual dysfunction, and autonomic dysfunction may negatively impact this modality of care. There are limited studies on effectiveness of vestibular therapy in concussed individuals. Available evidence, although weak, shows promise in this population [14].

References

1. McCrory P, et al. Consensus statement on concussion in sport—the 5th international conference on concussion in sport held in Berlin, October 2016. Br J Sports Med. 2017;51(11):838–47.
2. Harmon KG, et al. American Medical Society for Sports Medicine position statement on concussion in sport. Br J Sports Med. 2019;53(4):213–25. Meaney, D. F., & Smith, D. H. (2011). Biomechanics of concussion. *Clinics in Sports Medicine*, 30(1), 19–vii. https://doi.org/10.1016/j.csm.2010.08.009.
3. Tator CH. Concussions and their consequences: current diagnosis, management and prevention. CMAJ. 2013;185(11):975–9. https://doi.org/10.1503/cmaj.120039.
4. Guskiewicz KM, McCrea M, Marshall SW, et al. Cumulative effects associated with recurrent concussion in collegiate football players: the NCAA Concussion Study. JAMA. 2003;290:2549–55.
5. Prins ML, Alexander D, Giza CC, Hovda DA. Repeated mild traumatic brain injury: mechanisms of cerebral vulnerability. J Neurotrauma. 2013;30(1):30–8. https://doi.org/10.1089/neu.2012.2399. PMID: 23025820; PMCID: PMC4047842
6. Ferry B, DeCastro A. Concussion. [Updated 2021 Apr 30]. In: StatPearls [Internet]. Treasure Island: StatPearls Publishing; 2021. Available from: https://www.ncbi.nlm.nih.gov/books/NBK537017/.
7. Haider MN, Leddy JJ, Du W, Macfarlane J, Alexander, Viera KB, Willer BS. Practical management: brief physical examination for sport-related concussion in the outpatient setting. Clin J Sport Med. 2020;30(5):513–7. https://doi.org/10.1097/JSM.0000000000000687.
8. Leong DF, Balcer LJ, Galetta SL, Liu Z, Master CL. The King-Devick test as a concussion screening tool administered by sports parents. J Sports Med Phys Fitness. 2014;54(1):70–7. PMID: 24445547.
9. Papa L, Edwards D, Ramia M. Exploring serum biomarkers for mild traumatic brain injury. In: Kobeissy FH, editor. Brain neurotrauma: molecular, neuropsychological, and rehabilitation aspects. Boca Raton: CRC Press/Taylor & Francis; 2015. Chapter 22.
10. McCrea MA, Asken B, Nelson LD. Neuropsychological screening of sport-related concussion. Neurol Clin. 2017;35(3):487–500. https://doi.org/10.1016/j.ncl.2017.03.005. Epub 2017 May 30. PMID: 28673411.
11. Centers for Disease Control and Prevention. Accessed 6/2/2020. Traumatic brain injury & concussion.
12. McNally KA, Patrick KE, LaFleur JE, Dykstra JB, Monahan K, Hoskinson KR. Brief cognitive behavioral intervention for children and adolescents with persistent post-concussive symptoms: a pilot study. Child Neuropsychol. 2018;24(3):396–412. https://doi.org/10.1080/09297049.2017.1280143. Epub 2017 Jan 26. PMID: 28125932.
13. Murray DA, Meldrum D, Lennon O. Can vestibular rehabilitation exercises help patients with concussion? A systematic review of efficacy, prescription and progression patterns. Br J Sports Med. 2017;51(5):442–51. https://doi.org/10.1136/bjsports-2016-096081. Epub 2016 Sep 21. PMID: 27655831.
14. Feld JA, Rabadi MH, Blau AD, Jordan BD. Berg balance scale and outcome measures in acquired brain injury. Neurorehabil Neural Repair. 2001;15(3):239–44. https://doi.org/10.1177/154596830101500312. PMID: 11944746.
15. Petit KM, Savage JL, Bretzin AC, Anderson M, Covassin T. The sport concussion assessment tool-5 (SCAT5): baseline assessments in NCAA division I collegiate student-athletes. Int J Exerc Sci. 2020;13(3):1143–55. Published 2020 Aug 1.
16. Giza CC, Hovda DA. The neurometabolic cascade of concussion. J Athl Train. 2001;36(3):228–35.
17. Pattinson CL, Meier TB, Guedes VA, Lai C, Devoto C, Haight T, Broglio SP, McAllister T, Giza C, Huber D, Harezlak J, Cameron K, McGinty G, Jackson J, Guskiewicz K, Mihalik J, Brooks A, Duma S, Rowson S, Nelson LD, Pasquina P, McCrea M, Gill JM, CARE Consortium Investigators. Plasma biomarker concentrations associated with return to sport following sport-related concussion in collegiate athletes-a concussion assessment, research, and education (CARE) consortium study. JAMA Netw Open. 2020;3(8):e2013191. https://doi.org/10.1001/jamanetworkopen.2020.13191. PMID: 32852552; PMCID: PMC7453307.
18. Chen C-L, Lin M-Y, Huda MH, Tsai P-S. Effects of cognitive behavioral therapy for adults with post-concussion syndrome: a systematic review and meta-analysis of randomized controlled trials. J Psychosom Res. 2020;136:110190.

Part II

Spine

Section Editor

S. Ali Mostoufi

Back Pain: Strain and Myofascial Pain

3

Ryan Budwany, Carolyn Poston, and Tony K. George

3.1 Synonyms

- Myofascial Pain Syndrome
- Myofascial Pain
- Strain of muscle, fascia and tendon

3.2 ICD-10 Codes

M79.18, M79.10, S39.012A

New Brunswick	
Fibromyalgia	Spondylolysis
Sacroiliac Joint Pain	Spondylolisthesis
Facet Joint Pain	Spondylosis
Discogenic Back Pain	Diffuse Idiopathic Skeletal Hyperostosis
Cluneal Neuropathy	Lumbar Insufficiency Fracture
Postherpetic Neuralgia	Pelvic Insufficiency Fracture
Polymyalgia Rheumatica	Ankylosing Spondylitis

3.3 Description

Myofascial pain and muscle strain are common in musculoskeletal and pain clinics. They both occur in skeletal muscle. While both involve improper mechanics, myofascial pain is duration-dependent creating muscle fatigue and muscle strain is force-dependent with micro or macro tears.

Myofascial pain is a focal or regional skeletal muscle pain involving muscle and connective tissue. It evokes a combination of sensory, motor, and autonomic symptoms, a hallmark summation of which is trigger point.

Muscle strain is defined as an acute hyperextension injury caused by forceful eccentric stretching of the muscle beyond its tolerable tensile limits. It may involve a partial or complete tear of the muscle from extensive mechanical stress that overwhelms its capacity to adapt.

Anatomy In general, the lumbar spinal muscles work to counter the effect of gravity. In an upright position, the back muscles are quiescent. In positions of flexion and extension, the influence of gravity causes concentric and eccentric contraction of opposing muscles to maintain stability. The line of gravity lies in front of the L4 vertebral body in 75% of individuals [1]. A tilt forward or backward, activates the abdominal or erector spinae muscles. Lumbar discs play a critical role in redistributing pressure and aiding the lumbar muscles in flexion, extension, side bending, and rotatory positions. A degenerated or herniated disc would increase load borne by the muscles potentially increasing risk for fatigue and altered biomechanics across the segment. Tight hip flexors and hamstrings could also create muscle imbalance predisposing to myofascial pain [2]. A flexed and rotated position of the spine puts maximum pressure, increasing the likelihood for a lumbar strain.

Epidemiology More than 80% of people will experience low back pain in their lifetime [3]. Low back pain is more common in females than in males [4]. Back pain due to muscle strain and myofascial pain is more common than back pain due to some other causes such as trauma, infection or malignancy [4]. Lumbar strain is the cause of 70% of uncomplicated low back pain and seen between the ages 20 and 50 [5]. Myofascial pain is estimated to occur in around 85% of patients visiting pain clinics. The most common age group for myofascial pain is between 27 and 50 years [6, 7].

R. Budwany
WVU Center for Integrative Pain Medicine,
Morgantown, WV, USA
e-mail: ryan.budwany@hsc.wvu.edu

C. Poston
The Spine and Nerve Center of the Virginias,
Charleston, WV, USA
e-mail: cposton@centerforpainrelief.com

T. K. George (✉)
Restorative Orthopaedics Spine & Sports (ROSS) Institute,
Somerset, NJ, USA

Department of Orthopaedics, Rutgers-Robert Wood Johnson
Medical School, New Brunswick, NJ, USA

© The Author(s), under exclusive license to Springer Nature Switzerland AG 2022

S. A. Mostoufi et al. (eds.), *Clinical Guide to Musculoskeletal Medicine*, https://doi.org/10.1007/978-3-030-92042-5_3

Etiology Overuse syndrome and alterations in biomechanics are common etiologies of myofascial pain and muscle strain. Overuse syndrome includes increased exercise activity and overload from work postures [8]. Poor work ergonomics are an independent contributor to myofascial pain [8]. Structural changes such as spondylosis and age-related scoliosis are degenerative contributors of myofascial pain. Less common etiologies of myofascial pain include trauma-induced and systemic causes such as vitamin D, iron deficiency, and hypothyroidism. Eleven Studies show myofascial trigger points commonly appear in muscular structures used for posture maintenance [9]. In lumbar spine, muscle imbalances between the erector spinae groups, pelvic floor groups, and hips girdle muscles can trigger myofascial pain. Quadratus Lumborum and Gluteus Medius muscles may be more frequently involved than lumbar and gluteal muscles [2].

3.3.1 Trigger Point

Although the exact reason for trigger point is not well understood, the integrated hypothesis proposed by Travell and Simons explains the interplay of biomechanical, biochemical, and pain sensitization mechanisms giving rise to trigger points seen in myofascial pain. Biomechanical factors such as repetitive contraction and/or excessive muscle load cause buildup of acetylcholine, low acidic PH, and a low ATP energy state creating ischemia, hypoxia, and capillary constriction [10]. In an unprovoked state, biochemical changes in normal muscle activation are in equilibrium. This equilibrium is disturbed when repetitive eccentric contractions or submaximal or maximal concentric contractions create muscle imbalances [10]. An imbalance in acetylcholine required for muscle activation hinders its formation and breakdown leading to an inflammatory and noxious ischemic state [10]. Persistent contractions continue this process of inflammation and ischemia. Recurrent nociceptor activation caused by the noxious milieu modulates pain perception by converting peripheral sensitization to central sensitization [10].

3.4 Clinical Presentation

History is critical in differentiating myofascial pain over lumbar muscle strain as the latter may involve an acute inciting event.

3.4.1 Myofascial Pain

Myofascial pain is described as deep, aching, or sharp and its intensity can vary from minimal to incapacitating. The pain may be felt at rest or during activity. It is regional, often poorly localized and not well circumscribed. Distinct from cutaneous pain, myofascial pain refers highlighting the importance of ruling out other referral sources such as spinal radicular pain. The presence of muscle tenderness and reproduction of symptoms through palpation of "trigger points taut bands" are understood as diagnostic criteria for myofascial pain [7].

Table 3.1 Muscle strains grades and clinical presentation

Grade 1	Less than 5% of muscle fibers effected. Mild damage to individual muscle fibers without loss of strength and motion.
Grade 2	Between 5% and 50% of fibers affected. Partial muscle tear without complete rupture but with significant pain and loss of strength and motion.
Grade 3	Complete rupture of a muscle or tendon. Severe pain, swelling, and complete loss of function. May present with a palpable defect. May require surgery to reattach the damaged muscle and tendon.

3.4.2 Muscle Strain

A muscle strain is a mechanical impairment coinciding with pain. Much of the clinical presentation of strain would overlap with myofascial pain with similar functional deficits and hesitancy toward activity participation. There are three grades of strains as seen in Table 3.1 [11].

3.5 Physical Examination

Examination findings may overlap for myofascial pain and strain making it difficult to distinguish them with examination alone. A distinct feature for myofascial pain is the presence of palpable taut bands. Patients may present with posture asymmetry due to back spasm and demonstrate guarding or hesitancy during active range of motion testing in flexion, extension, side bending or rotation along with impaired function. Trunk movements could trigger symptomatic muscle spasm and patients may hesitate or defer manual strength testing. There should be no antalgic components although there may be an element of hesitation with ambulation. Leg length discrepancy, pelvic obliquity, and scoliosis create mechanical strain affecting lumbar muscles during ambulation. Hamstring and hip flexors should be judiciously examined for range of motion and strength deficits. Their tightness or weakness impacts muscles in its proximity [12].

Lumbar myofascial pain is characterized by palpable bands of muscle tissue called trigger points. Further classified as active and passive, active trigger points are painful at rest and latent trigger points are asymptomatic at rest [13]. They are asynchronous to the direction and texture of normally palpated tissue. They feel nonuniform, heterogenous, with a firm consistency, and refer pain. Sometimes a local twitch response is elicited upon transverse palpation or needle insertion. In the lower back, iliopsoas, piriformis, and quadratus lumborum are common causes of myofascial pain and trigger points in about 48% of the cases [14].

3.6 Diagnostic Workup

3.6.1 Myofascial Pain

Physical examination is all needed for myofascial pain, in particular palpation of taut bands with concordant pain. Imaging is not necessary in myofascial pain. EMG evaluations show increased activity with synergistic muscle contraction of taut muscles compared to normal muscles. These appear as increased frequency of miniature endplate potentials at neuromuscular junctions of taut bands with abnormal spontaneous activity creating endplate noise. Ultrasonography can differentiate taut band which has tissue texture changes and hypoechogenicity [15].

3.6.2 Muscle Strain

In addition to a physical exam, to determine the degree of injury to the muscle, advance imaging could be considered. Both US and MRI have utility in muscle strain. Ultrasound (US) is a first level diagnostic tool, affordable, fast to perform with 77% and 93% for nonstructural and structural injuries, respectively [27]. Ultrasound allows diagnosing a structural injury of the muscle 36–48 hours after the trauma. US appearance of a partial moderate lesion is characterized by a hyperechoic area which becomes markedly inhomogeneous, with evidence of structural disarray, and a wide anechoic area within and outside the muscle [27]. MRI, in particular fluid-sensitive (STIR and T2) sequences, allows detection of lower grade muscle strain and also deeper muscle injuries with sensitivity approaching 92% [27].

3.7 Treatments

3.7.1 Medical Management

3.7.1.1 Muscle Strain

Acute muscle strain should be managed immediately with Protection, Rest, Ice, Compression, and Elevation (PRICE formula). This will help reduce swelling and allow for appropriate healing of the tissue to begin. Bed rest may be appropriate for severe strain and only for a short duration of 1–2 days (prolonged bed rest can have poorer clinical outcome) [20]. NSAIDS are considered first line therapy and effective for nociceptive pain and inflammation associated with acute muscle strain [16]. Duloxetine and mild opioids could be utilized for short-term pain relief of acute muscle injury including strains [17].

3.7.1.2 Myofascial Pain

Acetaminophen and nonsteroidal anti-inflammatory medications are commonly used. Studies have shown topical lidocaine, topical diclofenac sodium, and lidocaine/tetracaine patches are more effective than a control patch [18, 19]. Muscle relaxants may be beneficial in managing myofascial pain but could result in sedation. There are no indications for narcotics in myofascial pain. Studies have shown low levels of vitamin D may have a role in myofascial pain etiology (and other chronic MSK conditions) [2], therefore supplementing it may be necessary.

3.7.2 Rehabilitation

Studies show exercise and patient education reduced the risk of a future episode of low back pain by 45%, whereas exercise alone reduced the risk by only 35% [4].

3.7.2.1 Myofascial Pain

Myofascial Release (MFR)

It is a hands-on soft tissue technique facilitating a stretch into the restricted fascia. The releasing technique addresses both superficial and deep restrictions that may be affecting all four layers of the connective tissue. This technique uses a sustained pressure of 90–120 seconds applied into the tissue barrier causing a histological length change allowing the first release to occur. This is followed by additional releases into the new barrier and can occur many times repetitively. The tissue will then become softer and pliable as the length of the myofascial tissue is restored and will take pressure off of the pain-sensitive structures including nerves and blood vessels allowing normal joint mobility and alignment. Some benefits of MFR include normalization of fluid flow and muscle function, improved nervous system, and proprioceptive function decreasing stress on tissue around the fascia and in other areas of the body.

Physical Therapy

PT can be effective through skilled therapy addressing both soft tissue and joint dysfunction enabling better and more efficient movement patterns. One common example of this would include iliopsoas dysfunction. Restrictions in the iliopsoas are observed in patients presenting with excessive anterior pelvic tilt (Fig. 3.1). This tilt will inhibit transverse abdominal recruitment and can easily be the driver of lumbar strain with activity. Myofascial release to the iliopsoas

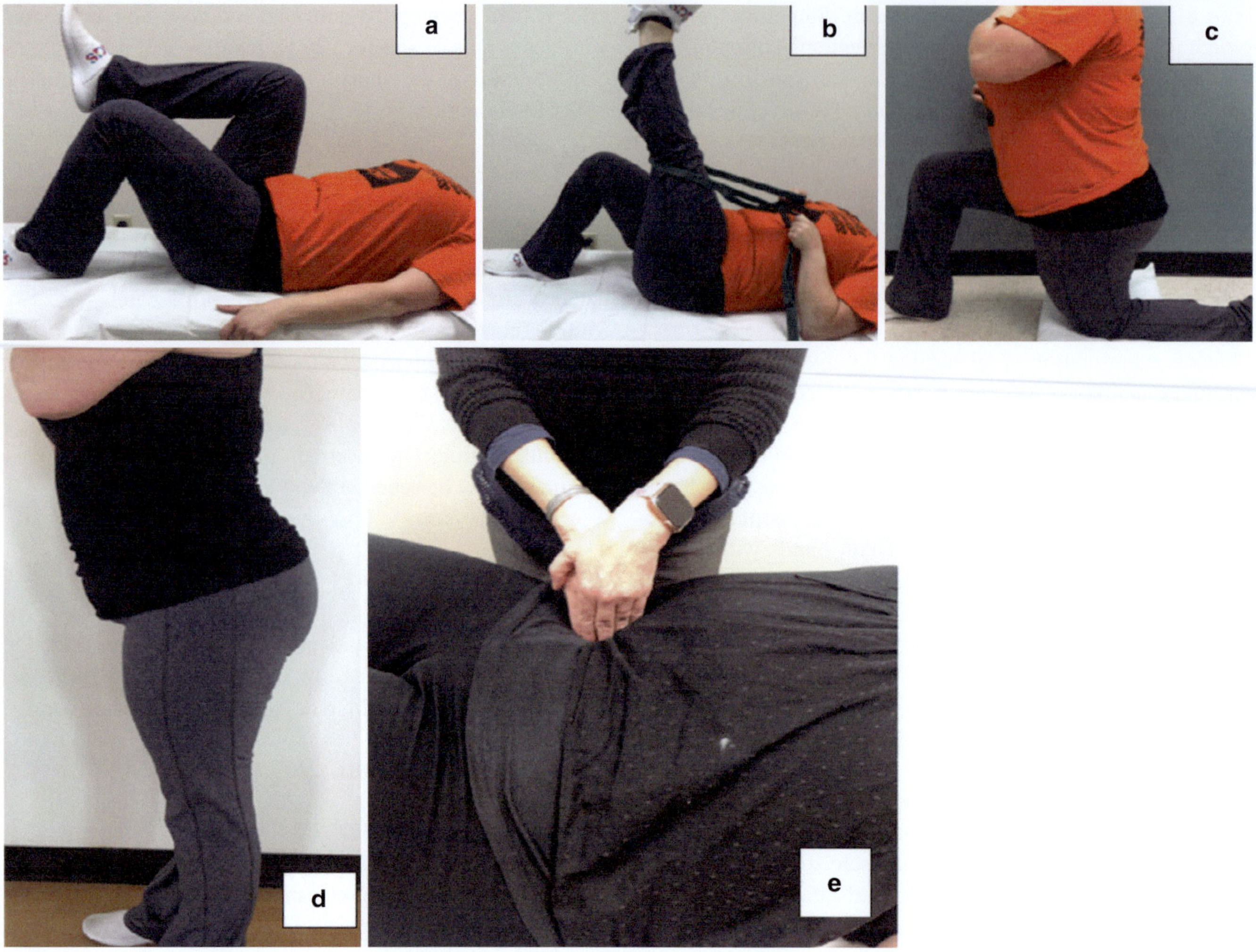

Fig. 3.1 (**a**) Lumbar stabilization exercise. (**b**) Hamstring Stretch. (**c**) Hip flexor stretching. (**d**) Anterior pelvic tilt due to restricted iliopsoas muscles. (**e**) MFR right psoas muscle

(Fig. 3.1) followed by hip flexor stretching (Fig. 3.1) and strengthening allow to strengthen the stabilizers and correct posture in weight bearing, thus reducing stress and strain on the lumbar tissues.

Spray and Stretch Technique

Using vapocoolant spray (e.g., Fluoromethane) along with stretching can facilitate taut muscle length restoration. Cool vapocoolant spray anesthetizes and inhibits cutaneous nociceptors permitting painless range of motion through passive stretch. The stretching motion inactivates myofascial trigger points by releasing muscle tension in the taut fibers and restoring muscle length [19].

3.7.2.2 Muscle Strain

Pain-free active range of motion can be encouraged once the inflammatory phase of healing is ending. As range of motion normalizes and does not elicit pain, strengthening can begin. As strength normalizes, progressions into sport or work-specific activities may commence. This process may take as little as four weeks or as long as three to six months depending upon grade of muscle strain, degree of injury, and the activity levels required from the individual.

In lumbar strain, limitations in hamstring flexibility and loss of adequate strength or recruitment of the stabilizers or inner core, specifically the transverse abdominis are observed. Initial treatments include passive modalities to help continue the healing process. For muscle strain, the passive modalities most commonly used include ultrasound and electrical stimulation (TENS), as well as ice or heat, depending on the stage of healing. Manual therapy including soft tissue and joint mobilization, myofascial release, and muscle energy techniques aid in tissue healing and improve muscular recruitment and balance. Active treatment should include lumbar stabilization exercises (Fig. 3.1) as well as hamstring stretching activities (Fig. 3.1). The stabilization activities typically begin with nonweight bearing but can progress to weight bearing as indicated. Individuals with work-related injuries or bending/lifting deficits, should eventually progress to instruction on proper lifting techniques and body mechanics. Depending on the individual, skilled therapy may be needed 1–2 times per week, for 4–12 weeks to adequately educate on a home exercise program and monitor progress to an appropriate level.

3.7.3 Procedures

3.7.3.1 Trigger Point Injection

Pain associated with myofascial trigger point (active and latent) responds to trigger point injections (TPI) of local anesthetic or dry needling [18, 22]. A physical muscle twitch (twitch response or jump sign) is often seen in TPI/dry needling. In the author's experience, when twitch response is noted, the trigger point injection is more effective. Use of steroids or botulinum toxin is not validated in TPI. US may be used for lower thoracic TPI, particularly in thin individuals to avoid iatrogenic pneumothorax.

3.7.3.2 Acupuncture

Acupuncture is considered one of the oldest medical procedures. Acupuncture stimulation results in the release of endorphins, interleukins, substance P, and adenosine which help to mitigate pain. Opioid antagonists can block the analgesic effects of acupuncture [23, 24]. A meta-analysis showed that acupuncture therapies in isolation or combined with other therapies, are effective in decreasing pain and improving physical function in patients with myofascial pain [25].

3.7.3.3 Orthobiologics

There is no evidence to support the use of orthobiologics in myofascial pain. Utility of PRP has been studied more in tendon disorders as opposed to muscle injury, although PRP may have some utility in Grade I or II muscle strains [21]. Application of orthobiologics in MSK medicine is discussed elsewhere in this book.

3.7.4 Surgery

3.7.4.1 Myofascial Pain

Surgery is not indicated for myofascial pain.

3.7.4.2 Muscle Strain

Surgery for muscle strain may involve reattachment of torn muscle or tendon particularly for a grade III injury. It is indicated for complete lesion of the muscle belly or of the myotendinous junction, and subtotal lesion associated with persistent pain and loss of strength after exhausting conservative management [26, 27]. Optimal suturing of the myotendinous muscle junction injuries should permit early rehabilitation with a low risk of rupture or stitch pullout [27].

References

1. Asmussen E, Klausen K. Form and function of the erect human spine. Clin Orthop. 1962;25:55–63.
2. Malanga GA, Cruz Colon EJ. Myofascial low back pain: a review. Phys Med Rehabil Clin N Am. 2010;21(4):711–24.
3. Rubin DI. Epidemiology and risk factors for spine pain. Neurol Clin. 2007;25(2):353–71.
4. Maher C, Underwood M, Buchbinder R. Non-specific low back pain. Lancet. 2017;389(10070):736–47.
5. Deyo RA, Weinstein JN. Low back pain. N Engl J Med. 2001;344(5):363–70.
6. Tantanatip A, Chang KV. Myofascial pain syndrome. In: StatPearls. Treasure Island (FL); 2021.
7. Nasirzadeh Y, Ahmed S, Monteiro S, Grosman-Rimon L, Srbely J, Kumbhare D. A survey of healthcare practitioners on myofascial pain criteria. Pain Pract. 2018;18(5):631–40.
8. Gerwin RD. A review of myofascial pain and fibromyalgia--factors that promote their persistence. Acupunct Med. 2005;23(3):121–34.
9. Rachlin ES. ISRE: History and physical examination for myofascial pain syndrome. In: Myofascial pain and fibromyalgia. 2nd ed. St Louis: Mosby; 2002. p. 217–30.
10. Gerwin RD, Dommerholt J, Shah JP. An expansion of Simons' integrated hypothesis of trigger point formation. Curr Pain Headache Rep. 2004;8(6):468–75.
11. Jarvinen TA, Kaariainen M, Jarvinen M, Kalimo H. Muscle strain injuries. Curr Opin Rheumatol. 2000;12(2):155–61.
12. Borenstein DG, Wiesel SW, Boden SD. Low back and neck pain: comprehensive diagnosis and management. 3rd ed. Philadelphia: Elsevier; 2004. p. 229–41.
13. Fernandez-de-Las-Penas C, Dommerholt J. International consensus on diagnostic criteria and clinical considerations of myofascial trigger points: a Delphi study. Pain Med. 2018;19(1):142–50.
14. Levene R, Gunther O, Rothkotter HJ, Bitterlich N, Buchmann J. Treatment of myofascial lumbar dorsal pain. Effective clinical diagnostics and therapy. Schmerz. 2014;28(6):573–83.
15. Sikdar S, Shah JP, Gebreab T, Yen RH, Gilliams E, Danoff J, Gerber LH. Novel applications of ultrasound technology to visualize and characterize myofascial trigger points and surrounding soft tissue. Arch Phys Med Rehabil. 2009;90(11):1829–38.
16. Dueweke JJ, Awan TM, Mendias CL. Regeneration of skeletal muscle after eccentric injury. J Sport Rehabil. 2017;26(2):171–9.
17. Qaseem A, Wilt TJ, McLean RM, Forciea MA. Clinical guidelines Committee of the American College of P: noninvasive treatments for acute, subacute, and chronic low back pain: a clinical practice guideline from the American College of Physicians. Ann Intern Med. 2017;166(7):514–30.
18. Urits I, Charipova K, Gress K, Schaaf AL, Gupta S, Kiernan HC, Choi PE, Jung JW, Cornett E, Kaye AD, et al. Treatment and management of myofascial pain syndrome. Best Pract Res Clin Anaesthesiol. 2020;34(3):427–48.
19. Han SC, Harrison P. Myofascial pain syndrome and trigger-point management. Reg Anesth. 1997;22(1):89–101.
20. Deyo RA, Diehl AK, Rosenthal M. How many days of bed rest for acute low back pain? A randomized clinical trial. N Engl J Med. 1986;315(17):1064–70.
21. Chellini F, Tani A, Zecchi-Orlandini S, Sassoli C. Influence of platelet-rich and platelet-poor plasma on endogenous mecha-

nisms of skeletal muscle repair/regeneration. Int J Mol Sci. 2019;20(3):683.
22. Zink W, Bohl JR, Hacke N, Sinner B, Martin E, Graf BM. The long-term myotoxic effects of bupivacaine and ropivacaine after continuous peripheral nerve blocks. Anesth Analg. 2005;101(2):548–54, table of contents.
23. White MC, J. Filshie. Eds. : An introduction to western medical acupuncture-2nd ed. Elsevier Sanders. 2019.
24. Engel GL. The clinical application of the biopsychosocial model. Am J Psychiatry. 1980;137(5):535–44.
25. Wang R, Li X, Zhou S, Zhang X, Yang K, Li X. Manual acupuncture for myofascial pain syndrome: a systematic review and meta-analysis. Acupunct Med. 2017;35(4):241–50.
26. Fernandes TL, Pedrinelli A, Hernandez AJ. Muscle injury - physiopathology, diagnosis, treatment and clinical presentation. Rev Bras Ortop. 2011;46(3):247–55.
27. Maffulli N, Del Buono A, Oliva F, et al. Muscle injuries: a brief guide to classification and management. Transl Med UniSa. 2014;12:14–8. Published 2014 Sep 1.

Back Pain: Discogenic

4

Ya-Ting Chen, Ashley Cotter, and Zacharia Isaac

4.1 Synonyms

- Axial back pain
- Discogenic low back pain
- Discogenic neck pain
- Low back pain without radiculopathy
- Degenerative intervertebral disc disease without herniation
- Annular disruption-induced low back pain
- Internal endplate disruption-induced low back pain

4.2 ICD 10 Code

- Cervical Discogenic Pain Syndrome M50.20
- Discogenic Cervical Pain M54.2
- Lumbar Discogenic Pain Syndrome M51.26
- Discogenic Thoracic Pain M54.6

4.3 Description

Discogenic low back pain is pain related to degenerative disc disease without herniation or other spinal deformities. It is a common etiology in the low back pain population with higher prevalence among younger adults [1–3]. Discogenic pain occurs from degenerative changes of the intervertebral disc in the setting of biomechanical instability and inflammation [1, 2]. Such changes result in central and peripheral nervous system sensitization through mechanisms discussed further below [4, 5, 6]. Diagnosis is predominantly clinical and presently lacks a sensitive and specific noninvasive gold standard test. Degenerative disc changes are commonly present in asymptomatic individuals with increasing incidence based on age. However MRI, CT, and X-ray imaging findings of degenerative disc changes are not sufficient to establish the diagnosis of discogenic pain. Invasive testing, such as provocative discography, has limitations including risk of accelerated disc degeneration [1, 7–9] and therefore is not part of standard medical workup. Additionally, treatment options such as surgical fusion have not demonstrated superiority in several randomized controlled trials compared to cognitive and exercise-oriented therapies [10].

Anatomy The disc is composed of the gel-like central nucleus pulposus containing proteoglycan and water surrounded by the annulus fibrosus consisting of concentric interwoven lamellar sheets, bordered by superior and inferior cartilaginous endplates. Common disc degenerative changes include disc desiccation (dehydration), loss of disc height, concentric bulging, annular tears, and Modic marrow changes of the vertebral endplate. Degenerated disc tissues have high concentrations of inflammatory cytokines and other proinflammatory substances which may contribute to Modic endplate changes; pain-sensitizing processes also occur involving nerve ingrowth into the endplates [4, 5, 6, 11, 12]. The body's attempt to repair annular tears through neovascularization and tissue granulation can further sensitize the new unmyelinated nerve endings of the disc and endplate [4]. Thus, discogenic pain is considered both nociceptive and neuropathic [1]. Discogenic pain originates from the degenerated posterior annulus and is distinct from vertebrogenic pain. Vertebrogenic pain is hypothesized to be nociceptive signals originating from the edematous vertebral endplate and transmitted via the basivertebral nerve [6, 11].

Y.-T. Chen
Department of Physical Medicine and Rehabilitation, Harvard Medical School, Boston, MA, USA
e-mail: ychen118@partners.org

Z. Isaac (✉)
Department of Physical Medicine and Rehabilitation, Harvard Medical School, Comprehensive Spine Care Center, Brigham and Woman's Hospital, Boston, MA, USA
e-mail: zisaac@mgh.harvard.edu

A. Cotter
MGH Brigham Rehabilitation Services, Harvard Medical School, Boston, MA, USA
e-mail: ahcotter@bwh.harvard.edu

© The Author(s), under exclusive license to Springer Nature Switzerland AG 2022

S. A. Mostoufi et al. (eds.), *Clinical Guide to Musculoskeletal Medicine*, https://doi.org/10.1007/978-3-030-92042-5_4

Etiology (Table 4.2) The incidence of discogenic lower back pain appears to be higher in patients who are obese, sedentary, smokers, and those with jobs exposed to frequent lifting and vibration [13]. Based on studies, MRI of individuals who smoke or have jobs requiring lifting shows a greater disc height reduction over the course of years. This suggests smoking and lifting as modifiable risk factors for discogenic pain [14]. Additionally, inflammatory reactions, infections, and metabolic disorders could also potentially accelerate disc degeneration [1]. A 16-year prospective cohort study also demonstrated cardiovascular risk factors including atherosclerosis to be significantly and independently associated with symptomatic lumbar disc herniation [15]. In a case-control study, genetic and familial risk factors as well as occupational risk factors were contributors to degenerative disc disease [14, 16]. Recent studies demonstrate intervertebral disc disease to be a common cause of chronic low back pain among younger adults (mean age of 44 years), while older patients are more likely to have facet joint or sacroiliac joint pain until age 70 [3].

4.4 Clinical Presentation

Discogenic pain is generally described as a midline, nonradiating, deep dull ache, provoked by forward flexion due to increased axial loading [17]. Coughing, sneezing, valsalva, jumping, and running may trigger an acute painful episode severe enough to warrant urgent care visit. Pain can radiate to the groin, buttocks or thigh, even without nerve compression [17]. Symptoms may improve with standing, lying flat, and lumbar extension [18]. Red flags must be ruled out including fever and chills, progressive weakness and numbness, bowel and/or bladder dysfunction, and weight loss, as they may indicate systemic disease, cancer, spinal abscess, osteomyelitis, or spinal cord compression. Discogenic pain can be difficult to diagnose as it may overlap with other back pain etiologies, including myofascial pain, fractures, facet-mediated pain, sacroiliac-mediated pain, proximal lumbar radiculopathy, and vertebrogenic pain.

4.5 Physical Examination

A comprehensive neurological and musculoskeletal examination helps narrow the differential diagnoses of low back pain (Table 4.1). There is no gold standard highly sensitive/specific examination for discogenic back pain. A reliable test is axial low back pain during forward flexion and should raise the suspicion for discogenic or vertebrogenic pathology [17]. As discogenic pain shares similar characteristics with many other spinal and skeletal disorders, examining patients to rule out the other common back pain etiologies is important.

4.6 Diagnostic Workup

4.6.1 X-Rays

Plain radiographs are poor in visualizing disc material but can identify deformities, spondylolysis, and spondylolisthesis, disc space narrowing, bony endplate changes, calcification in soft tissue, and other degenerative changes of spine structure including the facets. X-ray is often the first diagnostic test in a symptomatic spine without red flags.

4.6.2 MRI

Currently there is no gold standard for diagnosing discogenic back pain. MRI is the most frequently used diagnostic imaging modality in evaluating discogenic pain [19]. Despite different MRI techniques, it is important to know that many people with imaging findings of disc degeneration are asymptomatic. MRI is only moderately effective in identifying the etiology of back pain.

MRI can assess disc desiccation (decreased water concentration and decreased proteoglycan content), loss of disc height, disc herniations, and marrow endplate abnormality (Modic changes) [9, 14]. In research, the MRI-based Pfirrmann grading (I-V) is typically used to provide both semiquantitative and subjective assessment of the disc structures and signal intensities on a sagittal T2-weighted MRI

Table 4.1 Differential diagnosis of discogenic low back pain

Spinal stenosis with back pain	Spondylolisthesis
Compression fracture	Failed back surgery syndrome
Proximal extent of radiculopathy	Sacroiliac joint dysfunction syndrome
Facet joint pain	Myofascial pain
Kyphosis/scoliosis-related mechanics	Ligamentous injury

Table 4.2 Risk Factors for Discogenic back pain

Cardiovascular risks (Age <60)	Genetic risks	Occupational risks	General risks
Hypertension	Polymorphisms of matrix metalloproteinase 3	Smokers with a lifting job	Smokers
Atherosclerosis	Polymorphisms of vitamin D receptor	Jobs with twisting	BMI >30
Diabetes	Family history of LBP	Jobs with bending	Previous Back injury
MI	Familial obesity	Jobs with whole body vibration	Sedentary people

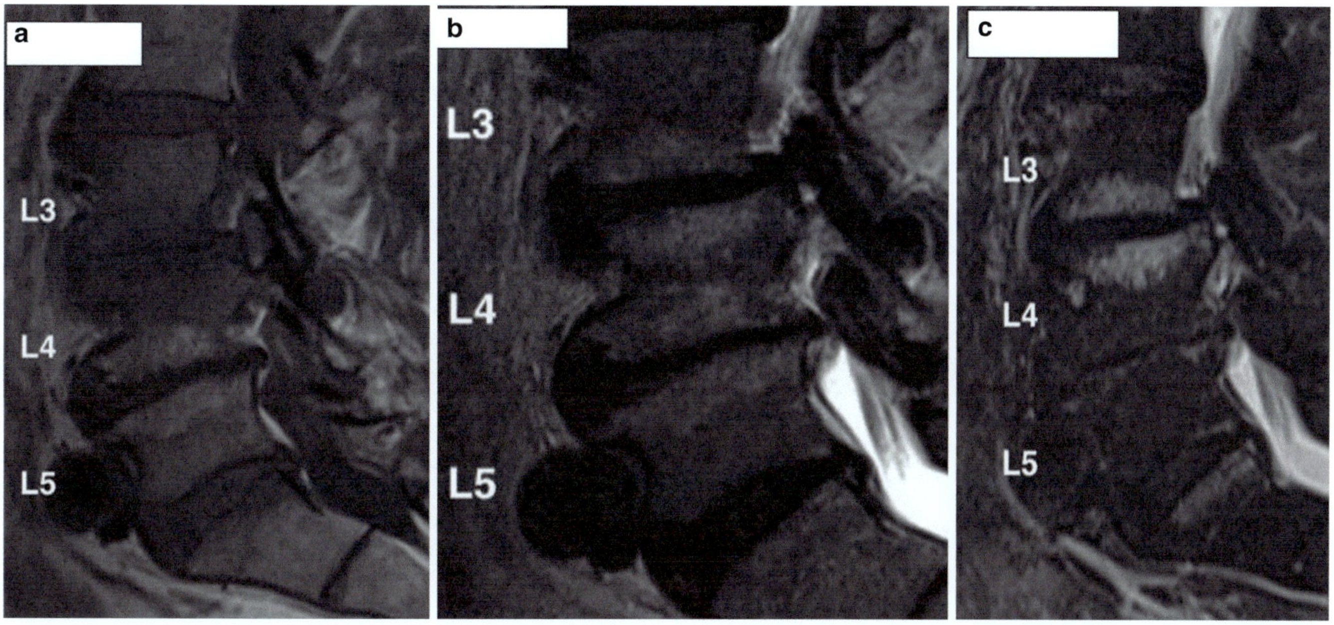

Fig. 4.1 Modic type 1 changes at L3-4 hallmarked by marrow edema (hypointense on T1-weighted (**a**), hyperintense on T2-weighted (**b**), and hyperintense on STIR (**c**). Modic type 2 changes are present at L4-5 hallmarked by marrow signal changes being hyperintense on T1 (**a**), hyperintense on T2 (**b**), and isointense on STIR (**c**)

Table 4.3 The Modic classification based on MRI sequence [20]

Modic Type	Endplate changes	T1-weighted Sequence	T2-weighted Sequence
1	Edema	Hypointense	Hyperintense
2	Fat infiltration	Hyperintense	Isointense or hyperintense
3	Sclerotic changes	Hypointense	Hypointense

[1]. The Modic classification (types 1–3) is also commonly used to describe the endplate-related signal changes (Fig. 4.1 and Table 4.3) and is based on findings seen in both T1-weighted and T2-weighted MRI [20]. Modic 1 change in particular is highly associated with discogenic back pain [21]. Additionally, the high-intensity zone (HIZ), a hyperintense signal located in the posterior annulus fibrosus is clearly distinct from the signal from the nucleus pulposus on MRI and correlates with increased level of annulus damage and back pain [1].

Hyperintensity zone (HIZ) has been shown to be particularly easy to recognize on T2-weighted MRI of the lumbosacral spine [1, 22, 23]. Both type 1 Modic changes and HIZ have shown to correlate to positive findings on discography [1, 24, 25]. On conventional T2-weighted MRI, morphology and water content of the disc can be assessed, but this modality is not sensitive to detecting the proteoglycan content found in nucleus pulposus [26]. Alternatively, $T1_\rho$ MRI is a different technique shown to correlate well with nucleus pulposus' proteoglycan content [27]. In a study with a sample size of 28 patients, the $T1_\rho$ value was significantly lower in the painful discs among patients who received multilevel provocative discography [27].

4.6.3 Discography

According to a systematic review, discography was the second most commonly utilized diagnostic test for this diagnosis [19]. Image-guided provocative discography can be performed to elicit concordant back pain by injecting contrast dye into the nucleus pulposus of the disc and pressurizing the degenerated disc while comparing the result to injection of contrast into a control disc which is normal on MR and pain-free with the injection (Fig. 4.2). An asymptomatic disc (control) is required to determine whether this test has specificity. When pain is generated by discography, it is either *concordant* (familiar in location and diagnostic) or *discordant* (different location and nondiagnostic). Discography is considered positive if it elicits concordant pain. Further characterization of the disc degeneration requires postdiscography CT scan which defines internal disc derangement including annular tear and fissures.

The risks for provocative discography include discitis, neurologic injury, reaction to contrast dye, increased risk of accelerated disc degeneration, and ipsilateral herniation [8, 9]. Despite these potential risks, it was estimated that about 70,000 patients had received lumbar provocative discography in 2013 [8]. It is therefore important to have an informed discussion with the patient regarding the limitations, benefits, and risks of discography in the diagnostic workup for discogenic back pain.

A recent systematic review found the diagnostic accuracy of lumbar discography for chronic discogenic back pain to have a fair level of evidence when the International Association for the Study of Pain (IASP) criteria were applied [28]. The IASP criteria are met when a patient's back

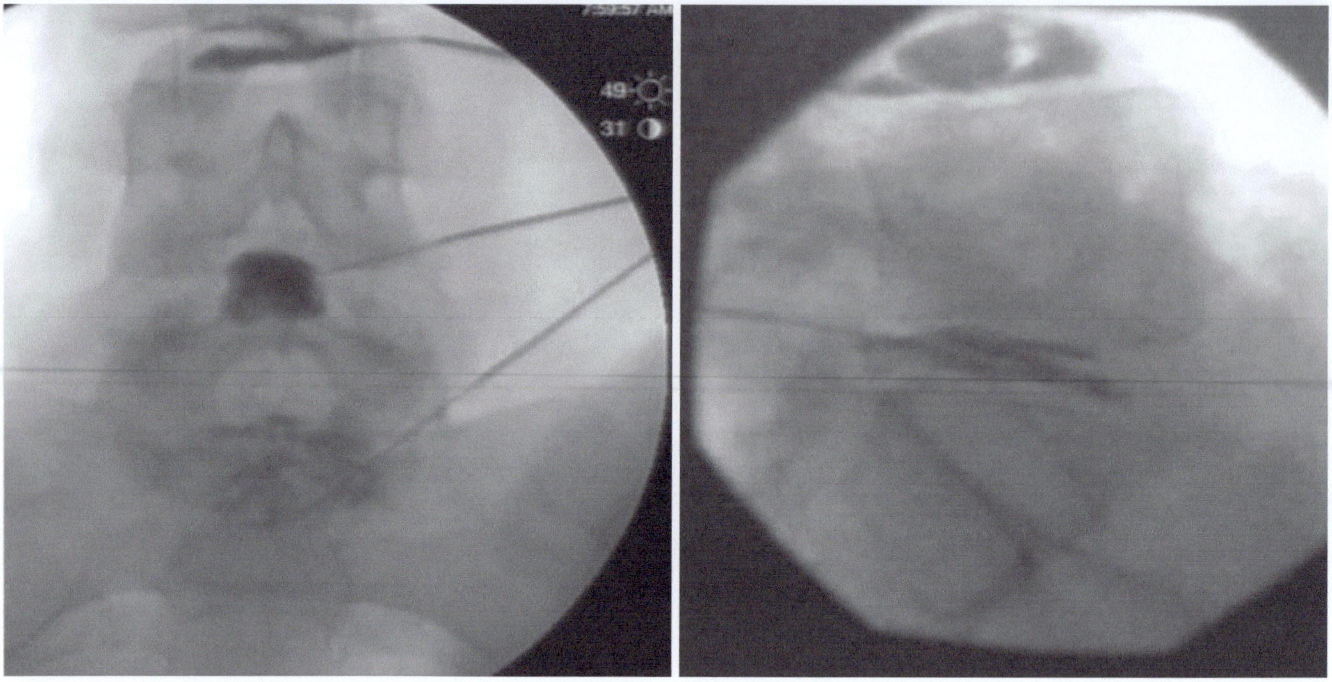

Fig. 4.2 AP and lateral X-rays of L3-5 discography. L3/4 and L5/S1 are both desiccated. L4/5 and L5/S1 disc both appear fissured

pain is reproduced with disc stimulation without pain provocation at two adjacent discs, and when no other pain generator could be identified [19]. The systemic review demonstrated Level 3 evidence for the prevalence and diagnostic accuracy of lumbar discography, and Level 4 evidence for cervical discography utilizing IASP criteria [28]. Though a strong correlation between positive discography and positive imaging for disc degeneration has been demonstrated, discography does not appear to improve spinal fusion outcomes [7, 8].

Serum Biomarkers Many serum biomarkers are being studied as a new way to determine the source of back pain and they include but are not limited to tumor necrosis factors, interleukins, type 2 collagen, fibrinogen, substance P, and complement C3. These biomarkers can be indicative of specific biologic processes contributing to discogenic pain, but the major diagnostic challenge is in increasing their specificity as many of these biological factors are also involved in systemic disorders [1].

4.7 Treatments

4.7.1 Medical Management

To date, there is no well-established treatment that is consistently effective for managing discogenic pain [1, 2, 19]. Nonoperative and nonpharmacological therapies are recommended as first-line treatments including acetaminophen, nonsteroidal anti-inflammatory agents (NSAIDs), and short-term opioids [1, 2, 29]. Oral steroids have minimal role in managing discogenic pain [2]. Use of muscle relaxants is common but causes sedation with limited benefit [1, 29]. As discogenic pain consists of both nociceptive and neuropathic pain, duloxetine, a selective serotonin and norepinephrine reuptake inhibitor, may be useful in managing discogenic pain (FDA approved for chronic low back pain in adults) [1, 2, 30].

4.7.2 Rehabilitation

Therapeutic PT exercises include range-of-motion, stretching, core stabilization, motor control, strengthening, and general conditioning. Individualized exercises prescribed to match the directional preference have been shown to promote centralization for radiating lower extremity pain, improve mobility, and reduce medication use [31, 32]. Discogenic low back pain typically follows an extension directional preference, such as repeated standing or prone lumbar extension, and can reduce radicular symptoms and low back pain (Fig. 4.3). Lumbar core stabilization instruction can be individualized according to the patient's directional preference, with emphasis on appropriate recruitment patterns of the deep core spinal stabilizers, such as bird-dog exercise (Fig. 4.4) and prone trunk (Fig. 4.5) extension exercise [33, 34]. Stretching of tight lower extremity and core musculature can be beneficial in relieving local myofascial symptoms, but not recommended if the stretch increases radicular symptoms.

Physical therapists also provide general education on body mechanics, behavioral education, and pain physiology

[32]. This includes but is not limited to functional movement training, home exercise program, strategies to prevent recurrence, cognitive behavioral therapy, and pain education. Current evidence supports pain education with chronic musculoskeletal conditions and has been shown to reduce psychosocial factors, increase patient knowledge of pain, decrease disability and pain, and minimal healthcare utilization [35].

The physical therapy management of discogenic low back pain is most effective with a multimodal treatment approach with a combination of McKenzie Method of Mechanical Diagnosis and Therapy, therapeutic PT exercise, manual therapy, traction, modalities, and pain neuroscience education.

Manual therapy for the lumbar spine includes spinal manipulative therapy (SMT), spinal mobilization, soft tissue mobilization, and myofascial release. Studies have shown patients with discogenic low back pain undergoing lumbar mechanical traction in combination with manual therapy had statistically significant improvement in low back pain and lumbar range of motion [36, 37].

4.7.3 Procedures

4.7.3.1 Steroid Injections

There is no indication for the routine use of epidural steroid injections for discogenic low back pain, and there is also a lack of evidence for intradiscal steroid injections [1, 7, 38]. In low power studies, patients with discogenic axial back pain appear to benefit from transforaminal epidural delivery in terms of pain and physical function [39].

4.7.3.2 Intradiscal PRP

Platelet-rich plasma (PRP) is a concentrated solution of platelet, fibrin, and growth factors that may promote cellular repair or replacement of the diseased annulus fibrosus, nucleus pulposus, and intervertebral discs [1, 40]. Based on a recent meta-analysis, intradiscal PRP has been shown to significantly improve discogenic pain (visual analog scale) and disability (Oswestry Disability Index score) by 2 months and 6 months after intradiscal injections [40, 41]. While intradiscal PRP (Fig. 4.6) carries similar risks to discography

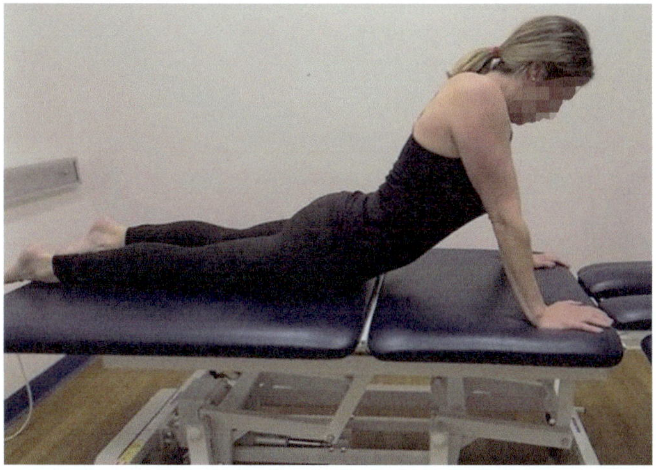

Fig. 4.3 Prone lumbar extension

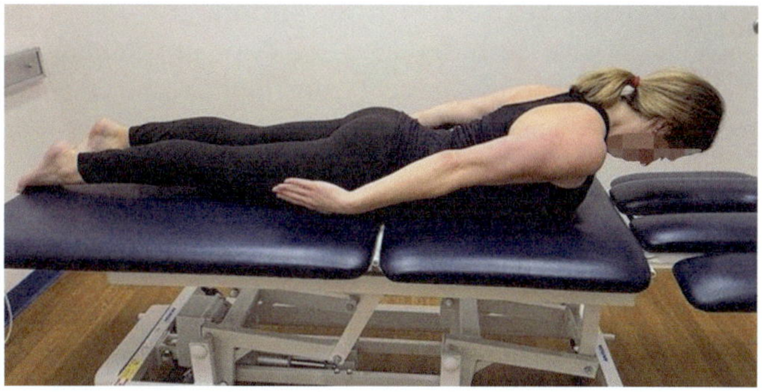

Fig. 4.5 Prone lumbar extension hold

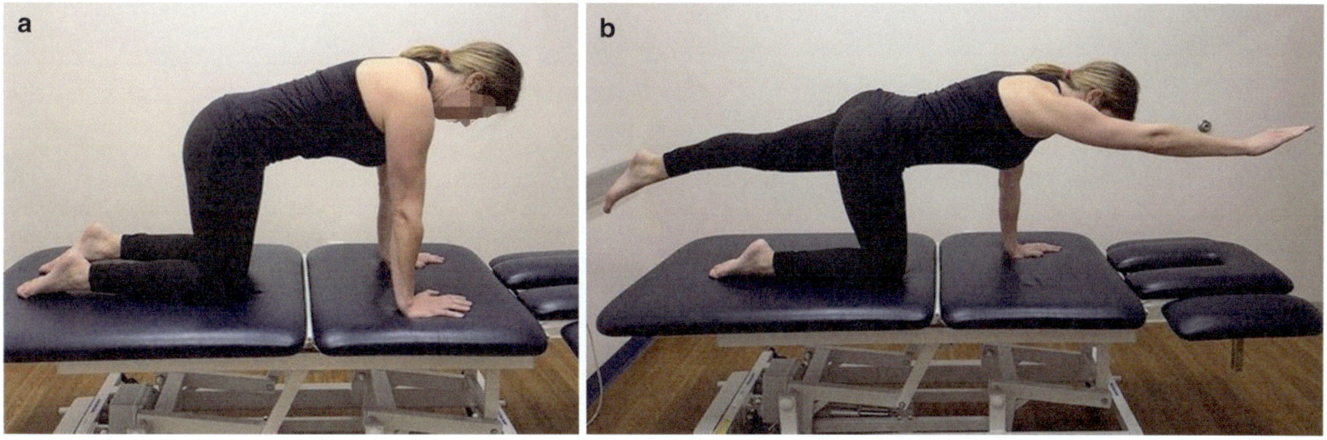

Fig. 4.4 (**a**) Deep core stabilization. (**b**) Bird-dog exercise

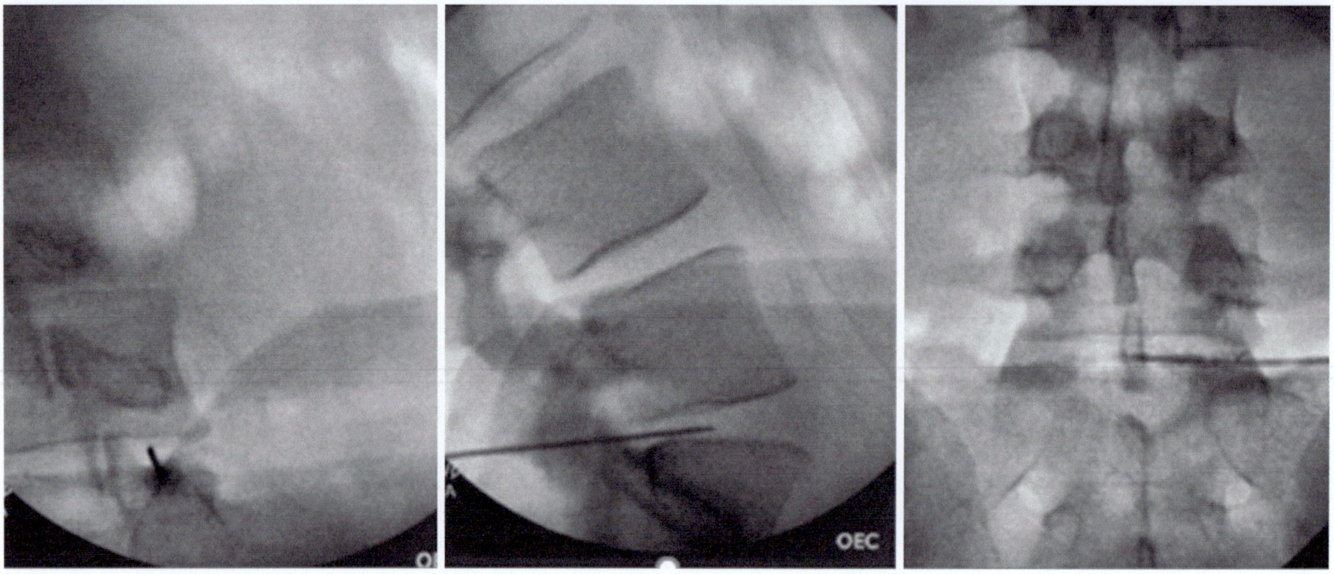

Fig. 4.6 Intradiscal access for regenerative disc treatments

given its invasive nature (Fig. 4.6), no adverse event was reported in aforementioned meta-analysis [2]. Further research is needed to evaluate PRP's long-term safety and outcome [2].

4.7.3.3 Other Intradiscal Interventions

Techniques have been developed to thermally (intradiscal electrothermal therapy) or chemically (intradiscal methylene blue injection) ablate the newly grown nerve fibers and/or inflammatory structures at the involved disc, but these interventions overall have poor evidence and therefore are rarely used [1, 2].

4.7.3.4 Intraosseous Radiofrequency Ablation of the Basivertebral Nerve

As vertebrogenic low back pain can also occur due to increased nociceptive transmission via the basivertebral nerve in the setting of discogenic endplate degenerative changes, a transpedicular delivery system (Intracept System, Relievant Medsystems, Sunnyvale, CA, USA) has been developed with the goal to interrupt the pain transmission by thermally ablating the basivertebral nerve [11]. This minimally invasive technique has recently gained level 1 evidence based on a double-blinded, randomized clinical trial with 2-year outcome among patients with chronic lumbar back pain and Type 1 or 2 Modic changes who had not responded to nonoperative management [11]. For details on this topic, refer to chapter *Vertebrogenic back pain.*

Spinal cord stimulation (SCS) While SCS is not indicated for treating discogenic pain in nonoperated spine, it is a growing neuromodulation therapy utilized for refractory chronic back or leg pain in the postoperative failback conditions. Paresthesia-free high frequency SCS is shown to be superior to the traditional paresthesia-based SCS in two randomized clinical trials [42].

4.7.4 Surgery

Pursuing interbody fusion surgeries to remove the painful disc is considered as a second-line option for those who did not respond to nonoperative therapies [1]. Long-term clinical studies so far have seen fusion failure, persistent chronic pain, and adjacent segment disease (ASD) as potential complications after the surgery [2]. Total or artificial disc replacement is a newer technology that may avoid ASD and maintain segmental mobility, but its long-term outcome is still being investigated [1, 7]. For details of surgical options, refer to chapter *Surgeries in Spine*.

References

1. Fujii K, Yamazaki M, Kang JD, Risbud MV, Cho SK, Qureshi SA, Hecht AC, Iatridis JC. Discogenic back pain: literature review of definition, diagnosis, and treatment. JBMR Plus. 2019; https://doi.org/10.1002/jbm4.10180.
2. Zhao L, Manchikanti L, Kaye AD, Abd-Elsayed A. Treatment of discogenic low Back pain: current treatment strategies and future options—a literature review. Curr Pain Headache Rep. 2019; https://doi.org/10.1007/s11916-019-0821-x.
3. DePalma MJ, Ketchum JM, Saullo T. What is the source of chronic low Back pain and does age play a role? Pain Med. 2011;12:224–33.
4. García-Cosamalón J, del Valle ME, Calavia MG, García-Suárez O, López-Muñiz A, Otero J, Vega JA. Intervertebral disc, sensory

nerves and neurotrophins: who is who in discogenic pain? J Anat. 2010;217:1–15.
5. Yang G, Liao W, Shen M, Mei H. Insight into neural mechanisms underlying discogenic back pain. J Int Med Res. 2018;46:4427–36.
6. Fischgrund JS, Rhyne A, Franke J, et al. Intraosseous basivertebral nerve ablation for the treatment of chronic low back pain: a prospective randomized double-blind sham-controlled multi-center study. Eur Spine J. 2018;27:1146–56.
7. Chou R, Loeser JD, Owens DK, et al. Interventional therapies, surgery, and interdisciplinary rehabilitation for low back pain: an evidence-based clinical practice guideline from the American pain society. Spine. 2009;34:1066–77.
8. Cuellar JM, Stauff MP, Herzog RJ, Carrino JA, Baker GA, Carragee EJ. Does provocative discography cause clinically important injury to the lumbar intervertebral disc? A 10-year matched cohort study. Spine J. 2016;16:273–80.
9. Carragee EJ, Don AS, Hurwitz EL, Cuellar JM, Carrino J, Herzog R. 2009 ISSLS prize winner: does discography cause accelerated progression of degeneration changes in the lumbar disc: a ten-year matched cohort study. Spine. 2009;34:2338–45.
10. Mannion AF, Brox JI, Fairbank JCT. Comparison of spinal fusion and nonoperative treatment in patients with chronic low back pain: long-term follow-up of three randomized controlled trials. Spine Journal. 2013;13:1438–48.
11. Fischgrund JS, Rhyne A, Franke J, et al. Intraosseous basivertebral nerve ablation for the treatment of chronic low back pain: 2-year results from a prospective randomized double-blind sham-controlled multicenter study. Int J Spine Surg. 2019;13:110–9.
12. Brown MF, Hukkanen MVJ, McCarthy ID, Redfern DRM, Batten JJ, Crock HV, Hughes SPF, Polak JM. Sensory and sympathetic innervation of the vertebral endplate in patients with degenerative disc disease. J Bone Joint Surg. 1997;79-B:147–53.
13. Urits I, Burshtein A, Sharma M, et al. Low back pain, a comprehensive review: pathophysiology, diagnosis, and treatment. Curr Pain Headache Rep. 2019; https://doi.org/10.1007/s11916-019-0757-1.
14. Videman T, Battié MC, Parent E, Gibbons LE, Vainio P, Kaprio J. Progression and determinants of quantitative magnetic resonance imaging measures of lumbar disc degeneration: a five-year follow-up of adult male monozygotic twins. Spine. 2008;33:1484–90.
15. Jhawar BS, Fuchs CS, Colditz GA, Stampfer MJ. Cardiovascular risk factors for physician-diagnosed lumbar disc herniation. Spine J. 2006;6:684–91.
16. Zawilla NH, Darweesh H, Mansour N, Helal S, Taha FM, Awadallah M, el Shazly R. Matrix metalloproteinase-3, vitamin D receptor gene polymorphisms, and occupational risk factors in lumbar disc degeneration. J Occup Rehabil. 2014;24(2):370–81. https://doi.org/10.1007/s10926-013-9472-7.
17. Park WM, Kim K, Kim YH. Effects of degenerated intervertebral discs on intersegmental rotations, intradiscal pressures, and facet joint forces of the whole lumbar spine. Comput Biol Med. 2013;43:1234–40.
18. Chou R, Cotton D, Rao JK, Taichman D, Williams S. Low back pain. Ann Intern Med. 2014; https://doi.org/10.7326/0003-4819-160-11-201406030-01006.
19. Malik KM, Cohen SP, Walega DR, Benzon HT. Diagnostic criteria and treatment of discogenic pain: a systematic review of recent clinical literature. Spine J. 2013;13:1675–89.
20. Herlin C, Kjaer P, Espeland A, Skouen JS, Leboeuf-Yde C, Karppinen J, Niinimäki J, Sørensen JS, Storheim K, Jensen TS. Modic changes—their associations with low back pain and activity limitation: a systematic literature review and meta-analysis. PLoS One. 2018; https://doi.org/10.1371/journal.pone.0200677.
21. Dudli S, Fields AJ, Samartzis D, Karppinen J, Lotz JC. Pathobiology of Modic changes. Eur Spine J. 2016;25:3723–34.
22. Teraguchi M, Samartzis D, Hashizume H, et al. Classification of high intensity zones of the lumbar spine and their association with other spinal MRI phenotypes: the Wakayama spine study. PLoS One. 2016; https://doi.org/10.1371/journal.pone.0160111.
23. Carragee EJ, Paragioudakis SJ, Khurana S. Lumbar high-intensity zone and discography in subjects without low back problems. Spine. 2000;25:2987–92.
24. Dongfeng R, Hou S, Wu W, Wang H, Shang W, Tang J, Li Z, Lei G. The expression of tumor necrosis factor-α and CD68 in high-intensity zone of lumbar intervertebral disc on magnetic resonance image in the patients with low back pain. Spine. 2011; https://doi.org/10.1097/BRS.0b013e3181dfce9e.
25. Thompson KJ, Dagher AP, Eckel TS, Clark M, Reinig JW. Modic changes on MR images as studied with provocative diskography: clinical relevance-a retrospective study of 2457 disks. Radiology. 2009;250:849–55.
26. Pfirrmann CWA, Metzdorf A, Zanetti M, Hodler J, Boos N. Magnetic resonance classification of lumbar intervertebral disc degeneration. Spine. 2001;26:1873–8.
27. Borthakur A, Maurer PM, Fenty M, Wang C, Berger R, Yoder J, Balderston RA, Elliott DM. T1ρ magnetic resonance imaging and discography pressure as novel biomarkers for disc degeneration and low back pain. Spine. 2011;36:2190–6.
28. Manchikanti L, Soin A, Benyamin RM, Singh V, Falco FJE, Calodney AK, Grami V, Hirsch JA. An update of the systematic appraisal of the accuracy and utility of discography in chronic spinal pain. Pain Physician. 2018;21:91–110.
29. Chou R, Deyo R, Friedly J, Skelly A, Weimer M, Fu R, Dana T, Kraegel P, Griffin J, Grusing S. Systemic pharmacologic therapies for low back pain: a systematic review for an American College of physicians clinical practice guideline. Ann Intern Med. 2017;166:480–92.
30. Schukro RP, Oehmke MJ, Geroldinger A, Heinze G, Kress HG, Pramhas S. Efficacy of duloxetine in chronic low back pain with a neuropathic component: a randomized, double-blind, placebo-controlled crossover trial. Anesthesiology. 2016;124:150–8.
31. Lam OT, Strenger DM, Chan-Fee M, Pham PT, Preuss RA, Robbins SM. Effectiveness of the McKenzie method of mechanical diagnosis and therapy for treating low back pain: literature review with meta-analysis. J Orthop Sports Phys Ther. 2018;48:476–90.
32. Delitto A, George SZ, Van Dillen LR, Whitman JM, Sowa G, Shekelle P, Denninger TR, Godges JJ, Orthopaedic Section of the American Physical Therapy Association. Low back pain. J Orthop Sports Phys Ther. 2012; https://doi.org/10.2519/jospt.2012.42.4.a1.
33. MacDonald DA, Lorimer Moseley G, Hodges PW. The lumbar multifidus: does the evidence support clinical beliefs? Man Ther. 2006;11:254–63.
34. Kelly M, Jacobs D, Wooten ME, Edeer AO. Comparison of electromyographic activities of lumbar iliocostalis and lumbar multifidus muscles during stabilization exercises in prone, quadruped, and sitting positions. J Phys Ther Sci. 2016;28:2950–4.
35. Louw A, Zimney K, Puentedura EJ, Diener I. The efficacy of pain neuroscience education on musculoskeletal pain: a systematic review of the literature. Physiother Theory Pract. 2016;32:332–55.
36. Mohamed HE, Wadida, Elsayed H, Aneis YM. The combined effect of maitland spinal mobilization with mechanical lumbar traction in patients with chronic nonspecific low back pain. Egypt J Appl Sci. 2020;35:136–50.
37. Lee Y, Lee CR, Cho M. Effect of decompression therapy combined with joint mobilization on patients with lumbar herniated nucleus pulposus. J Phys Ther Sci. 2012;24:829–32.
38. Foster NE, Anema JR, Cherkin D, et al. Prevention and treatment of low back pain: evidence, challenges, and promising directions. Lancet. 2018;391:2368–83.
39. Kumar K, Taylor RS, Jacques L, et al. Spinal cord stimulation versus conventional medical management for neuropathic pain: a

multicentre randomised controlled trial in patients with failed back surgery syndrome. Pain. 2007;132:179–88.
40. Chang MC, Park D. The effect of intradiscal platelet-rich plasma injection for management of discogenic lower back pain: a meta-analysis. J Pain Res. 2021;14:505–12.
41. Jain D, Goyal T, Verma N, Paswan AK, Dubey RK. Intradiscal platelet-rich plasma injection for discogenic low back pain and correlation with platelet concentration: a prospective clinical trial. Pain Med (United States). 2020;21:2719–25.
42. Caylor J, Reddy R, Yin S, et al. Spinal cord stimulation in chronic pain: evidence and theory for mechanisms of action. Bioelectr Med. 2019; https://doi.org/10.1186/s42234-019-0023-1.
43. Tuakli-Wosornu YA, Terry A, Boachie-Adjei K, Harrison JR, Gribbin CK, LaSalle EE, Nguyen JT, Solomon JL, Lutz GE. Lumbar intradiskal platelet-rich plasma (PRP) injections: a prospective, double-blind, randomized controlled study. PM & R. 2016;8:1–10.
44. Levi D, Horn S, Tyszko S, Levin J, Hecht-Leavitt C, Walko E. Intradiscal platelet-rich plasma injection for chronic discogenic low back pain: preliminary results from a prospective trial. Pain Med (United States). 2016;17:1010–22.
45. Kapural L, Yu C, Doust MW, et al. Novel 10-kHz high-frequency therapy (HF10 therapy) is superior to traditional low-frequency spinal cord stimulation for the treatment of chronic back and leg pain. Anesthesiology. 2015;123:851–60.
46. Cameron T. Safety and efficacy of spinal cord stimulation for the treatment of chronic pain: a 20-year literature review. J Neurosurg. 2004;100:254–67.

Back Pain: Facet Syndrome

5

Paragi Rana

5.1 Synonyms

- Facet joint arthropathy
- Facet joint arthritis
- Facet joint pain
- Zygapophyseal joint pain
- Spondylosis (Cervical, Thoracic, or Lumbar)

5.2 ICD 10 – Code

- ***Cervical*** – M47.812 Spondylosis without myelopathy or radiculopathy cervical region; M47.892 Other spondylosis, cervical region; M54.2 cervicalgia
- ***Thoracic*** – M47.814 Spondylosis without myelopathy or radiculopathy thoracic region; M47.894 Other spondylosis, thoracic region; M54.6 Pain in thoracic spine
- ***Lumbar*** – M47.817 Spondylosis without myelopathy or radiculopathy; M47.896 Other spondylosis, lumbar region, M54.5 Low back pain

5.3 Description

Spine facet syndrome (unilateral or bilateral) occurs when facet or zygapophyseal joints become the source of pain. The reported prevalence of facet pain in the population is both variable and controversial ranging from cervical 25–66%, thoracic 34–48%, and lumbar 22–45% [1, 2]. Overall, its incidence increases with advancing age.

Facetogenic pain most commonly occurs in the setting of degenerative disease, repetitive sprain, poor ergonomics, and trauma. Intervertebral disc degeneration will also alter stress forces on the facet joints and vice versa. The presence of concurrent disc height narrowing is associated a nearly two-fold increased risk of facet joint osteoarthritis [3]. Other etiologies of facet pain, include synovial cyst, inflammatory arthritis, and trauma particularly deceleration injuries; this includes whiplash injuries which can account for more than 50% of cases of chronic axial neck pain following motor vehicle accidents [4]. In the lumbar spine, Body Mass Index (BMI) has been found to be an independent risk factor. BMI of 25–30 and BMI of 30–35 are associated with a three- and five-fold higher risk of developing facet arthropathy respectively [5].

In the cervical spine, the C2-3 is the most common cervical facet pain generator followed by C5-6 [6]. The C1-2 and C2-3 joints are generally implicated in cervicogenic headaches. In the lumbar spine, the greatest degree of strain and motion occurs at L4-5 and L5-S1.

5.3.1 Anatomy

There are 23 pairs of facet joints from C2 to S1. Facets and intervertebral discs combined provide stability to the spinal column. Each facet joint is formed by the articulation of the inferior and superior articular processes of adjacent vertebral bodies. Facets are synovial joints and its articulation processes are covered by cartilage and synovial lining, and the joint is surrounded by a fibrous capsule and ligaments [7]. The orientation of the facet joint is variable based on location. In the cervical spine, the joints are inclined approximately 45 degrees from the axial plane. Thoracic facet joints are the most vertically orientated; they have an approximate 60-degree incline and 20-degree rotation in the axial plane. In the lumbar spine, upper lumbar facet joints are more aligned with the sagittal plane; in contrast, lower lumbar facet joints are more parallel to the coronal plane [3]. The volume capacity of the joint is 0.5–1 mL in the cervical/thoracic spine and 1–1.5 mL in the lumbar spine.

The facet joint is well innervated by encapsulated, unencapsulated, and free nerve endings. The synovial lining contains small C-type nerve fibers [8]. In general, facets have a

P. Rana (✉)
Anesthesiology, Yale School of Medicine, New Haven, CT, USA
e-mail: rana.paragi@yale.edu

© The Author(s), under exclusive license to Springer Nature Switzerland AG 2022
S. A. Mostoufi et al. (eds.), *Clinical Guide to Musculoskeletal Medicine*, https://doi.org/10.1007/978-3-030-92042-5_5

Table 5.1 Differential diagnosis of cervical facet syndrome

Cervical discogenic pain	Myofascial/soft tissue pain, fibromyalgia
Cervical radiculopathy	Cervical spine strain/sprain
Inflammatory arthritis/rheumatoid arthritis	Discitis/osteomyelitis/fractures

Table 5.2 Differential diagnosis of thoracic facet syndrome

Thoracic discogenic pain	Myofascial/soft tissue pain, fibromyalgia
Thoracic radiculopathy	Thoracic spine strain/sprain
Rib fracture	Discitis/osteomyelitis/fractures

Table 5.4 Lumbar facet joint pain referral patterns [9]

Location	Implicated Joint
Low back	L3-4, L4-5, L5-S1
Buttock	L3-4, L4-5, L5-S1
Lateral thigh	L2-3, L3-4, L4-5, L5-S1
Posterior thigh	L3-4, L4-5 L5-S1
Greater trochanter	L2-3, L3-4, L4-5, L5-S1
Groin	L1-2, L2-3, L3-4, L4-5, L5-S1
Lateral lower leg	L3-4, L4-5, L5-S1
Upper back	L1-2, L2-3, L3-4
Flank	L1-2, L2-3
Foot	L4-5, L5-S1

Table 5.3 Differential diagnosis of lumbar facet syndrome (spondylosis)

Lumbar discogenic pain	Myofascial/soft tissue pain, fibromyalgia
Lumbar radiculopathy	Lumbar strain/sprain
Sacroiliac joint pain	Piriformis muscle pain
Vertebral/sacral fracture	Discitis/osteomyelitis/fractures
Inflammatory arthritis	Diffuse idiopathic skeletal hyperostosis

bisegmental innervation from the medial branch of the dorsal rami of the same level and the level above. Exceptions include innervation of *atlanto-occipital and atlanto-axial joints* which are derived from the C1 and C2 nerve roots, the *C2–3 facet* which is supplied by the third occipital nerve (and an articular branch of the posterior ramus of C3), and the *L5-S1 facet* joint which is innervated by the L5 dorsal ramus and the L4 medial branch. In the lumbar spine, each medial branch travels underneath the mamillo-accessory ligament. Lumbar medial branch also innervates the interspinal ligaments, periosteum of the neural arch, and multifidus muscle.

Tables 5.1, 5.2, and 5.3 provide the differential diagnosis for facet-mediated pain in the cervical, thoracic, and lumbar spine.

5.4 Clinical Presentation

While presenting symptoms and pain referral patterns can assist clinicians in diagnosing facetogenic pain, specificity of such clinical information has not been demonstrated to be reliable [6, 9].

Cervical Facet Syndrome Patient will present with axial unilateral > bilateral dull, aching pain. This neck pain often has a particular referring pattern depending on which specific facets are involved. Upper facet joints produce pain in the proximal neck and occiput/headache (in particular C2/3). Middle cervical facet joints tend to be localized with referral toward shoulder tip and upper traps while lower cervical facet pain refers to the scapula.[28] Sometimes facet pain may refer toward the arm but in contrary to radiculopathy, it does not follow a particular dermatome. Motor, sensory, and reflexes are normal in facetogenic pain [10].

Thoracic Facet Syndrome Patients will often describe thoracic/mid-back pain. This pain may be heightened by rotating the trunk and extending the spine and may refer along the adjacent rib. Pain is often associated with thoracic paraspinal muscle tightness [10].

Lumbar Facet Syndrome In the lumbar spine, facetogenic pain is often axial with associated stiffness. It has an insidious unprovoked onset, to most part localized, but can present with a nondermatomal radiculitis. It is common to describe stiffness upon getting up to walk, and resolution of stiffness after a few minutes of moving around [10]. Upper lumbar facet can refer to the flank, lateral hip, and upper lateral thigh. Lower lumbar facets tend to produce back pain, buttock/hip/groin, and posterolateral thigh pain (Table 5.4). Symptoms will be exacerbated by extension, lateral flexion, and combination which are referred to as "Facet loading". Prolonged sitting and standing may trigger facet pain. Pain will often be relieved with forward flexion, walking, and intermittent rest.

5.5 Physical Examination

All patients should undergo an appropriate musculoskeletal and neurologic examination to identify deficits which may indicate the presence of critical diagnosis like myelopathy, cauda equina, or severe spinal stenosis. Sensation, motor strength, and deep tendon reflexes will be normal unless patients have coexisting diagnosis of nerve root impingement or stenosis. In some instances, strength may be functionally limited secondary to pain. Physical examination should be appropriately expanded based on abnormal findings. Other more concerning yet rare etiologies such as infection, fracture, or neoplasm should also be ruled out.

ROM should be tested and often has limitation due to pain or DJD. Pain may be reproduced by localizing pressure against painful facet(s) and may reproduce patient's usual referral pattern. There are no physical exam maneuvers that are specific for the diagnosis of cervical, thoracic or lumbar facet syndrome, although "facet loading" may have some value. Extension, rotation, lateral flexion may reproduce symptoms [11]. Palpation of the segmental muscles overlying the facet joints may reveal tenderness and/or spasm. Tenderness of the lumbar paraspinal muscle have been found to have a positive predictive value in two large RCTs [12, 13].

5.6 Diagnostic Workup

5.6.1 Imaging

Radiologic imaging (X-ray, MR, CT) may show DJD in the facets of 40–85% of volunteered individuals, whether symptomatic or not [14]. Imaging may assist with other causes of low back pain including degenerative disc disease, spondylolysis, spondylolisthesis, spinal stenosis, spondyloarthropathy, fractures, tumors, and infection. Primary findings of facet joint osteoarthritis on advance imaging (CT/MR) include joint space narrowing, sclerosis, cartilage thinning, subchondral sclerosis, erosion, joint capsule calcification, joint. MRI will better assess sequela of facet arthritis such as neural impingement, and facetitis with periarticular inflammatory soft tissue changes. Single-photon emission computed tomography (SPECT) utilizing 99mTc labeled bisphosphonates provides the ability to identify areas of increased osteoblastic activity or synovial changes caused by hyperemia or inflammation which may prove to be more clinically useful. It has been demonstrated that SPECT may help in the identification of patients who would benefit from facet injection [16]. Many studies have failed to show a clear correlation between radiographic finding of facet DJD and response to diagnostic facet injections [15].

5.6.2 Diagnostic Injections

Given the inability to accurately diagnose the presence of facet-mediated pain by history, physical examination, and imaging, clinicians have used diagnostic injection as a practical tool to identify specific facets as a source of pain. Medial branches that innervate target facets are blocked with low-volume (0.5 cc) anesthetics and pain relief as well as functional gain is tracked for the half-life of the anesthetic used. Controversy does exist regarding the threshold of relief and number of diagnostic blocks which should be performed prior to establishing the diagnosis of spine facet syndrome and considering more definitive therapy. Most clinicians perform two sequential blocks with two different anesthetics (short- acting vs. long-acting) to minimize false-positive response. Recent systematic review of lumbar MBB and RF showed that patient selection based on 70–80% pain relief over two diagnostic blocks can expect 50% pain relief in 50–60% of patients, 50% chance of obtaining 80% relief, and 25% chance of 100% relief. When the selection threshold is raised to 100%, the probability of resolution of pain was stated to increase to 56% [19]. The incidence of false-negative blocks is estimated to be 11% and false-positive is approximately 25% [9, 17, 18].

5.7 Treatment

5.7.1 Medical Management

Nonsteroidal anti-inflammatories, muscle relaxants, and acetaminophen have been utilized for symptom management in spine DJD, particularly in acute flare-ups. Topical over the counter or compounded medication in cream/lotion or patch format may provide effective pain relief. Adjunct medications can be considered including anticonvulsants, gabapentinoids, serotonin norepinephrine reuptake inhibitors (SNRI), and tricyclic antidepressants (TCA). Both osteopathic manipulation and acupuncture have been demonstrated to provide benefit in patients with axial low back pain in comparison to placebo [9]. Concurrent psychopathology such as depression, anxiety, substance use disorder should also be adequately treated. Studies have demonstrated that untreated mood disorders have a negative predictive value for interventional therapies utilized in the management of facet-mediated pain [9].

5.7.2 Rehabilitation

Patients with spine facet syndrome will benefit from self-directed exercise, as well as formal flexion-biased rehabilitation programs. If there is spondylolisthesis with evidence of instability on dynamic films, aggressive ROM exercises and manipulation should be avoided. Based on American Physical Therapy Association (APTA), evidence-based practice guidelines for orthopedic physical therapy management of patients with musculoskeletal impairments, in facetogenic pain, clinicians should provide a multimodal approach care including spinal manipulation/mobilization, neuromuscular exercise (coordination, proprioception, and postural training), stretching, strengthening, endurance training, aerobic conditioning, and cognitive affective elements. Physical therapist may include dry needling, laser treatment for photobiomodulation or intermittent mechanical/manual traction as part of treatment. Patient education and ergonomic consideration are important in preventing chronicity of spinal axial pain [22].

5.7.3 Procedures

There are two primary interventional therapies which can be considered for the management of spine facet syndrome: intra-articular injections (steroid vs. biologics) and radiofrequency denervation of medial branches.

5.7.3.1 Intra-Articular Steroid Injection

The cervical facet injections (Image 5.2) can be performed both from posterior or lateral approach. Intra-articular placement in thoracic facet pain can be challenging due to its orientation, and X-ray/CT-guided posterior approach is the preferred technique. Orientation of the facet joints changes from L1 to L5 requiring adjustment to fluoroscopic angle (Image 5.1). There is controversy regarding the utility of intra-articular steroid injection in the management of spine facet syndrome. Pain relief from facet steroid injection is expected to be short lived. There is some evidence to suggest that intra-articular steroid injection may provide intermediate-term pain relief to a specific subset of patients who demonstrate an active inflammatory process on SPECT imaging [9]. Since steroid is introduced, and steroid has systemic effect, the facet steroid injection may not serve as ideal diagnostic tool for facetogenic pain. When used as a prognostic tool before lumbar facet radiofrequency, medial branch block is associated with a higher success rate than intra-articular steroid injection [23].

5.7.3.2 Intra-Articular Biologics

In the past few years, with increased application of orthobiologics in MSK medicine, platelet-rich plasma, mesenchymal stem cell, and prolotherapy have been applied to treat painful facets with DJD. PRP is derived from centrifugation of whole blood to augment platelet concentration while removing other unneeded cellular components. Currently, PRP preparation with high platelet count and low neutrophil content is preferred. A small number of prospective trials have suggested that there may be some benefit to using PRP injection in the treatment of pain or functional decline caused by facet joint arthropathy. Wu et al. administered intra-articular PRP in 19 patients with facet syndrome diagnosed by history, physical exam, and lumbosacral radiographs [21]. At 4 and 8 weeks, 15 of 19 patients reported "good" or "excellent" relief, statistically significant changes were observed on the Roland-Morris Disability Questionnaire; a 10% improvement in ODI was demonstrated, and a clinically significant improvement in VAS was reported from 6.68 to 2.63 [21]. There is a need for large-scale randomized controlled trials to determine the efficacy, safety, and long-term effects of regenerative therapies in facet-mediated pain [24].

5.7.3.3 Radiofrequency Medial Branch Ablation (RFA)

If a patient has significant pain relief (70% or more) from two diagnostic medial branch blocks (Image 5.1), the treating physician may recommend proceeding to RF ablation (Image 5.1) of the same medial branches. Denervation of the medial branch is achieved by placement of the active tip of the radiofrequency cannula parallel to the nerve. Sensory and motor stimulation of the medial branch is done to evaluate the distance to the target nerve and to avoid denervating ventral nerve root. Conventional radiofrequency (Image 5.2)

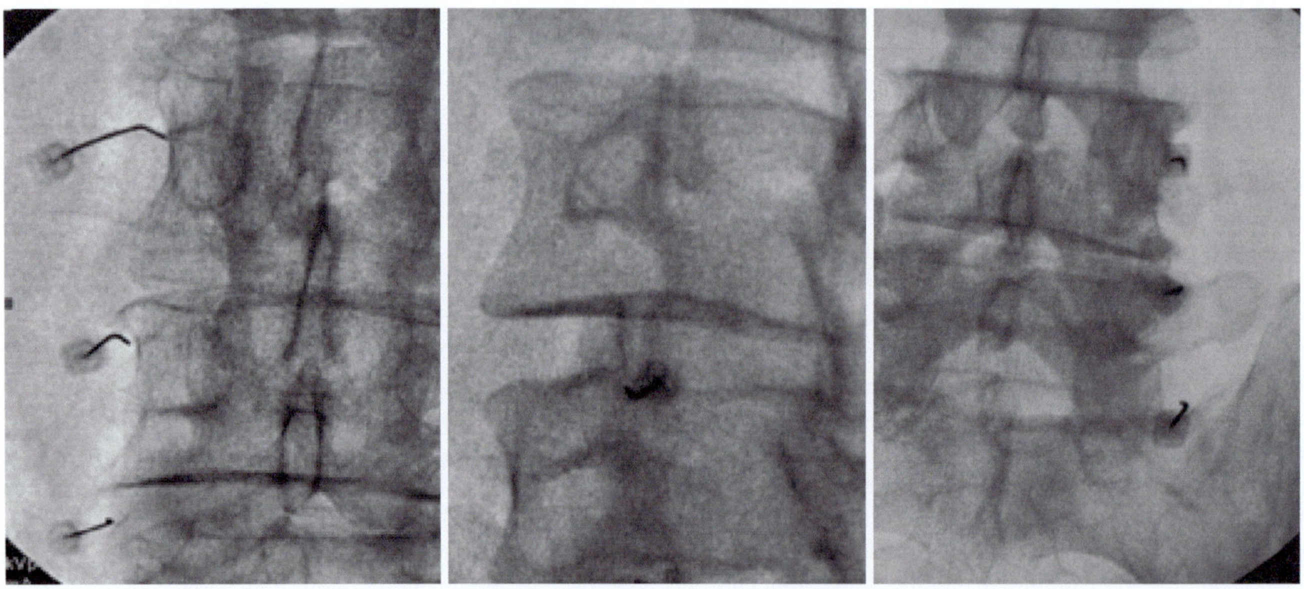

Image 5.1 Lumbar Medial Branch Block needle placement (left), Left L4-5 Facet joint Injection (middle), and Right Lumbar Medial Branch RF needle placement (right). (Images courtesy of S. Ali Mostoufi, MD, New England Spine Care Associates)

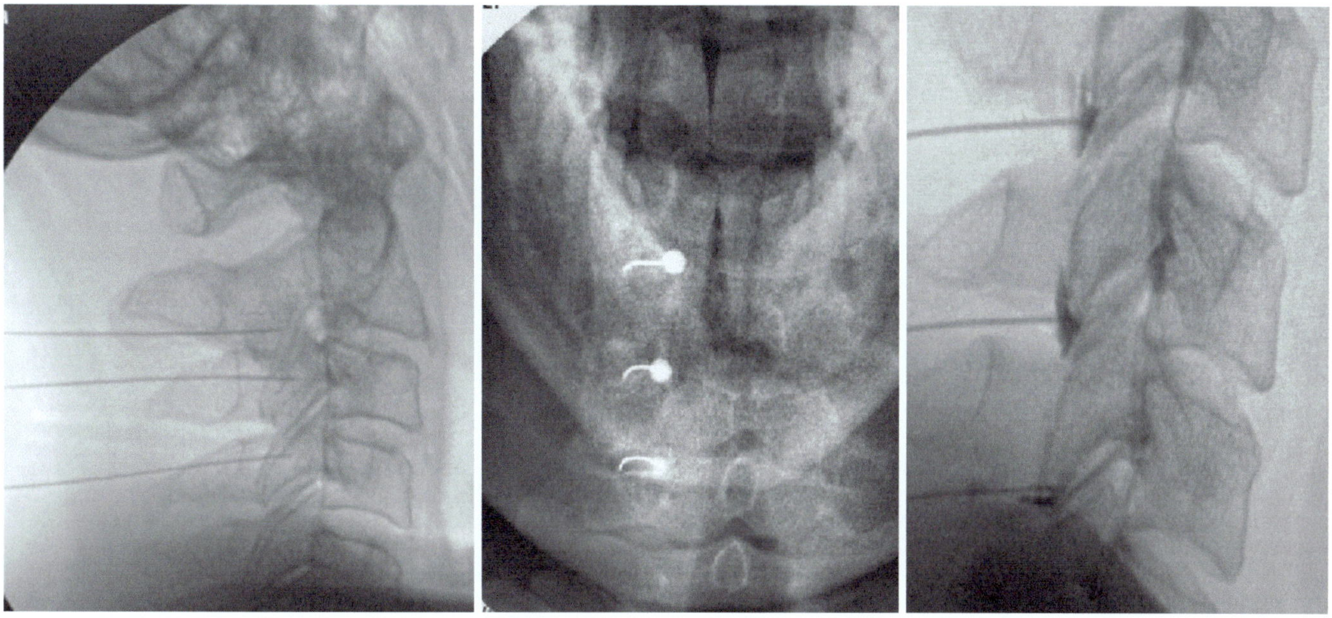

Image 5.2 Lateral views of TON, C3, C4 Medial Branch Injection (left), Cervical Facet Joint Injection with contrast enhancing each joint space (linear intra-articular flow) as well as filling of the capsular recess on both dorsal and ventral joint (middle and right). (Images courtesy of S. Ali Mostoufi, MD, New England Spine Care Associates)

will produce small pear-shaped tissue coagulation along the uninsulated length of a radiofrequency cannula. In studies examining the efficacy of RFA in the lumbar and cervical spine, data are overall positive for its utilization in appropriately selected patients. Durability of relief is also variable in the literature ranging from 6 to 12 months, but often there is a correlation with age (longer effect in elderly). Radiofrequency denervation may be repeated as clinically indicated with reproducible success rates in pain relief. The most catastrophic and feared complication of radiofrequency denervation is inadvertent thermal damage of the ventral root, or the cord which should be largely avoidable with proper needle placement and neuromuscular testing (sensory at 2 Hz and motor at 50 Hz). Neuritis is the most commonly reported complication following radiofrequency ablation occurring in 5–10% of patients, and patients may describe as a "sunburn" pain.

5.7.3.4 Prolotherapy

This treatment involves the administration of a nonbiologic proliferant to promote repair of connective tissue and alleviate pain through recruitment of inflammatory cells. There are three primary classes, irritants, osmotic agents, and chemotactic agents. Currently hypertonic dextrose is the most commonly used [20]. To date, the application of prolotherapy for facet pain is not well studied.

5.7.4 Surgery

There is no definite surgical management for facet-mediated pain without spondylolisthesis. Spinal fusion immobilizes the disc space and same segment facet joint and may lead to decreased pain [9]. Current North American Spine Society Evidence-Based Clinical Guidelines for treatment of spinal pain in the setting of degenerative spondylolisthesis largely support operative treatment of patients' refractory to conservative measures. However, the optimal manner of operative treatment remains poorly established.

References

1. Kirpalani D, Mitra R. Cervical facet joint dysfunction: a review. Arch Phys Med Rehabil. 2008;89(4):770–4.
2. Pdf TP, Disorders BMCM, Manchikanti L, Boswell MV, Singh V, Pampati V, et al. Prevalence of facet joint pain in chronic spinal pain of cervical, thoracic, and lumbar regions thoracic, and lumbar regions. BMC Musculoskelet Disord [Internet]. 2018;30(3):133–43. Available from: https://doi.org/10.1016/j.neucir.2018.05.004.
3. Gellhorn AC, Katz JN, Suri P. Osteoarthritis of the spine: the facet joints. Nat Rev Rheumatol. 2013;9(4):216–24.
4. Aprill C, Bogduk N. The prevalence of cervical zygapophyseal joint pain-a first approximation. Spine. 1992;17:744–7.
5. Suri P, Katz JN, Rainville J, Kalichman L, Guermazi A, Hunter DJ. Vascular disease is associated with facet joint osteoarthri-

tis. Osteoarthr Cartil [Internet]. 2010;18(9):1127–32. https://doi.org/10.1016/j.joca.2010.06.012.
6. Brummett CM, Cohen SP. Facet Syndrome: Facet Joint Injections, Medial Branch Blocks, and Radiofrequency Denervation. In: Essentials of Pain Medicine. 2011. p. 322–9.
7. Tournade A, Patay Z, Krupa P, Tajahmady T, Million S, Braun M. A comparative study of the anatomical, radiological and therapeutic features of the lumbar facet joints. Neuroradiology. 1992;34(4):257–61.
8. Cavanaugh JM, Ozaktay AC, Yamashita HT, King AI. Lumbar facet pain: biomechanics, neuroanatomy and neurophysiology. J Biomech. 1996;29(9):1117–29.
9. Cohen SP, Raja SN. Pathogenesis, diagnosis, and treatment of lumbar zygapophysial (facet) joint pain. Anesthesiology. 2007;106(3):591–614.
10. Chiravuri S, Brummett CM, Kohn L. Facet joint pain. America Society of Regional Anesthesia; 2019.
11. Schneider GM, Jull G, Thomas K, Smith A, Emery C, Faris P, et al. Derivation of a clinical decision guide in the diagnosis of cervical facet joint pain. Arch Phys Med Rehabil [Internet]. 2014;95(9):1695–701. https://doi.org/10.1016/j.apmr.2014.02.026.
12. Cohen SP, Bajwa ZH, Kraemer JJ, Dragovich A, Williams KA, Stream J, et al. Factors predicting success and failure for cervical facet radiofrequency denervation: a multi-center analysis. Reg Anesth Pain Med. 2007;32(6):495–503.
13. Cohen SP, Hurley RW, Christo PJ, Winkley J, Mohiuddin MM, Stojanovic MP. Clinical predictors of success and failure for lumbar facet radiofrequency denervation. Clin J Pain. 2007;23(1):45–52.
14. Wood KB, Garvey TA, Gundrey C, Heithoff KB. Magnetic resonance imaging of the thoracic spine. J Bone Jt Surg Am. 1995;77-A(11):1631–8.
15. Schwarzer AC, Wang S, O'Driscoll D, Harrington T, Bogduk N LR. CT ability to ID painful zygapophysial joint LBP.pdf. 1995. p. 907–12.
16. Pneumaticos SG, Chatziioannou SN, Hipp JA, Moore WH, Esses SI. Low pain: prediction of short-term outcome of facet joint injection with bone scintigraphy. Radiology. 2006;238(2):693–8.
17. Barnsley L, Lord S, Wallis B, Bogduk N. False-positive rates of cervical zygapophysial joint blocks. Clin J Pain. 1993;9:124–30.
18. Kaplan M, Dreyfuss P, Halbrook B, Bogduk N. The ability of lumbar medial branch blocks to anesthetize the zygapophysial joint: a physiologic challenge. Spine. 1998;23:1847–52.
19. Schneider BJ, Doan L, Maes MK, Martinez KR, Gonzalez Cota A, Bogduk N. Systematic review of the effectiveness of lumbar medial branch thermal radiofrequency neurotomy, stratified for diagnostic methods and procedural technique. Pain Med (United States). 2020;21(6):1122–41.
20. Valimahomed AK, Haffey PR, Urman RD, Kaye AD, Yong RJ. Regenerative techniques for neuraxial back pain: a systematic review. Curr Pain Headache Rep. 2019;23(3):20.
21. Wu J, Du Z, Lv Y, Zhang J, Xiong W, Wang R, et al. A new technique for the treatment of lumbar facet joint syndrome using intra-articular injection with autologous platelet-rich plasma. Pain Physician. 2016;19(8):617–25.
22. Blanpied PR, Gross AR, Elliott JM, Devaney LL, Clewley D, Walton DM, Sparks C, Robertson EK. Neck pain: revision 2017. J Orthop Sports Phys Ther. 2017;47(7):A1–A83.
23. Cohen SP, Moon JY, Brummett CM, White RL, Larkin TM. Medial branch blocks or intra-articular injections as a prognostic tool before lumbar facet radiofrequency denervation: a multicenter, case-control study. Reg Anesth Pain Med. 2015;40(4):376–83. https://doi.org/10.1097/AAP.0000000000000229.
24. Urits I, Viswanath O, Galasso AC, Sottosani ER, Mahan KM, Aiudi CM, Kaye AD, Orhurhu VJ. Platelet-rich plasma for the treatment of low Back pain: a comprehensive review. Curr Pain Headache Rep. 2019;23(7):52.

6 Back Pain: Sacroiliac Joint Pain

S. Ali Mostoufi, Mo Hamouda, and Ariana Mostoufi

6.1 Synonyms

Sacroiliac pain
Sacroiliac dysfunction
Sacroiliac arthropathy
Sacroiliac joint disease
Sacroiliitis
Sacroiliac Sprain

6.2 ICD-10

- Disorders of Sacrum M53.1
- Sacroiliitis M46.1
- Sprain of sacroiliac joint S33.6xxA

6.3 Definition

Sacroiliac joint (SIJ) syndrome is defined as pain originating from the sacroiliac joint and its ligamentous support due to osteoarthritis, trauma, altered joint mobility, or inflammatory arthropathy. The SI joint is on the differential diagnosis of any low back and buttock pain presentation. The controlled diagnostic blocks utilizing the International Association for the Study of Pain (IASP) criteria demonstrated sacroiliac joint pain prevalence of 15–30% [8].

6.3.1 Anatomy [1, 17]

The sacroiliac joint is an articulation of the sacrum with the medial edges of both ilium. This boot-shaped joint is critical for effective load transfer between the spine and legs. The bony anatomy is variable in size, shape, and contour, and its shape changes from infancy to adulthood. The sacral auricular part is generally concave, and the iliac part is predominantly convex, with the highest coefficient of friction of any diarthrodial joint. It is a true diarthrodial joint, which consists of both fibrocartilage and hyaline cartilage [2]. The sacral surface remains smooth until after puberty, when roughening occurs creating unevenness on the articular surface and thereby providing more stability with weight bearing. In late life, particularly in males, SI joint could fully ankylose. Mobility of this joint is controversial but current research supports limited motion in the average range of 2° in all three planes of the SI joint [1]. Its motion is nonlinear as it occurs simultaneously in multiple planes [5].

Short and long dorsal sacroiliac ligaments complement the interosseous ligaments in stabilizing the joint. Ventrally, the anterior sacroiliac ligament stretches between the ventral surface of the sacral alar and that of the ilium. The inferior synovial portion of the joint is of most interest to pain interventionalists since it is a common access point for intra-articular procedures. The ventral SIJ capsule is relatively thin and frequently has defects. Fortin reported 61% of 76 joints reviewed demonstrated leakage of injected contrast which may result in ineffective therapeutic injections [3]. Many researchers have published studies on the innervation of the SI joint but current research suggests that the innervation includes ventral rami of L4 and L5, superior gluteal nerve, and dorsal rami of L5-S2 [4].

S. A. Mostoufi (✉)
Department of Orthopedics and Rehabilitation, Tufts University School of Medicine, Boston, MA, USA

New England Spine Care Associates & Boston Regenerative Medicine, Cambridge, MA, USA
e-mail: ali.mostoufi@tufts.edu

M. Hamouda
Department of Anesthesia, University of Colorado School of Medicine, Denver, CO, USA

A. Mostoufi
Concord Carlisle High School, Concord, MA, USA

© The Author(s), under exclusive license to Springer Nature Switzerland AG 2022
S. A. Mostoufi et al. (eds.), *Clinical Guide to Musculoskeletal Medicine*, https://doi.org/10.1007/978-3-030-92042-5_6

Table 6.1 Differential Diagnosis of Sacroiliac pain

Differential Diagnosis of Sacroiliac pain	
Myofascial pain	Piriformis syndrome
Hip pathology	S1 radiculopathy
Facet Joint Pain	Sacral Insufficiency Fracture
Pelvic Floor dysfunction	Cluneal neuropathy
Sciatic mononeuropathy	Proximal Hamstring Tendinopathy

6.3.2 Etiology

Solonen was the first to propose that the SI joint has all the usual elements of an articulation, and should be considered as a source of subjective pain presentation with objective findings [1].

Pain can origin from both intra-articular and extra-articular causes. Extra-articular cause is often a ligamentous injury. Intra-articular causes include osteoarthritis, inflammatory arthritis (psoriasis, ankylosing spondylitis), and infection. It was found that one-third of psoriatic arthritis patients developed sacroiliitis after 5 years of illness and that half of patients developed sacroiliitis by 10 years [9].

Biomechanical factors including scoliosis with pelvic obliquity and leg length discrepancy, antalgic gait due to lower extremity joint disease, abnormal foot arches, pregnancy, previous pelvic fracture, poor body mechanics, lumbar immobilization with fusion, all could contribute to sacroiliac-mediated back pain. High-impact athletic endeavors, with repetitive stress of the pelvic structures can lead to sacroiliac strain and associated pain. Differential diagnosis of sacroiliac pain is in Table 6.1.

6.3.3 Symptoms

Patients complain about regional pain around the sacrum and PSIS and into the mid to lower buttock, especially the top one-third of the gluteal region. Short or prolonged sitting and transition pain such as sit to stand motion or getting in and out of vehicles are common parts of the history. Symptomatic sacroiliac joint can present as lower back pain, sacral pain, and often with referral to the ipsilateral groin. Although it could present bilaterally, it is often unilateral. Pain originating from the SIJ can refer to the ipsilateral posterior leg but often does not extend beyond the posterior knee.

6.3.4 Physical Examination

Full musculoskeletal and neurological examination is indicated to assist with diagnosis.

Inspection Examination includes looking for scoliosis, pelvic obliquity, exaggerated lumbar lordosis, muscle atrophy, and evidence of skin disease pointing to inflammatory arthropathies. Examiners should assess any biomechanical explanation for symptomatic sacroiliac joint including deformity of foot arches and pronated feet.

Neurological examination In general, neurological examination should be unremarkable in this diagnosis.

Skeletal examination Manual muscle testing, sensory testing as well as reflexes should be normal. Examiners should evaluate lumbar and lower extremity joint range of motion including the hips, and also assess for abnormal gait.

Lab test HLA-b27 should be ordered in suspected cases of Rh-negative spondyloarthropathy and sacroiliitis [19]. If infection is suspected, full blood panel and cultures are indicated.

Special Testing Current research suggests no single test is both specific and sensitive to detect sacroiliac joint as a pain generator. Cumulative effect of adding simultaneous testing will increase sensitivity and can lead to a more accurate diagnosis [17, 18]. FABER maneuver, Gaenslen test, femoral thrust test, pelvic distraction, pelvic compression, and sacral thrust have been utilized to diagnose sacroiliac pain. A recent systematic review determined there was significant evidence to constitute a clinical diagnostic rule for SIJ pain based upon three of five positive tests [6]. Another study suggests combination of Patrick's test and Gaenslen test may carry a 94% sensitivity based on recent study [7].

6.3.5 Diagnostic Workup

X-Ray Plain radiographs will identify pathology in the hip and changes in the sacroiliac joint.

The changes in ankylosing spondylitis are subchondral bony erosion, sclerosis, and fusion of the sacroiliac joints.

MRI MRI is useful in diagnosis of sacroiliitis, pelvic stress fractures, infection infiltration, but is not as helpful in degenerative causes of sacral pain.

CT Scan CT scans provide detailed anatomy of the bony architecture including erosion, fractures, periarticular bleeding.

Bone Scan If infection is suspected, blood work, PET scan, and bone scans are indicated.

Diagnostic Injections Diagnostic blocks identify the source of persistent pain related to adjacent level facet joints, sacroiliac joints, degenerative disc, annular disc tear, piriformis muscle, or nerve root impingements. Performing procedures on an operated back may pose technical challenges requiring the expertise of a skilled interventionalist.

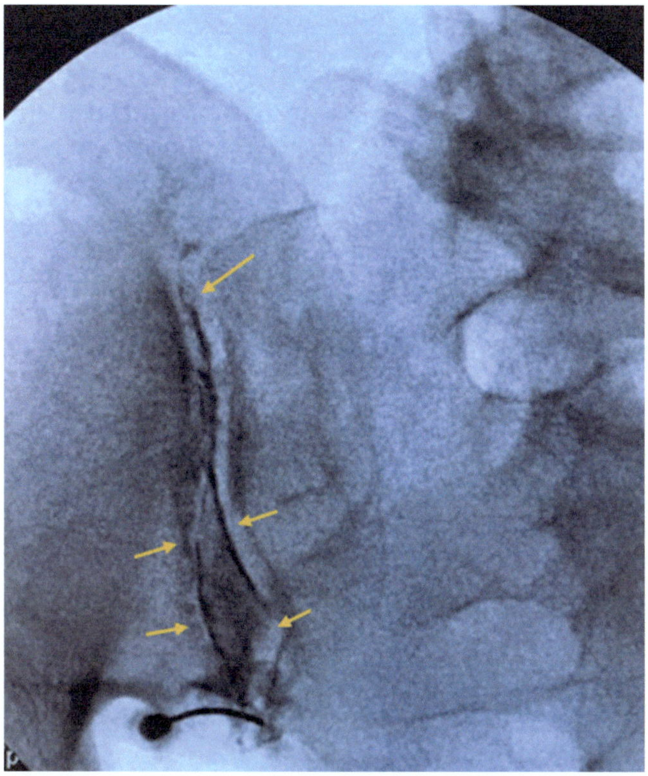

Fig. 6.1 SI joint injection with needle penetrating distal joint and contrast injection demonstrating a cephalad spread with an ideal medial (dorsal) and lateral (Ventral) flow pattern

Intra-articular anesthetic injection The validity of intra-articular injection as a single diagnostic test has been debated but in combination with physical exam maneuvers, it can lead to higher chance of correct diagnosis. Image guidance is necessary for accurate needle placement and along with contrast dye should confirm intra-articular spread (Fig. 6.1).

6.4 Treatment

6.4.1 Medical Management

Clinicians take different approaches to manage a symptomatic sacroiliac joint depending on its etiology which includes pregnancy, degeneration, scoliosis with pelvic obliquity, and traumatic or rheumatologic. In the acute phase, rest from pain-provoking activities (running, single-leg stance or jumps, or twisting activities) may be advised to help with quicker recovery.

Medications If the pain and dysfunction are related to sacroiliitis, primary attention emphasizes treating this rheumatologic disorder with appropriate medications outlined in chapter "Rheumatological and Soft Tissue Disorders". Often the first choice of treatment for pain is an NSAID such as a Cox-II inhibitor. Tylenol is recommended in patients with NSAIDS intolerance or pregnant women. In patients with associated myofascial pain or muscle spasms, muscle relaxants as needed can add value. For acute and disabling sacroiliac strain, a few days of short-acting opioids may be advisable but as a chronic treatment option, it carries typical opioid-related risks including dependency and abuse.

Modalities and bracing Thermodalities including ice or heat are often advised by physicians to help with temporary pain relief, lasting from few minutes to few hours after use. Patients should protect skin against burn, particularly in diabetics and those with peripheral vascular disease. Many patients try managing SI joint pain with a TENS unit, a treatment based on gate control theory of pain relief [10]. In patients experiencing muscle spasm, a muscle stimulator may provide additional benefits. For support and pain relief, sacroiliac brace can be prescribed, and its small profile increases patient's tolerance and compliance. In individuals developing sacroiliac pain due to scoliosis with pelvic obliquity and leg length discrepancy, corrective shoe lift (with arch support) should be considered.

Manipulation Chiropractic or osteopathic adjustments are often part of the treatment of back pain including those originating from SI joint and may be one of the few good options in pregnant females with symptomatic SI back pain during last trimester [11].

6.4.2 Rehabilitation

Improving function is an important step in managing sacroiliac pain. Exercise-based treatments are combined with patient education and ergonomic corrections to achieve functional gains. In general, physical therapy treatments include a mix of manual treatments, improving range of motion, stretching exercises, strengthening exercises, gait training, and balance training. Often associated with SI joint pain, a degree of strength deficit in pelvic girdle muscles including gluteus medius can in turn affect hip movement, balance, and walking. Also included in strengthening protocol are lumbar paraspinals, hamstrings, and other muscles affecting the mobility of the sacroiliac joint [12]. Physical therapists may instruct the patient on stretches to lengthen muscles that attach to the ilium and sacrum directly and/or indirectly, especially those that limit hip internal rotation [16].

6.4.3 Procedure

Steroid Injections Injecting medication into the sacroiliac joint is often the first line of procedural treatment (Image 1). Intra-articular injection may be done as a diagnostic step (contrast and anesthetic only), or therapeutic (contrast, steroid, and anesthetic). Standard of care is an X-ray-guided injection, but CT or US-guided sacroiliac injections are alternative options. US-guided treatment is safe (even during in pregnancy), low cost, and its portability allows for point of care access to treatment.

RF denervation Clinicians have attempted to study the exact innervation of the SI joint so that RF procedure can be attempted. L5 dorsal rami, S1 and S2 lateral branches have the most contribution to the SI joint. The L5 dorsal rami anatomy is consistent in both female and male but the S1 and S2 lateral branches have variable extraforaminal course, therefore it impacts the outcome of the RF procedure. Both thermal and pulsed RF for SI denervation have been tried. Some practitioners advocate for bipolar RF treatment and others advocate for cooled RF which creates larger lesions and may increase the success rate for S1 and S2 lateral branch treatment.

Orthobiologics There is a growing interest in utilizing orthobiologics in MSK medicine and this includes treating the stabilizing ligaments across the SI joint as well as injecting the SI joint itself. To date, there are no large-scale double-blind studies in support of orthobiologics in SI-mediated pain but smaller studies suggest sustainable pain relief and perhaps superiority as compared to SI joint steroid injection [13, 14].

SI joint Percutaneous Fusion See below.

6.4.4 Surgery

- *Open SI joint Fusion:*

Open SI joint fusion has been performed since the 1920s but is no longer the preferred approach to SI joint fusion.

- *Percutaneous SI joint Fusion:*

Percutaneous sacroiliac fusion treatments whether through direct dorsal approach (Fig. 6.2) or lateral transiliac method are now available as a minimally invasive procedure performed in outpatient settings under conscious sedation and fluoroscopic guidance. Multiple minimally invasive SI fusion devices exist, details of which are beyond the scope of this chapter.

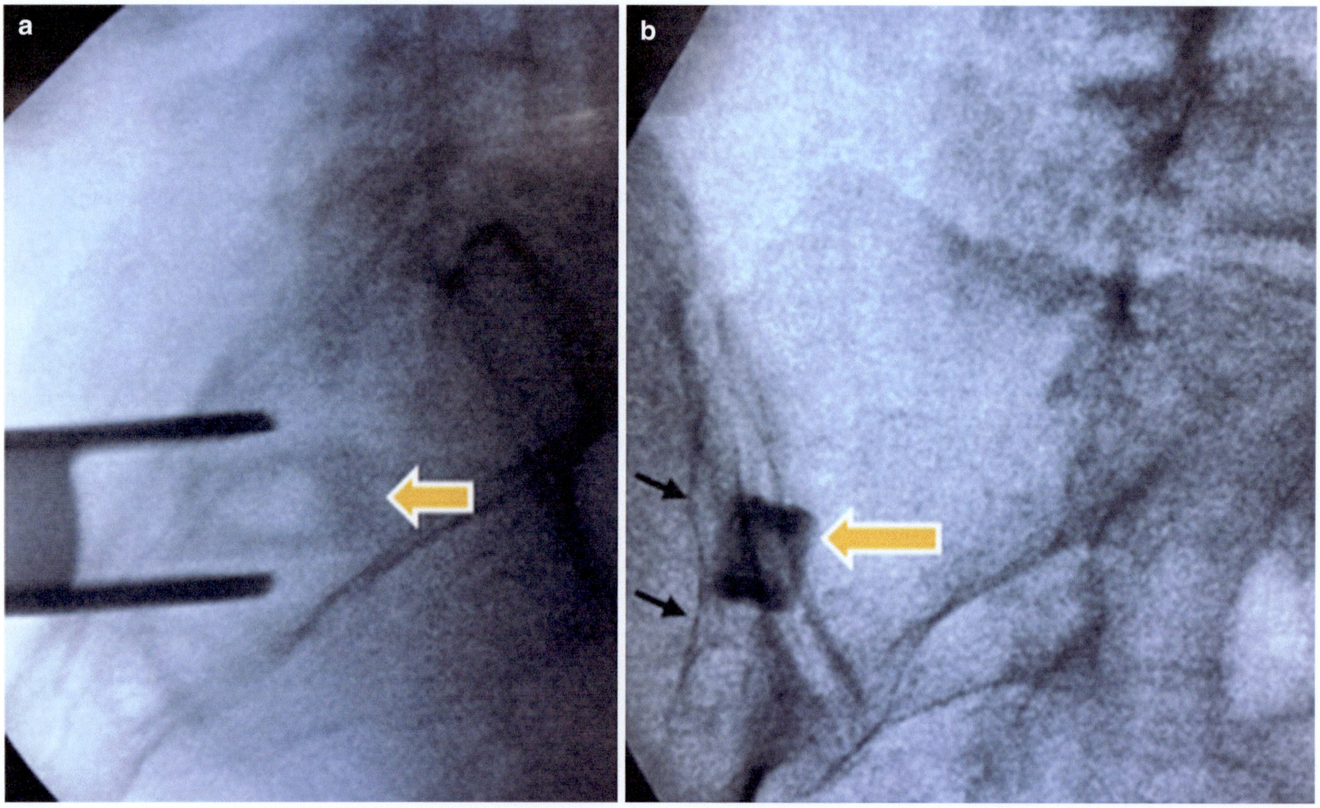

Fig. 6.2 Percutaneous Sacroiliac fusion. (**a**) demonstrates implantation of the bony allograft (arrow) on a lateral view. (**b**) demonstrates contralateral oblique view of the SI joint, approximating posterior and anterior joint, and visualizing square-shaped allograft (thick arrow) within the SI joint. The thinner arrows are pointing to PSIS. (Image from authors cases)

Overall, the quality of available evidence is mixed and in general consists of level 4 retrospective studies, level 2 prospective studies, and only two level 1 prospective clinical trials [15]. In a level 1 study of triangular implants by month 24, 82% received substantial clinical benefit in VAS SI joint pain score, and 66% had received substantial clinical benefit in ODI score [20]. This topic is covered in more detail in the chapter "Minimally Invasive Spine Procedure".

References

1. Vleeming A, Schuenke MD, Masi AT, Carreiro JE, Danneels L, Willard FH. The sacroiliac joint: an overview of its anatomy, function, and potential clinical implications. J Anat. 2012;221(6):537–67. https://doi.org/10.1111/j.1469-7580.2012.01564.x.
2. Forst SL, Wheeler MT, Fortin JD, Vilensky JA. The sacroiliac joint: anatomy, physiology, and clinical significance. Pain Physician. 2006 Jan;9(1):61–7.
3. Fortin JD, Washington WJ, Falco FJ. Three pathways between the sacroiliac joint and neural structures AJNR. Am J Neuroradiol. 1999;20(8):1429–34.
4. Wong M, Sinkler MA, Kiel J. Anatomy, abdomen and pelvis, sacroiliac joint. [Updated 2020 Aug 10]. In: StatPearls [Internet]. Treasure Island: StatPearls Publishing; 2021.
5. Falowski S, Sayed D, Pope J, et al. A review and algorithm in the diagnosis and treatment of sacroiliac joint pain. J Pain Res. 2020;13:3337–48. Published 2020 Dec 8. https://doi.org/10.2147/JPR.S279390.
6. Petersen T, Laslett M, Juhl C. Clinical classification in low back pain: best-evidence diagnostic rules based on systematic reviews. BMC Musculoskelet Disord. 2017;18(1):188. https://doi.org/10.1186/s12891-017-1549-6.
7. Mekhail N, Saweris Y, Sue Mehanny D, Makarova N, Guirguis M, Costandi S. Diagnosis of sacroiliac joint pain: predictive value of three diagnostic clinical tests. Pain Pract. 2021;21(2):204–14. https://doi.org/10.1111/papr.12950. Epub 2020 Oct 24. PMID: 32965780.
8. Cohen SP. Sacroiliac joint pain: a comprehensive review of anatomy, diagnosis, and treatment. Anesth Analg. 2005;101:1440–53. https://doi.org/10.1213/01.ANE.0000180831.60169.EA.
9. Chandran V, Barrett J, Schentag CT, Farewell VT, Gladman DD. Axial psoriatic arthritis: update on a long-term prospective study. J Rheumatol. 2009;36(12):2744–50.
10. Melzack R, Wall PD. Pain mechanisms: a new theory. Science. 1965;150:971–9.
11. Hensel KL, Buchanan S, Brown SK, Rodriguez M, Cruser dA. Pregnancy research on osteopathic manipulation optimizing treatment effects: the PROMOTE study. Am J Obstet Gynecol. 2015;212(1):108.e1–108.e1089. https://doi.org/10.1016/j.ajog.2014.07.043.
12. Lee DG, Vleeming A. Impaired load transfer through the pelvic girdle- a new model of altered neutral zone function. In: Proceedings from the 3rd interdisciplinary world congress on low back and pelvic pain. Vienna, Austria; 1998.
13. Singla V, Batra YK, Bharti N, et al. Steroid vs. platelet-rich plasma in ultrasound-guided sacroiliac joint injection for chronic low back pain. Pain Pract. 2017;17:782–91.
14. Ko GD. Platelet-rich plasma injections for sacroiliac joint pain: case series with preliminary screening tool and literature review. Pract Pain Manage. 2010;10:55–67.
15. Martin CT, Haase L, Lender PA, Polly DW. Minimally invasive sacroiliac joint fusion: the current evidence. Int J Spine Surg. 2020;14(Suppl 1):20–9. Published 2020 Feb 10. https://doi.org/10.14444/6072.
16. Vleeming A, Van Wingerden JP, Snijders CJ, Stoeckart R, Stijnen T. Load application to the sacrotuberous ligament; influences on sacroiliac joint mechanics. Clin Biomech (Bristol, Avon). 1989;4(4):204–9.
17. Poilliot AJ, Zwirner J, Doyle T, Hammer N. A systematic review of the normal sacroiliac joint anatomy and adjacent tissues for the pain physicians. Pain Physician. 2019;22(4):247–74.
18. Telli H, Telli S, Topal M. The validity and reliability of provocative tests in the diagnosis of sacroiliac joint dysfunction. Pain Physician. 2018;21:E376. Wei Zhu, et al. Ankylosing spondylitis: etiology, pathogenesis, and treatment. Bone Res; 2019.
19. Lee DW, Patterson DG, Sayed D. Review of current evidence for minimally invasive posterior sacroiliac joint fusion. Int J Spine Surg. 2021;15(3):514–24. https://doi.org/10.14444/8073.
20. Polly DW, Swofford J, Whang PG, et al. Two-year outcomes from a randomized controlled trial of minimally invasive sacroiliac joint fusion vs. non-surgical management for sacroiliac joint dysfunction. Int J Spine Surg. 2016;10:28.

Back Pain: Vertebrogenic

7

Steven Falowski and Dawood Sayed

7.1 Synonyms

Vertebral Endplate Pain

7.2 ICD-10 Codes

- Nonspecific Low Back Pain codes currently in use: (2020)
- M47.816 Spondylosis w/o myelopathy or radiculopathy, lumbar region
- M47.817 Spondylosis w/o myelopathy or radiculopathy, lumbosacral region
- M51.36 Other intervertebral disc degeneration, lumbar
- M54.5 Low back pain

7.3 Description

Vertebrogenic pain is a condition in which damaged or degenerated vertebral endplates result in chronic axial lower back pain.

Anatomy The vertebral endplate (VEP) is a bilayer of cartilage and bone separating the intervertebral discs (IVD) and the adjacent vertebrae. Endplate subchondral bone is innervated by the basivertebral nerve (BVN), a branch of the sinuvertebral nerve. The BVN fibers enter the vertebral bone marrow along with nutrient arteries through the posterior basivertebral foramen and become thinly or nonmyelinated after entering the bone marrow [1, 2]. Endplate damage has been shown to result in densification of the basivertebral nerves. In fact, vertebral endplate pathologies are more innervated than intervertebral disc pathologies, both in terms of the incidence and extent of innervation [1].

Biomechanically, the endplate is subjected to significant loads during activities of daily living as the trunk muscles contract to stabilize posture. The IVD nucleus becomes pressurized in response to these forces, and the endplate distributes these intradiscal pressures onto the adjacent vertebrae, preventing the pressurized disk nucleus from bulging into the underlying trabecular bone. At the same time, the endplate also serves as a primary pathway for nutrient transport between vertebral capillaries and cells within the disk nucleus. The endplate's dual roles of nutritional support for the disc and structural support for the spine are at odds, making it vulnerable to damage [2].

The vertebral endplates become further susceptible to damage as a normal part of physiological aging, with gradual endplate thinning and calcification, and from pathological degeneration due to high tensile strains associated with disc degeneration [3]. Once damaged, the VEP allows for biologic communication, or "crosstalk", between the bone marrow and proinflammatory disc material, leading to hydraulic, inflammatory, and fibrogenic coupling between the two compartments. The persistent autoinflammatory response that ensues, with up-regulation of inflammatory mediators, creates the predisposing condition for the development of bone marrow intensity changes (BMIC), or Modic Changes (MC), seen on magnetic resonance imaging (MRI) of patients with damaged and degenerated VEPs [4].

The presence of Modic type 1 or 2 changes (Fig. 7.1) is strongly associated with disabling chronic low back pain, making them an excellent biomarker for treatment [5–8]. Weishaupt et al. reported 100% specificity to discography in individuals with extensive Type 1 and Type 2 Modic changes [9] and Kuisma et al. found a 2.28 odds ratio for the presence of Modic changes at L5-S1 in individuals with chronic low back pain [10]. Modic changes are more prevalent and more severe at the lower lumbar levels (L4–S1) [2, 10, 11].

S. Falowski (✉)
Functional Neurosurgery Neurosurgical Associates of Lancaster, Lancaster, PA, USA

D. Sayed
Anesthesiology and Pain Medicine, The American Society of Pain and Neuroscience (ASPN), The University of Kansas Health System, Kansas City, KS, USA

© The Author(s), under exclusive license to Springer Nature Switzerland AG 2022

S. A. Mostoufi et al. (eds.), *Clinical Guide to Musculoskeletal Medicine*, https://doi.org/10.1007/978-3-030-92042-5_7

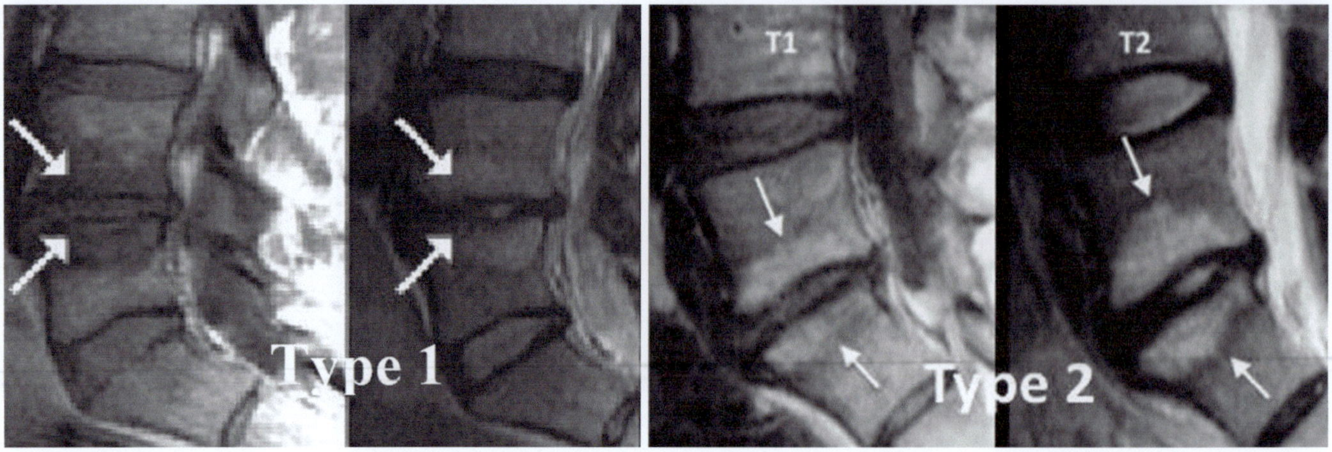

Fig. 7.1 Type 1 MC (left) with decreased signal intensity on T1-weighted images, and increased signal intensity on T2-weighted images. Type 2 MC (right) with increased signal intensity on T1-weighted images and T2-weighted images. (Adapted from Dudli et al. "Pathobiology of Modic Changes," 2016)

7.4 Clinical Presentation

A thorough clinical history, musculoskeletal and neurologic examination are indicated in the evaluation of vertebrogenic pain to exclude alternate or coexisting sources of axial low back pain, including the presence of symptoms that might indicate more serious conditions such as malignancy, infection, or trauma.

Patients with vertebrogenic pain generally describe a midline, deep, aching, pain of progressive nature. It is less commonly associated with burning or electrical shock sensations. Although somatic referred pain can be present in some patients, there is no radicular expression, unless the patient has coexisting nerve root entrapment. The pain tends to be worse with forward flexion, sitting for prolonged periods, and general physical activity [10–15]. To provide additional insight on vertebrogenic pain symptomatology, Relievant Medsystems Inc (Minneapolis, MN) aggregated pain location data from independent mapping of 410 clinical trial patient-completed pain body diagrams revealing 69% of patients had midline pain only; 86% of patients had midline pain, including paraspinal pain; and only 9.5% of patients had pain below the mid-gluteal line.

7.5 Physical Examination

If there is suspicion of other system involvement, the physical examination should be expanded.

Visual Inspection The clinical examination of patients with vertebrogenic lower back pain should include visual inspection of the thoraco-lumbar and lumbo-sacral spine with special attention paid toward abnormal curvature, such as flat-back, exaggerated lumbar lordosis, or significant scoliosis. With episodes of acute pain, the patient may demonstrate spasmodic scoliosis.

Palpation Tenderness should be elicited, and specific areas of tenderness should be correlated with imaging findings. Muscular hypertonicity or spasm should also be noted. Palpation of the lumbosacral spine in vertebrogenic pain patients often reveals midline tenderness, although paravertebral tenderness can occur. Pain over the sacral sulcus or posterior-superior iliac spine might indicate the presence of sacroiliac joint pain.

Gait The gait examination in patients with vertebrogenic pain is most often normal. An abnormal gait should be investigated, and the source determined.

Range of Motion Alleviating and exacerbating maneuvers often reveal increased pain on flexion (greater than with extension), and pain that is relieved by standing and walking. There might be limited range of motion in forward flexion.

Neurological Examination Absence of a coexisting radicular pain syndrome should be noted for Vertebrogenic pain and the neurological examination is typically normal.

7.6 Diagnostic Workup

X-Ray: Plain radiographs are often the initial imaging modality used in patients with LBP to identify degenerative and traumatic changes, including facet spondylosis, loss of disc height, vertebral body fractures, and spondylolysis. Plain radiographs are sensitive to evaluate curvature and alignment of the lumbar vertebrae (scoliosis and lordosis) and to detect spondylolisthesis. They can identify instability by means of flexion-extension views. They have less utility in identifying Modic changes or pathologic changes in the endplates.

Magnetic Resonance Imaging MRI is the gold standard imaging for patients with vertebrogenic pain. The diagnostic biomarker for vertebrogenic pain is Modic Changes, which are readily visible on T1- and T2-weighted MRI. To further delineate MRI features of vertebrogenic pain, 296 vertebrogenic patients' MRIs were evaluated by an independent physician for Modic bone marrow characteristics. Bone marrow Intensity Changes (BMIC) were most often located in the lumbosacral region (69% at L5/S1) and Modic I changes were twice as prevalent as Modic 2. BMICs were typically localized to the vertebral endplates (VEP) with 75% of endplates evaluated having <25% of the vertebral body height involved and only 3% with BMIC that entailed more than 50% of the vertebral body height. In approximately 50% of the VEPs evaluated, BMIC extended to more than 2/3 of the endplate surface area and 69% had VEP defects. Using the International Society for the Study of the Lumbar Spine (ISSLS) Spine Phenotype Workgroup nomenclature, 91% of VEP defects were irregular in shape. Pfirrmann grades were III in 23%, grade IV in 42%, and grade V in 33% of motion segments [16, 17].

Computer Tomography (CT) Although not sensitive for Modic changes, CT scans of the lumbosacral spine can detect vertebral endplate changes, disruption and fissuring of the endplate, and endplate defects that are associated with Modic changes. In patients who have a contraindication to MRI, CT scans are a useful surrogate when determining treatment.

Bone SPECT/CT The diagnosis of vertebrogenic pain is based on Modic 1 (MC1) or Modic 2 (MC2) on MRI. However, De Vivo et al. describe outcomes of basivertebral nerve ablation (BVN) for vertebrogenic pain in patients with MC 1 or mixed MC 1 and MC 2 with additional positive bone SPECT/CT scans [18]. The patients also underwent additional CT-guided medial branch injections to exclude facet joint-mediated pain. The patients had a high responder rate to treatment with BVN ablation, as well as a large improvement in pain (VAS). A high positive correlation between Modic changes on MRI and increased metabolic activity on Bone SPECT/CT imaging has previously been noted [19]. Modic type I changes were the best binary predictor for positivity on bone SPECT/CT, with a high metabolic activity in 96.1% of endplates in patients showing Modic type I changes on MRI, and 77.8% in cases of Modic type II changes. Given this high correlation between MRI and Bone SPECT/CT scans, and given the similar responder rates between comparative single arm studies using MC 1 or 2 alone versus the addition of Bone SPECT/CT scan, the incremental benefit of adding Bone SPECT/CT scanning has not been clearly established [20].

Provocation Discography (PD) Provocation discography is a test that attempts to correlate low back pain with disc degeneration in the diagnosis of discogenic pain (painful disc degeneration). The rationale behind PD is that disc pressurization with contrast results in stimulation of nociceptors in the posterior annulus in patients with discogenic pain. However, discography has also been demonstrated to result in deflection of the vertebral endplates during pressurization, potentially leading to stimulation of painful nociceptors in the endplate as well as the posterior annular [20]. Currently, there is no evidence that discography can differentiate vertebrogenic pain from discogenic pain.

7.7 Treatment

To date, only basivertebral nerve ablation has demonstrated consistent clinical efficacy in the treatment of vertebrogenic low back pain [18, 20–31]. Two ablation techniques have been studied, intraosseous RF ablation [18, 20–27] and transforaminal epiduroscopic laser ablation [29–31]. However, only intraosseous RF ablation has been studied in Level I RCTs [22, 25]. Collectively, studies on interosseous RF ablation of the basivertebral nerve ablation demonstrate consistent, statistically significant, clinically meaningful, and durable improvements in pain and function, and an excellent safety profile.

The most widely used and studied technique (The Intracept Procedure®, Relievant Medsystems Inc) involves a unilateral transpedicular access to each vertebral body (L3-S1) with Modic Type 1 or 2 changes at the vertebral endplates (Fig. 7.2). A channel to the base of the basivertebral nerve ablation is then created using a curved cannula assembly, and a bipolar RF probe is positioned across the BVN (Figs. 7.3 and 7.4). Ablation is performed using radiofrequency energy at 85 degrees Celsius for a specific amount of time (Figs. 7.2, 7.3, and 7.4).

Except for intraosseous basivertebral nerve ablation, there are very few clinical studies describing the outcomes of other surgical or nonsurgical treatments in patients with vertebrogenic pain. The available studies on patients with MC types 1 or 2 are too few and too heterogeneous to reach definitive conclusions, and no diagnostic or therapeutic treatment algorithm has been established [32, 33].

One hypothesized mechanism for the development of Modic changes and low back pain is low-grade bacterial infection by *Cutibacterium acnes* (formerly known as *Propionibacterium acnes*). Using this hypothesis, several studies have examined the role of antibiotic treatment using amoxicillin with conflicting results. One randomized,

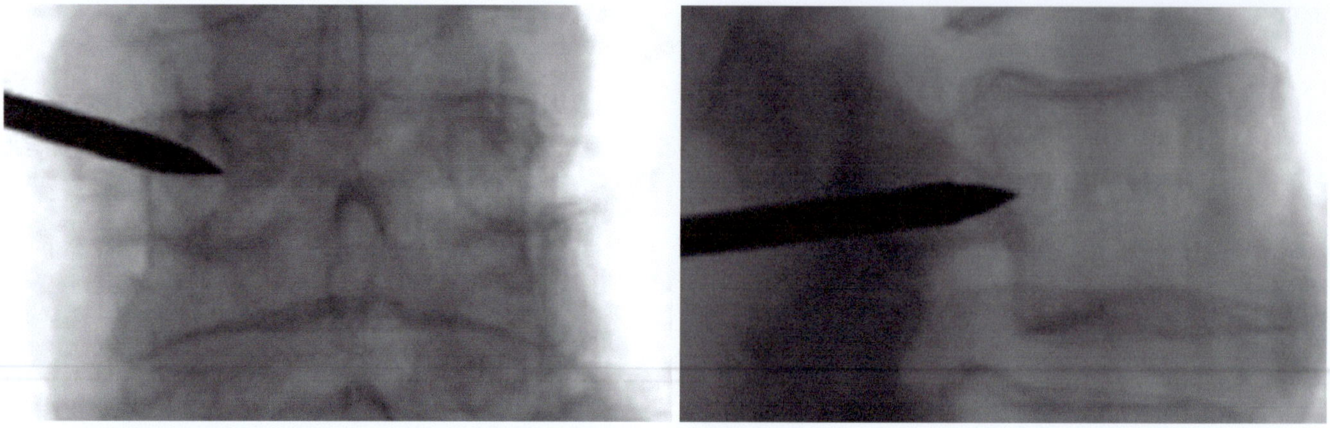

Fig. 7.2 AP and lateral views of the introducer trocar as it traverses the pedicle, ending at the posterior wall of the vertebral body

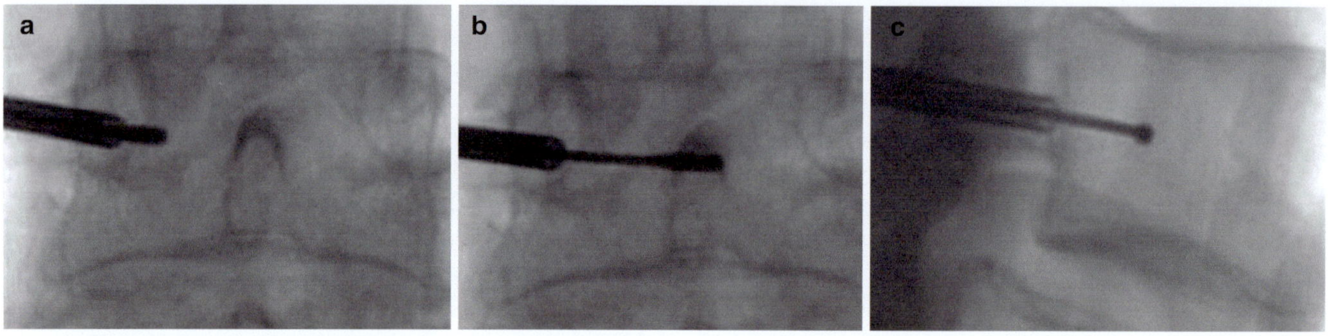

Fig. 7.3 AP and lateral views of the creation of a curved path through the vertebral body using the curved cannula assembly. Start of curved tunneling (**a**), mid-way across (**b**), and final position just across the midline (**c**)

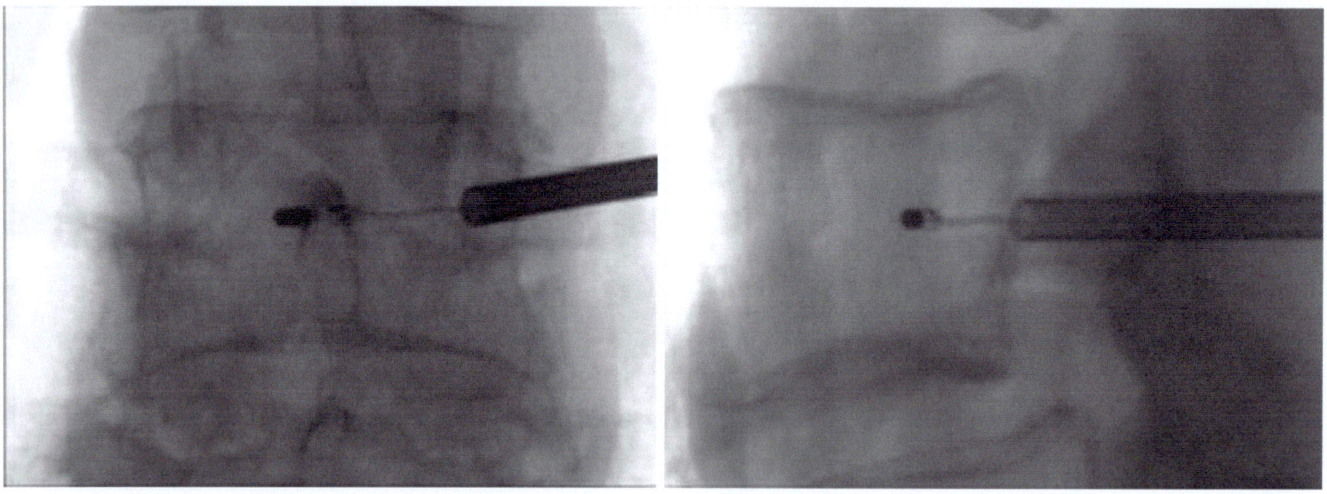

Fig. 7.4 Final position of the RF probe, with the distal electrode just past the midline as observed on an AP image (left) and pointed toward the observer at the predetermined relative distance from the posterior wall (right)

placebo-controlled trial by Albert et al. reported a statistically significant between group difference of 8.3 points on the Roland-Morris Disability Questionnaire (RMDQ) at 1-year follow-up in patients with chronic low back pain, prior disc herniation, and type 1 Modic changes treated for three months with amoxicillin [34]. However, a more recent randomized, placebo-controlled trial (the AIM Study) failed to show any clinically important benefits of three months of amoxicillin in patients with chronic low back pain and Modic changes using similar inclusion/exclusion criteria and similar trial design [35]. Further analysis of the AIM Study data demonstrated no evidence of cost-effectiveness in patients treated with amoxicillin with chronic LBP and Modic changes during 1-year follow-up [36].

References

1. Fields AJ, Liebenberg EC, Lotz JC. Innervation of pathologies in the lumbar vertebral end plate and intervertebral disc. Spine J. 2014;14(3):513–21. https://doi.org/10.1016/j.spinee.2013.06.075.
2. Lotz JC, Fields AJ, Liebenberg EC. The role of the vertebral end plate in low back pain. Global Spine J. 2013;03(3):153–64. https://doi.org/10.1055/s-0033-1347298.
3. Fields AJ, Lee GL, Keaveny TM. Mechanisms of initial endplate failure in the human vertebral body. J Biomech. 2010;43(16):3126–31. https://doi.org/10.1016/j.jbiomech.2010.08.002.
4. Dudli S, Fields AJ, Samartzis D, Karppinen J, Lotz JC. Pathobiology of Modic changes. Eur Spine J. 2016;25(11):3723–34. https://doi.org/10.1007/s00586-016-4459-7.
5. Luoma K, Vehmas T, Kerttula L, Grönblad M, Rinne E. Chronic low back pain in relation to Modic changes, bony endplate lesions, and disc degeneration in a prospective MRI study. Eur Spine J. 2016;25(9):2873–81. https://doi.org/10.1007/s00586-016-4715-x.
6. Schistad EI, Espeland A, Rygh LJ, Røe C, Gjerstad J. The association between Modic changes and pain during 1-year follow-up in patients with lumbar radicular pain. Skelet Radiol. 2014;43(9):1271–9. https://doi.org/10.1007/s00256-014-1928-0.
7. Jensen RK, Leboeuf-Yde C. Is the presence of modic changes associated with the outcomes of different treatments? A systematic critical review. BMC Musculoskelet Disord. 2011;12:183. https://doi.org/10.1186/1471-2474-12-183.
8. Jensen OK, Nielsen CV, Sørensen JS, Stengaard-Pedersen K. Type 1 Modic changes was a significant risk factor for 1-year outcome in sick-listed low back pain patients: a nested cohort study using magnetic resonance imaging of the lumbar spine. Spine J. 2014;14(11):2568–81. https://doi.org/10.1016/j.spinee.2014.02.018.
9. Weishaupt D, Zanetti M, Hodler J, Min K, Fuchs B, Pfirrmann CW, et al. Painful lumbar disk derangement: relevance of endplate abnormalities at MR imaging. Radiology. 2001;218(2):420–7. https://doi.org/10.1148/radiology.218.2.r01fe15420. PMID: 11161156.
10. Kuisma M, Karppinen J, Niinimäki J, Ojala R, Haapea M, Heliövaara M, et al. Modic changes in endplates of lumbar vertebral bodies: prevalence and association with low back and sciatic pain among middle-aged male workers. Spine (Phila Pa 1976). 2007;32(10):1116–22. https://doi.org/10.1097/01.brs.0000261561.12944.ff. PMID: 17471095.
11. Järvinen J, Karppinen J, Niinimäki J, Haapea M, Grönblad M, Luoma K, et al. Association between changes in lumbar Modic changes and low back symptoms over a two-year period. BMC Musculoskelet Disord. 2015;16:98. https://doi.org/10.1186/s12891-015-0540-3. PMID: 25897658; PMCID: PMC4413535.
12. Kjaer P, Korsholm L, Bendix T, Sorensen JS, Leboeuf-Yde C. Modic changes and their associations with clinical findings. Eur Spine J. 2006;15(9):1312–9. https://doi.org/10.1007/s00586-006-0185-x.
13. Urits I, Noor N, Johal AS, Leider J, Brinkman J, Fackler N, et al. Basivertebral nerve ablation for the treatment of vertebrogenic pain. Pain Ther. 2021;10(1):39–53. https://doi.org/10.1007/s40122-020-00211-2. Epub 2020 Oct 31. PMID: 33128702; PMCID: PMC8119576.
14. Francio TV, Sherwood D, Twoehy E, et al. Developments in minimally invasive surgical options for vertebral pain: basivertebral nerve ablation - a narrative review. J Pain Res. 2021;14:1887–907.
15. Nguyen KML, Nguyen DTD. Minimally invasive treatment for degenerative lumbar spine. Tech Vasc Interv Radiol. 2020;23(4):100700. https://doi.org/10.1016/j.tvir.2020.100700.
16. Zehra U, Bow C, Lotz JC, Williams FMK, Rajasekaran S, Karppinen J, et al. Structural vertebral endplate nomenclature and etiology: a study by the ISSLS Spinal Phenotype Focus Group. Eur Spine J. 2018;27(1):2–12. https://doi.org/10.1007/s00586-017-5292-3. Epub 2017 Sep 12. PMID: 28900744.
17. McCormick Z, Boody B. Vertebrogenic pain characteristics from aggregated data of three clinical trials. Relievant Medsystems Inc. Unpublished.
18. De Vivo AE, D'Agostino G, D'Anna G, Al Qatami H, Gil I, Ventura F, Manfrè L. Intra-osseous basivertebral nerve radiofrequency ablation (BVA) for the treatment of vertebrogenic chronic low back pain. Neuroradiology. 2021;63(5):809–15. https://doi.org/10.1007/s00234-020-02577-8. Epub 2020 Oct 13. PMID: 33051706.
19. Russo VM, Dhawan RT, Dharmarajah N, Baudracco I, Lazzarino AI, Casey AT. Hybrid bone single photon emission computed tomography imaging in evaluation of chronic low Back pain: correlation with Modic changes and degenerative disc disease. World Neurosurg. 2017;104:816–23. https://doi.org/10.1016/j.wneu.2017.03.107.
20. Truumees E, Macadaeg K, Pena E, Arbuckle J 2nd, Gentile J 2nd, Funk R, et al. A prospective, open-label, single-arm, multi-center study of intraosseous basivertebral nerve ablation for the treatment of chronic low back pain. Eur Spine J. 2019;28(7):1594–602. https://doi.org/10.1007/s00586-019-05995-2. Epub 2019 May 21. PMID: 31115683.
21. Becker S, Hadjipavlou A, Heggeness MH. Ablation of the basivertebral nerve for treatment of back pain: a clinical study. Spine J. 2017;17:218–23.
22. Fischgrund JS, Rhyne A, Franke J, Sasso R, Kitchel S, Bae H, et al. Intraosseous basivertebral nerve ablation for the treatment of chronic low back pain: a prospective randomized double-blind sham-controlled multi-center study. Eur Spine J. 2018;27(5):1146–56. https://doi.org/10.1007/s00586-018-5496-1.
23. Fischgrund JS, Rhyne A, Macadaeg K, Moore G, Kamrava E, Yeung C, et al. Long-term outcomes following intraosseous basivertebral nerve ablation for the treatment of chronic low back pain: 5 year treatment arm results from a prospective randomized double-blind sham-controlled multi-center study. Eur Spine J. 2020;29(8):1925–34. https://doi.org/10.1007/s00586-020-06448-x.
24. Fischgrund JS, Rhyne A, Franke J, Sasso R, Kitchel S, Bae H, et al. Intraosseous basivertebral nerve ablation for the treatment of chronic low back pain: two-year results from a prospective randomized double-blind sham- controlled multi-center study. Int J Spine Surg. 2019:13(2).
25. Khalil J, Smuck M, Koreckij T, Keel J, Beall D, Goodman B, et al. A prospective, randomized, multi-center study of intraosseous basivertebral nerve ablation for the treatment of chronic low Back pain. Spine J. 2019; https://doi.org/10.1016/j.spinee.2019.05.598. pii: S1529-9430(19)30800-9.
26. Smuck M, Khalil JG, Barrett K, Hirsch JA, Kreiner S, Koreckij T, et al. A prospective, randomized, multi-center study of intraosseous basivertebral nerve ablation for the treatment of chronic low back pain: 12-month results. Society of Interventional Spine Online Annual Meeting. Sep 2020.
27. Macadaeg K, Truumees E, Boody B, Pena E, Arbuckle A, Gentile J, et al. A prospective, open-label, single-arm, multi-center study of intraosseous basivertebral nerve ablation for the treatment of chronic low back pain: 12-month results. NASSJ. 2020;3(100030) E-pub 18 Sept 2020. https://doi.org/10.1016/j.xnsj.2020.100030.
28. Markman J, Rhyne A, Sasso R, Patel A, Hsu W, Fischgrund J, et al. Association between opioid use and patient-reported outcomes in

a randomized trial evaluating basivertebral nerve ablation for the relief of chronic low back pain. Neurosurgery. 2019;0:1–5.
29. Kim HS, Adsul N, Yudoyono F, Paudel B, Kim KJ, Choi SH, et al. Transforaminal epiduroscopic basivertebral nerve laser ablation for chronic low Back pain associated with Modic changes: a preliminary open-label study. Pain Res Manag. 2018;2018:6857983. https://doi.org/10.1155/2018/6857983. PMID: 30186540; PMCID: PMC6112211.
30. Kim HS, Wu PH, Jang IT. Lumbar degenerative disease part 1: anatomy and pathophysiology of intervertebral discogenic pain and radiofrequency ablation of basivertebral and sinuvertebral nerve treatment for chronic discogenic back pain: a prospective case series and review of literature. Int J Mol Sci. 2020;21(4):1483. https://doi.org/10.3390/ijms21041483. PMID: 32098249; PMCID: PMC7073116.
31. Kim HS, Kashlan ON, Singh R, Adsul NM, Yong Z, Oh SW, et al. Percutaneous transforaminal endoscopic radiofrequency ablation of the sinuvertebral nerve in an olympian with a left L5 pedicle/pars interarticularis fracture-associated left L5-S1 disk desiccation. World Neurosurg X. 2019;3:100032. https://doi.org/10.1016/j.wnsx.2019.100032. PMID: 31225524; PMCID: PMC6584597.
32. Viswanathan VK, Shetty AP, Rajasekaran S. Modic changes – an evidence-based, narrative review on its patho-physiology, clinical significance and role in chronic low back pain. J Clin Orthop Trauma. 2020;11(5):761–9. https://doi.org/10.1016/j.jcot.2020.06.025. Epub 2020 Jun 18. Erratum in: J Clin Orthop Trauma. 2020;11(6):1169–1171. Erratum in: J Clin Orthop Trauma. 2020;11(6):1178. Erratum in: J Clin Orthop Trauma. 2020;11(6):1172–1174. PMID: 32879563; PMCID: PMC7452231.
33. Jensen RK, Leboeuf-Yde C. Is the presence of modic changes associated with the outcomes of different treatments? A systematic critical review. BMC Musculoskelet Disord. 2011;12:183. https://doi.org/10.1186/1471-2474-12-183. PMID: 21831312; PMCID: PMC3162945.
34. Albert HB, Sorensen JS, Christensen BS, Manniche C. Antibiotic treatment in patients with chronic low back pain and vertebral bone edema (Modic type 1 changes): a double-blind randomized clinical controlled trial of efficacy. Eur Spine J. 2013;22:697–707. https://doi.org/10.1007/s00586-013-2675-y. PMID: 23404353.
35. Bråten LCH, Rolfsen MP, Espeland A, Wigemyr M, Aßmus J, Froholdt A, et al; AIM Study Group. Efficacy of antibiotic treatment in patients with chronic low back pain and Modic changes (the AIM study): double blind, randomised, placebo-controlled, multicentre trial. BMJ. 2019;367:l5654. https://doi.org/10.1136/bmj.l5654. Erratum in: BMJ. 2020;368:m546. PMID: 31619437; PMCID: PMC6812614.
36. Grotle M, Bråten LC, Brox JI, Espeland A, Zolic-Karlsson Z, Munk Killingmo R, et al; AIM-Study Group. Cost-utility analysis of antibiotic treatment in patients with chronic low back pain and Modic changes: results from a randomised, placebo-controlled trial in Norway (the AIM study). BMJ Open. 2020;10(6):e035461. https://doi.org/10.1136/bmjopen-2019-035461. PMID: 32546490; PMCID: PMC7299049.

8 Neck Pain: Whiplash and Cervicogenic Headache

Sagar S. Parikh, Tomas Salazar, and Roy Taborda

8.1 Synonyms

C2 neuralgia, cervical facet syndrome, whiplash-associated syndrome.

8.2 ICD-10 Codes

- G44.89—cervicogenic headache
- M47.812—cervical spondylosis without radiculopathy
- S13.4—whiplash injury

8.3 Description

Anatomy The cervical spine consists of C1 to C7 vertebrae, separated by intervertebral disks between C2 and T1, and 8 pairs of spinal nerves existing intervertebral foramina. Joints in the c-spine consist of occiput to C1 and C1–C2 articulations, and six pairs of di-arthrodial facet joints. The specific orientation of these joints allows for flexion, extension, and lateral tilt of the cervical spine. Spinal nerves exit each cervical level via left and right lateral foraminal openings. Medial branches originate from the dorsal rami of each exiting cervical spinal nerve, innervating the facet joint capsules (Fig. 8.1).

There are three nerves from the C2 and C3 spinal nerves, which supply the posterior scalp of the head up to the vertex.

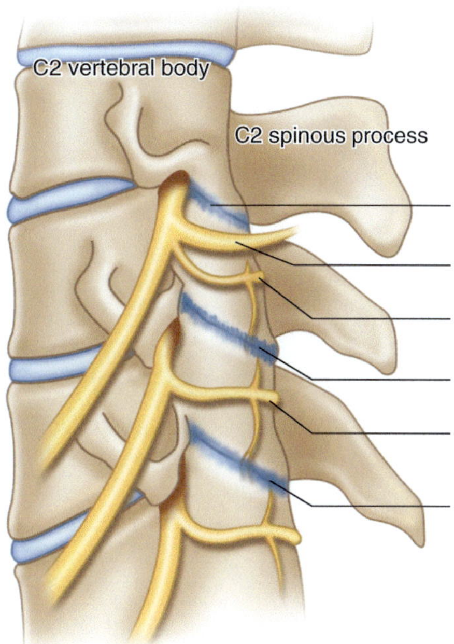

Fig. 8.1 Innervation of cervical facet joints. (Author's illustration)

1. The greater occipital nerve (GON) arises from the medial division of the dorsal ramus of C2 spinal nerve and moves across the inferior capitis oblique and semispinalis capitis [1]. In the course of the GON, it pierces the semispinalis capitis and may even penetrate the trapezius and inferior oblique, which may predispose the nerve to entrapments and irritations. The GON supplies the scalp up to the vertex and ear (Fig. 8.2).
2. The lesser occipital nerve (LON) originates from the ventral rami of C2 and C3 spinal nerves and has three branches, namely the auricular, mastoid, and occipital branches. It travels along the posterior border of the sternocleidomastoid muscle. After penetrating the cervical fascia, it then moves superior to the occiput where it communicates with the GON. It primarily supplies the lateral and superior aspects of the head behind the ears.

S. S. Parikh (✉)
Hackensack Meridian School of Medicine, Nutley, NJ, USA
e-mail: sagar.Parikh@hmhn.org

T. Salazar
JFK Johnson Rehabilitation Institute, Edison, NJ, USA

R. Taborda
Department of Physical Medicine & Rehabilitation, JFK Johnson Rehabilitation Institute, Edison, NJ, USA

© The Author(s), under exclusive license to Springer Nature Switzerland AG 2022

S. A. Mostoufi et al. (eds.), *Clinical Guide to Musculoskeletal Medicine*, https://doi.org/10.1007/978-3-030-92042-5_8

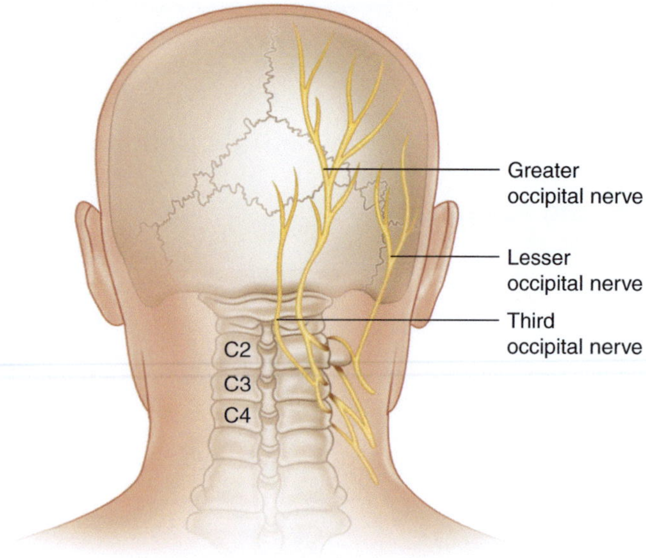

Fig. 8.2 Anatomy of greater, lesser, and third occipital nerve. (Author's illustration)

Table 8.1 Differential diagnosis of cervicogenic headache

Vascular	Giant cell arteritis and aberrant vasculature causing irritation
Neurogenic	C2 radiculopathy, C2 myelitis, multiple sclerosis, schwannomas, occipital neuralgia, migraine headache, other headache disorders, and whiplash-related injury
Osteogenic	C1–C2 arthrosis, osteolytic lesion, subluxation of atlantoaxial joint, and rheumatoid arthritis
Other	Myofascial pain syndrome and Arnold Chiari malformation

3. The third occipital nerve (TON) is a superficial branch of the dorsal ramus of the C3 spinal nerve. It courses to the dorsolateral C2–C3 facet joint where it may branch with the contralateral TON [1]. It may pierce the splenius capitis, trapezius, and semispinalis capitis to communicate with the GON. It primarily innervates the skin below the superior nuchal line.

Clinical criteria of cervicogenic headache include unilateral proximal neck, occiput, and frontal headache without crossing midline to the contralateral side [2]. In case of whiplash injury, pain presentation may be more diffuse and bilateral. The differential diagnosis for CGH is outlined in Table 8.1. For the purposes of this chapter, we will be focusing on cervicogenic headache as it pertains to cervical facet disease and whiplash injury.

Cervicogenic headache (CGH) is a term encompassing headache syndromes originating from the anatomic upper cervical spine and its exiting nerve structures detailed below. When discussing cervicogenic headache, we are mainly referencing structures within the upper cervical spine including facets, soft tissue structures, and exiting spinal nerves and its branches. Cervicogenic headaches typically arise from irritation of cervical structures innervated by spinal nerves C1, C2, and C3 and its relay of pain signals centrally to the trigeminocervical nucleus (the nociceptive nucleus of the head and neck) that is thought to be the reason for referred pain sensations to the occiput and eyes [3, 4].

Cervical spondylosis, in particular proximal facets (C2–C4), contributes to cervicogenic headache. These arthritic changes are frequently due to progressive and degenerative wear and tear or breakdown of the facet joints [5]. This degeneration can occur through the normal aging process or be a consequence of a traumatic event such as whiplash injury (acceleration–deceleration injury) [6]. Cervical spondylosis or facet disease is the most common progressive aging process in the neck and usually begins after the age of 40 [7]. Close to 50% of patients, over the age of 50 will show some degree of cervical degenerative changes radiographically [7]. Changes in cervical range of motion and radiographic findings may pre-date the onset of persistent pain. Spondylosis relating to trauma will present with pain more profoundly.

Whiplash-associated disorder (WAD) describes injuries due to a sudden acceleration–deceleration movements [8]. It is considered a common outcome after "non-catastrophic" motor vehicle accidents where the patient's head and neck and thrusted forward and backward (into flexion and extension) suddenly and violently causing bony or soft tissue injury. Symptomatic cases of whiplash have a global incidence of between 16 and 200 per 100,000 individuals [9]. Prevalence of traumatic cervical facet disease after whiplash injury has been estimated at between 54% and 60% making it a significant contributor in the post-traumatic pain setting [10] where there can be a component of headache pain originating from mild brain trauma or damage to cervical facet structure. Other symptoms of whiplash-associated disorder apart from general biomechanical neck strain and headache include decreased pain thresholds and central hypersensitivity [11]. When comparing pain thresholds in chronic age-related neck pain and whiplash, patients with WAD demonstrated more widespread painful hypersensitivity to mechanical and thermal stimuli diffusely [12]. There has also been evidence of altered or lost motor recruitment patterns in the neck musculature, altered eye movements control, proprioceptive challenges, and in some cases muscle weakness, especially in the cervical paraspinal, trapezius, and adjacent neck musculature [11]. Traumatic WAD can also lead to irritation of the occipital nerves causing a neuralgia and lancination pain, which is also a source of headache and in the differential diagnosis [13].

8.4 Clinical Presentation

8.4.1 Cervicogenic Headache Presentation

Patients present with chronic neck pain with occiput and frontal headache and at times shoulders (Fig. 8.3). The pain can be improved with rest and worsened with movement of the neck especially in extension rotation and lateral flexion.

8.4.1.1 Diagnostic Criteria

The International Headache Society established diagnostic criteria for both occipital neuralgia and cervicogenic headaches. These guidelines were last updated in 2018 and are used to guide the diagnostic workup [13].

1. Imaging or clinical evidence of cervical spine or neck soft tissue disease known to cause a headache.
2. The headache must also fulfill at least two of the following:
   (a) Commencement of headaches with a temporal relationship to the beginning of the cervical spine or neck disease.
   (b) The headache improves/resolves if the cervical disorder improves or is treated.
   (c) Reduced cervical range of motion and worsened headache with provocative maneuvers.
   (d) Diagnostic block of the cervical structure leads to improvement in the headache.
3. Headache is not better explained by another diagnosis [13].

8.4.2 Whiplash-Associated Injury Presentation

Whiplash-associated injury classically presents after a motor vehicle accident during which there is sudden neck extension and flexion. Typically, the collision involves the patient being rear-ended, but other mechanisms of sudden movement can also occur. Neck pain or headache is the usual presenting symptom after the accident as well as decreased neck range of motion and guarding; symptoms can occur immediately or several days later but must present within 7 days [13]. Patients can also complain of shoulder pain, changes in muscle strength, vision changes, alterations in memory and concentration, dizziness, tinnitus, numbness, and hypersensitivity [6]. A classification system for WAD has been devised by the Quebec task force as follows: [8]

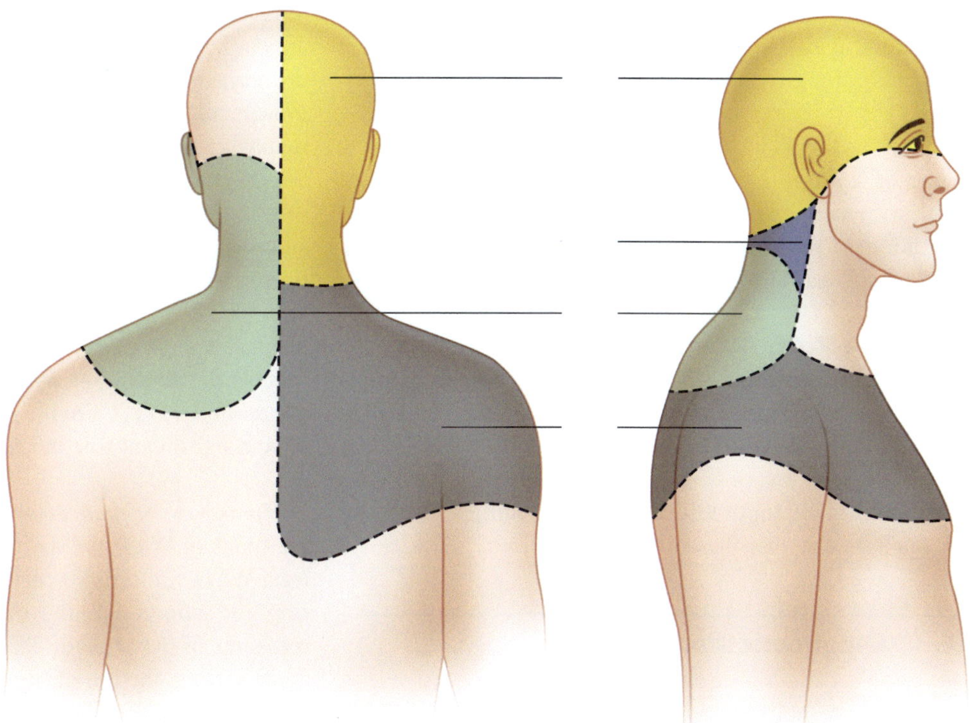

Fig. 8.3 Cervical facet pain referral pattern. (Author's illustration)

- Grade 0: No complaints of neck pain. No physical signs
- Grade I: Neck complaint of pain, stiffness, or tenderness only. No physical signs
- Grade II: Neck complaint AND musculoskeletal sign. Musculoskeletal signs include decreased range of motion and point tenderness.
- Grade III: Neck complaint AND neurological signs. Neurological signs include decreased range of motion and point tenderness
- Grade IV: Neck complaint AND fracture or dislocation

8.5 Physical Examination

A full MSK, spine, and neurologic examination should be concocted.

Inspection The patient's head, shoulder, and neck positioning should be noted as posture can be a source of pain. Loss of normal lordosis of the cervical spine, neck guarding, and stiffness can be assessed on presentation.

Palpation In addition to palpating the cervical facets, tenderness with cervical paraspinal palpation has been found to be a strong indicator of facet-mediated pain [14]. The examiner should thus palpate the spinous processes, paraspinals muscles, and facet joints carefully. Palpation of the neck musculature can also trigger cervicogenic headaches in the setting of myofascial pain, so trigger points should also be identified [13]. Palpation may detect tenderness along the course of the GON in occipital neuralgia [15].

Range of motion Neck pain and headache may be triggered by neck extension, rotation, and lateral flexion. Limitation in ROM may be noted due to DJD, pain, and muscle tighness [14]

Sensory and Reflex testing Reflexes and sensory tests are normal in this diagnosis. Patient with dysesthesia or allodynia or positive Tinel's sign of greater occipital nerve may have occipital neuralgia [13].

Motor testing Strength testing in the extremities should be full, but pain can alter these findings.

8.6 Diagnostic Workup

X-ray It may help reveal an osseous and hypertrophic pathology. Findings are not definitive, though, as many patients with CGH have asymptomatic cervical spine pathology.

CT scan As compared to x-rays, CT scan provides a better definition of bony changes of the facet joints, vertebrae, C1/2 articulation, and any bleeding and dislocation and may be indicated in traumatic cases.

MRI Magnetic resonance helps visualize cervical facets and identify other causes of neck pain such as discogenic changes, stenotic central canal, cord myelomalacia, demyelinating disease, and bony infiltration.

Diagnostic blocks Diagnostic medial branch block is specific to facet-generated spinal pain and can be utilized in cervicogenic headache. Fluoroscopic-guided C2 and C3 medial branch + TON block is the most common diagnostic test for cervicogenic headache from C2/3 facet. Greater occipital nerve block can differentiate between occipital neuralgia versus other etiologies of headache. Soft tissue muscle pain may improve with trigger point injections. C3 radiculopathy can be differentiated by means of a selective C3 nerve root block (low-volume anesthetic).

8.7 Treatment

8.7.1 Medical Management

Cervical spondylosis There is a paucity of studies evaluating the true efficacy of medication management on long-term cervicogenic headaches relief [16]. Non-steroidal anti-inflammatory drugs (NSAIDs), oral steroids, and muscle relaxants can be used initially for their anti-inflammatory, muscle relaxation, and pain relief. Additionally for headache management, a trial of antidepressants (such as amitriptyline, Cymbalta) and anticonvulsants (such as gabapentin or pregabalin) for their membrane-stabilizing effect can be considered. A double-blind randomized control trial of pregabalin in the setting of CGH caused by C2 nerve irritation did show a statistically significant decrease in the number of headache days per month, along with long-term improvements in headache intensity, sleep, and levels of anxiety and depression [17]. Chronic opioid usage generally does not have a significant role in CGH management [18].

Whiplash-associated disorder Initially, the pharmacological focus of WAD will be to decrease pain. Though one can treat WAD similarly to cervical spondylosis in the acute setting for pain relief, the evidence for NSAIDs or muscle relaxants in the acute or chronic setting is scarce [19]. In the acute setting, the use of high-dose steroids is correlated with fewer sick days, fewer disabling symptoms, and overall decrease in pain intensity [20]. Benzodiazepines and opioids are generally discouraged in chronic WAD patients. Though antidepressants and anticonvulsants have a role in treating neuropathic pain conditions, there is a lack of good evidence for its role in WAD treatment [19].

8.7.2 Rehabilitation

Cervical trauma, whiplash, or C2–C3 facet arthritis may result in ensuing inflammation with sensitization of C-fibers and lower pain threshold, thus increasing symptom severity [21]. For this reason, early rehabilitation is important to improve function and help with pain relief [22]. A systematic review and meta-analysis of physical therapy in headaches did demonstrate a statistically significant reduction in intensity, frequency, and duration of cervicogenic headaches [23]. A study comparing early mobilization and range of motion exercise to rest and immobilization in whiplash population demonstrated that early intervention (within 96 hours after injury) and mobility significantly reduced pain intensity, sick leave, and almost complete resolution of pre-injury cervical range of motion [22]. Specific attention is placed on neck and scapular strengthening and range of motion as well as dynamic and static neck stabilizing exercises [8]. Some theorize that establishment of a foundation of self-efficacy in the patient with early intervention improves recovery. Self-efficacy and confidence in movement patterns is a highly predictive factor in the persistence of disability in the WAD population [24]. The benefit of mobilization and range of motion exercises are less robust in the chronic WAD population. Acute WAD is treated with neck stabilization exercises including chin tucks, side-to-side rotation, side bending, and isometric exercises (Fig. 8.4). In the setting of chronic WAD, a good deal of attention must be placed on muscle tension relaxation (i.e., massage, myofascial release) before neck stabilization exercises are initiated.

Based on American Physical Therapy Association (APTA) evidence-based practice guidelines for patients with musculoskeletal impairments, in facetogenic pain, a multimodal approach care including spinal manipulation /mobilization, neuromuscular exercise (coordination, proprioception, and postural training), stretching, strengthening, and cognitive-affective elements should be provided. Physical therapists may include dry needling, laser treatment for photobiomodu-

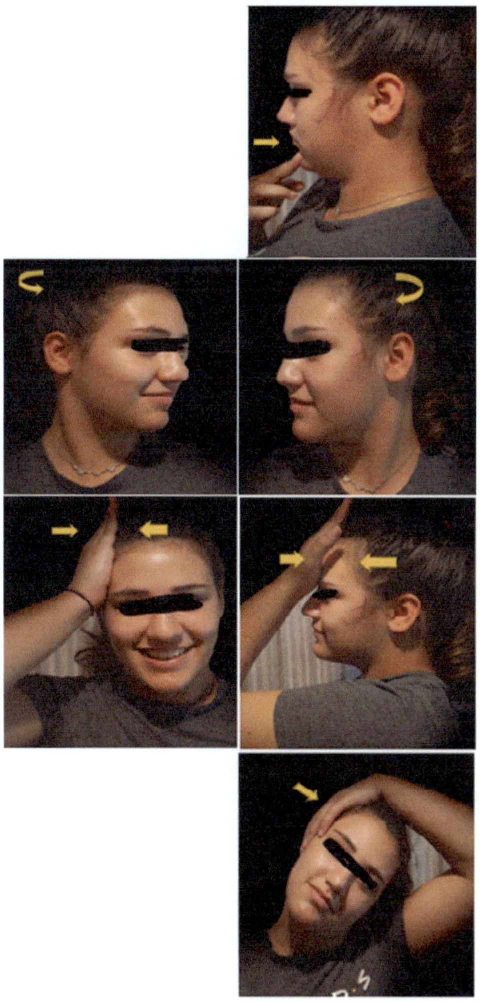

Fig. 8.4 Physical therapy exercises for neck pain and headache in patients without instability

lation, or intermittent mechanical/manual traction as part of treatment. A randomized control trial found that both manipulative therapy (low and high velocity) and low-load exercise designed to improve muscle control in the cervical–scapular area reduced headache frequency and intensity. High-velocity manipulation of the cervical spine comes along with significant vascular risks including arterial dissection, and caution must be taken [25]. Patient education and ergonomic consideration are important in preventing chronicity of spinal axial pain [26].

8.7.3 Procedures

8.7.3.1 Cervical Medial Branch Radiofrequency Ablation (RFA)

Targeting the C2 and C3 medial branches and TON can be effective in blocking the afferent pain signal from C2–C3 and C3–C4 facet joints. Before committing to RFA, these nerves are anesthetized, and if there is at least 70–80% neck pain and headache relief, RF can be recommended [27]. Thermal RFA provides an average of 6–12 months of pain relief and has self-limiting potential complications including dysesthesia and prolonged cutaneous anesthesia in a specific sensory distribution [1].

8.7.3.2 Occipital Nerve Blocks

Greater occipital nerve (GON) blocks may be an effective strategy in differentiating occipital neuralgia from facet-mediated headaches. Using anesthetic, only (diagnostic) or a mixture of local anesthetic and corticosteroid, with 70% or more reduction in pain, is a desirable outcome [28]. Ultrasound guidance increases accuracy and avoids injury to adjacent vasculature. GON neuromodulation (based on gate theory of pain) may be an effective modality of care, once diagnosis of refractory occipital neuralgia is confirmed by diagnostic block and less invasive treatments have been exhausted [29].

8.7.3.3 Trigger Point Injection and Botulinum Toxin

In cervicogenic headaches (CH), trigger point injection and botulinum toxin may provide significant relief by targeting specific muscles (i.e., semispinalis, splenius capitis, trapezius) that may entrap the nerves. In a placebo-controlled trial, a significant difference was found among the group treated with botulinum neurotoxin type A when compared to the saline-treated placebo group at 6- and 12 weeks post-treatment. Given the relatively acceptable safety profile, botulinum toxin is a viable option to help reduce frequency and the number of painful days [30].

8.7.3.4 Regenerative Medicine/Biologics

Multiple guidelines exist from the Food and Drug Administration, potentially limiting the use of stem cells (bone marrow or fat origin) in MSK conditions. There is an increased affinity for the application of PRP for arthritic joint pain. Intra-articular zygapophyseal joint injection could be the target of PRP treatment. At the time of this publication, the body of evidence to support regenerative medicine in the spine is limited.

8.7.4 Surgery

Surgery is not commonly recommended for cervicogenic headaches. In rare cases of headache related to occipital nerve compression by adjacent vascular structure, decompression may be considered. In rare cases of intractable cervicogenic headaches, proximal cervical fusion may be considered, but risk versus benefits should be carefully evaluated due to the invasive nature of this treatment.

References

1. Yu M, Wang SM. Anatomy, head and neck, occipital nerves. [Updated 2020 Nov 12]. In: StatPearls [Internet]. StatPearls Publishing.
2. Antonaci F, et al. Cervicogenic headache: evaluation of the original diagnostic criteria. Cephalalgia. 2001;21(5):573–83.
3. Khalili Y, et al. Cervicogenic headache STATPEARLS [Internet] Last Update: March 8, 2021. Treasure Island (FL): StatPearls Publishing,
4. Wang E, et al. Treatment of cervicogenic headache with cervical epidural steroid injection. Curr Pain Headache Rep. 2014;18(9):442.
5. Theodore N. Degenerative cervical spondylosis. N Engl J Med. 2020;383(2):159–68.
6. Bogduk N. The anatomy and pathophysiology of whiplash. Clin Biomech. 1986;1(2):92–101.
7. Singh S, et al. Risk factors in cervical spondylosis. J Clin Orthop Trauma. 2014;5(4):221–6.
8. Pastakia K, et al. Acute whiplash associated disorders (WAD). Open Access Emerg Med. 2011;3:29–32.
9. Pato U, Stefano GD, Fravi N, et al. Comparison of randomized treatments for late whiplash. Neurology. 2010;74:1223–30.
10. Manchikanti L, et al. Prevalence of cervical facet joint pain in chronic neck pain. Pain Physician. 2002;5(3):243–9.
11. Sterling M. Whiplash-associated disorder: musculoskeletal pain and related clinical findings. J Man Manip Ther. 2011;19(4):194–200.
12. David S, et al. Widespread sensory hypersensitivity is a feature of chronic whiplash-associated disorder but not chronic idiopathic neck pain. Clin J Pain. 2005;21(2):175–81.
13. Arnold M. Headache classification committee of the international headache society (IHS) the international classification of headache disorders. Cephalalgia. 2018;38(1):1–211.
14. Frontera WR, Silver JK, Rizzo TD. Essentials of physical medicine and rehabilitation e-book. Elsevier Health Sciences; Elsevier: Amsterdam, The Netherlands. 2018.
15. Loukas M. Identification of greater occipital nerve landmarks for the treatment of occipital neuralgia. Folia Morphol (Warsz). 2006;65(4):337–42.

16. Mazanec D, Reddy A. Medical management of cervical spondylosis. Neurosurgery. 2007;60(suppl_1):S1–43.
17. Boudreau GP, Marchand L. Pregabalin for the management of cervicogenic headache: a double blind study. Can J Neurol Sci. 2014;41(5):603–10.
18. Barmherzig R, Kingston W. Occipital neuralgia and cervicogenic headache: diagnosis and management. Curr Neurol Neurosci Rep. 2019;19:20.
19. Curatolo M. Pharmacological and interventional management of pain after whiplash injury. J Orthop Sports Phys Ther. 2016;46(10):845–50.
20. Petterson K, Toolanen G. High-dose methylprednisolone prevents extensive sick leave after whiplash injury. A prospective, randomised, double-blind study. Spine. 1998;23:984–9.
21. Al Khalili Y, Ly N, Murphy PB. Cervicogenic headache. [Updated 2021 Mar 8]. In: StatPearls [Internet]. Treasure Island (FL): StatPearls Publishing; 2021.
22. Borchegrevnik GE, Kaasa A, McDonagh D, et al. Acute treatment of whiplash neck sprain injuries. Spine. 1998;23:25–31.
23. Luedtke K, et al. Efficacy of interventions used by physiotherapists for patients with headache and migraine—systematic review and meta-analysis. Cephalalgia. 2016;36(5):474–92.
24. Bunketorp L, Lindh M, Carlsson J, Stene-Victorin E. The perception of pain and pain related cognition in subacute whiplash associated disorders: its influence on prolonged disability. Disabil Rehabil. 2006;28:271–9.
25. Jull G, et al. A randomized controlled trial of exercise and manipulative therapy for cervicogenic headache. Spine. 2002;27(17):1835–43.
26. Allen SM, Mookadam F, Cha SS, Freeman JA, Starling AJ, Mookadam M. Greater occipital nerve block for acute treatment of migraine headache: a large retrospective cohort study. J Am Board Fam Med. 2018;31(2):211–8.
27. Mehnert M, et al. Focused clinical review - update on the role of Z-joint injection and radiofrequency neurotomy for cervicogenic headache. PM R. 2013;5(3):221–7.
28. Juškys R, Šustickas G. Effectiveness of treatment of occipital neuralgia using the nerve block technique: a prospective analysis of 44 patients. Acta Med Litu. 2018;25(2):53–60.
29. Lambru G, Matharu MS. Occipital nerve stimulation in primary headache syndromes. Ther Adv Neurol Disord. 2012;5(1):57–67. https://doi.org/10.1177/1756285611420903.
30. Karadaş O, Oztürk B, Ulaş UH, Kütükçü Y, Odabaşı Z. The efficacy of botulinum toxin in patients with cervicogenic headache: a placebo-controlled clinical trial. Balkan Med J. 2012;29(2):184–7. https://doi.org/10.5152/balkanmedj.2012.003.

Spinal Stenosis

9

Augustine Lee, Derek Miles, and David J. Kennedy

9.1 Synonyms

Neurogenic claudication; spondylosis, spondylitis, myelopathy, central canal stenosis, lumbar canal stenosis

9.2 ICD-10

- M48.01-04 Spinal stenosis cervical region.
- M48.04 Spinal stenosis thoracic region.
- M48.05 Spinal stenosis thoracolumbar region.
- M48.061 Spinal stenosis lumbar region without neurogenic claudication.
- M48.062 Spinal stenosis lumbar region with neurogenic claudication.

9.3 Description

Spinal stenosis is a condition of reduced spinal canal space and resultant compression of its neural and vascular elements, secondary to acquired or hereditary changes in the spinal canal [1]. When symptomatic, spinal stenosis commonly manifests as insidious-onset pain, sensory, or motor dysfunction in a pattern consistent with the corresponding spinal nerves affected, and is biomechanically exacerbated by activities that further reduce space in the spinal canal. In addition, the clinical presentation of this condition can be further influenced by the timing of disease duration, extent of stenosis, disease progression, presence of multisegmental involvement, complications in pain perception and pain processing, and associated physical or psychological comorbidities. Hence, spinal stenosis can clinically present on a spectrum of variable signs and symptoms, ranging from asymptomatic to severe cervical or thoracic myelopathy or cauda equina syndrome [1, 2].

Spinal stenosis is most commonly found in the lumbar vertebral region of the spine (fourfold higher than cervical stenosis) and will therefore be the focus of this chapter [3]. Cervical and thoracic stenosis differs from lumbar stenosis in the potential for progression to myelopathy, the latter of which would warrant urgent surgical evaluation. Thoracic stenosis is less common than its cervical or lumbar counterparts, and can be challenging to diagnose as its associated myotomal distribution is relatively limited.

Etiologies of spinal stenosis have been commonly classified as hereditary vs acquired. *Acquired spinal stenosis* is the most common and can be further classified as one or a combination of degenerative, traumatic, or deformity. Further anatomic classification of spinal stenosis specifies areas of focal narrowing, including the central canal, lateral recess, or exiting neuroforamina [2]. *Congenital spinal stenosis* is rare and results from abnormal development of spinal canal bone structure, including congenitally short pedicles and laterally directed laminae [4, 5]. These abnormalities result in a reduced anterior–posterior spinal canal diameter. Symptoms are suspected to manifest at a younger age than degenerative stenosis, classically presenting as young athletes with temporary neurological deficits following physical contact that subsequently resolves. Data on prevalence estimates are sparse, but suspected to affect far less than 25% of the patient population with spinal stenosis. Symptomatic presentation of congenital stenosis is similar to that of acquired spinal stenosis, but anatomically has been more frequently observed to be multisegmental [5].

A. Lee (✉)
Department of Physical Medicine and Rehabilitation, Vanderbilt University Medical Center, Vanderbilt University School of Medicine, Nashville, TN, USA

D. Miles
Department of Physical Therapym Barbell Medicine, Cincinnati, OH, USA
e-mail: Derek@barbellmedicine.com

D. J. Kennedy
Spine Interventional Society, Department of Physical Medicine and Rehabilitation, Vanderbilt University, Nashville, TN, USA
e-mail: David.j.kennedy@vumc.org

© The Author(s), under exclusive license to Springer Nature Switzerland AG 2022

S. A. Mostoufi et al. (eds.), *Clinical Guide to Musculoskeletal Medicine*, https://doi.org/10.1007/978-3-030-92042-5_9

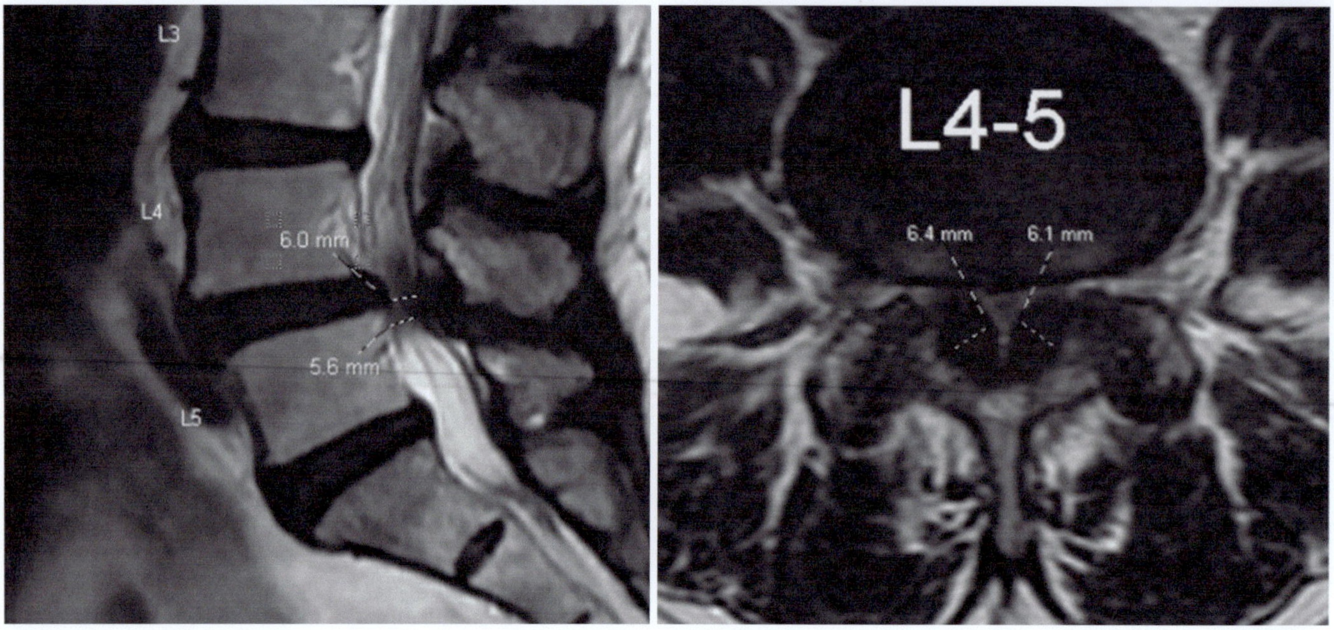

Fig. 9.1 Degenerative L4/5 spinal stenosis due to facet arthropathy and thickening of ligamentum flavum and grade 1 spondylolisthesis. Milder L3-4 narrowing also noted. (Courtesy of Ali Mostoufi, MD, New England Spine Care)

Degenerative spinal stenosis (Fig. 9.1) is prevalent and tends to increase with age. Radiographically degenerative spinal stenosis is present in up to 80% of patients over the age of 70 and, in some estimates, up to 77% of adults over the age of 40 [5]. The high prevalence of degenerative spinal stenosis is also costly as it is the most common indication for surgery among patients older than 65 years of age [6]. The estimated total Medicare costs for spinal stenosis in 2007 were 1.65 billion dollars, primarily as a result of surgery [2]. Other risk factors associated with the development of stenosis include male gender, obesity, tobacco use, and occupational hazard of repetitive spinal stress [7].

Common mechanisms of pathology Narrowing of the spinal canal can occur anteriorly from the disk desiccation/bulge, laterally from facet joint hypertrophy, and posteriorly from ligamentum flavum thickening. Furthermore, mechanical narrowing of the spinal canal can result from spinal column deformity, including spondylolisthesis (i.e., pathologic anterior displacement of the vertebral body) and scoliosis (abnormal lateral curvature of the spine) [8].

The degenerative process leading to stenosis starts with disk degeneration [1, 2]. Progressive desiccation of the nucleus pulposus results shortens the anterior spine, which shifts stress toward the posterior elements of the spine, including the facet joints, interspinous ligaments, ligamentum flavum, and subarticular ligaments. This chronically increased stress subsequently results in the reactive development of facet osteophytes, hypertrophy, cystic changes, and ligamentum flavum redundancy [2, 9, 10]. Symptoms of canal narrowing are primarily the result of neural elements compression, including the thecal sac or traversing spinal roots. However, a vascular contribution to spinal stenosis has also been theorized to also contribute to symptomatic pathogenesis via either arterial insufficiency (i.e., reduced arterial flow to the nerve roots) or venous engorgement (i.e., inadequate oxygenation of the capillary bed of the cauda equina and accumulation of toxic metabolites) [2, 9, 10].

Research has only supported a weak-to-moderate correlation between radiographic/anatomic pathology and severity of symptoms [2, 4, 11]. Some of the variance between radiographic vs. symptom severity is suspected to be explained in part by complexities in pain processing. The underlying mechanism for spinal stenosis is likely multifactorial. Emerging research on the complex nature of multiple descending and ascending pain processing pathways between the spinal cord and brain has shaped the conceptualization of pain sensitization, i.e., hyper-excitability of pain perception [12]. There is also a substantial contribution from psychological and cognitive factors, including depression/anxiety, self-efficacy, and pain catastrophizing [13].

9.4 Clinical Presentation

Lumbar spinal stenosis and acute lumbar radiculopathy from a herniated disk can have overlapping aspects of underlying pathology and even co-occur. When comparing the two, however, signs of dural tension (e.g., straight leg raise, femoral nerve stretch, and slump test) are more classically seen in the setting of acute radiculopathy [2]. Furthermore, acute radiculopathy tends to occur more frequently in patients under 50 years of age, have focal motor weakness (as opposed to gait disturbance or positive Romberg test), and have an acute/sudden onset of symptoms (as opposed to insidious) when relatively compared with spinal stenosis [2]. Another key distinction is that acute radiculopathy is more likely to symptomatically worsen with sitting, whereas spinal stenosis is more likely to improve with sitting and worsen with walking/spinal extension. Vascular claudication is another important clinical syndrome to distinguish from stenosis. Vascular claudication also worsens with walking, but differs from stenosis in that symptoms are relieved with rest while standing and occur below the knee (most commonly the calf). Furthermore there are signs of pallor, foot/shin skin breakdown, distal extremity hair loss, and diminished distal pulses [14]. Findings concerning vascular claudication could warrant referral to primary care or vascular specialist.

The hallmark of lumbar spinal stenosis is neurogenic claudication; numbness, pain, heaviness, and/or weakness in the legs radiate from the spine to the buttocks and legs while walking or prolonged standing. Neurogenic claudication is often relieved with sitting or stooping. Patients may also note pain while walking, relief of symptoms with forward flexion, relief of symptoms with bicycle/shopping cart, motor/sensory disturbance while walking, the presence of low back pain, the presence of lower extremity weakness, and the presence of pulses in the feet.

Studies support the presentation of pain radiating into the buttocks or distal leg having a sensitivity of 88% for the diagnosis of lumbar spinal stenosis but a specificity of only 34%. Moreover, a history of back pain while the patient was standing but no pain at all when the patient was sitting had a specificity for lumbar spinal stenosis of 93%, but a sensitivity of only 46% [1].

Cervical spinal stenosis can present with pain in the neck, arm pain, and numbness, and at times focal myotomal weakness and muscle atrophy. In cervical or thoracic myelopathy, gait disturbance, bowel or bladder dysfunction, clumsiness, dropping items, and gross muscle weakness can occur from cord comparison, often correlating with cord signal abnormality on MRI [1, 2]. Cervical and thoracic myelopathy would have upper motor neuron signs, while mostly lower motor neuron signs are observed in cauda equina syndrome and conus medullaris syndrome, except increased muscle tone can be seen in conus [10].

9.5 Physical Examination

The physical examination of a patient with suspected spinal stenosis involves a comprehensive neurologic, musculoskeletal, and vascular examination. A broad goal of the examination is to evaluate a pattern of signs consistent with spinal stenosis, nerve root irritation, red flag signs indicating the need for urgent further workup (e.g., fracture, myelopathy, cauda equina syndrome, or neoplasm), or other pathologies commonly known to mimic spinal stenosis (Table 9.1) [2].

Table 9.1 Differential diagnosis of lumbar spinal stenosis

Vascular claudication	Sacroiliac dysfunction
Peripheral neuropathy	Spinal canal tumor/metastatic disease
Hip osteoarthritis	Spondylolisthesis
Hip trochanteric bursitis	Arteriovenous malformations
Facet arthropathy (+/− facet synovial cyst)	Epidural hematoma
Discogenic pain	Epidural lipomatosis

Inspection is important to observe any asymmetry, discoloration, abnormal posturing, muscle wasting, or bony deformity.

Spine range of motion should be observed in the sagittal, coronal, and axial planes with notation of any restriction or provocation of symptoms. Palpation should be done along the midline spine and paraspinal areas and pelvis.

Gait Evaluation: Gait disturbance classically described in spinal stenosis is a slow, wide-based gait [1]; however, gait may also be normal. Scissoring gait can be observed in the setting of myelopathy.

Manual muscle testing can aid the evaluation for specific nerve root pathology based on myotomal weakness: shoulder abduction (C5), elbow extension (C5–C6), wrist extension (C6–C7), wrist flexion (C7–C8), distal finger flexion (C8), and finger abduction (T1), hip flexion (L2), knee extension (L3), ankle dorsiflexion (L4–L5), and ankle plantar flexion (S1). Given the strength of the plantar flexors, if weakness is a concern the patient should be able to perform 10 single leg calf raises as the standard for normal strength.

Sensory testing can include light touch, pinprick, and proprioception/vibration along corresponding dermatomal areas of the extremities.

Deep Tendon Reflex is helpful in the assessment for signs of upper (UMN) or lower motor neuron (LMN) pathology. UMN typically presents with hyperreflexia, increased muscle tone, and upward-going toes on plantar response. LMN typically presents with hyporeflexia, fasciculations, reduced muscle tone, and downward-going toes on plantar response. Reflexes are typically graded on a scale from 0 to 4, reflecting increasing strength of response. Lumbar stenosis presents as LMN dysfunction, except conus involvement. Thoracic and cervical stenosis can present as UMN if the cord is affected or LMN if the nerve roots are affected.

Clonus is a rhythmic series of muscle contractions induced by stretching the tendon and the highest level of reflex response.

Hoffman's sign is an involuntary flexion movement of the thumb/index finger. This is performed when the examiner flicks the patient fingernail of the middle finger down (58% sensitive, 78% specific) [15]. It can be a normal finding in those with hyperreflexia, but could also indicate an UMN issue.

Signs of cauda equina/conus medullaris/cervical myelopathy are also important to identify, including saddle anesthesia and upper motor neuron findings in cervical or thoracic myelopathy.

9.5.1 Special Maneuvers

Note these maneuvers are primarily to evaluate for other sources of pathology and are frequently negative in those with spinal stenosis or are a secondary cause of pain.

Dural Tension signs are typically negative for stenosis, but positive for acute radiculopathy. Sensitivity and specificity numbers are for radiculopathy, as they do not exist for spinal stenosis.

- Straight leg raise/Lasegue (*SLR*): (72% sensitive, 66% specific) [16].
  Technique: While supine and knee fully extended, the hip is passively fully flexed and subsequently the ankle dorsiflexed.
- *Seated Slump Test:* (84% sensitive, 83% specific) [10].
  Technique: Neck is flexed while slumped forward at the thoracic and lumbar spine while seated. One knee is extended, and subsequently, the ankle is dorsiflexed.
- *Femoral Nerve Tension:* (84% sensitivity for high lumbar disk herniation) [16].
  Technique: While prone the knee is fully flexed and subsequently the hip is passively fully extended, while the examiner uses one hand to maintain pelvic stability.
- *Hip Pelvic Tests* for hip and or pelvic pathology. Sensitivity and specificity are not for stenosis but for hip or pelvic pathology.
- *Log Roll:* Evaluates hip pathology. (90% sensitive, 36% specific) [17].
  Technique: Involves passive alternating external and internal rotation of the hip to the ends of its range of motion while the patient is supine.
- *FADDIR* (flexion adduction internal rotation): Evaluates femoroacetabular impingement/anterior labrum pathology (60% sensitive, 52% specific) [18].
  Technique: Hip is full-flexed and adducted with combined internal hip rotation while supine.
- *Patrick's/FABER test* (flexion abduction external rotation): Evaluates hip joint or sacroiliac pathology (71% sensitive, 100% specific) [10].
  Technique: Hip is full-flexed and abducted with combined external hip rotation, while the patient is supine.
- *Spurling:* Evaluates cervical root impingement.
  Technique: The patient's neck is slightly laterally rotated and extended with or without axial compression (40% sensitive, 92% specific) [16].
- *Romberg test*: Evaluates balance.
  Technique: Patient stands with feet together, arms crossed, and eyes closed [10] (40% sensitive, 91% specific).

9.6 Diagnostic Workup

Plain X-rays Plain films may demonstrate abnormalities suggestive of lumbar stenosis, including spondylolisthesis, disk narrowing, facet joint hypertrophy, and end-plate sclerosis, but lack assessment of soft tissue, spinal cord, or spinal canal diameter.

MRI MRI without contrast is the most widely used radiographic modality for the diagnosis of spinal stenosis [2]. MRI with contrast is often used in postoperative cases or suspected bony infiltration or infection, or in patients with prior operative spinal intervention as it is perceived to better display postoperative adhesions [9]. Five MR criteria that should be used as a minimum standard in the evaluation of stenosis (central and foraminal) are as follows: (1) compromise of the central spinal canal; (2) relation between fluid and cauda equina (in central canal stenosis); (3) nerve root compression in the lateral recess (for lateral recess stenosis); (4) foraminal nerve root impingement (for lateral recess stenosis); and (5) compromise of the foraminal zone (for foraminal stenosis) [19]. There is a substantial body of evidence demonstrating the lack of significant correlation between radiographic severity of stenosis and clinical symptom severity [2]. In addition, an estimated 21% of people with radiographic stenosis on MRI are asymptomatic [20].

CT-based studies CT without contrast can be useful to appraise bony pathology, pars fractures, extent of facet degeneration, and calcified ligaments and disk space [2]. CT myelography has been suggested as an alternative for MRI when cannot be performed (e.g., post-instrumentation with metallic artifact). CT myelography has been shown to have similar diagnostic capacity as MRI, although it is associated with radiation and the myelogram is an invasive procedure [4].

Furthermore, emerging research has suggested a potential nocebo role for the routing wording of radiographic reports when directly read by the patient. These negative effects included symptom catastrophizing and poor functional response to conservative management, and adjustments to avoid anxiety-provoking terminology on radiographic reports were suggested [21].

Electromyography (EMG/NCS) Electrodiagnostic studies are helpful when suboptimal correlation exists between radiographic and clinical findings [2]. EMG also assists with differentiating spinal origin complaints from alternative diagnoses like neuropathy and plexopathy. Sensory nerve conduction studies are typically expected to be normal unless the dorsal root ganglion is also affected. Motor nerve conduction studies may or may not be normal at L5 or S1 pathology, and H-reflexes may be abnormal in S1 pathology. Needle EMG usually involves a sampling of lumbar paraspinal muscles and 5–7 muscles of the affected limb that are innervated by different peripheral nerves and nerve roots [22]. Haig et al. demonstrated high specificity and moderate-to-low sensitivity for many electrodiagnostic elements, including fibrillations (47% sensitivity, 87% specificity) and H-wave (36% sensitivity, 91% specificity) [23]. Paraspinal mapping, an advanced needle localization EMG protocol for the paraspinal muscles, has shown promising diagnostic utility (30–90% sensitivity, 100% specificity) for lumbar spinal stenosis [24].

9.7 Treatments

9.7.1 Medical Management

A myriad of nonoperative non-procedural treatments exists including lifestyle modification, therapy, medications, injections, and even multidisciplinary rehabilitation. There is no specific medication for spinal stenosis. Patients often try over-the-counter medications including acetaminophen and nonsteroidal anti-inflammatories when tolerated. Topical anti-inflammatories/capsaicin may be used with lower GI and renal/cardiovascular side effects. Prescribed gabapentin may reduce pain (spinal and radicular) with limited literature support [25]. Some practitioners prescribed antidepressants including tricyclic and norepinephrine reuptake inhibitors with very limited literature support [26]. Neither muscle relaxants nor opioids have superiority over NSAIDs and acetaminophen. Muscle relaxants have anticholinergic side effects, and opioids may have CNS and GI side effects and could result in dependency and abuse. Other medications (e.g., prostaglandins, calcitonin, and vitamin B1) have potential to improve pain and walking distance, but evidence was low quality [2].

9.7.2 Rehabilitation

Main goals of rehabilitation in spinal stenosis are reduction in pain, improvement of function including walking, improvement of range of motion, gait training, and patient education and fall prevention. Exercise programs vary dramatically with strengthening, range of motion, stretching, proprioception, and various other forms all represented but none emerging as superior to the other [27]. Means of increasing compliance such as shared decision-making and individualized programs can help people experiencing symptomatic spinal stenosis regain function. The overall aim is to increase activity in these individuals and have exercise/movement become habitual.

9.7.2.1 Lumbar Spinal Stenosis

Exercise-based programs including strength training have demonstrated the ability to increase physical function and reduce risk of falls, a common functional deficit in individuals with symptomatic lumbar stenosis [28]. In a symptomatic population, gauging intensity of exercise is crucial as an activity at too low a threshold or at too high may deter continued participation and adaptation may not take place. The majority of individuals experiencing symptomatic lumbar spinal stenosis are sedentary (up to 75% in one study being entirely inactive) so increasing physical activity in any fashion is more beneficial than a specific program.

Multiple studies have demonstrated a significant, small effect with the addition of manual therapy to an exercise program in the treatment of stenosis. The effects of manual therapy on patient outcomes have been demonstrated to be nonspecific and not directed at specific tissue structure. If manual therapy is to serve as an adjunct to exercise, the narrative-associated needs to be taken into account so as to encourage movement and a belief of resilience in patients. Manual therapy should not serve as a stand-alone treatment in patients with spinal stenosis.

9.7.2.2 Thoracic Spinal Stenosis

With thoracic spinal stenosis being exceedingly rare, there is a paucity of high-quality information on management. The course of rehabilitation would follow that of either cervical or lumbar stenosis in a focus on symptom management and increasing capacity for activity.

9.7.2.3 Cervical Spinal Stenosis

Rehabilitation for cervical spinal stenosis should include movement strategies to increase tolerance for physical activity as well. This may be inclusive of strengthening exercises to address identified weakness or specific grip work and task-specific activities of daily living issues such as placing objects on shelves and fine motor skill training. It could also include aerobic activity or aquatic exercises to encourage movement from a systemic level. Current clinical practice guidelines from the American Physical Therapy Association advocate exercise and advice to stay active per patient tolerance as the cornerstones of rehabilitation. If a patient is experiencing frequent radicular symptoms, clinicians may utilize nerve glides as a means of graded exposure to work on tolerance.

9.7.2.4 Treatment Modalities

Exercise programs vary dramatically with strengthening, range of motion, stretching, proprioception, and various other forms all represented but non-emerging as superior to the other. Each program should be tailored to the individual in order to find a starting point for movement according to their tolerance, the equipment to which they have access, and their goals. There is no good evidence for the utilization of passive modalities such as ice, heat, ultrasound, or transcutaneous electrical nerve stimulation (TENS). There is low-level evidence for utilization of acupuncture as an adjunct to exercise, but the narrative associated with utilization needs to be taken into account.

9.7.3 Procedures

Epidural steroid injections (Fig. 9.2) Widely used in the treatment of spinal stenosis recalcitrant to a trial of less invasive care, including medications and PT [2]. In an attempt to reduce nerve tissue inflammation, glucocorticoid is injected in the epidural space in proximity of the identified stenotic segment. The procedure is most commonly done percutaneously via needle insertion to the epidural space under fluoroscopic guidance. Epidural steroid delivery can be interlaminar (cervical, thoracic, or lumbar), transforaminal, or caudal approach (although data are lacking for the caudal approach, and it should have a limited role in a modern medical practice). Potential complications include infection, allergic reaction to injectate, nerve root damage, dural puncture, hematoma, transient cortisol suppression, transiently altered glucose metabolism, and in rare cases spinal cord ischemia secondary to inadvertent intra-arterial injection of particulate corticosteroid [29]. A large portion of the existing literature has shown short-term (<3 months) symptomatic improvements.

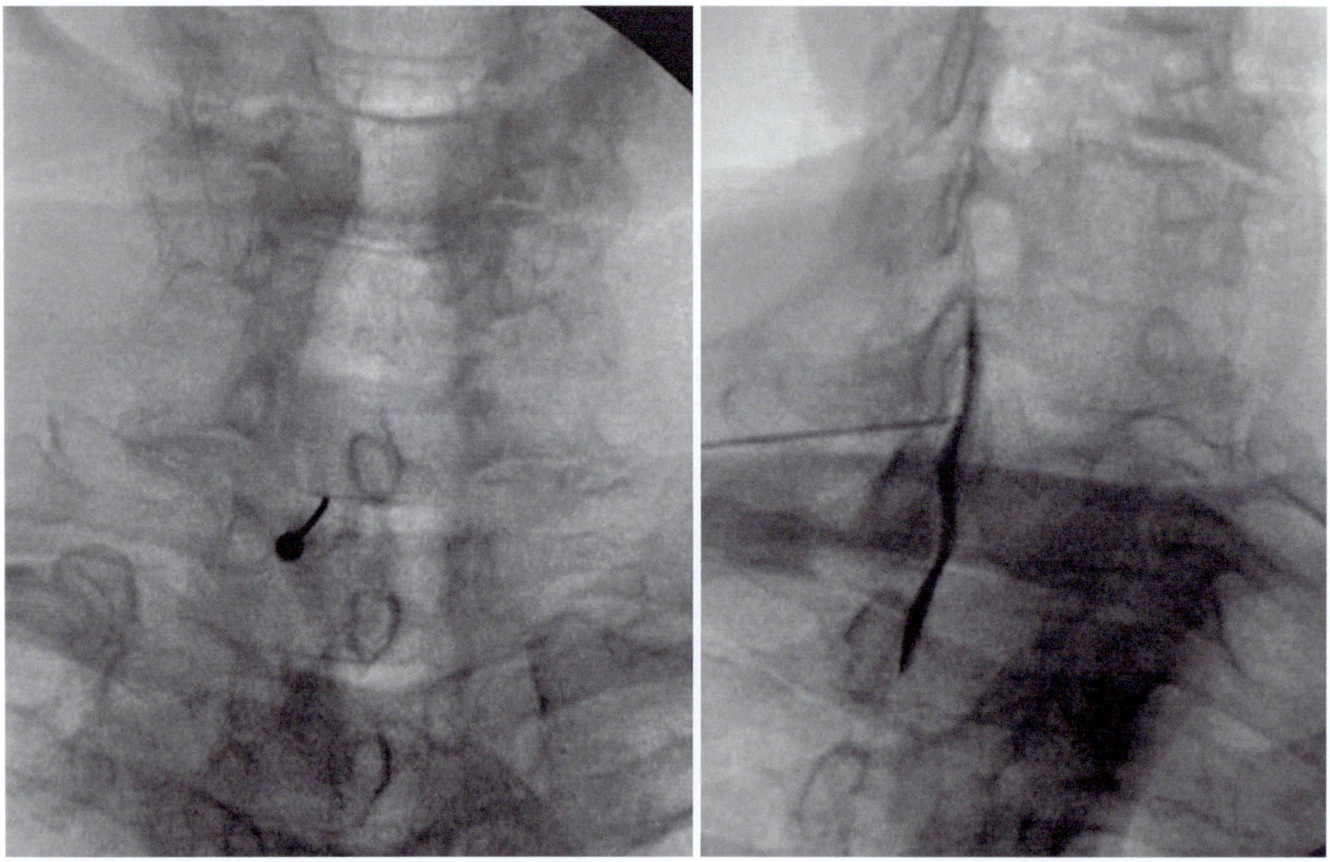

Fig. 9.2 Cervical interlaminar epidural Injection with contrast material enhancing posterior epidural space. (Image courtesy of Ali Mostoufi, MD, New England Spine Care Associates)

9.7.4 Minimally Invasive Percutaneous Procedures

There are also percutaneous minimally invasive procedures that are available to treat patients with spinal stenosis, including MILD procedure (Vertos Medical Inc., USA) and Vertiflex procedure (Superion® Indirect Decompression System by Boston Scientific, Marlborough, MA, USA). Both of these procedures have published 5-year safety and outcome data. These treatments represent exciting advances in our ability to treat lumbar spinal stenosis and will likely continue to expand our ability to appropriately treat patients suffering from this condition. They are covered in greater depth in Chap. 14.

9.7.5 Surgery

Indications for referral include failure of conservative nonoperative management or signs of progressive neurological deficit or myelopathy. The specific details of the surgical approach vary according to the location of the stenosis, number of segments affected, associated deformity or spinal instability, history of previous surgery, and surgeon's preferences [2, 29, 30]. Depression, cardiovascular comorbidity, impaired gait, and scoliosis were patient factors found on systematic reviews to be predictors of poorer postoperative outcomes. Conversely, better walking ability, better perceived health, and higher income predicted better postoperative outcomes [31].

The primary goal of surgery is to decompress the stenotic neural structures, relief of symptoms, and improved functioning. Operative options include traditional laminectomy, bilateral laminotomies, bilateral decompression through unilateral laminotomy, and laminoplasty (cervical stenosis). Fusion is considered if there are any instabilities, unstable spondylolisthesis, or deformity in addition to or contributing to stenosis. The Spine Patient Outcomes Research Trial (SPORT) compared surgery and nonoperative treatment in lumbar stenosis. It found no differences in intent-to-treat analyses, but due to substantial crossover, per-protocol analyses did show early benefit to surgery [32]. However, per-protocol analyses sacrifice the preservation of randomization. For more details on spine surgery, see Chaps. 15 and 16.

References

1. Suri P, Rainville J, Kalichman L, Katz JN. Does this older adult with lower extremity pain have the clinical syndrome of lumbar spinal stenosis? JAMA [Internet]. 2010 Dec 15 [cited 2021 Jul 24];304(23):2628–36. Available from: https://jamanetwork-com.ezproxy.library.tufts.edu/journals/jama/fullarticle/187077.
2. Lurie J, & Tomkins-Lane C. Management of lumbar spinal stenosis. BMJ : British Medical Journal (Online). 2016;352. http://dx.doi.org/10.1136/bmj.h6234.
3. Lee MJ, Cassinelli EH, Riew KD. Prevalence of cervical spine stenosis: anatomic study in cadavers. J Bone Jt Surg - Ser A [Internet]. 2007 [cited 2021 Jul 26];89(2):376–80. Available from: https://pubmed-ncbi-nlm-nih-gov.ezproxy.library.tufts.edu/17272453/.
4. Maus TP. Imaging of spinal stenosis. Neurogenic intermittent claudication and cervical spondylotic myelopathy. Radiol Clin N Am [Internet]. 2012;50(4):651–79. Available from: https://doi.org/10.1016/j.rcl.2012.04.007.
5. Kalichman L, Cole R, Kim DH, Li L, Suri P, Guermazi A, et al. Spinal stenosis prevalence and association with symptoms: the Framingham study. Spine J. 2009;9(7):545–50.
6. Deyo RA, Mirza SK, Martin BI, Kreuter W, Goodman DC, Jarvik JG. Trends, major medical complications, and charges associated with surgery for lumbar spinal stenosis in older adults. JAMA. 2010;303(13):1259–65.
7. Yabuki S, Fukumori N, Takegami M, Onishi Y, Otani K, Sekiguchi M, et al. Prevalence of lumbar spinal stenosis, using the diagnostic support tool, and correlated factors in Japan: a population-based study. J Orthop Sci [Internet]. 2013 [cited 2021 Jul 26];18(6):893–900. Available from: https://pubmed-ncbi-nlm-nih-gov.ezproxy.library.tufts.edu/23963588/.
8. Ilyas H, Udo-Inyang I, Savage J. Lumbar spinal stenosis and degenerative spondylolisthesis: a review of the SPORT literature [Internet]. Clin Spine Surg. 2019 [cited 2021 May 3];32:272–8. Available from: https://pubmed-ncbi-nlm-nih-gov.ezproxy.library.tufts.edu/31145150/. Lippincott Williams and Wilkins.
9. Ross JS, Moore K. Diagnostic imaging: spine. Fourth ed. Ross JS, Moore K, editors. Philadelphia: Elsevier; 2021.
10. Cifu DX. Braddom's physical medicine & rehabilitation. Fifth ed. Cifu DX, editor. Philadelphia: Elsevier; 2016.
11. Burgstaller J, Schüffler P, Buhmann J, Andreisek G, Winklhofer S, Del Grande F, et al. Is there an association between pain and magnetic resonance imaging parameters in patients with lumbar spinal stenosis? Spine (Phila Pa 1976) [Internet]. 2016 Sep 1 [cited 2021 Jul 25];41(17):1053–62. Available from: https://pubmed.ncbi.nlm.nih.gov/26953669/.
12. Clauw DJ. Diagnosing and treating chronic musculoskeletal pain based on the underlying mechanism(s). Best Pract Res Clin Rheumatol. 2015;29(1):6–19.
13. Crofford LJ. Psychological aspects of chronic musculoskeletal pain [Internet]. Best Pract Res Clin Rheumatol. 2015 [cited 2021 Jul 26];29:147–55. Available from: https://pubmed-ncbi-nlm-nih-gov.ezproxy.library.tufts.edu/26267008/.
14. Conte MS, Pomposelli FB, Clair DG, Geraghty PJ, McKinsey JF, Mills JL, et al. Society for Vascular Surgery practice guidelines for atherosclerotic occlusive disease of the lower extremities: management of asymptomatic disease and claudication. J Vasc Surg [Internet]. 2015 Mar 1 [cited 2021 Jul 26];61(3):2S–41S.e1. Available from: https://pubmed-ncbi-nlm-nih-gov.ezproxy.library.tufts.edu/25638515/.
15. Grijalva RA, Hsu FPK, Wycliffe ND, Tsao BE, Williams P, Akpolat YT, et al. Hoffmann sign. Spine (Phila Pa 1976) [Internet]. 2015 Feb 17 [cited 2021 Jul 29];40(7):475–9. Available from: https://www.ncbi.nlm.nih.gov/books/NBK545156/.
16. Malanga G, Nadler S. Musculoskeletal physical examination: an evidenced based approach. Malanga G, Nadler S, editors. Philadelphia: Elsevier; 2006. 340 p.
17. Rahman LA, Adie S, Naylor JM, et al. A systematic review of the diagnostic performance of orthopedic physical examination tests of the hip. BMC Musculoskelet Disord 14, 257 (2013). https://doi.org/10.1186/1471-2474-14-257.

18. Casartelli NC, Brunner R, Maffiuletti NA, Bizzini M, Leunig M, Pfirrmann CW, et al. The FADIR test accuracy for screening cam and pincer morphology in youth ice hockey players. J Sci Med Sport [Internet]. 2018 Feb 1 [cited 2021 Jul 29];21(2):134–8. Available from: https://pubmed.ncbi.nlm.nih.gov/28669665/.
19. Andreisek G, Deyo RA, Jarvik JG, Porchet F, Winklhofer SFX, Steurer J. Consensus conference on core radiological parameters to describe lumbar stenosis - an initiative for structured reporting. Eur Radiol. 2014;24(12):3224–32.
20. Boden SD, Davis DO, Dina TS, Patronas NJ, Wiesel SW. Abnormal magnetic-resonance scans of the lumbar spine in asymptomatic subjects. A prospective investigation. J Bone Joint Surg Am. 1990;72(3):403–8.
21. Rajasekaran S, Dilip Chand Raja S, Pushpa BT, Ananda KB, Ajoy Prasad S, Rishi MK. The catastrophization effects of an MRI report on the patient and surgeon and the benefits of 'clinical reporting': results from an RCT and blinded trials. Eur Spine J [Internet]. 2021;30(7):2069–81. Available from: https://doi.org/10.1007/s00586-021-06809-0.
22. Preston D, Shapiro B. Electromyography and neuromuscular disorders. Second edition. Preston D, Shapiro B, editors. Elsevier Amsterdam, The Netherlands; 2013.
23. Haig AJ, Tong HC, Yamakawa KSJ, Quint DJ, Hoff JT, Chiodo A, et al. The sensitivity and specificity of electrodiagnostic testing for the clinical syndrome of lumbar spinal stenosis. Spine (Phila Pa 1976). 2005;30(23):2667–76.
24. Chiodo A, Haig AJ, Yamakawa KSJ, Quint D, Tong H, Choksi VR. Needle EMG has a lower false positive rate than MRI in asymptomatic older adults being evaluated for lumbar spinal stenosis. Clin Neurophysiol. 2007;118(4):751–6.
25. Diwan S, Sayed D, Deer TR, Salomons A, Liang K. An algorithmic approach to treating lumbar spinal stenosis: an evidenced-based approach. Pain Med [Internet]. 2019 Dec 1 [cited 2019 Dec 27];20(Supplement_2):S23–31. Available from: https://academic.oup.com/painmedicine/article/20/Supplement_2/S23/5661171.
26. Bussières A, Cancelliere C, Ammendolia C, Comer CM, Zoubi F Al, Châtillon C-E, et al. Non-surgical interventions for lumbar spinal stenosis leading to neurogenic claudication: a clinical practice guideline. J Pain [Internet]. 2021 [cited 2021 Jul 25];0(0):2021–2. Available from: http://www.jpain.org/article/S1526590021001887/fulltext.
27. Owen PJ, Miller CT, Mundell NL, Verswijveren SJJM, Tagliaferri SD, Brisby H, et al. Which specific modes of exercise training are most effective for treating low back pain? Network meta-analysis [Internet]. Br J Sports Med. 2020 [cited 2021 Jul 26];54:1279–87. Available from: https://pubmed-ncbi-nlm-nih-gov.ezproxy.library.tufts.edu/31666220/.
28. Ciolac EG, Rodrigues-da-Silva JM. Resistance training as a tool for preventing and treating musculoskeletal disorders [Internet]. Sports Med. 2016 [cited 2021 Jul 27];46:1239–48. Available from: https://pubmed-ncbi-nlm-nih-gov.ezproxy.library.tufts.edu/26914266/.
29. Kreiner DS, Hwang SW, Easa JE, Resnick DK, Baisden JL, Bess S, et al. An evidence-based clinical guideline for the diagnosis and treatment of lumbar disc herniation with radiculopathy. Spine J [Internet]. 2014;14(1):180–91. Available from: https://doi.org/10.1016/j.spinee.2013.08.003.
30. Ammendolia C, Kj S, Rok E, Rampersaud R, Ca K, Pennick V, et al. Nonoperative treatment of lumbar spinal stenosis with neurogenic claudication: a systematic review. Spine (Phila Pa 1976). 2013;37(10):E609–16.
31. Stevens-Lapsley JE, Schenkman ML, Dayton MR. Comparison of self-reported knee injury and osteoarthritis outcome score to performance measures in patients after total knee arthroplasty. PM R. 2011;3(6):541–9.
32. Weinstein JN, Lurie JD, Tosteson TD, Hanscom B, Tosteson ANA, Blood EA, et al. Surgical versus nonsurgical treatment for lumbar degenerative spondylolisthesis. N Engl J Med [Internet]. 2007;356(22):2257–70. Available from: http://www.pubmedcentral.nih.gov/articlerender.fcgi?artid=2553804&tool=pmcentrez&rendertype=abstract.

10 Disk Herniation and Radiculopathy

Savion Johnson, S. Ali Mostoufi, Peter K. Yi, Abby Dillard, Amanda Nelli, and Padma Gulur

10.1 Cervical Radiculopathy

10.1.1 Synonyms

Cervical disk disease with radiculopathy; cervical radiculitis; cervical neuritis

10.1.2 ICD-10 Codes

M54.11- M54.13

10.1.3 Description

Cervical radiculopathy is a condition in which dysfunction of a cervical nerve root results in a painful neck or arm with associated sensory, motor, and reflex abnormality. Cervical radicular pain is not necessarily associated with loss of sensation, motor function, or reflex abnormality. In radiculopathy, the involvement of the ventral root of the spinal nerves may result in motor weakness, and involvement of the dorsal root of the spinal nerve may result in sensory deficits; involvement of either may result in abnormal reflexes on examination.

S. Johnson · P. K. Yi · P. Gulur (✉)
Department of Anesthesiology, Duke University School of Medicine, Durham, NC, USA
e-mail: Padma.Gulur@Duke.edu

A. Nelli
Duke Anesthesiology, Durham, NC, USA

S. A. Mostoufi
Department of Orthopedics and Rehabilitation, Tufts University School of Medicine, Boston, MA, USA

New England Spine Care Associates & Boston Regenerative Medicine, Cambridge, MA, USA

A. Dillard
Department of Physical Therapy and Occupational Therapy, Duke University Health System, Durham, NC, USA

Anatomy The cervical spine consists of 7 vertebrae, 5 cervical disks (C2–C6), and 8 pairs of cervical nerve roots. The C1 vertebrae are ring-shaped, do not have a central body, and connect with the occipital condyle of the skull via lateral masses [15]. C1 articulates with the C2 vertebrae through atlantoaxial joints, and the primary articulation points for neck rotation. The C2 vertebrae body has a unique cephalad extension called the dens, which is tightly secured in place against the C1 arch by a transverse ligament, allowing for a majority of the cervical rotation at the C1–C2 junction. Dorsally, each vertebra connects through cervical facet joints, which are situated in a coronal plane with inferior angulation. Cervical facets allow for flexion, extension, and lateral tilt of the cervical spine. Unique to the cervical spine is the uncinate processes and associated uncovertebral joints between C3 and C7, which is rudimentary at birth but evolves with age, stabilizing the spine but also prone to degenerative changes [16, 17].

Cervical nerve roots exit through the inferior portion of the cervical intervertebral foramina [1] and are named for the corresponding vertebral body below them, except the C8 nerve, which exists at the C7-T1 foramen. The cervical neuroforamina is bordered anteriorly by the disk, posterior laterally by the facet joint, anteromedial by the uncovertebral joint, and the superior and inferior pedicle of the adjacent vertebrae. Facet arthropathy and uncovertebral arthropathy both may result in nerve impingement and radicular pain. C1–C3 spinal nerves have dorsal innervations including suboccipital (C1), greater occipital (C2), and third occipital nerve (C3) [2]. C1–C4 ventral primary rami form the cervical plexus, and C5–C8 ventral primary rami contribute to the brachial plexus.

The most common cervical radiculopathy is the C7 nerve followed by C6 and C8. The most common etiology for cervical radiculopathy is a posterolateral disk herniation with nerve root impingement or narrowing of the neuroforamina as a result of facet spondylosis, uncinate hypertrophy, or spondylolisthesis. Less common causes include facet synovial cysts, extradural masses, spinal tumors, and abscesses. Differential diagnosis of cervical radiculopathy is in Table 10.1.

© The Author(s), under exclusive license to Springer Nature Switzerland AG 2022
S. A. Mostoufi et al. (eds.), *Clinical Guide to Musculoskeletal Medicine*, https://doi.org/10.1007/978-3-030-92042-5_10

Table 10.1 Differential diagnosis of cervical radiculopathy

Brachial plexopathy	Peripheral neuropathy
Cervical myelopathy	Thoracic outlet syndrome
Demyelinating disease	Upper extremity arthralgia
Peripheral nerve entrapment	Upper extremity tendinopathy
Neuromuscular conditions	Upper extremity bursopathy

10.1.4 Clinical Presentation

Classic presentation of cervical radiculopathy is neck and unilateral arm pain in a specific nerve root pattern with sensory, motor, or reflex abnormalities. Sensory complaints follow a dermatomal pattern, and weakness follows the same anatomic level myotome. Of the subjective complaints, the distribution of hand paresthesias appears to have the greatest localizing value [3]. There is level 1 evidence that suprascapular (C5–C6), interscapular (C7), and scapular (C8) pain suggests radiculopathy [4]. Common aggravating factors include motion of the head toward the painful side, hanging of the arm, cough, sneeze, or Valsalva. Often pulling, pushing, and lifting items are not tolerated in the acute phase. Pain may improve when the head is tilted away from the painful side or if the affected arm is placed over the head. Clumsiness and deficits in fine motor movements (grip or pinch force) may precede gross weakness. Cervical myelopathy due to cord compression should also be ruled out, which often is associated with poor balance, bowel or/and bladder dysfunction, and bilateral sensory or motor abnormalities, along with distinct upper motor neuron examination findings.

10.1.5 Physical Examination

Full musculoskeletal and neurologic examination is indicated in the evaluation of cervical radicular pain.

Visual observation Clinicians should be trained to notice poor posture, abnormal body mechanics, spinal deformity, muscle atrophy, gait anomaly, use of an assistive device, skin abnormalities, and nonverbal cues or behaviors.

Palpation Ipsilateral tenderness and muscle tightness (taut bands) in trapezius and periscapular muscles are common findings.

Range of motion (ROM) C-spine ROM should be examined in all planes. The normal cervical ROM is as follows: extension: 55°, flexion: 45°; lateral bending: 40°; and rotation: 70° [5]. Among common ADLs, backing up a car requires the most combined ROM maneuvers.

Sensory testing Radiculopathy results in specific dermatomal abnormality in sensory examination of the shoulder girdle and the symptomatic arm. Light touch, pinprick, and proprioception/vibration should be tested in the symptomatic and asymptomatic arms. Based on the dermatomal deficits, clinicians can localize the anatomic level of nerve root impingement. To date, the most standardized sensory testing guideline is published by the *International Standards for Neurological Classification of Spinal Cord Injury* [6].

Table 10.2 Key reflexes, muscle group, and sensory point testing in cervical radiculopathy

Root	Reflex	Key muscle group	Key Sensation point
C2	Normal reflexes	Neck flexion	1 cm lateral to occipital protuberance
C3	Normal reflexes	Neck extension Neck lateral flexion	Supraclavicular fossa, mid-clavicle line
C4	Normal reflexes	Shoulder elevation	Skin over AC joint
C5	Diminished biceps DTR	Elbow flexor	Radial side of the antecubital fossa
C6	Diminished brachioradialis DTR	Wrist extension	Dorsal surface, proximal phalanx of thumb
C7	Diminished Triceps DTR	Elbow extension	Dorsal surface, proximal phalanx of third digit
C8	Normal reflexes	Long finger flexors	Dorsal surface, proximal phalanx of 5th digit

Deep tendon reflexes The following reflexes should be tested bilaterally as part of a standard radiculopathy examination. Hyporeflexia or areflexia indicates lower motor neuron involvement. Hyperreflexia is an indication of CNS involvement (Table 10.2, Fig. 10.1).

Motor Testing Patterns of weakness can help localize a lesion to a particular spinal cord level, nerve root, peripheral nerve, or muscle. Comparing the strength of each muscle group with its contralateral counterpart allows for the detection of any asymmetries. The degree of pain and the patient's effort can be a limiting factor in examination of the strength. For cervical radiculopathy, strength testing is often focused on C4–C8 nerve roots. The *International Standards for Neurological Classification of Spinal Cord Injury* recommends testing five key muscles in the upper extremity [6]. Muscle strength is rated on a scale of 0/5 to 5/5 (Table 10.3).

Joint Examination Careful examination of the cervical facets, shoulder, elbow, and wrist is also important in differentiating radicular neck pain from other musculoskeletal causes.

10.1.5.1 Special Maneuvers

Spurling Maneuver It is a classic test to identify nerve root irritation (Fig. 10.1). It is a combination of ipsilateral neck tilt, forward flexion, and exerting axial load. A modified Spurling maneuver is a combination of the ipsilateral rotation, extension, and exerting axial load (Fig. 10.2). Reproduction of the patient's radicular symptoms in either maneuver is considered

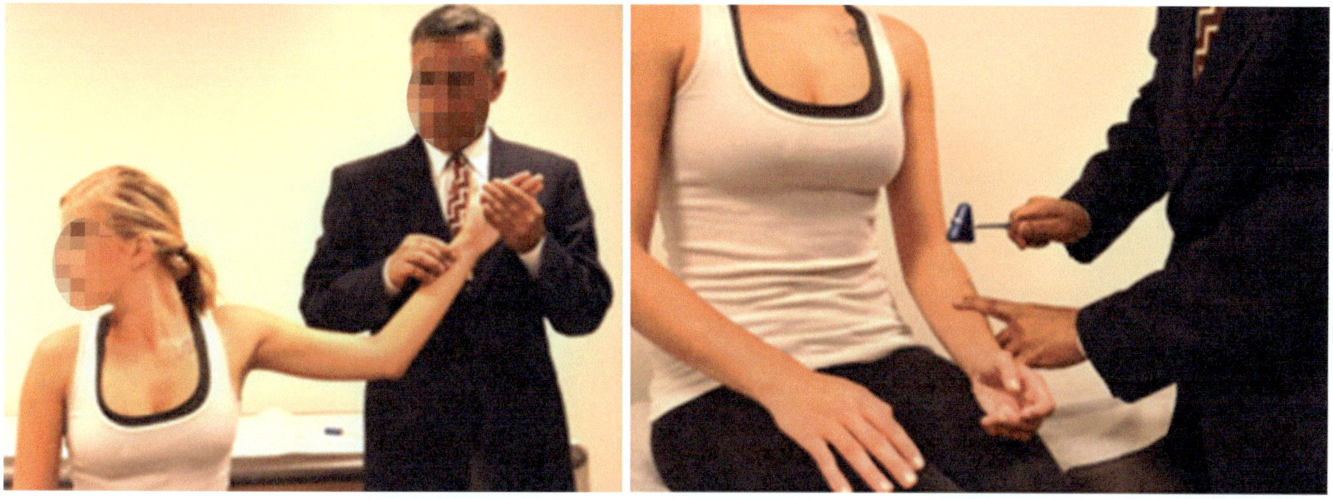

Fig. 10.1 Adson's test (left) and brachioradialis reflex testing (right)

Table 10.3 Cervical root-innervated muscles in c-spine and arm

C2	Sternocleidomastoid, rectus capitis, longus colli
C3	Trapezius, splenius capitis
C4	Trapezius, levator scapulae
C5	Deltoid, biceps, supraspinatus, infraspinatus
C6	Wrist extensors, biceps, brachioradialis, supinator
C7	Wrist flexors, triceps
C8	Thumb extensor and adductors. Wrist ulnar deviators, flexor digitorum superficialis

a positive test. The spurling maneuver has low sensitivity (40–50%), high specificity (greater than 80%), and fair to good interexaminer reliability [7]. This maneuver is contraindicated when fractures or instability is suspected.

Adson's test and Roos test Pain, weakness, and neurovascular deficits are associated with thoracic outlet syndrome that is in the differential diagnosis of cervical radiculopathy. Clinicians should be familiar with these tests when examining patients with neck and arm pain (Fig. 10.1).

Babinski response, Hoffmann sign, Lhermitte's sign, and clonus are also part of examination for cervical radiculopathy as they may point to cervical myelopathy and cord compression instead of single nerve root impingement.

10.1.6 Diagnostic Workup

Plain Films X-rays are the initial imaging modality used electively or in acute trauma to identify anatomic changes in bony structure of cervical spine including facet/uncovertebral spondylosis, loss of disk height, and vertebral body or dens fractures. It evaluates the alignment of the cervical vertebrae (scoliosis and kyphosis) and detects spondylolisthesis. It can identify instability of the C-spine by means of flexion–extension and open mouth views. It has less utility in identifying the cause of radicular pain except for the evaluation of bony neuroforamina narrowing in static or dynamic films.

Computed Tomography CT is the best modality to evaluate the bony anatomy and bleeding. Since it is cross-sectional imaging, it can identify bony narrowing of the central canal or neuroforamina and thickening of the ligamentum flavum. CT is an excellent modality in multitrauma workup of fractures and bleeding in or around the spinal canal. CT with 2D axial and coronal reconstruction is used to identify proper fusion of the adjacent vertebrae after spinal fusion surgery. Although CT is less sensitive as compared to MRI, it can identify disk herniation. CT is the modality of choice in patients with implanted pacemakers and other devices that are not compatible with MRI. Finally, CT is used after performing discography to better visualize internal disk derangements including radial tears.

MRI MRI is the gold standard imaging modality for patients with radicular symptoms. It can identify normal and abnormal changes in soft tissue (muscle, nerve, DRG, cord, disk, ligaments, adipose, etc.). MRI can visualize the caliber of the spinal canal and the neuroforamina (Fig. 10.3). With MRI, one can evaluate any spinal cord or bone marrow signal abnormality. MRI can determine acuity of fractures, presence of infection, and primary or metastatic tumors of the spinal column. Pre- and post-contrast MRI images are necessary to further define certain conditions such as cancerous and vascular lesions, postsurgical scarring, and nerve sheath tumors.

NCS/EMG Electrodiagnosis is considered an extension of the physical examination. In patients with clear cervical

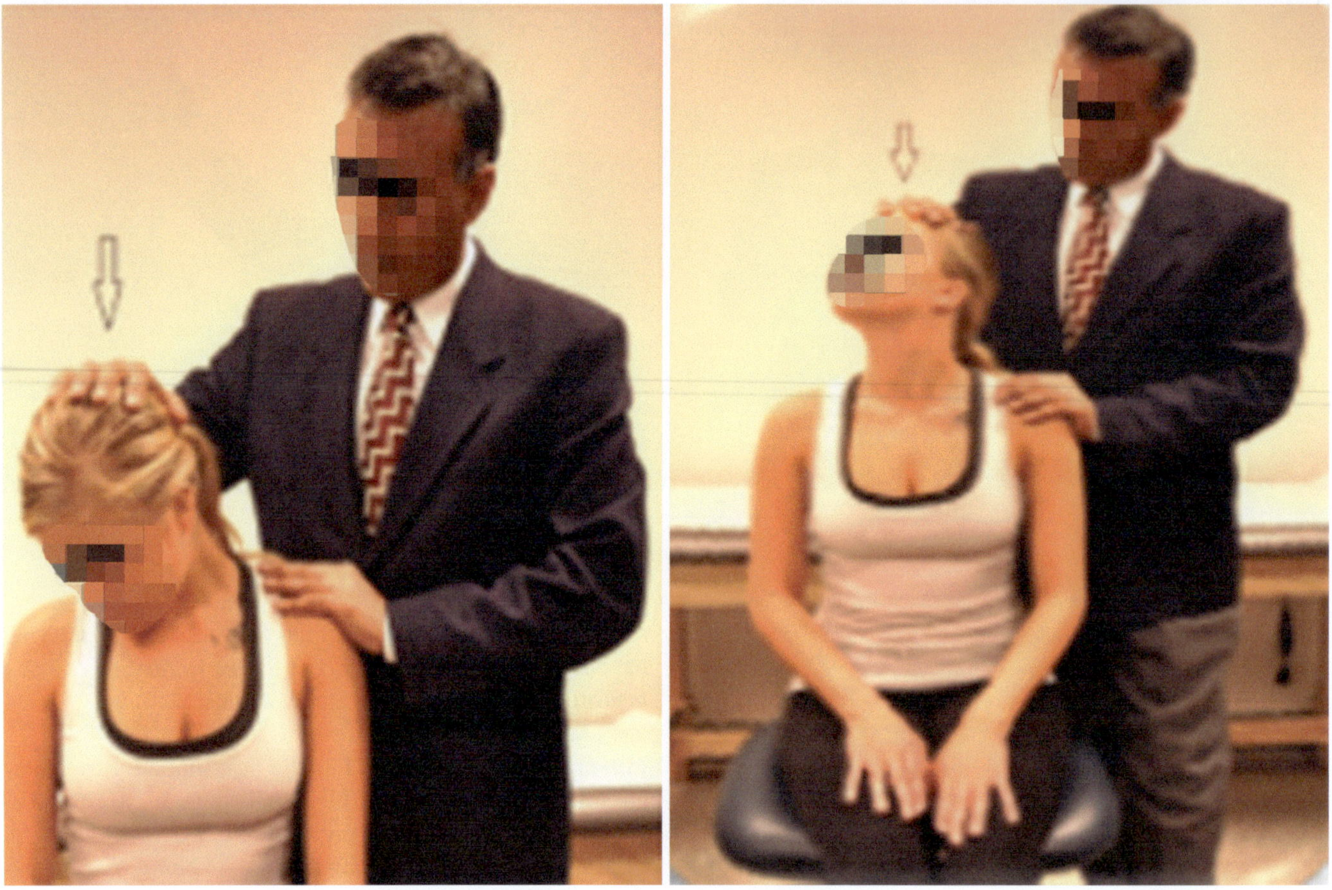

Fig. 10.2 Spurling maneuver (left) and modified Spurling maneuver (right)

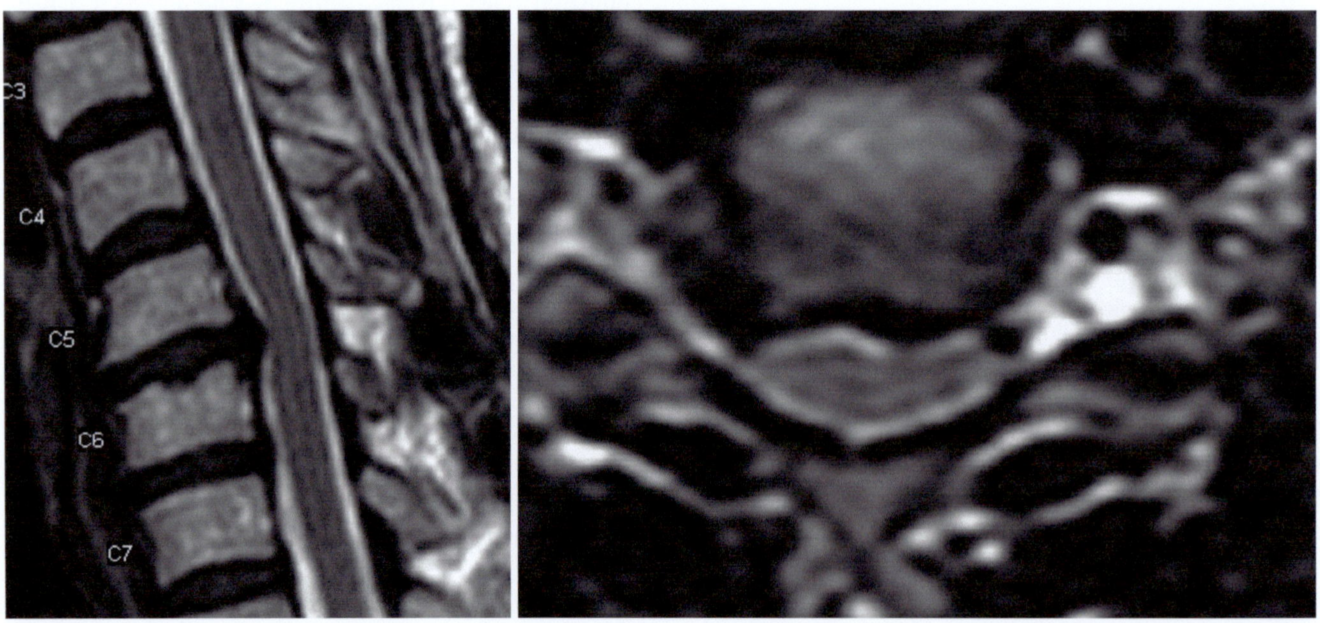

Fig. 10.3 Cervical herniated disk at C5–6 with central thecal sac impression and left foraminal stenosis and normal cord signal. (Image courtesy of Ali Mostoufi, MD, New England Spine Care Associates)

radicular signs and symptoms and supportive MRI, there is no indication for EMG. It can be a useful tool in clinical scenarios in which symptoms, physical examination, and imaging are not concordant [10]. If there is a suspicion of coexisting medical conditions along with cervical radiculopathy (peripheral neuropathy or peripheral entrapment), then confirmatory EMG results can lead to specific and better treatment outcomes.

Myelogram Before MRI was developed, the CT myelogram was highly utilized to identify caliber of the central canal and intervertebral foramen and help determine existing nerve root or spinal cord compression. In modern medicine, CT myelograms continue to be valuable when MRI is contraindicated or when there is poor visibility on MRI. In complex postsurgical cases or surgical revisions or spinal tumors, a myelogram may also be utilized as a diagnostic tool. *Diagnostic spinal injections*: Fluoroscopic-guided procedures can deliver certain medications to a desired target for diagnostic or therapeutic purposes. In complex cases in which multilevel degenerative changes are seen, and there is a question as to which segment is contributing to the patient's pain, spine surgeons may ask for a diagnostic selective nerve root injection. Properly trained interventionalists can deliver anesthetics to a specific nerve root. The degree of pain relief (depending on the half-life of the local anesthetic) can provide valuable preoperative information to the surgeon and increase likelihood of a successful surgical outcome.

10.1.7 Treatment

10.1.7.1 Medical Management

About 70–80% of patients with cervical radicular pain improve with conservative care [8]. Pain reduction and patient education are important initial goals. For the acute phase, one can consider ice and passive treatments consisting of a cervical collar and rest from activities that aggravate the condition. If tolerated, prescribed medications can reduce acute-phase symptoms including NSAIDs, muscle relaxants, and short tapering course of oral steroids. In acute cervical radiculopathy, if NSAIDs do not provide adequate analgesia, opioid pain medications are indicated for 7–14 days. In chronic cases, adjunct medications such as anticonvulsants, tricyclic antidepressants, or select norepinephrine reuptake inhibitors may be used. Experienced clinicians can educate patients with methods to prevent worsening and recurrence by activity modification, correct body mechanics (neutral spine), proper lifting techniques, use of a proper pillow and mattress, and suitable exercises.

10.1.7.2 Rehabilitation

Early involvement of physical therapy and occupational therapy is encouraged in the management of cervical radicular pain. Rehabilitation treatment should focus on reduction in muscle tension and improvement in ROM and strength. Cervical stabilization, stretching (passive and active), isometric strengthening, and progressive resistive exercises (Fig. 10.4) are incorporated in the rehabilitation phase and should be transitioned to a home exercise program [9]. If there is no contraindication, cervical traction can be effective in reducing radicular symptoms and can be incorporated into the treatment plan. Moist heat, ultrasound, manual traction, and TENS treatment are often used by PT and OT for temporary pain relief. Cervical spine manipulation can be a helpful adjunct treatment, but complications including cervical arterial dissection are of concern and premanipulative cervical instability testing and arterial integrity tests appear to be unreliable in identifying patients at risk for this adverse event [18]. Interventional procedures and medications can reduce pain and in turn increase patient compliance with rehabilitation treatment. Within the context of rehabilitation, the patient is educated on body mechanics, proper desk ergonomics, and use of adaptive equipment like a book stand, a hands-free phone or headset, and a document holder.

10.1.7.3 Procedures

Interlaminar Cervical Epidural steroid injections (C-ESI): An C-ESI is indicated in persistent painful cervical radiculopathy despite appropriate initial medical and rehabilitation treatments. In the hands of trained physicians, when performed with image guidance, it is a safe and effective treatment. Based on a systematic review of literature, the evidence for treating cervical radicular pain with interlaminar epidural steroid injection is good (Fig. 10.5) [11, 12].

Cervical Selective Nerve Root Block (SNRB): This is a diagnostic procedure. If a patient has substantial decrease in pain with image-guided contrast-enhanced injection of anesthetics at a specific nerve root, the clinician can consider that specific nerve root to be the main cause of arm pain. Selectivity of such injection is lost if there is epidural spread of the injectate. Spine surgeons use SNRB diagnostic information for surgical planning.

10.1.7.4 Surgery

A progressive neurologic deficit, myelopathy, and failed conservative care for over 6 months are indications for spinal surgery. Factors such as severity of degenerative changes, previous spine surgery, spine instability, and cervical spondylolisthesis are used to decide what type of surgery would benefit the patient. The most common surgical techniques are anterior cervical discectomy and fusion (ACDF), foraminotomy, and disk arthroplasty.

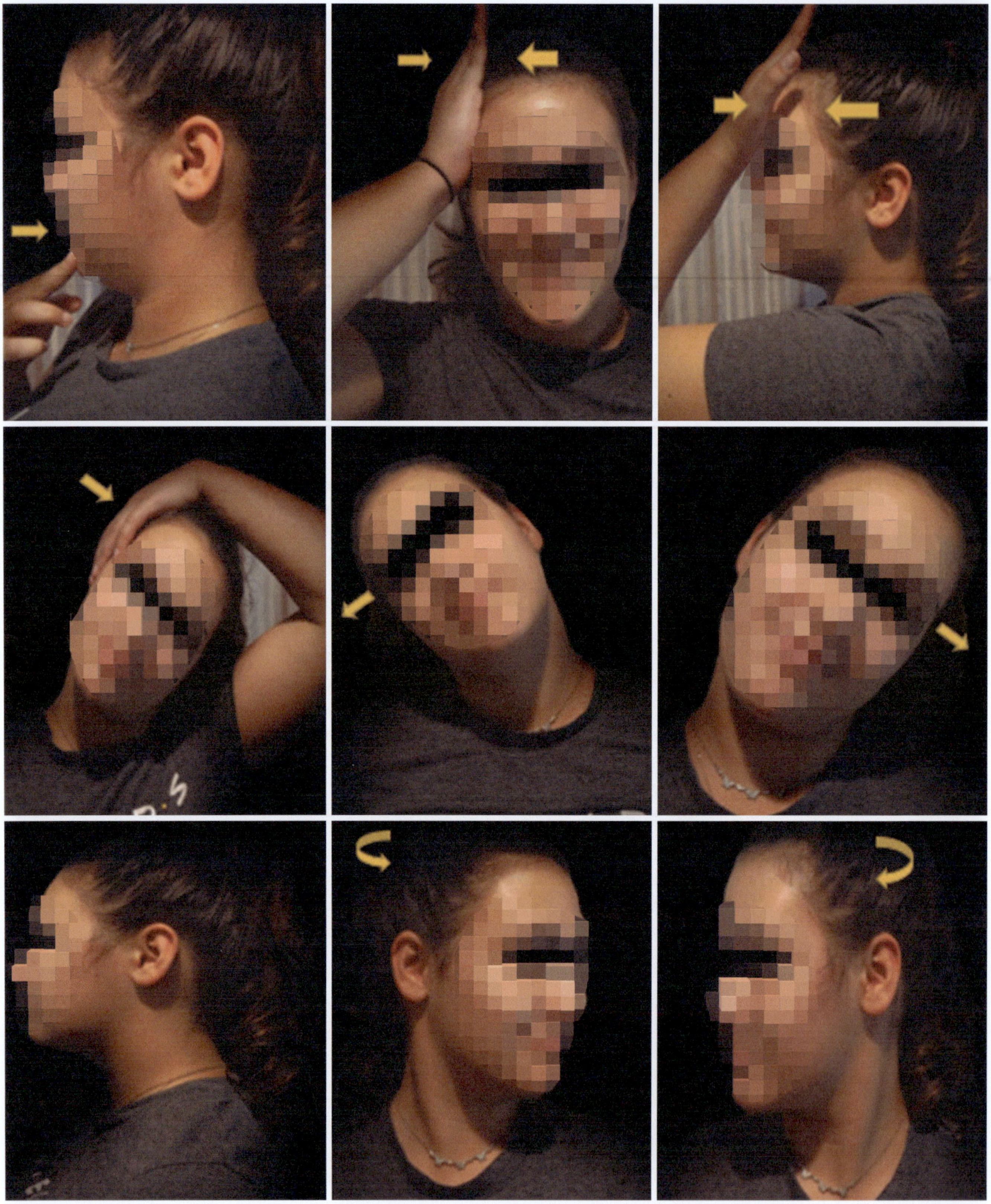

Fig. 10.4 Strengthening and ROM exercises for cervical spine including isometrics. (Image courtesy of Ali Mostoufi, MD, New England Spine Care Associates)

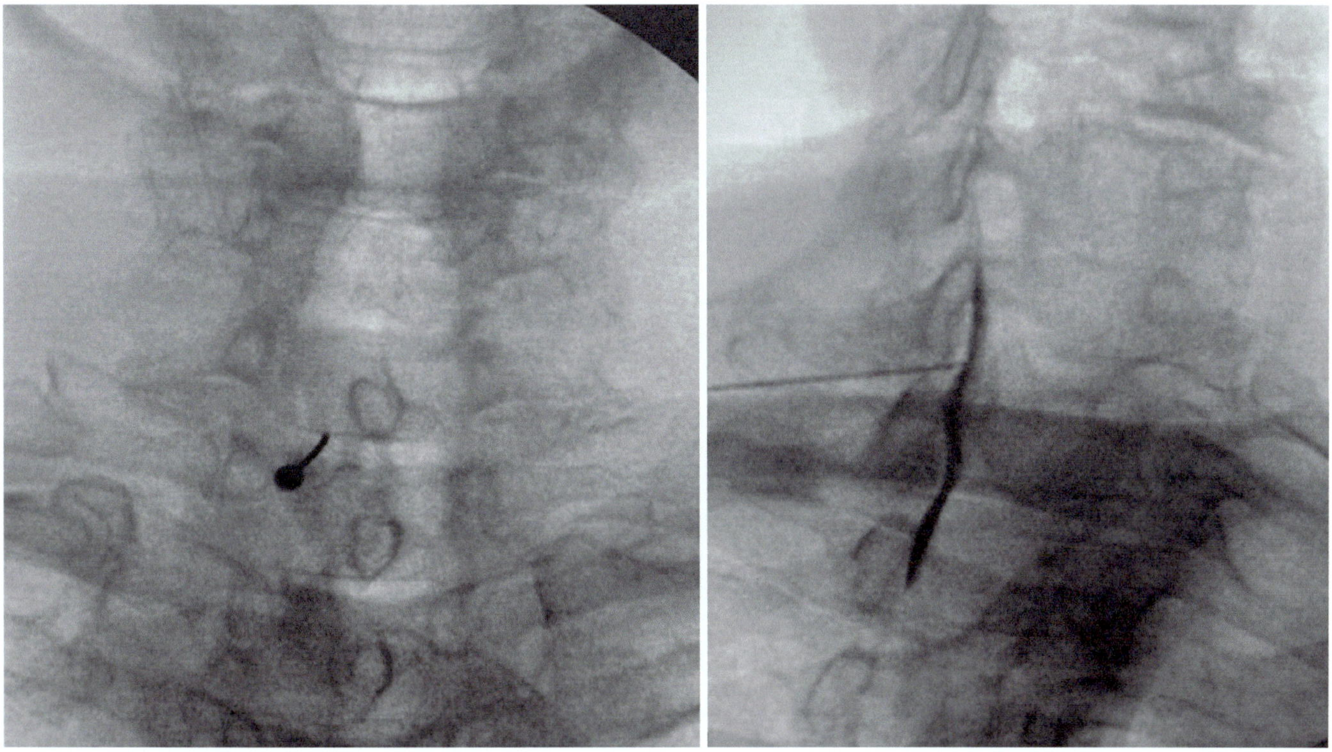

Fig. 10.5 Cervical interlaminar epidural injection with contrast material enhancing posterior epidural space. (Image courtesy of Ali Mostoufi, MD, New England Spine Care Associates)

ACDF is the most common surgical treatment for cervical radiculopathy. Surgical intervention has been shown to provide faster improvement in pain intensity, sensory disturbance, and muscle strength, but one-year outcome comparisons between surgical and nonsurgical groups are statistically similar [14, 21]. Meta-analysis studies show that in patients with symptomatic cervical disk disease, cervical disk arthroplasty is superior over ACDF in terms of overall success, neurological improvement, the incidence of implant/surgery-related serious adverse events, need for secondary procedures, functional outcomes, patient satisfaction, and adjacent segment degeneration [13, 18–20]. See Chaps. 15 and 16 for more details on spine surgery.

10.2 Thoracic Radiculopathy

10.2.1 Synonyms

Thoracic radiculitis; neuropathy, thoracic; thoracic radiculopathy due to degenerative disk disease of the spine

10.2.2 ICD-10 Codes

M54.14, M47.24

10.2.3 Description

Thoracic radiculopathy is a condition in which dysfunction of the thoracic nerve root results in pain and sensory abnormalities in the chest and upper back. This radiculopathy can also result in severe pain with coughing or sneezing, feeling of weakness in the chest, and shortness of breath.

Anatomy Thoracic spine consists of 12 vertebrae, which correspond with the 12 ribs, 12 thoracic disks (T1–T12), 12 pairs of thoracic nerve roots, which innervate the chest. Thoracic nerves are named corresponding to the vertebral body above them.

Thoracic radiculopathy is the least common radiculopathy. The most common etiology for thoracic radiculopathy is a posterolateral disk herniation with nerve root impingement or narrowing of the neuroforamina as a result of aging. Less common causes include ossification of the spinal ligaments and trauma, such as car accidents. Table 10.4 outlines differential diagnosis of thoracic radiculopathy.

10.2.4 Clinical Presentation

Classic presentation of thoracic radiculopathy is unilateral band-like pain in a specific nerve root (dermatomal) pattern.

Table 10.4 Differential diagnosis of thoracic radiculopathy

Thoracic myelopathy
Demyelinating disease
Chest wall injury
Neuromuscular disease
Intercostal neuralgia
Post-herpetic neuralgia
Rib fracture
Costochondritis (Tietze disease)
Costovertebral joint pain

There may also be complaints of shortness of breath, especially with deep breathing, or sharp pain with coughing or sneezing. Thoracic myelopathy due to cord compression needs to be ruled out, which often is associated with bilateral sensory or motor abnormalities, lower extremity hyperreflexia, gait disturbance, upper motor neuron disease examination finding (clonus), dysreflexia, and neurogenic bowel and bladder dysfunction.

10.2.5 Physical Examination

Full musculoskeletal and neurologic examination is indicated in the evaluation of thoracic radicular pain.

Visual observation Clinicians should be trained to notice spinal deformities, skin abnormalities, and nonverbal cues or behaviors.

Palpation Ipsilateral tenderness and muscle tightness in paraspinals and intercostal muscles are common findings.

Range of motion (ROM) Thoracic spine ROM should be examined in all planes, and deficits should be documented. The normal thoracic ROM are as follows: flexion: 50° and rotation: 30° [22].

Sensory testing Radiculopathy results in specific dermatomal abnormality in sensory examination of the chest, sides, and back. Light touch, pinprick, and proprioception/vibration should be tested on the symptomatic and asymptomatic sides. Based on the dermatomal deficits, clinician can localize the anatomic level of nerve root impingement. Nipple line in males correlates with T5, bellybutton correlates with T10, and inguinal line correlates with L1.

Motor Testing Thoracic nerves have motor innervation of the intercostal muscles, which do not have specific motor nerve examinations. In high thoracic myelopathy, engaging intercostal muscles in active deep breathing may be impaired.

10.2.6 Diagnostic Workup

- *X-Ray:* X-rays are used to identify anatomic changes in bony structure of thoracic spine, loss of disk height, and vertebral body fractures. It is essential to evaluate coronal and sagittal alignment of the vertebrae (scoliosis/rotation/kyphosis)).
- *Computed Tomography*: CT is the best modality to evaluate the bony anatomy and bleeding. CT is an excellent modality in multitrauma workup of fractures and bleeding in or around spinal canal. Although CT is less sensitive compared to MRI, it can identify disk herniation.
- *MRI:* MRI is the gold standard imaging for patients with radicular symptoms. MRI can visualize the caliber of the spinal canal and the neuroforamina and can determine acuity of fractures, presence of infection, and primary or metastatic tumors of the spinal column.
- *Myelogram*: CT myelogram provides valuable information when MRI is contraindicated or when there is a metallic artifact from artificial disk or previous thoracic fusion instrumentation leading to poor visibility on MRI.

10.2.7 Treatment

10.2.7.1 Medical Management

Many patients with thoracic radicular pain improve with conservative care. For the acute phase, one can consider ice and rest from activities that aggravate the condition. If tolerated, prescribed medications can reduce acute-phase symptoms including NSAIDs, acetaminophen, and muscle relaxants. In acute thoracic radiculopathy, if NSAIDs do not provide adequate analgesia, a short course of opioid pain medications can be an option. In chronic cases, adjunct medications like anticonvulsants, tricyclic antidepressants, or select norepinephrine reuptake inhibitors may be used.

10.2.7.2 Rehabilitation

Improved ROM, reduced pain, enhanced function, development of a home exercise program, and postural/ergonomic education are the goals of PT. Both active and passive exercises (including thoracic and lumbar paraspinal strengthening, modalities, Tens unit, and soft tissue treatments) should be considered.

10.2.7.3 Procedures

Thoracic interlaminar epidural steroid injections (T-ESI): An T-ESI (Fig. 10.6) can be helpful in persistent painful thoracic radiculopathy despite appropriate medical and rehabilitation treatments. Utilizing contralateral oblique X-rays while

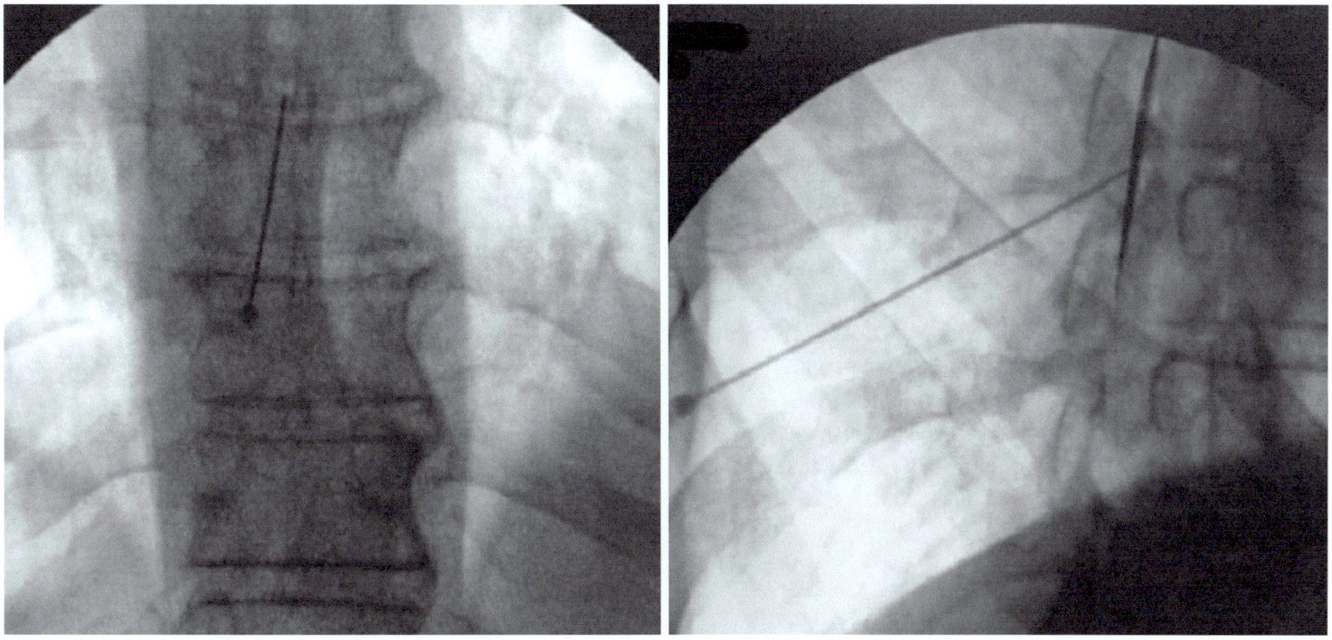

Fig. 10.6 Thoracic interlaminar epidural Injection. PA and contralateral oblique images assist in delivering steroid injectate safely to the epidural space. Linear contrast flow seen highlighting posterior epidural space. (Image courtesy of Ali Mostoufi, MD, New England Spine Care Associates, Cambridge, MA, USA)

performing thoracic ESI (and cervical) provides excellent visualization for needle placement and reduces risks and complications.

10.2.7.4 Surgery

Progressive neurologic deficit, myelopathy, and failed conservative care are indications for spinal surgery. Factors such as severity of degenerative changes, previous spine surgery, and spine instability are used to decide what type of surgery would benefit the patient. Posterior approach, posterolateral approach (costotransversectomy), anterior approach via thoracotomy, or MIS VATS (video-assisted thoracic surgery) can be options depending on location of the herniation, surgeons' experience, and availability of technology as well stability of the patient.

10.3 Lumbar Radiculopathy

10.3.1 Synonyms

Lumbar radicular syndrome; lumbar radiculitis; lumbar radicular pain; lumbar disk disease with radiculopathy; lumbar disk herniation with radiculopathy

10.3.2 ICD-10 Codes

M54.16, M51.16

10.3.3 Description

Lumbar radiculopathy is a condition characterized by irritation of a particular lumbar nerve root, resulting in unilateral pain, numbness, paresthesias, or weakness in the buttock or a leg. It is usually secondary to dysfunction of the dorsal root ganglia or lumbar sensory spinal nerve roots. The most common cause of lumbar radiculopathy is lumbar disk herniation (younger adults) or disk–osteophyte complex (older adults). Lumbar radiculopathy is often used interchangeably with sciatica even though sciatica best describes pain in the distribution of the S1 nerve. Another term used is lumbar radiculitis. Lumbar radiculitis, an inflammatory condition, has similar pain presentation as lumbar radiculopathy but lacks motor, sensory, or reflex abnormalities. Differential diagnosis of lumbar radiculopathy is in Table 10.5.

Anatomy The lumbar spine consists of five vertebrae with the vertebral canal bound anteriorly by the vertebral body and intervertebral disk and dorsally by lamina. The pedicles and the facet joints bind the vertebral canal posterolaterally. Pedicle width normally increases gradually from L1 to L5. The nerve roots exit in the foramen below the pedicles at each level. The facet joints (zygapophysial) are synovial joints formed from the superior and inferior articular processes of contiguous vertebral levels. The pars interarticularis unites the superior and inferior articular processes at each spinal level. A pars fracture, commonly called spondylolysis, affects adolescents, in particular athletes (gymnast,

Table 10.5 Differential diagnosis of lumbar radiculopathy

Piriformis syndrome	SI joint pain
IT band tendinopathy	Meralgia paresthetica
Femoral mononeuropathy	Lumbar spinal stenosis
Spinal tumor and abscess	Lumbar facet joint pain
Ischiofemoral impingement	HIP or knee OA
Peripheral neuropathy	Demyelinating disease
Diabetic amyotrophy	Cauda equine syndrome
Lumbar or sacral plexopathy	CRPS

divers, cheerleaders), but can happen in falls, work injury, and motor vehicle accidents. The most common level affected is spondylolysis of L5. The ventral roots form the lumbar plexus, terminating at various peripheral nerves. The spinal cord ends most commonly at L1 with the distal part of the spinal cord forming the conus medullaris. This is followed by the cauda equina.

The lumbar spine's blood supply is derived from the segmental arteries with each segmental artery dividing into a spinal branch, which supplies the vertebrae, spinal cord, and cauda equina.

10.3.4 Clinical Presentation

The clinical presentation of lumbar radiculopathy consists of pain as the primary symptom along with a constellation of symptoms of the involved nerve root including paresthesias, numbness, and weakness. Radicular pain travels along a narrow band, with a shooting, lancinating quality often described like an electric shock. Objective findings include gait disturbance, antalgia, dermatomal loss of sensation, myotomal weakness, and hyporeflexia. Radicular pain from L1, L2, and L3 is normally felt in the lower abdomen, groin, and anterior thigh. Lumbosacral radicular pain from the involvement of the L4 and L5 nerve roots is usually felt in the back of the thigh, down into the leg and foot (see Fig. 10.3). With L4 radicular symptoms, one can see difficulty with knee extension and reduced patellar tendon reflex. With L5 radicular symptoms, one can see difficulty with heel walking and reduced strength of the ankle and extension of the toe.

10.3.5 Physical Examination

Evaluation of lumbar radiculopathy involves a thorough musculoskeletal and neurologic. This includes evaluation for abnormal posture, asymmetry, deformity, abnormal range of motion of spine, and lower extremity joints.

Range of motion (ROM) L-spine ROM should be examined in all planes. The normal lumbar ROM is extension: 25°, flexion: 60°; lateral bending: 25°; and rotation: 20°.

Neurologic examination This includes assessment of sensation (light touch, two-point discrimination, pinprick, dermatomes in Fig. 10.7) reflexes (Table 10.6), muscle strength, and pain. Tenderness to touch and cutaneous findings may suggest alternative diagnosis. The patellar and Achilles reflexes should be tested, pointing to L4 and S1 radiculopathy. Sensory examination can be subjective, but assessing dermatomal changes for light touch, temperature, and pain can be useful and should correlate with MR findings.

10.3.5.1 Special Maneuvers

Straight leg raise test The straight leg raise test is when the clinician raises the patient's extended leg on the symptomatic side with the foot dorsiflexed. The presence or worsening of radicular pain with this maneuver is termed Lasegue's sign. The straight leg raise test is sensitive but variable specificity for radiculopathy caused by disk herniation and is best for the L5 and S1 levels.

Contralateral straight leg raise test This is done by the clinician lifting the patient's asymptomatic leg in an attempt to produce radicular pain in the symptomatic leg. It is specific for radiculopathy due to disk herniation [23].

Patrick's test The clinician externally rotates the hip with the ipsilateral knee flexed at 90°, and the heel is placed on the opposite knee. If hip or buttock pain ensues, the test is positive. It is nonspecific for radicular disease but does raise a higher suspicion for hip OA or sacroiliac disease.

10.3.6 Diagnostic Workup

X-rays This is often the initial imaging modality of choice, due to availability and low cost. X-rays identify abnormal alignment and anatomic changes in the bone and joints of the lumbar spine due to degeneration or trauma (Fig. 10.8).

CT As with the cervical spine, computed tomography is the best modality to evaluate the bony anatomy and bleeding in the lumbar spine. It is particularly superior to MRI for facet joints, DJD, synovial cyst, and lateral recesses bony stenosis. When utilized with myelography, it can be used as an alternative if MRI cannot be done.

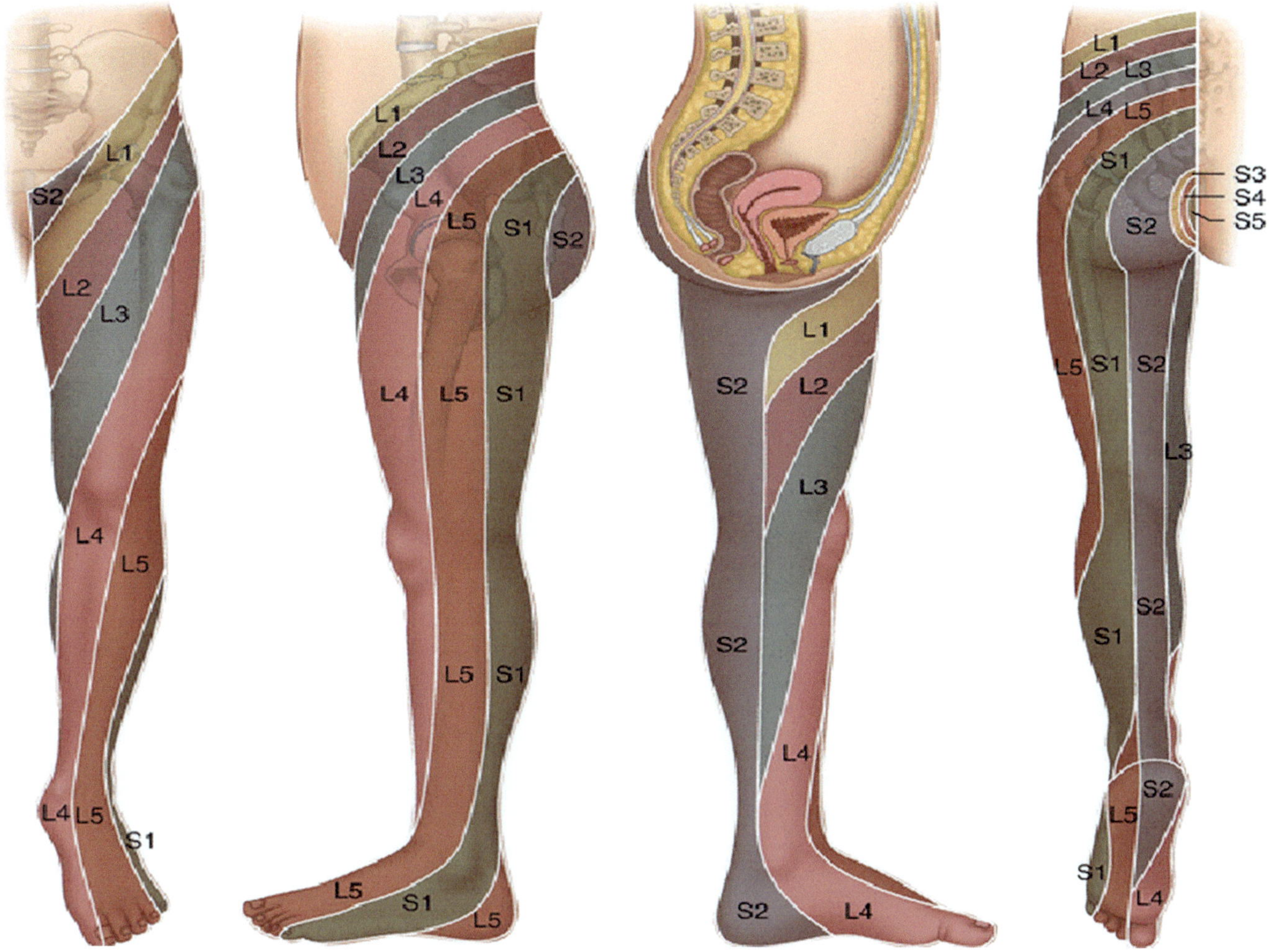

Fig. 10.7 Lumbar–sacral plexus dermatomes. (Copyright © 2018, Springer International Publishing AG)

Table 10.6 Key reflexes, muscle group, and sensory point testing in lumbar radiculopathy

Root	Reflex	Key muscle group	Key sensation point
L1/ L2		Psoas, iliacus, sartorius, gracilis, pectineus, adductor longus, adductor brevis	Anterior aspect of upper thigh
L3		Quadriceps, adductor longus, magnus, brevis	Anterolateral thigh
L4	Patellar reflex	Quadriceps	Anterior thigh, medial shin
L5	Posterior tibial	Peroneal, anterior tibial, extensor hallucis longus	Great toe, dorsum of foot
S1	Achilles reflex	Gluteus maximus, gastrocnemius, plantar flexors of toes	Lateral foot, small toe

MRI MRI is the gold standard imaging for patients with radicular symptoms (Fig. 10.9). It can identify normal and abnormal changes in soft tissue (muscle, nerve, DRG, cord, disk, ligaments, adipose, etc.). MRI can visualize the caliber of the spinal canal and the neuroforamina. With MRI, one can evaluate any spinal cord or bone marrow signal abnormality. MRI can determine acuity of fractures, presence of infection, and primary or metastatic tumors of the spinal column. The use of pre- and post-contrast MRI images is necessary to further define certain conditions like cancerous and vascular lesions, postsurgical scarring, and nerve sheath tumors.

EMG/NCV Electrodiagnostic modalities such as electromyography, nerve conduction velocity, and somatosensory-evoked potentials are beneficial in confirming radicular symptoms when distinguishing between lumbar radicular symptoms and peripheral neuropathy.

Myelogram Before MRI was developed, myelogram was highly utilized to identify caliber of the central canal and intervertebral foramen and help determine exiting nerve root or spinal cord compression. In modern medicine, CT myelogram continues to provide valuable information regarding the caliber of the canal or intervertebral foramen when MRI is contraindicated or when there is a metallic artifact from

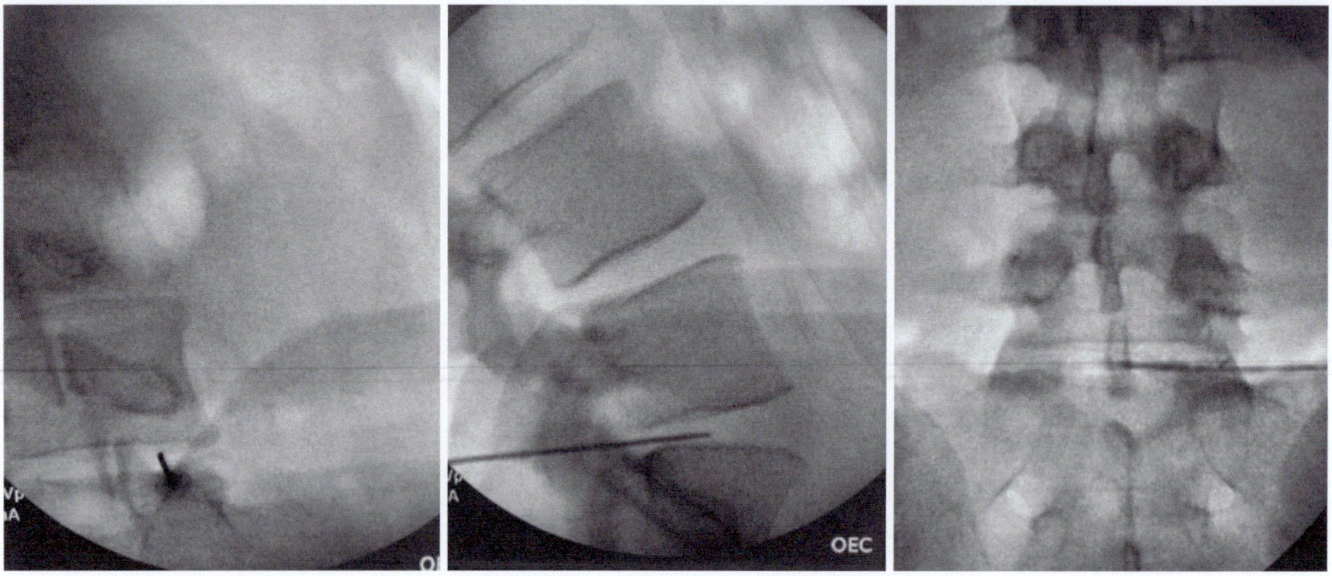

Fig. 10.8 X-ray-guided mechanical percutaneous discectomy. (Image courtesy of Ali Mostoufi, MD, New England Spine Care)

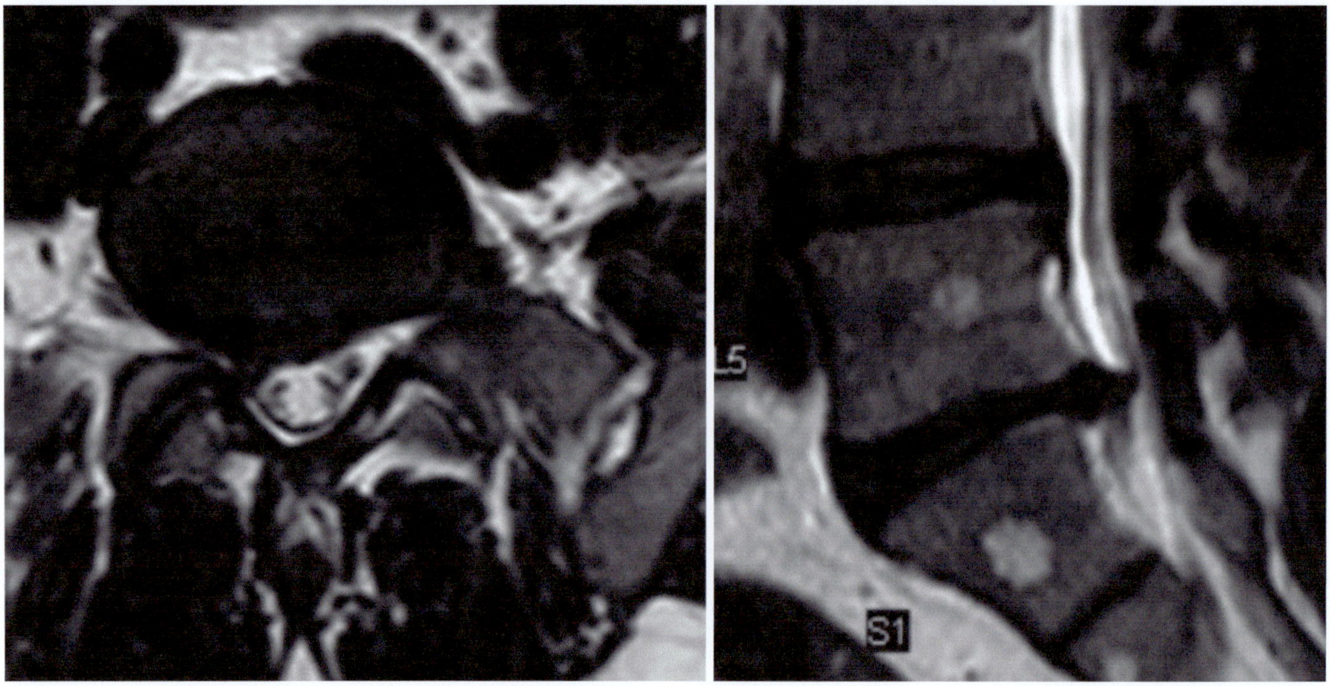

Fig. 10.9 L5 disc protrusion in right paramedian space impinging on traversing nerve roots with right L5/S1 radicular signs and symptoms

artificial disk or previous fusion instrumentation leading to poor visibility on MRI. In complex postsurgical cases or surgical revisions or spinal tumors, myelogram may also be utilized as a diagnostic tool.

Diagnostic spinal injections Fluoroscopic-guided, contrast-enhanced procedures (selective nerve root injection—Fig. 10.9) can deliver certain medications to a desired target for diagnostic or therapeutic purpose. In complex cases in which multilevel degenerative changes are seen, and there is a question of which segment is contributing to the patient's leg pain, spine surgeons may ask for a diagnostic selective nerve root injection. Properly trained interventionalists deliver anesthetics to a specific nerve root in question, and the degree of pain relief (depending on the half-life of the local anesthetic used) can provide valuable preoperative information to the surgeon and increase likelihood of successful surgical outcome.

10.3.7 Treatments

10.3.7.1 Medical Management

Medical management of lumbar radiculopathy starts with patient education, activity modification, and establishment of goals. Initially, patients should be managed conservatively with exercise, physical therapy, and NSAIDs as first-line therapy. In the acute phase, back brace and tapering dose of corticosteroids can be prescribed. Other therapies that can be used as adjuncts when conservative treatments fail include opioids, muscle relaxants, and neuroleptic medications though there is less evidence for their effectiveness. In acute radiculopathy, a short course of opioid medication is acceptable.

10.3.7.2 Rehabilitation

Physical therapy is indicated in the management of acute, subacute, and chronic thoracic and lumbar radiculopathy. Pathoanatomical explanations for pain consistent with thoracic and lumbar radiculopathy should be assessed and relevant psychological, behavioral, social, and/or environmental factors also known to contribute negatively to pain and disability. An individualized plan of care is developed based on shared decision-making between clinician and patient in synchrony with the best available evidence-based literature, clinician expertise, and patient preference. Rehabilitation will likely focus on a combination of active and passive forms of treatment including but not limited to manual therapy, mechanical or manual traction, neurodynamic interventions, therapeutic activity, therapeutic exercise, aquatic therapy, cognitive-behavioral informed techniques, and/or patient education. Passive modalities, such as ice, heat, and/or electrical stimulation, may be utilized to modulate pain; however, it is important to note that passive forms of treatment are generally not effective for long-term symptom management. Passive modalities, if utilized, should be employed to promote more active forms of treatment and self-management. Patients are educated on the physiology of pain, and fear-avoidance beliefs are addressed if necessary. Extended bed rest and prolonged periods of inactivity due to pain should be discouraged. Limited evidence is available related to the management of thoracic radiculopathy as this condition is generally less prevalent compared to radiculopathy of the cervical and lumbar regions; however, the evaluation and treatment of thoracic radiculopathy are similar to that described above.

10.3.7.3 Procedures

Lumbar epidural steroid injections (interlaminar or transforaminal) are indicated for persistent painful lumbar radiculopathy that has failed conservative care (therapy and NSAIDs). Paramedian interlaminar approach (Fig. 10.10) delivers steroids to the dorsal epidural space. Transforaminal injections have the advantage of delivering medication to the anterior epidural space and the specific impinged nerve root (Fig. 10.11). Studies have shown ESIs to be more beneficial than control treatments, especially in the short term [2]. A selective nerve root block is also used to relieve lumbar radicular pain by reducing inflammation of the nerve root through steroid injection. Recurrence can be expected however as the irritant pathology is still present.

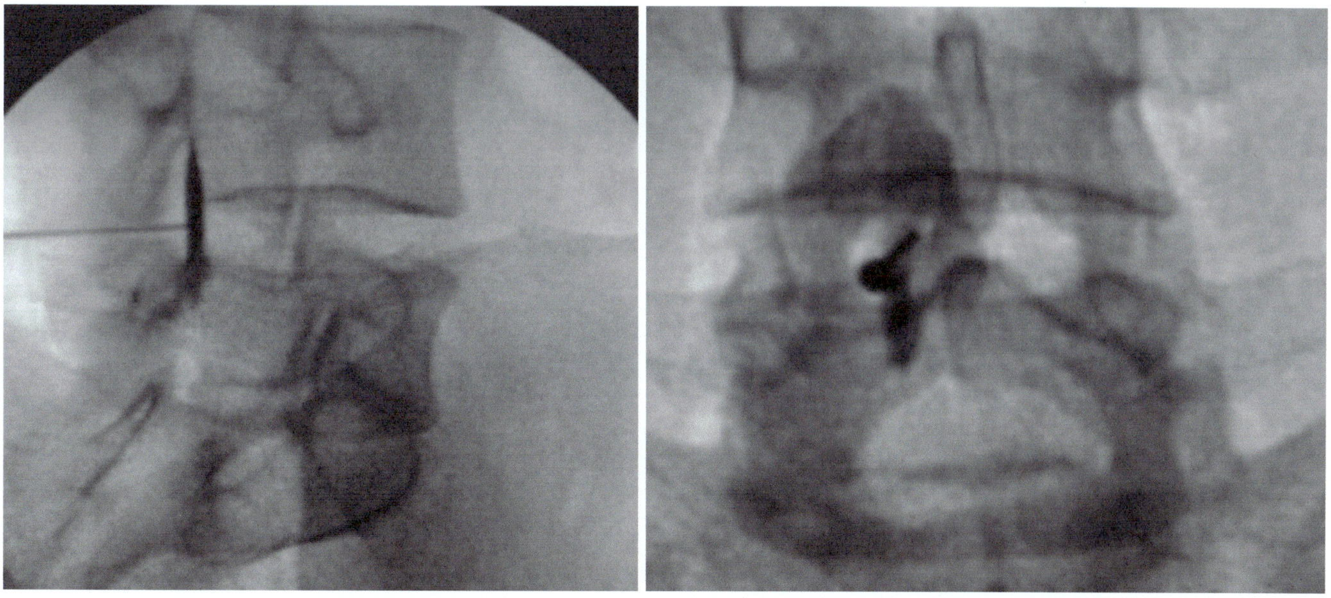

Fig. 10.10 Lumbar interlaminar epidural injection delivering steroids to the dorsal epidural space. (Image courtesy of Ali Mostoufi, MD, New England Spine Care)

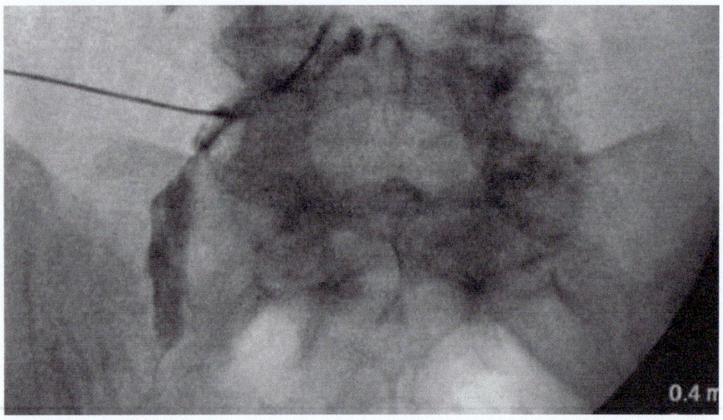

Fig. 10.11 Left L5 selective nerve root block. Contrast enhances the exiting left L5 nerve with some flow of the contrast toward L5 dural sleeve. (Image courtesy of Ali Mostoufi, MD, New England Spine Care)

Emerging Therapies

Percutaneous endoscopic lumbar discectomy via transforaminal posterolateral approach is an emerging therapy for the treatment of lumbar disk herniations. It has advantages over open lumbar surgery and microdiscectomy, which include low morbidity, minimal blood loss, and low complication rates, and it can be done under local anesthesia, allowing patients to undergo the procedure who historically would not have been surgical candidates. Other minimally invasive techniques for the treatment of lumbar disk herniation are mechanical percutaneous disk decompression or thermal percutaneous disk decompression. The later technique utilizes a laser fiber placed in the center of the nucleus pulposus, and energy from the laser is used to reduce intradiscal pressure. Lastly, another minimally invasive treatment for lumbar herniated disk is chemical percutaneous discectomy. One chemical utilized for this technique is ozone, where ozone gas is injected into the nucleus pulposus of the herniated disk, which leads to a reduction in disk size, relieving mechanical nerve root compression. For more reading on these newer treatment options, please go to Chap. 14.

10.3.7.4 Surgery

Surgery for lumbar radiculopathy is indicated if there is progressive neurologic deficit or if there is no relief in symptoms over a chronic period. The gold standard surgical treatment for lumbar radiculopathy is microdiscectomy with techniques improving from more invasive to minimally invasive techniques (endoscopic). Microdiscectomy has been shown to be superior to open surgical techniques. Minimally invasive lateral foraminotomy with partial lateral facetectomy is effective for foraminal stenosis causing nerve root compression and radiculopathy. Lumbar fusion is recommended for patients with failed back syndrome, degenerative instability, deformity, and symptomatic spondylolysis. More details regarding surgical options are discussed in Chaps. 15 and 16.

References

1. Caridi J, Pumberger M, Hughes A. Cervical radiculopathy, a review. HSSJ. 2011;7(3):265–72.
2. O'Rahilley R, Muller F, Carpernter S, Swanson R. Basic human anatomy, muscles, vessels, nerve and joints of the back, Chapter 40. Online version published by Dartmouth Medical School (Dartmouth.edu/~humananatomy).
3. Yoss RE, Corbin KB, MacCarty CS, et al. Recent data on significance of symptoms and signs in localization of involved root in cervical disc protrusion. Neurology. 1957;7:673–83.
4. Tanaka Y, Kokubun S, Sato T, Ozawa H. Cervical roots as origin of pain in the neck or scapular regions. Spine. 2006;31(17):E568–73.
5. Murphey F, Simmons JCH, Brunson B. Ruptured cervical discs 1939-1972. Clin Neurosurg. 1973;20:9–17.
6. International standards for neurological classification of spinal cord injury. J Spinal Cord Med. 2011;34(6):547–54.
7. Gutrecht J, Murphy DK. Lhermitte's sign in cavernous angioma of the cervical spinal cord. J Neurol Neurosurg Psychiatry. 1998;65:954–5.
8. Sampath P, Bendebba M, Davis JD, et al. Outcome in patients with cervical radiculopathy: prospective, multicenter study with independent clinical review. Spine. 1999;24:591–7.
9. Michael W, Wolff M, Levine L. Cervical radiculopathies: conservative approaches to management. Phys Med Rehabil Clin N Am. 2002;13:589–608.
10. Nardin RA, Patel MR, Gudas TF, Rutkove SB, Raynor EM. Electromyography and magnetic resonance imaging in the evaluation of radiculopathy. Muscle Nerve. 1999;22(2):151–5.
11. Diwan S, Manchikanti L, Benyamin RM, et al. Systematic review, effectiveness of cervical epidural injections in the management of chronic neck and upper extremity pain. Pain Physician. 2009;12(1):137–57.
12. Abdi S, Datta S, et al. Epidural steroids in the management of chronic spinal pain: a systematic review. Pain Physician. 2007;10:185–212. ISSN 1533-3159
13. Coric D, Nunley PD, Guyer RD, et al. Prospective, randomized, multicenter study of cervical arthroplasty: 269 patients from the Kineflex|C artificial disc investigational device exemption study with a minimum 2-year follow-up. J Neurosurg Spine. 2011;15(4):348–58.
14. Persson LC, Moritz U, Brandt L. Cervical radiculopathy: pain, muscle weakness and sensory loss in patients with cervical radiculopathy treated with surgery, physiotherapy or cervical collar. A prospective, controlled study. Eur Spine J. 1997;6:256.
15. Anatomy of Atlas, Wheeler Text Book of Orthopedics, Online edition, 2017.
16. Hartman J. Anatomy and clinical significance of the uncinate process and uncovertebral joint: a comprehensive review. Clin Anat. 2014;27(3):431–40.
17. Nguyen C, Sanchez K, et al. Anatomical specificities of the degenerated cervical spine: a narrative review of clinical implications, with special focus on targeted spinal injections. Ann Phys Rehabil Med. 2016;59(4):276–81.
18. Kranenburg HA, et al. Adverse events associated with the use of cervical spine manipulation or mobilization and patient

characteristics: a systematic review. Musculoskelet Sci Pract. 2017;28:32–8.
19. Xie L, et al. Cervical disc arthroplasty versus anterior cervical discectomy and fusion in symptomatic cervical degenerative disc diseases: an updated meta-analysis of prospective randomized controlled trials (RCTs). Springerplus. 2016;5(1):1188.
20. Hu Y, et al. Mid- to long-term outcomes of cervical disc arthroplasty versus anterior cervical discectomy and fusion for treatment of symptomatic cervical disc disease: a systematic review and meta-analysis of eight prospective randomized controlled trials. PLoS One. 2016;11(2):e0149312.
21. Maurits W, et al. Surgery versus conservative care for neck pain: a systematic review. Eur Spine J. 2013;22(1):87–95.
22. Services CaB. Spinal (thoracic) range of motion DCBS: WCD; 2020.
23. Van der Windt DAWM, Simons E, Riphagen II, Ammendolia C, Verhagen AP, Laslett M, Deville W, Deyo RA. Physical examination for lumbar radiculopathy due to disc herniation in patients with low-back pain. Cochrane Database Syst Rev. 2010;(2):CD007431.

Failed Back Syndrome

11

Ryan Budwany, Tony K. George, and Timothy R. Deer

11.1 ICD-10 Codes

M96.1

11.2 Definition

The International Association for the Study of Pain defines failed back syndrome as lumbar spinal pain of unknown origin either persisting despite surgical intervention or appearing after surgical intervention for spinal pain originally in the same topographical location [1]. Patients with FBS have chronic back pain, with or without referred or radicular symptoms, and have had one or more surgical interventions that have failed to treat the original pain. The word "back" in failed back syndrome refers to any segment of the spine where surgical intervention has occurred. Open surgery has been a default corrective action to address spine complaints, but in the recent years, advances in minimally invasive interventions have resulted in improvement of function, mitigating pain, and reduced risk of failed back pain syndrome [2].

Low back pain is the leading cause of disability and the second most common presentation to primary care physicians [3, 4]. When compared to other chronic health conditions (i.e., angina pectoris, diabetes mellitus), low back pain is the third most expensive condition for employers in the USA. Lower back pain has many causes, but most patients present with nonspecific mechanical back pain. Rare causes including infection, fractures, and malignancies are always in differential diagnosis [3]. Despite its large prevalence, initial approach for treating nonspecific low back pain is not surgical, whereas instability and progressive neurological deficits require early surgical intervention. Two adjacent column or middle column fractures and high-grade spondylolisthesis lead to instability and potential neurologic deficits requiring surgery. Radiculopathy, a nerve root impingement caused by spinal stenosis or disk herniation (traumatic or nontraumatic) leads to pain and functional loss. Radicular pain can be addressed with an epidural injection; however, radiculopathy with muscle weakness may require surgery.

FBS is the unforeseeable result of a surgical attempt(s) to alleviate low back or radicular pain in patients who have not responded to conservative care. FBS has a prevalence of 5–30% in 2-year postoperative phase [1]. FBS has a significant clinical and economic impact. Pain and functional limitations continue in these patients and require further care. Appropriately identification and treatment of pain generator could prevent surgery and potential complications including FBS [5].

11.3 Etiology

Failed back syndrome etiologies include multiple spine surgeries, spine surgery complicated by bleeding or infection, or aggressive surgical management combined with a poorly defined pain generator [6]. Back pain can be debilitating; therefore, the severity of pain may force early surgical intervention as compared to pursuing conservative management. In addition to its indication for segmental instability, high-grade spondylolisthesis, and spinal tumors/fractures, the prevalence of spinal fusion for treatment of axial back pain has increased over the past several years [6]. Despite advancement in technology and modification in surgical techniques, spinal fusion is associated with higher cost of care and limited clinical outcome [7–9].

R. Budwany
WVU Center for Integrative Pain Medicine, Morgantown, West Virginia, USA
e-mail: ryan.budwany@hsc.wvu.edu

T. K. George
Restorative Orthopaedics Spine & Sports (ROSS) Institute, Somerset, NJ, USA

Department of Orthopaedics, Rutgers-Robert Wood Johnson Medical School, New Brunswick, NJ, USA

T. R. Deer (✉)
West Virginia School of Medicine, Charleston, WV, USA
e-mail: tdeermd@centerforpainrelief.com

© The Author(s), under exclusive license to Springer Nature Switzerland AG 2022

S. A. Mostoufi et al. (eds.), *Clinical Guide to Musculoskeletal Medicine*, https://doi.org/10.1007/978-3-030-92042-5_11

One-third of patients undergoing spine surgery do not achieve satisfactory outcomes [10]. Success rates decrease with sequential spine surgery, falling from 50% after the first surgery to 30% after the second surgery, 15% after the third surgery, and 5% after the fourth surgery [11]. Additionally, diagnostic evaluations such as lumbar discography, medial branch blocks, or selective nerve blocks have limited utility and are poor predictors of surgical success. The utility of provocative discography for discogenic back pain carries a positive predictive value of 50–60%, and its utility is debated in the literature leading to its decline over the past decade [12, 13]. Medial branch blocks are strictly diagnostic for facet-generated neck or back pain and should not be utilized as a predictor of surgical outcome. Best practices recommend an algorithmic approach to identify the pain generator, allowing effective treatment through surgical or nonsurgical means (Fig. 11.1).

Risk factors for FBS are many (Table 11.1), including patient-sensitive factors, surgeon operative factors, and tissue responsive factors [14]. Patient-sensitive risk factors include anxiety, depression, smoking, obesity, secondary gain, litigation, and workers' compensation cases. Surgeon operative risk factors include misdiagnosis of the pain generator, poor surgical technique, and successive surgical procedures. Tissue responsive risk factors include recur-

Table 11.1 Risk factors for developing FBS

Preoperative factors	Intraoperative factors	Postoperative factors
Improper selection criteria Premorbid psychological risk factors Litigation, workers' compensation cases Improper communication of goals Unrealistic expectations of patients	Misdiagnosis Wrong spinal-level surgery Inadequate decompression Improper screw placement Fusion instability	Stenosis (residual/new) Epidural fibrosis Herniated disk (residual/new) Worsening degenerative disk

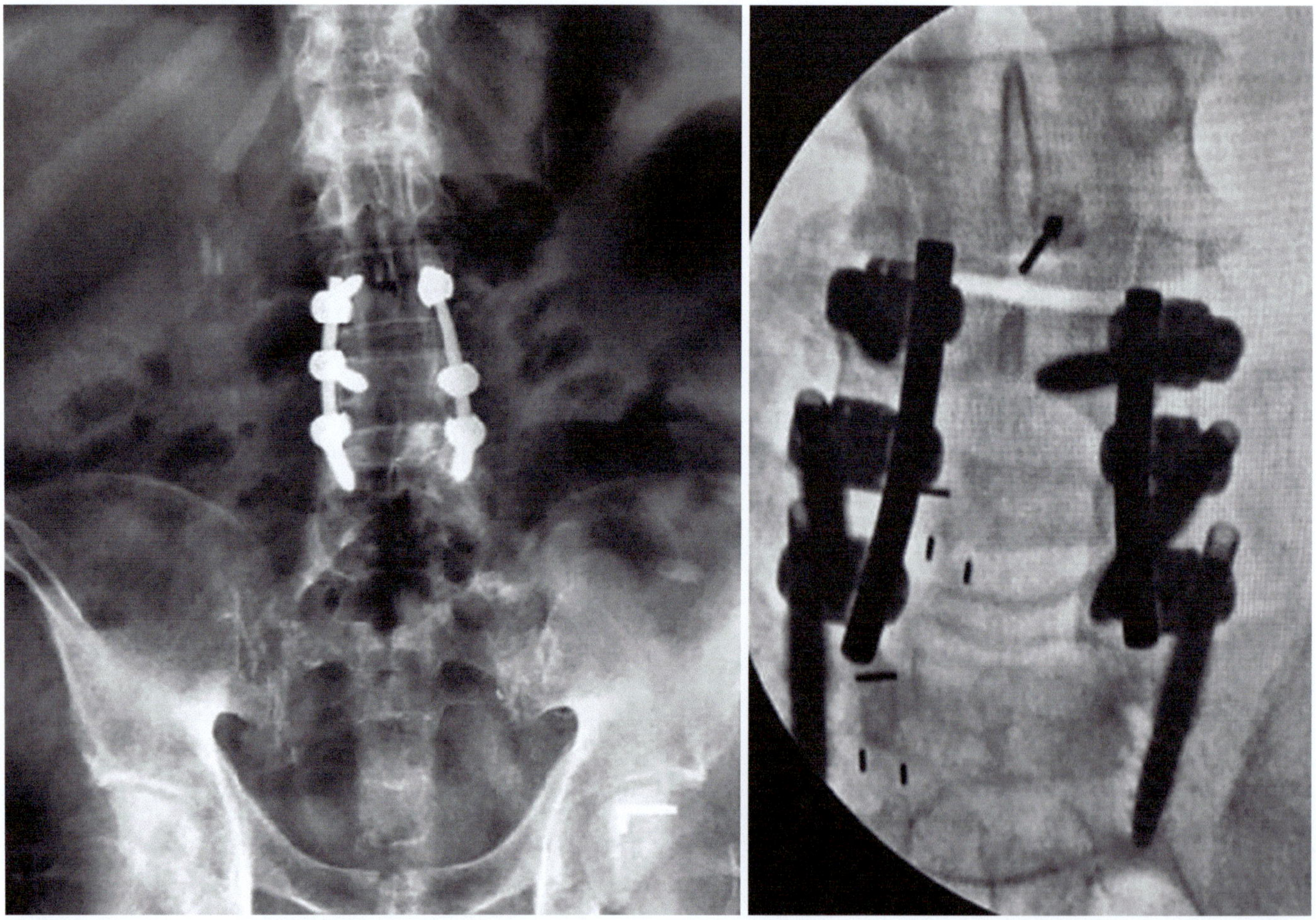

Fig. 11.1 72-year-old man who had surgery for chronic back pain in 2015 without prior conservative care. Pain did not resolve and progressively worsened. In 2019, revision surgery was performed; however, pain and dysfunction persisted (FBS). In 2021, he responded to a simple interlaminar epidural injection with 80% sustainable pain relief

rent disk herniation, spondylolisthesis, epidural fibrosis, nerve injury, infection, hematoma, progressive spinal stenosis, altered biomechanics, myofascial pain, and adjacent-level disease or pain sensitization [14]. Psychosocial factors have the strongest association with poor surgical outcome and potentially FBS [15, 16]. Surgical invasiveness correlates with FBS, with higher reports of failure after lumbar fusion as opposed to a minimally invasive microdiscectomy [17].

11.4 Symptoms

Pain is localized to the back with or without a radicular component to the lower extremities (Table 11.2). Paresthesia and numbness must be differentiated from underlying medical issues, such as diabetes mellitus or causes of diffuse or focal neuropathy. Activities of daily living may be compromised due to pain, and the present symptoms should be compared to the preoperative state to confirm similarities, differences, and possible psychological overlay.

11.5 Physical Examination

Examination findings are nonspecific, and the findings elicited from its interdependent parts and associated mechanical dysfunctions provide supportive clues [17].

Inspection and palpation Skin examination will show scar from previous spine surgery. Reduction in lumbar or cervical lordosis is often seen due to implants and hardware (flat back). Myofascial pain is common after dissection of muscle tissue, pedicle screw fixation, or chronic paraspinal muscle atrophy. In case of fusion, facet loading could elicit segmental pain above or below the fusion. Another classic finding is spondylolisthesis presenting as an indentation or step-off at the affected level.

Range of motion Restriction in active and passive range of motion is evident due to surgical fixation or soft tissue limitations. Limitations may also occur from adjacent segment disease or spondylosis.

Motor testing Strength is diminished at the involved myotome, and weakness could be from disuse, pain, or other spinal disease like foraminal stenosis or herniation.

Sensory testing Sensory deficits are apparent at the involved dermatome with hypoesthesia or in cases of CRPS, hyperalgesia, and allodynia. Symmetric deficits could suggest diffuse or metabolic etiology.

Reflexes Abnormal hyporeflexia may be related to previous preoperative disease (stenosis, nerve compression) or related to new herniation and stenosis. Hyperreflexia should alarm clinician to potential myelopathy or other central nervous disease and should be expeditiously explored.

Special tests Neural tension signs including straight leg raise test, spurling maneuver, and femoral stretch are part of a standard examination. However, these tests may not differentiate between a new disk herniation and impingement from scar tissue surrounding a spinal nerve root.

Table 11.2 Differential dx of FBS and presentation

Source of pain	Characteristics	Examination	Tests
Degenerative disk disease	Axial pain May radiate out to gluteal/groin Non-dermatomal leg pain Increases with sitting, bending lifting Improves with rest or walking around	Pain with flexion Decrease ROM Normal neuro-examination	X-rays: Disk space narrowing MRI: Reduced disk T2 signal changes (dehydration) and modic changes of vertebral endplate Discogram
Disk herniation	Dermatomal pain in lower extremity Myotomal weakness	+ SLR (Lasegue) + Femoral stretch test	+ MR or CT + EMG in radiculopathy Both MR and EMG should correlate with examination
Facet pain	Pain with extension, rotation, lateral flexion Can be unilateral or bilateral Refers to buttock/groin	Pain on facet loading (extension and lateral flexion)	X-ray/CT and MR show facet arthropathy Lumbar diagnostic medial branch block
Spinal stenosis	LBP with neurogenic claudication (pseudo-claudication) Walking and standing limitation. Pain relief with sitting Pain relief with forward bending (shopping cart)	Abnormal sensation or strength Hyporeflexia Positive slump test	CT scan, MRI, or myelography can diagnose central stenosis
Multifidus dysfunction	Dynamic segmental stabilizer Weakness and atrophy are associated with chronic low back pain	Myofascial pain	CT/MRI

11.6 Diagnostic Workup

X-ray After spine surgery, clinicians rely on X-rays to evaluate fusion status, new bony fracture, hardware position, pedicular screw loosening, or fracture [18]. Dynamic X-rays evaluate for segmental instability and are superior to magnetic resonance imaging (MRI) for evaluation of spondylolisthesis.

MRI MRI with contrast provides supporting evidence for persistent pain such as new herniation, progressive stenosis, and synovial cyst.

CT scan Computed tomography (CT) is the modality of choice if MRI is incompatible (defibrillator, other metallic implants). CT with 2-D reconstruction evaluates failed fusion, hardware loosening, bony abnormality, or fluid collection not identified otherwise. CT delineates bone and is superior for facet degeneration or pseudarthrosis but overall, less desirable than an MRI due to high level of radiation. In rare cases, CT myelogram is ordered, for nondiagnostic MRI findings such as for epidural fibrosis [18].

Bone scan If infection is suspected, blood work, pet scan, and bone scans are indicated.

Diagnostic injections Diagnostic blocks identify sources of persistent postoperative pain related to adjacent-level facet joints, sacroiliac joints, degenerative disk, annular disk tear, piriformis muscle, or nerve root impingements. Performing procedures on an operated back may pose technical challenges requiring the expertise of a skilled interventionalist.

11.7 Treatments

Consideration should at first hand be given to pharmacological therapy, physiotherapy, and management of psychological and social factors.

11.7.1 Medical Management

Medications address axial pain or radiculopathy. Neuropathic medications such as gabapentinoids and tricyclic antidepressants such as amitriptyline have fair evidence for managing radiculopathy [19]. Anti-inflammatory medications such as COX-1 and COX-2 inhibitors are effective for chronic back pain; however, its risk of cardiovascular, gastrointestinal, and renal events are high and should be used with caution. Opioid medications are effective for acute nociceptive pain but not recommended for chronic spinal pain due to lack of long-term benefit and potential for side effect, tolerance, and diversion .

11.7.2 Rehabilitation

The main goal of physical therapy in failed back syndrome is to improve function. Pain relief is not necessarily a goal of physical therapy, but if pain relief is achieved, it is a welcomed outcome. There is no standard protocol for rehabilitation in patients in this postoperative phase with chronic pain. Combining physical therapy with other modalities, in an interdisciplinary approach (PT, OT, Psych support, medical and procedural treatment), may result in better outcome. Goals of physical therapy is patient education, improve range of motion, working on soft tissue to relaxation tense muscles, therapeutical exercise to improve core strength, and functional gain in ADLs and in work environment. Over time, with supervised PT, strength, endurance, and function may improve resulting in patient satisfaction. Patient education will increase compliance and continue with the exercises despite occasional flare-ups. Combining PT with procedural treatment including neuromodulation can have the best long-term outcome.

11.7.3 Procedures

The goals of procedures are to reduce pain, improve function, and increase compliance with exercise-based treatment. Failed back syndrome is often a combination of back and neuropathic leg pain. Radiculitis could be treated with selective nerve blocks and coexisting mechanical pain from the facet joints, or the sacroiliac joints could be treated with facet and sacroiliac joint procedures. In patients that simple pain procedures are not effective; neuromodulation should be considered.

11.7.3.1 Sacral-Mediated Pain

Sacroiliac (SI) joint dysfunction is common after L5–S1 fusion. This is often thought to be related to immobility of the fused segment, transferring the stress to the adjacent tissues including the sacroiliac joint. If the SI joint is identified as the primary pain source, intra-articular injections or neuroablation treatments can be offered first. In recent years, percutaneous SI joint fusion has become available to patients suffering from intractable SI joint-mediated back pain.

11.7.3.2 Facet-Mediated Pain

In patients who have undergone fusion, adjacent facets both proximal and distal to immobilize disk space become responsible for the majority of the motion in the lumbar segment. As a result, facet joints can become a source of pain due to increased mechanical forces. In postoperative cases with facet-generated pain, concordant diagnostic medical branch blocks with subsequent radiofrequency ablation treatment can lead to successful pain relief. In recent years, advances in regenerative options have resulted in trial of intra-articular PRP for facet-generated pain. Such treatments warrant further research.

11.7.3.3 Radiculopathy

In failed back syndrome, radicular symptom can originate from re-herniation, intraoperative trauma to nerve root, wrong-level surgery, inadequate decompression, nerve root irritation by improper pedicular screw placement or osteophytosis, scarring in the surgical bed, and tissue adhesion. There is no standard of care in the treatment of radiculitis in failed back syndrome, but options include epidural injection, transforaminal ESI, caudal epidural injection, endoscopic or percutaneous adhesiolysis, and neuromodulation. There is evidence that treating radicular pain with caudal epidural injection has a better outcome over considering repeat lumbar surgery [20]. Some studies are suggesting mechanical, endoscopic, or percutaneous adhesiolysis versus chemical adhesiolysis with hyaluronidase to be superior to steroid alone in treating FBS pain [20–22].

11.7.3.4 Neuromodulation

Neuromodulation is based on the *gait theory* of pain (Melzack and Wall in 1965), stimulating the wide dynamic range of neurons and utilizing its powerful inhibitory effect on painful stimuli carried by A-delta and C fibers. Both dorsal column of the spinal cord (SCS) and dorsal root ganglion (Fig. 11.2) can be stimulated to achieve pain control. Parameters that are important in delivering effective stimulation include amplitude, frequency, and pulse width, all of which can be adjusted and optimized [23]. SCS types are traditional paresthesia-based, high-frequency stimulation, burst stimulation, or a combination of modalities. There is strong evidence supporting spinal cord stimulation (SCS) for managing failed back syndrome [23, 24]. There is level I evidence supporting SCS over reoperation for managing FBS symptoms [24]. Recent level 1 studies support high-frequency stimulation for treatment of axial back pain with or without leg pain [25, 26]. In regards to DRG stimulation, T12 stimulation may be an optimal method of controlling postoperative back pain [27]. Supporting research suggests the use of paddle leads to be superior to percutaneous leads with less incidence of lead migration (most common complication) [28].

A week-long trial of SCS or DRG stimulation before permeant placement is considered the standard of care. During this week, patient would evaluate pain relief and functional gain from the neuromodulation treatment before committing to a permanent device. Permanent SCS treatment involves implanting either a paddle or percutaneous leads in mid-lower thoracic spine (Fig. 11.2), anchoring to supraspinous ligament, and connecting the lead to a pulse generator, which is also implanted . For DRG stimulation, lead is placed dorsal to DRG (Fig. 11.3), and no anchoring is needed as the lead is looped in epidural space. After implantation of neuromodulation systems, further adjustments and programming are done to optimize the effect.

11.8 Surgery

The literature review suggests revision spine surgeries have limited success [11]. A decision to repeat surgery should weigh several factors where declining neurologic function should be the paramount consideration. For pain alone, SCS may be more effective than repeat surgery [29]. Absolute

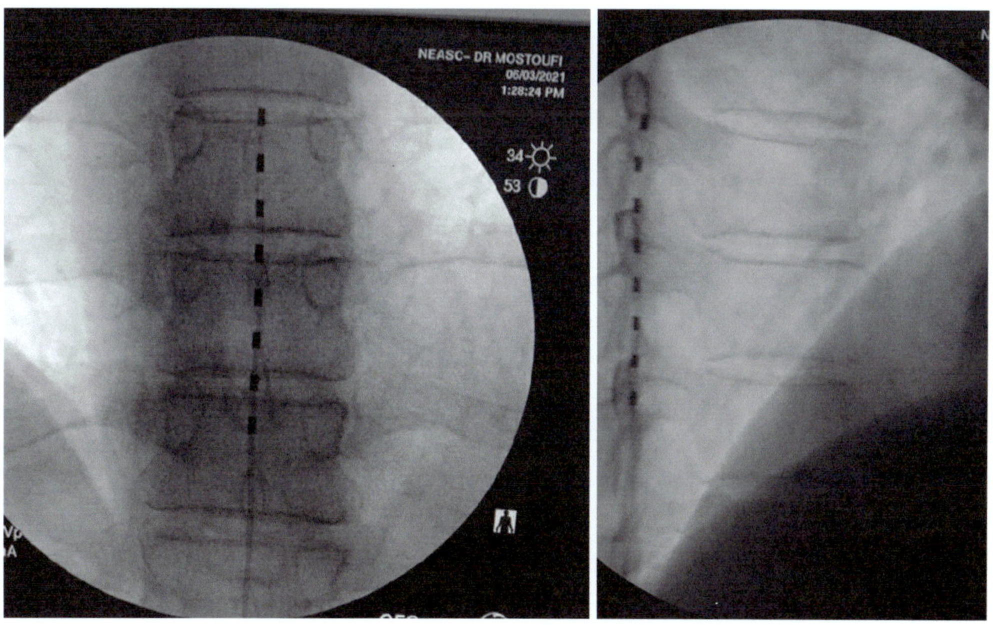

Fig. 11.2 Lead placement for spinal cord stimulator. Image demonstrates a single lead, with 8 contacts, placed midline with tip of the lead at T9. (Image courtesy of Ali Mostoufi, MD. New England Spine Care Associates)

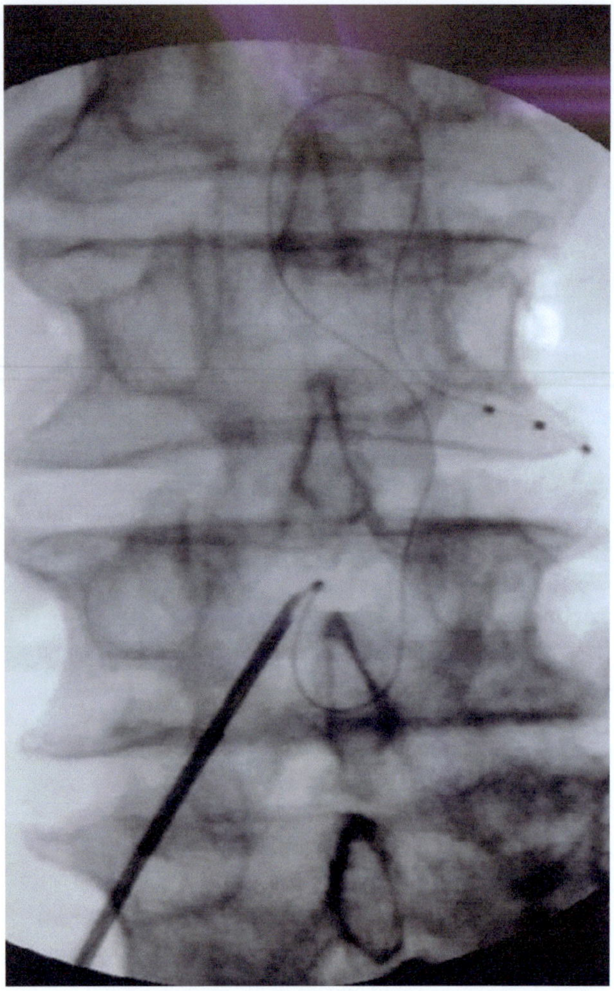

Fig. 11.3 Placement of DRG lead, demonstrating lead placed dorsal to L2 DRG, and the lead is looped in an S shape configuration in the dorsal epidural space. (Image courtesy of Ali Mostoufi, MD. New England Spine Care Associates)

indications for surgery include impaired bowel and bladder function, progressive or profound motor weakness, and continued neural deficit or interactable severe pain.

References

1. Parker SL, Mendenhall SK, Godil SS, Sivasubramanian P, Cahill K, Ziewacz J, McGirt MJ. Incidence of low back pain after lumbar discectomy for herniated disc and its effect on patient-reported outcomes. Clin Orthop Relat Res. 2015;473(6):1988–99.
2. Al-Kaisy A, Palmisani S, Smith TE, Carganillo R, Houghton R, Pang D, Burgoyne W, Lam K, Lucas J. Long-term improvements in chronic axial low back pain patients without previous spinal surgery: a cohort analysis of 10-kHz high-frequency spinal cord stimulation over 36 months. Pain Med. 2018;19(6):1219–26.
3. Deyo RA, Weinstein JN. Low back pain. N Engl J Med. 2001;344(5):363–70.
4. Global Burden of Disease Study C. Global, regional, and national incidence, prevalence, and years lived with disability for 301 acute and chronic diseases and injuries in 188 countries, 1990-2013: a systematic analysis for the Global Burden of Disease Study 2013. Lancet. 2015;386(9995):743–800.
5. Chou R, Shekelle P. Will this patient develop persistent disabling low back pain? JAMA. 2010;303(13):1295–302.
6. Deyo RA, Mirza SK. The case for restraint in spinal surgery: does quality management have a role to play? Eur Spine J. 2009;18 Suppl 3:331–7.
7. Krames E, Poree L, Deer T, Levy R. Implementing the SAFE principles for the development of pain medicine therapeutic algorithms that include neuromodulation techniques. Neuromodulation. 2009;12(2):104–13.
8. Martin BI, Mirza SK, Spina N, Spiker WR, Lawrence B, Brodke DS. Trends in lumbar fusion procedure rates and associated hospital costs for degenerative spinal diseases in the United States, 2004 to 2015. Spine (Phila Pa 1976). 2019;44(5):369–76.
9. Resnick DK, Choudhri TF, Dailey AT, Groff MW, Khoo L, Matz PG, Mummaneni P, Watters WC 3rd, Wang J, Walters BC, et al. Guidelines for the performance of fusion procedures for degenerative disease of the lumbar spine. Part 1: introduction and methodology. J Neurosurg Spine. 2005;2(6):637–8.
10. Thomson S. Failed back surgery syndrome - definition, epidemiology and demographics. Br J Pain. 2013;7(1):56–9.
11. Nachemson AL. Evaluation of results in lumbar spine surgery. Acta Orthop Scand Suppl. 1993;251:130–3.
12. Carragee EJ, Lincoln T, Parmar VS, Alamin T. A gold standard evaluation of the "discogenic pain" diagnosis as determined by provocative discography. Spine (Phila Pa 1976). 2006;31(18):2115–23.
13. Eck JC, Sharan A, Resnick DK, Watters WC 3rd, Ghogawala Z, Dailey AT, Mummaneni PV, Groff MW, Wang JC, Choudhri TF, et al. Guideline update for the performance of fusion procedures for degenerative disease of the lumbar spine. Part 6: discography for patient selection. J Neurosurg Spine. 2014;21(1):37–41.
14. Orhurhu VJ, Chu R, Gill J. Failed back surgery syndrome. In: StatPearls. Treasure Island (FL); 2021.
15. Kizilkilic O, Yalcin O, Sen O, Aydin MV, Yildirim T, Hurcan C. The role of standing flexion-extension radiographs for spondylolisthesis following single level disk surgery. Neurol Res. 2007;29(6):540–3.
16. Voorhies RM, Jiang X, Thomas N. Predicting outcome in the surgical treatment of lumbar radiculopathy using the Pain Drawing Score, McGill Short Form Pain Questionnaire, and risk factors including psychosocial issues and axial joint pain. Spine J. 2007;7(5):516–24.
17. Chan CW, Peng P. Failed back surgery syndrome. Pain Med. 2011;12(4):577–606.
18. Barrey C, Darnis A. Current strategies for the restoration of adequate lordosis during lumbar fusion. World J Orthop. 2015;6(1):117–26.
19. Attal N, Cruccu G, Haanpaa M, Hansson P, Jensen TS, Nurmikko T, Sampaio C, Sindrup S, Wiffen P, Force ET. EFNS guidelines on pharmacological treatment of neuropathic pain. Eur J Neurol. 2006;13(11):1153–69.
20. Manchikanti L, Singh V, Cash KA, Pampati V, Datta S. Management of pain of post lumbar surgery syndrome: one-year results of a randomized, double-blind, active controlled trial of fluoroscopic caudal epidural injections. Pain Physician. 2010;13(6):509–21.
21. Cho JH, Lee JH, Song KS, Hong JY, Joo YS, Lee DH, Hwang CJ, Lee CS. Treatment outcomes for patients with failed back surgery. Pain Physician. 2017;20(1):E29–43.
22. Manchikanti L, Singh V, Cash KA, Pampati V. Assessment of effectiveness of percutaneous adhesiolysis and caudal epidural injections in managing post lumbar surgery syndrome: 2-year follow-up of a randomized, controlled trial. J Pain Res. 2012;5:597–608.
23. Amirdelfan K, Webster L, Poree L, Sukul V, McRoberts P. Treatment options for failed back surgery syndrome patients with refractory chronic pain: an evidence based approach. Spine (Phila Pa 1976). 2017;42 Suppl 14:S41–52.

24. North RB, Kidd D, Shipley J, Taylor RS. Spinal cord stimulation versus reoperation for failed back surgery syndrome: a cost effectiveness and cost utility analysis based on a randomized, controlled trial. Neurosurgery. 2007;61(2):361–8; discussion 368–369.
25. Kapural L, Yu C, Doust MW, Gliner BE, Vallejo R, Sitzman BT, Amirdelfan K, Morgan DM, Brown LL, Yearwood TL, et al. Novel 10-kHz high-frequency therapy (HF10 therapy) is superior to traditional low-frequency spinal cord stimulation for the treatment of chronic back and leg pain: the SENZA-RCT randomized controlled trial. Anesthesiology. 2015;123(4):851–60.
26. Kapural L, Yu C, Doust MW, Gliner BE, Vallejo R, Sitzman BT, Amirdelfan K, Morgan DM, Yearwood TL, Bundschu R, et al. Comparison of 10-kHz high-frequency and traditional low-frequency spinal cord stimulation for the treatment of chronic back and leg pain: 24-month results from a multicenter, randomized, controlled pivotal trial. Neurosurgery. 2016;79(5):667–77.
27. Chapman KB, Groenen PS, Vissers KC, van Helmond N, Stanton-Hicks MD. The pathways and processes underlying spinal transmission of low back pain: observations from dorsal root ganglion stimulation treatment. Neuromodulation. 2021;24(4):610–21.
28. Babu R, Hazzard MA, Huang KT, Ugiliweneza B, Patil CG, Boakye M, Lad SP. Outcomes of percutaneous and paddle lead implantation for spinal cord stimulation: a comparative analysis of complications, reoperation rates, and health-care costs. Neuromodulation. 2013;16(5):418–26; discussion 426–417.
29. North RB, Kidd DH, Farrokhi F, Piantadosi SA. Spinal cord stimulation versus repeated lumbosacral spine surgery for chronic pain: a randomized, controlled trial. Neurosurgery. 2005;56(1):98–106; discussion 106-107.

Spinal Deformities: Kyphosis and Scoliosis

12

S. Ali Mostoufi, Tony K. George, and Yasmine Mostoufi

12.1 Kyphosis

12.1.1 ICD 10

Kyphosis deformity of spine M40.209.

12.1.2 Synonyms

Idiopathic spinal deformity, acquired spinal deformity, kyphoscoliosis, Scheuermann's disease.

12.1.3 Description

Kyphosis is an increase in the forward curvature of the spine seen in the sagittal view (Fig. 12.1).

Kyphosis is a physiologic curvature of the thoracic spine and its connection with cervical and lumbar lordosis curves above and below make up the length of the spine above the sacrum. In the sagittal view, thoracic kyphosis normal angular range falls between 20° and 40°. Hyperkyphosis is defined as a cobb angle greater than 50° (Fig. 12.3).

The thoracic spine is less flexible as compared to the cervical and lumbar spine where its attachment to the ribcage is a source for its immobility. The spine comprises 7 cervical vertebrae, 12 thoracic vertebrae, 5 lumbar vertebrae, a fused sacrum, and fused coccyx. From the age of 40, physiologic kyphosis progresses and the kyphotic angle increases with age [1]. Hyperkyphosis is prevalent in 20–40% of the population after age 60 (Fig. 12.1) [2]. It affects women more than men and progresses more in woman of menopausal age. Menopause accelerates bone turnover, and low bone mineral density is a risk factor for fracture and kyphotic progression. About a third of patients with osteoporosis have compression fractures [3]. Compression fractures cause wedging of the vertebral body putting pressure on additional segmental levels in the spine and increasing the risk of future fractures and progression of kyphotic angle (Fig. 12.2). Each vertebral fracture can increase kyphosis angle by 3.8° [4]. Conversely, nonmetabolic kyphosis may not be a risk fracture for compression fractures [5]. In kyphosis, postural imbalance with anterior displacement of the center of mass increases the risk of falls and nonspine fractures [6]. Other risk factors include degenerative disk disease, weakness of back extensor muscles, older age, and family history of hyperkyphosis (Table 12.1).

Kyphosis can occur in the pediatric and adult populations. There are three types of pediatric kyphosis, which include postural, juvenile, and congenital kyphosis.

Postural kyphosis is related to adolescent slouching and forward head tilt creating weakening of the extensor muscles of the upper back. The vertebral structures are normal in shape and form in this diagnosis. As the spine maintains flexibility, this deformity can be corrected.

Juvenile kyphosis, also known as Scheuermann's disease, is a thoracolumbar structural deformity occurring before puberty. The vertebral structures demonstrate anterior wedging due to aberrant bone mineralization. This spine is rigid compared to postural kyphosis and restrictive to correction.

Congenital kyphosis from anomalies is rare however disabling and rapidly progressing. The result of either lack of spinal segmentation or failure of segmental development is usually diagnosed during childhood.

S. A. Mostoufi (✉)
Department of Orthopedics and Rehabilitation, Tufts University School of Medicine, Boston, MA, USA

New England Spine Care Associates & Boston Regenerative Medicine, Cambridge, MA, USA
e-mail: ali.mostoufi@Tufts.edu

T. K. George
Restorative Orthopaedics Spine & Sports (ROSS) Institute, Somerset, NJ, USA

Department of Orthopaedics, Rutgers-Robert Wood Johnson Medical School, New Brunswick, NJ, USA

Y. Mostoufi
Medical Illustration and Image Optimization, Senior at Landmark High School, Beverly, MA, USA

© The Author(s), under exclusive license to Springer Nature Switzerland AG 2022

S. A. Mostoufi et al. (eds.), *Clinical Guide to Musculoskeletal Medicine*, https://doi.org/10.1007/978-3-030-92042-5_12

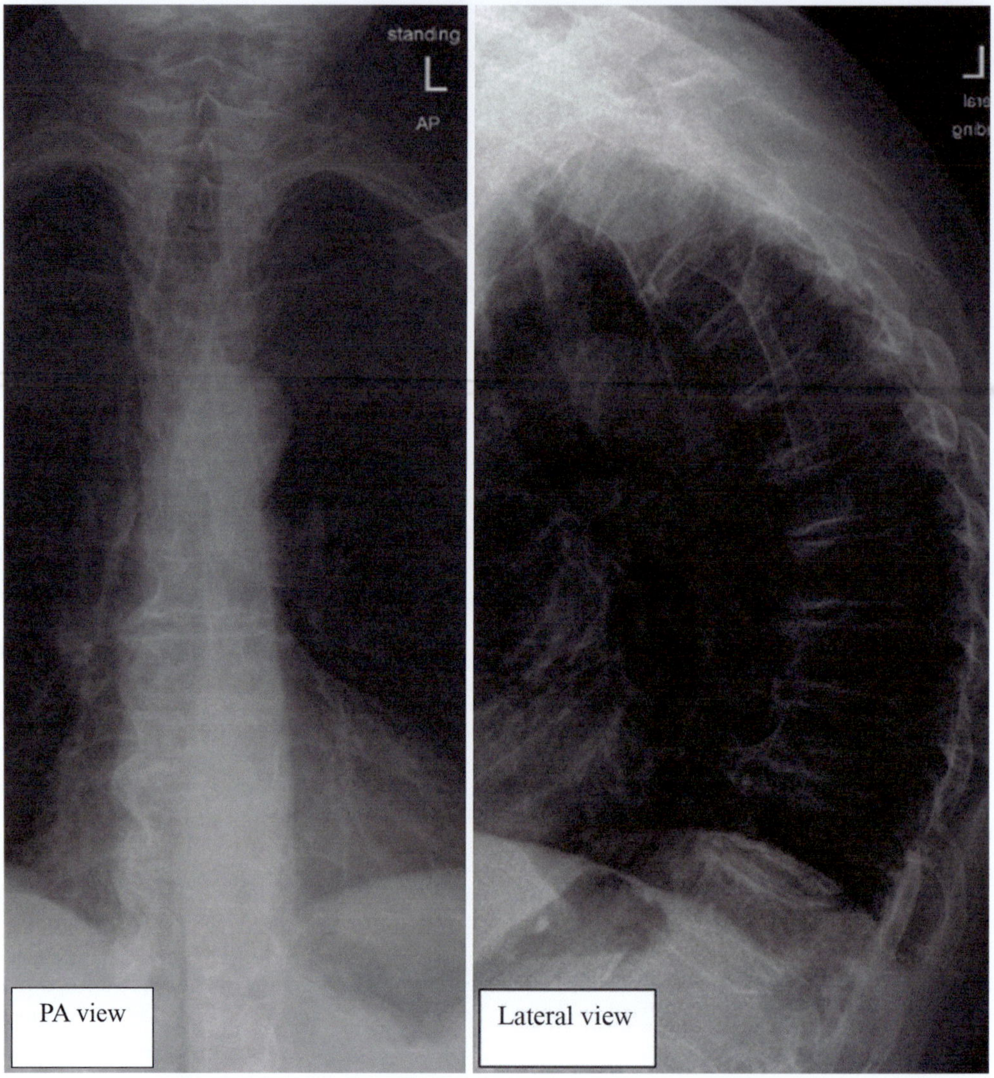

Fig. 12.1 PA and lateral views of Spine. On PA view, no lateral deformity is noted, but the lateral views demonstrate kyphosis

Adult kyphosis can be from degenerative, metabolic, iatrogenic, and post-traumatic, autoimmune from ankylosing spondylitis, neurologic from neurofibromatosis, and infectious from tuberculosis (Table 12.1). Metabolic causes are kyphosis from osteoporosis. Degenerative and metabolic etiologies comprise a majority of adult-related kyphosis. Potts kyphosis is vertebral infection from tuberculosis resulting in segmental damage causing severe thoracic or thoracolumbar kyphosis. Segmental junctional kyphosis is an iatrogenic kyphosis after spinal fusion surgery causing collapse of the proximal vertebral segments.

Complications of hyperkyphosis include pulmonary compromise with restricted vital capacity putting patients at risk of pneumonia and COPD. Kyphosis angulation increases energy expenditure making household chores and ADL activities cumbersome. Neurologic compromise can be expected in severe kyphotic angles >90°, and in some cases as early as beyond 50° [7].

12.1.4 Symptoms

Pain and stiffness are common symptoms from spinal stress due to kyphotic changes. Shortness of breath may be present due to reduced capacity, limited lung expansion, and rib immobility [8]. Fatigue is common from increased energy expenditure due to kyphotic angulation.

Cord compression should be suspected in cases of hyperkyphosis with bowel incontinence, bladder retention, and progressive gait deficits.

12.1.5 Physical Examination

Inspection Patients present with a forward head and neck tilt with a rounded back or humpback deformity. Increased lumbar lordosis and forward pelvic tilt are also present. Also, true height is reduced from forward riding head tilt and neck extension may be limited due to muscle weakness.

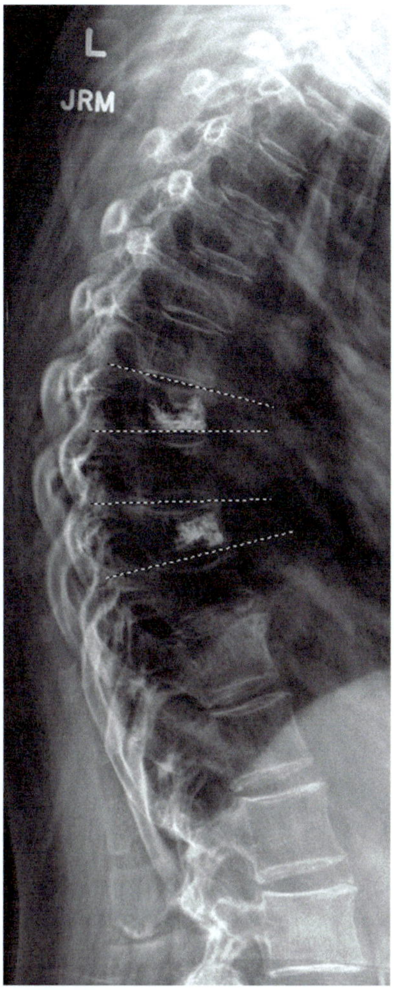

Fig. 12.2 Image demonstrates two thoracic vertebral fractures (augmented), each with anterior wedging, which has resulted in segmental kyphosis and increased overall kyphotic angulation of thoracic spine. (Image from author's library)

Table 12.1 Kyphosis and its possible etiologies

Adult kyphosis	Pediatric kyphosis
Degenerative, idiopathic, autoimmune	Postural
Post-traumatic (wedge fracture)	Juvenile (Scheuermann)
Neurologic, metabolic, iatrogenic	Congenital

MSK examination Muscle examination would reveal tight hamstrings and hip joint contractures with pelvic obliquity due to compensation efforts to correct sagittal imbalance. Patients would demonstrate tenderness to palpate the thoracolumbar paraspinal muscles including facet joints above and below the apex of the curve. Belly protrusion from weak abdominal muscle and chest wall collapse may be evident on observation.

Special tests Special tests to differentiate rigid and flexible kyphosis would be laying the patient in the supine position and observing flattening and correction of flexible kyphosis and retention of curvature for rigid kyphosis.

12.1.6 Diagnostic Studies

12.1.6.1 Plain Films

Standing X-ray in the lateral view is the gold standard for assessing kyphosis using imaging. Cobb angle is the gold standard to measure degree of kyphotic angle and wedging between vertebral segments. It is measured from the superior endplate of T2 to the inferior endplate of T12 (Fig. 12.3). Serial X-rays are useful to monitor the immature adolescent spine, especially during growth spurt for kyphosis correction. Advanced imaging modalities are considered if complications are suspected.

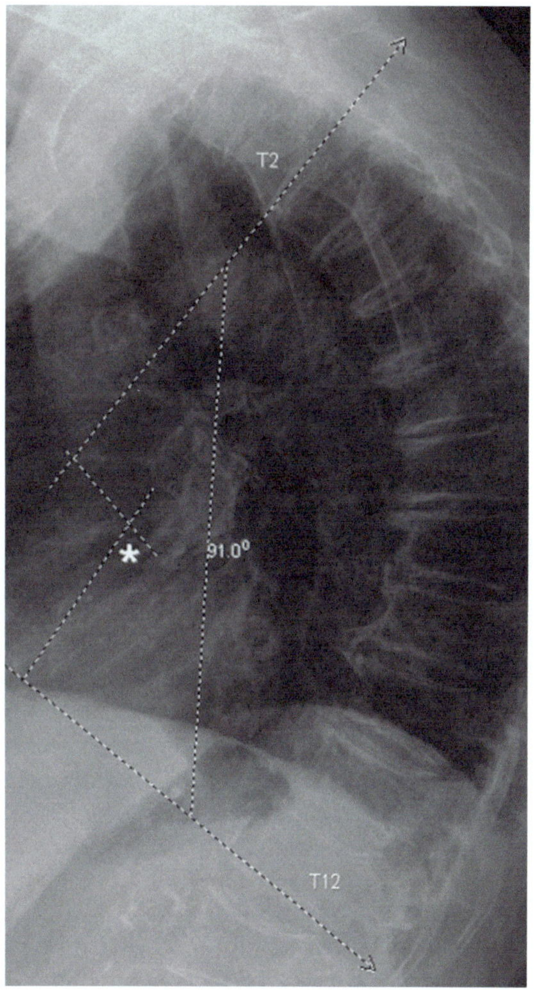

Fig. 12.3 Cobb angle measurement (Star) in a patient with kyphotic deformity. (Image from author's library)

12.1.6.2 MRI/CT

MRI with and without contrast or CT with myelogram (for MRI incompatibility) are considered if cord compression is suspected or for infectious etiologies such as Potts kyphosis. Advanced MRI or CT imaging is also useful if surgical correction is being considered.

Pulmonary function tests help measure lung compromise from the restrictive effect of progressing kyphosis.

12.1.7 Treatment

12.1.7.1 Medical Management

Bracing is appropriate for the adolescent child with kyphosis where corrective bracing can retard its progression [9]. Milwaukee brace is commonly worn for extended daily periods until skeletal maturity is reached. If kyphosis fails bracing, surgical correction may be required.

Modalities and TENS can assist in desensitizing pain. NSAIDs and Tylenol are first-line oral pain medication for general pain conditions and can be trialed for kyphosis-mediated pain. Topical lidocaine and Flector patches at the site of maximal tenderness can help reduce nociceptive-mediated pain. Opioids are not recommended due to long-term unfavorable sequelae from opioid dependence, and further compromise of respiratory function.

Bisphosphonate management is recommended for patients with osteoporosis and kyphosis.

Bisphosphonates stall osteoporosis progression, thereby stalling kyphosis progression and fractures. In addition, calcium and vitamin D reduce risk of osteoporosis-related fractures.

12.1.7.2 Rehabilitation

Physical therapy emphasizes improving flexibility and postural alignment and strengthening weak back extensors. In patients with osteoporosis, flexion exercises should be avoided as they could potentiate fractures. Studies suggest strengthening rather than stretching exercises are beneficial for kyphosis correction [10]. Prone-based exercises, which strengthen middle and lower trapezius, and scapular exercises including scapular retraction and trunk stabilization are emphasized. Studies suggest 2–3 physical therapy sessions per week for 8–12 weeks. Balance and gait training are integral as falls are a common predisposition in this population. Restrictive lung compromise is prevalent in advanced kyphosis, and diaphragmatic breathing should be encouraged to improve pulmonary function. Modern digital technologies with phone apps are useful for short exercise video clips for spine strengthening and posture at convenience of home.

12.1.7.3 Procedures

RF Ablation Progressive segmental degeneration present with neck and upper back pain from facet joints. If cervical and thoracic facet is suspected as a source of pain, medical branch block can aid with diagnoses and treatment including RF ablation could be offered.

Trigger point Myofascial pain in the cervical or thoracic region from compensation could be addressed with muscle relaxants and trigger point injections.

Bone Augmentation Acute vertebroplasty or kyphoplasty are indicated for acute pain management in the setting of recent compression fracture that may lead to exaggerated kyphosis. Kyphoplasty improves pain and may prevent further kyphotic angulation due to progressive anterior vertebral collapse.

12.1.7.4 Surgery

Age and comorbidities are factored into surgical considerations. Some indications in the juvenile and adolescent population include limited conservative relief for at least 6 months, progressive deformity and debility, kyphosis progression despite corrective bracing, and curves greater than 70° [11]. Corrective surgery is not recommended in the elderly due to comorbidities and unfavorable risk safety profile, however is considered on an individual basis. Other surgical indications include debilitating pain, severe disability from cardiopulmonary compromise, and progressing neurologic deficits.

Surgery involves pedicle screw fixation and osteotomy using a posterior, anterior, or combined approach. As long-term stabilization is the goal, these surgeries typically involve spinal fusion. The surgeries can be performed in single- or two-stage approaches for correction of deformity.

They involve restoration of segmental alignment, sagittal rod contouring, and osteotomies.

12.2 Scoliosis

12.2.1 ICD 10

- Scoliosis deformity of spine M49.1.
- Scoliosis, cervical M41.122.
- Scoliosis, thoracic M 41.124.
- Scoliosis, lumbar M41.126.

12.2.2 Synonyms

Idiopathic spinal deformity, acquired spinal deformity, dextroscoliosis, levoscoliosis, scoliotic deformity, kyphoscoliosis,

12.2.3 Description

A normal spine is generally straight and has no appreciable lateral curve on coronal radiographs. A lateral curvature of the spine is considered scoliosis. A leftward curved spine is levoscoliosis, and rightward curved spine is dextroscoliosis. A deviation from vertical line could also be combined with a spinal rotation defined as scoliosis with rotatory component. In some patients, segmental lateral listhesis is noted in addition to the abnormal scoliotic curve.

Scoliosis can develop in any segment of the spine although thoracic and lumbar scoliosis is more often recognized by clinicians. Patients may have an isolated levoscoliosis or isolated dextroscoliosis, but often on X-rays, a combination of levoscoliosis and dextroscoliosis is seen in the same patient as spine curves in one direction proximally and in the opposite direction distally (S or reversed S shape). According to the Scoliosis Research Society, at least 10° of scoliosis should be notable on the PA radiograph to be considered diagnostic (Figs. 12.4 and 12.5) [12].

In general, scoliosis is either congenital, idiopathic, secondary to other conditions, or degenerative (Table 12.2). In congenital cases, it is related to abnormally developed vertebrae resulting in scoliotic curve. Secondary causes of scoliosis could be related to neuromuscular/neurological disorders such as cerebral palsy, muscle abnormalities as in Duchenne muscular dystrophy, and some genetic disorders including Marfan syndrome and neurofibromatosis. Idiopathic scoliosis is by far the most commonly seen type in MSK clinics, and there is no underlying etiology for this type of scoliosis. Juvenile idiopathic scoliosis in ages 4–10 comprises 10–15% of all the idiopathic scoliosis in children, and if untreated may have cardiopulmonary consequences [14]. Furthermore, curvature of 30° or more in this age population tends to progress, of which 95% would likely require surgical intervention [14]. Scoliosis has a genetic component in which siblings have up to 7 times more frequency of developing scoliosis, children of patients with scoliosis have 3 times more prevalence of having scoliosis [15], and counseling pregnant females with scoliosis should include education on potential scoliosis and their offspring.

Pediatric orthopedist/physiatrist closely monitors the progression of the scoliosis in children, and clinical determination is made to monitor, brace, or operate depending on degree of curvature, the rapidity of the progression, patient's age, and the Tanner stage. Degenerative scoliosis often develops in the 6–8th decade of life, due to osteoarthropathy of the facet joints, vertebral compression fracture, and desiccated disk spaces with asymmetrical intervertebral spacing.

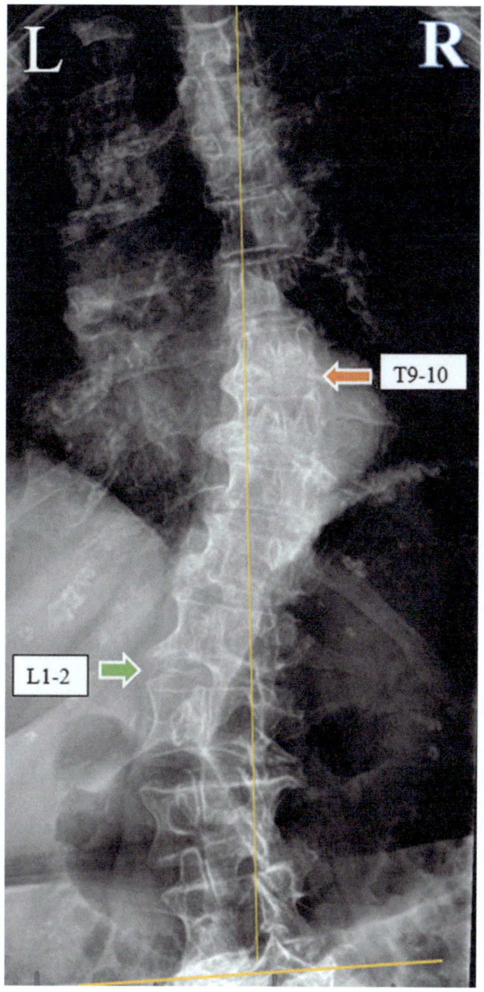

Fig. 12.4 Reversed S scoliotic curve with dextroscoliosis centered at T9–10 disk space and levoscoliosis centered at L1–2 disk space. (Image from author's library)

12.2.4 Clinical Presentation

Scoliosis is often symptom-free but can be associated with complaints such as asymmetrical shoulders, asymmetrical pelvis, leg length discrepancy, chest wall/breast asymmetry, back asymmetry, unilateral scapular protuberance, and in degenerative scoliosis complaint of getting shorter. Presenting symptoms may be pain at the apex of the scoliosis convexity. If a patient has an S-shaped scoliosis, pain may be on either of the two convexities of the curve. Unless the scoliosis is associated with severe rotation or lateral listhesis, numbness, tingling, or weakness is not a presenting symptom. In a severe scoliotic curve, when cardiopulmonary function is compromised, shortness of breath and early fatigue with activities could be a presenting symptom, which can be validated by pulmonary function testing.

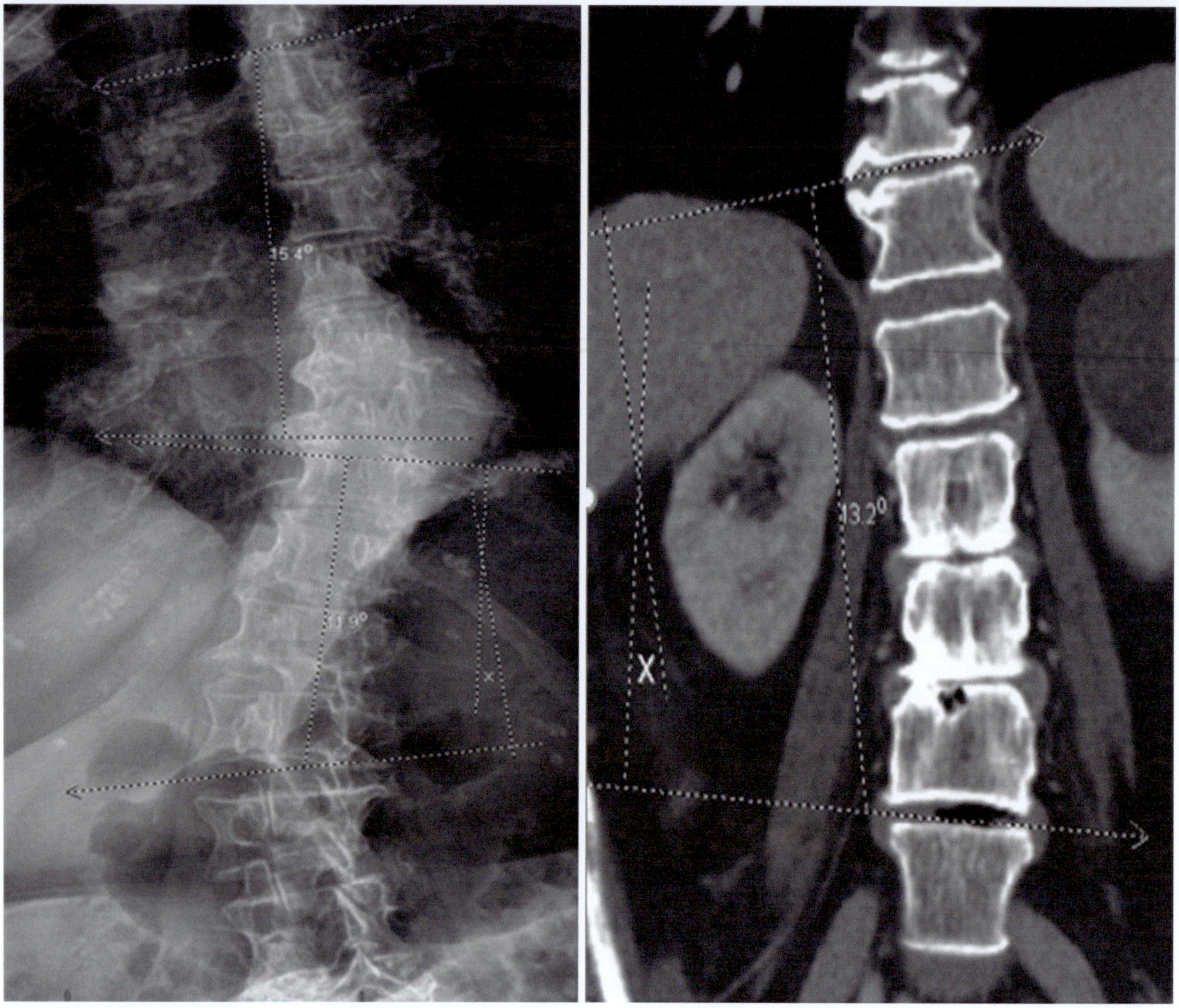

Fig. 12.5 Measurement of Cobb angle on CT or plain film. X = Cobb angle. (Image from author's library)

Table 12.2 Scoliosis can be a manifestation of neuromuscular disease and some of the rare syndromes, listed in this table [13]

Cerebral palsy	Marfan's syndrome	Muscular dystrophy
Charcot Marie tooth	Duchenne's dystrophy	Neurofibromatosis
Ehlers–Danlos syndrome	Congenital hypotonia	Myelomeningocele
Poliomyelitis	Osteogenesis imperfecta	Achondroplasia

12.2.5 Physical Examination

Thorough musculoskeletal examination is necessary. Height of the patient and the Tanner stage should be documented and followed in time as they are part of monitoring skeletal growth and risk of curve progression. Examination includes detection of out of norm findings including excessively tall patients with perhaps long fingers (signs of Marfan), any skin abnormalities that may relate to secondary scoliosis (such as neurofibromatosis), abnormal joint laxity (Ehlers–Danlos syndrome), evaluation of gait, and evaluation of the foot and its arch, which may point to genetic causes of scoliosis. In patients with severe scoliosis, auscultation of heart and lungs at both apex and distal lung is indicated and ventilation in all quadrants of the lung should be documented.

A thorough sensory/motor/reflex testing should be performed. Expectations are normal findings in scoliosis, unless there is any particular nerve root impingement in which dermatomal/myotomal deficits may be noted.

Skeletal examination includes identifying asymmetry in both coronal and sagittal planes. In the coronal plane, asymmetrical shoulders, asymmetrical pelvis, and asymmetry in the spine either S or reversed S curve are noted. In the sagittal plane, attention should be made to any rotation of the spine, and any asymmetry in chest wall, breast, scapular protuberance, and rib cage all should be documented and tracked in serial examinations. Observation should include side-to-side asymmetry in ASIS/PSIS, which leads to leg length discrepancy. Leg length discrepancy should be measured to aid with shoe lift prescription (measurement between ASIS and medial malleoli).

12.2.6 Diagnostic Workup

12.2.6.1 Plain Films

Plain radiograph is a standard diagnostic test for scoliosis. Scoliosis series include full-length AP and full-height left lateral spine views. It could be done in a standing or decubitus position. Cobb angle is measured when the patient is followed over time, repetitive Cobb angle measurement determines the progression of the curve (Fig. 12.5). Risser sign (ossification of the iliac apophysis) should be documented on X-ray as it identifies the degree of spinal skeletal maturity, which is the clinical information for the management of adolescent scoliosis [16].

12.2.6.2 CT Scan

This modality requires high-dose radiation. CT is reserved for patients prior to surgical planning, potential congenital anomalies, and in cases with spondylolisthesis and rotatory component. Sagittal and coronal reformatting would add additional value. In post-fusion state, if there is concern regarding nonfusion, CT with 2D coronal and sagittal reconstruction may be utilized.

12.2.6.3 Ultrasound

There is no indication for diagnostic ultrasound in scoliosis; however, it may avoid inadvertent pneumothorax while performing trigger point injections in the paraspinal muscles through visualization of the needle tip within muscle layers, in patients with significant rotatory scoliosis of the thoracic spine.

MRI: In degenerative spine with scoliosis, additional findings including stenotic central canal and foraminal impingement can be identified and the extent of degenerative disk disease could be fully evaluated.

12.2.7 Treatment

12.2.7.1 Medical Management

In degenerative scoliosis, facet arthropathy and asymmetrical muscle firing may lead to symptomatic scoliosis including pain. In this group in particular, anti-inflammatories (oral or topical) and muscle relaxants may be used. Latter treatment options include spinal manipulation, utilization of TENS unit, therapeutic massage, and rehabilitation efforts. Opioids are generally not indicated.

12.2.7.2 Bracing

Goal of bracing in scoliotic patients is to halt the progression of the curve before reaching skeletal maturity. Other goals include improving cosmetically and reducing the risk of prolonged symptomatic scoliosis (cardiopulmonary and pain). Examination, *Cobb angle*, *Risser sign* of skeletal maturity, *and Tanner stages* all play a role in the determination of bracing and the timing of it (Table 12.3).

Effectiveness of bracing in early nonoperative management has been established by BrAIST RTC study, level 1 research [17, 18]. It was demonstrated that 18 hours/day bracing was approximately 72% successful in halting curve progression as compared to 48% in the control arm that received no brace and was simply observed. There was a significant positive association between hours of brace wear and rate of treatment success.

Braces are customized to the patient. Brace type and extent of bracing depend on type of curvature (single versus L-shaped and with segment of spine). The most common type of brace is TLSO (thoracolumbosacral orthosis) appropriate for thoracolumbar S-shaped curvature. Several types are available, and research projects have been done to compare efficacy. These braces include the Boston brace, the Wilmington brace, Charleston brace, and the Providence brace. Ultimate success will lie on proper customization/fitting, proper monitoring, and compliance of the patient with the brace.

Table 12.3 Scoliosis Research Society recommended criteria for bracing in idiopathic scoliosis

RISSER sign	Curve (in degree)	Action
0–1	0–20	Observe
0–1	20–40	Brace
2–3	0–30	Observe
2–3	30–40	Brace
0–3	40–50	Gray
0–3	Over 50	Surgery

12.2.7.3 Rehabilitation

Several systematic reviews, including a Cochrane systematic review on the effects of exercises for scoliosis, report promising results, some showing improved neuromotor control, respiratory function, back muscle strength, and cosmetic appearance [19, 20]. Exercises are individualized according to patient needs, curve pattern, and treatment phase. A large cohort study of patients with scoliosis ($N = 813$) showed that after a course exercise program vital capacity and chest wall expansion were improved [20, 21]. Engagement in frequent and regular sport activity has been confirmed as a positive component in helping to minimize curves in young patients [20].

Physiotherapy Scoliosis Specific Exercises (PSSEs) have been used in the USA in conjunction with spinal orthotic management in the treatment of progressive idiopathic scoliosis. The combination of the two modalities may offer advantages over more simplified treatment plans. PSSEs have also been applied for adult patients with pain associated with scoliosis. According to the 2016 Society on Scoliosis Orthopaedic and Rehabilitation Treatment (SOSORT) consensus and guidelines, the common principles of PSSE involve autocorrection, elongation, and chest wall expansion with the integration of the "corrected" posture into daily life activities. SOSORT also endorses usage of exercises in the postsurgical rehabilitation period. It has been reported that patients who experience pain 10 or more years after scoliosis surgery can reduce the pain frequency through a multimodal treatment including stabilizing postural and respiratory exercises [22].

Other "schools" of scoliosis physiotherapy have evolved, Schroth technique, Schroth-Barcelona School, SEAS in Italy, and DoboMed and FITS in Poland all of which incorporate exercise-based treatment.

12.2.7.4 Procedures

Myofascial pain in the paraspinal muscles adjacent to the scoliotic region could be addressed with trigger point injections.

Pain from degenerative facet in the context of scoliosis can be treated with standard treatments for facet-mediated pain including RF ablation of medial branches.

12.2.7.5 Surgery

Severe and/or progressive scoliosis often needs surgery. Criteria for surgical care are outlined in Scoliosis Research Society Recommendations. This includes curves greater than 50° progressing even after skeletal maturity, curves of greater magnitude causing loss of pulmonary function, and much greater curves causing respiratory failure. Posterior fusion with instrumentation has been a standard surgical treatment for scoliosis using Harrington rods. In modern instrumentation systems, anchors are used to connect the rod and the spine, resulting in better correction and less frequent implant failures. Segmental pedicle screw constructs or hybrid constructs using pedicle screws, hooks, and wires are commonly done today [20]. For details for surgical management in spine, see Chaps. 15 and 16.

References

1. Roghani T, Zavieh MK, Manshadi FD, King N, Katzman W. Age-related hyperkyphosis: update of its potential causes and clinical impacts-narrative review. Aging Clin Exp Res. 2017;29(4):567–77.
2. Kado DM, Prenovost K, Crandall C. Narrative review: hyperkyphosis in older persons. Ann Intern Med. 2007;147:330–8.
3. Kado DM, Huang MH, Karlamangla AS, et al. Factors associated with kyphosis progression in older women: 15 years' experience in the study of osteoporotic fractures. J Bone Miner Res. 2013;28(1):179–87.
4. Kado DM, Huang MH, Karlamangla AS, Cawthon P, Katzman W, Hillier TA, Ensrud K, Cummings SR. Factors associated with kyphosis progression in older women: 15 years' experience in the study of osteoporotic fractures. J Bone Miner Res. 2013;28(1):179–87.
5. Kado DM, Lui LY, Ensrud KE, et al. Hyperkyphosis predicts mortality independent of vertebral osteoporosis in older women. Ann Intern Med. 2009;150(10):681–7. https://doi.org/10.7326/0003-4819-150-10-200905190-00005.
6. Kado DM, Miller-Martinez D, Lui LY, et al. Hyperkyphosis, kyphosis progression, and risk of non-spine fractures in older community dwelling women: the Study of Osteoporotic Fractures (SOF). J Bone Miner Res. 2014;29(10):2210–6.
7. Lonstein JE, Winter RB, Moe JH, et al. Neurologic deficits secondary to spinal deformity. A review of the literature and report of 43 cases. Spine (Phila Pa 1976). 1980;5:331–55.
8. Lorbergs AL, O'Connor GT, Zhou Y, Travison TG, Kiel DP, Cupples LA, Rosen H, Samelson EJ. Severity of kyphosis and decline in lung function: the Framingham study. J Gerontol A. 2017;72(5):689–94. https://doi.org/10.1093/gerona/glw124.
9. Weiss HR, Turnbull D, Bohr S. Brace treatment for patients with Scheuermann's disease - a review of the literature and first experiences with a new brace design. Scoliosis. 2009;4:22.
10. González-Gálvez N, et al. Effects of exercise programs on kyphosis and lordosis angle: a systematic review and meta-analysis. PLoS One. 2019;14(4):e0216180. https://doi.org/10.1371/journal.pone.0216180.
11. Loughenbury PR, Tsirikos AI. Scheuermanns kyphosis: diagnosis, presentation and treatment. Orthop Trauma. 2017;31(6):388–94. https://doi.org/10.1016/j.mporth.2017.09.010.
12. Morrissy RT, Weinstein SL. Lovell and Winter's pediatric orthopaedics. Philadelphia: Lippincott Williams & Wilkins; 2006. p. 693–762.
13. Janicki JA, Alman B. Scoliosis: review of diagnosis and treatment. Paediatr Child Health. 2007;12(9):771–6. https://doi.org/10.1093/pch/12.9.771.
14. Coillard C, Circo AB, Rivard CH. SpineCor treatment for juvenile idiopathic scoliosis: SOSORT award 2010 winner. Scoliosis. 2010;5:25.
15. Wynn-Davies R. Familial (idiopathic) scoliosis. A family survey. J Bone Joint Surg Br. 1968;50:24–30.

16. Risser JC. The iliac apophysis; an invaluable sign in the management of scoliosis. Clin Orthop. 1958;11:111–9.
17. Weinstein SL, Dolan LA, Wright JG, Dobbs MB. Effects of bracing in adolescents with idiopathic scoliosis. N Engl J Med. 2013;369:1512–21. https://doi.org/10.1056/NEJMoa1307337.
18. Kuroki H. Brace treatment for adolescent idiopathic scoliosis. J Clin Med. 2018;7(6):136. Published 2018 Jun 4. https://doi.org/10.3390/jcm7060136.
19. Otman S, Kose N, Yakut Y. The efficacy of Schroth s 3-dimensional exercise therapy in the treatment of adolescent idiopathic scoliosis in Turkey. Saudi Med J. 2005;26(9):1429–35.
20. Maruyama T, Takeshita K. Surgical treatment of scoliosis: a review of techniques currently applied. Scoliosis. 2008;3:6. Published 2008 Apr 18. https://doi.org/10.1186/1748-7161-3-6.
21. Weiss HR. The effect of an exercise program on vital capacity and rib mobility in patients with idiopathic scoliosis. Spine. 1991;16(1):88–93.
22. Weiss H-R. Rehabilitation of adolescent patients with scoliosis – what do we know? A review of the literature. Pediatr Rehabil. 2003;6(3–4):183–94.

Spine Dislocations and Fractures

13

Andrew Hecht and Jonathan S. Markowitz

13.1 Cervical Spine Trauma and Injuries

13.1.1 Synonyms

- Odontoid fracture
- Jefferson fracture
- Hangman's fracture
- Clay-shoveler fracture
- Facet dislocation

13.1.2 ICD 10 Code

- Dislocation of unspecified cervical vertebrae, initial encounter S13.101A
- Unspecified fracture of cervical vertebra S12.000A-S12.600A
- Spondylosis without myelopathy or radiculopathy, cervical region M47.812

13.1.3 Description

Cervical spine fractures often result in significant morbidity and mortality. The yearly incidence of cervical spine fractures has been reportedly increasing and is reported to be as high as 640 cases per one million individuals [1]. The most prevalent mechanisms of cervical spine injuries described in the literature are motor vehicle accidents (MVAs) and/or falls. Cervical spine injuries occur in a bimodal distribution with an increased incidence in patients younger than 25 and older than 65 years old. Cervical spine injuries occur in 3–5% of all blunt trauma victims of which less than 25% sustain a spinal cord injury (SCI) [2, 3]. Fractures of C2, the axis, make up 27% of all cervical spine injuries. Fractures of the odontoid process are the most common subtype of axis fractures and account for 35–78% of C2 fractures and 10–15% of all cervical spine fractures [4]. The most commonly injured levels in the subaxial cervical spine occur at C6 and C7 [2]. Utilizing a systematic approach to appropriately evaluate and treat those with suspected cervical spine injuries is critical to achieve the best possible outcomes.

Anatomy The cervical spine is comprised of 7 vertebral bodies and 8 pairs of cervical nerve roots and can be divided into two main regions: the craniocervical junction, from the occiput (C0) joint to the axis (C2), and the subaxial cervical spine, which encompasses injuries from C3 to C7. The axis has peg-like odontoid process, the dens, that projects itself superiorly from its body. The upper cervical spine contributes to a large proportion of overall cervical spine motion. The occipito-atlantal articulation contributes to approximately 50% of overall cervical flexion extension, while the atlantoaxial articulation contributes to approximately 50% of overall cervical spine rotation. The stability about the C1–C2 joint is provided by the odontoid process, transverse atlantal ligament (TAL), paired alar ligaments, and the apical ligament. The TAL limits anterior translation of C1 on C2, while both the apical and alar ligaments limit rotation of the upper cervical spine.

The subaxial cervical spine has an overall lordotic alignment that slightly decreases with age. Vertebral body sizes increase as you travel caudally in the cervical spine. The spinal ligaments are essential for both function and stability, and one must critically evaluate these structures when assessing a patient with a potential cervical spine injury. The anterior longitudinal ligament (ALL) and posterior longitudinal ligament (PLL) are ligaments that extend from C2 to the sacrum along the anterior and posterior vertebral bodies, respectively. While the ALL generally ends at C2, the PLL will travel

A. Hecht (✉)
Orthopedics and Neurosurgery, Icahn School of Medicine at Mount Sinai, New York, NY, USA
e-mail: Andrew.hecht@mountsinai.org

J. S. Markowitz
Department of Orthopaedic Surgery, Icahn School of Medicine at Mount Sinai, New York, NY, USA
e-mail: Jonathan.markowitz@mountsinai.org

© The Author(s), under exclusive license to Springer Nature Switzerland AG 2022
S. A. Mostoufi et al. (eds.), *Clinical Guide to Musculoskeletal Medicine*, https://doi.org/10.1007/978-3-030-92042-5_13

cephalad as the tectorial membrane and attaches at the base of the skull. The posterior ligamentous structures include the ligamentum flavum, facet joint capsule, and nuchal ligament, all of which are essential for cervical spine stability. The paired vertebral arteries typically run in the foramen transversarium of C1 through C6 on both sides of vertebral bodies. The apex of the odontoid process is generally supplied by branches of internal carotid artery, while the base is often supplied from branches of vertebral artery. Due to this unique blood supply, a vascular watershed area exists between the apex and base of the odontoid, thus affecting the healing potential of certain odontoid fractures [5].

13.1.4 Clinical Presentation

The most prevalent mechanisms of cervical spine injuries described in the literature are motor vehicle accidents (MVAs) and/or falls. Classically, MVAs are high-energy injuries and patients often present with multiple injuries including head trauma, pelvic ring fractures, long bone fractures, and chest contusions. Cervical spine injuries result from hyperflexion, hyperextension, axial loading, or rotational forces. While higher velocity mechanisms usually equate with a greater risk of injury, low-energy falls in the elderly have been shown to have a mortality rate as high as 25% [6]. Significant injuries can occur in patients with an ankylosed spine, and one should have a high degree of suspicion for cervical spine fractures in this patient population, even after minimal trauma.

An alert and oriented patient with a cervical spine injury will often endorse neck stiffness or pain with or without neurologic deficits. Fractures of C1, the atlas, account for 10% of all cervical spine fractures [7]. These fractures are generally classified based on the fracture location in the anterior arch, posterior arch, or lateral masses. A Jefferson fracture has a characteristic pattern of fractures in both the anterior and posterior arches of C1.

Odontoid fractures can be seen in low-energy falls in elderly patients and high-energy traumatic injuries in younger patients. Fractures of the odontoid process pose a unique challenge given a vascular watershed exists between the apex and the base of the odontoid. Odontoid fractures have been divided into 3 major types according to the classification of Anderson and D'Alonzo [8]. Type I is an avulsion of the odontoid tip by the alar ligaments. Type II occurs at the base of the odontoid process and represents the most common fracture type. Type III extends into the body of the axis and has good healing potential.

Traumatic spondylolisthesis of axis, colloquially referred to as a Hangman's fracture, is the result of a high-energy trauma. In this injury pattern, hyperextension and axial loading of the upper cervical spine cause bilateral fractures of the pars interarticularis, leading to anterior spondylolisthesis of the axis. This injury has been reported to make up 11–25% of all C2 fractures [9, 10].

Cervical facet dislocations most often occur as a result of a flexion/distraction injury to the cervical spine. This injury pattern causes failure of the posterior ligamentous elements and anterior displacement of the cephalad vertebral body relative to the caudal segment. Facet dislocation occurs when the inferior facet translates over the superior facet [Fig. 13.2].

Subaxial cervical spine injuries refer to injuries to the cervical spine that affect C3 to C7. These injuries can be osseous, ligamentous, or both. Fractures of the subaxial cervical spine include but are not limited to flexion teardrop and floating pillar fractures as well as cervical spinous process fractures, colloquially referred to as a clay-shoveler fracture. The most common classification used to describe cervical spine injuries is the subaxial injury classification system (SLIC)[11]. It takes into account 3 major aspects of injury; the morphology, the disco-ligamentous complex, and the patient's neurological status. In each category, points are awarded for abnormalities, where more points indicate a more severe injury, and the total score leads to a recommendation for surgical or non-surgical treatment.

13.1.5 Physical Examination

In acute severe trauma, Advanced Trauma Life Support (ATLS) guidelines should be followed. After the management of the airway, breathing, circulation, and all life-threatening injuries, a detailed history and physical examination should be performed. Paying particular attention to the mechanism of injury is important in identifying cervical injuries, as many injuries may be not be immediately evident. One should visually inspect the entire spine and palpate along the entire spinal column for tenderness, crepitus, and step-offs between spinous processes. A complete neurologic examination, one that examines cognitive function, cranial nerves, and motor and sensory functions of all extremities, which reflexes along with pathologic reflexes must be performed. The corresponding muscle group and sensory distribution for each cervical spinal root should be assessed. C3 to C4 contributes to breathing by controlling the muscles of the diaphragm and sensation to the lateral aspects of the face and posterior portion of the head. Patients with an injury to this area of the cervical spine can complain of difficulty breathing. Symptoms indicating neurological deficits at any level can include weakness or paralysis of innervated muscle group, decreased or absent reflexes, loss of sensation, and/or proprioception. Patient's neurologic function should be documented according to the American Spinal Injury Association (ASIA) standards (Fig. 13.1).

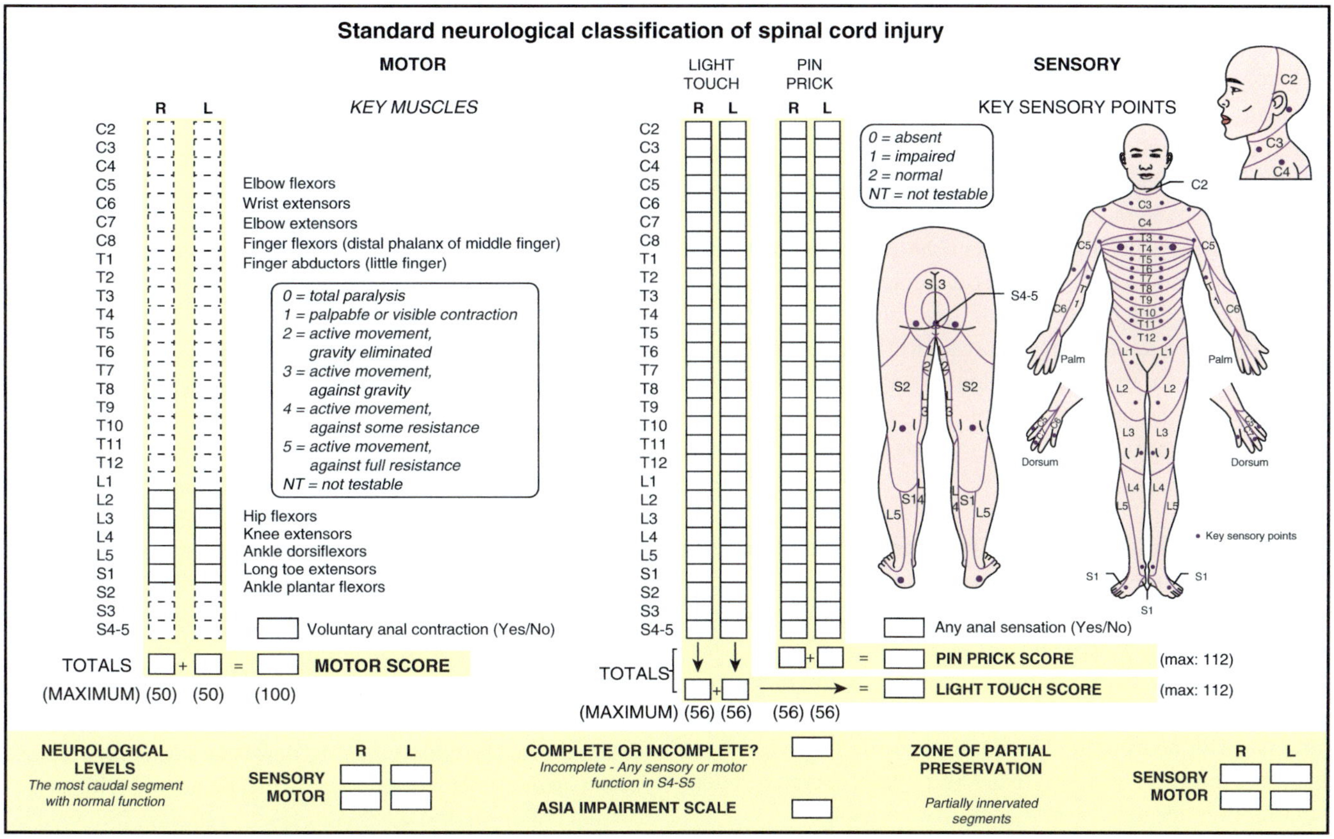

Fig. 13.1 American Spinal Injury Association (ASIA) form (From American Spinal Injury Association: International Standards for Neurological Classification of Spinal Cord Injury with permission of American Spinal Cord Injury Association, Chicago, IL)

Perianal and anal sensation, both volition and resting rectal tone assessed by a digital rectal examination, as well as the bulbocavernosus reflex must be assessed and documented in anyone presenting with a suspected spinal injury. An absent bulbocavernosus reflex indicates that spinal shock is still present and the true extent of neurologic impairment may not be fully appreciated.

13.1.6 Diagnostic Workup

X-Ray Historically, a single cross-table lateral radiograph was commonly used as a screening tool for cervical spine trauma. A major limitation in using plain radiographs as a screening tool includes the inherent difficulty in assessing discoligamentous injuries and the cervicothoracic junction (C7 to T1). This is particularly difficult in patients with a large body habitus, as it is often hard to visualize anatomy at this level. When evaluating a lateral cervical spine radiograph, one should pay close attention to prevertebral soft tissue swelling and overall sagittal alignment. Sagittal alignment can be assessed by critically evaluating four imaginary parallel lines; the anterior vertebral line, which is formed by the anterior margin of the vertebral bodies, the posterior vertebral line, which is formed by the posterior margin of the vertebral bodies, the spinolaminar line, which is formed by the posterior margin of the spinal canal or the anterior cortical margin of the lamina, and lastly the posterior spinous line, which is a continuous line about the tips of the spinous processes. These four radiographic lines should follow a smooth, slightly lordotic curve without step-offs. Any malalignment should be considered evidence of bony or ligamentous injury. While flexion–extension radiographs are commonly used to evaluate cervical spine instability, they are not generally obtained in the acute setting. In an alert patient, an open-mouth odontoid view can be obtained to assess for odontoid fractures and a compromised TAL. Combined lateral mass displacement should be <6.9 mm, otherwise a TAL injury is assumed and the injury pattern is considered unstable [11]. Unilateral facet dislocations are often associated with facet fractures. In a unilateral facet dislocation, plain radiographs may demonstrate up to 25% vertebral body subluxation, whereas in bilateral facet dislocations, one can see about 50% vertebral subluxation.

Computer Tomography Studies have demonstrated that plain radiographs were missing a significant number of injuries [12, 13], and as a result, CT with sagittal and coronal reconstruction has largely replaced plain radiograph in the initial assessment of cervical spine trauma. Careful attention must be paid to the presence of fractures and altered relationships between the basion, occipital condyles, dens, atlas, and axis. Craniocervical instability can be evaluated using the Harris lines rule of 12 [14]. Transverse atlantal ligament (TAL) injury and C1–C2 instability can be evaluated by measuring the atlantodental interval (ADI), measured as the distance between the anterior odontoid cortex and the posterior cortex of the anterior arch of C1. An ADI > 3.5 mm in adults or 5 mm in children indicates possible C1–C2 instability.

MRI MRI is useful in assessing the intervertebral disc, ligamentous structures, and spinal cord. Magnetic resonance is not recommended as an initial screening tool in the workup of patients with cervical spine trauma as it has been shown that MRI is not cost-effective as a screening device in patients without neurologic deficits [15]. An MRI is indicated for patients with neurologic deficits, those with suspected ligamentous injuries and those that will require operative intervention in order to help with operative planning.

13.1.7 Treatments

Treatment algorithms for cervical spine injuries take into consideration the stability of the fracture pattern, potential for healing, fracture displacement, patient age, associated injuries, and the patient's neurological status. Generally, in the acute setting patients should be placed in a cervical collar and transfers should be minimized.

13.1.7.1 Medical Management

Non-operative treatment with a cervical spine orthosis is a common, definitive treatment for many spine injuries. This treatment modality is indicated for those with stable fractures that are likely to heal without surgical fixation or those patients who are not surgical candidates. Various cervical orthosis options exist, including soft collar, hard collar (i.e. Aspen Collar [Aspen Medical Products], Miami J [Össur]) cervicothoracic brace, and halo vests. When utilizing an orthosis to definitively treat a cervical spine injury, one should follow some general principles. A trained orthotist should fit the patient for the brace. The orthosis must control head mandible motion relative to the thorax. Twice daily skin checks should be ordered to assess for any skin irritation or breakdown. The patient, family, and nursing staff should be educated on the intricacies of the brace. Prolonged use of a poorly fitted collar can cause pressure ulcers. The use of halo vests in the elderly population should be used with caution as this treatment option has been associated with significant complications such as aspiration, pneumonia, and death [16]. Serial radiographs should be obtained while in the brace to assess for overall alignment, increasing cervical kyphosis, and/or subluxation. We generally recommend that follow-up radiographs are obtained at the 2-, 6-, and 10-week marks. Any change in the patient's neurological status or overall alignment on serial radiograph may be an indication to pursue operative intervention.

TAL injuries are often subclassified into intrasubstance tears vs. bony avulsion injuries at TAL insertion [17]. Bony avulsion injures of the TAL are generally treated non-operatively in a rigid cervical collar for up to 3 months. The optimal treatment for odontoid fractures remains controversial as there are many contributing factors, including fracture location and risk for non-union and patient age. Avulsion fractures of the odontoid apex and fractures through its base when treated with a cervical orthosis generally have good outcomes. Treatment of bilateral fractures of the pars interarticularis of C2, a traumatic spondylolisthesis of axis, is based on both the fracture displacement and whether there is intervertebral disc disruption making it grossly unstable. Fracture patterns that do not require surgery can be treated with a rigid cervical collar for 4–6 weeks or closed reduction followed by halo immobilization for 8–12 weeks. Cervical spinous process fractures are generally treated non-operatively with NSAIDs, rest, and immobilization in hard collar for comfort.

13.1.7.2 Rehabilitation

Physical therapy is important for those who sustain cervical spine trauma. Rehab protocols for cervical spine injuries vary drastically, and there is insufficient research on specific structured exercise programmes. Physical therapist will work with patients on range of motion and strengthening exercises, functional training, and postural education. Therapists will also provide patients with aerobic conditioning and home exercises programmes. In cases where patients sustain spinal cord injuries, therapists help maximize sensory and motor function recovery, prevent secondary complications, and help patients reintegrate into society.

13.1.8 Procedures

Closed reduction of cervical facet dislocation: The treatment of unilateral facet dislocations remains somewhat controversial, although most agree that closed reduction should be attempted. The ultimate goal of a closed reduction of a facet dislocation is to realign the facets and relieve any compression on the spinal cord or nerve roots. A closed reduction is usually attempted in an awake and cooperative individual where serial neurologic assessments can be performed throughout the procedure. Close reduction requires pharmacological sedation and muscle relaxation, mechanical traction, and repetitive radiographic evaluation. The patient is placed supine, and Gardner wells tongs are applied in the appropriate position. Traction weights of 10–15 lb are initially used to help with distraction. Gradual increase in axial traction is accomplished with the addition of weights in 5–10 lb. increments until a successful reduction is visualized (Fig. 13.2). It is important to perform serial neurologic and radiographic examinations after the addition of each weight. The procedure should be aborted with any change in a patient's neurologic status, and an MRI should be obtained immediately. After successful closed reduction, patients are generally treated with a cervical orthosis or a halo vest.

13.1.9 Surgery

Surgical intervention is indicated in unstable fracture patterns and those with neurologic injuries. Occipitocervical dissociation requires a posterior occipitocervical fusion. Combined lateral mass displacement that is >6.9 mm generally indicates an TAL injury that is considered unstable. These patients require a posterior C1–C2 fusion or an occipitocervical fusion. C1–C2 fusion can be achieved in a variety of ways, either through posterior wiring or transarticular screw fixation. Fractures through the odontoid waist have a more tenuous healing potential given that it is a true synovial joint and any amount of displacement in this area significantly decreases bony apposition. Generally, fractures through the odontoid waist are treated with surgical fixation via anterior odontoid screw or a C1–C2 posterior fusion depending on the fracture morphology. Bilateral fractures of the pars interarticularis of C2 that do require surgery either undergo a C2–C3 ACDF, posterior C1–C3 fusion, or bilateral C2 pars screw osteosynthesis. In unilateral facet fracture dislocations, displacement may occur when there is a fracture that is >40% of the facet. These fracture dislocations are generally considered unstable and require open reduction and surgical stabilization usually via an anterior cervical discectomy and fusion. Bilateral facet dislocations are associated with disruption of the posterior osteoligamentous complex and by definition are considered unstable. Open vs. closed reduction must be performed, and operative stabilization is achieved with an anterior or posterior fusion. Flexion teardrop injuries are almost universally considered unstable and generally require surgical intervention with both anterior and posterior fusions with or without a corpectomy. Cervical spinous process fractures that experience a symptomatic non-union, surgical excision of the affected spinous processes can be considered. Chapters 15 and 16 contain more information on spine surgery.

13.2 Thoracic and Lumbar Vertebral Fractures

13.2.1 Synonyms

Compression fracture
Burst fracture
Chance fracture

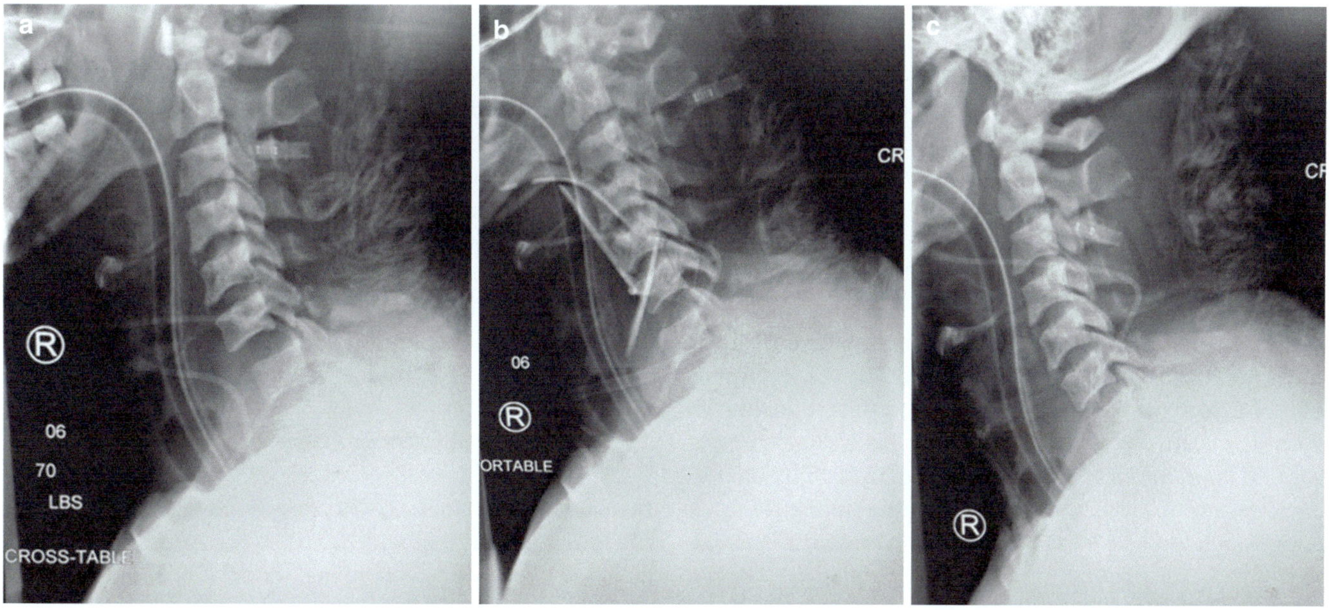

Fig. 13.2 Closed reduction of C6–C7 facet dislocations: (**a**) distraction with 30 pounds of weight, (**b**) complete distraction at 60 pounds, (**c**) successful reduction of C6–C7 facet dislocation

13.2.2 ICD 10 Code

Unspecified fracture of thoracic vertebra S22.019A-S22.089A

Unspecified fracture of unspecified lumbar vertebra S32.009A - S32.059A

Age-related osteoporosis with current pathological fracture, vertebra(e) M80.08XA

13.2.3 Description

Thoracolumbar (TL) spine fractures are common injuries that can result in significant disability, deformity, and neurological deficits. TL fractures range from low-energy insufficiency and fragility fractures to high-energy fractures and dislocations. In one series, 4.4% of all patients arriving at a level I trauma centre were eventually diagnosed with a TL fracture [18]. Injuries of the thoracic and lumbar spine are generally grouped anatomically, as pure thoracic (T1–T9), thoracolumbar (T10–L2), and low lumbar (L3–L5). Among TL injuries, about 50–60% affect the transitional zone (T11–L2), 25–40% affect the thoracic spine, and 10–14% involve the lower lumbar spine and sacrum [19]. TL fractures are generally classified by fracture morphology including compression, distraction, or translational-rotational injuries. Utilizing a systematic approach to appropriately evaluate and treat those with suspected thoracolumbar spine injuries is critical to achieve the best possible outcomes.

Anatomy The thoracic spine is composed of 12 vertebra and 12 paired spinal roots, while the lumbar spine is composed of 5 vertebra and 5 paired spinal roots. The thoracic spine is kyphotic and has some inherent stability afforded to it from the surrounding rib cage making this region of the spine relatively rigid. The narrow spinal canal in the region of the thoracic spine influences the high incidence of neurological deficits when an injury occurs at this level. Facet orientation dictates the principal motion of both the thoracic and lumbar spine. In the thoracic spine, the facets are generally oriented in the coronal plane allowing for mainly axial rotation. The lumbar spine exhibits an overall lordotic sagittal alignment. The facets in the lumbar spine are generally oriented in the sagittal plane allowing for maximal flexion and extension. The PLC, composed of the facet joint capsule, the interspinous ligament, supraspinous ligament, and ligamentum flavum, is important in overall spinal column stability, and its integrity must be assessed when evaluating patients with TL injuries. This soft tissue complex limits the spine from excessive flexion, distraction, translation, and rotation. The TL junction, T12–L1, is a transition point from the relatively rigid thoracic spine to the more mobile lumbar spine. As a result, this junction experiences a lot of stress and is more susceptible to injury than other levels.

13.2.4 Clinical Presentation

TL injuries range from low-energy insufficiency and fragility fractures to high-energy fractures and dislocations. Patients who present after a ground-level fall often complain of back pain and pain with ambulation. Those who experience TL injuries due to high-energy blunt trauma are often present with other distracting injuries such as head trauma, long bone fractures, pelvic ring injuries, intra-abdominal visceral injuries, rib fractures, and pneumo-hemothoraxes. The incidence of missed injuries of the TL spine has been reported to be as high as 20%, especially in those who present with an altered mental status after high-energy blunt trauma [20].

The most commonly used classifications to assess TL injuries include the thoracolumbar injury classification and severity (TLICS) scale [21] and the AO spine classification of thoracolumbar injuries. Both these classification systems attempt to predict the injury pattern's overall stability, natural history, and need for surgery. A numerical score is given to each category based on the injury morphology, neurologic status, and competency of the posterior ligamentous complex (PLC) (Fig. 13.3).

Compression fractures are the result of axial compression and subsequent failure of the anterior column of the vertebral body. In this injury pattern, the posterior column is generally spared. If an injury to the posterior column is present, one should consider a more significant injury such as a flexion–distraction injury. Burst fractures also result from an axial compression mechanism but are characterized by failure of both the anterior and middle columns with retropulsion of bone fragments into the spinal canal. This fracture pattern is distinguished from compression fractures in that the middle column, which includes the posterior portion of the vertebral body, is fractured as well (Fig. 13.4). Flexion-distraction injuries, also referred to as chance fractures or chance variants, are characterized by a horizontal fracture extending through the spinous process, the lamina, and pedicle into the vertebral body [22]. Flexion-distraction injuries may be entirely osseous, entirely discoligamentous or a combination of the two. This injury classically occurs in MVA due to lap-belt restraints and is often associated with intra-abdominal injuries. The incidence of neurologic deficits in flexion-distraction injuries is estimated to be between 10% and15% [20].

13.2.5 Physical Examination

In acute severe trauma, Advanced Trauma Life Support (ATLS) guidelines should be followed. After the management of the airway, breathing, circulation, and all life-threatening injuries, a detailed history and physical examination should be performed. Patients should be log rolled onto their side in a controlled manner and one should inspect and palpate the back for any swelling, palpable

Fig. 13.3 Thoracolumbar injury classification and severity score (TLICS) is a classification system for thoracolumbar spine injuries, designed to assist in clinical management

The Thoraco-Lumbar Injury Classification and Severity score (TLICS) 3 Independent Predictors				
1	Morphology	- Compression - Burst - Translation/rotation - Distraction	1 2 3 4	- Assess on Xray or CT
2	Integrity of PLC	- Intact - Suspected - Injured	0 2 3	- Assess on MRI
3	Neurological Status	- Intact - Nerve root - Complete cord - Incomplete cord - Cauda Equina	0 2 2 3 3	- Assess on physical exam
	Predicts	- Need for surgery	0-3 4 >4	- Non-surgical - Surgeon's choice - Surgical

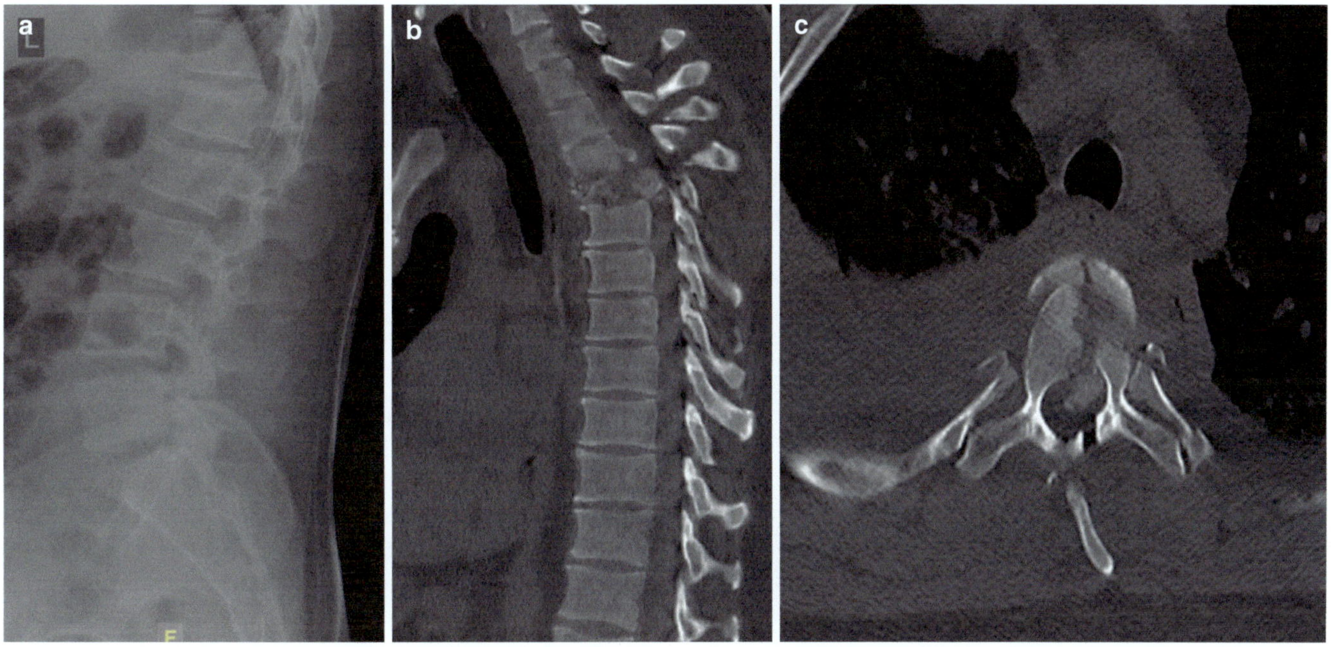

Fig. 13.4 (**a**) Lateral radiograph demonstrating compression fracture of the L1 and L2 vertebral bodies' superior endplate with approximately 25% vertebral body height loss, (**b**) sagittal CT scan demonstrating burst fractures of the T3 and T4 vertebral bodies, (**c**) axial CT scan demonstrating large T4 and retropulsed fracture fragments leading to central canal stenosis

subcutaneous fluid, crepitus, bony malalignment, and step-offs. A formal neurologic examination should examine strength, sensation, and reflexes of both the upper and lower extremities. Perianal and anal sensation, both volition and resting rectal tone assessed by a digital rectal examination, as well as the bulbocavernosus reflex must be assessed and documented in anyone presenting with a suspected spinal injury. The bulbocavernosus reflex is a well-known somatic reflex that is useful for gaining information about the state of the sacral spinal cord segments. An absent bulbocavernosus reflex indicates that spinal shock is still present and the true extent of neurologic impairment may not be fully appreciated. In high-energy trauma, one should pay careful attention to the presence of overt occult blood in the urethral meatus, rectum, or vaginal vault.

13.2.6 Diagnostic Workup

X-Ray AP and lateral radiographs of the thoracic and lumbar spine can be used as an initial screening tool for suspected TL spine trauma. The anteroposterior radiograph should be used to assess the interpedicular distance, overall coronal alignment, and the presence or absence of rib and transverse process fractures. When evaluating the lateral radiograph, one should examine the vertebral body height/width and overall sagittal alignment. The anterior and posterior vertebral body margins should have an overall contiguous alignment with the cranial and caudal vertebral bodies. One should also pay close attention to the radiographic findings commonly seen in patients with an ankylosed spine such as ankylosing spondylitis (AS) or diffuse idiopathic skeletal hyperostosis (DISH). In this patient population, if there is not an obvious fracture on plain radiographs, advanced imaging such as a CT should be obtained.

Computed Tomography Similar to cervical spine trauma, CT has generally supplanted XR in the initial evaluation of TL trauma. Studies have shown that CTs more reliably diagnose TL spine fractures than XR [23].

MRI MRI is generally used as an adjunct to CT given the cost and logistics associated with obtaining one. MRI can aid in understanding the severity of one's injury and should be obtained in a patient with neurological deficits. This imaging modality is particularly useful in assessing the extent of spinal cord, disc, and ligament injury and delineates the presence of oedema, hematoma, cord compression, and neural root compression. MRI is used to help assess the integrity of the PLC. Definite PLC injury is defined as loss of low signal intensity of the ligamentum flava or supraspinous ligaments on T1 and T2, while high signal intensity of the interspinous ligaments or along the facet joint on T2 STIR may be indicative of PLC injury.

13.2.7 Treatments

13.2.7.1 Medical Management

The appropriate type of non-operative treatment, the indications for surgical management, the timing of surgery, surgical approach, and the role of spinal canal decompression are debated. The use of steroids in the acute treatment of those with spinal cord injuries is controversial, and the initial positive results presented in the North American Spinal Cord Injury Study (NASCIS) have been criticized.

The role of bracing in thoracolumbar trauma is controversial. When bracing is indicated, it provides relative immobilization of the spine above and below the level of the injury. Injuries to the mid-to-low thoracic and upper lumbar spine that are amenable to non-operative intervention can be treated with a standard thoracolumbar orthosis. Injuries to the lower lumbar spine are more difficult to immobilize because of the difficulty immobilizing the segments caudal to the lumbosacral junction. These injuries often require a thoracolumbosacral orthosis that occasionally incorporates one of the thighs in order to maximize stability. When utilizing an orthosis to definitively treat a TL injury, one should follow some general principles. A trained orthotist should fit the patient for the brace. Once the brace is fitted, erect radiographs should be obtained to assess fracture stability and alignment in the brace. Serial radiographs should be obtained while in the brace to assess for overall alignment, increasing kyphosis, and/or subluxation. We generally recommend that follow-up radiographs are obtained at the 2-, 6-, and 10-week marks. Any change in the patient's neurological status or overall alignment on serial radiograph may be an indication to pursue operative intervention. We strongly advise patients to wear the brace whenever out of bed and to refrain from any bending, lifting, and twisting (BLT). We begin weaning the brace once there is both clinical and radiographic evidence of fracture healing. Upon discontinuation of the brace, we obtain flexion extension radiographs to ensure that there is no evidence of dynamic instability.

Compression fractures are inherently stable and generally not associated with severe neurological insult. As a result, these fractures are commonly treated non-operatively. In these injuries, bracing is not needed for stability but can be used for comfort. The severity of burst fractures exists on a spectrum from stable to unstable burst fractures. While the definition of stability is controversial, factors that guide treatment include the presence or absence of neurological injury, degree of angular kyphosis, and vertebral body height loss at the level of the injury, the integrity of the PLC, and the extent of spinal canal compromise. Some authors have advocated for bracing treatment in patients who are neurologically intact with less than 30° of angular kyphosis and 50% vertebral body height loss at the injured level and no injury to the PLC [24, 25]. Other randomized controlled trials assessing bracing in stable thoracolumbar burst fractures in neurologically intact patients have shown that bracing may not offer any clinical or radiographic advantage over mobilization without a brace [26, 27]. Osseous flexion distraction injuries are generally amenable to bracing in TLSO brace, while discoligamentous injuries are more likely to require surgery as the PLC does not reliably heal well.

13.2.7.2 Rehabilitation

There is no consensus on the rehabilitation protocols for patients with thoracolumbar trauma. Physical therapists will work with patients on range of motion and strengthening exercises of the back, and abdominal and leg musculature. Functional training, postural education, aerobic conditioning, and home exercises programmes will be provided for patients. Therapists will also assist patients with soft tissue mobilization as needed for areas of soft tissue restriction or muscle guarding. In cases where patients sustain spinal cord injuries, therapists help maximize sensory and motor function recovery, prevent secondary complications, and help patients reintegrate into society.

13.2.8 Procedures

Vertebroplasty/kyphoplasty: Both vertebroplasty and kyphoplasty have been used in the treatment of osteoporotic compression fractures to address both progressive kyphotic deformity and persistent pain that is refractory to nonsurgical management. While both of these modalities involve percutaneous fluoroscopic or CT-guided injection of polymethylmethacrylate (PMMA) into the vertebral body, kyphoplasty attempts to elevate the endplate and restore vertebral height. These interventions are described in detail in the osteoporosis chapter.

13.2.9 Surgery

The goals of surgical intervention for TL injuries are to achieve and maintain anatomic reduction and stability of the fracture, minimize construct length while providing sufficient stability to allow for early mobilization, achieve neural element decompression when necessary, and minimize complications. While non-operative treatment is generally recommended for compression fractures, surgical intervention for this fracture pattern can be considered in the setting of significant kyphosis and/or vertebral height loss, although the degree of deformity or vertebral body height loss is debated in the literature. When surgery is indicated, posterior spinal fusion with pedicle screw and rod fixation is the traditional mode of treatment. Patients who experience a burst fracture with associated neurologic injury or PLC disruption are best treated surgically in order to maximize the chance for neurologic recovery, prevent further neurologic deterioration, and allow for early mobilization. Surgical approaches vary depending on the fracture morphology and need for decompression but can be accomplished from both anterior and posterior approaches. Unstable flexion-distraction injuries are generally treated via a posterior spinal fusion with pedicle screw and rod constructs.

13.3 Spondylolysis and Spondylolisthesis

13.3.1 Synonyms

Vertebral body slippage
Pars interarticularis fracture

13.3.2 ICD 10 Code

Spondylolisthesis, acquired M43.10
Spondylolisthesis, congenital Q76.2
Spondylolysis, lumbosacral region M43.07

13.3.3 Description

Lumbar spondylolysis and spondylolisthesis are often identified in the evaluation of patients with low back pain. Spondylolysis refers to an anatomical defect or fracture of the pars interarticularis of the vertebra. The pathology seems to be rare in patients under 5 years old, but by the age of 6 the reported prevalence of isthmic spondylolysis is 4.4%, which increases to 6% by adulthood [28]. While studies have demonstrated that there may be a mechanical aetiology to the development of isthmic spondylolysis, other studies suggest that spondylolysis may have a genetic predisposition as spondylolysis occurs in 15–70% of first-degree relatives of individuals with this disorder [29, 30]. Spondylolysis can progress to spondylolisthesis, which is defined as anterior displacement of the vertebral body in reference to the bordering vertebral bodies. The risk of progression to spondylolisthesis is greater if the pars interarticularis defect is bilateral rather than unilateral. There are six broad categories of spondylolisthesis, which include dysplastic, isthmic, degenerative, traumatic, pathologic, and iatrogenic [31]. Both spondylolysis and spondylolisthesis vary in their presentations and require the application of both conservative and surgical treatment strategies.

Anatomy The lumbar spine is composed of 5 vertebra and 5 paired spinal roots. The lumbar spine exhibits an overall lordotic sagittal alignment, and their facets are generally oriented in the sagittal plane, allowing for maximal flexion and extension. The pars interarticularis is a small segment of bone that lies between the superior and inferior articular processes bilaterally at each vertebral level.

13.3.4 Clinical Presentation

Spondylolysis is usually asymptomatic and may be found incidentally on standard radiographic imaging. Those who are symptomatic tend to endorse pain after an inciting event and usually present with focal, dull, aching, non-radiating lower back pain that is exacerbated with back extension. Biomechanical studies have shown that repetitive hyperextension stress to the pars interarticularis is a risk factor for spondylolysis, and as a result, this pathology is commonly seen in athletes such as football linemen, divers, gymnasts, and weight lifters. Spondylolysis occurs at the L5 vertebrae between 85% and 95% of the time and at L4 vertebrae between 5% and15% of the time [32]. Degenerative spondylolisthesis occurs mostly at the L4–L5 level, as opposed to isthmic spondylolisthesis, which occurs most often at L5–S1 [31]. Progression of spondylolisthesis after the age of 20 years is much less common than progression during childhood and adolescence. Patients with degenerative spondylolisthesis often complain of axial back pain and endorse bilateral radicular symptoms more commonly than unilateral radiculopathy. Classically, patients present with symptoms associated with L5 nerve root compression, including pain radiating to the buttocks and posterior thigh and/or weakness of the extensor hallucis longus. Spondylolysis with spondylolisthesis may result in significant neuroforaminal compression. Those with low-grade slips may present with intermittent radiculopathy. In patients who have central stenosis, neurogenic claudication may be their presenting symptom. These patients often report their claudicatory or radicular symptoms are relieved with forward flexion, and therefore, they prefer to stand with a kyphotic lumbar posture in order to relieve pressure off of the nerve roots.

13.3.5 Physical Examination

Patients should undergo a comprehensive neurologic examination that examines strength, sensation, and reflexes of both the upper and lower extremities. In acute cases of spondylolysis, palpation of the lumbar spine may reveal focal tenderness. Patients generally maintain full painless flexion, but hyperextension tends to exacerbate one's symptoms. A single leg hyperextension test can be performed to help differentiate between unilateral and bilateral lysis. This test is performed by asking the patient to bear weight on one leg while flexing the hip and knee of the contralateral leg and hyperextending the lumbar spine. If the patient experiences asymmetrical lower back pain, this generally indicates a unilateral spondylolysis. Patients with spondylolysis generally present with a grossly unremarkable neurological examination.

Patients with high-grade spondylolisthesis often ambulate and stand with increased flexion at the hips and knees due to hamstring tightness. Scoliosis is often associated with spondylolisthesis, and the evaluation of both the patient's global coronal and sagittal alignment should be included in the physical examination. Those with high-grade spondylolisthesis may present with a palpable step-off over the spinous processes.

13.3.6 Diagnostic Workup

X-ray: Standing posteroanterior and lateral radiographs of the thoracolumbar spine are most useful in performing an initial assessment to evaluate for potential spondylolysis or spondylolisthesis. The standard posteroanterior radiographic view allows evaluation of coexisting scoliosis and overall coronal alignment. The standing lateral view is useful in identifying spondylolytic defects and documenting the degree of spondylolisthesis. Isthmic spondylosis is visualized as lucency in the region of the pars interarticularis. This lucency is commonly described as a broken neck of the Scotty dog (Fig. 13.5). The Meyerding classification quantifies the amount of forward translation of the vertebral body in relation to the caudal vertebra based on the standing lateral radiograph. There are five grades of spondylolisthesis, with grade I < 25 per cent slippage, grade II 26–50% slippage, grade III 51–75% slippage, grade IV 76–100% slippage, and grade V over 100% slippage, and are referred to as spondyloptosis [33] (Fig. 13.6). The standing lateral radiograph is used to assess the slip angle, which quantifies the degree of lumbosacral kyphosis that has occurred in association with this anterior translation. Standing lateral flexion–extension views assess for the presence of any instability and are essential for further treatment planning.

Computed Tomography In patients whose plain radiographs are normal but the history and physical examination are strongly suggestive of the spondylolysis, thin-cut axial CT is highly effective for detecting such pathology. Thin section CT scans can aid with defining the bony anatomy, identifying dysplastic facets, quantifying the degree of cortical disruption, and identifying sclerosis at the pars, lamina, or pedicle.

MRI MRI is recommended in all cases with neurologic findings. MRI is useful in assessing nerve root compression, lumbar disc, and spinal cord abnormalities. MRI offers the

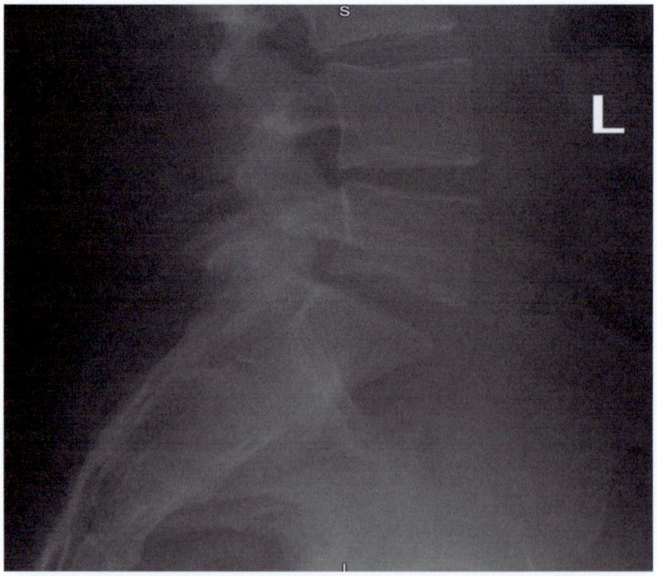

Fig. 13.5 Lateral radiograph of the lumbosacral spine demonstrating an L5 spondylolysis

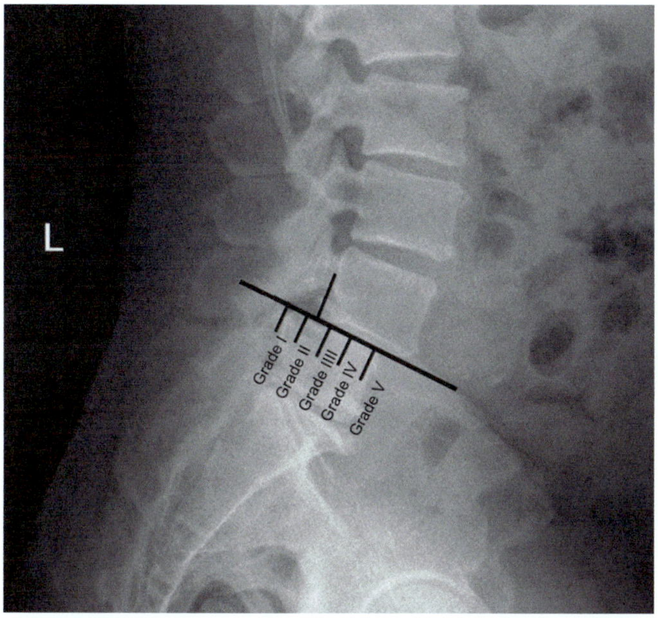

Fig. 13.6 L4–L5 grade II spondylolisthesis based on the Meyerding classification. The Meyerding classification of spondylolisthesis classifies the grade based on the amount of slippage of the superior vertebral body on the vertebral body below. Grade I indicates slippage from 5% to 25%; grade II is 26% to 50%; grade III is 51% to 75%; grade IV is more than 75%; and grade V is complete dislocation of adjacent vertebrae, also called spondyloptosis

distinct advantage of identifying stress reactions at the par interarticularis early on in the disease process prior to the end-stage bony defect.

13.3.7 Treatments

Few clinical trials exist that focus on the treatment of spondylolysis making it difficult to determine a proper treatment algorithm for conservative and surgical treatment. Young patients with spondylolysis generally receive conservative management as their initial treatment, although the specific non-operative protocol depends on several factors including the degree of spondylolisthesis, laterality of the defect, duration of symptoms, and the patients' age.

13.3.7.1 Medical Management

The initial treatment for spondylolysis focuses on rest to reduce pain and allow for bony union. We recommend that patients refrain from participating in sporting activities for at least 3 months. The effectiveness of antilordotic orthotics is debated. These braces are fabricated to prevent excessive hyperextension and rotation. Our preferred orthosis is a modified Boston brace, which is an anti-lordotic, total contact, low-profile polyethylene orthosis that extends from just below the nipples to 1 inch above the trochanters. We recommend the brace be worn for 23 hours/day for 6–12 weeks [34]. Early treatment with brace immobilization and PT has been shown to be more effective than bracing and beginning PT after an initial trial period of activity restriction [35, 36]. Studies have shown that in young patients with spondylolysis, there are no significant differences in functional outcomes and pain levels at 1 year between those who undergo non-operative vs. operative treatment [37]. After patients experience complete symptom relief and no pain with lumbar hyperextension, we wean them out of the orthosis and allow them to ease back into sports over a 2-month course while progressing with physical therapy.

While patients with low-grade dysplastic spondylolisthesis due to facet hypoplasia and high-grade isthmic spondylolisthesis are less likely to respond to conservative management than patients with low-grade isthmic spondylolisthesis, conservative therapy should still be initially attempted.

13.3.7.2 Rehabilitation

Early involvement of physical therapy is encouraged in the management of patients with lower back pain, neurogenic claudication, and/or radiculopathy. The goals of physical therapy are to reduce pain, to restore range of motion and function, and to strengthen and stabilize the spine.

Physical therapy activities may be active or passive. In the acute setting passive techniques such as massages, thermal therapy, and ultrasound are used to help ameliorate acute symptoms and encourage participation in active portion of physical therapy. The Watkins–Randall protocol is our preferred physical therapy protocol. Both passive and active ranges of motion exercises are encouraged. We generally recommend flexion exercises rather than extension exercises [38, 39] and isometric back and deep abdominal musculature strengthening [40].

13.3.8 Procedures

Epidural steroid injections (ESIs): ESIs should be considered in those who fail a reasonable course of therapy. ESI involves delivery of a corticosteroid solution, such as methylprednisolone, either in the interlaminar space or the transforaminal nerve root. While no studies have evaluated the effectiveness of epidural steroid injections in patients with degenerative spondylolisthesis alone, multiple studies have shown that patients with spinal stenosis can expect improvement in their pain and functional measures [41].

13.3.9 Surgery

Surgical management is indicated for patients with persistent pain, progressive spondylolisthesis, and neurologic symptoms despite conservative management. The goal of surgical intervention is to achieve neural decompression and stabilization of the unstable segment with an instrumented fusion. While the treatment approach is influenced by the degree of slippage, expected progression, patient's activity level, and symptomatology, the two broad categories of surgical options are a direct repair of the pars defect or fusion of the lumbar segment. Isolated repair of the pars defect can be achieved via multiple techniques including the Buck technique, Scott wiring [42, 43], or repair with an ipsilateral pedicle screw and hook. Isolated repair of the pars interarticularis defect is preferred in cases of L1 to L4 isthmic defect without disc degeneration and/or spondylolisthesis that have failed non-operative management. Direct repair of the pars interarticularis preserves motion while avoiding fusion and the potential for adjacent segment degeneration in the future. We recommend a posterolateral fusion without or without an anterior interbody fusion for patients with a progressive grade I or II spondylolisthesis, dysplastic spondylolisthesis, or an L5 isthmic spondylolysis who have failed conservative treatment. Treatment of high-grade spondylolisthesis, defined as Meyerding grades III, IV, and V, is more controversial. While conservative measures should initially be attempted, these patients tend to not respond as well as patients with lower-grade spondylolisthesis. If conservative treatment fails, a posterolateral fusion, with or without an anterior interbody fusion, is widely recommended in patients with high-grade spondylolisthesis. Reduction of the spondylolisthesis is more controversial with no widely accepted guidelines. Most authors attempt to correct the slip angle rather than the degree of anterior listhesis.

13.4 Sacral/Coccyx Fractures

13.4.1 Synonyms

Sacral insufficiency fracture
Lumbopelvic disassociation

13.4.2 ICD 10 Code

Unspecified fracture of sacrum S32.10XA
Fracture of coccyx S32.2XXA

13.4.3 Description

The sacrum acts as the keystone of the pelvic ring, as it maintains stability while transmitting forces from the lumbosacral articulation across the sacroiliac joints to the pelvis. As a result, injuries to the sacrum can potentially compromise the stability of the pelvic ring, the spinopelvic junction, or both. Sacral fractures may result in altered spinal sagittal alignment, chronic pain, loss of lower extremity motor and/or sensory function, sexual dysfunction, and urinary and bowel dysfunction. The severity of sacral and coccyx fractures varies widely from insufficiency fractures seen in the elderly, to complex fracture patterns seen in those who sustain high-energy injuries, or falls from significant heights. The incidence of non-osteoporotic sacral fractures has been reported as 21 cases per a million individuals, while osteoporotic fractures have been reported to have an incidence of 1–5% in elderly patients at risk [44]. In the USA, between 2002 and 2011, there has been a reported three-fold increase in traumatic sacral fractures from 0.7 to 2.9 per 100,000 in the population [45]. Treatment algorithms for sacral fractures are nuanced and require an understanding of both non-operative and operative treatment options.

Anatomy The sacrum is the lowest functional portion of the spinal column and is composed of 5 kyphotically aligned fused vertebra and 5 paired spinal nerve roots. The coccyx is the terminal segment of the spine that consists of 3 to 5 fused segments. The sacrum has 4 paired ventral and dorsal neuroforamina through which the ventral and dorsal nerve roots exit. The sacrum acts as an anchor point for the mobile lumbar spine and forms the posterior segment of the pelvic ring through the sacroiliac joints. Biomechanically, the sacrum functions to transfer loads from the spinal column to the pelvis. Variation in the upper sacral anatomy exists including transitional vertebra and sacral dysplasia. Several ligaments that are essential for maintaining the stability of the pelvic ring originate on the sacrum. These include the sacrospinous and sacrotuberous ligaments, anterior and posterior sacroiliac ligaments, along with the iliolumbar and lateral lumbosacral ligaments. A large number of neurovascular structures, including the cauda equina, the filum terminale, the sacral plexus, and the sciatic nerve are positioned within close proximity to the sacrum and may be injured in association with sacral fractures. The L5 nerve root lies on the anterosuperior surface of the S1 vertebral body and sacral ala. The common iliac arteries bifurcate at the lumbosacral junction giving rise to the internal and external iliac arteries, which course anterolateral to the iliac veins.

13.4.4 Clinical Presentation

Close to 75% of patients who present to the emergency room with sacral fractures are neurologically asymptomatic, making these fractures difficult to clearly diagnosis [45]. The rate of missed or delayed diagnosed sacral fractures ranges from 25% to 70% [44]. Sacral fractures occur in two distinctly different patient populations. Firstly, insufficiency fractures occur in those with suboptimal bone quality and typically occur in post-menopausal women due to osteoporosis. Sacral insufficiency fractures are estimated to occur in 1% of women older than age 55 years [46]. Other risk factors for sacral insufficiency fractures include chronic corticosteroid therapy, rheumatoid arthritis, radiation, and other endocrinopathies such as hyperparathyroidism. These insufficiency fractures often occur after a fall onto the buttock from a standing or sitting position. Patients often present with vague and poorly localized lower back pain without or without lumbosacral radiculopathy. In contrast, complex sacral fracture patterns are seen in those who sustain high-energy injuries or who fall from significant heights. Sacral fractures associated with high-energy trauma often co-exist with other injuries including pelvic ring injuries, head, and thoracoabdominal trauma. Various classification schemes exist to describe sacral fractures. These classifications schemes can be categorized into classifications that are based on the energy of injury, fracture morphology, location, and association with pelvic ring injuries. The Denis classification categorizes sacral fractures into 3 zones according to the location of the fracture relative to the sacral foramina and correlates the fracture location with the incidence of neurologic injury (Fig. 13.7). In zone 1, or the alar zone, fractures remain lateral to the neuroforamina throughout their course. In zone 2, or the foraminal zone, fractures involve one or more neuroforamina but remain lateral to the spinal canal. Zone 3 fractures, described as fractures medial to neuroforamina, are reported to have the highest risk of neurological injury and worse prognosis. Denis and colleagues found that zone 1 fractures had 5.9% incidence of neurologic injury, while zone 3 fractures had a 56.7% incidence of neurologic injury [47]. Descriptive classifications of sacral fractures include the H, Y, and lambda fracture patterns and the sacral U variant, which leads to inherent spinopelvic instability.

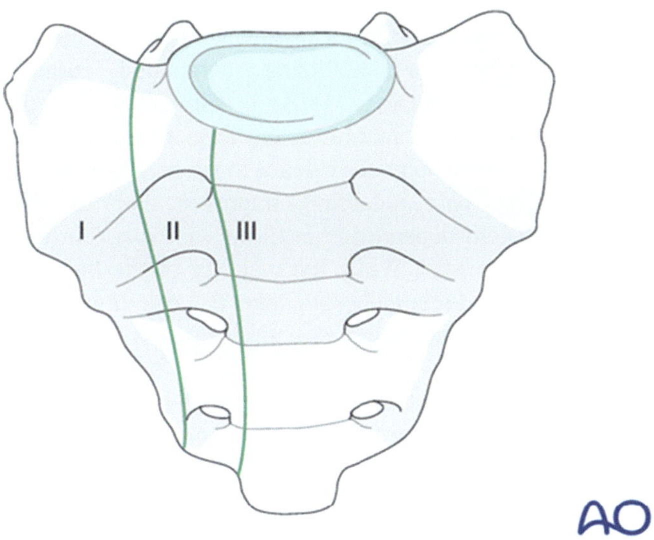

Fig. 13.7 Denis classification sacral fractures: In zone 1, fractures remain lateral to the neuroforamina throughout their course and have a 5.9% incidence of neurologic injury. In zone 2, fractures involve one or more neuroforamina but remain lateral to the spinal canal and have a 28.4% incidence of neurologic injury. In zone 3 fractures, fractures are medial to neuroforamina and are reported to have up to a 56.7% incidence of neurological injury and worse prognosis. Copyright of AO Foundation, Switzerland

Coccyx fractures generally occur after a backwards fall onto the buttocks. Patients often present complaining of "tailbone pain". The pain will usually be worse with prolonged sitting, leaning back while seated, prolonged standing, and rising from a seated position.

13.4.5 Physical Examination

In acute severe trauma, Advanced Trauma Life Support (ATLS) guidelines should be followed. After the management of the airway, breathing, circulation, and all life-threatening injuries are stabilized, a detailed history and physical examination should be performed. The initial physical examination should include visual inspection for ecchymosis and lacerations along the entire vertebral column. Palpation should then be performed along the entire spinal column for any areas of tenderness or step-offs. Particular attention should be paid to the pelvic ring. Manual compression over the iliac crests may help identify pelvic ring instability and the need for temporary methods of pelvic ring stabilization. Next, a comprehensive neurological examination should be performed that assesses the overall severity of neurologic injury according to the ASIA score. The majority of the nerves that exit through the sacral foramina are involved in urogenital and anal sphincter control and perineal sensation. Therefore, a thorough neurological examination should include an evaluation of one's anal sphincter tone, resting and volitional perianal contraction, perianal sensation, and the bulbocavernosus reflex. An absent bulbocavernosus reflex indicates that spinal shock is still present and the true extent of neurologic impairment may not be fully appreciated. Once one's spinal shock has resolved, an absent bulbocavernosus reflex may indicate an injury to the S2–S4 nerve roots.

13.4.6 Diagnostic Workup

X-ray Plain radiographs with an anteroposterior pelvis view and inlet/outlet views are generally used as the first line of investigation and should be carefully scrutinized for the presence of sacral and coccyx fractures. Identification of sacral fractures on plain radiographs can be challenging for a number of reasons including juxtaposition of the iliac wings, sacral dysmorphism, and osteoporotic bone. Associated signs on plain radiographs that should raise concern for a possible sacral fracture include L4 or L5 transverse process fractures and anterior pelvic ring disruptions. A lateral radiograph of the sacrum can be obtained and is useful in evaluating the presence of transverse fractures. The Ferguson view, a true anterior–posterior view of the sacrum, is obtained with a 30 degree cranially inclined projection. Advanced imaging as opposed to plain radiographs is often recommended when assessing sacral fractures, as the overall detection rate in plain radiographs has been reported to be as low as 30%. The evaluation of patients with persistent coccyx pain following a coccyx fracture should include dynamic radiographs taken with the patient standing and sitting to assess for coccyx hypermobility or non-union.

Computed tomography CT scan is considered the gold standard given its high sensitivity and specificity. CT scans of the abdomen and pelvis are also being used more routinely in the initial assessment of trauma patients and contribute a more sophisticated view of the sacrum for evaluation. Sagittal and coronal reconstructions should be obtained for adequate characterization of the fracture pattern. Three-dimensional CT reconstructions can help surgeons to assess the fracture patterns prior to surgery.

Magnetic resonance MRI is recommended in all cases with neurologic findings as it can be helpful in demonstrating areas of neural compression. If both radiographs and CT are inconclusive and suspicion remains high for an insufficiency fracture, then MRI should be performed and is considered the gold standard to diagnose occult fractures.

13.4.7 Treatments

13.4.7.1 Medical Management

The decision between non-operative vs operative treatment of sacral fractures must take into account the fracture pattern, location, presence of instability, or malalignment and the neurologic status of the patient. Sacral fractures are commonly defined as stable or unstable, with unstable fractures being those that are likely to shift or displace with physiological loads.

Non-operative treatment of sacral fractures is generally reserved for osteoporotic and minimally displaced fractures without neurologic injury. In those with non-displaced fractures, mobilization with a walker or crutches is generally recommended to allow for touch toe weight bearing on the injured side. These patients should be followed clinically to assess for new or worsening neurologic symptoms. Serial radiographs should be obtained to assess for fracture displacement.

Osteoporotic compression fractures are also generally amenable to non-operative treatment, which consists of rest, pain relief with NSAIDs, physical therapy, and early mobilization as tolerated. Treating the underlying cause of the patient's osteoporosis is crucial to decrease the risk of another insufficiency fracture. Vitamin D and calcium supplementation should be initiated to slow further bone loss. The use of bisphosphonates should be considered and discussed with one's primary care physician.

Conservative treatment of coccyx fractures is successful in the majority of individuals. We recommend patients use modified over-the-counter wedge-shaped cushions to relieve the pressure on the coccyx while the patient is seated. A limited course of NSAIDs along with the application of heat and/or cold packs can be used for symptomatic pain control.

13.4.7.2 Rehabilitation

Physical therapists will work with patients on range of motion and strengthening exercises of the back, abdominal, and leg musculature. Functional training, postural education, aerobic conditioning, and home exercise programmes will be provided for the patients. Therapists will also assist patients with soft tissue mobilization as needed for areas of soft tissue restriction or muscle guarding. In cases where patients sustain spinal cord injuries, therapists help maximize sensory and motor function recovery, prevent secondary complications, and help patients reintegrate into society.

13.4.8 Procedures

Sacroplasty: Sacroplasty is a percutaneous, image-guided technique where a stabilizing compound, usually polymethyl-methacrylate (PMMA), is administered into the cancellous portion of sacrum at the level of the fracture. There is a growing body of evidence to support its potential for significant pain reduction, improved mobility, and decreased opioid dependence in those with sacral insufficiency fractures [48]. While the majority of the literature has shown it to be relatively safe, there is a risk of extrusion of cement around the neural structures that could result in neural compromise.

Coccyx injections: Coccyx injections utilizing a combination of steroid and anaesthetic can be considered in those with persistent coccyx pain who have failed non-operative treatment.

Ganglion impar sympathetic nerve block: Ganglion impar sympathetic nerve blocks can be considered for patients with persistent coccydynia following coccyx fractures. In this treatment option, local injection of an anaesthetic is administered to the ganglion impar, which is usually located anterior to the sacrococcygeal junction or the first coccygeal vertebra. This technique has been reported to provide relief in 50–75% of patients [49].

13.4.9 Surgery

Although various classification schemes exist to help facilitate decision-making in those with sacral injuries, it is important to consider these classification systems within the context of the overall condition of the patient and their associated injuries. The timing of surgical intervention is determined by various factors including the patient's overall physiologic status, presence of open fractures, neurologic deficits, and overall soft tissue envelope. Surgical intervention is generally indicated for patients with sacral fractures with severe fracture displacement, fracture instability, and/or neurologic compromise. The goals of surgical treatment are neurological decompression in those with neurologic deficits and fracture reduction and stabilization in the cases of significant displacement or instability. Surgical fixation for these fractures is ideally percutaneous and utilizes a low implant profile to prevent skin breakdown and soft tissue compromise while providing enough biomechanical stability to allow for early mobilization. When sacral fractures are associated with a pelvic ring injury, anterior pelvic fixation techniques can be performed. Most fractures involving the pelvis, specifically the sacrum, can be effectively stabilized with posterior pelvic fixation. Posterior pelvic fixation connects the ilium to the sacrum, most commonly through an iliosacral screw. In this fixation pattern, a cannulated screw is inserted through the safe corridor of the S1 and/or S2 bodies. Another method of posterior pelvic fixation is a transiliac–transsacral screw, in which a long-threaded implant passes across the entirety of S1 or S2 corridor to the contralateral ilium. Significantly unstable fractures that create spinopelvic instability, as seen in vertical shear and U-type variants, require the addition of lumbopelvic fixation. Postoperative complications of sacral fracture fixation include infection, delayed wound healing, instrumentation failure, and soft tissue irritation requiring implant removal. The indication for coccygectomy is significant, disabling coccygodynia with radiographic subluxation or instability. This should only be considered after a significant trial of non-operative intervention has been pursued. The current literature suggests that a coccygectomy may provide relief in the appropriate patient who has failed all other non-operative treatments [50, 51]. However, this procedure can be associated with a high complication rate and failure to relieve the pain.

References

Cervical Spine Trauma and Injuries

1. Passias PG, Poorman GW, Segreto FA, Jalai CM, Horn SR, Bortz CA, Vasquez-Montes D, Diebo BG, Vira S, Bono OJ, De La Garza-Ramos R. Traumatic fractures of the cervical spine: analysis of changes in incidence, cause, concurrent injuries, and complications among 488,262 patients from 2005 to 2013. World Neurosurg. 2018;1(110):e427–37.
2. Goldberg W, Mueller C, Panacek E, Tigges S, Hoffman JR, Mower WR, NEXUS Group. Distribution and patterns of blunt traumatic cervical spine injury. Ann Emerg Med. 2001;38(1):17–21.
3. Oliver M, Inaba K, Tang A, Branco BC, Barmparas G, Schnüriger B, Lustenberger T, Demetriades D. The changing epidemiology of spinal trauma: a 13-year review from a level I trauma centre. Injury. 2012;43(8):1296–300.
4. Robinson AL, Olerud C, Robinson Y. Epidemiology of C2 fractures in the 21st century: a national registry cohort study of 6,370 patients from 1997 to 2014. Adv Orthoped. 2017;1:2017.
5. Schiff DC, Parke WW. The arterial supply of the odontoid process. JBJS. 1973;55(7):1450–6.
6. Damadi AA, Saxe AW, Fath JJ, Apelgren KN. Cervical spine fractures in patients 65 years or older: a 3-year experience at a level I trauma center. J Trauma Acute Care Surg. 2008;64(3):745–8.
7. Levine AM, Edwards CC. Treatment of injuries in the C1-C2 complex. Orthop Clin North Am. 1986;17(1):31–44.
8. Anderson LD, D'Alonzo RT. Fractures of the odontoid process of the axis. J Bone Joint Surg Am. 1974;56(8):1663–74.
9. Hadley MN, Dickman CA, Browner CM, Sonntag VK. Acute axis fractures: a review of 229 cases. J Neurosurg. 1989;71(5):642–7.
10. Wang H, Coppola M, Robinson RD, Scribner JT, Vithalani V, de Moor CE, Gandhi RR, Burton M, Delaney KA. Geriatric trauma patients with cervical spine fractures due to ground level fall: five years experience in a level one trauma center. J Clin Med Res. 2013;5(2):75.
11. Spence KF, Decker S, Sell KW. Bursting atlantal fracture associated with rupture of the transverse ligament. JBJS. 1970;52(3):543–9.
12. Bohlman HH. Acute fractures and dislocations of the cervical spine. An analysis of three hundred hospitalized patients and review of the literature. JBJS. 1979;61(8):1119–42.
13. Platzer P, Jaindl M, Thalhammer G, Dittrich S, Wieland T, Vecsei V, Gaebler C. Clearing the cervical spine in critically injured patients: a comprehensive C-spine protocol to avoid unnecessary delays in diagnosis. Eur Spine J. 2006;15(12):1801–10.
14. Harris JH Jr, Carson GC, Wagner LK. Radiologic diagnosis of traumatic occipitovertebral dissociation: 1. Normal occipitovertebral relationships on lateral radiographs of supine subjects. AJR Am J Roentgenol. 1994;162(4):881–6.
15. Vaccaro AR, Kreidl KO, Pan W, Cotler JM, Schweitzer ME. Usefulness of MRI in isolated upper cervical spine fractures in adults. J Spinal Disord. 1998;11(4):289–93.
16. Dickman CA, Greene KA, Sonntag VK. Injuries involving the transverse atlantal ligament: classification and treatment guidelines based upon experience with 39 injuries. Neurosurgery. 1996;38(1):44–50.
17. Majercik S, Tashjian RZ, Biffl WL, Harrington DT, Cioffi WG. Halo vest immobilization in the elderly: a death sentence? J Trauma Acute Care Surg. 2005;59(2):350–7.

Thoracic and Lumbar Vertebral Fractures

18. Cooper C, Dunham CM, Rodriguez A. Falls and major injuries are risk factors for thoracolumbar fractures: cognitive impairment and multiple injuries impede the detection of back pain and tenderness. J Trauma Acute Care Surg. 1995;38(5):692–6.
19. Gertzbein SD. Scoliosis Research Society. Multicenter spine fracture study. Spine. 1992;17(5):528–40.
20. Keene JS. Radiographic evaluation of thoracolumbar fractures. Clin Orthop Relat Res. 1984;189:58–64.
21. Vaccaro AR, Lehman RA Jr, Hurlbert RJ, Anderson PA, Harris M, Hedlund R, Harrop J, Dvorak M, Wood K, Fehlings MG, Fisher C. A new classification of thoracolumbar injuries: the importance

of injury morphology, the integrity of the posterior ligamentous complex, and neurologic status. Spine. 2005;30(20):2325–33.
22. Chance GQ. Note on a type of flexion fracture of the spine. Br J Radiol. 1948;21(249):452–3.
23. Hauser CJ, Visvikis G, Hinrichs C, Eber CD, Cho K, Lavery RF, Livingston DH. Prospective validation of computed tomographic screening of the thoracolumbar spine in trauma. J Trauma Acute Care Surg. 2003;55(2):228–35.
24. Cantor JB, Lebwohl NH, Garvey T, Eismont FJ. Nonoperative management of stable thoracolumbar burst fractures with early ambulation and bracing. Spine. 1993;18(8):971–6.
25. Mumford J, Weinstein JN, Spratt KF, Goel VK. Thoracolumbar burst fractures. The clinical efficacy and outcome of nonoperative management. Spine. 1993;18(8):955–70.
26. Bailey CS, Urquhart JC, Dvorak MF, Nadeau M, Boyd MC, Thomas KC, Kwon BK, Gurr KR, Bailey SI, Fisher CG. Orthosis versus no orthosis for the treatment of thoracolumbar burst fractures without neurologic injury: a multicenter prospective randomized equivalence trial. Spine J. 2014;14(11):2557–64.
27. Shamji MF, Roffey DM, Young DK, Reindl R, Wai EK. A pilot evaluation of the role of bracing in stable thoracolumbar burst fractures without neurological deficit. Clin Spine Surg. 2014;27(7):370–5.

Spondylolysis and Spondylolisthesis

28. Fredrickson BE, Baker D, McHolick WJ, Yuan HA, Lubicky JP. The natural history of spondylolysis and spondylolisthesis. JBJS. 1984;66(5):699–707.
29. Albanese M, Pizzutillo PD. Family study of spondylolysis and spondylolisthesis. J Pediatr Orthop. 1982;2(5):496–9.
30. Wynne-Davies R, Scott JH. Inheritance and spondylolisthesis: a radiographic family survey. J Bone Joint Surg Br. 1979;61(3):301–5.
31. Wiltse LL, Newman PH, Macnab IA. Classification of spondylosis and spondylolisthesis. Clin Orthop Relat Res. 1976–2007;117:23–9.
32. Hu SS, Tribus CB, Diab M, Ghanayem AJ. Spondylolisthesis and spondylolysis. JBJS. 2008;90(3):656–71.
33. Meyerding HW. Spondylolisthesis. Surg Gynecol Obstet. 1932;54:371–7.
34. Steiner ME, Micheli LJ. Treatment of symptomatic spondylolysis and spondylolisthesis with the modified Boston brace. Spine. 1985;10(10):937–43.
35. Blanda J, Bethem D, Moats W, Lew M. Defects of pars interarticularis in athletes: a protocol for nonoperative treatment. J Spinal Disord. 1993;6(5):406–11.
36. Selhorst M, Fischer A, Graft K, Ravindran R, Peters E, Rodenberg R, Welder E, MacDonald J. Timing of physical therapy referral in adolescent athletes with acute spondylolysis: a retrospective chart review. Clin J Sport Med. 2017;27(3):296–301.
37. Lee GW, Lee SM, Ahn MW, Kim HJ, Yeom JS. Comparison of surgical treatment with direct repair versus conservative treatment in young patients with spondylolysis: a prospective, comparative, clinical trial. Spine J. 2015;15(7):1545–53.
38. Gramse RR, Sinaki M, Ilstrup DM. Lumbar spondylolisthesis: a rational approach to conservative treatment. Mayo Clin Proc. 1980;55(11):681–6.
39. Sinaki M, Lutness MP, Ilstrup DM, Chu CP, Gramse RR. Lumbar spondylolisthesis: retrospective comparison and three-year follow-up of two conservative treatment programs. Arch Phys Med Rehabil. 1989;70(8):594–8.
40. O'Sullivan PB, Phyty GD, Twomey LT, Allison GT. Evaluation of specific stabilizing exercise in the treatment of chronic low back pain with radiologic diagnosis of spondylolysis or spondylolisthesis. Spine. 1997;22(24):2959–67.
41. Riew KD, Yin Y, Gilula L, Bridwell KH, Lenke LG, Lauryssen C, Goette K. The effect of nerve-root injections on the need for operative treatment of lumbar radicular pain: a prospective, randomized, controlled, double-blind study. JBJS. 2000;82(11):1589.
42. Johnson GV, Thompson AG. The Scott wiring technique for direct repair of lumbar spondylolysis. J Bone Joint Surg Bri. 1992;74(3):426–30.
43. Nicol RO, Scott JH. Lytic spondylolysis. Repair by wiring. Spine. 1986;11(10):1027–30.

Sacral/Coccyx Fractures

44. Santolini E, Kanakaris NK, Giannoudis PV. Sacral fractures: issues, challenges, solutions. EFORT Open Rev. 2020;5(5):299–311.
45. Bydon M, De la Garza-Ramos R, Macki M, Baker A, Gokaslan AK, Bydon A. Lumbar fusion versus nonoperative management for treatment of discogenic low back pain: a systematic review and meta-analysis of randomized controlled trials. J Spinal Disord Tech. 2014;27:297–304.
46. Mehta S, Auerbach JD, Born CT, Chin KR. Sacral fractures. JAAOS J Am Acad Orthopaedic Surg. 2006;14(12):656–65.
47. Mahmood B, Pasternack J, Razi A, Saleh A. Safety and efficacy of percutaneous sacroplasty for treatment of sacral insufficiency fractures: a systematic review. J Spine Surg. 2019;5(3):365.
48. Buttaci CJ, Foye PM, Stitik TP. Poster board 56: Coccydynia successfully treated with ganglion impar blocks: a case series. Am J Phys Med Rehabil. 2005;84(3):218.
49. Perkins R, Schofferman J, Reynolds J. Coccygectomy for severe refractory sacrococcygeal joint pain. Clin Spine Surg. 2003;16(1):100–3.
50. Trollegaard AM, Aarby NS, Hellberg S. Coccygectomy: an effective treatment option for chronic coccydynia: retrospective results in 41 consecutive patients. J Bone Joint Surg Br. 2010;92(2):242–5.
51. Browner BD, editor. Skeletal trauma: basic science, management, and reconstruction. Elsevier Health Sciences; 2009.

Minimally Invasive Spine Procedures

14

S. Ali Mostoufi and Cameron Mostoufi

14.1 Minimally Invasive Lumbar Decompression (Mild® Procedure)

14.1.1 CPT

0275T

14.1.2 Description

Lumbar Spinal Stenosis is an acquired or congenital condition in which the spinal canal diameter is reduced resulting in compression of neural and vascular elements. The hallmark of lumbar spinal stenosis is neurogenic claudication; numbness, pain, heaviness, and/or weakness in the legs radiate from the spine to the buttocks and legs while walking or prolonged standing. Neurogenic claudication is often relieved with sitting or stooping. Spinal stenosis is most commonly found in the lumbar vertebral region of the spine [1].

Traditional nonoperative management of spinal stenosis varies from rehabilitation, medical management, and utilization of assistive devices such as cane and walker, back brace, activity modification, and procedural treatment. Procedural treatment in general is indicated when less aggressive treatments fail. Traditional spinal injections are designed to improve neurogenic claudication by injecting corticosteroid into the epidural space via a transforaminal or interlaminar approach. Effectiveness and duration of efficacy for epidural injection vary from patient to patient. Such intervention often requires repetitive treatments over the course of the disease.

In the past, beyond physical therapy (PT), medication management, and steroid injections, nonoperative spine/pain specialist choices were limited except referring to spine surgery for isolated laminectomy or laminectomy with fusion (depends on the pathology and concerns regarding stability). Open laminectomy remains the gold standard operative care for spinal stenosis. With the advancement in technology, percutaneous minimally invasive lumbar decompression has become available to patients presenting with neurogenic claudication associated with walking and standing and resolves with sitting. Percutaneous decompression options may be desirable for patients averse to open surgery or for elderly patients with complicated medical history intolerant to anesthesia or open surgery (ASA III or above).

The criteria for percutaneous lumbar decompression (MILD procedure) are ligamentum flavum thickening of over 2.5 mm, neurogenic claudication, and resolution of neuroclaudication with sitting. If there is weakness associated with spinal stenosis, it is encouraged to seek surgical consultation for open surgical care.

To date, two randomized controlled trials, together with 11 other controlled clinical studies, have established the efficacy of *mild* procedure. MIDAS-I study, a multicenter, nonblinded, prospective clinical study evaluating Visual Analog Score (VAS), Oswestry Disability Index (ODI), Zurich Claudication Questionnaire (ZCQ), and SF-12 Health Survey after performing MILD procedure, showed statistically and clinically significant reduction in all metrics. There were no major mild device or procedure-related complications reported in this patient cohort, with major complications defined as dural tears, nerve root injury, post-op infection, and hemodynamic instability. For claudication symptoms, at 6 weeks, the mean patient satisfaction response was 2.02, on a scale of 1–4 (50%). With respect to disability index, this study showed a 17.9-point improvement in mean ODI from baseline to 6 weeks post. The average baseline VAS was 7.3

S. A. Mostoufi (✉)
Department of Orthopedics and Rehabilitation, Tufts University School of Medicine, Boston, MA, USA

New England Spine Care Associates & Boston Regenerative Medicine, Cambridge, MA, USA
e-mail: ali.mostoufi@tufts.edu

C. Mostoufi
Department of Mechanical Engineering, Purdue University, West Lafayette, IN, USA
e-mail: cmostouf@Purdue.edu

© The Author(s), under exclusive license to Springer Nature Switzerland AG 2022

S. A. Mostoufi et al. (eds.), *Clinical Guide to Musculoskeletal Medicine*, https://doi.org/10.1007/978-3-030-92042-5_14

(range 3/10–10/10), which improved to 3.7/10 (approximately 53% reduction) in a 6-week follow-up [2].

MIDAS ONCORE study examined the long-term durability of the minimally invasive lumbar decompression (MILD) procedure in terms of functional improvement and pain reduction for patients with lumbar spinal stenosis and neurogenic claudication due to hypertrophic ligamentum flavum. This prospective, multicenter, randomized controlled clinical study compared outcomes for minimally invasive lumbar decompression (MILD) procedure versus epidural steroid injections. Follow-up occurred at 6 months and at 1 year for the randomized phase and at 2 years for MILD subjects. Oswestry Disability Index, Numeric Pain Rating Scale, and Zurich Claudication Questionnaire were used to evaluate function and pain. Safety was evaluated by assessing incidence of device−/procedure-related adverse events. At 2 years, ODI improved by 22.7 points (95% CI, 18.5–26.9), NPRS improved by 3.6 points (95% CI, 3.1–4.2), and ZCQ symptom severity and physical function domains improved by 1.0 (95% CI, 0.8–1.2) and 0.8 points (95% CI, 0.6–0.9), respectively. During 2-year follow-up, 5.6% of patients required a subsequent surgical procedure (6–7.5% reoperation rate in traditional laminectomy) [3].

There were no serious device−/procedure-related adverse events, and 1.3% experienced a device−/procedure-related adverse event. MIDAS Encore study concluded that Mild procedure has excellent long-term durability, and there was no evidence of spinal instability through 2-year follow-up [4].

14.1.3 Surgical Technique

Minimally invasive lumbar decompression (*Mild*® procedure) is performed as an outpatient procedure in an ASC or hospital. Procedure is done in full surgical sterile technique following surgical standards. The *Mild*® procedure is performed percutaneously through a 5-mm port with specially designed surgical instruments and can be done unilaterally or bilaterally, and at multiple levels through a single midline skin entrance. After skin anesthesia, the path for *Mild*® trocar is anesthetized to the depth of the targeted laminas. Epidural space is accessed with the loss of resistance technique, and an epidurogram (Fig. 14.1) is performed to highlight posterior epidural space and the space between the dura and the lamina at the treatment level (Fig. 14.2). The *Mild*® Trocar and portal are then inserted (5 mm skin incision) and advanced to the inferior lamina of the level above and superior lamina of the level below, using a bone rongeur biopsy-sized fragments of bone for the purpose of widening the interlaminar space to allow further advancement of the cannula. Often partial removal of the lamina is also associated with removing the ligamentum flavum that is in its proximity. Once three passes at the superior lamina and three passes

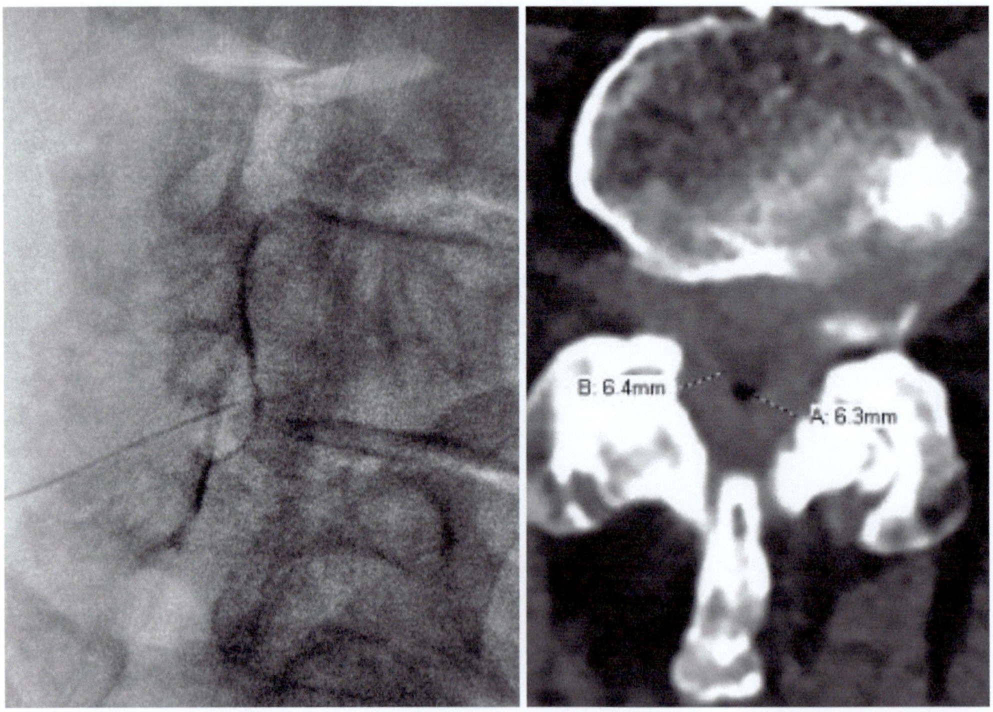

Fig. 14.1 Contralateral oblique view of epidurogram enhancing posterior epidural space highlighting safe space between the epidural line and lamina. The anterior displacement of dura is due to thickened ligamentum flavum resulting in central spinal canal stenosis. CT scan of the same patient showing spinal stenosis and thickening of ligamentum flavum, measured at 8.6 mm on right and 6.3 mm on left. (Image courtesy of Ali Mostoufi, MD, New England Spine Care, Cambridge, MA, USA)

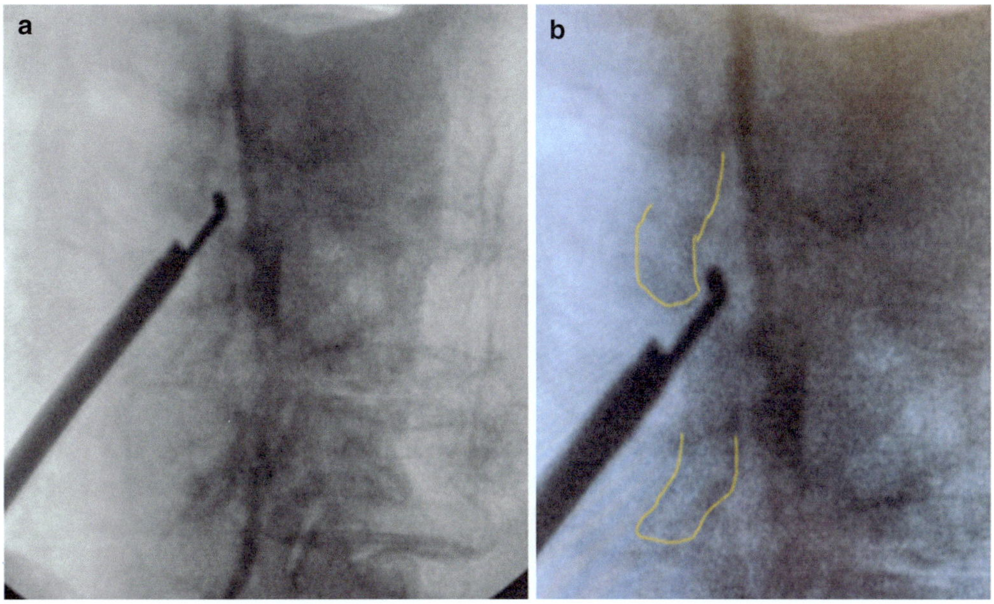

Fig. 14.2 (**a**) Removal of biopsy size bone from posterior lamina along with ligamentum flavum while the blunt side of the bone rongeur is away from posterior epidural line, highlighted by epidurogram. (**b**) Magnified image of the same patient, highlighting the superior and inferior lamina. (Image courtesy of Ali Mostoufi, MD, New England Spine Care, Cambridge, MA, USA)

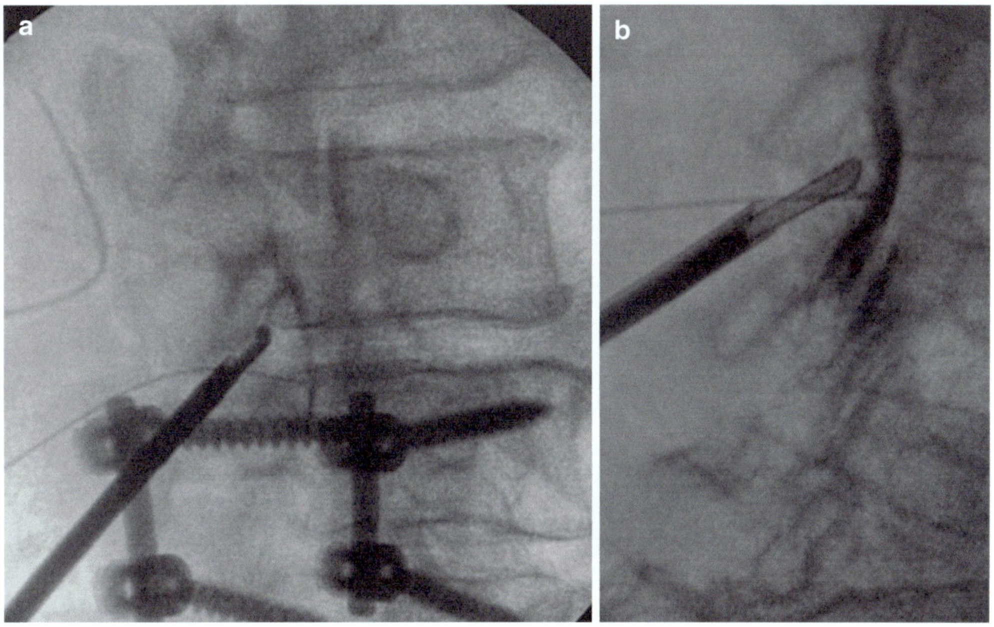

Fig. 14.3 (**a**) demonstrates challenges in proper placement of laminectomy tools to the desired depth in patients with previous fusion instrumentation. (**b**) Image shows the epidurogram highlighting posterior dura and removal of ligamentum flavum superficial to it. (Image courtesy of Ali Mostoufi, MD, New England Spine Care, Cambridge, MA, USA)

at the inferior lamina are completed, ligamentum flavum is debulked using tissue sculptor under contralateral views. Additional removal of ligamentum flavum allows for increased spinal canal space and ultimately reduction in neurogenic claudication (Fig. 14.3). The procedure can be complex if there is scoliotic curve, spondylolisthesis, or in patients with previous adjacent level fusion hardware Fig. 14.2a). There is very little downtime, and minimal post-operative pain was experienced. Patients are encouraged to pursue a daily walking program starting the very next day and a formal lumbar stabilization program in the subsequent weeks.

14.2 Vertiflex® Procedure (Interspinous Spacer)

14.2.1 CPT

22869, 22,870

14.2.2 Description

Lumbar spinal stenosis is an acquired or congenital condition in which spinal canal diameter is reduced, and as a result, neural and vascular elements are compressed. Although many patients are found with radiologic stenosis with no or minimal symptoms, the hallmark symptom is progressive neurogenic claudication (numbness, cramping, pain, heaviness, and/or weakness in the legs), relieved by sitting and worsening with standing and walking. Spinal stenosis may be combined with neuroforaminal stenosis, both of which can result in lower extremity symptoms. Many patients respond to physical therapy and localized facet and epidural blocks, but ultimately patients with worsening neurogenic claudication need to consider surgery.

Open laminectomy remains the gold standard operative care for spinal stenosis. The majority of patients with acquired spinal stenosis are elderly and have multiple comorbidities that can make open spinal surgery, an anesthesia risk, and vulnerable to the risk associated with hospitalization and recovery after spine surgery. Minimally invasive/percutaneous treatments provide an attractive alternative as it is performed in an ambulatory setting, utilizing fluoroscopic guidance under a light sedation with no hospitalization.

The use of the Superion™ Indirect Decompression System known as Vertiflex procedure (Boston Scientific, Boston MA, USA) is a recent addition to minimally invasive procedures to treat moderate spinal stenosis. It is used mostly by interventional pain/spine physicians who can also perform the minimally invasive lumbar decompression (*Mild®* procedure). Studies suggest that even the smallest incremental increase in overall spinal canal area without wide decompression can be effective in providing symptomatic relief in elderly patients [5].

Vertiflex procedure is indicated for L1/2–L4/5 moderate spinal stenosis with or without foraminal stenosis. L5/S1 spinal stenosis cannot be treated by this implant since the S1 spinous process is small and cannot be used to anchor the implant stabilizing arms (Table 14.1). Vertiflex® implant allows stabilization with mild adjacent level distraction and by preventing segmental extension. An ideal candidate presents with neurogenic claudication while standing and walking, which resolves as the patient sits. Patients should not have leg pain in sitting position and should not demonstrate myotomal weakness. Vertiflex should not be offered in patients with severe scoliosis and severe osteoporosis and in patients with unstable spondylolisthesis or greater than grade 2 spondylolisthesis (Table 14.1). Complications may include dislodged implant (poor surgical technique or due to spinous process fracture), spinous process fracture, infection, and invasion of spinal canal by the implant (poor surgical technique).

Table 14.1 Indication and contraindications for interspinous spacer implants to treat spinal stenosis

Vertiflex candidate	Vertiflex contraindications
Moderate spinal stenosis L1–L4 Neurogenic claudication with standing Neurogenic claudication with walking Able to sit continuously for 30 min	L5 spinal stenosis Claudication not resolved with sitting Leg symptom while sitting
Decline open laminectomy Unable to tolerate general anesthesia	Grade 2 or more spondylolisthesis/pars fracture Spinal instability Osteoporosis Moderate–severe scoliosis Cauda equina Previously ankylosed/fusion segment

Studies have shown the use of the Vertiflex® implant to be effective in both short-term relief and long-term relief of neurogenic claudication [6–9].

- *2-year* clinical outcomes for Superion -Vertiflex implant from a randomized controlled US Food and Drug Administration (FDA) to treat moderate lumbar spinal stenosis (n=391) showed neuroclaudication decreased in severity by 70% , back pain clinical success was 68%. Oswestry Disability Index clinical success was achieved in 65% of patients. [6]
- *4-year* clinical outcomes for Superion Vertiflex implant from a randomized controlled US Food and Drug Administration (FDA) to treat moderate lumbar spinal stenosis demonstrated sustained leg pain relief 78% and back pain reduction 66%, and Oswestry Disability Index clinical success was achieved in 62% of patients [7].
- *5-year* clinical outcomes for Superion Vertiflex implant from a randomized controlled US Food and Drug Administration (FDA) to treat moderate lumbar spinal stenosis demonstrated sustained leg pain decrease 80% and sustained back pain reduction 65%, and Oswestry Disability Index clinical success was achieved in 65% of patients. Percentage of improvements over baseline (before treatment) were leg pain 75%, lower back pain 66%, and ODO 58% ($P < 0.0001$) [8].

14.2.3 Surgical Technique

Vertiflex procedure (Superion™ Indirect Decompression System) can be done at a single segment or at two adjacent segments, which demonstrates moderate spinal stenosis. This surgical procedure is performed as an outpatient case following standard sterile surgical techniques. The operation is performed through a 2.5 cm skin incision to accommodate for surgical tools. Once optimal sedation is achieved, skin and subcutaneous tissues are anesthetized, and blunt tissue dissection is performed to the depth of the spinous process. The supraspinous/interspinous ligament is incised, and adjacent spinous processes are gently separated through provided surgical tools to allow for implant to be advanced in between two adjacent spinous processes. Using a proprietary tool, interspinous space is measured so the correct implant size can be selected. The implant is then inserted and advanced. Once the position of the implant is confirmed using PA and lateral views, the anchoring arms are deployed to engage with the two adjacent spinous processes (Fig. 14.4a). Once

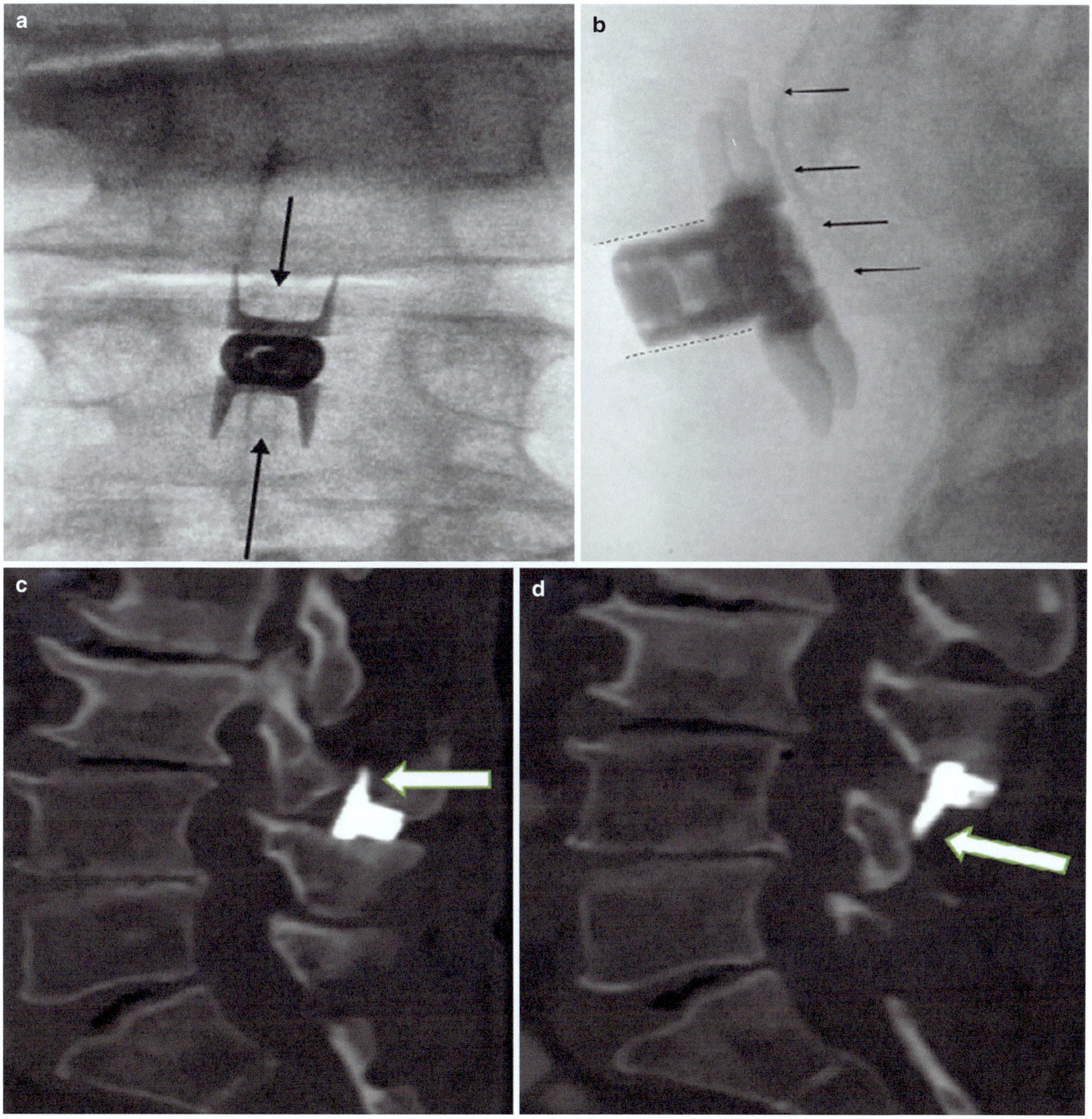

Fig. 14.4 (**a**) and (**b**) are in-procedure fluoroscopic pictures of the Vertiflex Superion implant on PA and lateral views. The anchors are seen in line with adjacent spinous processes on image **a**, and on lateral view resting in the final position in between spinous processes and placed against lamin (thin arrows on image **b**). Images **c**, **d**, **e**, and **f** are CT scan images on the same patient. In C and D, the deployed arms of the implants are seen against lamina (arrows). Images **e** and **f** show the implant in PA view with extended arms hugging the spinous process (arrows). In the axial images (image **f**), the implant's anchoring arms are seen against the lamina and in ideal position. (Image courtesy of Ali Mostoufi, MD, New England Spine Care, Cambridge, MA, USA)

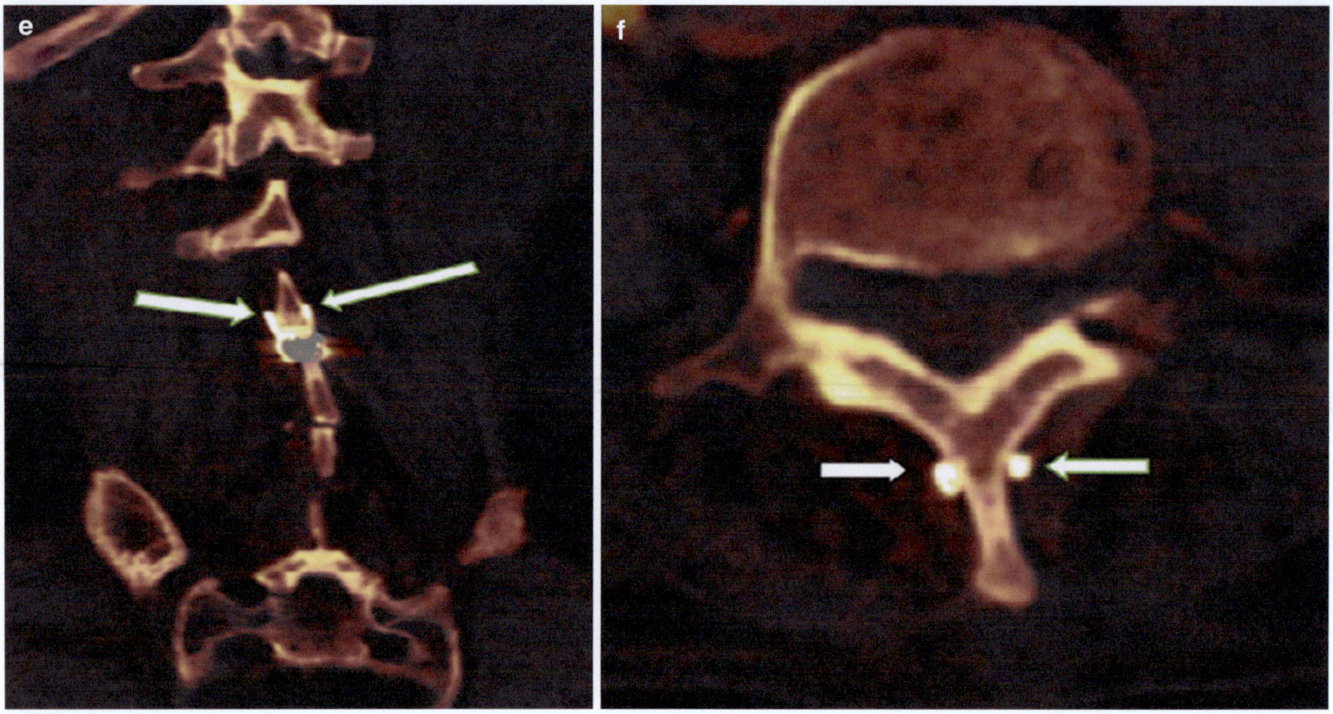

Fig. 14.4 (continued)

fully deployed, and both parallel pairs or superior and inferior anchors are hugging the spinous processes, the implant is further advanced to its final position (Fig. 14.4b), which should be dorsal and in contact with the adjacent lamina (Fig. 14.4c–e). The procedure is completed at this point, all instruments are removed, wound is irrigated, and deep/superficial sutures are used for closure.

14.2.4 Recovery and Rehabilitation

Postoperative care is minimal. Pain management is done by means of OTC or prescribed medications. Stitches are removed in 10 days, and no brace is necessary in the postoperative phase. Precautions include avoiding bending and twisting for 6 weeks to allow for the implant pocket to mature. In the first 6 weeks, a daily walking program is encouraged. This is followed by a formal PT program from weeks 6 to 12. Aggressive extension during the first 6–12 weeks is discouraged. Since the implant is an extension limiting device, there may be a small limitation in full extension noted by patients (in particular two-level implants). Improvement in neurogenic claudication is expected within the first 6–12 weeks after procedure.

14.3 Percutaneous Sacroiliac Fusion

14.3.1 CPT

27279

14.3.2 Description

Percutaneous sacroiliac fusion treatments through direct dorsal approach or lateral transiliac method are now available as a minimally invasive procedure performed in outpatient settings under conscious sedation and fluoroscopic guidance. Percutaneous sacroiliac fusion has become available in both academic and private settings as we have started to understand safety of this procedure and reproduction of the outcome. Dorsal approach is easier to perform with less chance of vascular or nerve injury, but its efficacy is less studied as compared to lateral approach.

In general, diagnosis of sacroiliac joint dysfunction is challenging. In addition to collecting history, and imaging, there are a number of clinical maneuvers that can point toward sacroiliac joint as a source of pain (see Chap. 6) [15]. Diagnostic intra-articular injection of anesthetic could also

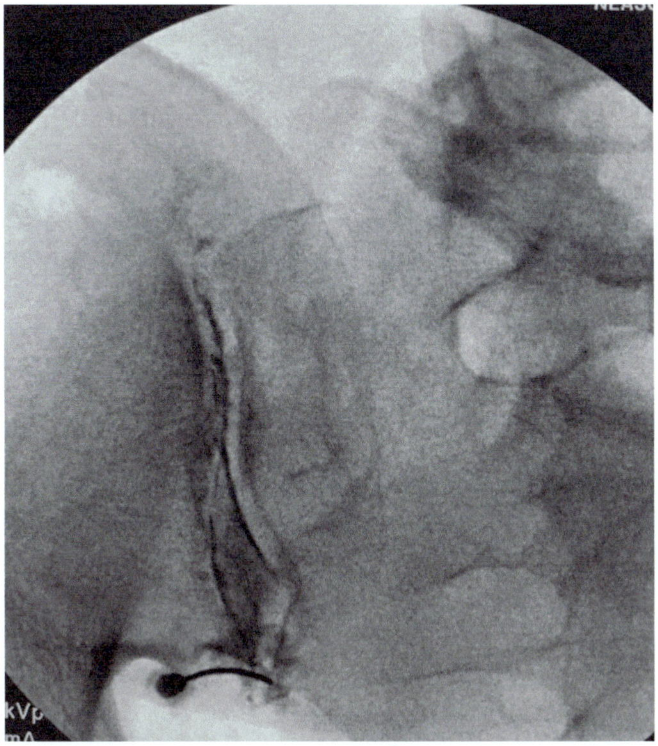

Fig. 14.5 Diagnostic injection of SI joint. Intra-articular placement of the needle through the most distal aspect of the sacroiliac joint, followed by administration of contrast within the joint prior to injection of anesthetics. (Image courtesy of Ali Mostoufi, MD, New England Spine Care, Cambridge, MA, USA)

be confirmatory (Fig. 14.5). Some clinicians choose to anesthetize L5 dorsal rami, and S1 and S2 lateral branches as a diagnostic step prior to offering therapeutic intervention for sacroiliac joint dysfunction.

If correct diagnosis of sacroiliac-mediated pain is established, *and* the patient is not responsive to less aggressive treatment, which includes physical therapy, sacroiliac belt, NSAIDs, chiropractic or osteopathic adjustments, TENS unit, and either corticosteroid injection or ablation treatment of innervating branches, then the interventionalist may choose to offer minimally invasive sacroiliac fusion to the patient.

Several comparisons of minimally invasive (MIS) SI joint fusion and open SI joint fusion have been reported. To date, the quality of available evidence is mixed and includes two level 1 prospective clinical trials and two level 4 retrospective studies, with some level 2 prospective studies [16]. In a level 1 studies of triangular implants by month 24, 82% received substantial clinical benefit in VAS SI joint pain score, and 66% had received substantial clinical benefit in ODI score [16].

14.3.3 Surgical Technique

Percutaneous sacroiliac (SI) fusion is performed in an ambulatory setting, utilizing fluoroscopic guidance and various joint stabilization systems. In the dorsal approach, once the SI joint is identified, a guidewire is placed within the joint, followed by gentle separation of the sacroiliac joint using specialized surgical instruments designed for a particular stabilization system. Bone decorticator is used to prepare the sacrum and ilium joint surface before implanting a bony allograft within the sacroiliac joint (Fig. 14.6).

14.3.4 Recovery and Rehabilitation

The patient is ambulatory after the procedure, requiring minimal downtime from work with 6 weeks precaution (avoiding aggressive bending and twisting), followed by 6 additional weeks of structural PT. Final fusion status is confirmed by serial X-rays or CAT scan, and depends on availability and coverage.

14.4 Percutaneous Lumbar Discectomy

14.4.1 CPT

62287

14.4.2 Description

Lumbar radiculopathy is a condition characterized by irritation of a particular lumbar nerve root, resulting in unilateral pain, numbness, paresthesias, or weakness in the buttock or a leg. The most common cause of lumbar radiculopathy is intervertebral disk herniation (younger adults) or disk–osteophyte complex (older adults). Initially, patients should be managed conservatively with exercise, physical therapy, and NSAIDs back brace and a tapering dose of corticosteroids or epidural injection. Early surgical referral may be necessary in patients with dense myotomal weakness or other red flags.

If symptomatic patients fail to improve with 6–12 weeks of conservative care, lumbar discectomy may be offered. Open microdiscectomy remains the gold standard of surgical care although new surgical training including minimally invasive open surgery (MIS) and endoscopic discectomy may result in even faster recovery and return to work.

X-ray-guided percutaneous lumbar discectomy is an emerging therapy for the treatment of lumbar disk hernia-

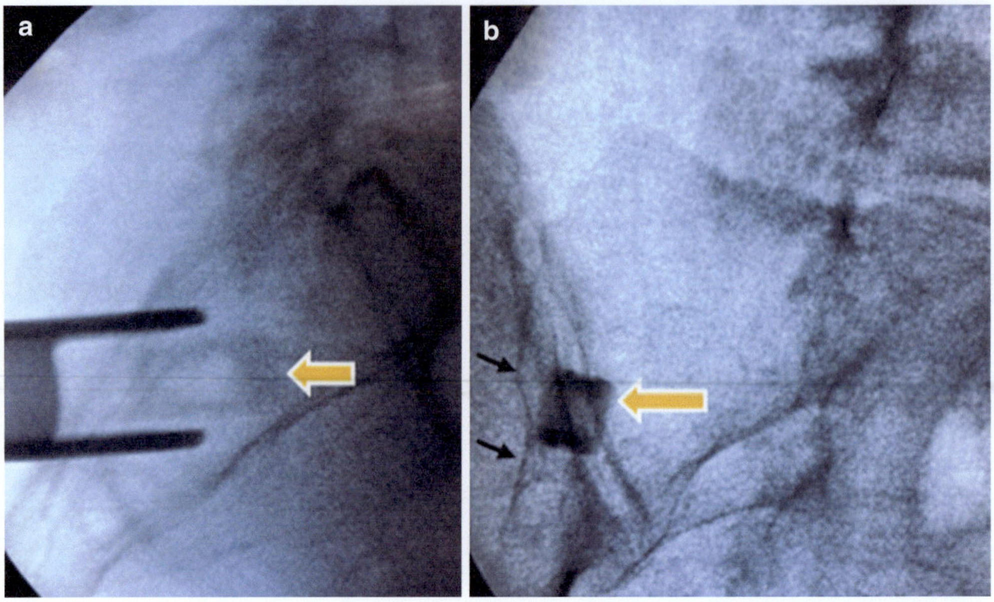

Fig. 14.6 Percutaneous sacroiliac fusion. (**a**) demonstrates implantation of the bony allograft (arrow) on a lateral view. (**b**) demonstrates contralateral oblique view of the SI joint, approximating posterior and anterior joint, and visualizing square-shaped allograft (thick arrow) within the SI joint. The thinner arrows are pointing to PSIS. (Image courtesy of Ali Mostoufi, MD, New England Spine Care, Cambridge, MA, USA)

Table 14.2 Different methods of percutaneous discectomy after access to the nucleus of the disk

Mechanical	Automated percutaneous discectomy (helical tip, Archimedes' screw principle) Pneumatic suction cutting probe Fluid jet cutting and suction-based removal probe
Thermal	Laser-based Radiofrequency-based Nucleoplasty Electrothermal
Chemical	Percutaneous ozone nucleolysis Percutaneous ethyl alcohol gel nucleolysis

tions. Many options are available, some are mechanical, some are chemical, and others utilize thermal technologies (Table 14.2).

There is limited research available on percutaneous discectomy.

- A randomized prospective trial with a noninferiority design for percutaneous laser disk decompression showed higher speed of recovery in favor of conventional surgery and significantly less reoperations in the conventional surgery group (38% vs. 16%). Overall, a strategy of percutaneous laser discectomy with delayed surgery if needed resulted in noninferior outcomes at 1 year [10].
- A systematic review of percutaneous lumbar mechanical disk decompression utilizing Dekompressor demonstrated level II evidence for short- and long-term relief [11]. They concluded that mechanical discectomy may provide appropriate relief in properly selected patients with contained lumbar disk prolapse.
- A meta-analysis study of the effectiveness and safety of percutaneous ozone nucleolysis for herniated lumbar disks (n = 8000) demonstrated that the mean improvement in radicular pain was 3.9 for VAS and 25.7 for ODI and predicted complication risk of 0.064%. The study concluded that pain and function outcomes are similar to the outcomes for lumbar disks treated with surgical discectomy, but the complication rate is much lower (<0.1%) and the recovery time is significantly shorter [12].
- A study of efficacy of percutaneous ethyl alcohol gel nucleolysis in symptomatic disk herniation [13] following patient for 1 year after treatment showed 65% reduction in ODI score, 50% reduction in analgesic use, and 63.5% in pain relief (sustained at 12 months). Another study compared the effectiveness of intradiscal injection of ethyl alcohol versus percutaneous laser disk decompression in patients with chronic radicular low back pain; both techniques were equivalent in pain reduction, but ethyl alcohol group had a greater effect on decreasing disability after 12 months, although the rate of progression to secondary treatments and/or surgery was almost equal in the two groups [14].

14.4.3 Surgical Technique

Procedure is performed in an outpatient setting, and often, no sedation is necessary. The common procedural portion in all the percutaneous discectomy options is access to the center of the disk using fluoroscopy or CT scan and utilizing either a mechanical, chemical, or thermal method for discectomy. Access to the disk is done in an identical method as discography, which has a complication risk of infection, nerve root injury, increase in herniation size, bleeding, and removal of annulus fibrosus instead of nucleus. Depending on the size of the probe and particular technology used, a small 1–2 mm skin incision may be needed to advance the probe through the "safe discography triangle" into the center of the disk (Fig. 14.6a). If fluoroscopy is used, PA/oblique and lateral views are used throughout the procedure to guide the needle/probe. Once the probe is in the center of the disk, a small amount of contrast can confirm intranucleus placement (Fig. 14.7).

If mechanical automated discectomy is chosen, a proprietary handle with spiral tip is placed through the probe into the disk and the discectomy is performed at high RPM (Fig. 14.8). In mechanical percutaneous discectomy, the

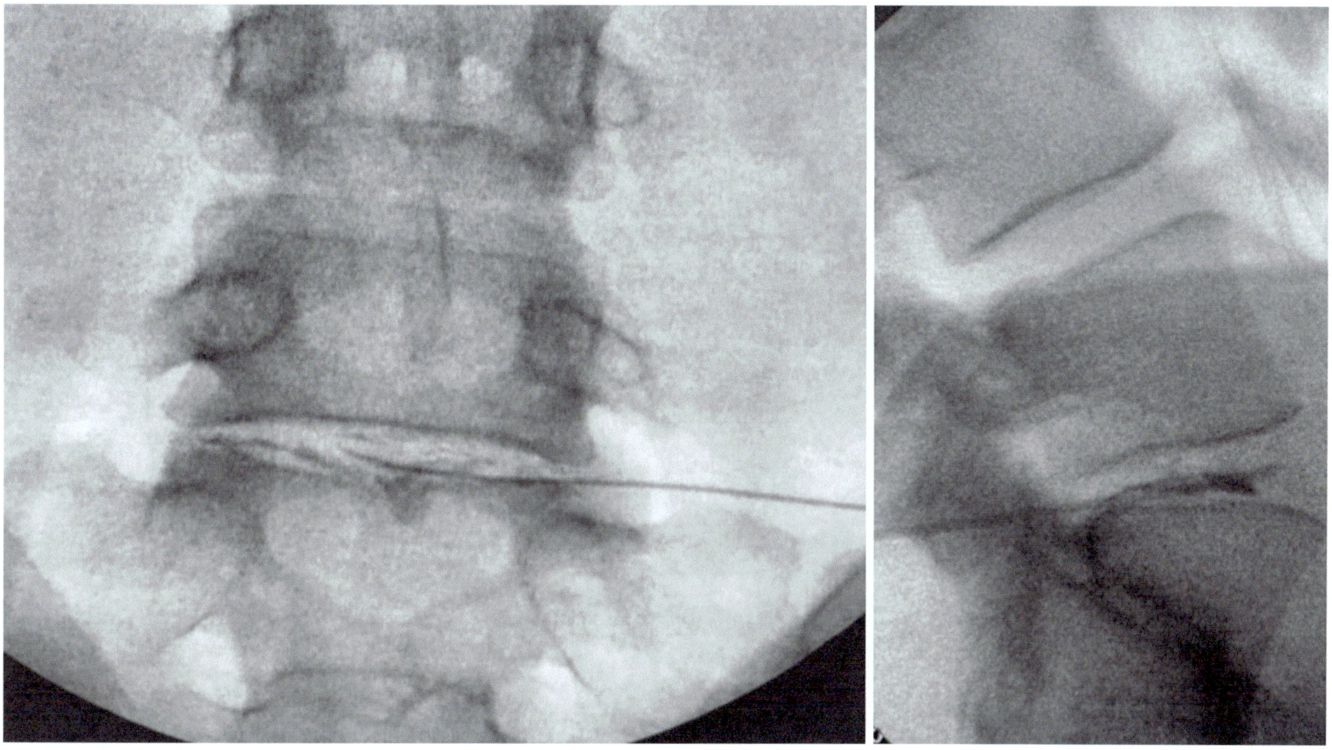

Fig. 14.7 Intradiscal placement of needle with contrast confirmation of nucleus placement. (Image courtesy of Ali Mostoufi, MD, New England Spine Care, Cambridge, MA, USA)

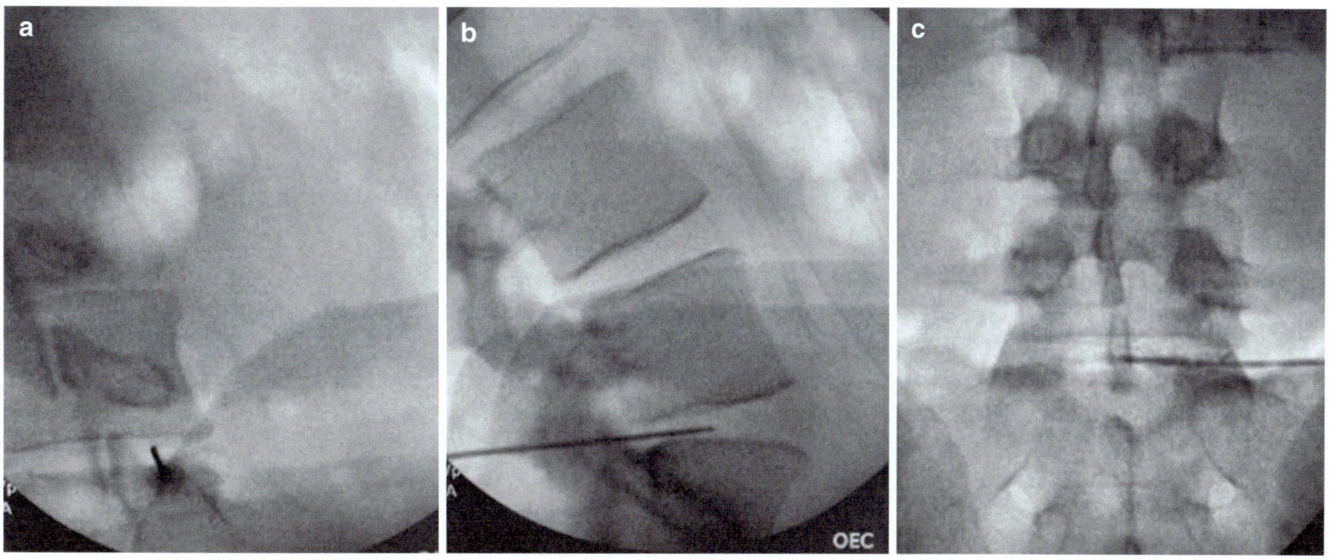

Fig. 14.8 X-ray-guided mechanical automated percutaneous discectomy. (**a**) Shows guiding the probe into the L5-S1 disk using standard discography technique. Image (**b**) and (**c**) showing proper probe placement in the center of the disk on lateral and PA images before performing mechanical discectomy. (Image courtesy of Ali Mostoufi, MD, New England Spine Care, Cambridge, MA, USA)

removed disk material is sent to pathology for confirmation and documentation.

In chemical discectomy, a 22 g spinal needle is placed in the center of the disk (two-needle technique) before delivering ozone or ethyl alcohol gel to the nucleus pulposus. Contrast is used prior to treatment to ensure intranucleus needle placement. Using a thin spinal needle is less damaging to the disk annulus as compared to thicker probes used for mechanical or thermal methods.

14.4.4 Recovery and Rehabilitation

The patient is ambulatory after the procedure, requiring minimal downtime from sedentary type work. A lumbar brace is advised for 2 weeks, as a reminder for patients to avoid aggressive bending. This allows natural healing of annulus, which was penetrated during the procedure. Pain management is necessary in rare cases, but nociceptive pain can respond to OTC or prescribed medications. Pain relief from percutaneous discectomy is gradual over several weeks, and this needs to be explained to the patient. A structured extension-biased PT program is advised 6–12 weeks after the procedure.

14.5 Vertebral Augmentation

14.5.1 Definition

Vertebral augmentation is a procedure in which fractured osteoporotic vertebrae are percutaneously injected with polymethyl methacrylate cement. The procedure is performed with or without creation of a cavity using an expandable balloon. The procedure can also be performed after partial height restoration through percutaneously placed implantable devices, followed by injection of cement. This procedure has been discussed in detail in Chap. 54.

References

1. Lee MJ, Cassinelli EH, Riew KD. Prevalence of cervical spine stenosis: anatomic study in cadavers. J Bone Joint Surg Ser A [Internet]. 2007 [cited 2021 Jul 26];89(2):376–80.
2. Chopko B, Caraway DL. MiDAS I (mild Decompression Alternative to Open Surgery): a preliminary report of a prospective, multi-center clinical study. Pain Phys. 2010;13(4):369–78. Erratum in: Pain Physician. 2012 Jul-Aug;15(4):349.
3. Weinstein JN, Tosteson TD, Lurie JD, et al. Surgical versus nonsurgical therapy for lumbar spinal stenosis. N Engl J Med. 2008;358(8):794–810.
4. Staats PS, Chafin TB, Golovac S, et al. Long-term safety and efficacy of minimally invasive lumbar decompression procedure for the treatment of lumbar spinal stenosis with neurogenic claudication: 2-year results of MiDAS ENCORE. Reg Anesth Pain Med. 2018;43(7):789–94.
5. Hartman J, Granville M, Jacobson RE. The use of Vertiflex® Interspinous spacer device in patients with lumbar spinal stenosis and concurrent medical comorbidities. Cureus. 2019;11(8):e5374. Published 2019 Aug 12. https://doi.org/10.7759/cureus.5374
6. Patel VV, Whang PG, Haley TR, Bradley WD, Nunley PD, Davis RP, Miller LE, Block JE, Geisler FH. Superion interspinous process spacer for intermittent neurogenic claudication secondary to moderate lumbar spinal stenosis: two-year results from a randomized controlled FDA-IDE pivotal trial. Spine (Phila Pa 1976). 2015;40(5):275–82. https://doi.org/10.1097/BRS.0000000000000735. PMID: 25494323
7. Nunley PD, Patel VV, Orndorff DG, Lavelle WF, Block JE, Geisler FH. Superion interspinous spacer treatment of moderate spinal stenosis: 4-year results. World Neurosurg. 2017;104:279–83. https://doi.org/10.1016/j.wneu.2017.04.163. Epub 2017 May 4
8. Nunley PD, Patel VV, Orndorff DG, Lavelle WF, Block JE, Geisler FH. Five-year durability of stand-alone interspinous process decompression for lumbar spinal stenosis. Clin Interv Aging. 2017;12:1409–17. https://doi.org/10.2147/CIA.S143503. PMID: 28919727; PMCID: PMC5593396.
9. Deer T, Grider J, Pope J, et al. The MIST guidelines: the lumbar stenosis consensus study group guidelines for minimally invasive spine treatment. Pain Pract. 2019;18:250–74.
10. Brouwer PA, Brand R, van den Akker-van Marle ME, Jacobs WC, Schenk B, van den Berg-Huijsmans AA, Koes BW, van Buchem MA, Arts MP, Peul WC. Percutaneous laser disc decompression versus conventional microdiscectomy in sciatica: a randomized controlled trial. Spine J. 2015;15(5):857–65. https://doi.org/10.1016/j.spinee.2015.01.020. Epub 2015 Jan 20. PMID: 25614151.
11. Hirsch JA, Singh V, Falco FJ, Benyamin RM, Manchikanti L. Automated percutaneous lumbar discectomy for the contained herniated lumbar disc: a systematic assessment of evidence. Pain Physician. 2009;12(3):601–20.
12. Steppan J, Meaders T, Muto M, Murphy KJ. A meta-analysis of the effectiveness and safety of ozone treatments for herniated lumbar discs. J Vasc Interv Radiol. 2010;21:534–48.
13. Marcia S, Bellini M, Hirsch JA, Chandra RV, Piras E, Marras M, Sanna AM, Saba L. Efficacy of an ethyl alcohol gel in symptomatic disc herniation. Eur J Radiol. 2018;109:101–7. https://doi.org/10.1016/j.ejrad.2018.10.029. Epub 2018 Oct 30. PMID: 30527290
14. Hashemi M, Dadkhah P, Taheri M, Katibeh P, Asadi S. Effectiveness of intradiscal injection of radiopaque gelified ethanol (DiscoGel®) *versus* percutaneous laser disc decompression in patients with chronic radicular low back pain. Korean J Pain. 2020;33(1):66–72.
15. Poilliot AJ, Zwirner J, Doyle T, Hammer N. A systematic review of the normal sacroiliac joint anatomy and adjacent tissues for the pain physicians. Pain Physician. 2019;22(4):247–74.
16. Martin CT, Haase L, Lender PA, Polly DW. Minimally invasive sacroiliac joint fusion: the current evidence. Int J Spine Surg. 2020;14(Suppl 1):20–9. Published 2020 Feb 10. https://doi.org/10.14444/6072.

Endoscopic and Minimally Invasive Spine Surgery

15

Grace X. Xiong, Harry M. Lightsey IV, Alexander M. Crawford, and Andrew K. Simpson

15.1 Description

The utilization of minimally invasive surgery (MIS) for spine applications has increased exponentially, spurred on by advances in technology and techniques permitting decreased soft tissue disruption with comparable anatomic outcomes and expedited recovery times. Specifically, the evolution of several procedural domains has fueled this growth: (1) improved soft tissue retractors, (2) leveraging less disruptive tissue planes, (3) adjuvant technologies to provide more intraoperative anatomic information, and (4) improved visualization technologies. Spinal endoscopy is one specific domain at the forefront of these efforts, transitioning the surgeon's perspective from direct external to indirect internal visualization and enabling improved demonstration of the surgical anatomy.

15.1.1 Minimally Invasive Spine Surgery

MIS of the spine denotes decreased soft tissue dissection with smaller incisions and less paraspinal muscle retraction. In contrast to an open surgical field in which spine surgeons retract the surrounding musculature to expose bony landmarks often with the aid of magnifying eyewear, or loupes, MIS techniques utilize specialized tubular retractors through which targeted dissection is carried out with microinstruments. Surgical visualization is either direct, with the use of an operating microscope, or indirect, with small cameras inserted into the retractor.

G. X. Xiong · H. M. Lightsey IV · A. M. Crawford
Harvard Combined Orthopaedic Residency Program, Harvard Medical School, Boston, MA, USA

A. K. Simpson (✉)
Department of Orthopaedic Surgery, Brigham and Women's Hospital, Harvard Medical School, Boston, MA, USA
e-mail: asimpson@bwh.harvard.edu

15.1.2 Microscopic Spine Surgery

Operating microscopes in spine surgery have been used since the 1970s as a means to permit microsurgical approaches [1]. Continual advancements in optical lens systems have bolstered their surgical utility. Microscopes are now routinely used to improve visualization across a wide variety of spine surgeries, such as anterior cervical discectomy and fusion procedures and posterior neural decompressions. Microscopic MIS techniques involve using the microscope to view a targeted surgical field through a retractor.

15.1.3 Endoscopic Spine Surgery

Endoscopic spine surgery entails the use of a small camera, i.e., the endoscope, inserted into a tubular retractor permitting indirect visualization of the surgical field. With the camera in place, microinstruments are inserted through a working channel, which may be the same tubular retractor or another point of access. Different endoscopic techniques are distinguished by the size and number of working channels; in most cases; however, incisions are typically less than 2 cm in length (Fig. 15.1).

15.1.4 Full Endoscopic Spine Surgery

In full endoscopic spine surgery, a single working channel houses both the endoscope and one instrument, which must be exchanged depending on the functionality needed. Full endoscopy is the least invasive endoscopic approach and requires an aqueous environment to assist in opening tissue planes and creating a clear surgical field. The primary limitation of this technique is the single working channel permitting a single instrument that must be moved in concert with the endoscope.

© The Author(s), under exclusive license to Springer Nature Switzerland AG 2022

S. A. Mostoufi et al. (eds.), *Clinical Guide to Musculoskeletal Medicine*, https://doi.org/10.1007/978-3-030-92042-5_15

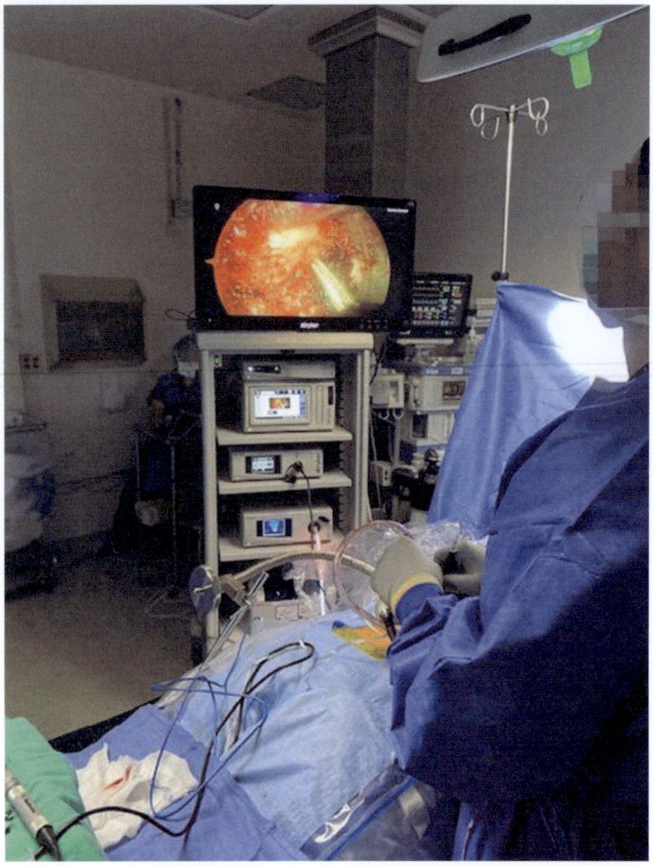

Fig. 15.1 Intraoperative set up for a microendoscopic decompression. The surgeon is able to independently manipulate two microinstruments concurrently, and the endoscope, situated along the inner side of the retractor, projects the working area onto a monitor

15.1.5 Microendoscopy Spine Surgery

Microendoscopic techniques rely on a single, slightly larger working channel that permits the use of multiple instruments and housing the endoscope (Figs. 15.1 and 15.2). The instruments can be moved independently, and the larger working channel size also allows for a broader range of tools and potential placement of interbody implants and bone graft for spinal fusions. Microendoscopy is currently predominantly performed in a dry environment.

15.1.6 Biportal Endoscopy

Biportal endoscopy utilizes two working channels, one for the endoscope and another for the instruments. The advantages of this approach include a greater degree of scope and instrument positioning, which can be critical for particularly difficult areas of access in the spine, and the incorporation of aqueous tissue dissection. Multiple portals do, however, create more tissue disruption and may make exchanging and triangulating instrumentation more challenging.

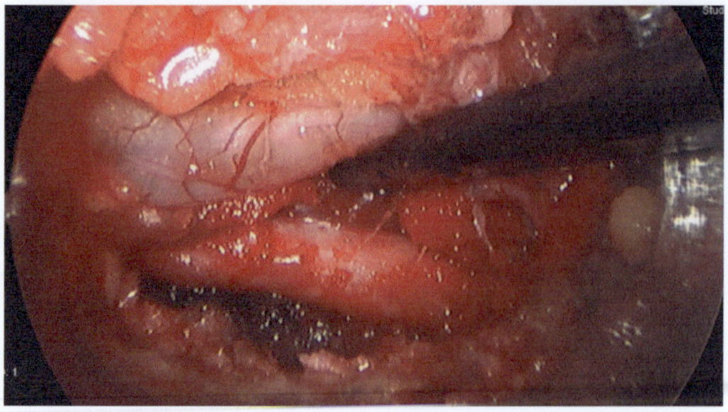

Fig. 15.2 Intraoperative image demonstrating the surgeon's view during a microendoscopic decompression for lateral recess stenosis with decompression of the dural sac and traversing nerve root

15.2 MIS and Endoscopic Surgeries in C-Spine

Cervical radiculopathy is often caused by a disk herniation or uncovertebral hypertrophy narrowing the neuroforamina.

15.2.1 Cervical Microscopic Foraminotomy

The mainstay MIS technique is microscopic foraminotomy, which first gained widespread exposure when Williams published his case series of 235 patients in 1983 [2]. In his cohort, he claimed that all patients achieved resolution of their radicular pain following surgical intervention. In the years since, microscopic foraminotomy has demonstrated similarly encouraging results when compared directly against open foraminotomy [3]. In their systematic review of MIS versus open foraminotomy, Clark et al. found that MIS technique delivered equivalent clinical results while also providing decreased blood loss, shorter postoperative stays, and reduced opioid requirements postoperatively [4].

15.2.2 Cervical Endoscopic Decompression

Posterior endoscopic cervical foraminotomy (PECF) or percutaneous endoscopic cervical discectomy (PECD), is another minimally invasive alternative to open treatment of cervical radiculopathy. In their prospective randomized controlled trial, Ruetten et al. provided level I evidence suggesting that PECF is noninferior to anterior cervical discectomy and fusion (ACDF), which is commonly considered the mainstay in open surgical management of cervical radiculopathy [5]. Further, PECF carried the benefit of maintaining segmental motion through the level operated upon, which is not the case with an ACDF. Similarly, in their prospective analysis, Ahn et al. demonstrated similar outcomes between PECF and ACDF in the treatment of cervical radiculopathy caused by soft cervical disk herniations [6]. In this study, the authors also found that PECF was associated with significantly decreased operative time, hospital stay, and time to return to work as compared to the ACDF cohort.

15.2.3 Cervical Myelopathy

Cervical myelopathy often involves multiple levels of the cervical spine. Mainstays of operative treatment include multilevel dorsal decompressions with laminoplasty or open laminectomy and fusion. While laminoplasty does maintain cervical motion, traditional techniques still require substantial muscular dissection.

MIS techniques have evolved to allow for single or multilevel dorsal decompression via an endoscopic approach. In their review of 61 cases, Minamide et al. compared the outcomes of patients with cervical spondylotic myelopathy treated with microendoscopic laminotomy versus laminoplasty [7]. Overall, the endoscopic group demonstrated similar functional outcomes at 5-year follow-up, with improved preservation of cervical alignment and less postoperative axial neck pain compared to traditional laminoplasty.

15.3 MIS and Endoscopic Surgeries in L-Spine

15.3.1 Lumbar Discectomy

Lumbar disk herniation is one of the most common indications for minimally invasive procedural solutions, ranging from less invasive retractors to microtubular approaches to endoscopy.

15.3.1.1 Lumbar Microdiscectomy

A microdiscectomy refers to any removal of a disk fragment performed with the use of an operating microscope. Some approaches modify a traditional open posterior midline exposure with the assistance of a surgical microscope, which allows for a smaller surgical incision. These make use of a standard dissection through musculotendinous insertions around the spine and are not considered minimally invasive.

15.3.1.2 Lumbar MIS Discectomy

A true minimally invasive approach further decreases the size of the incision and makes use of a tubular retractor to maintain consistent visualization into the specific surgical field.

MIS techniques typically exploit an intramuscular approach through a small paraspinal incision, which preserves musculotendinous insertions and further limits local soft tissue trauma. Specialized instruments facilitate discectomy in a small working area. Some studies have demonstrated benefits such as decreased blood loss and lower length of stay with tubular microdiscectomy compared with traditional open or mini-open discectomy [8], while other studies have demonstrated no difference [9]. The overall literature has not demonstrated a longer-term clinical advantage or difference in complication rates for either approach [9]. One randomized controlled trial of 325 patients showed no differences in patient-reported outcomes or reoperation rates at five years [10]. Nonetheless, the decreased soft tissue trauma and expedited postoperative recovery make this an attractive option.

15.3.1.3 Lumbar Endoscopic Discectomy

This option is becoming increasingly utilized for lumbar disk herniations and in many areas around the world is becoming the predominant treatment modality. Depending on the location of the herniated disk anatomically, this technique may be used to target more central or paracentral herniations via an interlaminar window (posteriorly between the dorsal aspect of the lamina), or more laterally via the foramen for more laterally based or extraforaminal herniations (transforaminal approach).

Studies comparing endoscopic approaches with both minimally invasive and open approaches have found relatively equivalent longer-term outcomes, with shorter-term benefits and more expedited recovery. For example, Ruetten randomized 178 patients with lumbar disk herniations to either an endoscopic or microscopic approach and found no difference in patient-reported outcomes as assessed by the visual analog scale (VAS), Oswestry Disability Index (ODI), or NASS scores, as well as no difference in recurrence or complication rates [11]. They did, however, show a shorter operative time (22 versus 43 minutes, $p < 0.0001$), lower postoperative pain medication use, and shorter time to return to work (25 versus 49 days, $p < 0.01$) in the endoscopic group. These findings were mirrored in other RCTs which demonstrated no difference in longer-term patient-reported outcomes between patients undergoing an endoscopic compared with microendoscopic or endoscopic compared with open approach [12].

15.3.2 Lumbar Spinal Stenosis

Lumbar spinal stenosis is another common diagnosis that is amenable to minimally invasive solutions. Under the umbrella of lumbar spinal stenosis, several anatomic areas contribute to neural compression and symptoms. The hypertrophied ligamentum flavum and degenerative facet joints and associated bony growth contribute to dorsal compression and lateral recess stenosis. Complete dorsal and lateral recess decompression is essential for a good clinical result. This standard open decompression for lumbar spinal stenosis consists of a midline tissue dissection involving the release of musculotendinous insertions. Minimally invasive techniques have the same surgical goals while minimizing collateral musculoligamentous tissue damage.

15.3.2.1 MIS Lumbar Decompression

Minimally invasive approaches to lumbar decompression typically include a unilateral paraspinal approach in order to preserve the midline musculotendinous structures, while still achieving a bilateral decompression. Termed a unilateral laminotomy with bilateral decompression (ULBD), this approach utilizes a partial removal of the lamina (the laminotomy) to remove the hypertrophied ligamentum flavum and parts of the facet joints, which are typically overgrown and causing significant compression in its advanced degenerative state [13]. One meta-analysis found higher patient satisfaction scores and lower pain scores with this approach compared to a traditional open approach [14].

15.3.2.2 Endoscopic Lumbar Decompression

Options also exist that use endoscopy for decompression in spinal stenosis. The interlaminar approach provides direct access to the posterior spine and is more commonly used in endoscopic decompression of lumbar spinal stenosis. This approach facilitates decompression of the posterior elements while still allowing access to the lateral recess, as the surgical goals remain the same as an open or minimally invasive approach. Randomized controlled trials have demonstrated equivalent one-year outcomes between endoscopic decompression for spinal stenosis compared with microscopic laminectomy [15]. The literature has also demonstrated similar complication rates between traditional MIS and endoscopic surgery for spinal stenosis [16, 17].

15.3.3 Lumbar Spinal Instability

Although minimally invasive techniques are most commonly used for pathology such as disk herniations, expanding indications have allowed for its use in spinal fusions for a variety of clinical indications.

15.3.3.1 MIS Lumbar Fusion

In general, indications for spinal fusion include degenerative changes causing axial pain, spondylolisthesis and stenosis causing neural compression, or spinal deformity. It is important to note that spinal fusion is both a mechanical process and a biologic process and that in the native spine the intervertebral disk and cartilaginous endplates act as natural barriers to osseous ingrowth. Therefore, during a surgical fusion, adequate debridement and preparation of any surface meant to participate in fusion are paramount to the long-term clinical success [18]. Failure to do this sufficiently will result in lack of fusion, termed a pseudarthrosis , which can lead to persistent or recurrent symptoms of instability or neural compression. Minimally invasive approaches offer a multitude of benefits as previously discussed; however, the particular challenge posed in minimally invasive fusions is adequate debridement and preparation of the fusion area. Despite these initial concerns, good fusion results have still been achieved with minimally invasive approaches through careful surgical technique [19, 20]. In many cases, more potent biologic materials are used as adjuncts to spinal fusion. These may be osteoconductive materials that act as a scaffold such as autograft or allograft or osteoinductive materials that facilitate the biologic process such as bone morphogenic protein.

- *Posterior Approaches—MIS Fusion*

One of the most common uses of minimally invasive interbody fusions is the utilization of a posterior approach through a transforaminal window. Unlike traditional open posterior approaches, which utilize a midline incision, an MIS transforaminal interbody fusion (MIS TLIF) is achieved via small incisions off the midline using an intramuscular approach (known as the Wiltse approach). This intramuscular plane is utilized both for decompression and for disk space access, as well as pedicle screw placement. MIS TLIF approaches have consistently been shown to have benefits over an open approach including decreased blood loss, less perioperative pain, and shorter length of stay, with equivalent long-term clinical outcomes [21]. Furthermore, the term "minimally invasive," as with previously described surgeries, may encapsulate a variety of techniques. Techniques utilizing both tubular systems and endoscopic systems have been described with similar fusion rates with a variety of implants [22, 23].

- *Anterior and Lateral approaches—MIS fusion*

Interbody fusions can also be performed via anterior, oblique, or lateral approaches, where restoration of the disk height and improvement in vertebral alignment provides indirect decompression of the neural elements. These approaches to fusion maximize intervertebral distraction to achieve increased height of the foramen and opening of the lateral recesses in order to avoid the need for direct visualization and exposure of the neural elements.

There are three broad areas for approaches to the anterior vertebral column: anterior, via an anterior abdominal incision and retroperitoneal access; oblique, between the vessels and anterior to the psoas; and lateral, through the psoas muscle (transpsoas). The majority of these cases also include concurrent posterior stabilization and fusion via the Wiltse approach described previously. As with other minimally invasive surgeries, the challenge lies in adequate debridement and preparation of the vertebral endplates. Advantages of these procedures include avoiding retraction and dissection around the thecal sac and nerve roots, as would be required with a posterior approach. Disadvantages include the proximity to the great vessels and the potential for abdominal or vascular complications [24]. Some approaches such as the lateral transpsoas approach also necessitate neuromonitoring due to proximity to nerves within the psoas muscle [25]. Clinical outcomes and fusion rates are comparable between the multiple approaches and certain nuances such as body habitus, history of prior abdominal or spinal surgery, and other factors can influence a surgeon's decision to perform one approach versus another, but are outside the scope of this chapter [26, 27].

15.4 Postoperative Rehabilitation

Patients with chronic spine complaints often become more and more deconditioned, given the limitation of activity due to pain. When pain is relieved with spine surgery, after the expected course of tissue healing, physical therapy is started with the goal of improvement of function, ROM, strengthening, and patient education to prevent further injury in the future. If there was any weakness prior to the surgery, physical therapy could assist with functional recovery although the degree of recovery depends on chronicity of weakness. There is no uniform consensus regarding physical therapy after minimally invasive surgeries for spine, but in general, spine stabilization program is what most patients postoperatively pursue [27]. Physical therapy can include soft tissue treatment. Manual therapy can assist with soft tissue mobilization, and thermal modalities could reduce pain and increase compliance with exercises. Some patients develop either postoperative flat back or swayback posture, and physical therapy may assist with the improvement of symptom and strengthening paraspinal muscles. Multifidus muscle, hamstrings, and transverse abdominis become important targets for PT programs, and some therapists used surface EMG for biofeedback during strengthening exercises [28]. There is also an effort to increase stamina and endurance in the postoperative phase, and progress could be tracked by means of 6-minute or 12-minute walk testing. Finally, improving in range of motion and flexibility becomes a part of the rehabilitation program. In patients who have interbody fusions, depending on the level and number of levels treated, there may be a plateau in the improvement of range of motion. Improving range of motion of hip and knee and ankle will improve patient's function and is as important as improving the spine range of motion.

References

1. Williams RW. Microlumbar discectomy: a conservative surgical approach to the virgin herniated lumbar disc. Spine (Phila Pa 1976). 1978;3(2):175–82.
2. Williams RW. Microcervical foraminotomy. A surgical alternative for intractable radicular pain. Spine (Phila Pa 1976). 1983;8(7):708–16.
3. Platt A, Gerard CS, O'Toole JE. Comparison of outcomes following minimally invasive and open posterior cervical foraminotomy: description of minimally invasive technique and review of literature. J Spine Surg (Hong Kong). 2020;6(1):243–51.
4. Clark JG, Abdullah KG, Steinmetz MP, Benzel EC, Mroz TE. Minimally invasive versus open cervical foraminotomy: a systematic review. Glob Spine J. 2011;1(1):9–14.
5. Ruetten S, Komp M, Merk H, Godolias G. Full-endoscopic cervical posterior foraminotomy for the operation of lateral disc herniations using 5.9-mm endoscopes: a prospective, randomized, controlled study. Spine (Phila Pa 1976). 2008;33(9):940–8.
6. Ahn Y, Keum HJ, Shin SH. Percutaneous endoscopic cervical discectomy versus anterior cervical discectomy and fusion: a comparative cohort study with a five-year follow-up. J Clin Med. 2020;9(2):371.
7. Minamide A, Yoshida M, Simpson AK, Yamada H, Hashizume H, Nakagawa Y, et al. Microendoscopic laminotomy versus conventional laminoplasty for cervical spondylotic myelopathy: 5-year follow-up study. J Neurosurg Spine. 2017;27(4):403–9.
8. Barber SM, Nakhla J, Konakondla S, Fridley JS, Oyelese AA, Gokaslan ZL, et al. Outcomes of endoscopic discectomy compared with open microdiscectomy and tubular microdiscectomy for lumbar disc herniations: a meta-analysis. J Neurosurg Spine. 2019:1–14.
9. Li X, Chang H, Meng X. Tubular microscopes discectomy versus conventional microdiscectomy for treating lumbar disk herniation: systematic review and meta-analysis. Medicine (Baltimore). 2018;97(5):e9807.
10. Overdevest GM, Peul WC, Brand R, Koes BW, Bartels RH, Tan WF, et al. Tubular discectomy versus conventional microdiscectomy for the treatment of lumbar disc herniation: long-term results of a randomised controlled trial. J Neurol Neurosurg Psychiatry. 2017;88(12):1008–16.
11. Ruetten S, Komp M, Merk H, Godolias G. Full-endoscopic interlaminar and transforaminal lumbar discectomy versus conventional microsurgical technique: a prospective, randomized, controlled study. Spine (Phila Pa 1976). 2008;33(9):931–9.
12. Teli M, Lovi A, Brayda-Bruno M, Zagra A, Corriero A, Giudici F, et al. Higher risk of dural tears and recurrent herniation with lumbar micro-endoscopic discectomy. Eur Spine J Off Publ Eur Spine Soc Eur Spinal Deform Soc Eur Sect Cerv Spine Res Soc. 2010;19(3):443–50.
13. Mobbs R, Phan K. Minimally invasive unilateral laminectomy for bilateral decompression. JBJS Essent Surg Tech. 2017;7(1):e9.
14. Phan K, Mobbs RJ. Minimally invasive versus open laminectomy for lumbar stenosis: a systematic review and meta-analysis. Spine (Phila Pa 1976). 2016;41(2):E91–100.
15. Park S-M, Park J, Jang HS, Heo YW, Han H, Kim H-J, et al. Biportal endoscopic versus microscopic lumbar decompressive laminectomy in patients with spinal stenosis: a randomized controlled trial. Spine J. 2020;20(2):156–65.
16. Choi D-J, Kim J-E. Efficacy of biportal endoscopic spine surgery for lumbar spinal stenosis. Clin Orthop Surg. 2019;11(1):82–8.
17. Hasan S, McGrath LB, Sen RD, Barber JK, Hofstetter CP. Comparison of full-endoscopic and minimally invasive decompression for lumbar spinal stenosis in the setting of degenerative scoliosis and spondylolisthesis. Neurosurg Focus. 2019;46(5):E16.

18. Gum JL, Reddy D, Glassman S. Transforaminal lumbar interbody fusion (TLIF). JBJS Essent Surg Tech. 2016;6(2):e22.
19. Tatsumi R, Lee Y-P, Khajavi K, Taylor W, Chen F, Bae H. In vitro comparison of endplate preparation between four mini-open interbody fusion approaches. Eur Spine J Off Publ Eur Spine Soc Eur Spinal Deform Soc Eur Sect Cerv Spine Res Soc. 2015;24 Suppl 3:372–7.
20. Rihn JA, Gandhi SD, Sheehan P, Vaccaro AR, Hilibrand AS, Albert TJ, et al. Disc space preparation in transforaminal lumbar interbody fusion: a comparison of minimally invasive and open approaches. Clin Orthop Relat Res. 2014;472(6):1800–5.
21. Lee MJ, Mok J, Patel P. Transforaminal lumbar interbody fusion: traditional open versus minimally invasive techniques. J Am Acad Orthop Surg. 2018;26(4):124–31.
22. Kim J-E, Yoo H-S, Choi D-J, Park EJ, Jee S-M. Comparison of minimal invasive versus Biportal endoscopic Transforaminal lumbar interbody fusion for single-level lumbar disease. Clin Spine Surg. 2021;34:E64.
23. Morgenstern R, Morgenstern C. Percutaneous transforaminal lumbar interbody fusion (pTLIF) with a posterolateral approach for the treatment of denegerative disk disease: feasibility and preliminary results. Int J Spine Surg. 2015;9:41.
24. Mobbs RJ, Phan K, Malham G, Seex K, Rao PJ. Lumbar interbody fusion: techniques, indications and comparison of interbody fusion options including PLIF, TLIF, MI-TLIF, OLIF/ATP, LLIF and ALIF. J Spine Surg (Hong Kong). 2015;1(1):2–18.
25. Mandelli C, Colombo EV, Sicuri GM, Mortini P. Lumbar plexus nervous distortion in XLIF(®) approach: an anatomic study. Eur Spine J Off Publ Eur Spine Soc Eur Spinal Deform Soc Eur Sect Cerv Spine Res Soc. 2016;25(12):4155–63.
26. Nakashima H, Kanemura T, Satake K, Ito K, Tanaka S, Ouchida J, et al. Patient-reported quality of life following posterior lumbar interbody fusion or indirect decompression using lateral lumbar interbody fusion. Spine (Phila Pa 1976). 2020;45(18):E1172–8.
27. Xu DS, Walker CT, Godzik J, Turner JD, Smith W, Uribe JS. Minimally invasive anterior, lateral, and oblique lumbar interbody fusion: a literature review. Ann Transl Med. 2018;6(6):104.
28. Richardson C, Jull G, Hodges P, Hides J. Therapeutic exercise for spinal segmental stabilization in low Back pain. Scientific basis and clinical approach. Churchill Livingstone; 1999.

16 Spine Surgeries

Rojeh Melikian and Kirkham B. Wood

16.1 Lumbar Decompression

16.1.1 Introduction

Lumbar spinal stenosis is a condition resulting from narrowing of the lumbar spinal canal, usually from facet and ligamentum flavum hypertrophy resulting in compression of spinal nerves and resultant neurogenic claudication. The initial treatment for many patients is conservative; however, surgical intervention is indicated in those with refractory leg pain and/or neurological deficit. The more severe the symptoms and the more severe the neurological compression, the more likely symptoms will progress and the less likely they will respond to conservative management. Decompressive lumbar laminectomy involves the removal of some of the posterior elements of the spine in order to relieve the neural impingement (Fig. 16.1).

16.1.2 Indications

Operative intervention in lumbar spinal stenosis is considered after failed nonoperative care (physical therapy, medications, and injections) [1]. However, patients with weakness or severe, intractable pain are candidates for early intervention. Patients with rapidly progressive neurological deficit or cauda equina syndrome should undergo urgent operative intervention. A relative contraindication for laminectomy alone is patients with spondylolisthesis. Patients with this accompanying spinal instability may need to undergo fusion in addition to decompressive laminectomy.

R. Melikian (✉)
DISC Spine and Sports, Marina Del Ray, CA, USA

K. B. Wood
Stanford University School of Medicine, Palo Alto, CA, USA
e-mail: kbwood@stanford.edu

16.1.3 Technique

Lumbar laminectomy can be done through a traditional midline approach to the lumbar spine. The lamina is exposed while being careful to preserve the facet joint capsules. Following this, the spinous process of the cranial level (i.e., the L4 spinous process for L4–5 level) can be removed

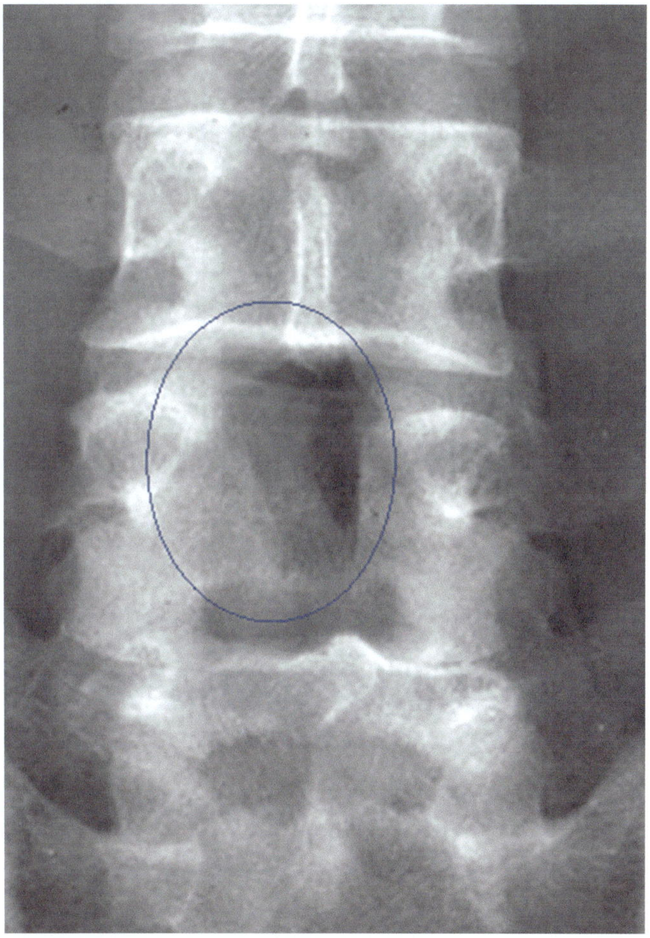

Fig. 16.1 Image shows postoperative PA views of L4–5 laminectomy. (Images courtesy of Ali Mostoufi, MD, New England Spine Care)

© The Author(s), under exclusive license to Springer Nature Switzerland AG 2022

S. A. Mostoufi et al. (eds.), *Clinical Guide to Musculoskeletal Medicine*, https://doi.org/10.1007/978-3-030-92042-5_16

followed by the lamina bilaterally, heading cranial to the insertion of the ligamentum flavum but being careful to excessively thin out the area of the pars interarticularis. Once the ligamentum flavum is freed cranially, a curette can then be used to free it laterally and distally from its insertion on the caudal lamina. The ligamentum can then be left in place as a barrier between the surgeon and the dura. The decompression is then carried laterally into the area of the lateral recess, resecting the medial portion of the facet joint out to where the pedicle of the caudal level is palpable. The ligamentum flavum can then be removed to expose the underlying thecal sac.

In a similar fashion, several different variations of lumbar laminectomy have been developed in an attempt to preserve more of the native anatomy. One such approach is the attempt at using a unilateral laminar window to decompress not only the ipsilateral side but then reach across and decompress the contralateral side, allowing for preservation of the spinous process, interspinous ligaments, and muscle insertions on the contralateral side. However, the goal is the same, to achieve adequate lateral recess and central decompression.

16.1.4 Complications

The most common complication after lumbar laminectomy surgery is dural tear, with a rate of 9 [2]. The 8-year reoperation rate in the SPORT trial was 18%. Iatrogenic instability may occur if the area of the pars interarticularis is thinned out too much and fractures.

16.1.5 Outcomes

In patients with symptomatic lumbar stenosis, lumbar laminectomy demonstrates an overall advantage over nonoperative care until at least 5 years out from surgery for pain, function, satisfaction, and self-rated progress scores. The outcomes between surgery and nonsurgical care tend to converge after 5 years or so, with some groups in the SPORT trial maintaining an advantage for surgery out to 8 years [2].

16.2 Laminoplasty

16.2.1 Introduction

Cervical spondylotic myelopathy is the result of degenerative compression on the cervical cord, eventually resulting in deterioration of neurological function. The initial approach to this issue was posterior decompression with laminectomy; however, multilevel laminectomy without stabilization often led to postoperative kyphosis and instability [3]. Cervical laminoplasty is a technique designed to avoid this issue by retaining the posterior elements. It is a posterior-based, lamina-preserving technique that expands the spinal canal in order to alleviate cervical stenosis (Fig. 16.2). It was first described as a technique for the management of cervical myelopathy and can be used in cases of myelopathy secondary to ossification of the posterior longitudinal ligament (OPLL), congenital stenosis, and cervical spondylosis [4]. It serves as an alternative to laminectomy with or without

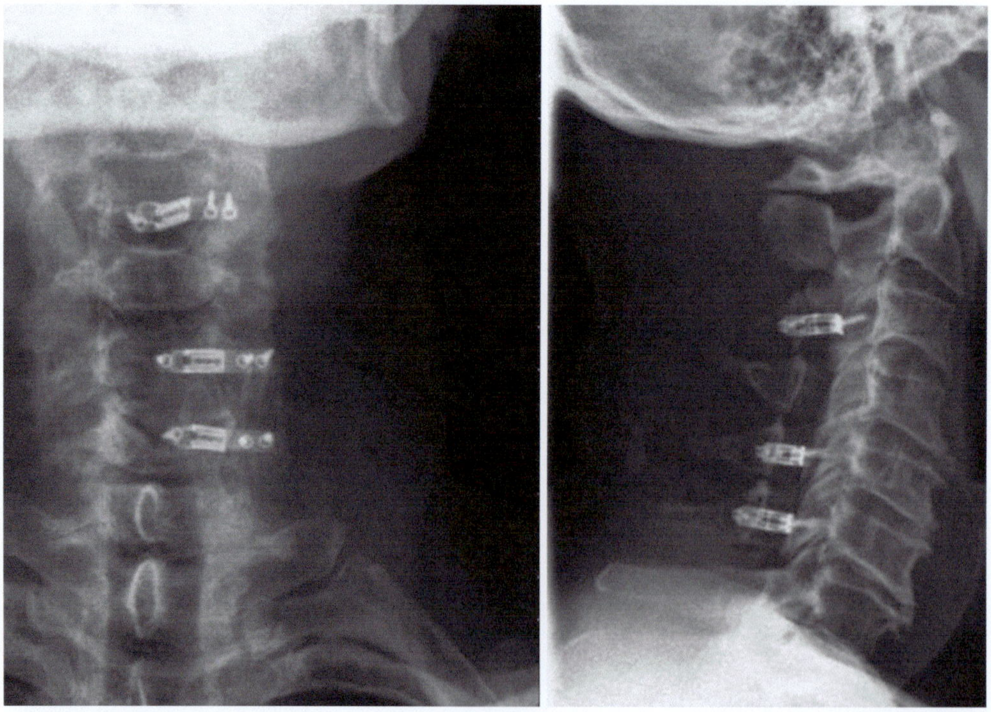

Fig. 16.2 Postoperative images of multilevel cervical laminoplasty. (Images from author's library)

fusion. Because it relies on posterior drift of the spinal cord, it is ideally performed in a patient with a lordotic cervical spine where the alignment allows the spinal cord to drift backward posteriorly.

16.2.2 Indications

Laminoplasty was originally developed as a way to decompress the cervical spinal cord across multiple segments without having to perform a fusion and while trying to avoid the complication of post-laminectomy kyphosis, which comes with laminectomy alone. The ideal patient for patients with multilevel stenosis needs ≥3 level decompression with preserved cervical lordosis; however, up to 10 degrees of cervical kyphosis has been shown to produce adequate spinal cord decompression [5]. It should be avoided in patients with ossification of the ligamentum flavum as the dural adhesions make posterior opening more difficult. If patients have significant axial neck pain as a portion of their complaints, surgeons may choose to avoid laminoplasty as it is not intended to treat neck pain. While earlier studies had warned of increasing axial neck pain with laminoplasty, more modern studies have demonstrated that laminoplasty does not increase axial neck pain postoperatively [6]. That being said, if axial neck pain is a significant portion of their complaint complex, laminoplasty may not fare as well as the alternatives. If patients have significant foraminal stenosis requiring foraminotomy, laminoplasty typically allows for a more thorough foraminotomy on the open-door side as opposed to the hinge side.

16.2.3 Technique

Intubation should be performed with caution to not extend the cervical spine past where the patient can comfortably extend prior to surgery. A Mayfield head holder can be applied to provide a stable mechanism for holding onto the head while leaving the eyes and face free. Depending on the severity of the stenosis, some patients may receive arterial line placement in order to ensure mean arterial pressures >80 mm to ensure adequate cord perfusion. Neural monitoring is routinely set up in myelopathy cases, which can help identify problems during positioning and during the canal expansion phases. The patient is then placed prone on the operating table and the head was secured via the Mayfield to the table. The arms are tucked at the side taking care to pad the ulnar nerves and the bed was placed in reverse Trendelenburg to minimize the bleeding.

Once the patient is prepped and draped, a midline incision is made over the spinous process spanning whichever segment needs to be addressed. Electrocautery is used to dissect down to the spinous processes taking care to stay in the midline avascular plane. Fluoroscopy is then used to localize the correct levels intraoperatively. Once on the spinous processes, the dissection is carried out laterally to the lateral mass/lamina junction. Any muscle insertions onto the C2 spinous process should be preserved as this decreases the risk of postoperative kyphosis. If performing a laminoplasty to decompress C2 to T1, the interlaminar ligaments at C2–3 and C7-T1 are removed. A high-speed burr is then used to prepare the opening troughs. The burr is placed along the lamina/lateral mass junction, and the bone is thinned down to the remaining cortex at the bottom. The opening trough can then be completed using the same burr or by switching to a Kerrison Rongeur. Once all the opening troughs are created, the hinge-side trough is prepared on the opposite side. In a similar fashion, the burr is placed along the lateral mass/lamina junction and the bone is thinned down to the ventral cortex but not through it. The hinge stiffness can be checked periodically, and the thinness of the ventral cortex is adjusted until you have a hinge, which is malleable enough to open yet still thick enough not to break completely during the opening. Using two small curettes, the lamina is then elevated on the opening side and any remaining ligamental attachments are resected. Care must be taken not to allow the hinges to suddenly close back shut. The opening is done in sequence heading from C3 down to C7 until adequate spinal canal expansion is achieved.

The lamina on the opening side can then be held in place using plate fixation, sutures, allograft struts, or autograft struts made from the spinous processes. The spinous processes can then be trimmed to allow for decreased prominence or left in place. A deep drain is then placed, and the wound was then closed in layers. Patients are then placed in a soft collar with the goal of quick return to motion to prevent postoperative discomfort and range of motion loss [3, 7].

16.2.4 Complications

The complications for cervical laminoplasty tend to focus on segmental nerve root palsies, axial neck pain, loss of range of motion, and loss of cervical lordosis. The most common motor deficit is the C5 nerve root palsy, which can have an incident of 5–11% and tends to occur on post-op day number 2 or 3 [8, 9]. While the C5 root is the most common, these nerve palsies can occur in any of the segmental nerve roots and have also been described after laminectomy and fusion and anterior cervical procedures [3, 10]. Loss of cervical motion has been reported after laminoplasty of 15.4 ± 8.4°l; however, this is less than laminectomy and fusion [11]. Loss of cervical lordosis is about 35%, with 10% of patients going on to develop post-laminoplasty kyphosis [12]. Loss of cervical lordosis has also been reported, with kyphosis rates ranging from 2% to 6%. However, early removal of cervical orthoses, early initiation of postoperative neck exercises, and modifications of surgical technique have been shown to preserve cervical lordosis [13] .

Axial neck pain following laminoplasty has a range of 6 to 60% in meta-analyses [12]. Axial neck pain has been shown to be significantly higher in laminoplasty than after fusion [14]. However, more recent studies suggest there is no worsening in axial neck pain symptoms following laminoplasty [6]. Postoperative axial symptoms may be limited by correct patient selection and adjustment of surgical techniques, including avoiding those prone to developing postoperative kyphosis, preservation of facet capsules, and C3 and C7 laminectomies instead of laminoplasty and early postoperative rehabilitation [15, 16].

16.2.5 Outcomes

Neurological outcomes following laminoplasty are excellent, with multiple studies and meta-analyses showing 80% of patients with improved neurological outcomes [12, 17, 18]. When comparing neurological outcomes to those after laminectomy and fusion, there are no significant differences; however, other complications were higher in the fusion group including myelopathy progression, nonunion, instrumentation failure, subjacent segment degeneration, reoperations, and infection [9]. Using pre- and postoperative Japanese Orthopedic Association (JOA) scores, neurologic recovery rate is 72% in a study of 25 patients after a 34-month follow-up [19].

16.3 Microdiscectomy

16.3.1 Introduction

Lumbar disk herniation is one of the most common causes of lumbar radiculopathy. Symptoms from the herniated disk result from a multifactorial mechanism comprised of mechanical compression of nerve roots by extruded material, inflammatory signaling, and an acidic microenvironment within the herniated lumbar disk [20]. The majority of patients with radiculopathy from lumbar disk herniations are treated conservatively; however, for those with continued symptoms microdiscectomy is a consideration. Microdiscectomy provides excellent, long-term outcomes for radiculopathy due to lumbar disk herniations. The 8-year outcomes of the Spine Patient Outcomes Research Trial (SPORT) demonstrated better outcomes with regard to pain and functional status when comparing operative versus non-operative management of lumbar disk herniation [21].

16.3.2 Indications

Absolute indications for lumbar microdiscectomy include bowel and bladder dysfunction due to massive disk herniation (i.e., cauda equina syndrome) and progressive neurological deficit. More relative indications include failure of conservative measures for 6–12 weeks and those who present with profound neurological deficits. Though surgery is commonly performed for the relative indications, there is no consensus on when conservative care should be abandoned and patients are referred to surgery. There are studies demonstrating prolonged symptom duration to have adverse effects on outcomes after microdiscectomy; however, the duration of symptoms in these studies ranges from 2 to 12 months [22, 23, 24].

16.3.3 Technique

After intubation, patients are positioned prone on a Wilson frame, Andrews table, or Jackson table. The hips and knees are flexed to decrease lumbar lordosis and allow for increased access through the interlaminar window. The interlaminar window is used for the vast majority of lumbar disk herniations within the central canal or subarticular zones. Far lateral herniations may be treated with the intertransverse window.

For the interlaminar approach, an incision is made directly over the midline posteriorly over the spinous processes. Dissected is carried down to the spinous processes and then subperiosteal approach is undertaken on the side of the spinous process ipsilateral to the herniation. A retractor is then placed, and fluoroscopy was used to confirm the operative level. A laminotomy of the cephalad lamina and minimal medial facetectomy is performed using a burr and Kerrison Rongeur, being careful to preserve at least 5 mm of the lateral pars interarticularis. The laminotomy should be wide enough to allow for palpation of the pedicle and mobilization of the traversing nerve root. The ligamentum flavum is then freed from its lateral insertion, and the lateral edge of the traversing root was identified. The traversing root is then mobilized medially allowing for access to the disk space in the safe zone lateral to the traversing root and in the axilla of the exiting root. Once the disk herniation is visualized, free fragments can be removed with a pituitary rongeur. If the disk herniation is contained, the annulus can be incised with a 15- or 11-blade scalpel and the disk space itself is entered. The disk fragment can be teased out with a nerve hook. Within the disk space, any remaining free fragments can be removed and the disk space was irrigated with angiocath to ensure no other free fragments remain.

For far lateral herniations, the intertransverse window can be used to gain access to the herniated disk fragment. The dissection is carried off midline in a plane between the multifidus and longissimus muscles. A retractor is placed, and an intraoperative radiograph was taken to confirm the correct level. The transverse processes are then exposed, and the intertransverse membrane lifted off the transverse process and retractor cranially. Gentle blunt dissections are used to identify the disk space and ensure you are below the exiting nerve root. A nerve hook and pituitary rongeur are then used to tease out the herniated disk fragments while minimizing nerve root retraction. This technique places the surgery on close proximity to the dorsal root ganglion, and so, retraction may result in postoperative radiculitis and/or complex regional pain syndrome.

Following both techniques, the disk space is irrigated using angiocath irrigation to ensure there are no other free fragments. The wound is then closed in layers.

16.3.4 Complications

Microdiscectomy complications include durotomy surgeon-dependent complications such as durotomy, nerve root injury, instability, and missed pathology and environment-dependent complications such as recurrent disk herniation, wound infection, and hematoma. Durotomy rates range from 0.7% to 4% for primary microdiscectomies [25]. A 2015 meta-analysis demonstrates nerve root injury rates of 1.1–2.6%, wound complication rates from 0.5% to 2%, hematoma rates of 0.5–0.6%, and reoperation rates of 7.1–10.2% [26]. Instability can result from excessive resection of the lamina, which results in a thin pars interarticularis, which fractures postoperatively or > 50% resection of the facet joint. 8-year SPORT data demonstrated 9.1% of patients who had primary discectomy undergoing revision surgery for re-herniation within the 8-year follow-up period. 37.8% of those procedures were during the first year after surgery [27].

16.3.5 Outcomes

In patients with lumbar radiculopathy due to disk herniation with leg symptoms persisting at least 6 weeks, surgery was superior to conservative treatment in relieving sciatic symptoms and improving function. At 8-year follow-up, surgical patients in the SPORT trial demonstrated significant advantages in sciatica bothersomeness, satisfaction with symptoms, and self-rated improvement [21]. Patients with significant medical comorbidities such as diabetes or smoking and those with ongoing litigation, worker's compensation claims, or depression are less likely to experience favorable outcomes with surgery [28, 29].

16.4 Anterior Cervical Discectomy and Fusion (ACDF)

16.4.1 Introduction

Degenerative conditions resulting in radiculopathy and myelopathy are frequently encountered in the cervical spine. Anterior cervical discectomy and fusion (ACDF) is the most common operation used to decompress the neurological structures and restore disk height. It has been shown to have excellent clinical results and has a relatively safe track record. It offers the advantage of directly visualizing anterior compressive structures such as the disk and/or anterior osteophytes, this allows for their removal of the spinal cord and nerve roots.

16.4.2 Indications

Current indications for ACDF are patients with cervical spondylosis, presenting with cervical radiculopathy or myelopathy that has been unresponsive to conservative care. It can also be indicated in cases of cervical degenerative disk disease It is generally done for 1–3 levels of cervical disk disease. Posterior cervical surgery should be considered in cases in which compressive lesions extend to >3 levels. Contraindications to ACDF include approach-related concerns that preclude anterior access (including the previous history of anterior neck radiation).

16.4.3 Technique

Patients are positioned supine on standard operating table with their cervical spine in neutral position. Their shoulders may be taped down to facilitate the X-rays, although great care should be taken as to the amount of force applied through the tape. A standard Smith–Robinson approach to the anterior cervical spine is then undertaken, coursing between the strap muscles and sternocleidomastoid superficially and the esophagus and carotid sheath more deeply. Once the correct level is localized via fluoroscopy, the longus colli muscles are elevated and a retractor placed underneath them. A knife is then used to enter the disk space, and a complete discectomy is then performed. The posterior longitudinal ligament can then be resected, and a Kerrison was used to decompress the foramen. Once the decompression is complete, the trials are brought in for the cervical disk arthroplasty. The appropriate size is then picked both by how it feels and by fluoroscopy images. Some surgeons utilize allograft bone for the implant, while others utilize synthetic cages, which can then be filled with demineralized bone matrix or synthetic materials for fusion. Once the implant is placed, an anterior plate is then

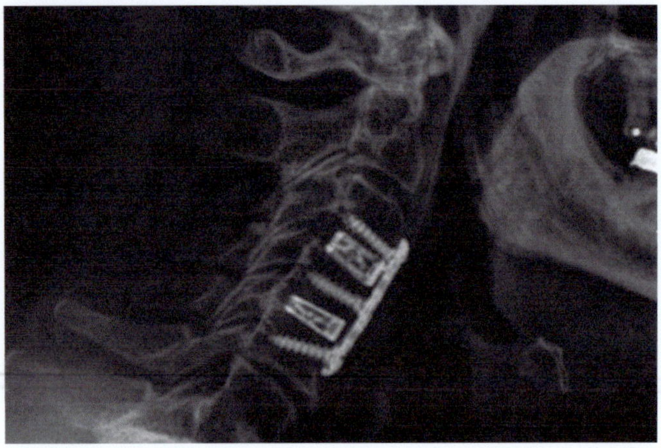

Fig. 16.3 Lateral views of postoperative C4–5 and C5/6 ACDF. (Images from author's library)

added with screws fixated into the bone on either side of the disk to be fused. The top of the plate is kept >5 mm away from the adjacent disk space so as to minimize the risk of adjacent level ossification (Fig. 16.3).

16.4.4 Complications

Complications of ACDF can include approach-related issues such as esophageal perforation, dysphagia, vertebral artery injury, and recurrent laryngeal nerve injury. Esophageal perforation is an uncommon complication with a rate of 0.3–0.9% [59, 60]. Surgeons should have a high index of suspicious for this as the late consequences of this can result in mediastinitis and sepsis. Immediate postoperative dysphagia is relatively common after ACDF, with some series documenting anywhere between 2% and 67% incidence; however, this tends to decrease over time [61]. Vertebral artery injury is uncommon with an incidence of 0.1–0.5% but can result in stroke and severe postoperative neurological deficit. The vertebral artery is generally located 1–2 mm lateral to the uncovertebral joint and can be injured by excessive lateral bone removal. Vocal cord paralysis due to recurrent laryngeal nerve injury has an incidence of 2–3% [62]. The etiology is usually due to compression of the nerve against the larynx.

Degeneration of adjacent disks after ACDF has been known to occur. In systematic reviews, asymptomatic adjacent segment degeneration had an incidence of 16–96% with symptomatic degeneration having a range of 1.8–36% [63].

16.4.5 Outcomes

Long-term clinical outcomes for ACDF tend to be very favorable. In a study on >10-year clinical outcomes of ACDF, there were significantly improved outcomes for all diagnoses that were sustained out to 10 years [57]. In another study of patients with substantial preoperative neck pain undergoing ACDF, there were significant reductions in neck pain, disability, and physical function scores after ACDF [58].

16.5 Cervical Foraminotomy

16.5.1 Introduction

The use of a posterior approach for the treatment of cervical radiculopathy was first described by Mixter [30]. Posterior cervical foraminotomy can be used to treat foraminal stenosis and/or foraminal disk herniation causing a radiculopathy. The borders of the neural foramen are the disk and uncovertebral joint ventrally, the pedicles above and below, and the superior articular facet of the caudal segment (i.e., the C5 superior articular facet for the C4–5 foramen). The concept of foraminotomy is the posterior unroofing of the neural foramen by removing the medial portion of superior articular process and allowing the nerve root to float dorsally away from anterior pathology.

16.5.2 Indications

Posterior cervical foraminotomy can be done in patients with foraminal stenosis and foraminal disk herniations resulting in cervical radiculopathy, which fails to respond to nonsurgical treatments.

16.5.3 Technique

Patients are positioned prone for the foraminotomy. Their head may be placed into Mayfield head holder or Gardner Wells tongs. The table is then placed into reverse Trendelenburg, and the shoulder is taped down slightly to facilitate fluoroscopy. The head should be flexed to unshingle the facet joint and allow more visualization of the superior articular facet. Once the patient is prepped and draped, a small midline incision can be made and subperiosteal dissection is carried down to the cervical lamina and facet joint. Intraoperative X-ray should then be taken to confirm that this is the appropriate level.

Following that, a high-speed burr can be used to resect the medial portion of the inferior articular process, which is overlying the superior articular process. Once the superior articular process is visible, this can be thinned down with the burr and then resected with a Kerrison Rongeur out to the lateral margin of the pedicles. The lateral walls of the cranial and caudal pedicles can then be palpated with a nerve hook to ensure there is no residual bony overlying the area of the foramen. Hemostasis can then be achieved with hemostatic agents such as Gelfoam Thrombin or Floseal. The wound is then irrigated, and multilayer closure is undertaken.

16.5.4 Complications

Special attention should be paid when performing the foraminotomy at C4–5 as C5 palsy is a well-known complication of any posterior cervical surgery, with incidences ranging from 4.7% to 6.4%. Incidental durotomy rates tend to be low (1–1.7%) [33].

16.5.5 Outcomes

Most studies show good or excellent outcomes of about 85–95% for posterior cervical foraminotomy [31]. The incidence of revision surgery is about 2.3% [32]. Instability can result from overaggressive resection of the facet joint and resultant lateral mass fracture. Manipulation of the nerve can cause worsening radiculopathy and/or neurological deficit postoperatively.

16.6 Lumbar Fusion

16.6.1 Introduction

Lumbar fusion can be used to treat a wide variety of pathologies. It is most commonly done for patients with spondylolisthesis with motion on their flexion/extension films or patients with spinal deformities requiring reconstruction. It can be used to treat patients with discitis and/or discogenic low back pain. The choice of fusion type to perform is decided upon by approach-related factors and a variety of patient factors. Types of fusion include anterior lumbar interbody fusion (ALIF), transforaminal lumbar interbody fusion (TLIF), and posterior lumbar interbody fusion (Figs. 16.4 and 16.5).

16.6.2 ALIF

For *anterior lumbar interbody fusion* (Fig. 16.4), patients are positioned supine, with either an inflatable pillow or fold blankets placed underneath them to facilitate lordosis. The break in the table can also be used to provide more lordosis. An anterior retroperitoneal approach is then undertaken to the anterior lumbar spine, staying outside the peritoneum, moving laterally to until the psoas muscle is visible, and then retracting the peritoneum toward the midline until the lumbar spine and great vessels are seen. For the L5-S1 segment, the middle sacral vessels will be found traversing the disk space from cranial to caudal and should be clipped prior to beginning the discectomy. To expose the L4–5 segment, identification of the iliolumbar vein on the left is necessary to ensure it does not get injured with movement of the vascular structures when they are retracted to the right.

A knife is used to begin the discectomy, and in a similar fashion to other procedures, the disk is removed with curettes, cobb, and other instruments while being careful to avoid violating the endplate. The posterior longitudinal ligament is not routinely resected but can be freed up from the back of the vertebral bodies with a curette. A distractor can be placed into the disk space to allow for better visualization. Anterior neural foraminotomies can then be completed with a Kerrison Rongeur.

Once the discectomy is completed, the disk space distractors can be removed, and the trial implants were brought in. Once the appropriate size is found, the final graft can be packed with the surgeon's choice of bone graft/substitutes and then impacted into place under fluoroscopic guidance (Fig. 16.4).

16.6.3 TLIF and PLIF

Transforaminal lumbar interbody fusion (TLIF) or posterior lumbar interbody fusion (PLIF) is performed on a Jackson table, allowing the patient's abdomen to hang free in order to minimize venous congestion and bleeding. The hips should be extended to maximize positional lordosis. Once the area is prepped and draped, the standard midline approach is undertaken and the correct level was localized using fluoroscopy.

TLIF—After the exposure is completed the facet joint on the side is completely resected using a burr and kerrisons. This provides access to the triangular working zone between the exiting root, traversing root, and the caudal pedicle. With the nerve roots protected, the annulus of the disk is then incised and the disk space preparation begun. Several types of curettes and pituitaries have been designed for disk space preparation for TLIF. The disk on the ipsilateral side is first cleaned out, and then, longer instruments can be used to reach the contralateral portions of the disk. Great care should be taken not to violate the anterior or anterolateral annulus, as this could result in vascular injury. Lateral fluoroscopy can be used to assess the depth of the instruments in the disk space. Once the disk space has been cleared out, the trial implants can be brought in to assess the appropriate height of the cage. After that has been decided, the final implant can be packed with the surgeon's choice of graft material and impacted into place. The implant should be placed as anterior and central as possible under fluoroscopic guidance. Pedicle screws can then be placed for stabilization.

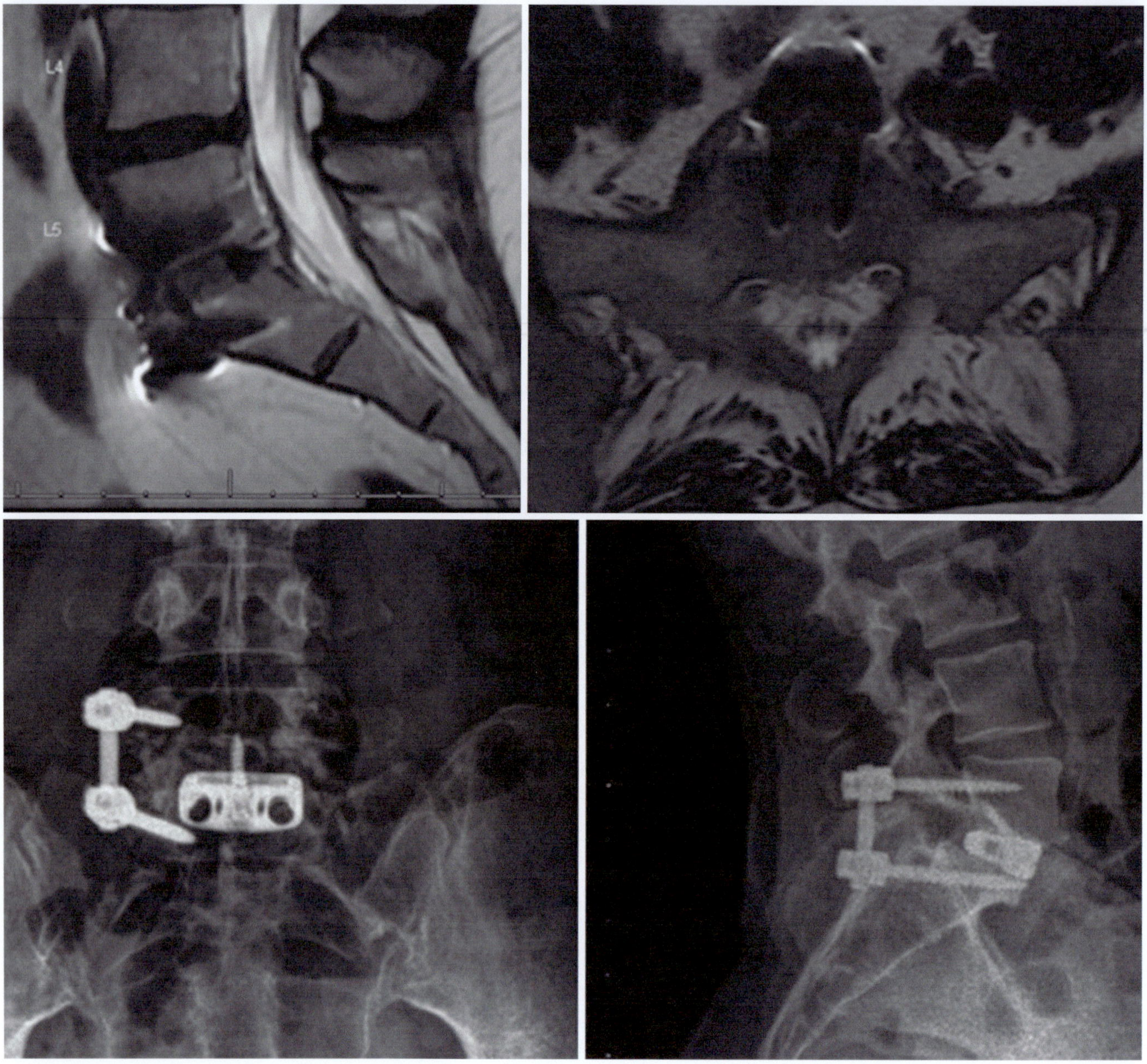

Fig. 16.4 MR imaging of patients with L5-S1 ALIF and X-ray imaging of patient with ALIF and unilateral posterior pedicular screw fixation. (Images from author's library)

PLIF (Fig. 16.5)—The PLIF procedure is essentially identical to a TLIF other than bilateral annular windows that are made, and these windows are more medial than they would be for TLIF. The remainder of the procedure is identical with disk space clean out, trialing, and impacting the final implants into position. These tend to go in straighter than the TLIF cages because of the trajectory available.

XLIF (Fig. 16.5)—It is an increasingly popular lateral trans-psoas interbody fusion technique, which utilizes a minimally invasive approach, sparing the anterior longitudinal ligament, and allowing sufficient visualization of the intervertebral disks and bodies to debride and place a large, lordotic cage. It is indicated for thoracolumbar spine and enables surgical debridement of the disk space and facilitates fusion. In vast majority, it is coupled with posterior pedicle screws fixation.

16.6.4 Complications

ALIF: Approach-related complications tend to be the most common with ALIF, with vascular or visceral injury being the result. The vascular injury rate with ALIFs is cited at

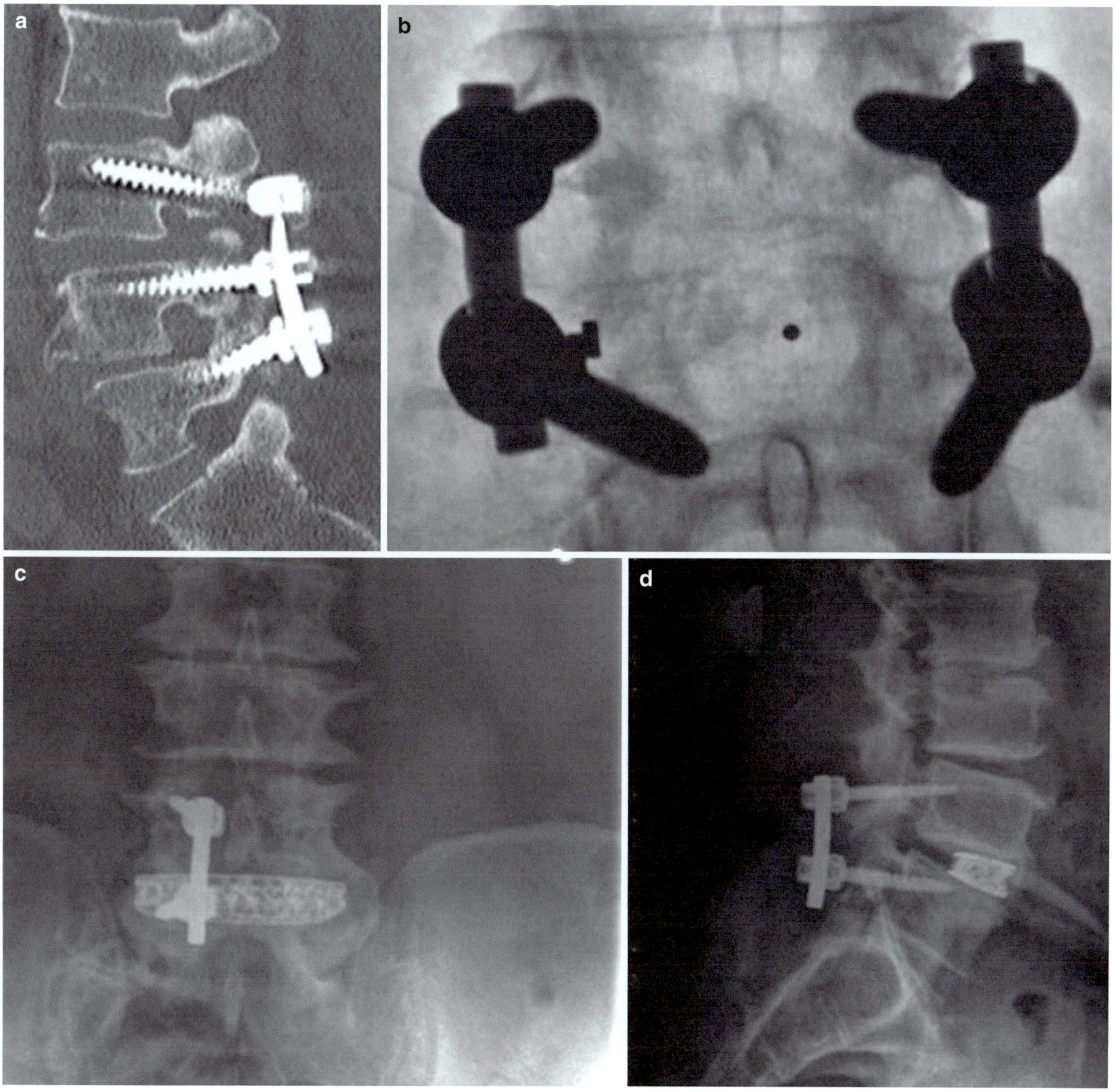

Fig. 16.5 (**a**) Postoperative CT of a patient after L3/4 and L4/5 PLIF. (**b**) AP X-rays of a patient after L4–5 PLIF. (Image courtesy of Ali Mostoufi, MD). Images **c** and **d** demonstrate XLIF. Extreme lateral interbody fusion (XLIF) is a minimally invasive lateral trans-psoas approach, which is coupled with pedicle screw fixation. (Images from author's library)

anywhere between 1.9% and 20% and is most common at the L4–5 level, where the bifurcation of the great vessels requires greater retraction of the vessels to see the disk space [34]. Incidence of deep vein thrombosis following ALIF ranges from 0% to 12.2% [35]. Retrograde ejaculations in men can occur as a result of parasympathetic fiber disruption. It occurs up to 5% in ALIF cases [34].

TLIF: Dural tear can occur as a result of passing multiple instruments and cages near the dura and has an incident rate ranging from 5.1% to 14.3% [35, 36]. Instrumentation failure and interbody cage migration can also occur at a rate ranging from 1.8% to 2.3%. Cases of revision TLIF also demonstrate higher infection rates than primary TLIF.

PLIF: As compared to TLIF for treating multilevel stenosis, PLIF was equivalent in terms of VAS of back pain, VAS of leg pain, SF-36 scores, and ODI. However, the TLIF group has less blood loss and shorter hospital stays [37].

16.6.5 Outcomes

ALIF—ALIF has a biomechanical advantage over the posterior approaches, particularly for restoration of disk height and lumbar lordosis [38]. It also accesses a much larger portion of the disk space, allowing for placement of a larger implant. It also accomplishes all this without dissecting the posterior spinal musculature. The rate of dural injury is much lower in ALIF as compared with posterior approaches (TLIF and PLIF) [39]. Conversely, the rate of vascular injury is higher than in posterior approaches.

TLIF–TLIF allows for interbody fusion without the need for a separate anterior approach; however, the trade-off is more limited access to the disks space for placement of the interbody cage. This results in smaller disk height, less segmental lordosis, and lower whole spine lordosis as compared to ALIF [39]. However, in terms of outcomes, meta-analyses have shown no difference between ALIF and TLIF for leg or back pain scores nor in terms of fusion rates [40, 41].

PLIF—As compared to TLIF, the PLIF approach may provide higher immediate stability, especially in lateral bending as it does not require resection of the facet joint to gain a more lateral entry to the disk space [42]. However, the more central approach requires great retraction of the dura and resultant higher rates of neurological injury as compared to TLIF (7.8 in PLIF vs 2% in TLIF) [43]. Similar to TLIF, cage migration can occur but is uncommon.

16.7 Disk Replacement

16.7.1 Introduction

Degenerative spondylosis resulting in radiculopathy and myelopathy is frequently encountered in the cervical spine. Traditionally, anterior cervical discectomy and fusion (ACDF) has been the most common operation used to decompress the neurological structures and restore disk height. However, adjacent segment deterioration and limitation in range of motion spurred an interest in cervical disk arthroplasty. These allow for maintained motion at the surgical levels and theoretically lower rates of adjacent segment degeneration.

In parallel, lumbar disk replacement has also become increasingly common as a treatment option for degenerative disk disease.

16.7.2 Indications

Current indications for cervical disk arthroplasty are patients with cervical spondylosis presenting with cervical radiculopathy or myelopathy that has been unresponsive to conservative care. Cervical disk arthroplasty (Fig. 16.6) is currently only approved for 1 or 2 levels in the cervical spine. Dynamic instability (>3.5 mm of motion on flexion–extension X-rays) and ossification of the posterior longitudinal ligament are contraindications for cervical disk arthroplasty. A relative contraindication in patients with axial neck pain is due to facet arthrosis as their axial symptoms may not improve or may worsen with cervical disk arthroplasty. Osteoporosis is also a relative contraindication due to risk of implant subsidence.

16.7.3 Technique

Patients are positioned supine on a standard operating table with their cervical spine in neutral position. Their shoulders may be taped down to facilitate the X-rays, although great care should be taken as to the amount of force applied through the tape. A standard Smith–Robinson approach to the anterior cervical spine is then undertaken, coursing between the strap muscles and sternocleidomastoid superficially and the esophagus and carotid sheath more deeply. Once the correct level is localized via fluoroscopy, the longus colli muscles are elevated and a retractor was placed underneath them. A knife is then used to enter the disk space, and a complete discectomy is then performed. The posterior longitudinal ligament can then be resected, and a Kerrison was used to decompress the foramen. Once the decompression is complete, the trials are brought in for the cervical disk arthroplasty. The appropriate size is then picked both by how it feels and by fluoroscopy images. Great care must be taken to ensure the trials are in the midline of the disk space and to get trials wide and deep enough to provide as much coverage to the endplate as possible. Following this step, once the implant size is selected, some systems may necessitate a keel cut, which can then be completed under fluoroscopy. Following this, the final implant can be placed, and final X-rays are taken to ensure the implant sits in the middle of the disk space.

16.7.4 Complications

Complications from cervical disk arthroplasty include subsidence of the implant, device dislocation, osteolysis, and heterotopic ossification (HO). Radiographic subsidence has a range of 0% to 33%, with clinically significant subsidence being around 3% [46]. Arthroplasty should be performed with caution in patients with osteoporosis, and great care should be taken with the endplates at the time of surgery. Risk of subsidence and implant dislocation can be reduced by avoiding drilling and preserving the endplates during disk space preparation. Subsidence risk can also be lessened by avoiding placement of an implant with too large a height for the disk space.

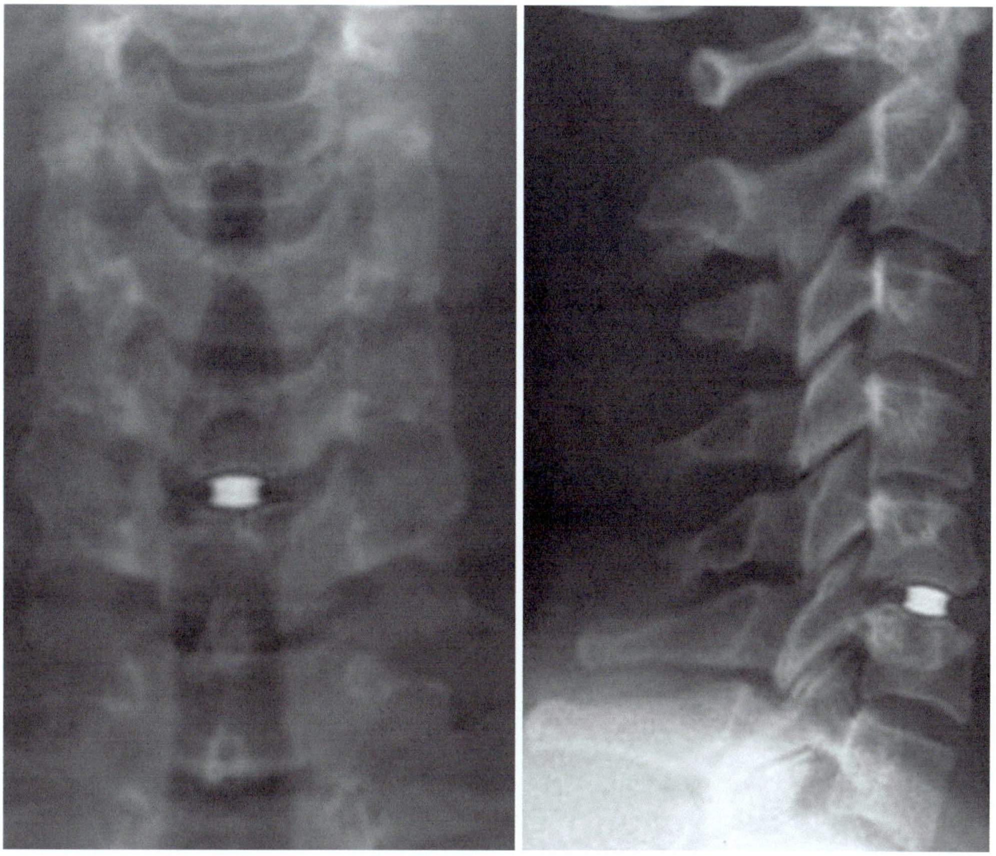

Fig. 16.6 Image shows example of C5/6 disk replacement surgery

Heterotopic ossification can also occur after cervical disk arthroplasty, ranging from minimal to inadvertent arthrodesis. Male sex and older age have been shown to be risk factors for HO [47]. Some degree of HO is common after cervical disk arthroplasty, with rates approaching 53.6% at the 5- to 10-year range [48]. The risk can be decreased by avoiding excessive drilling and appropriate sizing of the implant to provide near-complete endplate coverage. Similar to hip arthroplasty, patients can be placed on nonsteroidal anti-inflammatory drugs during the early postoperative period to try and reduce the risk of HO.

16.7.5 Outcomes

In a study of 2-level degenerative disease, Fay et al. demonstrated cervical disk arthroplasty to preserve mobility at the operative levels and provide similar outcomes to ACDF. Another prospective study on 2-level cervical disk arthroplasty vs ACDF demonstrated significantly greater improvements in neck disability index, patient satisfaction, and perceived overall success in the arthroplasty group [44]. The ACDF patients also had a higher rate of subsequent surgeries (15.2% vs 4%) and radiographic adjacent disk degeneration. However, when comparing cervical arthroplasty to ACDF, most studies have not shown a difference in adjacent segment pathology [45].

16.8 Coccygectomy

16.8.1 Introduction

Coccydynia can occur as a result of acute or cumulative trauma to the coccyx. The majority of patients are treated conservatively; however, in refractory cases coccygectomy can be considered. This pain can be quite debilitating, particularly while sitting. Patients who fail treatments such as NSAIDs, sitting aids, and warm compresses can undergo injection of local anesthetic and steroids. Those who fail to achieve good long relief can consider coccygectomy.

16.8.2 Technique

Patients are positioned in the prone position and both gluteal regions held out of the way with adhesive tape. A longitudinal incision is made over the coccyx, taking great care to avoid the rectal sphincter. The disk between the sacrum and coccyx is then exposed and removed. A towel clamp can then be used to grab the coccyx and pull it forward. The surrounding soft tissues are then elevated and dissected free. Once the coccyx is removed, rectal integrity can be checked from inside the incision and then the wound was thoroughly irrigated and closed in layers.

16.8.3 Complications

The most common complication of coccygectomy is infection. Overall wound infection rates were 10% [50]. E. coli and S. aureus were the most frequently recorded bacteria. Other wound complications such as hematoma, persistent drainage, and wound dehiscence can occur and necessitate surgical management; however, they are less common than wound infection.

16.8.4 Outcomes

A study by Cebesoy et al. demonstrated high patient satisfaction rates with coccygectomy [49]. At 24 months, mean VAS scores had decreased to 2.76. In another meta-analysis, 84% of patients had an excellent or good outcomes [50].

16.9 Deformity Surgery

16.9.1 Introduction

The adult human spine has a carefully balanced sagittal profile, which functions to position the head directly over the sacrum and pelvis. This balance allows for less energy usage in maintaining forward gaze and has been described as the cone of economy [51]. When misalignment of the spinal column leads to the spinal column existing outside of this cone, increased energy is required to maintain upright posture. The resulting increased energy expenditure and asymmetric loading of motions segments lead to pain, which can be debilitating.

16.9.2 Indications

For patients with sagittal imbalance who continue to be symptomatic despite conservative care, surgical deformity correction can be considered (Figs. 16.7 and 16.8). Due to the nature of these surgeries, imperative patients are carefully screened and ruled out for osteoporosis, smoking, and nutritional abnormalities.

16.9.3 Technique

The technique chosen for deformity correction depends in part on the pathology driving the deformity. For regional sagittal balance deformities (i.e., one driven by mostly thoracic spine), most deformity corrections will occur via a posterior-based approach. For global sagittal balance defor-

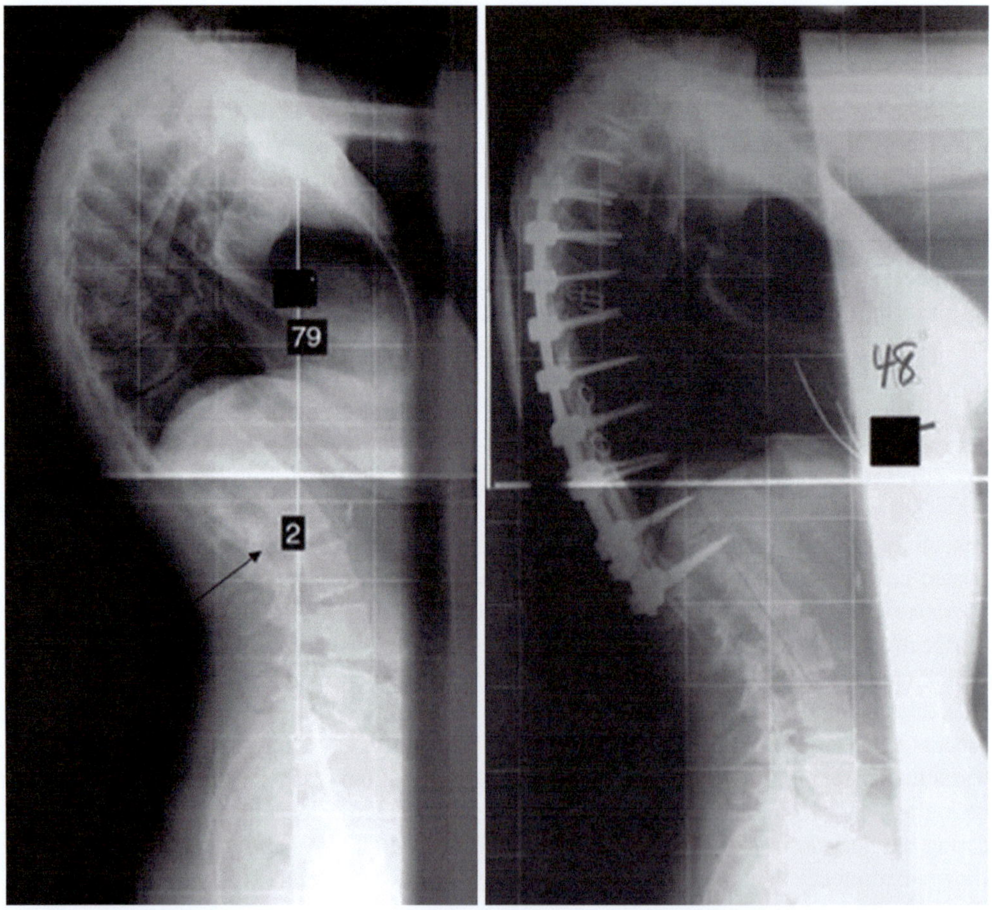

Fig. 16.7 Preoperative and postoperative plain films of a patient with thoracic kyphosis

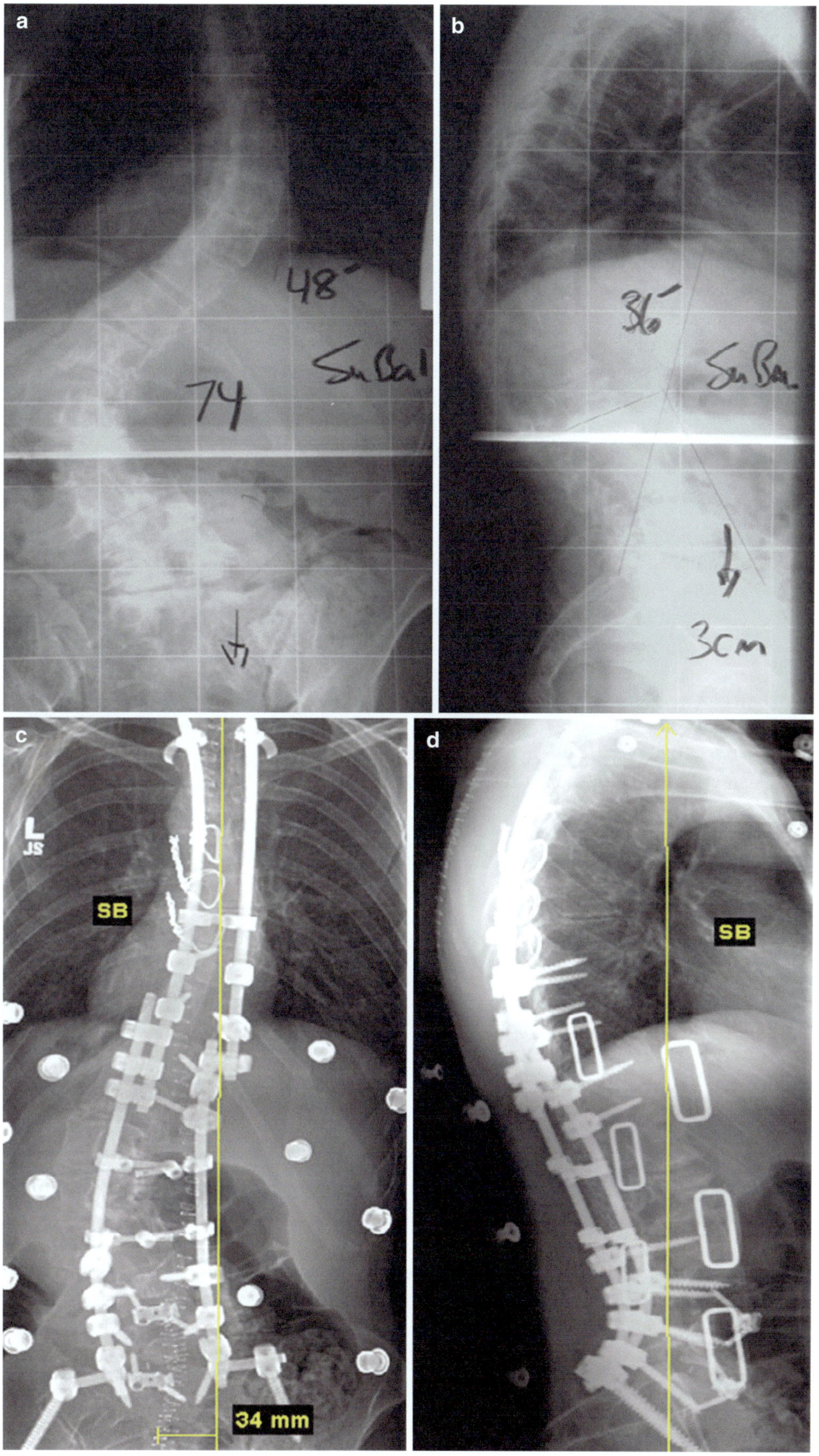

Fig. 16.8 Preoperative and postoperative images of a 49-year-old woman with painful thoracolumbar scoliosis. Images **a** and **b** show preoperative AP and lateral views. **c** and **d** are postoperative films, with the patient wearing a brace to reduce motion and lessen pain

mities, the patient's deformity can be classified as to how flexible and correctable it is and then a treatment plan involves *posterior-only* or *combined anterior–posterior* approach.

If there is a flexible deformity at the disk level, a Smith–Peterson type osteotomy (SPO) can be done at multiple levels to achieve correction. The SPO involves a wedge-shaped osteotomy, which removes part of the facets, posterior arch, and ligamentum flavum and allows for approximately 9–10 degrees of deformity correction per level [52]. SPOs are thus best suited for long-sweeping thoracic kyphosis where multiple levels can be done to achieve correction.

For fixed deformities, pedicle subtraction osteotomy (PSO) can be considered. This involved removing a wedge of bone from the vertebral body along with the entire posterior arch and pedicles. The procedure consists of initially removing the posterior bony elements and then resecting the pedicles down to the vertebral body. A wedge from the vertebral body is then removed with osteotomes, taking care not to remove the anterior wall itself. Once the bone elements are resected, compression can be delivered through the pedicle screws and/or the surgical table was extended to achieve closure of the osteotomy. Most PSOs can achieve 30–45 degrees of correction [53].

The most severe and rigid deformities may require total vertebral column resection (VCR). This involves resection of the entire posterior column and vertebral body from the posterior approach. An interbody cage can then be placed to fill the defect created by resection of the vertebral body.

16.9.4 Complications

The rate of complications ranges from 20% to more than 50% in some series for adult deformity correction. The most common complications are dural tear (5.9%), wound infections (3.8%), neurological deficit (3.6%), and instrumentation failure (1.7%) [54]. Proximal junctional kyphosis (PJK) or forward bending at the upper end of the spinal fusion is also a well-known complication in adult deformity surgery. Most cases occur within 2 years of the index surgery, and the incidence ranges from 5% to 46% [55].

16.9.5 Outcomes

Despite the relatively high rate of complications, outcomes after adult deformity correction tend to be relatively good, resulting in decreased pain and longer ambulation distances for patients. Even in those over the age of 70, one study showed significant benefit with ODI scores decreased from 49 to 25 [56].

References

1. Amundsen T, Weber H, Nordal HJ, Magnaes B, Abdelnoor M, Lilleâs F. Lumbar spinal stenosis: conservative or surgical management? A prospective 10-year study. Spine. 2000;25:1424.
2. Lurie JD, Tosteson TD, Tosteson A, Abdu WA, Zhao W, Morgan TS, Weinstein JN. Long-term outcomes of lumbar spinal stenosis: eight-year results of the Spine Patient Outcomes Research Trial (SPORT). Spine. 2015;40(2):63–76. https://doi.org/10.1097/BRS.0000000000000731.
3. Braly BA, Lunardini D, Cornett C, Donaldson WF. Operative treatment of cervical myelopathy: cervical laminoplasty. Adv Orthoped. Article ID 508534. https://doi.org/10.1155/2012/508534.
4. Oyama M, Hattori S, Moriwaki N, Nitta S: [A new method of cervical laminectomy]. *Chuubu Nippon Seikeigeka Gakkai Zasshi* 16: 792–794, 1973. (Japanese).
5. Uchida K, Nakajima H, Sato R, et al. Cervical spondylotic myelopathy associated with kyphosis or sagittal sigmoid alignment: outcome after anterior or posterior decompression—clinical article. J Neurosurg. 2009;11(5):521–8.
6. Stephens BF, Rhee JM, Neustein TM, et al. Laminoplasty does not lead to worsening axial neck pain in the properly selected patient with cervical myelopathy: a comparison with laminectomy and fusion. Spine. 2017;42:1844–50.
7. Yoneunobu K, Wada E, Ono K. Treatment of cervical myelopathy. Part B: laminoplasty. In: Clark CR, et al., editors. The cervical spine. 4th ed. Philadelphia: Lippincott Williams & Wilkins; 2005. p. 1057–71.
8. Imagama S, Matsuyama Y, Yukawa Y, et al. C5 palsy after cervical laminoplasty: a multicentre study. J Bone Joint Surg. 2010;92B(3):393–400.
9. Heller JG, Edwards CC, Murakami H, Rodts GE. Laminoplasty vs laminectomy and fusion for multilevel cervical myelopathy. Spine. 2001;26:1330–6.
10. Yoneunobu K, Wada E, Ono K. Treatment of cervical myelopathy. Part B: laminoplasty. In: Clark CR, Benzel EC, editors. The cervical spine. 4th ed. Philadelphia: Lippincott Williams & Wilkins; 2005. p. 1057–71.
11. Hyun SJ, Riew KD, Rhim SC. Spine J. 2013;13(4):384–90. https://doi.org/10.1016//j.spinee.2012.10.037. Epub 2012 Dec 6
12. Sani S. A critical review of laminoplasty. Neurosurg Q. 2004;14:5–16.
13. Machino M, Yukawa Y, Hida T, Ito K, Nakashima H, Kanbara S, Morita D, Kato F. Cervical alignment and range of motion after laminoplasty. Spine. 2012;37(20):E1243–50.
14. Woods BI, Hohl J, Lee J, Donaldson W 3rd, Kang J. Laminoplasty versus laminectomy and fusion for multilevel cervical spondylotic myelopathy. Clin Orthop Relat Res. 2011;469(3):688–95. https://doi.org/10.1007/s11999-010-1653-5.
15. Michael KW, Neustein TM, Rhee JM. Where should a laminoplasty start? The effect of proximal level on post-laminectomy loss of lordosis. Spine J. 2016;16(6):737–41.
16. Riew KD, Raich AL, Dettori JR, Heller JG. Neck pain following cervical laminoplasty: does preservation of the C2 muscle attachments and/or C7 matter? Evid Based Spine Care J. 2013;4(1):42–53.
17. Tomita K, Kawahara N, Toribatake Y, Heller JG. Expansive midline T-saw laminoplasty (modified spinous process-splitting) for the management of cervical myelopathy. Spine. 1998;23:32–7.
18. Hirabayashi K, Satomi K. Operative procedure and results of expansive open-door laminoplasty. Spine. 1988;13:870–6.
19. Tetreault L, Kopjar B, Nouri A, Arnold P, Barbagallo G, Bartels R, Qiang Z, Singh A, Zileli M, Vaccaro A, Fehlings MG. The modified Japanese Orthopaedic association scale: establishing criteria for mild, moderate and severe impairment in patients with degenerative cervical myelopathy. Eur Spine J. 2017;26:78–84.

20. Amin RM, Andrade NS, Neuman BJ. Lumbar disc herniation. Curr Rev Musculoskelet Med. 2017;10(4):507–16. https://doi.org/10.1007/s12178-017-9441-4).
21. Lurie JD, Tor DT, Tosteson ANA, Zhao W, Morgan TS, Abdu WA, Herkowitz H, Weinstein JN. Surgical versus nonoperative treatment for lumbar disc herniation: eight-year results for the spine patient outcomes research trial [published correction appears in Spine (Phila Pa 1976). 2015 Jan;40(1):E59]. Spine (Phila Pa 1976). 2014;39(1):3–16. https://doi.org/10.1097/BRS.0000000000000088.
22. Beck J, Westin O, Brisby H, Baranto A. Association of extended duration of sciatic leg pain with worse outcome after lumbar disc herniation surgery: a register study in 6216 patients. J Neurosurg Spine. 2021;12:1–9. https://doi.org/10.3171/2020.8.SPINE20602. Online ahead of print.
23. Schoenfeld AJ, Bono CM. Does surgical timing influence functional recovery after lumbar discectomy? A systematic review. Clin Orthop Relat Res. 2015;473(6):1963–70. https://doi.org/10.1007/s11999-014-3505-1. PMID: 24526298; PMCID: PMC4419004.
24. Nygaard OP, Romner B, Trumpy JH. Duration of leg pain as a predictor of outcome after lumbar disc surgery. Acta Neurochir. 1994;128:53–6.
25. Desai A, Ball PA, Bekelis K, Lurie JD, Mirza SK, Tosteson TD, Weinstein JN. Outcomes after incidental durotomy during first-time lumbar discectomy. J Neurosurg Spine. 2011;14(5):647–53.
26. Shriver MF, Xie JJ, Tye EY, Rosenbaum BP, Kshettry VR, Benzel EC, Mroz TE. Lumbar microdiscectomy complication rates: a systematic review and meta-analysis. Neurosurg Focus. 2015;39(4):E6.
27. Abdu RW, Abdu WA, Pearson AM, Zhao W, Lurie JD, Weinstein JN. Reoperation for recurrent intervertebral disc herniation in the spine patient outcomes research trial: analysis of rate, risk factors, and outcome. Spine (Phila Pa 1976). 2017;42(14):1106–14. https://doi.org/10.1097/BRS.0000000000002088.
28. Zeeni C, Carabini LM, Gould RW, Bebawy JF, Hemmer LB, Moreland NC, Koski TR, Koht A, Schafer MF, Ondra SL, Gupta DK. The implementation and efficacy of the Northwestern High Risk Spine Protocol. World Neurosurg. 2014;82(6):e815–23. https://doi.org/10.1016/j.wneu.2014.06.020. Epub 2014 Jun 17.PMID: 24947117.
29. Dewing CB, Provencher MT, Riffenburgh RH, Kerr S, Manos RE. The outcomes of lumbar microdiscectomy in a young, active population: correlation by herniation type and level. Spine (Phila Pa 1976). 2008;33(1):33–8. https://doi.org/10.1097/BRS.0b013e31815e3a42.
30. Mixter WJ. Rupture of the intervertebral disk; a short history of this evolution as a syndrome of importance to the surgeon. J Am Med Assoc. 1949;140(3):278–82.
31. Kim KT, Kim YB. Comparison between open procedure and tubular retractor assisted procedure for cervical radiculopathy: results of a randomized controlled study. J Korean Med Sci. 2009;24(4):649–53.
32. Song Z, Zhang Z, Hao J, Shen J, Zhou N, Xu S, Ni W, Hu Z. Microsurgery or open cervical foraminotomy for cervical radiculopathy? A systematic review. Int Orthop. 2016;40(6):1335–43. https://doi.org/10.1007/s00264-016-3193-4. Epub 2016 Apr 25
33. Oshina, Masahito; Segawa, Tomohide; Oshima, Yasushi; Tanaka, Sakae ; Inanami, Hirohiko. C5 palsy after C5/6/7 posterior foraminal decompression, Medicine: 2020; 99(3): e18817 i: https://doi.org/10.1097/MD.0000000000018817.
34. Mobbs, Ralph J , , Kevin Phan, Daniel Daly, Prashanth J Rao; Andrew Lennox. "Approach-related complications of anterior lumbar interbody fusion: results of a combined spine and vascular surgical team." Global Spine J 6,2 (2016): 147–154. doi:https://doi.org/10.1055/s-0035-1557141.
35. Wong AP, Smith ZA, Nixon AT, Lawton CD, Dahdaleh NS, Wong RH, Auffinger B, Lam S, Song JK, Liu JC, Koski TR, Fessler RG. Intraoperative and perioperative complications in minimally invasive transforaminal lumbar interbody fusion: a review of 513 patients. J Neurosurg Spine. 2015;22(5):487–95. https://doi.org/10.3171/2014.10.SPINE14129. Epub 2015 Feb 20
36. Tormenti MJ, Maserati MB, Bonfield CM, Gerszten PC, Moossy JJ, Kanter AS, Spiro RM, Okonkwo DO. Perioperative surgical complications of transforaminal lumbar interbody fusion: a single-center experience. J Neurosurg Spine. 2012;16(1):44–50. https://doi.org/10.3171/2011.9.SPINE11373. Epub 2011 Oct 14
37. Fan G, Wu X, Yu S, Sun Q, Guan X, Zhang H, Xin G, He S. Clinical outcomes of posterior lumbar interbody fusion versus minimally invasive transforaminal lumbar interbody fusion in three-level degenerative lumbar spinal stenosis. BioMed Res Int. 2016; Article 540298, 7 pages, 2016. https://doi.org/10.1155/2016/9540298.
38. Pradhan BB, Nassar JA, Delamarter RB, Wang JC. Single-level lumbar spine fusion: a comparison of anterior and posterior approaches. J Spinal Disord Tech. 2002;15(5):355–61.
39. Phan K, Thayaparan GK, Mobbs RJ. Anterior lumbar interbody fusion versus transforaminal lumbar interbody fusion – systematic review and meta-analysis. Br J Neurosurg. 2015;29:705–11.
40. Kim JS, Lee KY, Lee SH, Lee HY. Which lumbar interbody fusion technique is better in terms of level for the treatment of unstable isthmic spondylolisthesis? J Neurosurgery Spine. 2010;12:171–7. Epub 2010/02/04. Eng
41. Crandall DG, Revella J. Transforaminal lumbar interbody fusion versus anterior lumbar interbody fusion as an adjunct to posterior instrumented correction of degenerative lumbar scoliosis: three year clinical and radiographic outcomes. Spine. 2009;34:2126–33. Epub 2009/09/16. Eng)
42. Sim HB, Murovic JA, Cho BY, Lim TJ, Park J. Biomechanical comparison of single-level posterior versus transforaminal lumbar interbody fusions with bilateral pedicle screw fixation: segmental stability and the effects on adjacent motion segments: laboratory investigation. J Neurosurg Spine. 2010;12(6):700–8.
43. Mehta VA, McGirt MJ, G. L., Ambrossi G, et al. Trans-foraminal versus posterior lumbar interbody fusion: comparison of surgical morbidity. Neurol Res. 2011;33(1):38–42.
44. Fay LY, Huang WC, Tsai TY, Wu JC, Ko CC, Tu TH, Wu CL, Cheng H. Differences between arthroplasty and anterior cervical fusion in two-level cervical degenerative disc disease. Eur Spine J. 2014;23:627–34. https://doi.org/10.1007/s00586-013-3123-8.
45. Maldonado CV, Paz RD, Martin CB. Adjacent-level degeneration after cervical disc arthroplasty versus fusion. Eur Spine J. 2011;20 Suppl 3:403–7.
46. Parish JM, Asher AM, Coric D. Complications and complication avoidance with cervical total disc replacement. Int J Spine Surg. 2020;14(s2):S50–6. https://doi.org/10.14444/7091).
47. Leung C, Casey AT, Goffin J, Kehr P, Liebig K, Lind B, Logroscino C, Pointillart V. Clinical significance of heterotopic ossification in cervical disc replacement: a prospective multicenter clinical trial. Neurosurgery. 2005;57(4):759–63.
48. Kong L, Ma Q, Meng F, Cao J, Yu K, Shen Y. The prevalence of heterotopic ossification among patients after cervical artificial disc replacement: a systematic review and meta-analysis. Medicine. 2017;96(24):e7163.
49. Cebesoy O, Guclu B, Kose KC, Basarir K, Guner D, Us AK. Coccygectomy for coccygodynia: do we really have to wait? Injury. 2007;38(10):1183–8. https://doi.org/10.1016/j.injury.2007.01.022. Epub 2007 Apr 6
50. Kwon HD, Schrot RJ, Kerr EE, Kim KD. Coccygodynia and coccygectomy. Korean J Spine. 2012;9(4):326–33. https://doi.org/10.14245/kjs.2012.9.4.326.
51. Duval-Beaupère G, Schmidt C, Cosson P. A barycentremetric study of the sagittal shape of spine and pelvis: the conditions required for an economic standing position. Ann Biomed Eng. 1992;20(4):451–62. https://doi.org/10.1007/BF0236813.

52. Enercan M, Ozturk C, Kahraman S, Sarıer M, Hamzaoglu A, Alanay A. Osteotomies/spinal column resections in adult deformity. Eur Spine J. 2013;22 Suppl 2(Suppl 2):S254–64. https://doi.org/10.1007/s00586-012-2313-0. Epub 2012 May 11
53. Bridwell KH, Lewis SJ, Lenke LG, Baldus C, Blanke K. Pedicle subtraction osteotomy for the treatment of fixed sagittal imbalance. J Bone Joint Surg Am. 2003;85(3):454–63.
54. Smith JS, Sansur CA, Donaldson WF 3rd, Perra JH, Mudiyam R, Choma TJ, Zeller RD, Knapp DR Jr, Noordeen HH, Berven SH, Goytan MJ, Boachie-Adjei O, Shaffrey CI. Short-term morbidity and mortality associated with correction of thoracolumbar fixed sagittal plane deformity: a report from the Scoliosis Research Society Morbidity and Mortality Committee. Spine (Phila Pa 1976). 2011;36(12):958–64.
55. Lee J, Park Y-S. Proximal junctional kyphosis: diagnosis, pathogenesis, and treatment. Asian Spine J. 2016;10(3):593–600. https://doi.org/10.4184/asj.2016.10.3.593.
56. Daubs MD, Lenke LG, Cheh G, Stobbs G, Bridwell KH. Adult spinal deformity surgery: complications and outcomes in patients over age 60. Spine (Phila Pa 1976). 2007;32(20):2238–44.
57. Buttermann GR. Anterior cervical discectomy and fusion outcomes over 10 years. Spine. 2018;43(3):207–14.
58. Stull JD, Goyal DKC, Mangan JJ, Divi SN, et al. The outcomes of patients with neck pain following ACDF. Spine. 2020;45(21):1485–90.
59. Bertalanffy H, Eggert HR. Complications of anterior cervical discectomy without fusion in 450 consecutive patients. Acta Neurochir. 1989;99(1–2):41–50.
60. Tasiou A, Giannis T, Brotis AG, Siasios I, Georgiadis I, Gatos H, Tsianaka E, Vagkopoulos K, Paterakis K, Fountas KN. Anterior cervical spine surgery-associated complications in a retrospective case-control study. J Spine Surg. 2017;3(3):444–59.
61. Epstein NE. A review of complication rates for Anterior Cervical Diskectomy and Fusion (ACDF). Surg Neurol Int. 2019;10:100. Published 2019 Jun 7. https://doi.org/10.25259/SNI-191-2019.
62. Kilburg C, Sullivan HG, Mathiason MA. Effect of approach side during anterior cervical discectomy and fusion on the incidence of recurrent laryngeal nerve injury. J Neurosurg Spine. 2006;4(4):273–7.
63. Carrier CS, Bono CM, Lebl DR. Evidence-based analysis of adjacent segment degeneration and disease after ACDF: a systematic review. Spine J. 2013;13(10):1370–8.

Part III

Trunk and Pelvis

Section Editor

Tony K. George

Chest Wall Disorders

17

Bobby Oommen, Tricia Prince, Omar Walli,
Armando Alvarez, Magda Aldousany, Luis Feigenbaum,
and Timothy Tiu

17.1 Sternoclavicular Joint Dislocations

17.1.1 Synonyms

Clavicular dislocations, sternoclavicular sprain, sternoclavicular subluxation

17.1.2 ICD-10 Codes

S43.20-S43.216

B. Oommen
Champlain Spine & Pain Management, Champlain Valley Physicians Hospital, The University of Vermont Health Network, Plattsburgh, NY, USA
e-mail: boommen@cvph.org

T. Prince
Department of Physical Medicine & Rehabilitation, University of Miami Miller School of Medicine, Miami, FL, USA
e-mail: tap134@med.miami.edu

O. Walli · A. Alvarez
Department of Physical Medicine & Rehabilitation, University of Miami Miller School of Medicine, Miami, FL, USA
e-mail: omar.walli@jhsmiami.org; a.alvarez1818@med.miami.edu

M. Aldousany
Senior Associate Athletics Director for Performance, Health and Wellness, Miller School of Medicine, University of Miami, Miami, FL, USA
e-mail: m.aldousany@umiami.edu

L. Feigenbaum
Performance, Health and Wellness, Miller School of Medicine, University of Miami, Miami, FL, USA
e-mail: lfeigenbaum@med.miami.edu

T. Tiu (✉)
Department of Physical Medicine & Rehabilitation, University of Miami Miller School of Medicine, Miami, FL, USA

Christine E. Lynn Rehabilitation Center Outpatient Clinics, Miami, FL, USA
e-mail: ttiu@miami.edu

17.2 Description

17.2.1 Anatomy

The sternoclavicular joint (SCJ) is a saddle-type of synovial joint between the clavicle and manubrium of the sternum and involves part of the 1st costal cartilage. The SCJ is a synovial joint where the epiphysis does not fuse until age 22–25. Therefore, in young people, dislocations in this area tend to have concomitant fractures through the growth plate. The SCJ is the single true attachment of the upper limb and axial skeleton. Fibrocartilage overlays the articular surfaces, and a fibrocartilaginous articular disk separates the joint into two compartments. A synovial membrane lines the inner surface of the joint capsule, thereby reducing friction between structures with its production of synovial fluid. Although the SCJ is a fairly mobile joint, there are four stabilizing ligaments: anterior and posterior sternoclavicular, interclavicular, and the costoclavicular ligaments. The sternoclavicular and interclavicular ligaments stabilize the joint, whereas the costoclavicular ligament provides stability with rotation and during shoulder elevation. The suprascapular and internal thoracic arteries are the vascular supply, while the medial supraclavicular nerve (C3–C4) and nerve to the subclavius (C5–C6) innervate the area [1]. The movements that involve the SCJ are shoulder elevation, depression, protraction, retraction, and rotation.

SCJ injuries are rare compared to acromioclavicular joint (ACJ) injuries despite its lack of osseous support and ligamentous attachments. In regard to dislocations, posterior dislocations are rare, but considered medical emergencies, as the presence of the airway and great vessels posterior to the joint are at high risk of injury. The more common anterior dislocations involve disruption of the sternoclavicular and costoclavicular ligaments and are graded I through III depending on the level of capsular disruption (Table 17.1) [2].

Mechanisms of injury for dislocations range from a fall on an outstretched arm to a direct blow to the shoulder in a likely single traumatic event. An athlete getting driven into

© The Author(s), under exclusive license to Springer Nature Switzerland AG 2022

S. A. Mostoufi et al. (eds.), *Clinical Guide to Musculoskeletal Medicine*, https://doi.org/10.1007/978-3-030-92042-5_17

Table 17.1 Grading of anterior sternoclavicular joint dislocations

Type I	Sprain with no ligamentous damage or instability
Type II	Strain or partial rupture of sternoclavicular or costoclavicular ligaments; partial joint displacement
Type III	Dislocation with complete disruption of capsule and ligaments

the mat during a wrestling match on the posterolateral aspect of the shoulder or the player at the bottom of a pile-up in football would be some examples. A less common but important mechanism is a posteriorly directed force directly over the SCJ, for example, the impact of the steering wheel to the chest in a motor vehicle accident. Typically, injury to the SCJ requires a considerable high energy force.

17.3 Clinical Presentation

The patient presentation is with swelling over the SCJ and severe pain with any arm movement. With anterior dislocations, there is a firm palpable mass from the medial clavicular prominence. Posterior dislocations may have SCJ swelling but are often misdiagnosed because of the absence of the medial prominence on palpation.

17.4 Physical Examination

There may be complaints of upper extremity paresthesias, weakness, venous congestion, diminished pulses, or dysphonia on the ipsilateral side. Some patients may have neck muscle spasms resulting in the head being titled toward the ipsilateral injured side. Posterior dislocations may complain of dysphagia and dyspnea. Alertness and appropriate monitoring of vitals, and neurological and vascular status are paramount to recognize compression of adjacent structures. While elevating the shoulder on examination, there may be a subluxation accompanied by a "pop" or "click" [3].

17.5 Diagnostic Workup

Plain radiographs in the AP and lateral chest X-ray views may help rule out associated injuries, but are limited in viewing the SCJ. The "serendipity" view is the most helpful and involves 40–45 degrees of cephalic tilt AP of the chest centered on the SCJ [2]. Tube distance for children should be 45 inches and for thicker-chested athletes, a distance of 60 inches is appropriate [4]. The gold standard diagnostic examination is a spiral CT as it can differentiate fractures vs. dislocations and assess adjacent mediastinal structures with IV contrast. If vascular injury is suspected, then angiography is utilized.

17.6 Treatment

17.6.1 Medical Management

Anterior dislocations (acute and chronic) are mainly managed nonoperatively. Type I dislocations can be managed with rest, ice, and a sling for 4–5 days given that there is no ligamentous damage or instability. After the rest period, activity is advanced as tolerated. Type II dislocations may be managed with rest, ice, NSAIDs and Fig. 17.8 harness immobilization for 6–8 weeks. There must be full, pain-free motion before resuming activity and advancing as tolerated. Full return may take up to 3 months. Type III dislocations are immobilized for 6–8 weeks and then advanced as tolerated after intraoperative reduction. Again, pain-free motion must be established prior to resuming activity [5].

17.6.2 Rehabilitation

Depending on the severity and direction (anterior or posterior) of the dislocation, conservative or postsurgical rehabilitative management will ensue [6]. Both conservative management and surgical management of SCJ dislocations will require the use of a shoulder sling for several weeks. Caution should be exercised in elevating the arm to 90° in the early stages of recovery. Conservative management will include soft tissue mobilization of the neck, upper chest wall, and shoulder musculature, improving thoracic mobility through joint mobilizations and exercises, and strengthening of the scapulothoracic and scapulohumeral musculature (Figs. 17.1, 17.2, and 17.3) [6–8].

After reconstruction of the SC joint, patients must avoid scapular protraction, retraction, depression, and elevation during the initial six weeks [6, 8]. Lifting or carrying objects with the affected extremity is not permitted for approximately two months, whereby tolerance to this activity will be monitored. Active range of motion exercises of the upper extremity should be incorporated during the early postoperative phases to avoid contractures and mobility limitations. Cervical and glenohumeral joint range of motion exercises are also encouraged to avoid stiffness and muscular spasm. Glenohumeral joint motion will likely begin after four weeks postoperatively. Passive and active-assisted range of motion exercises begins at approximately six weeks, with active range of motion commencing at eight weeks. Once clinically appropriate, rehabilitative care will emphasize strengthening of the scapulothoracic and scapulohumeral musculature, stretching, and progressive loading of the upper extremity in open and closed chains [6].

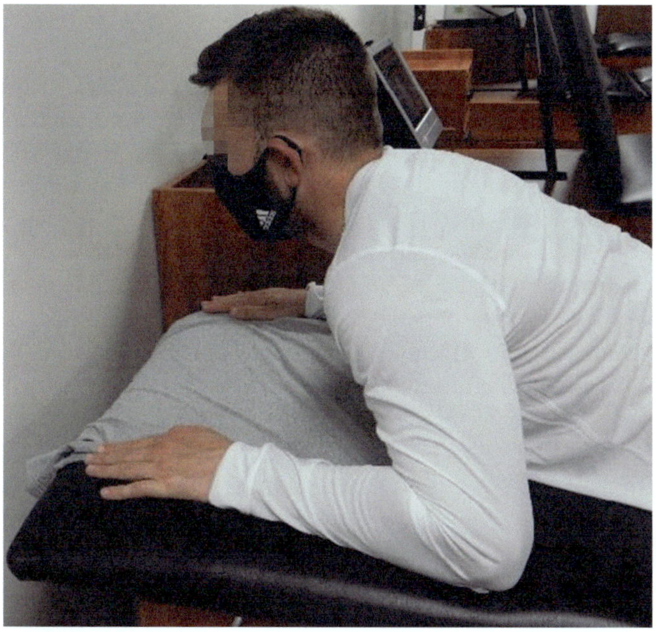

Fig. 17.1 Sternal lift exercise

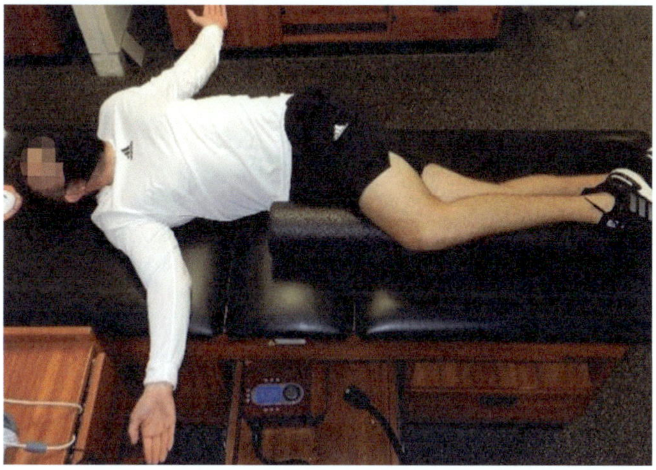

Fig. 17.2 Thoracic spine mobility series: "open book" exercise

17.6.3 Procedures

Reductions are best performed within the first week of injury for both anterior and posterior dislocations. There is a high rate of recurrence post-reduction. A standard sling increases the medial load on the clavicle increasing risk, and therefore, the Fig. 17.8 harness is used instead.

Anterior dislocation reduction involves placing the patient in a supine position with the arm abducted and extended while applying axial traction and direct pressure over the medial clavicle. The medial clavicle can be manipulated with a towel clip or fingers.

As mentioned, posterior dislocations are emergent given the risk to nearby structures. The preference is for reduction in an OR with a cardiothoracic surgeon. In case

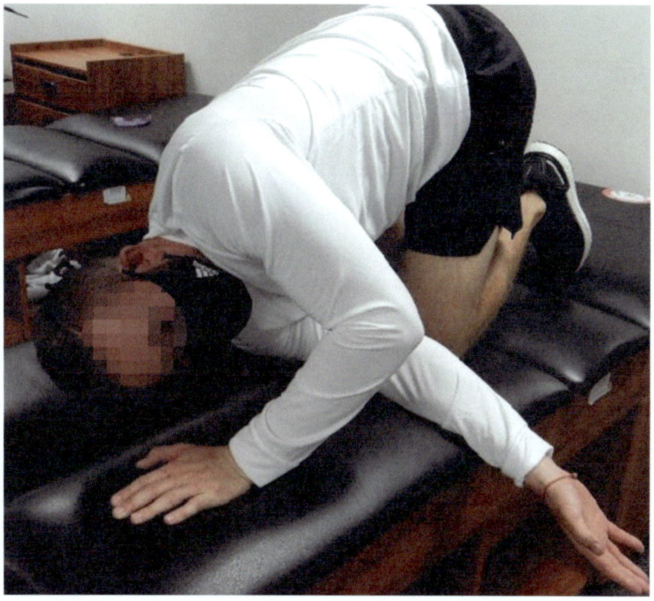

Fig. 17.3 Thoracic spine mobility series: "thread the needle" exercise

of neurovascular compromise with no availability for emergent transfer, reduction should be considered. With the patient in supine position, the arm is abducted and extended, axial traction is applied, and the medial clavicle with a towel clip is manipulated [9–11]. The shoulder should then be immobilized for 6–10 weeks following reduction.

17.6.4 Surgery

Chronic anterior dislocations tend to be managed with activity modification and support treatment for 6–12 months. Continued symptoms are referred for medial clavicle resectional arthroplasty and stabilization. Chronic posterior dislocations are treated with open reduction and resectional arthroplasty of the medial clavicle when more than 7–10 days postinjury [5, 12].

17.7 Pectoralis Major Tear

17.7.1 Synonyms

Pectoralis major rupture, pectoralis major strain, pulled chest muscle.

17.7.2 ICD 10 Codes

S29.011A—Strain of muscle and tendon of front wall of thorax, initial encounter.

17.7.3 Description

Pectoralis major tears are a rare injury where the pectoralis major muscle ruptures leading to pain, weakness, and impaired function.

Anatomy The pectoralis major is a fan-shaped muscle of the anterior chest composed of two heads: the superior clavicular head and the inferior sternal head. The clavicular head arises from the anterior medial half of the clavicle, while the sternal head arises from the anterior sternum, costal cartilage of the 1st–6th ribs, and the abdominal external oblique aponeurosis. Both heads course laterally and combine into the pectoralis major tendon, which inserts into the lateral lip of the bicipital (intertubercular) groove of the humerus. This tendon consists of an anterior and posterior lamina with the anterior lamina consisting of the clavicular head and part of the sternal head, and the posterior lamina consisting of the rest of the sternal head. Of note, the posterior lamina inserts higher on the humerus than the anterior lamina. The pectoralis major muscle is responsible for adduction, internal rotation, and flexion of the humerus. It is also used for dynamic stabilization of the shoulder [14, 16, 18–22]. The pectoralis major muscle is innervated by the lateral (C5–C7) and medial (C8–T1) pectoral nerves [14, 18, 20–22].

Etiology Pectoralis major tears most commonly occur during eccentric contraction under excess tension, as is done during bench presses [14, 16, 21, 22]. It can also occur due to direct trauma, but is much less common. The most common population is physically active males between 20 and 40 years of age [14, 21, 22]. Men are more susceptible to this tear, and several possibilities exist in the literature including smaller tendon to muscle diameter and reduced elasticity; however, no specific cause has been proven thus far [23]. There has also been some correlation of pectoralis major tears with anabolic steroid use [14, 17, 20, 22]. Pectoralis major tears most frequently occur at the humeral insertion with the tendon rupturing directly off the humerus. Less common sites, from most to least common, include at the myotendinous junction, muscle belly tears, and very rarely directly off the sternal origin [16, 19, 20, 22, 23].

Classification A classification system was created by Tietjen for pectoralis major injuries based on the location and severity of the injury. Type I injuries consist of muscle contusions and sprains, type II injuries consist of partial tears, and type III injuries consist of complete tears. Type III injuries are then further divided by the following tear locations: (a) muscle origin, (b) muscle belly, (c) myotendinous junction, and (d) muscle insertion [24].

17.7.4 Clinical Presentation

Presentation of a pectoralis major tear is a sudden, sharp chest pain with a tearing or popping sensation. Most patients will also be able to recall a specific incident associated with the pain. Associated symptoms will include the limited motion of the arm due to pain, asymmetry of the chest wall, ecchymosis, edema, and weakness. Patients may delay medical treatment as many initially treat tears as a common muscle sprain, and only seek out further treatment due to prolonged or worsening symptoms [14, 16, 18, 21, 22]. Differential diagnoses are listed in Table 17.2.

17.7.5 Physical Examination

A complete musculoskeletal examination is used to evaluate pectoralis major muscle tears.

Visual Observation: Inspection of the chest wall will demonstrate swelling and ecchymosis during the acute phase of the injury. The location of the findings will differ on the location of injury. More proximal injuries will have swelling and ecchymosis over the anterior chest wall, while more distal tears will have these signs over the arm or axilla area. Inspection will also reveal an asymmetric chest wall or a thinned-out, webbed appearance of the anterior axilla, accentuated by abduction of the arm to 90 degrees [18, 20–22].

Palpation: Tenderness can occur over the site of the tear. A palpable defect may be present, however can be difficult to detect in the acute phase due to swelling.

Range of Motion: Limited ROM with adduction, flexion, and internal rotation due to pain.

Motor Testing: Strength of adduction, flexion, and internal rotation of the humerus will be decreased compared to the noninjured side; however, full evaluation may be limited due to pain.

17.7.6 Diagnostic Workup

X-Ray Conventional radiography is of limited use for the diagnosis of a pectoralis major tear, but is routinely used to rule out other pathology including fractures, dislocations, or bony avulsion [14, 18, 21, 22].

Table 17.2 Differential diagnoses of anterolateral chest pain

Costochondritis	Proximal humerus fracture
Atypical myocardial infarct	Rotator cuff tendon tear
Rupture of the long head of biceps tendon	Subscapularis muscle tear
Shoulder dislocation	Medical pectoral nerve entrapment

Ultrasound Ultrasound is a low cost and easily accessible imaging technique used to evaluate pectoralis major tears. Tears are identified by hetero-echogenicity, presence of intramuscular hematoma, disruption of muscle fibers, or thinning compared to the uninjured side [16, 18, 20–22].

CT scan CT scan may be able to detect a pectoralis major muscle tear, however is not routinely used due to poor soft tissue visualization [21].

MRI scan MRI is the imaging modality of choice to evaluate pectoralis major tears. MRI can accurately evaluate the location, severity, and chronicity of tears, and has good correlation with surgical findings [15, 16, 18, 20–22].

17.8 Treatment

17.8.1 Medical Management

During the acute phase of injury, patients are treated with rest, icing, and pain control with NSAIDs or other analgesics. A sling is also used initially for immobilization of the arm in adduction and internal rotation. Conservative management is only recommended for proximal tears at the origin of the muscle and some partial tears. Complete tears may also be managed conservatively in older or sedentary individuals as the pectoralis major muscle is not needed for activities of daily living [14, 20–22].

17.8.2 Rehabilitation

Nonoperative rehab For conservative management patients are instructed to begin early shoulder mobilization. Patients should start with a partial passive range of motion exercises and then progress to active range of motion exercises in the first 2 weeks as tolerated (Fig. 17.4). Patients will then begin a full range of motion exercises from 2 to 6 weeks. Partial resistance exercises can be added at 6–8 weeks and will progress to full resistance exercise at 3–4 months from the initial injury [18, 20–22].

Postoperative rehab Please see surgical care below for post-operation rehab discussion.

17.8.3 Procedures

Although orthobiologics may have some utility in muscle injuries, a significant amount of further research is warranted to determine the optimal growth factor milieu that promotes muscular regeneration and healing.

17.8.4 Surgery

Early surgical intervention is the treatment of choice for most tears of the pectoralis major and should be done for complete tears at the myotendinous junction or muscle insertion site [18]. A meta-analysis of pectoralis major muscle injuries reported that patient with surgically

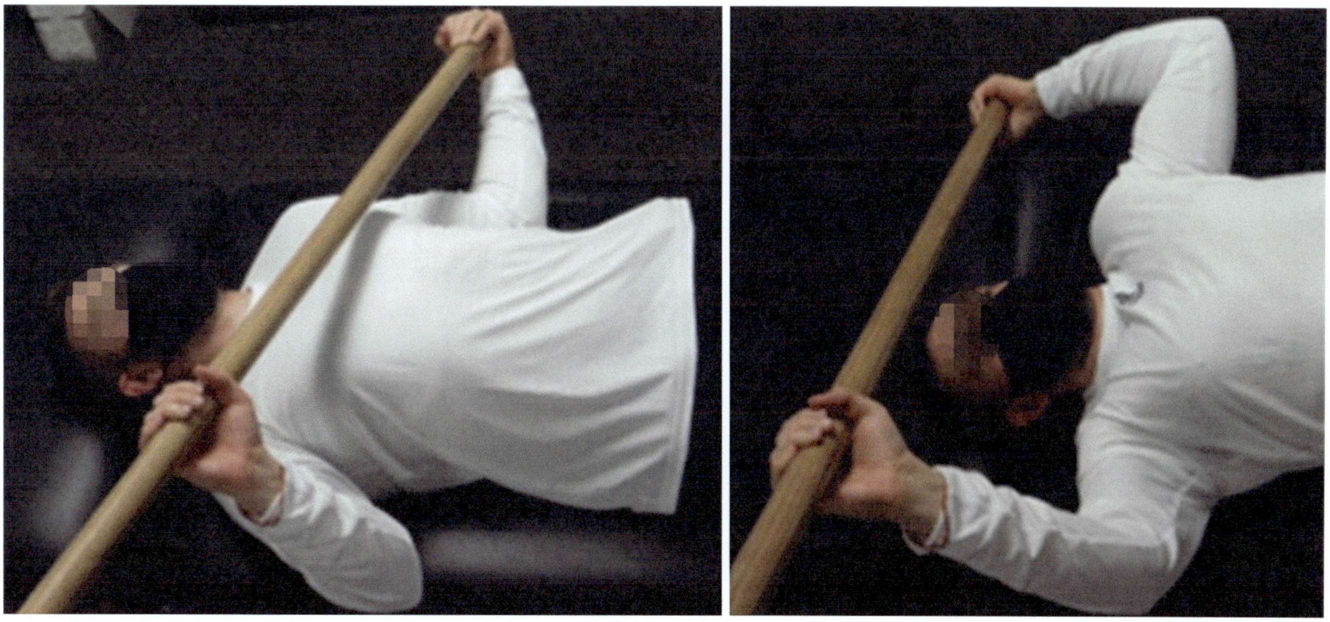

Fig. 17.4 Active-assisted range of motion exercises. Left—start position and right—end position

repaired pectoralis major muscle injuries had superior results compared to nonsurgical patients [13, 24]. Patients generally report better outcomes with surgery including reduced pain, higher postinjury strength, patient satisfaction, and return to prior activities compared to nonoperative management. Surgical repair can be done either in the acute (<6 weeks) or chronic (>6 weeks) stage of injury, and comparable results have been reported [14, 22, 23]. The most common surgical technique is a deltopectoral approach with suturing done through drill holes, as well as the anterior axillary approach [18, 20, 22].

Postoperative Rehabilitation Patients are given a sling to wear for 4–6 weeks after surgery; however, early mobilization of the shoulder is important. Rehabilitation should start with a focus on early mobilization immediately after surgery with shoulder pendulum exercises. Patients are also allowed to flex the shoulder to 130 degrees while the arm is adducted. During this time, patients should avoid active abduction, flexion, or external rotation. At 6 weeks, patients can progress to full passive range of motion exercises. Periscapular and isometric shoulder strengthening programs are also initiated at 6 weeks with avoidance of shoulder adduction and internal rotation. At 3 months, patients should be near full range of motion and can incorporate a pectoralis major muscle strengthening program including adduction, internal rotation, and flexion. At 6 months, patients may begin doing pushups and can perform dumbbell bench presses. Care must be taken that patients only perform low weight and high repetition bench press exercises. At 9–12 months, the patient can return to all prior activities; however, they should be advised against any heavyweight, and low repetition bench presses indefinitely due to the increased risk of re-rupture [20–22].

17.9 Costochondral Pain

17.9.1 Synonyms

Chest wall pain, costochondritis, Tietze syndrome, sternalis syndrome, xiphoidalgia, osteoarthritis of the sternoclavicular joint

17.9.2 ICD 10

M94, R07.9

17.9.3 Description

Costochondral pain is pain and discomfort on the anterior chest wall over the articulation of the sternum and ribs [25]. Ribs are composed of bone and cartilage. The cartilaginous portion connects the bony aspects of the rib and the sternum. The chest wall contains 12 ribs, of which 1–7 are referred to as true ribs, and 8–10 are false ribs. The difference between true and false ribs is that the former articulate anteriorly with the sternum and the latter articulate with the adjacent ribs through the costochondral cartilage. Ribs 11 and 12 do not articulate with any structure anteriorly and are referred to as floating ribs [26, 27]. The prevalence and incidence of chest pain secondary to musculoskeletal etiology are difficult to assess. One study assessing chest pain in the emergency room setting found that 30% of the 122 patients had a musculoskeletal etiology. Additionally, 69% of those with musculoskeletal chest pain were women, and 47% are Hispanic [28].

17.9.4 Clinical Presentation

Costochondritis Costochondritis often presents with point tenderness over the affected articulation between the sternum and attaching rib. The pain is not associated with warmth, visible edema, or signs of erythema. The key component of diagnosis is palpation with elicited pain over the affected joint [29].

Sternalis syndrome Similar to costochondritis, sternalis syndrome presents with pain around the costochondral articulations and over the body of the sternum. Palpatory pain over the body of the sternum can result in radiation of the pain bilaterally. Sternalis syndrome is often self-limited [30].

Tietze's syndrome Tietze's syndrome is a painful condition with focal swelling of the costosternal, sternoclavicular, or costochondral joints. The most commonly affected ribs are the second and third ribs. Although the etiology is idiopathic, it has been associated with viral upper respiratory infections [31].

Xiphodynia Xiphodynia presents with focal pain over the inferior portion of the sternum known as the xiphoid. Patients often complain of pain on forward flexion and rotational movements [32].

17.9.5 Physical Examination

The physical examination begins with inspection followed by palpation [26]. Tietze syndrome will have visible swelling, edema, and point tenderness over the affected articulation [31]. The precise location of pain and tenderness will guide diagnosis (Table 17.3). Pain over the articulation between the ribs and sternum is secondary to costochondritis, while pain over the body of the sternum may be from sternalis syndrome. Similarly, pain on palpation over the xiphoid will likely be secondary to xiphodynia [29–32].

Table 17.3 Differential for costochondral pain

Costochondritis	Point tenderness over the affected articulation with no swelling
Tietze's syndrome	Painful and localized swelling of the affected costochondral joint
Sternalis syndrome	Tenderness over the body of the sternum, affecting the sternalis muscle
Xiphoidalgia	Point tenderness over the inferior sternum (xiphoid)
Sternoclavicular OA	Focal pain of the sternoclavicular joint

17.9.6 Diagnostic Workup

Practitioners should exclude serious cardiac and pulmonary conditions of chest pain, by being mindful of the past medical history of the patient. Imaging modalities, starting with X-rays, are useful for clinical suspicion of a fracture of the ribs or sternum. There are no relevant laboratories to delineate the cause of costochondral pain, unless there is swelling, and erythema is noted on a physical examination. Laboratories at this point should include a CBC to rule out infection [33].

17.9.7 Treatments

17.9.7.1 Medical Management

The disease processes for xiphodynia, Tietze's syndrome, costochondritis, and sternalis syndrome are often self-limiting. Common treatments for costochondral pain include NSAIDs, physical therapy, and intra-articular corticosteroid injections [34].

17.9.7.2 Rehabilitation

Studies show an improvement in patient-reported outcome measures from consistent physical therapy as part of the initial plan of care [35] and are more effective when combined with pharmacotherapy than either alone [36]. Therapy interventions include manual therapy, stretching, and strengthening exercises [37]. Manual therapy techniques, including posterior–anterior glide joint mobilizations to the upper thoracic spine, were found to increase hypomobile joints and decrease pain (Fig. 17.5) [35]. In acute cases, instrument-assisted soft tissue mobilization may be effective at decreasing pain but further study is needed to determine if inflammatory changes or pain reduction is occurring (Fig. 17.6) [38]. Furthermore, stretching of tight postural muscles, including (but not limited to) the pectoralis major, the pectoralis minor, and the trapezius, was found to improve patients' posture and reduce pain (Figs. 17.7 and 17.8) [35, 37].

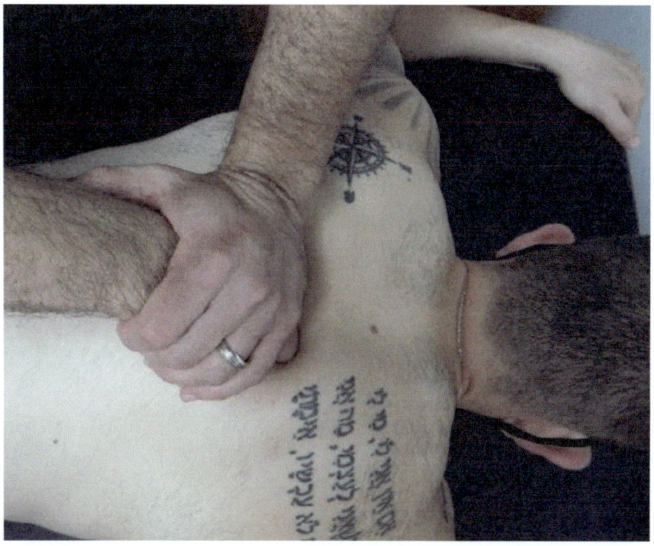

Fig. 17.5 Posterior–anterior mobilization manual therapy

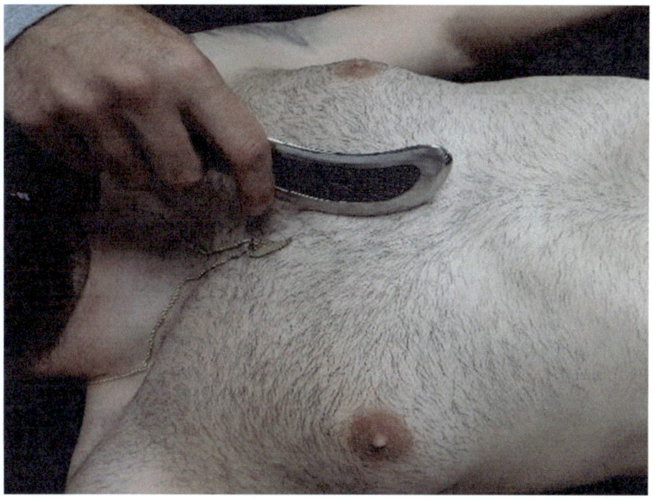

Fig. 17.6 Instrument-assisted soft tissue mobilization

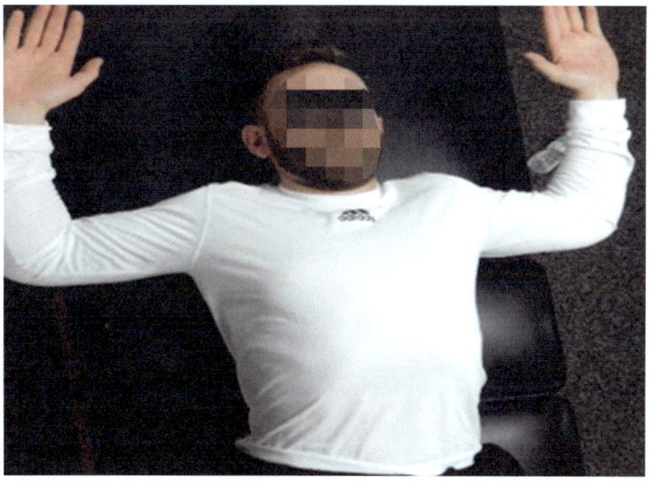

Fig. 17.7 Chest wall stretching exercise

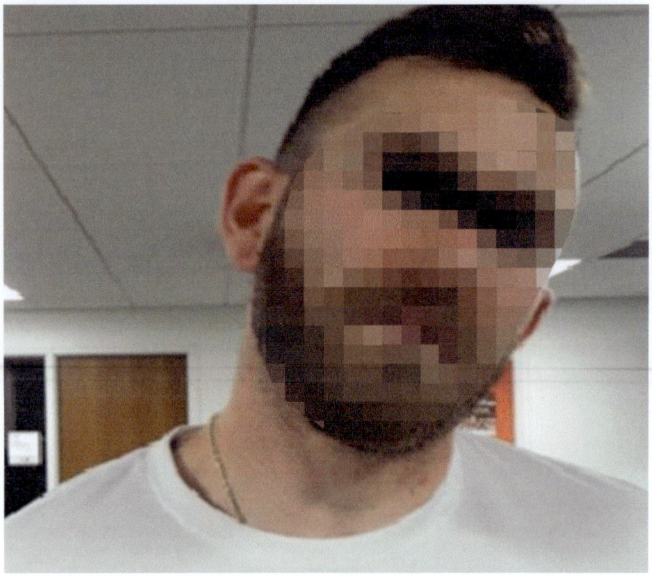

Fig. 17.8 Trapezius stretching exercise

17.9.8 Procedures

Corticosteroid injections into the affected costochondral joints can be considered for pain relief. The procedure should be done with image guidance (US or X-ray) to avoid complications such as pneumothorax.

17.9.9 Surgery

Surgery is not indicated for costochondritis.

17.10 Rib Fractures

Synonyms None

ICD 10 S22.3, S22.4, S22.5

17.10.1 Description

There are 12 pairs of ribs in the thoracic region. The first 7 are attached anteriorly to the sternum and posteriorly to the thoracic vertebrae. Ribs 8 to 10 are attached posteriorly to the corresponding thoracic vertebrae and anteriorly to the costal cartilage. Ribs 11 and 12 are attached posteriorly to the thoracic vertebrae only and are called floating ribs.

Rib fractures can be traumatic or atraumatic. The most common cause of traumatic fracture is a frontal crash sustained by restrained vehicle occupants. Fracture of upper ribs signifies severe trauma, possibly involving great vessels, while lower rib fractures may result in injury to the spleen, liver, or kidneys [39]. Atraumatic fractures may be secondary to osteoporosis or metastatic disease. Rib fractures are uncommon in children due to increased bone cartilage and elasticity. If found, child abuse should be suspected [40]. Rib fractures are indicative of the severity of trauma. Mortality and morbidity increase as the number of fractured ribs increases [41]. They are associated with pulmonary complications including pneumothorax, hemothorax, and pulmonary contusion. Rib fractures are associated with increased mortality and morbidity in the elderly. When a rib fractures in a contiguous fashion with 2 or more breaks per rib, it can result in a separate segment moving paradoxically to the rest of the chest and is termed as flail chest.

17.10.2 Clinical Presentation

Patients will report a history of trauma with rib pain aggravated with chest movements. Bruising maybe seen at the fracture site. Severe pain may result in shallow breathing, causing hypoventilation and pneumonia. Differential diagnoses of rib fractures include chest wall contusion, sternal fracture, clavicular fracture, and costochondritis/Tietze syndrome.

17.10.3 Physical Examination

Chest tenderness and deformity had the most sensitivity on physical examination tests [42].

Contusion and crepitus may be noted at the fracture site. Abnormal chest movements should be observed, and flail chest may result in paradoxical breathing. Breath sounds could be normal, but clinicians should be watchful for pneumothorax or hemothorax.

17.10.4 Diagnostic Workup

Plain chest X-rays in anteroposterior, lateral, and rib views are the initial diagnostic modality, but may detect only around 15% of rib fractures. Point of care ultrasound can detect rib fractures and pneumothorax. Griffith et al. found that sonography is more sensitive than radiographs in detecting rib fracture [43]. CT scan is the gold standard for detecting rib fractures, however is not mandatory in all cases, as there were no improvements in clinical outcome. Radionuclide scanning such as scintigraphy may rarely be required to confirm fracture.

17.10.5 Treatment

17.10.5.1 Medical Management

Pain control is important to normalize respiratory function [44]. Analgesia, ice, and rest are the initial treatment for simple rib fracture. The use of an incentive spirometer should be encouraged to prevent pulmonary atelectasis and splinting.

17.10.5.2 Rehabilitation

Rehabilitation will include a variety of breathing exercises (active breathing techniques, diaphragmatic breathing, localized breathing on the affected side, and bilateral lateral costal breathing) (Fig. 17.9), active coughing, and mobility exercises for the upper quarter, cervical, and thoracic spine(s). Education on strategies for applying support to the injured ribs during coughing and sneezing is important in the early phases of rehabilitation [45–47]. Clinicians need to balance the benefits of restrictive bracing techniques through wraps and compressive garments, to allow patients the opportunity to maximize full inspiration/expiration as tolerated (Fig. 17.10). Noninvasive pain management modalities include transcutaneous electrical nerve stimulation (TENS) and elastic taping (i.e., kinesiotaping).

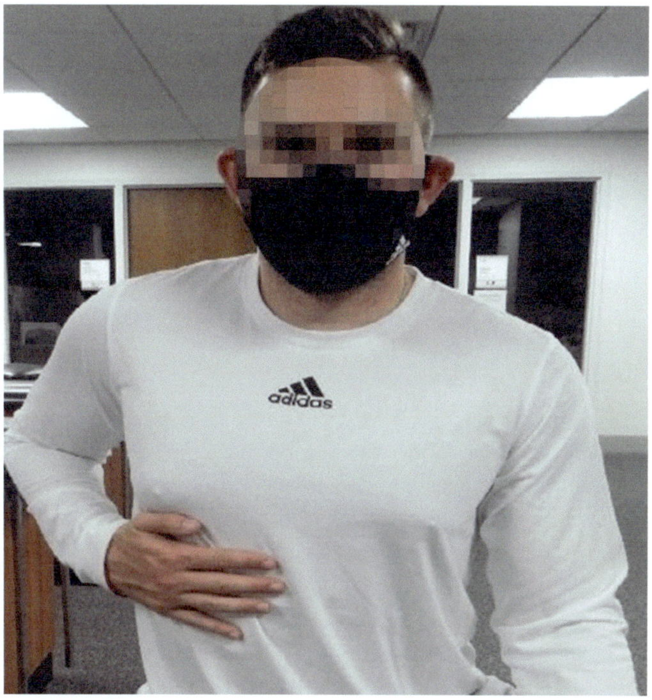

Fig. 17.9 Localized active breathing on the affected side

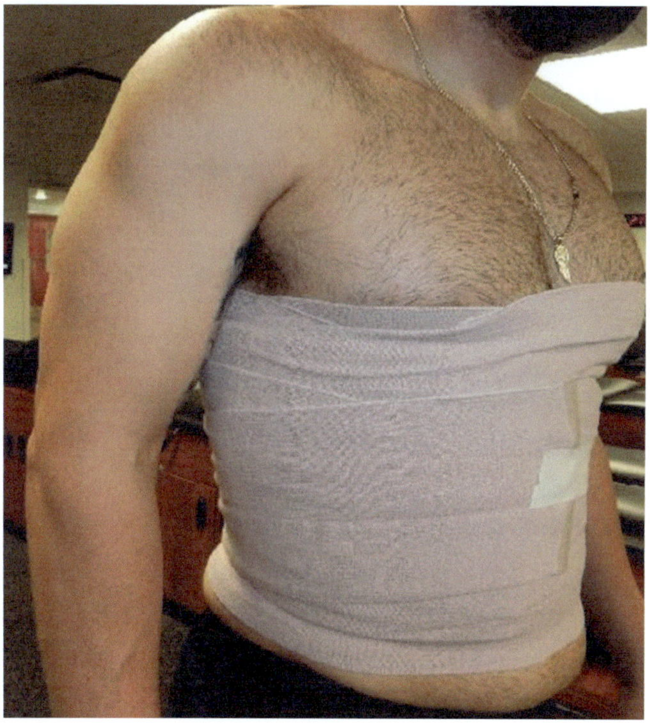

Fig. 17.10 Padded bracing for rib fracture

17.10.6 Procedures

If oral or topical agents fail, an intercostal nerve block (US or X-ray guided), patient-controlled analgesia, or continuous epidural analgesia may be considered [48, 49]. Catheter-based analgesia including epidural and paravertebral nerve catheters has been associated with decreased mortality rate [49].

17.10.7 Surgical

Surgery is considered when conservative management has failed, for pain control and to improve long-term quality of life. The consensus on surgical indications for rib fixation can be found in Table 17.4 [50].

17.11 Costovertebral Joint Dysfunction

Synonyms Costovertebral joint syndrome, costovertebral arthropathy

ICD-10 M99.08

17.11.1 Description

Anatomy: Costovertebral joints are arthrodial joints connecting the proximal ends of the ribs with the corresponding

Table 17.4 Consensus on clinical indications for rib fixation (9)

3 or more rib fractures with rib displacement of more than 1 rib cortical diameter
Flail segment
Pulmonary worsening with progressive volume loss on X-ray
Intubation/mechanical ventilation
Use of IV narcotics
Uncontrolled pain when using analgesia or visual analog scale score > 6 /10
Lung impalement
Open chest defect
Stabilization on the retreat of thoracotomy
Pulmonary herniation

thoracic vertebra. They are divided into 2 subsets, one connecting the heads of the ribs to the vertebral body and the other connecting the rib neck and tubercles with the transverse processes. The 2nd to 9th ribs have a superior and inferior articulating surface connecting the corresponding vertebrae and the one above [27]. The transverse process has a costal facet that forms the costotransverse joint with the articular surface of the costal tubercle. Branches of intercostal nerves innervate the two joints. The differential diagnosis includes thoracic disk herniation, thoracic stenosis, facet joint arthropathy, and slipping rib syndrome.

17.11.2 Clinical Presentation

Costovertebral joint dysfunction presents clinically as localized pain, a few centimeters lateral to the thoracic spine, with possible radiation along the ribs. The pain is increased on deep inspiration, radiating laterally with lateral flexion and rotation. Costovertebral pain may mimic cardiopulmonary causes. Common causes of dysfunction include trauma or overuse but may be caused by ankylosing spondylitis or osteoarthritis [51]. Occasionally, patients may complain of a "clicking" sound in their mid-back.

17.11.3 Physical Examination

On physical examination, the costovertebral joints may be tender to touch, or may show signs of inflammation, including localized swelling. Clinicians should be astute in performing a chest and abdominal examination to rule out non-musculoskeletal causes of pain.

17.11.4 Diagnostic Workup

Diagnosis is usually clinical, and imaging studies are nonspecific. In significant trauma, X-rays or CT imaging is done to rule out life-threatening conditions.

17.11.5 Treatment

17.11.5.1 Medical Management

Nonsteroidal anti-inflammatory medications are the initial treatment. Physical modalities such as heat and cold help in reducing the pain.

17.11.5.2 Rehabilitation

Joint mobilization and thrust manipulation of the ribs, thoracic spinal facet joints, and costosternal joints have shown benefit in treating costovertebral joint dysfunction (Fig. 17.11) [52–54]. Modalities such as acupuncture, laser therapy (Fig. 17.12), soft tissue mobilization, and trigger point release can help decrease muscle guarding

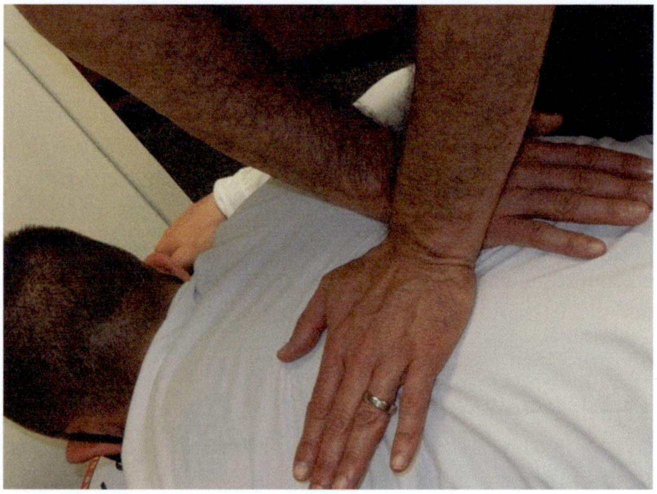

Fig. 17.11 Thoracic joint mobilization

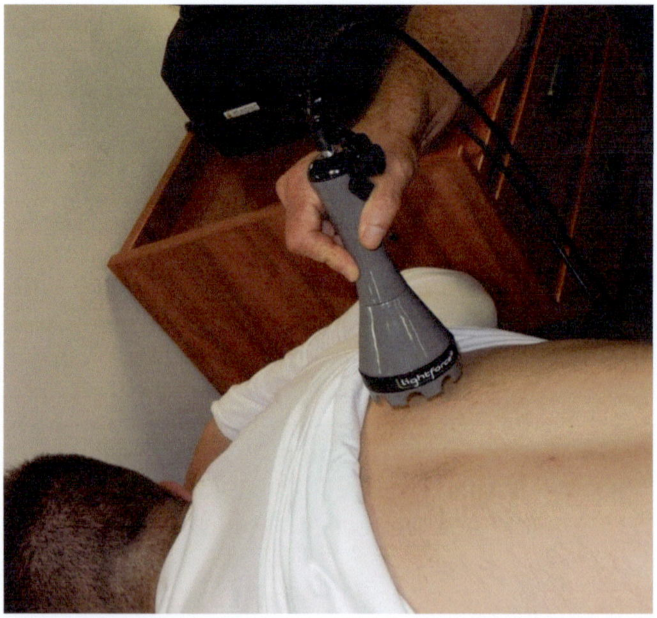

Fig. 17.12 Laser therapy

and pain in the region [52, 55]. Exercises emphasizing chest wall and thoracic spine mobility, scapulothoracic and scapulohumeral strength, and postural endurance should be included in the plan of care (Fig. 17.13) [55, 56].

17.11.6 Procedures

Costovertebral and costotransverse joint injection with steroid and lidocaine are effective and are done under fluoroscopic or sonographic guidance.

17.11.7 Surgery

Resection arthroplasty has been described to give intermediate relief for costovertebral joint osteoarthritis. Postoperatively, patients are allowed to mobilize without restriction [67].

17.12 Chest Wall Deformities

17.12.1 Synonyms

Pectus excavatum, pectus carinatum, Poland syndrome, cleft sternum, congenital malformation of sternum, other congenital deformities of chest, pigeon chest, sunken chest, funnel chest

17.12.2 ICD-10 Codes

Q67.6, Q67.7, Q67.8, Q76.7, Q798

17.12.3 Description

Chest wall deformities are malformations found in isolation or as a symptom of a syndrome [57]. Depending on its severity, there may be cardiopulmonary implications [58, 59]. These deformities can be categorized as either rib cage overgrowth or inadequate growth (aplasia or dysplasia) [60]. The two most common types, pectus excavatum (PE) (sternal depression, most common) and pectus carinatum (PC) (sternal protrusion), which account for 90% of congenital chest wall deformities, are due to rib cage overgrowth, or an abnormal elongation of costal cartilage [58, 60]. Syndromes associated with chest wall deformities include Marfan syndrome (up to two thirds of patients are affected) and Noonan syndrome [57, 60]. There is evidence of up to a 37% pattern of inheritance, with boys being three times more affected than girls [58, 60].

17.12.4 Clinical Presentation

Chest wall deformities are typically asymptomatic, unless severe enough to impact cardiopulmonary function, which may lead to exercise intolerance or respiratory infections. Individuals with syndromes such as Marfan or Noonan syndrome will have complaints specific to those conditions. Noonan syndrome has variability in anomalies, but consistently has hypoplasia or aplasia of the pectoralis muscles [60]. These deformities may have significant social and psychological impact [59].

17.12.5 Physical Examination

On inspection, there will be a visible symmetric or asymmetric deformity of the chest wall [61]. Severity of the deformity

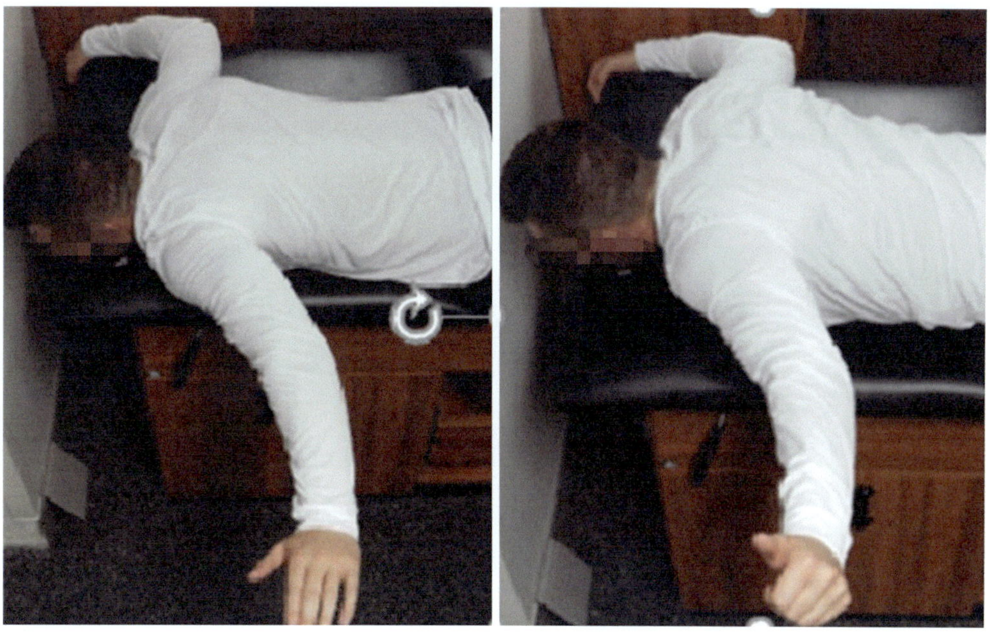

Fig. 17.13 Scapulothoracic and scapulohumeral exercises; left—prone abduction and right—prone abduction with external rotation

may vary from superficial to such where sternum approaches the spine [60]. If a deformity is identified, additional workup should explore for Marfan syndrome and other conditions associated with chest deformities.

17.12.6 Diagnostic Workup

Imaging is not diagnostically necessary or recommended in asymptomatic individuals; however, insurance companies may require imaging prior to surgical intervention [60]. Imaging can be used to calculate the *Haller index,* which is used to evaluate the severity of a deformity and is calculated as a ratio between transverse and anteroposterior chest diameters. Plain radiography is a viable initial imaging modality. Given the exposure to radiation, CT scanning in children should be avoided if possible. In severe cases, CT and MRI may be required to evaluate the underlying organs [59].

17.12.7 Treatment

17.12.7.1 Medical Management

If there is any suspicion of a genetic syndrome, the patient should be referred for genetic counseling for further evaluation and workup [57].

17.12.7.2 Rehabilitation

Pectus excavatum may cause cardiopulmonary dysfunction in patients. These patients often present with excessive thoracic kyphosis and decreased exercise tolerance. Typically, a rehabilitation program is between 3 and 4 months in length. From the outset of the program, patients should be educated on therapy goals to improve exercise tolerance, decrease pain, and/or increase cardiorespiratory fitness, and not resolution of their condition [62, 63]. Exercises for pectus excavatum include strengthening of the back extensors and abdominal muscles, as well as stretching the anterior chest muscles, diaphragmatic breathing, and cardiorespiratory fitness testing [63] (Figs. 17.14 and 17.15). Activities to increase cardiopulmonary functioning include the use of a treadmill, a cycle ergometer, or an upper body cycle ergometer (Fig. 17.16). Physical therapists may use fitness measurements such as cycle ergometry, spirometry readings, and the 6-minute walk test to determine if improvements in cardiorespiratory function have occurred throughout the rehabilitation program. Several studies have found that adherence to physical therapy exercises is equated with better patient outcomes [64].

In the case of patients with pectus carinatum, the physical therapist may work alongside the physician to educate and implement a home exercise program for bracing. In addition to bracing, exercises to stretch and strengthen the back extensors and anterior chest muscles should be performed. The rehabilitation program should focus on exercises such as rear deltoid raises, pushups, and planks.

17.12.8 Procedures

A vacuum bell may be applied to the chest wall in a depressive deformity. This requires daily application for an indefinite duration to allow for reformation. Bracing in protrusive deformities may result in progressive remodeling but must be worn for 14 hours daily for at least 2 years [60]. Physical therapy coupled with bracing was found to improve patient outcomes compared to bracing alone [65]. Bracing was found to be more effective in a younger patient population with high compliance to the bracing protocol [66].

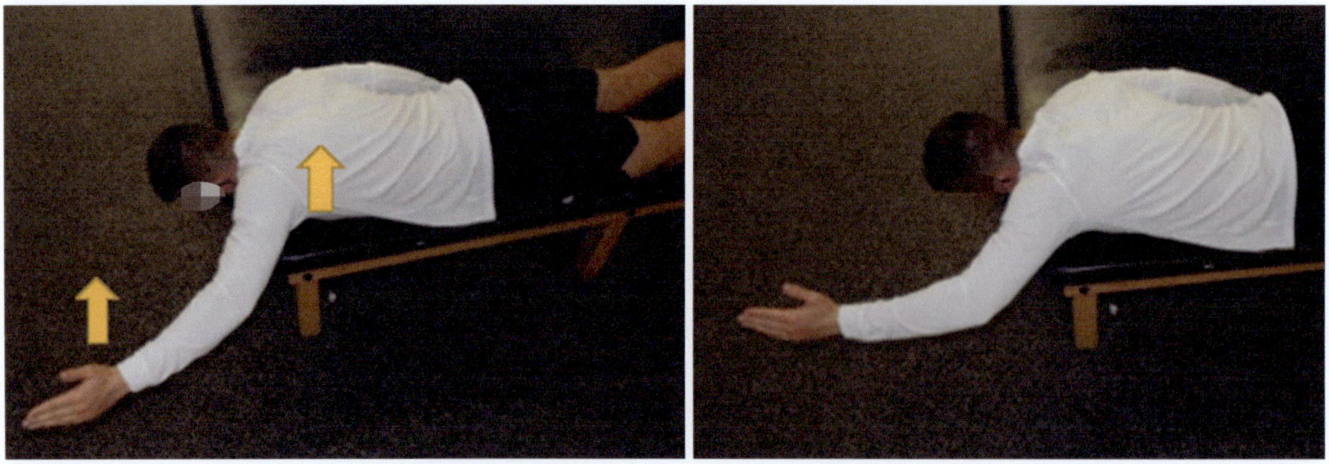

Fig. 17.14 Strengthening exercise for back extensors. Left—start position and right—end position with arm and torso lifted off the table

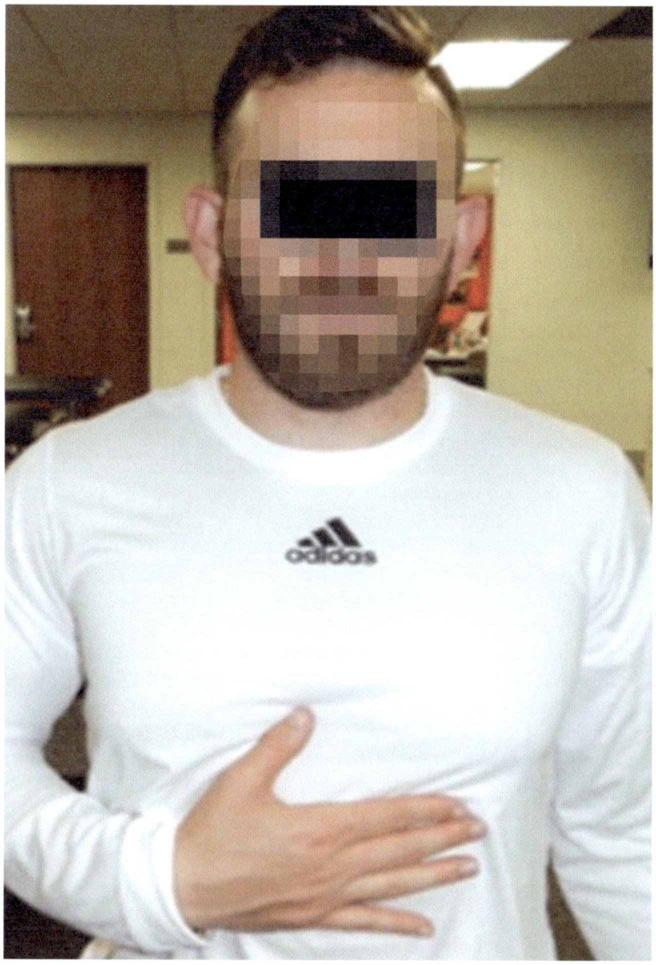

Fig. 17.15 Diaphragmatic breathing

17.12.9 Surgery

Surgical reconstruction may be indicated for cosmesis, but also for preserving deficits in cardiopulmonary function. Pectus excavatum may be treated with minimally invasive repair via the *Nuss procedure*, in which a pectus bar is implanted for 2–3 years. Potential adverse effects include wound infection, pneumothorax, bar displacement, allergy to the bar, and overcorrection leading to pectus carinatum. Pectus carinatum can be treated with a modified Nuss procedure, correcting a protrusion defect rather than a depression [60]. A structured course of rehabilitation (MSK rehab and Pulmonary rehab) follows the surgical repair.

17.13 Intercostal Neuralgia

This topic is discussed in Chap. 54 *Common Plexopathies and Neuropathies.*

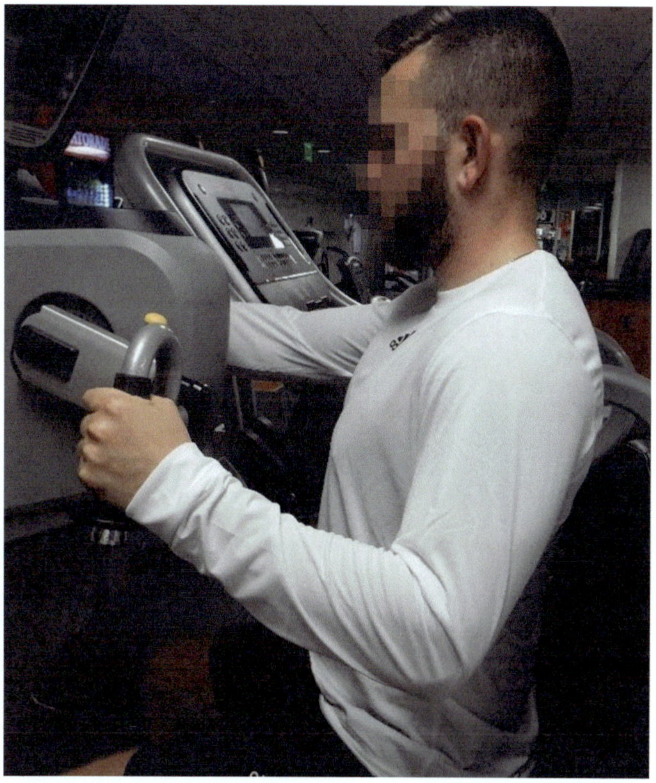

Fig. 17.16 Upper body ergometer

References

1. Schuenke M, Schulte E, Schumacher U. The upper limb. In: Ross LM, editor. Thieme atlas of anatomy: general anatomy and musculoskeletal system. New York: Thieme Medical; 2010.
2. Chang CJ, Dixit S. Ch. 46 Thorax and abdominal injuries. In: Madden CC, Putukian M, Young CC, McCarty EC, editors. Netter's sports medicine. Philadelphia: Saunders; 2010. p. 380–1.
3. Bytomski J, Moorman CT. Sternoclavicular joint sprains and dislocations. In: Oxford American handbook of sports medicine. Oxford, England: Oxford University Press; 2010.
4. Ciftdemir M, Copuroglu C, Ozcan M. Posterior dislocation of the sternoclavicular joint. Hippokratia. 2011;15(3):284.
5. Basamania CJ. Ch. 46 Sternoclavicular, clavicular, and acromioclavicular injuries. In: O'Connor FG, Sallis RE, Wilder RP, St. Pierre P, editors. Sports medicine just the facts. New York: McGraw-Hill; 2005. p. 273–5.
6. Logan C, Shahien A, Altintas B, Millett PJ. Rehabilitation following sternoclavicular joint reconstruction for persistent instability. Int J Sports Phys Ther. 2018;13(4):752–62.
7. Calderazzi F, Menozzi M, Valenti P, et al. A rare case of complicated pure posterior sternoclavicular dislocation in a young athlete. Acta Biomed. 2020;91(14-S):e2020015.
8. Cruz MF, Erdeljac J, Williams R, Brown M, Bolgla L. Posterior sternoclavicular joint dislocation in a division I football player: a case report. Int J Sports Phys Ther. 2015;10(5):700–11.
9. Morell DJ, Thyagarajan DS. Sternoclavicular joint dislocation and its management: a review of the literature. World J Orthop. 2016;7(4):244–50.

10. Colbenson K. Ch. 32 Chest trauma: thoracic injuries and conditions. In: Harrast MA, Finnoff JT, editors. Sports medicine study guide and review for boards. New York: Demos Medical Publishing; 2016. p. 372.
11. Nettles JL, Linscheid RL. Sternoclavicular dislocations. J Trauma Injury Infect Crit Care. 1968;8(2):158–64. Jougon JB, Lepront DJ, Dromer CEH. Posterior dislocation of the sternoclavicular joint leading to mediastinal compression. Ann Thorac Surg. 1996;61(2):711–3.
12. Äärimaa V, Rantanen J, Heikkilä J, Helttula I, Orava S. Rupture of the pectoralis major muscle. Am J Sports Med. 2004;32(17):1256–62.
13. Bodendorfer BM, et al. Treatment of pectoralis major tendon tears: a systematic review and meta-analysis of operative and nonoperative treatment. Orthop J Sports Med. 2020;8(2):2325967119900813.
14. Butt U, et al. Pectoralis major ruptures: a review of current management. J Shoulder Elbow Surg. 2015;24(4):655–62.
15. Carrino JA, Chandnanni VP, Mitchell DB, Choi-Chinn K, DeBerardino TM, Miller MD. Pectoralis major muscle and tendon tears: diagnosis and grading using magnetic resonance imaging. Skeletal Radiol. 2000;29(18):305–13.
16. Chiavaras MM, et al. Pectoralis major tears: anatomy, classification, and diagnosis with ultrasound and MR imaging. Skeletal Radiol. 2015;44(2):157–64.
17. de Castro PA, Andreoli CV, Belangero PS, Figueiredo EA, Terra BB, Cohen C, Andrade Mdos S, Cohen M, Ejnisman B. Clinical considerations for the surgical treatment of pectoralis major muscle ruptures based on 60 cases: a prospective study and literature review. Am J Sports Med. 2014;42(25):95–102.
18. Durant EJ, De Cicco FL. Pectoralis major tear. [Updated 2020 Dec 25]. In: StatPearls [Internet]. Treasure Island: StatPearls Publishing; 2021.
19. ElMaraghy AW, Devereaux MW. A systematic review and comprehensive classification of pectoralis major tears. J Shoulder Elbow Surg. 2012;21(15):412–22. https://doi.org/10.1016/j.jse.2011.04.035. Epub 2011 Aug 10. PMID: 21831661.
20. Haley CA, Zacchilli MA. Pectoralis major injuries: evaluation and treatment. Clin Sports Med. 2014;33(4):739–56.
21. Petilon J, Carr DR, Sekiya JK, Unger DV. Pectoralis major muscle injuries: evaluation and management. J Am Acad Orthop Surg. 2005;13(1):59–68.
22. Provencher CDRMT, et al. Injuries to the pectoralis major muscle: diagnosis and management. Am J Sports Med. 2010;38(8):1693–705.
23. Schepsis AA, Grafe MW, Jones HP, Lemos MJ. Rupture of the pectoralis major muscle: outcome after repair of acute and chronic injuries. Am J Sports Med. 2000;28:9–15.
24. Tietjen R. Closed injuries of the pectoralis major muscle. J Trauma. 1980;20(15):262–4.
25. Chicarilli ZN, Ariyan S, Stahl RS. Costochondritis: pathogenesis, diagnosis, and management considerations. Plast Reconstr Surg. 1986;77(1):50–9.
26. Gregory PL, Biswas AC, Batt ME. Musculoskeletal problems of the chest wall in athletes. Sports Med. 2002;32:235–50. https://doi.org/10.2165/00007256-200232040-00003.
27. Saker E, Graham RA, Nicholas R, et al. Ligaments of the costovertebral joints including biomechanics, innervations, and clinical applications: a comprehensive review with application to approaches to the thoracic spine. Cureus. 2016;8(11):e874. Published 2016 Nov 11. https://doi.org/10.7759/cureus.874.
28. Disla E, Rhim HR, Reddy A, Karten I, Taranta A. Costochondritis: a prospective analysis in an emergency department setting. Arch Intern Med. 1994;154(21):2466–9. https://doi.org/10.1001/archinte.1994.00420210106012.
29. Bösner S, Becker A, Hani MA, Keller H, Sönnichsen AC, Karatolios K, Schaefer JR, Haasenritter J, Baum E, Donner-Banzhoff N. Chest wall syndrome in primary care patients with chest pain: presentation, associated features and diagnosis.
30. Raikos A, Paraskevas GK, Tzika M, et al. Sternalis muscle: an underestimated anterior chest wall anatomical variant. J Cardiothorac Surg. 2011;6:73. Published 2011 May 16. https://doi.org/10.1186/1749-8090-6-73.
31. Rokicki W, Rokicki M, Rydel M. What do we know about Tietze's syndrome? Kardiochir Torakochirurgia Pol. 2018;15(3):180–2. https://doi.org/10.5114/kitp.2018.78443.
32. Dorn P, Kuhn MA, Schweizer BA, Schmid RA, Kocher GJ. Xiphoidectomy for intractable xiphodynia. World J Surg. 2018;42(11):3646–50. https://doi.org/10.1007/s00268-018-4668-9. PMID: 29770873.
33. Fam AG. Approach to musculoskeletal chest wall pain. Prim Care. 1988;15(4):767–82.
34. Proulx AM, Zryd TW. Costochondritis: diagnosis and treatment. Am Fam Physician. 2009;80(6):617–20. PMID: 19817327.
35. Zaruba RA, Wilson E. Impairment based examination and treatment of costochondritis: a case series. Int J Sports Phys Ther. 2017;12(3):458.
36. Ayloo A, Cvengros T, Marella S. Evaluation and treatment of musculoskeletal chest pain. Prim Care. 2013;40(4):863–87.
37. Rovetta G, Sessarego P, Monteforte P. Stretching exercises for costochondritis pain. G Ital Med Lav Ergon. 2009;31(2):169–71.
38. Kim J, Sung DJ, Lee J. Therapeutic effectiveness of instrument-assisted soft tissue mobilization for soft tissue injury: mechanisms and practical application. J Exercise Rehab. 2017;13(1):12.
39. Sırmalı M, Tastepe I, Kaya S, Yazici U, Gulhan E, Topcu S, et al. A comprehensive analysis of traumatic rib fractures: morbidity, mortality and management. Eur J Cardiothorac Surg. 2003;24(1):133–8.
40. Kemp A, Dunstan F, Harrison S, Morris S, Mann M, Rolfe K, et al. Patterns of skeletal fractures in child abuse: systematic review. BMJ. 2008;337(oct02 1):a1518.
41. Sırmalı M, Turut H, Topcu S, Gulhan E, Yazici U, Kaya S, Tastepe I. A comprehensive analysis of traumatic rib fractures: morbidity, mortality and management. Eur J Cardiothorac Surg. 2003;24(1):133–8.
42. Kalani N, Habibzadeh SR, Ghahremanizadeh R, Tavakolian A, Hatami N, Barazandehpour S, Abiri S. Diagnostic accuracy of physical examination and history taking in traumatic rib fracture; a single center experience. Bull Emerg Trauma. 2020;8(2):111.
43. Griffith JF, Rainer TH, Ching AS, Law KL, Cocks RA, Metreweli C. Sonography compared with radiography in revealing acute rib fracture. AJR Am J Roentgenol. 1999;173(6):1603–9.
44. Pettiford BL, Luketich JD, Landreneau RJ. The management of flail chest. Thorac Surg Clin. 2007;17(1):25–33. https://doi.org/10.1016/j.thorsurg.2007.02.005. PMID: 17650694.
45. van Aswegen H. Physiotherapy management of patients with trunk trauma: a state-of-the-art review. S Afr J Physiother. 2020;76(1):1406.
46. Kourouche S, Buckley T, Munroe B, Curtis K. Development of a blunt chest injury care bundle: an integrative review. Injury. 2018;49(6):1008–23.
47. Unsworth A, Curtis K, Asha SE. Treatments for blunt chest trauma and their impact on patient outcomes and health service delivery. Scand J Trauma Resusc Emerg Med. 2015;23:17.
48. Simon B, Ebert J, Bokhari F, et al. Management of pulmonary contusion and flail chest: an Eastern Association for the Surgery of Trauma practice management guideline. J Trauma Acute Care Surg. 2012;73:S351–61.
49. Flagel BT, Luchette FA, Reed RL, Esposito TJ, Davis KA, Santaniello JM, Gamelli RL. Half-a-dozen ribs: the breakpoint for mortality. Surgery. 2005;138(4):717–25.
50. Diaz JSAM, Gasparri M LL, Pohlman T. Special report: integrating surgical rib fixation into clinical practice: a report from the rib fracture consensus meeting. General Surgery News; 2013.

51. Erosa S, Erosa SC, Sperber K. Costovertebral pain syndromes. In: Kahn S, Xu R, editors. Musculoskeletal sports and spine disorders. Cham: Springer; 2017. https://doi.org/10.1007/978-3-319-50512-1_84.
52. Johnson K, et al. Thoracic region self-mobilization: a clinical suggestion. Int J Sport Phys Ther. 2012;7(2):252–6.
53. Hislop HJ, Avers D, Brown M. Daniels and Worthingham's muscle testing: techniques of manual examination and performance testing. 9th ed. PA: WB Saunders Co; 2014.
54. Walter R. Essentials of physical medicine and rehabilitation. Philadelphia: Elsevier Saunders; 2008. p. 576.
55. Heiderscheit B. Reliability of joint mobility and pain assessment of the thoracic spine and rib cage in asymptomatic individuals. J Man Manip Ther. 2008;16(4):210–6.
56. Fruth SJ. Differential diagnosis and treatment in a patient with posterior upper thoracic pain. Phys Ther. 2006;86(2):254–68.
57. Kotzot D, Schwabegger AH. Etiology of chest wall deformities—a genetic review for the treating physician. J Pediatr Surg. 2009;44(10):2004–11.
58. Fokin AA, et al. Anatomical, histologic, and genetic characteristics of congenital chest wall deformities. Semin Thorac Cardiovasc Surg. 21(1). WB Saunders; 2009.
59. Lain A, et al. New methods for imaging evaluation of chest wall deformities. Front Pediatr. 2017;5:257.
60. Blanco FC, Elliott ST, Sandler AD. Management of congenital chest wall deformities. Seminars in Plastic Surgery. 25(1). Thieme Medical Publishers; 2011.
61. Willital GH, et al. Chest-deformities: a proposal for a classification. World J Pediatr. 2011;7(2):118–23.
62. Jaroszewski D, Notrica D, McMahon L, Steidley DE, Deschamps C. Current management of pectus excavatum: a review and update of therapy and treatment recommendations. J Am Board Family Med. 2010;23(2):230–9.
63. Schoenmakers MA, Gulmans VA, Bax NM, Helders PJ. Physiotherapy as an adjuvant to the surgical treatment of anterior chest wall deformities: a necessity?: a prospective descriptive study in 21 patients. J Pediatr Surg. 2000;35(10):1440–3.
64. Berazaluce AM, Jenkins TM, Garrison AP, Hardie WD, Foster KE, Alsaied T, Tretter J, Moore RA, Fleck RJ, Garcia VF, Brown RL. The chest wall gender divide: females have better cardiopulmonary function and exercise tolerance despite worse deformity in pectus excavatum. Pediatr Surg Int. 2020;36(11):1281–6.
65. Alaca N, Alaca İ, Yüksel M. Does physiotherapy applied in conjunction with compression brace treatment in patients with pectus carinatum have efficacy? A preliminary randomized-controlled study. Pediatr Surg Int. 2020;36:789–97.
66. Lee RT, Moorman S, Schneider M, Sigalet DL. Bracing is an effective therapy for pectus carinatum: interim results. J Pediatr Surg. 2013;48(1):184–90.
67. Sales JR, Beals RK, Hart RA. Osteoarthritis of the costovertebral joints: the results of resection arthroplasty. The journal of bone and joint surgery. British Volume. 2007;89(10):1336–9.

Pubalgia and Groin Pain in Athletes

18

George Ross Malik, John Avila, and Monica E. Rho

18.1 Synonyms

Athletic pubalgia (AP), Core muscle injury (CMI), Inguinal disruption (ID), Osteitis pubis (OP), Sports hernia, Adductor tendinopathy, Hockey groin, Gilmore's groin

18.2 ICD-10 Codes

- S39 "Injury of muscle, fascia and tendon of abdomen, lower back and pelvis"
- S76 "Strain of adductor muscle, fascia and tendon of unspecified thigh, initial encounter"
- K40 "Inguinal hernia"
- R10.30 "Lower abdominal pain, unspecified"

18.3 Description

Groin pain is a nebulous term that has many connotations. Often, pain in this area is commonly referred to as simply a groin pull or strain. It has created a confusing clinical picture for medical professionals due to its broad anatomical location and constellation of symptoms and pathology. Groin pain has been described in athletes who participate in sports involving sudden changes in direction, kicking, and core torsion such as soccer, American football, Australian rules football, track and field, and hockey [1–4]. Recent trends have labeled groin pain as "core muscle injury" (CMI) encompassing muscular pathology in the anatomic region between the lower chest and middle thigh [4]. While some may think of CMI as an acute injury in these athletes, its origin is more often attributed to chronic overuse resulting from repetitive extreme athletic activity [5]. However, this pathology can also occur in recreational athletes and less commonly in more sedentary individuals as well.

Many groin injuries also involve concomitant hip pathology. This is most commonly seen with straight-line activities, whereas cases with focused pubic pathology are mostly demonstrated with kicking activities [1]. On MRI, the most common sites of anatomic pathology in these patients include the pubic symphysis (93%), rectus abdominis (76%), adductor longus (46%), pectineus (38%), adductor brevis (20%), and iliopsoas (6%) [4]. However, other studies have demonstrated greater involvement of adductor injuries in up to 66% of CMI, with the majority of adductor injuries involving the adductor longus. The iliopsoas and rectus femoris also exhibited pathology in 15–25% of CMI [6].

In patients presenting with groin pain, it is important to maintain a broad differential due to referred pain patterns, especially with hip involvement such as femoral acetabular impingement (FAI), avascular necrosis (AVN), pelvic stress fracture, and hip osteoarthritis (Table 18.1). If hip pathology is identified, the subject is less likely to return to the pre-injury sporting level compared to pubic pathology alone [1]. If pain at the adductors is identified, return-to-play (RTP) time is more than double that when groin pain, not specific to the adductors, is present. Identifying concomitant abdominal and adductor pain will quadruple the RTP time [7]. In a cohort of 998 sub-elite male soccer players, 54 reported 58 groin injuries spanning one season; adductor pathology (52% of injured players) was dominant followed by iliopsoas (31%) and abdominal (19%) pathology; and 30% of athletes with adductor pathology had concurrent abdominal pathology [7].

G. R. Malik (✉) · M. E. Rho
Shirley Ryan Ability Lab & Department of Physical Medicine and Rehabilitation, Northwestern University Feinberg School of Medicine, Chicago, IL, USA
e-mail: george.malik@northwestern.edu

J. Avila
Department of Physical Medicine and Rehabilitation, Northwestern University Feinberg School of Medicine, Chicago, IL, USA

© The Author(s), under exclusive license to Springer Nature Switzerland AG 2022

S. A. Mostoufi et al. (eds.), *Clinical Guide to Musculoskeletal Medicine*, https://doi.org/10.1007/978-3-030-92042-5_18

Table 18.1 Differential diagnosis for groin pain

Upper lumbar radiculopathy/ radiculitis	Meralgia paresthetica
Inguinal hernia (direct/indirect)	Genitofemoral entrapment
Hip stress fracture	Snapping hip syndrome
Hip labral tear	Femoral acetabular impingement (FAI)
Hip adductor strain/tear	Rectus abdominis aponeurosis strain/tear

In 2014 at the British Hernia Society, it was proposed that three out of the five following elements are necessary to diagnose core muscle injury (CMI): (1) pinpoint tenderness over the pubic tubercle at the point of insertion of the conjoint tendon, (2) palpable tenderness over the deep inguinal ring, (3) pain and/or dilation of the external ring with no obvious hernia evident, (4) pain at the origin of the adductor longus tendon, and (5) dull, diffuse pain in the groin, often radiating to the perineum and inner thigh or across the midline [8]. Establishment of this diagnostic criterion helped limit ambiguity in diagnosing CMI and focus therapeutic interventions on the specific area of pathology.

18.3.1 Groin Anatomy/Biomechanics

Core muscle injury (CMI) has been difficult to characterize due to the various anatomical structures in the area. While there are no official boundaries for the groin, typically it includes the lower abdomen, inguinal region, pubic symphysis, and proximal hip flexors and hip adductors [9]. The anterior pelvis contains the pubic symphysis, which is composed of the inferior and superior pubic rami bilaterally, separated by a fibrocartilaginous disc. This symphysis acts to stabilize the anterior pelvis as well as evenly distribute compressive and shear forces. It is also the focal point of multiple muscular attachments: the hip adductors including the adductor longus, adductor brevis, and adductor magnus and the anterior abdominal musculature including the rectus abdominis, transversus abdominis, internal obliques, and external obliques [10].

The adductor group works synergistically with the hip flexor group (iliopsoas and rectus femoris) as well as the hip external rotators to stabilize the anterior pelvis and assist during gait (swing phase). The adductor longus is anterior to the adductor brevis and magnus and acts in hip flexion and medial rotation, in addition to adduction. This muscle originates at the pubic/ischial bones and is most commonly injured at the proximal 2–4 cm myotendinous junction. This is due to decreased blood supply from the deep femoral artery compared with the more caudal portion inserting onto the linea aspera of the femur [10].

The rectus abdominis is three times wider at its origin on the lower ribs compared to its attachment on the pubic bone contributing to the concentration of forces at the pubic symphysis. This muscle group provides trunk flexion and tone to the anterior abdominal wall as well as assists with forceful exhalation [10]. These two muscle groups exist as antagonists during extension and rotation at the waist: adductors (inferior, anterior vector) and rectus abdominis (posterior, superior vector). Both muscles fuse together into a common aponeurosis over the anterior pubis [10]. With the abdominal musculature runs the cutaneous nerves that are susceptible to entrapment or impingement including the iliohypogastric nerve, ilioinguinal nerve, genitofemoral nerve, and lateral femoral cutaneous nerve. Nerve injuries can occur with pathology such as fascial hypertrophy or mass effect secondary to tissue herniation [10].

The inguinal canal can also cause groin pain as it envelopes the spermatic cord. The canal is bordered medially and laterally by the external obliques with the medial fibers becoming the superficial inguinal ring. The floor of the inguinal canal is formed by the inguinal ligament, which connects the anterior superior iliac spine (ASIS) to the pubic tubercle. The transversalis fascia becomes the deep inguinal ring. The posterior wall of the inguinal canal contains the transversalis fascia and the internal obliques. Any defects to these structures make the posterior wall susceptible to direct herniation (medial to inferior epigastric vessels); indirect herniation occurs within the inguinal canal itself (lateral to inferior epigastric vessels [9].

18.3.2 Epidemiology

Groin pain is quite prevalent in athletics such as those involving change of direction, twisting, and turning. In a study involving 218 patients in England, males were four times more likely to experience groin pain than females. For the male injuries in the study, 22% involved participation in soccer and 21% involved rugby; for the female injuries in the study, 40% involved running. Certainly, this can be a reflection of the sports played by different genders in England; however, it is important to note which sports can potentially lead to this type of chronic repetitive overuse in both genders. A retrospective review of almost 9000 patients over a 20-year span at an American surgical practice saw referrals for sports hernia increase almost ten times over that span, likely due to increased awareness of the pathology. The number of female patients increased from 1% initially to 15.2% over the last 5 years of the study. Additionally, the average age of the subjects increased from 24.7 initially to 28.6 in the last 3 years of the study (range of 8–88). Athletes comprised 82.8% of this population with an increase in non-athlete population from 0% initially to 24.9% in the final 5 years. The most prominent sports included soccer (44.6%), American football (22.3%), hockey (8.1%), baseball (6.3%), basketball (6.2%), and distance running (1.2%) [4].

18.3.3 Nomenclature/Taxonomy

Medical care for groin injuries has been hindered by inconsistent taxonomy over the years with regional and sport-specific biases. In 2015, the DOHA convention took the umbrella term "athletic pubalgia" and created three major categories of groin pain to be used in nomenclature: (1) defined clinical entities for groin pain (adductor-related, iliopsoas-related, inguinal-related, and pubic-related groin pain), (2) hip-related groin pain, and (3) other causes of groin pain in athletes [11].

Alternatively, Meyers et al. proposed the term "core muscle injury" using the term "core" taken from health and fitness literature, which traditionally involves the area inferior to the nipple line and superior to the middle thigh. This reduces the confusion associated with more focal anatomic terms such as athletic pubalgia (focusing on the pubic bone) and inguinal disruption (inguinal region), while allowing areas such as the lower abdominal musculature aponeurosis to be included [12].

18.3.4 Risk Factors

CMI is classically thought of as a clinical syndrome of overuse and has been noted more often in sports involving kicking and change of direction. A prospective cohort of 508 soccer players on 31 amateur teams exhibited an increased risk of groin injury during the season if they had a previous groin injury (OR 2.6) and weak adductor muscles (OR 4.28) [13]. Additionally, it has been shown that sport-specific training at higher competitive levels triples the risk of acquiring a groin injury [14]. Many athletes affected by CMI are believed to have weak posterior abdominal musculature and hip adductors, thereby making them more susceptible to injury. Subsequently, preseason strengthening protocols targeting these areas are being implemented to limit this hazard [3, 8].

18.4 Clinical Presentation

Patients diagnosed with core muscle injury frequently represent an active population comprising a variety of competitive levels from professional to recreational athletes. Commonly, pain is precipitated by increasing the activity level or change in training regimen. The pain is usually focal to the lower abdominal musculature or proximal adductor musculature, more often unilateral. Generally, the pain improves with cessation of activity. Pain may be non-radiating or occasionally radiates to the groin, thigh, or genitalia. If pain radiates to the genitalia, this may indicate involvement of the ilioinguinal, iliohypogastric, and/or genitofemoral nerves [15]. The most common symptoms include pain with side-to-side movement, pivoting, sprinting, jogging, and kicking [16]. In a study of 110 male athletes with groin pain, the most common mechanism of injury was kicking in soccer (40%), while in all other sports, change of direction was the most common (31%) [6]. Chronic CMI occurs three times more often than acute CMI. However, when acute, it can be attributed to abrupt trunk hyperextension or hip hyperabduction [15, 17].

18.5 Physical Examination

On physical examination, these patients may demonstrate tenderness over the pubic symphysis, superior pubic rami, proximal hip adductor tendons/origin, and/or rectus abdominis aponeurosis [15, 17]. Special tests that can be utilized to isolate CMI include the half sit-up, resisted sit-up (with palpation at the distal rectus abdominis), resisted hip adduction, and adductor squeeze test (Table 18.2) [17]. Valsalva maneuvers including coughing/sneezing may also illicit pain [15]. Kurowicki et al. demonstrated high sensitivity but poor specificity with maneuvers such as resisted cross-body sit-up and straight-leg sit-up (Table 18.2) [18]. Serner et al. did report high specificity (100% confirmed against MRI findings) for hip adductor muscle pathology with positive results for the following six tests: adductor palpation, squeeze test at 0° and 45°, resisted outer range adduction, passive adductor stretch, and FABER (flexion, abduction, and external rotation) (Table 18.2). The adductor squeeze test had the highest individual specificity at 94% [19]. It is also important to rule out confounding diagnoses, especially involving the hip and inguinal canal. FABER may also be positive if there is intra-articular hip involvement [17]. Palpation of the superficial and deep inguinal rings can aid in ruling out an inguinal hernia [15].

18.6 Diagnostic Workup

X-rays With suspicion of core muscle injury (CMI), standing AP pelvic radiographs are the standard imaging of choice. Flamingo series radiographs are also popular to evaluate potential instability within the pubic symphysis, which involves three views: (1) bilateral standing AP, (2) right leg standing AP, and (3) left leg standing AP (vertical displacement >2 mm on either side considered diagnostic) [20].

MRI Further imaging is typically helpful with MRI being the most common and ultrasound (US) becoming more prevalent. Many radiology departments utilize a pubalgia protocol for MRI which can improve detection of anatomic abnormalities. MRI has demonstrated a sensitivity of 68% and specificity of 100% with rectus abdominis injuries and

Table 18.2 Physical exam maneuvers

Test name	Sensitivity (%)	Specificity (%)	Demonstration	Description
Resisted cross-body sit-up	100	3	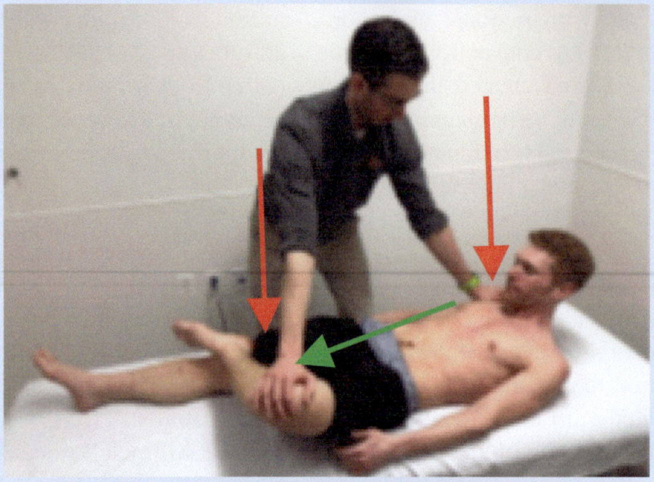	Patient is supine with ipsilateral hip flexed, abducted, and externally rotated. The patient then contracts core musculature to perform sit-up by bringing contralateral shoulder to ipsilateral knee (*green arrow*). The examiner provides resistance at the contralateral shoulder and ipsilateral knee (*red arrows*)
Straight-leg sit-up	74	20	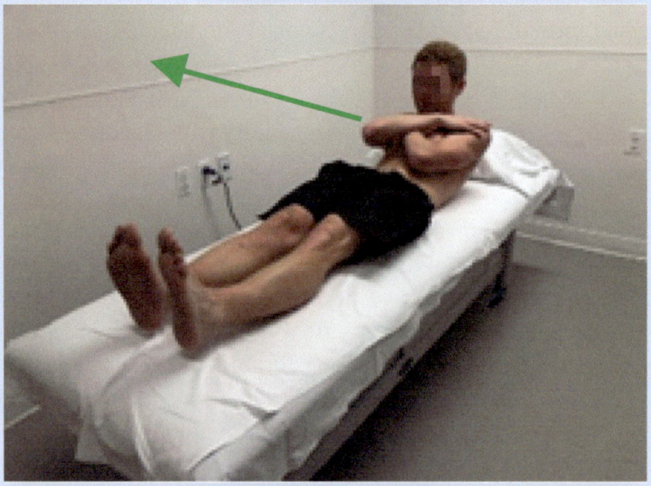	Patient is supine with knees extended and hips neutral. Bilateral knee extensors and hip flexors are contracted to lift heels off the bed. The patient then contracts core musculature to perform a sit-up (*green arrow*) while maintaining position of heels off the bed
Adductor palpation	96	78	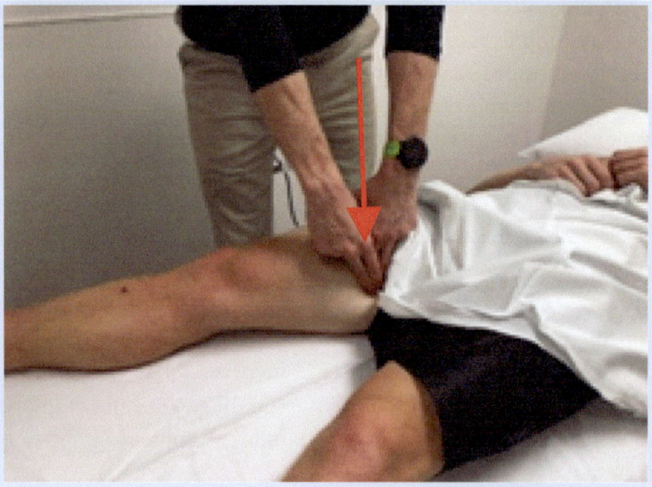	Patient is supine with knees extended and hips neutral. The ipsilateral hip can also be externally rotated. The examiner then applies pressure to the ipsilateral hip adductors (*red arrow*)

Table 18.2 (continued)

Test name	Sensitivity (%)	Specificity (%)	Demonstration	Description
Adductor squeeze test (0° and 45°)	80, 94	67, 78	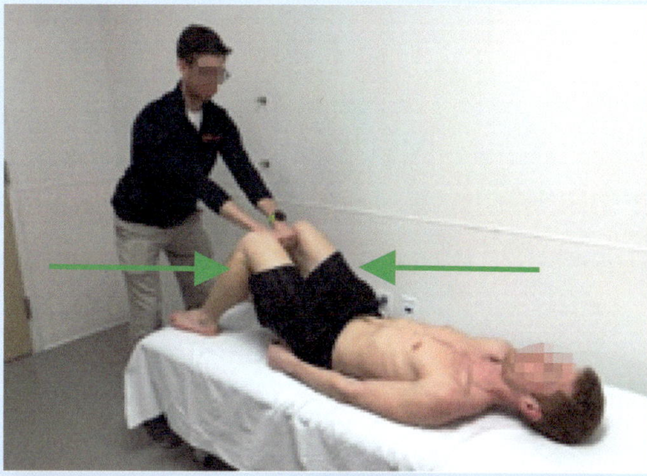	Patient is supine with hips either flexed to 45° or 0° (both have knees flexed to 90°). The patient then actively adducts bilateral hips (*green arrows*) against the examiner's fists which are positioned between the patient's knees
Resisted outer range adduction	85	89	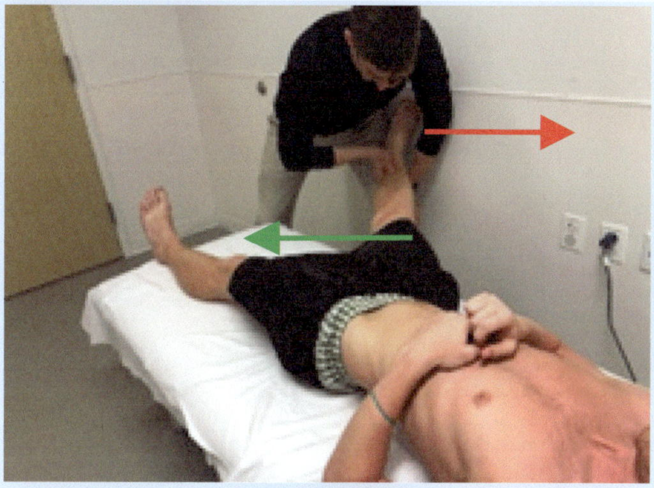	Patient is supine with knees extended and hips neutral. The patient begins with ipsilateral hip max abducted and actively adducts (*green arrow*) the ipsilateral limb against the examiner who applies a counteracting force (*red arrow*) to keep the limb adducted
Passive adductor stretch	61	89	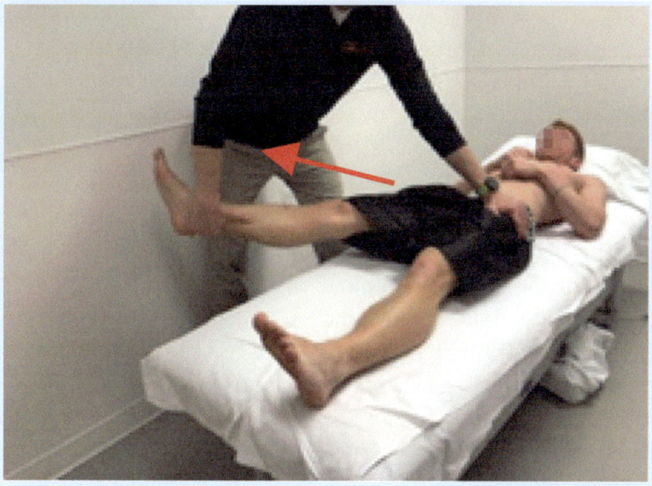	Patient is supine with knees extended. The examiner supports and abducts the ipsilateral limb (*red arrow*) and uses the other hand to stabilize the contralateral hip/pelvis

(continued)

Table 18.2 (continued)

Test name	Sensitivity (%)	Specificity (%)	Demonstration	Description
Flexion, abduction, external rotation (FABER)	46	72	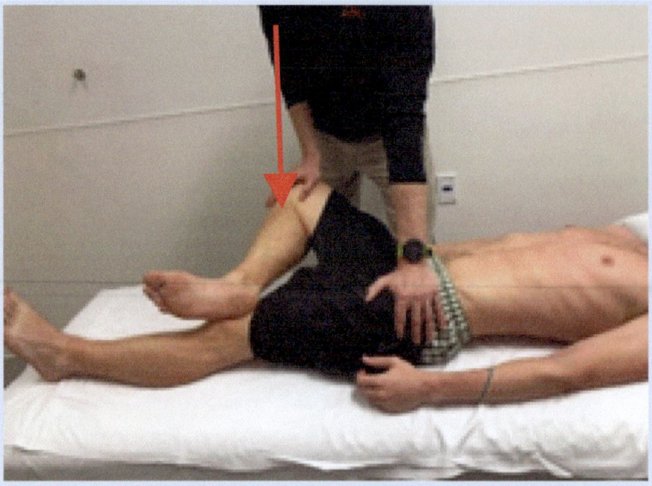	Patient is supine with ipsilateral hip flexed, abducted, and externally rotated. Examiner then applies pressure (*red arrow*) on the medial aspect of the distal femur/knee and stabilizes the contralateral hip/pelvis with the other hand

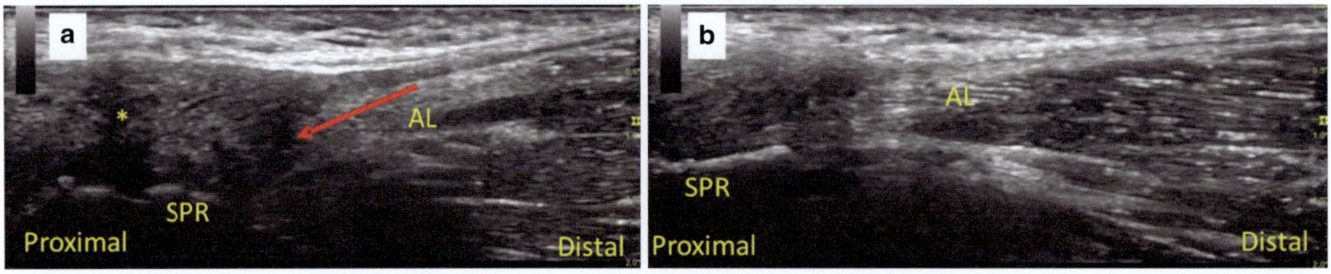

Fig. 18.1 Adductor longus (AL) sonography: (**a**) Left adductor longus in long axis; note the evidence of enthesopathy, loss of organized fibrillary architecture (red arrow), tendon hypertrophy at the muscle origin, cortical irregularity at the superior pubic ramus (SPR), hypoechogenicity which is reflective of tendinosis, and a partial tear (*). (**b**) Right adductor longus in long axis used for comparison (non-pathologic)

sensitivity of 86% and specificity of 89% for adductor longus injuries [10]. However, as much as 71% of athletes exhibit pathologic findings on MRI while being asymptomatic, so clinical context is essential [21].

US Sonographic evaluation has been increasingly employed as it allows evaluation of dynamic maneuvers, utilizing flexible fields of viewing and evaluating the patient in real time (Fig. 18.1). High-resolution views of the lower abdominal aponeurosis, hip flexor, and hip adductor musculature and ligaments are possible with US protocols [22]. The origins and insertions of the musculature can be visualized statically, as well as dynamically, allowing direct correlation to the patient's symptoms. US can also be quite useful for diagnostic and therapeutic injections. Pubic symphyseal, peritendinous, and nerve block injections under ultrasound guidance have been incorporated into patient care. Ultrasound can also aid in ruling out other diagnoses such as intra-articular hip pathology. If this is on the differential, a diagnostic injection into the hip capsule under ultrasound guidance can be performed as well.

18.7 Treatments

(a) *Medical Management*

Nonsteroidal anti-inflammatory medications are frequently used to treat core CMI. In a study of 35 soccer players with osteitis pubis (OP), subjects were treated conservatively with ibuprofen 300 mg TID for 14 days, in addition to other therapeutic modalities and rehabilitation therapy. All 35 athletes were able to return to play (RTP) on average between 3.8 (mild OP) and 10 weeks (severe OP) [23]. Additionally, for tendinosis, nitroglycerin transdermal patches may also be prescribed to increase blood flow to the tendon for recovery. There is an abundance of literature on the use of nitroglycerin patches for the Achilles tendon and common extensor tendon origin. However, there are no published studies on this pertaining to hip adductor tendons specifically.

(b) *Rehabilitation*

CMI is truly a diagnosis involving the kinetic chain. Understanding of the kinetic chain is integral in the treatment of this pathology. Interventions must be stratified based on the level of disability, symptom irritability, and pain severity. Manual therapy interventions may include joint or soft tissue mobilizations [24]. Joint mobilizations, which include ilium rotational mobilizations, sacroiliac regional thrust manipulations, femoral mobilizations, and lumbar mobilizations, can be used for pain modulation and to address joint hypomobility. Soft tissue mobilization may include cross-friction massage to the involved tendons, though this may not be tolerated in patients with highly volatile or severe symptoms [25, 26]. Modalities such as transcutaneous electrical nerve stimulation and thermal agents can also be utilized in such patients [27]. However, the use of modalities should be minimized as a supervised active approach to rehabilitation has achieved greater success in return to sport than passive modalities [28]. Addressing impairments in range of motion and muscle length in the trunk and proximal lower extremities can be accomplished through stretching exercises. Progressive trunk stabilization exercises should include isometric exercises in the supine (e.g., dead bug), prone (e.g., superman), quadruped (e.g., bird dog), and standing positions (e.g., wall squat) (Fig. 18.2a–c) [24, 27]. Exercises should begin

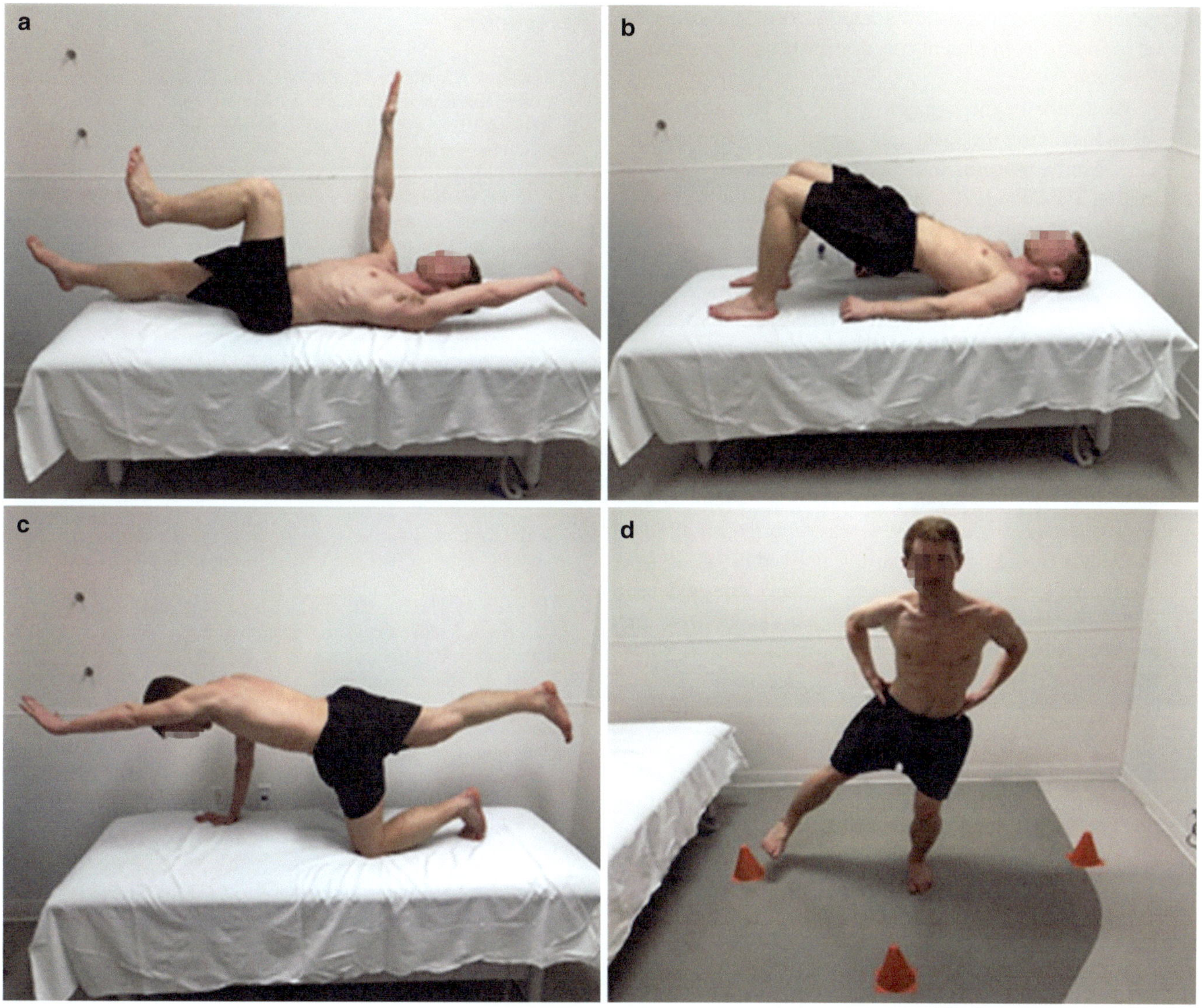

Fig. 18.2 Rehabilitation exercises for core muscle injury (CMI). (**a**) Dead bug (static): In supine, the trunk remains stationary as the arm and alternate leg are flexed and extended, respectively. (**b**) Bridge (static): The hips are elevated until in line with the shoulders and knees. (**c**) Bird dog (static): In quadruped, the trunk remains stationary as the arm and alternate leg are flexed and extended, respectively. (**d**) Single-leg stance with multidirectional lower extremity reaching (dynamic): The pelvis and stance leg remain stationary as the contralateral leg reaches to targets on the floor

with low-load versions and be advanced once the patient is able to perform an exercise pain-free and with proper form. Monitoring for optimal loading of the abdominals, hip adductors, and hip abductors is essential. Dynamic exercises should be incorporated after the patient has mastered isometrics. Such exercises include bridges, rotational planks, single-leg balance with upper or lower extremity reaching, and split squats (Fig. 18.2d) [24]. Aerobic exercise should begin with land- or water-walking. The patient can progress once pain-free to include cycling, water running, swimming, running, and stair climbing [24]. Once a patient is tolerating dynamic and aerobic exercise well, sport-specific drills can begin. When initiating sport-specific drills, monitor the patient's movement patterns and performance to derive an individualized plan of care for further progression.

(c) *Procedures*

As detailed earlier, diagnostic injections can be helpful in localizing the focal area of pathology in a patient. They can be performed at the rectus abdominis aponeurosis (CPT 20551), the pubic symphysis (CPT 20610), the hip adductor origins (CPT 20551), and between layers of the abdominal musculature or even local nerve blocks (CPT 64425). Popular non-surgical interventions addressing CMI include tendon fenestrations, platelet-rich plasma (PRP) injections, steroid/local anesthetic injections, and prolotherapy. There has been little evidence to suggest that corticosteroids have any benefit in the definitive treatment of CMI and could perhaps be tenocytotoxic. However, corticosteroid injections can be helpful in delaying surgical intervention as seen in athletes where an efficacy of 80% was reported for athletes in delaying surgical intervention until after the season concluded [29]. Limited positive evidence does exist for PRP injections for CMI in sports such as lacrosse and hockey with return to play ranging from 3.5 to 8 weeks [30, 31]. However more data is needed in the area of regenerative medicine and CMI.

(d) *Surgery*

Surgical interventions should be considered if conservative management fails. The specific intervention depends on the focal area of pathology involved with the CMI (e.g., adductor tendon stripping, rectus abdominis aponeurosis repair). However, as more patient-specific pathologies are understood, addressing only the focal area of injury versus other potential contributing sites has come into question. This has resulted in numerous specific or combinations of surgical procedures being performed including tenotomy, aponeurosis repair, mesh implantation, and hip labral repair [4].

Laparoscopic extraperitoneal repairs are more common than open repairs in today's medical world. Patients with chronic CMI undergoing laparoscopic repair had a 90% success rate with an average return to play of 3 months compared to a 50% success rate for chronic CMI patients pursuing physical therapy alone [32]. In a study of 27 patients who underwent surgical repair of CMI, 92.6% returned to their previous level of athletics after an average of 112 days and with 0% recurrence at 1 year. Interestingly, the cohort with only adductor pathology noted a prolonged RTP time compared to abdominal pathology alone (101.7 days vs 91.1 days). Additionally, when both adductor and abdominal pathologies were present, the RTP time was 30% longer than the adductor pathology alone [33].

References

1. Bradshaw CJ, Bundy M, Falvey E. The diagnosis of longstanding groin pain: a prospective clinical cohort study. Br J Sports Med. 2008;42(10):851–4. Orchard J, Best TM. The management of muscle strain injuries: an early return versus the risk of recurrence. Clin J Sport Med. 2002;12(1):3–5.
2. Tyler TF, Nicholas SJ, Campbell RJ, Donellan S, McHugh MP. The effectiveness of a preseason exercise program to prevent adductor muscle strains in professional ice hockey players. Am J Sports Med. 2002;30(5):680–3.
3. Orchard J, Seward H. Epidemiology of injuries in the Australian Football League, seasons 1997–2000. Br J Sports Med. 2002;36(1):39–44.
4. Meyers WC, McKechnie A, Philippon MJ, Horner MA, Zoga AC, Devon ON. Experience with "sports hernia" spanning two decades. Ann Surg. 2008;248(4):656–65.
5. MacMahon PJ, Hogan BA, Shelly MJ, Eustace SJ, Kavanagh EC. Imaging of groin pain. Magn Reson Imaging Clin N Am. 2009;17(4):655–66, vi.
6. Serner A, Tol JL, Jomaah N, Weir A, Whiteley R, Thorborg K, et al. Diagnosis of acute groin injuries: a prospective study of 110 athletes: a prospective study of 110 athletes. Am J Sports Med. 2015;43(8):1857–64.
7. Hölmich P, Thorborg K, Dehlendorff C, Krogsgaard K, Gluud C. Incidence and clinical presentation of groin injuries in sub-elite male soccer. Br J Sports Med. 2014;48(16):1245–50.
8. Sheen AJ, Stephenson BM, Lloyd DM, Robinson P, Fevre D, Paajanen H, et al. "Treatment of the sportsman's groin": British Hernia Society's 2014 position statement based on the Manchester Consensus Conference. Br J Sports Med. 2014;48(14):1079–87.
9. Koulouris G. Imaging review of groin pain in elite athletes: an anatomic approach to imaging findings. AJR Am J Roentgenol. 2008;191(4):962–72.
10. Omar IM, Zoga AC, Kavanagh EC, Koulouris G, Bergin D, Gopez AG, et al. Athletic pubalgia and "sports hernia": optimal MR imaging technique and findings. Radiographics. 2008;28(5):1415–38.
11. Weir A, Brukner P, Delahunt E, Ekstrand J, Griffin D, Khan KM, et al. Doha agreement meeting on terminology and definitions in groin pain in athletes. Br J Sports Med. 2015;49(12):768–74.
12. Meyers WC, Havens BK, Horner GJ. Core muscle injury (a better name than "athletic pubalgia" or "sports hernia"). Curr Orthop Pract. 2014;25(4):321–6.
13. Engebretsen AH, Myklebust G, Holme I, Engebretsen L, Bahr R. Intrinsic risk factors for groin injuries among male soccer players: a prospective cohort study. Am J Sports Med. 2010;38(10):2051–7.
14. Hölmich P, Larsen K, Krogsgaard K, Gluud C. Exercise program for prevention of groin pain in football players: a cluster-randomized

trial: exercise program for prevention of groin pain in football players. Scand J Med Sci Sports. 2010;20(6):814–21.
15. Larson CM. Sports hernia/athletic pubalgia: evaluation and management. Sports Health. 2014;6(2):139–44.
16. Schilders E, Talbot JC, Robinson P, Dimitrakopoulou A, Gibbon WW, Bismil Q. Adductor-related groin pain in recreational athletes: role of the adductor enthesis, magnetic resonance imaging, and entheseal pubic cleft injections. J Bone Joint Surg Am. 2009;91(10):2455–60.
17. Verrall GM, Slavotinek JP, Fon GT, Barnes PG. Outcome of conservative management of athletic chronic groin injury diagnosed as pubic bone stress injury. Am J Sports Med. 2007;35(3):467–74.
18. Kurowicki J, Kraeutler MJ, Dávila Castrodad IM, Hahn AK, Simone ES, Kelly MA, et al. Diagnostic accuracy of physical examination tests in core muscle injury. Am J Sports Med. 2020;48(8):1983–8.
19. Serner A, Weir A, Tol JL, Thorborg K, Roemer F, Guermazi A, et al. Can standardised clinical examination of athletes with acute groin injuries predict the presence and location of MRI findings? Br J Sports Med. 2016;50(24):1541–7.
20. Williams PR, Thomas DP, Downes EM. Osteitis pubis and instability of the pubic symphysis. When nonoperative measures fail: when nonoperative measures fail. Am J Sports Med. 2000;28(3):350–5.
21. Branci S, Thorborg K, Bech BH, Boesen M, Nielsen MB, Hölmich P. MRI findings in soccer players with long-standing adductor-related groin pain and asymptomatic controls. Br J Sports Med. 2015;49(10):681–91.
22. Morley N, Grant T, Blount K, Omar I. Sonographic evaluation of athletic pubalgia. Skelet Radiol. 2016;45(5):689–99.
23. Rodriguez C, Miguel A, Lima H, Heinrichs K. Osteitis pubis syndrome in the professional soccer athlete: a case report. J Athl Train. 2001;36(4):437–40.
24. Kachingwe AF, Grech S. Proposed algorithm for the management of athletes with athletic pubalgia (sports hernia): a case series. J Orthop Sports Phys Ther. 2008;38(12):768–81.
25. De Bruijn R. Deep transverse friction its analgesic effect. Int J Sports Med. 1984;5:35–6.
26. Gehlsen GM, Ganion LR, Helfst R. Fibroblast responses to variation in soft tissue mobilization pressure. Med Sci Sports Exerc. 1999;31(4):531–5.
27. Abouelnaga WA, Aboelnour NH. Effectiveness of active rehabilitation program on sports hernia: randomized control trial. Ann Rehabil Med. 2019;43(3):305–13.
28. Hölmich P, Uhrskou P, Ulnits L, Kanstrup IL, Nielsen MB, Bjerg AM, et al. Effectiveness of active physical training as treatment for long-standing adductor-related groin pain in athletes: randomised trial. Lancet. 1999;353(9151):439–43.
29. Poor AE, Roedl JB, Zoga AC, Meyers WC. Core muscle injuries in athletes. Curr Sports Med Rep. 2018;17(2):54–8.
30. Scholten PM, Massimi S, Dahmen N, Diamond J, Wyss J. Successful treatment of athletic pubalgia in a lacrosse player with ultrasound-guided needle tenotomy and platelet-rich plasma injection: a case report. PM R. 2015;7(1):79–83.
31. St-Onge E, MacIntyre IG, Galea AM. Multidisciplinary approach to non-surgical management of inguinal disruption in a professional hockey player treated with platelet-rich plasma, manual therapy and exercise: a case report. J Can Chiropr Assoc. 2015;59(4):390–7.
32. Paajanen H, Brinck T, Hermunen H, Airo I. Laparoscopic surgery for chronic groin pain in athletes is more effective than nonoperative treatment: a randomized clinical trial with magnetic resonance imaging of 60 patients with sportsman's hernia (athletic pubalgia). Surgery. 2011;150(1):99–107.
33. Kajetanek C, Benoît O, Granger B, Menegaux F, Chereau N, Pascal-Mousselard H, et al. Athletic pubalgia: return to play after targeted surgery. Orthop Traumatol Surg Res. 2018;104(4):469–72.

Pelvic Fracture

19

Jomar Aryee, John Stelmach, Chandler Berke, Steven Mennona, and Alfred J. Tria Jr

19.1 Pelvic Fractures

The bony articulations of the pelvis do not carry inherent stability, and the pelvic ring relies heavily on ligamentous support anteriorly and posteriorly to maintain its structure and perform its function. The most important determinant for surgical intervention is the stability of the pelvic ring after injury. Stable injuries are primarily bony, without posterior ligament disruption including isolated iliac wing fractures, isolated pubic ramus fractures, and small, isolated sacral ala fractures. These patterns are well managed non-operatively with a period of protected weight-bearing (weight-bearing with an assistive device) until full weight-bearing can be tolerated. Injuries affecting the posterior ligamentous complex of the pelvis disrupt the linkage of the iliac wings to the sacrum (posterior weight-bearing arch), causing vertical instability, rotational instability, or both [1]. These injuries are often of high energy and carry significant morbidity, and associated injuries are often a cause of mortality. When a patient sustains a completely unstable injury to the pelvic ring, early fixation – temporarily with binders or external fixators and definitively with internal fixation – is the key to reducing mortality and optimizing functional outcome [1].

19.2 Stable Pelvic Injuries

Traumatic injuries of the pelvis are categorized with the Young and Burgess classification [2]. The ring injuries are broken into two groups – anterior-posterior compression (APC) and lateral compression (LC) – based on the direction of the forces that cause the injury. These injuries are further divided into levels I, II, and III going from least to most severe. In APC I injuries, there is disruption of only the anterior ligamentous complex, which is stable for protected weight-bearing (PWB) immediately. The hallmarks of the LC I injury are fracture to the pubic ramus and sacral ala. Weight-bearing as tolerated can be instituted based upon the severity of the sacral ala component.

J. Aryee · J. Stelmach · C. Berke · S. Mennona
Department of Orthopaedics, Rutgers-Robert Wood Johnson Medical School, New Brunswick, NJ, USA
e-mail: cmi40@rwjms.rutgers.edu

A. J. Tria Jr (✉)
Department of Orthopaedics, Rutgers-Robert Wood Johnson Medical School, New Brunswick, NJ, USA

19.3 Unstable Injuries

APC levels II and III involve injury to the anterior and then anterior and posterior ligaments of the SI joint, respectively. The LC II injury involves an ilium fracture dislocation, and the LC III is a combination of both an LCII and APC III injuries on either side of the pelvis. What these injuries have in common is their disruption of the posterior pelvic arch and the rotational and vertical instability that they produce. For adequate function of the pelvis, these injuries require reduction of bony defects and joint dislocations and rigid internal fixation.

19.4 Rehabilitation

Recovery after pelvic fracture surgery varies with the severity of the injury and invasiveness of subsequent surgical procedure(s). The goal of recovery after these injuries should start with gentle, passive range of motion of the lower extremity and short transfers. No current consensus exists on the optimal postoperative rehabilitation strategy, so weight-bearing and activity status are typically progressed at the surgeon's discretion [3]. Recent investigations show that patients who sustain vertically and rotationally unstable injuries are typically restricted to toe-touch or touch-down weight-bearing (using a limb for balance but not bearing weight through the extremity) for about 8 or 9 weeks before

© The Author(s), under exclusive license to Springer Nature Switzerland AG 2022

S. A. Mostoufi et al. (eds.), *Clinical Guide to Musculoskeletal Medicine*, https://doi.org/10.1007/978-3-030-92042-5_19

progression [3]. Patients who have procedures for injuries that are vertically stable tend to have a more liberal weight-bearing status, protected or partial weight-bearing, for a similar amount of time.

19.5 Sacroiliac Fusion

Percutaneous sacroiliac joint fusion is discussed in detail in Chap. 14.

References

1. Kim W-Y. Treatment of unstable pelvic ring injuries. Hip Pelvis. 2014;26(2):79. https://doi.org/10.5371/hp.2014.26.2.79.
2. Young JWR, Burgess AR, Brumback RJ, Poka A. Pelvic fractures: value of plain radiography in early assessment and management. Radiology. 1986;160(2):445–51. https://doi.org/10.1148/radiology.160.2.3726125.
3. Rickman M, Link BC, Solomon LB. Patient weight-bearing after pelvic fracture surgery—A systematic review of the literature: what is the modern evidence base? Strateg Trauma Limb Reconstr. 2019;14(1):45–52. https://doi.org/10.5005/jp-journals-10080-1414.

Coccydynia

20

Marina Protopapas and Kelly Alhooie

20.1 Synonyms

- Tailbone pain
- Coccygodynia
- Sacrococcygeal pain
- Disorder of the coccyx
- Disorder of sacrococcygeal spine
- Pain in the coccyx

20.2 ICD-10 Codes

M50.0–M54.0

20.3 Description

Coccydynia is a pain syndrome that encompasses pain extending from the inferior most aspect of the sacrum, within the gluteal fold, to the anal sphincter. The word coccyx is derived from an ancient Greek word "kokku" because the coalesced tail bones resemble a cuckoo's moderately curved beak [1–3]. This pain syndrome usually affects women more than men, and it is often trauma/fall related, although it can be idiopathic. It is midline pain in the intergluteal cleft, typically associated with sitting, and exacerbated with having pressure over the coccyx. Other skeletal disorders like SI pain, piriformis pain, ischial pain, and disc-related pain can present with pain in the tailbone/pelvic region and should be in the differential diagnosis.

Bony Anatomy The coccyx, a midline bony structure, is a small triangulated os, composed of three to five fused coccygeal vertebrae that articulate with the inferior most aspect of the sacrum called the sacral cornua [4]. Coccyx bones share many similarities to lumbar vertebrae but on a smaller scale. It differs from lumbar vertebrae since it has no vertebral canal, no neuroforamina, and no cerebral spinal fluid present at the coccygeal level. Only mobile articulation is between the last sacral bone and first coccyx bone (Co1). Each consecutive coccygeal bone is typically smaller in height and width compared to the coccygeal bone above it. The female coccyx is more often shorter, straighter, and more retroverted [5].

Sacrococcygeal Joint Anatomy \Sacrococcygeal joint is formed by the lower end of the sacrum articulating with the upper end of the coccyx. This is illustrated in Fig. 20.1, where the sacrococcygeal facet joints comprised of bilateral inferior articular processes from S5, also known as the sacral cornua, form the lateral border of the sacral hiatus, and the bilateral SAPs from the first coccygeal segment, also known as the coccygeal cornua [6]. There is often intervertebral disc between sacrum and first coccyx bone. Balain et al. [7] reported that of 38 patients who underwent

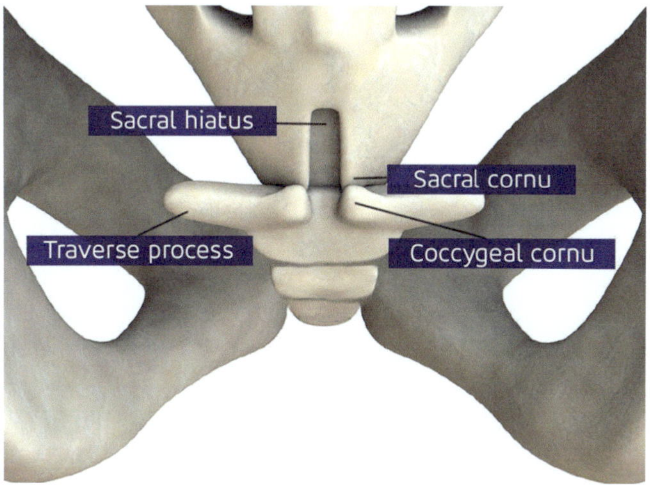

Fig. 20.1 Coccyx bony anatomy. (Illustrations by Sophie Asvesta)

M. Protopapas (✉)
National Spine and Pain Centers, Fairfax, VA, USA
e-mail: mprotopapas@treatingpain.com

K. Alhooie
OrthoPelvic Physical Therapy, Sterling, VA, USA
e-mail: Info@orthopelvicpt.com

© The Author(s), under exclusive license to Springer Nature Switzerland AG 2022
S. A. Mostoufi et al. (eds.), *Clinical Guide to Musculoskeletal Medicine*, https://doi.org/10.1007/978-3-030-92042-5_20

coccygectomy for coccydynia, 10 had at least two discs or moving joints, and 11 had only one disc or moving joint at histology.

Coccygeal Ligament Anatomy The anterior sacrococcygeal ligament and posterior longitudinal ligament span the length of the coccyx. The lateral sacrococcygeal ligaments bilaterally attach the lowest aspect of the sacrum to the ipsilateral transverse processes of the first coccygeal segment. The spinosacral ligaments bilaterally span the right and left ischial spines to the sacrum and coccyx. The sacrotuberous ligament extends from the sacrum and coccyx to the ischial tuberosity [8].

Surrounding Muscle Anatomy of the Coccyx The gluteus maximus originates from the posterior-inferior surface of the sacrum and coccyx, gluteal surface of the ilium, thoracolumbar fascia, and sacrotuberous ligament. The true pelvis is the area between the inlet and the outlet of the greater and lesser pelvis. The lower part of the pelvis is sealed off by a muscular diaphragm and perineal membrane known as the pelvic floor. Other borders of true pelvis consist of two lateral walls, a posterior wall (sacrococcygeal bones), and the pelvic floor. In Fig. 20.2, the muscles of the pelvic floor (or pelvic diaphragm) are depicted and are collectively referred to as the levator ani and coccygeus muscles. The coccygeus (also referred to as ischiococcygeus) is not part of the levator ani and supports the pelvic viscera and flexes the coccyx [9]. The levator ani is made up of the puborectalis, pubococcygeus, and iliococcygeus muscles. The pubococcygeus is also composed of the puboperinealis, puboprostaticus (males), pubovaginalis (female), and puboanalis. There are much more details related to coccyx and pelvic muscles that are beyond the scope of this chapter.

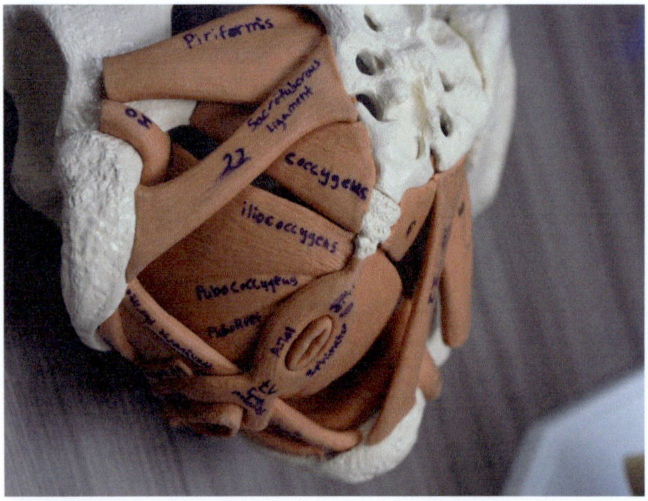

Fig. 20.2 Pelvic floor muscles

Vascular Supply The anterior division of the internal iliac artery is responsible for supplying the levator ani group of muscles. Its three terminal branches include the pudendal, inferior gluteal, and inferior vesical arteries. Venous drainage is achieved by the pudendal, inferior gluteal, and inferior vesical veins [9].

Innervation(S2–S4) Somatic nerves of the coccyx carry pain and other sensations from the coccygeal bones and ligaments. The sympathetic nervous system at the coccyx includes the ganglion impar, which appears to be involved in various forms of "sympathetically maintained pelvic pain." Branches from the sacral plexus S2–S4 contribute to the innervation of the levator ani muscles. The pudendal nerve directly innervates the pubococcygeus muscle [9, 10].

20.4 Etiology of Coccydynia

The most common cause of coccydynia is trauma, specifically single direct axial trauma such as a fall on the buttock, or cumulative trauma (prolonged suboptimal sitting position on a hard or uncomfortable surface). Aside from external trauma, the coccyx is susceptible to internal trauma such as difficult childbirth. The predominance of coccydynia in females is in part associated with pregnancy ligamentous laxity due to relaxin. BMI may be a risk factor for subluxation as proposed by Maigne et al., leading to painful coccyx [11]. Non-traumatic causes include sacrococcygeal joint hyper- or hypomobility, coccyx dislocation, coccyx DJD, infections, referred or radicular pain, and less commonly neoplasia [12]. Subluxation can also occur if the coccygeal bones fail to have their normal, slightly forward-flexed position (Table 20.1). In subluxation, the coccyx will extend posteriorly, and this can result in abnormal increased weight-bearing forces onto the coccyx while sitting [14]. There can also be morphological variations of the coccyx leading to bony spicule formation and coccygeal retroversion. Sympathetically mediated pain of the coccyx may occur due to hyperactivity or irritability of the ganglion impar [15, 16]. Non-organic causes such as somatization and psychiatric disorders have also been associated with coccydynia.

Table 20.1 Coccyx morphology types (modified Postacchini and Massobrio classification) [13]

I	Curved gently forward
II	Has a marked curve with the apex pointing straight forward
III	Angled forward sharply between Co1–Co2 and Co2–Co3
IV	Anteriorly subluxed at sacrococcygeal joint or Co1–Co2
V	Coccygeal retroversion with spicule
VI	Scoliotic deformity

20.5 Clinical Presentation

Coccydynia is midline pain in the intergluteal cleft, typically associated with sitting and exacerbated with having pressure over the coccyx. Patients often sit on their feet or on one buttock to avoid direct pressure against the coccyx. Pain can be present during defecation and intercourse, and there may be frequent urge to defecate [17]. Patients may have an inability to lay flat on the back and have greater comfort laying on her side. The history may reveal a recent axial load trauma or repeated prolonged episodes of sitting on hard uncomfortable surfaces [15, 16]. They often have favorite chairs to sit on or have many supportive cushions that they travel with.

20.6 Physical Examination

During examination, patients will often place their finger on the coccyx as a clue to diagnosis [18]. In visual inspection, the examiner is looking for any signs of redness, rash, fistula, hemorrhoids, or discharge that might suggest an underlying pilonidal cyst. With palpation, most patients with coccydynia will have focal reproduction of pain during external and posterior examination of the coccyx. In thin patients, a distal coccyx bone protuberance/sharp angle may be appreciated. Palpation of the anterior coccyx can be accomplished via digital rectal examination, particularly in patients in whom external palpation fails to reproduce their symptom. Rectal examination and bimanual manipulation of the coccyx will elicit pain and aid evaluation of any hypo- or hypermobility of the sacrococcygeal joint [19]. During intrarectal physical examination, pelvic floor muscles can be evaluated for hyperactivity and trigger points. Additionally, it is important to examine the adjacent structures such as the para-coccygeal muscles, anococcygeal ligament, ischiogluteal bursae, and piriformis muscles to rule out other musculoskeletal sources of pain.

20.7 Diagnostic Imaging

X-rays Radiographs can detect fracture, subluxation, and sharp coccyx angle. Seated radiographs may reveal abnormalities that were missed on standing radiographs [20]. The coccyx usually pivots between 5° and 25° between the sitting and standing positions. Coccydynia is commonly associated with coccygeal displacement, immobility (<5° of movement), or hypermobility (>25° of movement) [21]. Advanced imaging modalities and provocative tests will aid diagnosis but may not be as useful as dynamic radiographs obtained in the sitting and standing positions [21].

CT Sensitive test to detect malalignment, fractures, lytic lesion, and bleeding surrounding the coccyx.

MRI It can be used to assess the position or curvature of the coccyx, ligamentous injuries, soft tissue injury, fractures (marrow signal change), bony infiltration, and infection or tumors. MRI and technetium Tc-99m will also demonstrate inflammation associated with hypermobility and exclude other underlying pathologies [22].

Bone scan It can be used in patients with coccydynia in whom a search for malignancy or infection (e.g., osteomyelitis) is on the differential diagnosis [23].

Coccygeal discography Rarely used tool for diagnosing discogenic etiology of coccydynia [20].

Diagnostic injection A small volume anesthetic image guided injection of the coccyx, sacrococcygeal ligament, and the caudal space can confirm the diagnosis of coccydynia [24].

20.8 Treatment

20.8.1 Medical Management

Medical management includes non-steroidal anti-inflammatory drugs, ergonomic adaptation such as the use of doughnut/cutout cushions, extracorporeal shock wave therapy (ESWT), intrarectal medications, and intrarectal manipulation [19, 25]. In acute fracture, short course of mild opioids may be necessary.

20.8.2 Rehabilitation

On average it takes about 1–4 months of having a multifaceted approach with a physical therapist and pain management to get back to sitting without pain. In treating coccydynia, it is important to treat the pubococcygeus, iliococcygeus, coccygeus, glut max, and sacrospinous ligament because of the direct correlations to the coccyx.

Massage Massaging or stretching of the tonic muscle spasm to the anterior sacrococcygeal ligament, the gluteus maximus muscle, the coccygeus muscle, and the levator ani muscles attached to the coccyx can be performed to treat coccygeal pain [26].

Mobilization Maneuvers of the sacrococcygeal and intercoccygeal joints are performed to enhance coccygeal mobility. Maigne and Chatellier compared the effect of massage, mobilization, and stretching and reported that stretching methods had the highest success rate following by mobilization [27]. Seker et al. both studied patients that received transrectal manipulation and corticosteroid injections, and they determined that manual therapy combined with steroid injections would offer a successful alternative method for the management in cases of persistent coccydynia [19]. Lin et al. used extracorporeal shock wave therapy (ESWT) in the treatment of coccydynia and reported more satisfactory results compared with physical modalities [28].

20.8.3 Procedures

Sacrococcygeal Injection When conservative measures fail, patients may benefit from a local corticosteroid injection (Fig. 20.3b). Target will be junction of the sacrum with Co1 or over Co1–Co2 junction [19]. If there is a subluxation, often sacrococcygeal ligament dorsal to the subluxed segment will be the target for injection [19]. Studies suggest that patient who receives coccygeal steroid injections within 6 months of the onset of pain had better and longer outcomes (greater than 50% relief, $P = 0.055$) [29].

Caudal Epidural Steroid Injections On its own or in combination with sacrococcygeal injection, caudal injection can help with coccydynia pain (Fig. 20.3a). It may also be used to treat cases of coccygeal pain originating from Tarlov cysts and to treat lower sacral radicular pain.

Ganglion Impar Treatments The ganglion impar is found on the ventral surface of the sacrococcygeal joint and provides nociceptive and sympathetic innervation to the perineal and anal areas [30]. A ganglion impar block (Fig. 20.4a) can be used to also treat acute or chronic perineal pain [31]. The blocks are typically performed using the trans-sacrococcygeal and inter-sacrococcygeal approaches with the assistance of fluoroscopy [32]. Various medications can be injected such as local anesthetics and concomitant use of anesthetics and steroids, alcohol, phenol, and neurolysis by means of radiofrequency ablation.

Neuromodulation DRG stimulation for coccydynia in an off-label use. Giordano et al. proposed the use of a bilateral L1 and S2 DRG approach to the stimulator trial. They determined that since both neuropathic and nociceptive components are believed to contribute to chronic coccydynia [33], that there is an instrumental role of the DRG in both pain states may result in positive outcomes (Fig. 20.4b).

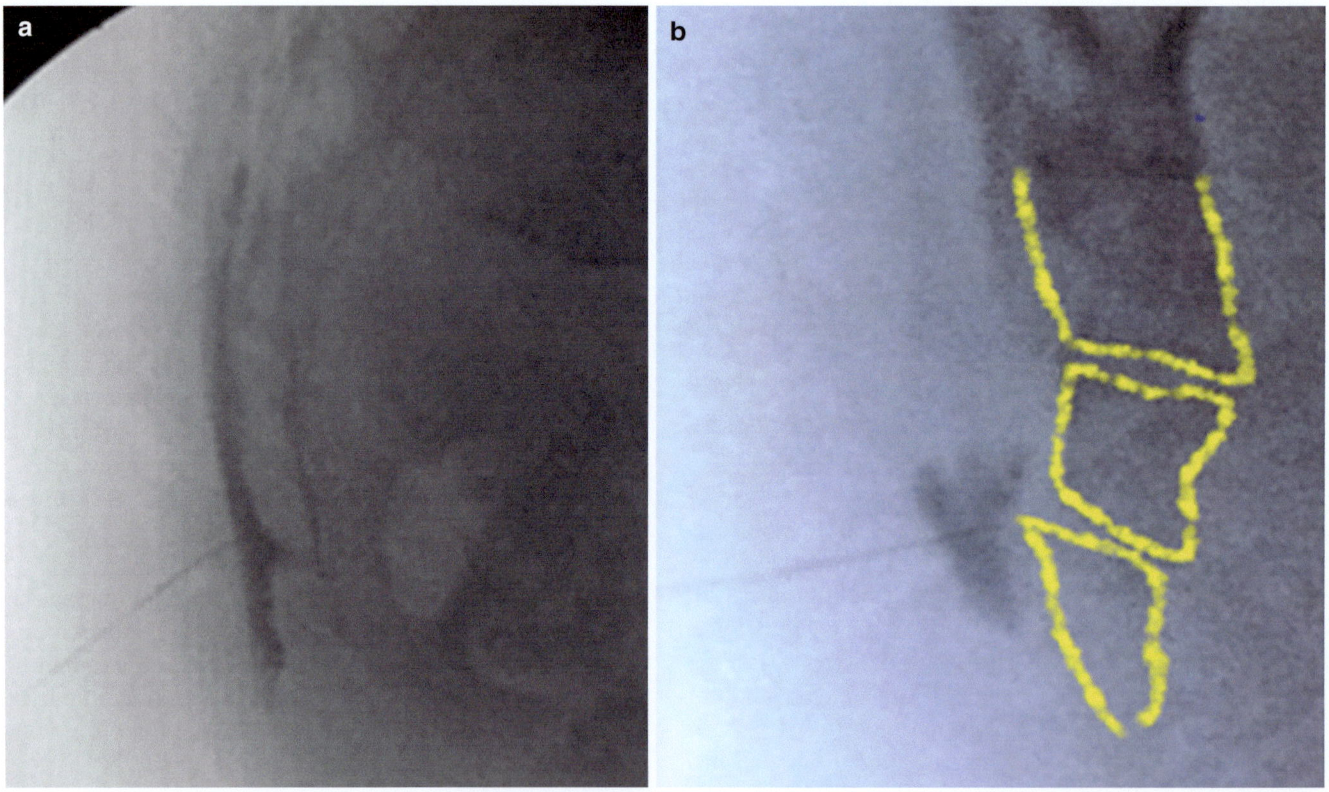

Fig. 20.3 Image (**a**) shows caudal injection of contrast, and image (**b**) shows sacrococcygeal injection (note subluxation of Co1–Co2 segment)

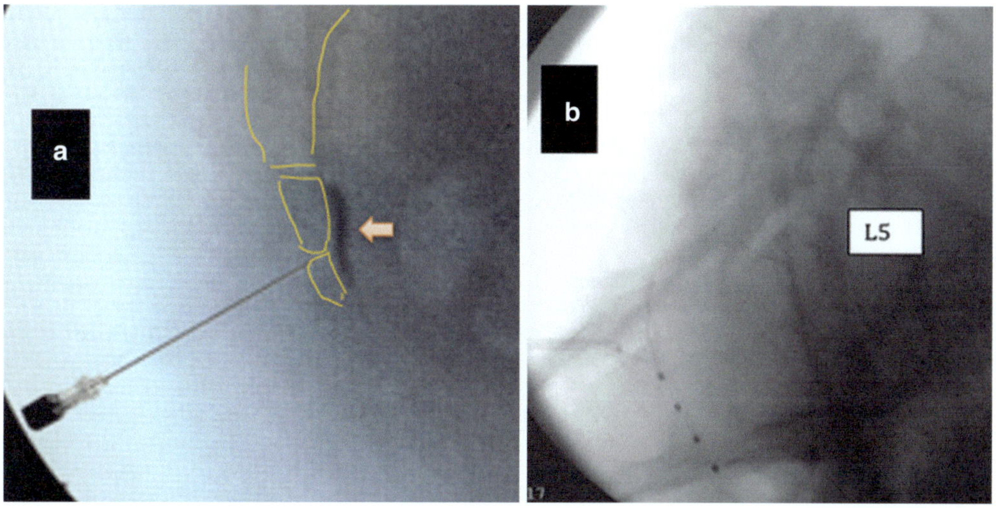

Fig. 20.4 Image (**a**) shows needle placement and contrast flow for ganglion impar block. Arrow points to linear flow of the contrast in the ventral surface of the coccyx. Image (**b**) shows placement of S2 dorsal root ganglion stimulator loop to treat pelvic pain via neuromodulation. (Images courtesy of Ali Mostoufi, MD, New England Spine Care, Cambridge, MA, USA)

Intrathecal Pain Pump In chronic and intractable cases of coccydynia, intrathecal pumps might also be considered.

Coccygeoplasty This intervention is recommended for retractable pain in the treatment of acute or subacute osteoporotic coccygeal fractures and coccydynia with edema [5].

20.8.4 Surgery

Coccygectomy The efficacy of coccygectomy for coccydynia has been variable, with studies reporting anywhere from 60% to 91% success rates [34]. Surgical outcome was shown to be increased by limiting coccygectomy to patients with instability and hypermobility of the sacrococcygeal junction (demonstrated by stress radiographs) [35]. Balain et al. [36] found that patients with moderate to severe coccyx DJD did better postoperatively than those with mild or no degenerative changes. Perkins et al. [37] indicated a success rate of 92% after coccygectomy for patients who had at least 75% pain relief after injection of local anesthetic into the sacrococcygeal joint. Coccygectomy remains an effective treatment for coccyx pain in severely disabled patients, although high risk of infection in postoperative phase should be carefully considered [36]. Coccygectomy is also discussed in Chap. 16.

References

1. Howorth B. The painful coccyx. Clin Orthop. 1959;14:145–60.
2. Kim NH, Suk KS. Clinical and radiological differences between traumatic and idiopathic coccygodynia. Yonsei Med J. 1999;40(3):215–20.
3. Sugar O. Coccyx. The bone named for a bird. Spine (Phila Pa 1976). 1995;20(3):379–83.
4. Drake R, Vogl AW, Mitchell A. Gray's anatomy for students. 2nd ed. Philadelphia: Churchill and Livingstone; 2009.
5. Akar E, Koban O, Öğrenci A, Yılmaz M, Dalbayrak S. Polymethylmetacrylate cement augmentation of the coccyx (coccygeoplasty) for fracture: a case report. Balkan Med J. 2020;37(6):348–50.
6. Woon JT, Maigne JY, Perumal V, Stringer MD. Magnetic resonance imaging morphology and morphometry of the coccyx in coccydynia. Spine (Phila Pa 1976). 2013;38(23):E1437–45.
7. Foye PM. Arthritis of the tailbone. Tailbone pain relief now! NJ: Top Quality Publishing Newark; 2015. p. 71–4.
8. Foye PM. Coccydynia: tailbone pain. Phys Med Rehabil Clin N Am. 2017;28(3):539–49.
9. Pelvic anatomy [Internet]. 2021. Cited 2021 Apr 4. https://www.kenhub.com/en/study/pelvic-floor-muscles.
10. Foye PM. Anatomy of tailbone pain. Tailbone pain relief now! NJ: Top Quality Publishing Newark; 2015. p. 29–36.
11. Maigne JY. Doursounian causes and mechanisms of common coccydynia: role of body mass index and coccygeal trauma. Spine. 2000;25:3072–9.
12. De Andres J, Chaves S. Coccygodynia: a proposal for an algorithm for treatment. J Pain. 2003;4:257–66.
13. Postacchini F, Massobrio M. Idiopathic coccygodynia: analysis of of fifty-one operative cases and a radiographic study of the normal coccyx. J Bone Joint Surg Am. 1983;65:1116–24. PMID: 6226668.
14. Foye PM. Abnormal position of the tailbone. Tailbone pain relief now! NJ: Top Quality Publishing Newark; 2015. p. 75–8.
15. Foye PM. Bone spurs of the tailbone. Tailbone pain relief now! NJ: Top Quality Publishing Newark; 2015. p. 65–70.
16. Foye PM. Sympathetic nervous system pain at the coccyx. Tailbone pain relief now! NJ: Top Quality Publishing Newark; 2015. p. 79–84.
17. Lirette LS, Chaiban G, Tolba R, Eissa H. Coccydynia: an overview of the anatomy, etiology, and treatment of coccyx pain. Ochsener J. 2014;14:84–7.
18. Fortin JD, Falco FJ. The Fortin finger test: an indicator of sacroiliac pain. Am J Orthop (Belle Mead NJ). 1997;26(7):477–80.
19. Nathan ST, Fisher BE, Roberts CS. Coccydynia: a review of pathoanatomy, aetiology, treatment and outcome. J Bone Joint Surg Br. 2010;92(12):1622–7. Rush J. Coccydynia. Curr Orthop. 1996;10(2):128–31.
20. Maigne JY, Guedj S, Straus C. Idiopathic coccygodynia. Lateral roentgenograms in the sitting position and coccygeal discography. Spine. 1994;19:930–4.

21. Maigne JY, Tamalet B. Standardized radiologic protocol for the study of common coccygodynia and characteristics of the lesions observed in the sitting position. Clinical elements differentiating luxation, hypermobility, and normal mobility. Spine. 1996;21:2588–93.
22. Prather H, Hunt D. Sacroiliac joint pain. Dis Mon. 2004;50:670–83.
23. Foye PM. Introduction. Tailbone pain relief now! 2015. Top quality.
24. Lirette LS, Chaiban G, Tolba R, Eissa R. Coccydynia: an overview of the anatomy, etiology, and treatment of coccyx pain. Ochsner J. 2014;14(1):84–7.
25. Fogel G, Cunningham P, Esses S. Coccygodynia: evaluation and management. J Am Acad Orthop Surg. 2004;12:49–54.
26. Emerson SS, Speece AJ 3rd. Manipulation of the coccyx with anesthesia for the management of coccydynia. J Am Osteopath Assoc. 2012;112:805–7.
27. Maigne JY, Chatellier G. Comparison of three manual coccydynia treatments: a pilot study. Spine (Phila Pa 1976). 2001;26:E479–83.
28. Lin SF, Chen YJ, Tu HP, Lee CL, Hsieh CL, Wu WL, Chen CH. The effects of extracorporeal shock wave therapy in patients with coccydynia: a randomized controlled trial. PLoS One. 2015;10(11):e0142475.
29. Mitra R, Cheung L, Perry P. Efficacy of fluoroscopically guided steroid injections in the management of coccydynia. Pain Physician. 2007;10(6):775–8.
30. Malec MM, Horosz B, Koleda I, et al. Neurolytic block of ganglion of Walther for the management of chronic pelvic pain. Wideochir Inne Tech Maloinwazyjne. 2014;9(3):458–62.
31. Wemm K Jr, Saberski L. Modified approach to block the ganglion impar (ganglion of Walther). Reg Anesth. 1995;20(6):544–5.
32. Patt RB, Plancarte R. RE: Yamada K, Ishihara Y, Saito T: Relief of intractable perineal pain by coccygeal nerve block in anterior sacrococcygeal ligament after surgery for rectal cancer. J Anesthesia (1994)8:52–54. J Anesth. 1997;11(2):170–1.
33. Giordano NL, van Helmond N, Chapman KB. Coccydynia treated with dorsal root ganglion stimulation. Case Rep Anesthesiol. 2018;2018:5832401.
34. Milosevic S, Andersen GØ, Jensen MM, Rasmussen MM, Carreon L, Andersen MØ, Simony A. The efficacy of coccygectomy in patients with persistent coccydynia. Bone Joint J. 2021;103-B(3):542–6.
35. Kwon HD, Schrot RJ, Kerr EE, Kim KD. Coccygodynia and coccygectomy. Korean J Spine. 2012;9(4):326–33.
36. Balain B, Eisenstein SM, Alo GO, Darby AJ, Cassar-Pullicino VN, Roberts SE, Jaffray DC. Coccygectomy for coccydynia: case series and review of literature. Spine (Phila Pa 1976). 2006;31(13):E414–20.
37. Perkins R, Schofferman J, Reynolds J. Coccygectomy for severe refractory sacrococcygeal joint pain. J Spinal Disord Tech. 2003;16(1):100–3. https://doi.org/10.1097/00024720-200302000-00016. PMID: 12571492.

Part IV

Shoulder

Section Editor
Jason L. Zaremski

Anterior and Lateral Shoulder Disorders

21

William A. Berrigan, Oluseun Olufade,
and Kenneth Mautner

21.1 Acromioclavicular (AC) Joint Injuries

21.1.1 Synonyms

- AC joint separation (S43.101A)
- Shoulder separation (S43.101A)
- Osteolysis of the distal clavicle (M89.519)
- Painful degeneration of the AC joint (M19.019)

21.1.2 Description

The AC joint is a common site for injury in athletes who fall onto the shoulder. The structure consists of the joint capsule and acromioclavicular ligaments which stabilize the joint in the anterior-posterior (AP) plane and coracoclavicular ligaments (conoid and trapezoid) that stabilize in the superior inferior plane.

AC joint injuries can be classified as acute or chronic. Acute injuries are often more straightforward and have focal tenderness, swelling, and deformity. Chronic injuries may be more difficult to diagnose given the frequency of association with concomitant shoulder pathology.

21.1.2.1 Acute AC Joint Injury

Acute injuries to the AC joint are often caused by a fall onto the point of the shoulder. They are classified into six different types of injuries based on the position of the clavicle with respect to the acromion and coracoid [1] (see Table 21.1).

21.1.2.2 Chronic AC Joint Injury

Repetitive motion and stress can lead to chronic inflammation of the AC joint. This occurs particularly with activities that involve an outstretched arm reaching overhead or across the body. This stress can lead to overuse injuries and such conditions as osteolysis of the clavicle and osteoarthritis of the joint.

21.1.3 Symptoms

Patients will often describe pain at the top of the shoulder with arms outstretched or movement across the body (such as reaching for a seat belt strap). It is one of the few sites within the shoulder where pain can radiate up into the trapezius muscle. Exercises that most commonly aggravate the AC joint include bench press, dips, and pushups [2].

Table 21.1 Rockwood classification of acromioclavicular joint injury

Acute AC Joint Injury	
Classification of injury	Description
Type I	Sprain of the acromioclavicular joint capsule
Type II	Complete tear of the acromioclavicular ligaments with sprain of the coracoclavicular ligaments
Type III	Complete tear of the acromioclavicular ligaments and coracoclavicular ligaments
Type IV	Complete tear of the acromioclavicular ligaments and coracoclavicular ligaments with the clavicle displaced posteriorly into the trapezius
Type V	Complete tear of the acromioclavicular ligaments and coracoclavicular ligaments with the clavicle displaced greater than 100% compared to contralateral side
Type VI	Complete tear of the acromioclavicular ligaments and coracoclavicular ligaments with inferior dislocation of the lateral clavicle

W. A. Berrigan
Clinical Sports Medicine Fellow, Department of Physical Medicine and Rehabilitation, Emory University School of Medicine, Atlanta, GA, USA

O. Olufade (✉)
Orthopaedics and Physical Medicine & Rehabilitation, Emory University School of Medicine, Atlanta, GA, USA

K. Mautner
Primary Care Sports Medicine, Emory University, Atlanta, GA, USA

Department of Orthopaedics and Physical Medicine and Rehabilitation, Emory University School of Medicine, Atlanta, GA, USA

© The Author(s), under exclusive license to Springer Nature Switzerland AG 2022

S. A. Mostoufi et al. (eds.), *Clinical Guide to Musculoskeletal Medicine*, https://doi.org/10.1007/978-3-030-92042-5_21

21.1.4 Physical Exam

There is a low level of statistical accuracy and precision of special tests for the AC joint when performed in isolation [3]. Therefore, it has been recommended to perform a combination of tests to better increase diagnostic value [4]. Still, physical examination maneuvers are not beneficial when pretest reliability is unequivocal. It is helpful then to have the patient point directly to the location of pain and attempt to localize the site of tenderness to the AC joint, which is important for diagnosis. The following provocative maneuvers can then be used to assist with diagnostic confirmation for the AC joint:

- Cross body adduction: Test is performed by passively adducting the arm across the body approximating the elbow to the contralateral shoulder (sensitivity 77%, specificity 79%) [3].
- Resisted arm extension: Test is performed by having the patient forward flex the arm 90° and flex the elbow 90°. The patient is then asked to extend the arm horizontally against resistance by the examiner. A positive test is pain at the AC joint (sensitivity 72%, specificity 85%) [3].
- Active compression test: Test is performed in two parts. First, the examiner asks the patient to flex forward the affected arm at 90° with the elbow in full extension and arm adducted at 10°–15°. The arm is then internally rotated so that the thumb is pointed downward. The examiner applies uniform downward force to the arm. The second part is performed with the arm in the same position, but the palm is supinated. A downward force is again applied. A positive test is pain with the first maneuver that is reduced or eliminated with the second maneuver. Pain should be localized over the AC joint or top of the shoulder (sensitivity 41%, specificity 95%) (Fig. 21.1) [3].

21.1.5 Diagnostic Workup

- *X-Rays in AC Joint Injury*
- Either a single AP view with both AC joints or one AP radiograph of each AC joint should be obtained for comparative evaluation. A Zanca view with 15–30 degrees of cephalic tilt can be helpful in evaluating for a Type II injury or distal clavicular fracture. Stress/weighted radiographs are no longer recommended. Coracoclavicular (CC) measurement should be done to evaluate for extent of injury. Normal distance is 11–13 mm, but the diagnostic value is in comparison to the contralateral side. An increase in CC distance of 25–50% indicates complete disruption. Type III injury can be distinguished from type V based on the amount of displacement. Type III has 25–100% greater coracoclavicular distance than the uninjured side, while type V is greater than 100% compared to the contralateral side [1, 5]. Axillary views help confirm anterior-posterior position of the distal clavicle in types III–VI.
- *X-Rays in Chronic AC Joint Injury*
- X-rays are often abnormal in adults with chronic injuries and can be identified by standard anterior-posterior (AP) shoulder, glenoid, and scapular Y views. A Zanca view can be obtained (15–30 degrees of cephalic tilt) to better visualize the AC joint above the acromion.
- *Ultrasound*
- Ultrasound can provide additional diagnostic information to identify degenerative joint disease, os acromiale, cysts,

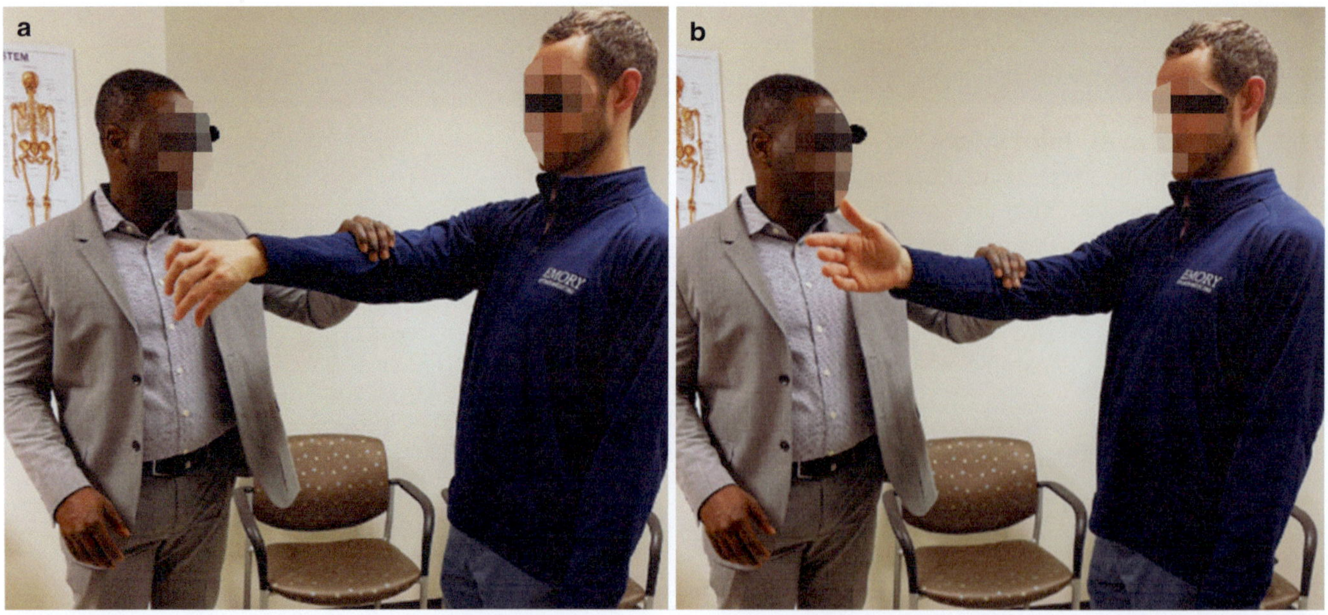

Fig. 21.1 The active compression test (**a**) is performed in the first position with the examiner applying a downward force on the arm with the patient's shoulder forward flexed and adducted. The test is then repeated with the patient's palm facing up (**b**). The pain should be decreased with the arm in the second position

and fluid within the joint as well as to look at the joint dynamically. It can also be used to enhance accuracy of injections [6, 7].

- *Magnetic Resonance Imaging (MRI)*
- MRI is not a routine method used for diagnosis of purely AC joint pathology. It can demonstrate degeneration of the AC joint and disruption of the ligamentous structures but is more helpful for ruling out other coinciding pathologies if clinically indicated [8].

21.1.6 Treatments

21.1.6.1 Acute Injury

Type I and II injuries do well with conservative management. Types IV through VI require surgical management for stabilization. Type III injuries are controversial, but the trend is toward conservative non-operative management [9].

Type I injuries often recover within 2 weeks, while type II can take 6–8 weeks. Type III may extend up to 12 weeks. The initial rehabilitation protocol should focus on a gentle range of motion exercises (pendulums). This should then be progressed to a limited strength program (2–6 weeks) followed by a challenging strength program that can progress to a return to sport (8–10 weeks) [9].

21.1.6.2 Chronic Injury

Chronic AC joint injury and degeneration can be treated with activity modifications, rest, ice, over-the-counter analgesics, and exercises to improve scapular retraction and stabilization. Injection with a corticosteroid may help provide short-term pain relief. Pain unresponsive to conservative measures may be indicated for surgical procedures as distal clavicle resection [10].

21.2 Adhesive Capsulitis (M75.0)

21.2.1 Synonyms

- Frozen shoulder
- Painful stiff shoulder
- Periarthritis of the shoulder
- Periarthritis scapulae
- Duplay disease
- Tendinitis of the short rotators

21.2.2 Description

Adhesive capsulitis is defined by the American Academy of Orthopaedic Surgeons as a "condition of varying severity characterized by the gradual development of global limitation of active and passive shoulder motion where radiographic findings other than osteopenia are absent" [11]. It can be classified as either primary or secondary. Primary, or idiopathic, is insidious in onset and often associated with other disease processes. The most prominent association is with diabetes mellitus (DM), with prevalence of DM in adhesive capsulitis reported at 30% and with those with DM to be at five times greater risk of developing adhesive capsulitis compared to controls [12]. Other risk factors include thyroid disease, dyslipidemia, prolonged immobilization, stroke, drugs such as anti-retrovirals, and Parkinson's disease [11]. Secondary adhesive capsulitis is usually caused by trauma or injury to the shoulder including rotator cuff tear, fracture, post-surgery, or prolonged immobilization.

The pathophysiology behind the disease process is not fully understood. It is hypothesized that there is an initial synovial inflammation within the joint capsule that leads to a subsequent reactive capsular fibrosis and adhesions within the synovial lining.

Differential diagnosis of shoulder adhesive capsulitis	
Common	Less common
Rotator cuff tendinopathy	Cervical degenerative disk disease
Subacromial bursitis	Referred pain from the cervical spine or diaphragm
Impingement syndrome	Polymyalgia rheumatica
Glenohumeral osteoarthritis	Malignancy (apical lung, metastasis)

21.2.3 Symptoms

Patients with adhesive capsulitis typically will present with insidious onset progressively worsening shoulder pain over weeks to months followed by significant limitation in range of motion of the shoulder. The mean age of onset is 55, more often affecting the non-dominant shoulder and women greater than men, with 20–30% having a recurrence of adhesive capsulitis on the contralateral shoulder [11]. The clinical manifestation is broken up into four phases [13]:

Phase 1: Pre-adhesive Stage

- Pathology: Diffuse glenohumeral synovitis without adhesions most prominent in the anterior-superior capsule
- Duration: 0–3 months
- Presentation: Full range of motion, non-specific pain particularly at night

Phase 2: Freezing Stage

- Pathology: Acute adhesive synovitis with proliferation of the synovium and early formation of adhesions, prominent in inferior capsular fold
- Duration: Symptoms present for 3–9 months
- Presentation: Pain is prominent, and motion loss is mild

Phase 3: Frozen Stage

- Pathology: Dense, proliferative hypervascular synovitis with more prominent fibrosis
- Duration: Symptoms present for 9–14 months
- Presentation: Report a previous history of a painful phase that resolved resulting in a pain-free but stiff shoulder

Phase 4: Thawing Stage

- Pathology: Capsular remodeling in response to continued use of the shoulder
- Duration: Symptoms present for 15–24 months
- Presentation: Minimal pain with progressive improvement in range of motion

21.2.4 Physical Exam

Patients with adhesive capsulitis demonstrate active and passive reduction in range of motion in two or more planes compared to the unaffected side. A mechanical restraint to passive motion is the hallmark of adhesive capsulitis and is best appreciated on passive external rotation with the arm at the side. Usually, range of motion is lost in the following order: external rotation, abduction, internal rotation, and forward flexion. Patients may demonstrate tenderness at the biceps tendon because its synovium is confluent with the glenohumeral joint. Rotator cuff strength is usually intact and does not cause significant pain with isometric testing. Often, the Neer and Hawkins test for impingement and the Speed's test for biceps tendinopathy are positive [12].

21.2.5 Diagnostic Workup

21.2.5.1 X-Rays

Plain radiographs are typically normal but are important in ruling out other causes of shoulder pathology including arthritis, calcific tendinopathy, and shoulder dislocation. Radiographs may also show diffuse osteopenia demonstrating long-standing disease.

21.2.5.2 Magnetic Resonance Imaging (MRI)

MRI is not needed to make a diagnosis of adhesive capsulitis, but can be useful in challenging cases and to rule out other coinciding pathologies. Findings on MRI include the following [14]:

- Rotator interval enhancement (Fig. 21.2)
- Axillary joint capsule enhancement
- Inferior glenohumeral ligament (IGHL) hyperintensity
- IGHL thickening
- Coracohumeral ligament thickening
- Fat obliteration of the rotator interval

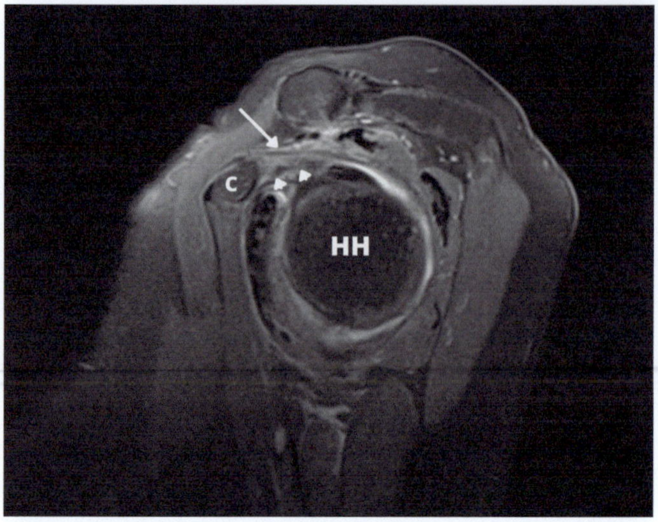

Fig. 21.2 T2 sagittal image demonstrating soft tissue thickening in the rotator interval (arrows) consistent with adhesive capsulitis. HH, humeral head; C, coracoid; Arrow, coracohumeral ligament (Image is from author's library)

21.2.5.3 Ultrasound

There are certain findings on ultrasound that may be useful as an adjunct for establishing the diagnosis. These include [15]:

- Limitation of the sliding movement of the supraspinatus tendon beneath the acromion with active arm elevation
- Abnormal hypoechogenicity and hyperemia in the rotator interval
- Thickening and increased stiffness of the coracohumeral ligament

21.2.6 Treatments

In most cases, adhesive capsulitis is a self-limiting disease with spontaneous recovery within 18–30 months. Treatment plans are focused on decreasing pain and improving range of motion and include medication, physical therapy, procedures, and surgical options [16].

21.2.7 Medical Management

- Non-steroidal anti-inflammatory drugs (NSAIDs) have been widely used for the treatment of adhesive capsulitis for pain control, especially during the initial inflammatory phases.
- Oral corticosteroids have been shown to improve pain and range of motion for short-term management of adhesive capsulitis [17].

21.2.8 Rehabilitation

Physical therapy with a home exercise program is one of the mainstay treatment options regardless of stage of adhesive capsulitis. Therapy should focus on gentle range of motion and as pain allows, stretching and strengthening exercises. Although a commonly used treatment, evidence for the effectiveness of physical therapy alone is lacking, but studies have shown that physical therapy with corticosteroid injection leads to a faster and significant improvement in function [18].

21.2.9 Procedures

No therapeutic intervention is universally accepted as the most effective treatment for adhesive capsulitis, but several options are available.

1. *Glenohumeral Corticosteroid Injection:* Injections have shown to decrease pain and improve range of motion and function. The effect has been described to last up to 6 weeks and is more effective when synovitis is present during the early stage of adhesive capsulitis [19].
2. *Glenohumeral Joint Hydrodistention:* In this procedure, the joint is injected with normal saline and corticosteroid to dilate the glenohumeral capsule. A summary of meta-analyses indicated that arthrographic hydrodistention with corticosteroid provides superior pain relief in the short term and improvement in range of motion across all time frames when compared to intra-articular corticosteroid or physiotherapy [20].
3. *Suprascapular Nerve Block:* A nerve block is a safe method for pain relief in refractory cases of adhesive capsulitis. The aim is to block the nerves to the glenohumeral joint as they branch from the suprascapular nerve near the suprascapular notch. One study suggested a suprascapular nerve block combined with intra-articular injection increased treatment efficacy at 1 year compared to intra-articular injection alone [21].

21.2.10 Surgery

Surgery is reserved for refractory cases that do not respond to conservative measures outlined above.

- *Manipulation Under Anesthesia*: A controlled, forced restoration of shoulder movements. The procedure is proven effective but does carry an increased risk of humerus fracture.
- *Surgical Capsular Release*: More commonly performed procedure involving the release of the capsule with improvement in long-term pain and functional outcome measures [22].

21.3 Proximal Biceps Tendinopathy (M75.22)

21.3.1 Synonyms

- Bicipital tendinitis (M75.22)
- Strain of the muscle, fascia, and tendon of other parts of the biceps (S46.211A)

21.3.2 Description

The biceps muscle is made up of a long and a short head. The long head originates from intraarticular superior glenoid tubercle, contributing to the formation of the glenoid labrum. The short head originates from the coracoid process. The short head attaches distally on the radial tuberosity, whereas the long head attaches proximally on the radial tuberosity.

The long head of the biceps tendon is the most common site of pathology. It is contained in the rotator interval that includes the coracohumeral ligament and superior glenohumeral ligament. It then sits in the bicipital groove between the greater and lesser tuberosities. Given the location, the long head of the biceps is rarely affected in isolation and is often associated with rotator cuff pathology, impingement/scapular dyskinesis, and glenohumeral joint instability. It can also be seen with disease processes that cause synovitis of the joint capsule given that the synovial lining of the biceps tendon sheath is continuous with the capsule [23].

The tendon can be affected either acutely or chronically and present throughout the full spectrum of tendinopathy with risk factors being repetitive movements such as lifting, reaching, and overhead throwing. Acute isolated injuries are more often seen in younger athletes, while chronic degenerative tendons present in older individuals [24].

Differential diagnosis of proximal biceps tendinopathy	
AC joint pathology	Adhesive capsulitis
Impingement syndrome	Glenohumeral instability
Rotator cuff tendinopathy	Cervical spine pathology
SLAP tears	Humeral head osteonecrosis
Subacromial bursitis	Glenohumeral osteoarthritis

21.3.3 Symptoms

Patients will often present with anterior-medial shoulder pain that may radiate down to the muscle belly of the biceps. Pain is worsened with flexion, lifting, pulling, and repetitive overhead activity. Isolated cases of biceps tendinopathy can occur in younger overhead athletes, but more often it coincides with other rotator cuff pathologies. A clicking or popping of the shoulder may occur and indicate instability and subluxation of the tendon which is most often associated with tears of the subscapularis tendon as the biceps tendon moves medially [25].

21.3.4 Physical Exam

Physical examination of the biceps tendon has its inherent challenges given that the tendon lies deep within the joint and the extra-articular portion within the biceps groove is adjacent to other structures. Findings, therefore, are similar to other pathological entities that may either be affecting the glenohumeral joint or rotator cuff. There are two tests for the bicep tendon that may aid with differential diagnosis [2, 25]:

- *Yergason's test:* The patient flexes the elbow to 90° with the forearm pronated. The examiner holds the patient's wrist to resist supination and has the patient actively supinate against the resistance of the examiner. The test is positive when pain is elicited within the bicipital groove (Fig. 21.3a) (sensitivity 43%, specificity 79%) [26].
- *Speed's test:* The patient flexes the shoulder against resistance, while the elbow is extended and the forearm supinated. The test is positive when pain is localized to the bicipital groove (Fig. 21.4b) (sensitivity 90%, specificity 13.8%) [27].

21.3.5 Diagnostic Workup

21.3.5.1 Ultrasound

Ultrasound can assist in delineating the spectrum of pathology for the biceps tendon, including tendinosis, tenosynovitis, and tendon tearing. A normal bicep tendon is tightly packed, fibrillar, and well defined as it sits in the bicipital groove (Fig. 21.4). An abnormal tendon can appear hypoechoic, thickened, and possibly with tendon fiber discontinuity or defect. Heterogeneous fluid surrounding the tendon can be suggestive of tenosynovitis. However, fluid surrounding the tendon may also be suggestive of rotator cuff pathology. Active subluxation of the tendon outside of the bicipital groove can be seen by having the patient supinate and pronate the forearm with active internal and external rotation of the shoulder. This is most commonly associated with tears of the subscapularis tendon [28].

21.3.5.2 MRI

Magnetic resonance imaging provides the ability to visualize the biceps tendon but with limited sensitivity and specificity for diagnosis of pathology [29, 30]. MRI should be reserved for advanced cases, suspected complete tear, and surgical planning and to further investigate the labrum. It can also be helpful in investigating coinciding pathology for those not responding to conservative measures.

21.3.6 Treatment

Initial treatment begins with activity modifications, a trial of NSAIDs and/or a corticosteroid injection. Ultrasound guidance should be used to enhance accuracy [31]. NSAIDs and corticosteroid injections should always be used for short-term pain relief in combination with a multi-phase rehabilitation program [32]. Other treatments that have been suggested for tendinopathy include topical nitroglycerine, iontophoresis, phonophoresis, therapeutic ultrasound, extracorporeal shock wave therapy, and low-level laser therapy [33].

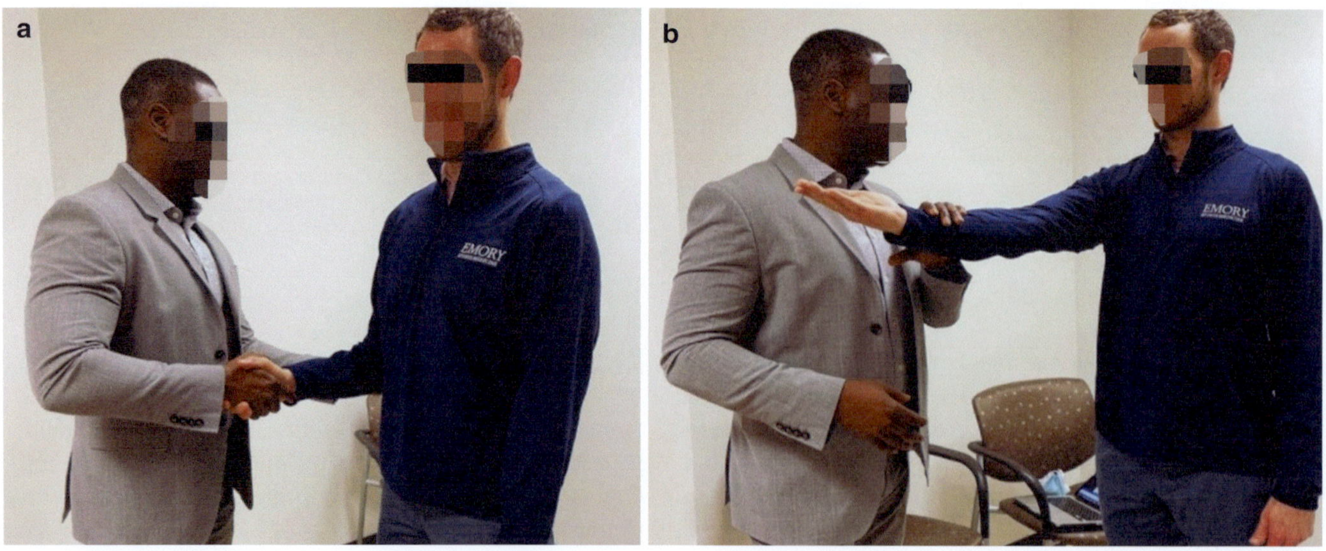

Fig. 21.3 (**a**) Yergason's test is performed by the examiner resisting forearm supination by the patient with the elbow bent. (**b**) Speed's test is performed by the examiner resisting shoulder flexion with the elbow extended and forearm supinated

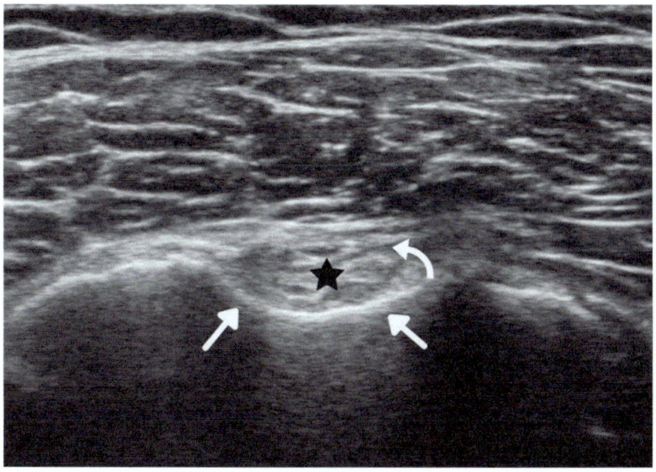

Fig. 21.4 Bicipital groove. 15–6 MHz transducer ultrasound image demonstrating the normal biceps tendon as a rounded and echogenic structure (star) within the bicipital groove (arrows). The transverse humeral ligament (curved arrow) bridges the greater and lesser tuberosity forming the bicipital sulcus into an osteofibrous tunnel

21.4 Shoulder Labral Tear (S43.43)

21.4.1 Synonyms

- SLAP (superior labral anterior-posterior) tears (S43.439)
- SLAP lesion of the right shoulder (S43.431)
- SLAP lesion of the left shoulder (S43.432)
- Humeral avulsion of the glenohumeral ligament (HAGL) (M24.419)
- Bankart lesion (M24.119)
- Bony Bankart lesion (M24.119)
- Reverse soft tissue Bankart lesion (M24.119)
- Other shoulder lesions, unspecified shoulder (M75.80)
- Other shoulder lesions, right shoulder (M75.81)
- Other shoulder lesions, left shoulder (M75.82)

21.4.2 Description

The labrum is a fibrocartilaginous ring located on the periphery of the glenoid that provides added depth, surface area, and stability to the glenohumeral joint. It serves as the primary attachment site for the shoulder capsule, glenohumeral ligaments, and biceps tendon. Injury can occur throughout all areas of the labrum, but the most studied is the superior labrum anterior posterior (SLAP) tear.

SLAP tears can occur via multiple mechanisms. An acute injury results from a forceful eccentric contraction exerted on the biceps tendon. Common mechanisms include falling on an outstretched arm, grabbing onto an object in an attempt to prevent oneself from falling, or suddenly attempting to lift a heavy object.

Chronically, SLAP tears can be seen in overhead throwing athletes. In throwing, the shoulder is forcefully abducted and externally rotated. Performing this motion with a weight in hand places stress on the labrum as shear forces from movement of the humeral head are resisted by the capsule. In addition, the anatomy of a thrower changes from adaptations over time. These athletes tend to have posterior capsular contractures with loose anterior structures and a retroverted humeral head. This increases external rotation and changes the torsional force on the bicep-labral complex, increasing the risk for tear [34].

Another common labral injury is a Bankart lesion. This occurs following an episode of anterior instability. As the humeral head moves anteriorly and inferiorly, damage occurs to the anterior-inferior labrum, glenohumeral ligaments, joint capsule, rotator cuff, and possible neurovascular structures. Ninety percent of patients less than 30 with an anterior dislocation will have a soft tissue Bankart lesion, and 5% will have an associated fracture, also known as a bony Bankart [35]. Bankart lesions lead to the risk of further instability as the labrum is no longer able to provide a suction seal with the glenoid.

21.4.3 Symptoms

The diagnosis relies on eliciting a history with the appropriate mechanism of injury in addition to the presentation listed below.

21.4.3.1 SLAP Tear

Patients complain of deep-seated sharp or dull pain localized to the posterior or posterosuperior joint line. The pain is exacerbated by abduction, overhead and behind the back arm motions, lifting, and pushing heavy objects. It can be associated with a popping, catching, or grinding sensation.

21.4.3.2 Bankart Lesions

Patients will have presented after an episode of anterior instability from being forced into excessive abduction and external rotation. The patient may not have had an overt injury, but could have had multiple episodes of instability. Often, these individuals will have their arm adducted and internally rotated for comfort, avoiding abduction and external rotation so as to not stress the injured structures. It is important to identify age at first dislocation, need for formal reduction, number of instability episodes, voluntary instability, and anticipated future sports activities [36].

21.4.4 Physical Examination

No current physical examination test is able to guarantee diagnostic value when used alone. A best-test combination is advised for the diagnosis. The following physical examination maneuvers can be used [2].

21.4.4.1 Active Compression (O'Brien) Test

This test is performed in two parts. First, the examiner asks the patient to forward flex the affected arm 90° with the elbow in full extension and arm adducted 10°–15°. The arm is then internally rotated so that the thumb is pointed downward. The examiner applies uniform downward force to the arm. The second part is performed with the arm in the same position, but the palm is supinated. A downward force is again applied. A positive test is pain with the first maneuver that is reduced or eliminated with the second maneuver. Pain should be localized as inside the glenohumeral joint itself.

21.4.4.2 Bicep Load Test

The patient is supine with the examiner adjacent to the patient on the same side as the shoulder. The examiner grasps the patient's wrist and elbow gently. The arm to be examined is elevated to 120° and externally rotated to its maximal point with the elbow at 90° flexion and the forearm in the supinated position. The patient is asked to flex the elbow while resisting elbow flexion by the examiner. The test is considered positive if the patient complains of more pain from the resisted elbow flexion regardless of the degree of pain before the elbow flexion maneuver. The test is negative if pain is not elicited by resisted elbow flexion or the preexisting pain during elevation and external rotation of the arm is unchanged or diminished (sensitivity 89%, specificity 96%) [36].

21.4.4.3 New Pain Provocation Test

The examiner is standing behind the patient with the arm in a position similar to the anterior apprehension test (abduction angle of the upper arm is maintained at 90–100 with the shoulder externally rotated). The patient is asked to resist pronation and supination of the forearm. The test is positive for a superior labral tear when pain is provoked only with the forearm in the pronated position or if pain is more severe in the pronated position than supinated (sensitivity 100%, specificity 90%) [37].

21.4.4.4 Crank Test

The arm is abducted greater than 100° in the scapular plane. The elbow is then flexed to 90°, and axial force is applied through the humerus onto the glenohumeral joint while externally and internally rotating the arm. A positive test is pain with the maneuver with or without a click or reproduction of symptoms (sensitivity 91%, specificity 93%) [38].

21.4.4.5 Anterior Slide Test

The patient is either standing or sitting with hands on the hip and thumbs pointing posteriorly. The examiner's hand is placed on top of the shoulder, and the other hand is placed behind the elbow; a forward and superior force is applied to the elbow and upper arm. The patient is asked to push back against the force. A positive test reproduces pain or a clicking sensation (sensitivity 78.4%, specificity 91.5%) [39].

21.4.4.6 Compression-Rotation Test

The patient is supine with the shoulder abducted to 90° and the elbow flexed at 90°. A compression force is applied to the humerus which is then rotated and attempts to trap the torn labrum. Pathology may be felt to catch and snap during the test (sensitivity 80%, specificity 19%) [40].

21.4.4.7 Dynamic Shear Test

With the examiner standing behind a patient, the patient's arm is placed in abduction of approximately 70°, and an anteriorly directed force is applied on the posterior shoulder. The arm is raised from 70° to 120°. In a positive test result, the patient experiences pain, particularly in the posterior and superior shoulder (sensitivity 72%, specificity 98%) [41],

21.4.5 Diagnostic Workup

21.4.5.1 X-Rays

Radiographs are often unrevealing for SLAP tears but can be used to assess other causes of shoulder pain including AC and GH joint osteoarthritis, calcific tendinopathy, osteochondral lesions, fracture, dislocation, and bony tumors. In acute shoulder dislocations causing a labral tear, radiographs can be used to exclude fracture and confirm reduction.

A *bony Bankart lesion* may be identified with a fracture of the anterior-inferior glenoid. A *Hill-Sachs defect*, or posterolateral humeral head depression fracture, may also be identified and is best appreciated on AP internal rotation view. When a Hill Sachs defect is identified, careful attention should be taken to assess for a Bankart lesion as they are up to 11 times more common in patients with a Hill-Sachs deformity [42].

21.4.5.2 MRI

MRI arthrogram is the diagnostic gold standard to evaluate the labrum (Fig. 21.5). Recently 3T MRI has also been used with similar accuracy and can avoid a contrast injection [43]. MRI to evaluate the labrum specifically is recommended in patients under the age of 35, but beyond 35, instability is often caused by rotator cuff pathology and is managed conservatively [44].

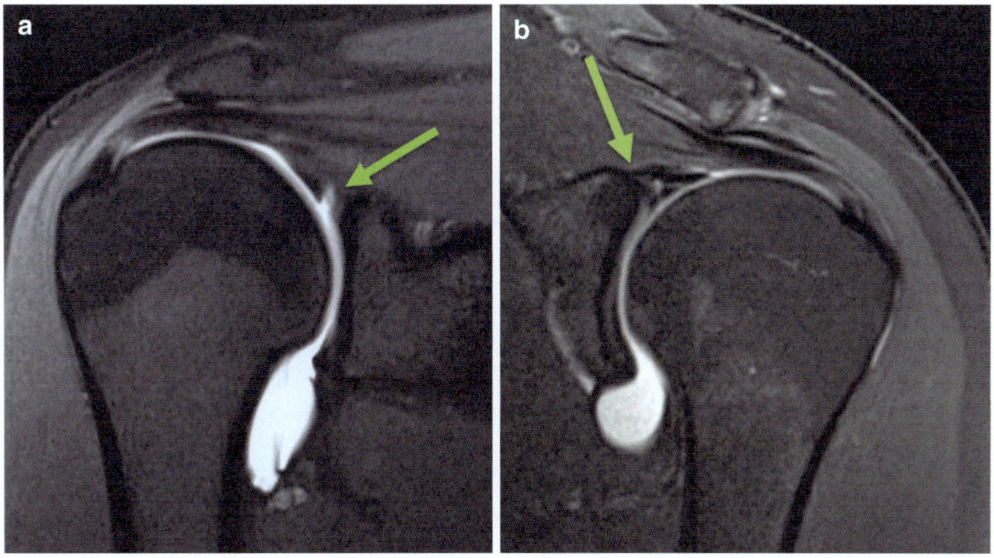

Fig. 21.5 SLAP tear. (**a**) MR arthrogram demonstrating high signal extending into the superior labrum, tracking into the labrum (**b**)

21.4.6 Treatment

21.4.6.1 SLAP Tear

Initial management includes avoiding aggravating activities such as overhead motions, abduction, and external rotation. Pain control can be achieved with the use of NSAIDs or non-opiate medications. Once the pain is controlled, a step-wise rehabilitation program should be started focusing on the following [45]:

- Improving pain-free range of motion
- Resolving posterior capsular tightness and internal rotation deficit (sleeper stretch, cross-arm adduction with forward elevation)
- Scapular stabilization
- Rotator cuff strengthening

Those that are not responsive to conservative management should be referred for surgical opinion. SLAP repair can be performed +/− biceps tenodesis and demonstrates good-excellent results in the proper patient selection [46]. Full return to play may take 3–6 months for recovery and rehabilitation. Surgical outcomes are less successful in adults over the age of 40 [47].

References

1. Rockwood CA, Williams, et al. Disorders of the AC join. In: The Shoulder, Vol. 1. Philadelphia: WB Saunders; 1998. p. 483.
2. McFarland EG. Musculoskeletal physical examination: an evidence-based approach. In: Gerard A. Malanga and Kenneth Mautner, 2nd ed. Elsevier: Amsterdam, The Netherlands; 2017. p. 31–71.
3. Chronopoulos E, Kim TK, Park HB, Ashenbrenner D, McFarland EG. Diagnostic value of physical tests for isolated chronic acromioclavicular lesions. Am J Sports Med. 2004;32(3):655–61. https://doi.org/10.1177/0363546503261723. PMID: 15090381.
4. Krill MK, Rosas S, Kwon K, Dakkak A, Nwachukwu BU, McCormick F. A concise evidence-based physical examination for diagnosis of acromioclavicular joint pathology: a systematic review. Phys Sportsmed. 2018;46(1):98–104. https://doi.org/10.1080/00913847.2018.1413920. Epub 2017 Dec 13. PMID: 29210329; PMCID: PMC6396285.
5. Kiel J, Kaiser K. Acromioclavicular Joint Injury. [Updated 2020 Aug 31]. In: StatPearls [Internet]. Treasure Island (FL): StatPearls Publishing; 2021. Available from: https://www.ncbi.nlm.nih.gov/books/NBK493188/
6. Sabeti-Aschraf M, Lemmerhofer B, Lang S, Schmidt M, Funovics PT, Ziai P, Frenzel S, Kolb A, Graf A, Schueller-Weidekamm C. Ultrasound guidance improves the accuracy of the acromioclavicular joint infiltration: a prospective randomized study. Knee Surg Sports Traumatol Arthrosc. 2011;19(2):292–5. https://doi.org/10.1007/s00167-010-1197-y. Epub 2010 Jun 19. PMID: 20563553.
7. Blankstein A, Ganel A, Givon U, Dudkiewicz I, Perry M, Diamant L, Chechik A. Ultrasonography as a diagnostic modality in acromioclavicular joint pathologies. Isr Med Assoc J. 2005;7(1):28–30. PMID: 15658142.
8. Jordan LK, Kenter K, Griffiths HL. Relationship between MRI and clinical findings in the acromioclavicular joint. Skelet Radiol. 2002;31(9):516–21. https://doi.org/10.1007/s00256-002-0530-z. Epub 2002 Jun 29. PMID: 12195504.
9. Cote MP, Wojcik KE, Gomlinski G, Mazzocca AD. Rehabilitation of acromioclavicular joint separations: operative and nonoperative considerations. Clin Sports Med. 2010;29(2):213–28, vii. https://doi.org/10.1016/j.csm.2009.12.002. PMID: 20226315.
10. Shaffer BS. Painful conditions of the acromioclavicular joint. J Am Acad Orthop Surg. 1999;7(3):176–88. https://doi.org/10.5435/00124635-199905000-00004. PMID: 10346826.
11. St Angelo JM, Fabiano SE. Adhesive capsulitis. [Updated 2020 Oct 27]. In: StatPearls [Internet]. Treasure Island (FL): StatPearls Publishing; 2020. Available from: https://www.ncbi.nlm.nih.gov/books/NBK532955/
12. Zreik NH, Malik RA, Charalambous CP. Adhesive capsulitis of the shoulder and diabetes: a meta-analysis of prevalence. Muscles Ligaments Tendons J. 2016;6(1):26–34. https://doi.org/10.11138/mltj/2016.6.1.026. Published 2016 May 19.

13. Hannafin JA, Chiaia TA. Adhesive capsulitis. A treatment approach. Clin Orthop Relat Res. 2000;372:95–109. PMID: 10738419.
14. Neviaser AS, Neviaser RJ. Adhesive capsulitis of the shoulder. J Am Acad Orthop Surg. 2011;19(9):536–42. https://doi.org/10.5435/00124635-201109000-00004. PMID: 21885699.
15. Suh CH, Yun SJ, Jin W, Lee SH, Park SY, Park JS, Ryu KN. Systematic review and meta-analysis of magnetic resonance imaging features for diagnosis of adhesive capsulitis of the shoulder. Eur Radiol. 2019;29(2):566–77. https://doi.org/10.1007/s00330-018-5604-y. Epub 2018 Jul 5. PMID: 29978436.
16. Jacobson J. Chapter 3: shoulder ultrasound. In: Jacobson J, editor. Fundamentals of musculoskeletal ultrasound. 3rd ed. Elsevier: Amsterdam, The Netherlands; 2018. p. 96–7.
17. Georgiannos D, Markopoulos G, Devetzi E, Bisbinas I. Adhesive capsulitis of the shoulder. Is there consensus regarding the treatment? A comprehensive review. Open Orthop J. 2017;11:65–76. https://doi.org/10.2174/1874325001711010065. Published 2017 Feb 28.
18. Buchbinder R, Hoving JL, Green S, Hall S, Forbes A, Nash P. Short course prednisolone for adhesive capsulitis (frozen shoulder or stiff painful shoulder): a randomised, double blind, placebo controlled trial. Ann Rheum Dis. 2004;63(11):1460–9. https://doi.org/10.1136/ard.2003.018218. PMID: 15479896; PMCID: PMC1754804.
19. Carette S, Moffet H, Tardif J, et al. Intraarticular corticosteroids, supervised physiotherapy, or a combination of the two in the treatment of adhesive capsulitis of the shoulder: a placebo-controlled trial. Arthritis Rheum. 2003;48:829–38.
20. Shah N, Lewis M. Shoulder adhesive capsulitis: systematic review of randomised trials using multiple corticosteroid injections. Br J Gen Pract. 2007;57(541):662–7. PMID: 17688763; PMCID: PMC2099674.
21. Lädermann A, Piotton S, Abrassart S, Mazzolari A, Ibrahim M, Stirling P. Hydrodilatation with corticosteroids is the most effective conservative management for frozen shoulder. Knee Surg Sports Traumatol Arthrosc. 2021. https://doi.org/10.1007/s00167-020-06390-x. Epub ahead of print. PMID: 33420809.
22. Jung TW, Lee SY, Min SK, Lee SM, Yoo JC. Does combining a suprascapular nerve block with an intra-articular corticosteroid injection have an additive effect in the treatment of adhesive capsulitis? A comparison of functional outcomes after short-term and minimum 1-year follow-up. Orthop J Sports Med. 2019. https://doi.org/10.1177/2325967119859277.
23. Berghs BM, Sole-Molins X, Bunker TD. Arthroscopic release of adhesive capsulitis. J Shoulder Elb Surg. 2004;13(2):180–5. https://doi.org/10.1016/j.jse.2003.12.004. PMID: 14997096.
24. Wilk KE, Hooks TR. The painful long head of the biceps brachii: nonoperative treatment approaches. Clin Sports Med. 2016;35(1):75–92. https://doi.org/10.1016/j.csm.2015.08.012. Epub 2015 Oct 17. PMID: 26614470.
25. Harwood MI, Smith CT. Superior labrum, anterior-posterior lesions and biceps injuries: diagnostic and treatment considerations. Prim Care. 2004;31(4):831–55. https://doi.org/10.1016/j.pop.2004.07.001. PMID: 15544823.
26. Nho SJ, Strauss EJ, Lenart BA, Provencher MT, Mazzocca AD, Verma NN, Romeo AA. Long head of the biceps tendinopathy: diagnosis and management. J Am Acad Orthop Surg. 2010;18(11):645–56. https://doi.org/10.5435/00124635-201011000-00002. PMID: 21041799.
27. Holtby R, Razmjou H. Accuracy of the Speed's and Yergason's tests in detecting biceps pathology and SLAP lesions: comparison with arthroscopic findings. Arthroscopy. 2004;20(3):231–6. https://doi.org/10.1016/j.arthro.2004.01.008. PMID: 15007311.
28. Bennett WF. Specificity of the Speed's test: arthroscopic technique for evaluating the biceps tendon at the level of the bicipital groove. Arthroscopy. 1998;14(8):789–96. https://doi.org/10.1016/s0749-8063(98)70012-x. PMID: 9848587.
29. Skendzel JG, Jacobson JA, Carpenter JE, Miller BS. Long head of biceps brachii tendon evaluation: accuracy of preoperative ultrasound. AJR Am J Roentgenol. 2011;197(4):942–8. https://doi.org/10.2214/AJR.10.5012. PMID: 21940583.
30. Malavolta EA, Assunção JH, Guglielmetti CL, de Souza FF, Gracitelli ME, Ferreira Neto AA. Accuracy of preoperative MRI in the diagnosis of disorders of the long head of the biceps tendon. Eur J Radiol. 2015;84(11):2250–4. https://doi.org/10.1016/j.ejrad.2015.07.031. Epub 2015 Jul 29. PMID: 26256048.
31. Carr RM, Shishani Y, Gobezie R. How accurate are we in detecting biceps tendinopathy? Clin Sports Med. 2016;35(1):47–55. https://doi.org/10.1016/j.csm.2015.08.002. Epub 2015 Sep 28. PMID: 26614468.
32. Hashiuchi T, Sakurai G, Morimoto M, Komei T, Takakura Y, Tanaka Y. Accuracy of the biceps tendon sheath injection: ultrasound-guided or unguided injection? A randomized controlled trial. J Shoulder Elb Surg. 2011;20(7):1069–73. https://doi.org/10.1016/j.jse.2011.04.004. Epub 2011 Jul 22. PMID: 21782470.
33. Schickendantz M, King D. Nonoperative management (including ultrasound-guided injections) of proximal biceps disorders. Clin Sports Med. 2016;35(1):57–73. https://doi.org/10.1016/j.csm.2015.08.006. Epub 2015 Sep 28. PMID: 26614469.
34. Childress MA, Beutler A. Management of chronic tendon injuries. Am Fam Physician. 2013;87(7):486–90. PMID: 23547590.
35. Kibler WB, Kuhn JE, Wilk K, Sciascia A, Moore S, Laudner K, Ellenbecker T, Thigpen C, Uhl T. The disabled throwing shoulder: spectrum of pathology-10-year update. Arthroscopy. 2013;29(1):141–161.e26. https://doi.org/10.1016/j.arthro.2012.10.009. PMID: 23276418.
36. Cleeman E, Flatow EL. Shoulder dislocations in the young patient. Orthop Clin North Am. 2000;31(2):217–29. https://doi.org/10.1016/s0030-5898(05)70142-5. PMID: 10736391.
37. Kim SH, Ha KI, Ahn JH, Kim SH, Choi HJ. Biceps load test II: a clinical test for SLAP lesions of the shoulder. Arthroscopy. 2001;17(2):160–4. https://doi.org/10.1053/jars.2001.20665. PMID: 11172245.
38. Mimori K, Muneta T, Nakagawa T, Shinomiya K. A new pain provocation test for superior labral tears of the shoulder. Am J Sports Med. 1999;27(2):137–42. https://doi.org/10.1177/03635465990270020401. PMID: 10102091.
39. Liu SH, Henry MH, Nuccion SL. A prospective evaluation of a new physical examination in predicting glenoid labral tears. Am J Sports Med. 1996;24(6):721–5. https://doi.org/10.1177/036354659602400604. PMID: 8947391.
40. Kibler WB. Specificity and sensitivity of the anterior slide test in throwing athletes with superior glenoid labral tears. Arthroscopy. 1995;11(3):296–300. https://doi.org/10.1016/0749-8063(95)90006-3. PMID: 7632305.
41. Holovacs TF, Osbahr D, Singh H, et al. The sensitivity and specificity of the physical examination to detect glenoid labrum tears. Presented at the specialty day meeting of the American Shoulder and Elbow Society, Orlando, March 2000.
42. Ben Kibler W, Sciascia AD, Hester P, Dome D, Jacobs C. Clinical utility of traditional and new tests in the diagnosis of biceps tendon injuries and superior labrum anterior and posterior lesions in the shoulder. Am J Sports Med. 2009;37(9):1840–7. https://doi.org/10.1177/0363546509332505. Epub 2009 Jun 9. PMID: 19509414.
43. Horst K, Von Harten R, Weber C, Andruszkow H, Pfeifer R, Dienstknecht T, Pape HC. Assessment of coincidence and defect sizes in Bankart and Hill-Sachs lesions after anterior shoulder dislocation: a radiological study. Br J Radiol. 2014;87(1034):20130673. https://doi.org/10.1259/bjr.20130673. PMID: 24452107; PMCID: PMC4064539.

44. Symanski JS, Subhas N, Babb J, Nicholson J, Gyftopoulos S. Diagnosis of superior labrum anterior-to-posterior tears by using MR imaging and MR arthrography: a systematic review and meta-analysis. Radiology. 2017;285(1):101–13. https://doi.org/10.1148/radiol.2017162681. Epub 2017 Jun 12. PMID: 28604236.
45. Neviaser RJ, Neviaser TJ. Recurrent instability of the shoulder after age 40. J Shoulder Elb Surg. 1995;4(6):416–8. https://doi.org/10.1016/s1058-2746(05)80032-1. PMID: 8665285.
46. Abrams GD, Safran MR. Diagnosis and management of superior labrum anterior posterior lesions in overhead athletes. Br J Sports Med. 2010;44(5):311–8. https://doi.org/10.1136/bjsm.2009.070458. PMID: 20371556.
47. Sayde WM, Cohen SB, Ciccotti MG, Dodson CC. Return to play after Type II superior labral anterior-posterior lesion repairs in athletes: a systematic review. Clin Orthop Relat Res. 2012;470(6):1595–600. https://doi.org/10.1007/s11999-012-2295-6.

Posterior Shoulder Disorders

22

Martin Weaver, Robert Bowers, and Kenneth Mautner

22.1 Rotator Cuff Tendinopathy (M67.919)

22.1.1 Synonyms

- Tendinosis of rotator cuff (M67.819)
- Rotator cuff injury (S46.099A)
- Rotator cuff strain (S46.012A)
- Unspecified rotator cuff tear/rupture (M75.100)
- Incomplete rotator cuff tear/rupture (M75.110)
- Calcific tendinitis (M65.2)
- Other shoulder lesions (M75.8)
- Injury of muscle(s) and tendon(s) of the rotator cuff of the shoulder (S46.0)
- Injury of unspecified muscle and tendon at the shoulder and upper arm level (S46.9)

22.1.2 Description

The rotator cuff is a common site for injury in patients who perform repetitive overhead activities. The structure consists of the supraspinatus, infraspinatus, teres minor, and subscapularis, which help range the shoulder joint through abduction, external rotation, adduction, and internal rotation, respectively.

Rotator cuff tendinopathies can be classified as acute or chronic. Acute injuries are more often traumatic, and the supraspinatus is the most commonly torn tendon [1]. Chronic injuries are more common [2] and may be more difficult to diagnose given the frequency of association with concomitant shoulder pathology [3]:

- Acute injury:
  - Acute injuries to the rotator cuff are often traumatic
  - Tears are classified into different subcategories with respect to location and severity [2]:
    Partial thickness versus full thickness
    Bursal sided versus articular sided versus intratendinous
- Chronic injury:
  - Repetitive motion and stress can lead to chronic inflammation of the rotator cuff tendons. This occurs particularly with activities that involve repetitive overhead use. This stress can lead to overuse injuries and such conditions as rotator cuff tendinopathy and calcific tendinitis. Chronic rotator cuff tears can progress to rotator cuff arthropathy.

22.1.3 Clinical Presentation

- Pain often described as dull and aching in anterolateral aspect of shoulder and lateral deltoid region which is exacerbated by overhead activities (shoulder abducted > 90°) [1].
- Pain may be worse after extended periods of activity and at night [1].
- Pain with sleeping on the affected side [1].
- Shoulder weakness is more apparent with full-thickness tears than partial-thickness tears [2].

22.1.4 Physical Exam

- *Painful arc test* – Patient actively abducts an internally rotated shoulder. Test is positive for impingement if it reproduces pain between approximately 70° and 120° of

M. Weaver
Department of Orthopaedics and Physical Medicine and Rehabilitation, Emory University School of Medicine, Atlanta, GA, USA
e-mail: martin.weaver@aya.yale.edu

R. Bowers (✉)
Department of Orthopaedics and Physical Medicine and Rehabilitation, Emory University School of Medicine, Atlanta, GA, USA
e-mail: rlbower@emory.edu

K. Mautner
Primary Care Sports Medicine, Emory University, Atlanta, GA, USA
e-mail: kmautne@emory.edu

© The Author(s), under exclusive license to Springer Nature Switzerland AG 2022

S. A. Mostoufi et al. (eds.), *Clinical Guide to Musculoskeletal Medicine*, https://doi.org/10.1007/978-3-030-92042-5_22

abduction that reduces after that level of elevation. This test is 67.4% sensitive and 47% specific for detecting partial-thickness rotator cuff tears. This test is 75.8% sensitive and 61.8% specific for detecting full-thickness rotator cuff tears [4].

- *Hawkins impingement test* – While patient is seated with elbow flexed to 90° and shoulder flexed to 90° examiner maximally internally rotates shoulder while stabilizing scapula. Test is positive if it reproduces pain at the anterior edge of acromion [5]. This test is 87.5% sensitive and 42.6% specific for detecting rotator cuff pathology [4].
- *Neer impingement test* – Examiner stands behind patient stabilizing scapula and passively elevates arm into full flexion with slight internal rotation and forearm pronation. Test is positive if it reproduces pain around 120° of glenohumeral flexion [5, 6]. This test is 83.3% sensitive and 50.8% specific for detecting rotator cuff pathology [4].
- *Yocum's test* – Patient adducts arm across chest with elbow flexed until hand overlies contralateral shoulder. Then, patient raises the elbow without moving the shoulder. Test is positive for impingement if pain reproduced [7]. This test is 79% sensitive and 79% specific for detecting rotator cuff pathology [4].
- *Empty can (Jobe) test* – Patient abducts shoulder to 90° and flexes shoulder to 30°. Examiner then internally rotates patient's arm until thumb points down and applies downward pressure onto arm. Test is positive for supraspinatus pathology if pain and weakness reproduced [8]. This test is 79.3% sensitive and 50% specific for detecting supraspinatus lesions [4].
- *Drop-arm rotator cuff test* – Examiner passively abducts patient's arm to 90° and then asks patient to slowly lower arm to his/her side. Test is positive for large rotator cuff tear if patient is unable to slowly lower arm and instead "drops" arm to side. This test is 10% sensitive and has a 100% positive predictive value for detecting rotator cuff tear [4].
- *Patte test* – Examiner supports patient's elbow in 90° of forward elevation in the scapular plane and asks the patient to actively rotate the arm laterally against resistance. Test is positive for tendonitis if pain is provoked, but strength is maintained or for infraspinatus tear if weakness is observed. This test is 70.5% sensitive and 90% specific for detecting infraspinatus lesions [4].
- *Lift-off test* – Patient places hand against mid-lumbar region with elbow flexed and then is asked to internally rotate the shoulder and lift the hand posteriorly off the back. Test is positive for subscapularis pathology if patient cannot lift hand off back without extending elbow or shoulder [6, 8]. This test is 35–40% sensitive and 75–79% specific for subscapularis pathology [4].
- *Bear hug test* – Patient places the hand of the affected shoulder onto the opposite shoulder and resists examiner's attempt to pull hand off shoulder. Test is positive for subscapularis pathology if the patient cannot maintain hand on shoulder. This test is 60% sensitive and 92% specific for subscapularis pathology [4].
- *Hornblower's test* – While patient is standing, examiner supports arm in 90° of abduction with elbow flexed to 90°, and then patient externally rotates arm against the examiner's resistance. Test is positive if arm cannot be externally rotated [6].

22.1.5 Diagnostic Workup

- *Plain Radiograph*
  - Chronic rotator cuff pathology may be demonstrated by cystic changes of the humeral head and sclerosis of the inferior acromion [8].
  - Complete rotator cuff tears may be diagnosed radiographically by visualization of a high-riding humeral head. Without the stabilization of the rotator cuff tendons maintaining the humeral head's seating within the glenoid, the humeral head may migrate superiorly and anteriorly approximating closer to the acromion [1].
- *Ultrasound*
  - Should be considered the first-line advanced imaging in most patients with atraumatic shoulder pain and normal plain radiographs with suspected rotator cuff disorder.
- *Magnetic Resonance Imaging*
  - MRI without intravenous contrast should be considered in patients with atraumatic shoulder pain and normal plain radiographs with suspected rotator cuff disorder and can be especially helpful for surgical planning.

22.1.6 Treatments

- *Medical Management*
- Rotator cuff tendinopathy treatment goals include resolution of pain including nightly pain and pain with overhead activities, while re-establishing range of motion and strength to regain upper extremity function and allow the patient's safe return to sport, employment, or activities of daily living.
- *Medications*
  - Acetaminophen [9]
  - NSAIDs [9]
  - Nitroglycerin:
    - While use is off-label, topical nitroglycerin has been shown to reduce pain and improve mobility, strength, and function at short-term and 6-month follow-up [10].

- *Rehabilitation*
  - Activity modifications and relative rest (no immobilization) for first 1–2 weeks [1].
  - Progressive shoulder stretching and strengthening program [1].
  - Manual therapy and exercise may be as effective as corticosteroid injection for improving pain and function in patients with chronic rotator cuff pathology [11].
- *Procedures*
  - Subacromial corticosteroid injection (Fig. 22.1) may provide short-term analgesia and functional improvement but no evidence of long-term benefit [3]. Single injection is preferred since repetitive injection may degrade integrity of rotator cuff and disadvantage subsequent repair.
  - Platelet-rich plasma (PRP) has been shown in systematic reviews to reduce pain associated with long-term rotator cuff injuries, improve healing rates and functional outcomes, and reduce pain when used adjunctively with rotator cuff repairs [12, 13].
  - Extracorporeal shock wave therapy (ESWT) has been shown to be an effective treatment strategy for calcific tendinopathy of the rotator cuff, but its use in noncalcific tendinopathy is not supported [14].
- *Surgery*
  - Surgery may be indicated for partial-thickness tears in active patients with traumatic injury, high-grade partial-thickness tears that have failed 3–6 months of nonoperative management, and full-thickness tears particularly in active patients [1].
  - Partial-thickness tears may be treated with tendon debridement and acromioplasty, arthroscopic repair, or mini-open repair [2]:
    - If tear <50% of tendon thickness, arthroscopic debridement with or without acromioplasty should be considered.
    - If tear >50% of tendon thickness, conversion or in situ repair should be considered.
  - Full-thickness tears may be treated with arthroscopic, mini-open, or open repair [15].
  - Randomized controlled trials have proven no significant difference in pain, disability, or function at a mean follow-up of 12 years between patients treated for rotator cuff tendinopathy with physical therapy alone versus combined with arthroscopic surgical decompression [16].

22.2 Subacromial Bursitis (M75.50)

22.2.1 Synonyms

- Subdeltoid bursitis
- Subacromial subdeltoid bursitis

22.2.2 Definition

A bursa is a thin, fluid-filled sac lined by synovial membrane positioned between mobile structures in the musculoskeletal system to facilitate smooth movement through expected

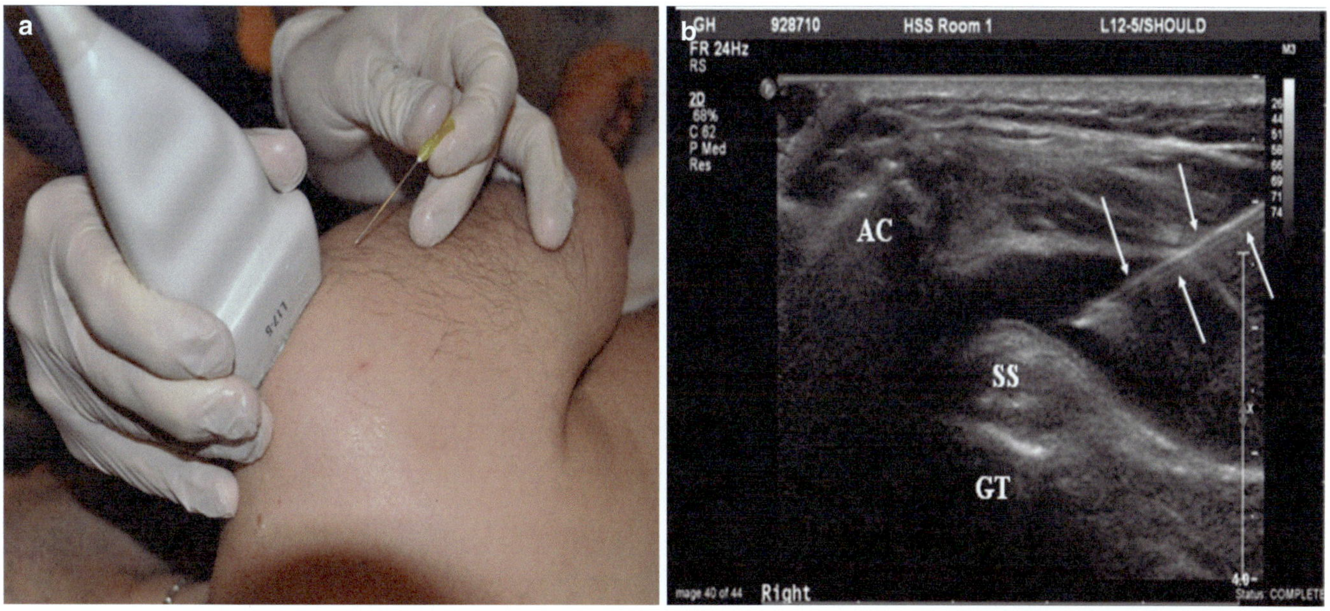

Fig. 22.1 Ultrasound-guided subacromial bursa injection. (**a**) Placement of probe and needle. (**b**) Ultrasound-guided in-plane injection approach of subacromial bursa. AC acromion, SS supraspinatus, GT greater tuberosity of humerus; arrows, needle. (Courtesy of Malanga and Mautner [68])

range of motion. Subacromial bursitis refers to inflammation of the bursa that lies between the bony acromion and the underlying supraspinatus tendon.

Bursitis can be caused by:

- Direct trauma
- Prolonged pressure
- Overuse or repetitive overhead activity
- Crystalline arthropathy
- Inflammatory arthropathy
- Infection

22.2.3 Clinical Presentation

- Pain present at rest and exacerbated by use.
- Pain refers to insertion of deltoid muscle about 10 cm distally along the lateral portion of the upper arm.
- Pain may impair sleep-related to side-lying applying local pressure to structure.
- Adhesive capsulitis may result from persistent immobility.

22.2.4 Physical Exam

- *Painful arc test* – This test is 70.6% sensitive and 46.9% specific for detecting subacromial bursitis [4].
- *Hawkins impingement test* – This test is 91.7% sensitive and 44.3% specific for detecting subacromial bursitis [4].
- *Neer impingement test* – This test is 75–85.7% sensitive and 47.5–49.2% specific for detecting subacromial bursitis [4].
- *Yocum's test*
- *Empty can (Jobe) test*
- *Drop-arm rotator cuff test*
- *Lift-off test*
- *Hornblower's test*

22.2.5 Diagnostic Workup

- *Plain Radiograph*
  - X-rays may reveal concomitant pathology such as acromion type predisposing to shoulder impingement syndrome or high-riding humeral head related to rotator cuff tear.
- *Ultrasound*
  - May reveal bursal thickening or increased fluid within the bursa sac representing bursitis
  - May also be helpful in determining if concomitant rotator cuff tear is involved
- *Magnetic Resonance Imaging*
  - MRI without intravenous contrast should be considered in patients with atraumatic shoulder pain and normal plain radiographs with suspected rotator cuff disorder.

22.2.6 Treatment

- *Medical/Rehabilitation Management*
- Subacromial bursitis treatment goals include resolution of pain including nightly pain and pain with overhead activities while re-establishing range of motion and strength to regain upper extremity function and allow the patient's safe return to sport, employment, or activities of daily living:
  - Medications: Nonsteroidal anti-inflammatory drugs (NSAIDs)
  - Physical therapy: Maintenance and/or restoration of range of motion
- *Procedures*
  - Subacromial corticosteroid injection (Fig. 22.2):
    Systematic review concluded patients may benefit from up to three injections in a 12-week period [17].
    Some data even suggests the frequency of steroid injections for subacromial bursitis does not impose the risk of developing rotator cuff tears [18].
    Limited data suggests ultrasound-guided injections may be more effective for treating subacromial bursitis than landmark-guided [19, 20], but these findings were not validated in a large systematic review [21].
- *Surgery*
  - *Subacromial bursectomy*: A surgical procedure designed to remove an inflamed pathologic bursa, thereby improving restricted movement of the rotator cuff tendons below. Randomized controlled trials suggest that bursectomy alone may be as effective as bursectomy followed by acromioplasty for improving pain and function up to 12 years in patients with primary subacromial impingement [22, 23].

22.3 Shoulder Impingement Syndrome (M75.40)

22.3.1 Synonyms

- Internal impingement of shoulder (M75.40)
- Bursitis of shoulder (M75.50)
- Other shoulder lesions (M75.80)

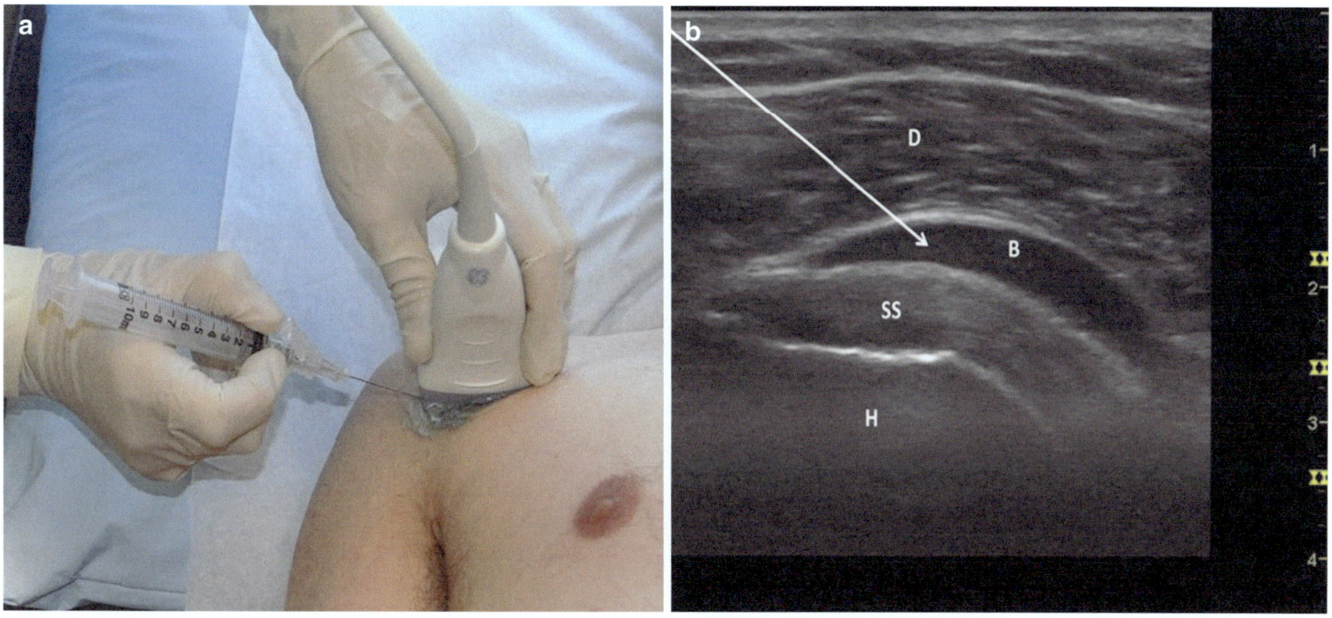

Fig. 22.2 Ultrasound-guided subcoracoid injection approach. (**a**) Placement of probe and needle. (**b**) Ultrasound of subcoracoid bursa demonstrating in-plane injection approach. D deltoid, B subcoracoid bursa, SS subscapularis, H humerus, arrow, needle trajectory. (Courtesy of Malanga and Mautner [68])

22.3.2 Definition

Impingement syndrome is common in patients who participate in sports or work requiring repetitive overhead or horizontal upper extremity activities. The etiology is typically multifactorial due to a combination of both functional and structural abnormalities such as weak rotator cuff stabilizers or acromial spurring, respectively.

Impingement syndrome is described as shoulder pain, weakness, and/or limited range of motion as a result of structural or functional changes of the shoulder joint.

The syndrome can be classified into two types [24, 25]:

- External shoulder impingement:
  - Subacromial impingement – The most common type due to compression of supraspinatus tendon, long head of biceps tendon, biceps interval, and/or subacromial bursa between coracoacromial arch and humeral head
  - Subcoracoid impingement – Compression of subscapularis tendon and subcoracoid bursa between coracoid process and humeral head
- Internal shoulder impingement:
  - Posterosuperior impingement – Compression of supraspinatus tendon, infraspinatus tendon, adjacent capsule, and/or bursa between the humeral head and posterosuperior glenoid labrum
  - Anterosuperior impingement – Compression of supraspinatus tendon, subscapularis tendon, long head of biceps tendon, coracohumeral ligament, and/or superior glenohumeral ligament between the humeral head and anterosuperior glenoid labrum

22.3.3 Clinical Presentation

- Subacromial Impingement
  - Patients typically experience anterolateral shoulder pain exacerbated by overhead activities or when rolling on symptomatic shoulder while sleeping.
- Subcoracoid Impingement
  - Patients typically experience anterior shoulder pain and coracoid tenderness exacerbated by repeated shoulder flexion and internal rotation.
- Posterosuperior Impingement
  - Patients typically experience posterior shoulder pain particularly in overhead athletes or occupations, exacerbated by overhead throwing, lifting, and hitting.
- Anterosuperior Impingement
  - Patients typically experience anterior shoulder pain exacerbated by shoulder flexion, adduction, and internal rotation.

22.3.4 Physical Exam

- *Painful arc test*
- *Hawkins impingement test*
- *Neer impingement test*
- *Yocum's test*
- *Empty can (Jobe) test*
- *Drop-arm rotator cuff test*
- *Lift-off test*
- *Hornblower's test*

- *Scapular assistance test* – The examiner stabilizes the upper medial border of the scapula and rotates the inferomedial border to assist the lower trapezius, while the patient actively abducts or adducts the arm. This test is positive for lower trapezius weakness as a cause of impingement if the examiner's support relieves pain, clicking, or weakness. This test is 100% sensitive and 33% specific for detecting lower trapezius weakness [4].

22.3.5 Diagnostic Workup

- *Plain Radiographs*
  - Plain radiographs may suggest predisposition to shoulder impingement syndrome based on anatomical variation of the acromion type [26]:
    1. Flat
    2. Curved – Parallel to the humeral head with concave undersurface, the most common type
    3. Hooked – The most anterior portion of the acromion has hooked shape; associated with increased incidence of shoulder impingement.
    4. Convex – Convex undersurface near the distal end of the acromion; no correlation with impingement syndrome.
- *Ultrasound*
  - Ultrasound is not needed to make a diagnosis of shoulder impingement syndrome but can be useful in challenging cases and to rule out other coinciding pathologies such as rotator cuff tears. Ultrasound also has the advantage of being able to view impingement dynamically to obtain more details on the pathologic structures.
- *Magnetic Resonance Imaging*
  - MRI is not needed to make a diagnosis of shoulder impingement syndrome but may be useful in challenging cases and to rule out other coinciding pathologies such as rotator cuff tears, abnormalities of supraspinatus outlet, or labral pathology.

22.3.6 Treatments

- *Medical Management*
- Shoulder impingement syndrome treatment goals include reducing pain and inflammation, improving range of motion, strengthening rotator cuff muscles, optimizing biomechanics, and facilitating return to activity. Conservative treatment with limiting painful activities, especially overhead, icing/heating, and analgesics are first-line treatments.
- *Medications*: The following medications can be prescribed:
  - Acetaminophen
  - NSAIDs
  - PO corticosteroids – may be considered in cases where alternatives are contraindicated (e.g., renal disease and liver disease)
- *Rehabilitation*
  - Rotator cuff strengthening
  - Scapular stabilization
  - Manual therapy
  - Kinesio taping
  - Acupuncture
  - Postoperative rehabilitation protocols described below as part of surgical care
- *Procedures*
  - *Subacromial corticosteroid injection* (Fig. 22.2): Injections have shown moderate evidence to decrease pain and improve range of motion and function short term, but multiple injections may compromise integrity of rotator cuff [3].
  - *Subcoracoid corticosteroid injection*
- *Surgery*
  - Surgery is reserved for refractory cases that do not respond to conservative measures outlined above.
  - Factors associated with poor outcomes following conservative management include the presence of rotator cuff tear >1 cm, pretreatment symptoms >1 year, and significant functional impairment at initial presentation [28]:
    - *Subacromial decompression:* A surgical procedure designed to release the coracoacromial ligament and shave away some undersurface of the acromion and/or osteophytes, thereby increasing the subacromial space to allow smooth movement of the rotator cuff tendons below. Systematic reviews have shown no difference between placebo and subacromial decompression surgery in improving shoulder pain, function, or quality of life at 1–2 years in adults with subacromial pain. They also suggest that improvements following subacromial decompression compared to exercise therapy may not be clinically significant [29]. A randomized controlled trial of arthroscopic subacromial decompression for subacromial shoulder pain also did not conclude improvement in pain or function [30].
    - *Subacromial bursectomy:* A surgical procedure designed to remove an inflamed pathologic bursa, thereby improving restricted movement of the rotator cuff tendons below. Randomized controlled trials suggest that bursectomy alone may be as effective as bursectomy followed by acromioplasty

for improving pain and function up to 12 years in patients with primary subacromial impingement [22, 23].

- Postoperative rehabilitation protocols may include [27]:
  1. No overhead activity for initial 6 weeks following surgery and caution with overhead activities up to 12 weeks following surgery.
  2. *Active assisted range of motion exercises immediately following surgery.*
  3. *Active range of motion and isotonic submaximal strengthening exercises at 2 weeks.*
  4. *Progression to eccentric, concentric, and isokinetic exercises at 6–12 weeks.*

22.4 Suprascapular Nerve Entrapment (G56.80)

22.4.1 Synonyms

- Other specified mononeuropathies of unspecified upper limb (G56.80)
- Suprascapular nerve compression (G56.80)
- Nerve entrapment syndrome, suprascapular (G56.80)
- Compression of suprascapular nerve (G56.80)
- Lesion of suprascapular nerve (G58.8)
- Suprascapular nerve injury (S44.8X9A)

22.4.2 Definition

The suprascapular nerve originates from the upper trunk of the brachial plexus and carries sensory fibers from the glenohumeral and acromioclavicular joints as well as motor fibers to the supraspinatus and infraspinatus muscles. Injuries occur most often due to entrapment at the suprascapular notch compared to at the spinoglenoid notch [31].

While direct trauma resulting from a football tackle, fall, motor vehicle accident, or rotator cuff tear is a common cause of injury, the nerve can also be injured during stretching, traction, or repetitive movements as seen in weightlifters, volleyball players, baseball players, and gymnasts [31–35]. Rarely, the suprascapular nerve can be compressed by ganglion cysts or tumors [36].

22.4.3 Clinical Presentation

- The patient typically presents with chronic and dull pain at the superior and posterolateral aspect of the shoulder often radiating to the neck or lateral arm [37].
- The patient may also complain of weakness or loss of function in either the infraspinatus alone (weak external rotation) if entrapped at the spinoglenoid notch or both infraspinatus and supraspinatus (weak external rotation and shoulder abduction between 90° and 180°) if entrapped at thte suprascapular notch [38].

22.4.4 Physical Exam

- *Suprascapular nerve stretch test* – The clinician stands behind the patient gently holding the head away and rotated laterally from the affected shoulder while retracting the affected shoulder with the other hand (Fig. 22.3). The test is positive if it reproduces posterior shoulder pain [37].
- *Crossed-body adduction test* – The patient adducts a forward flexed arm across the body which can be accentuated by external rotation of the humerus placing greater tension on the suprascapular nerve and increasing impingement of the suprascapular nerve on the medial border of the scapula at the spinoglenoid notch. This test is positive if it increases pain [39].

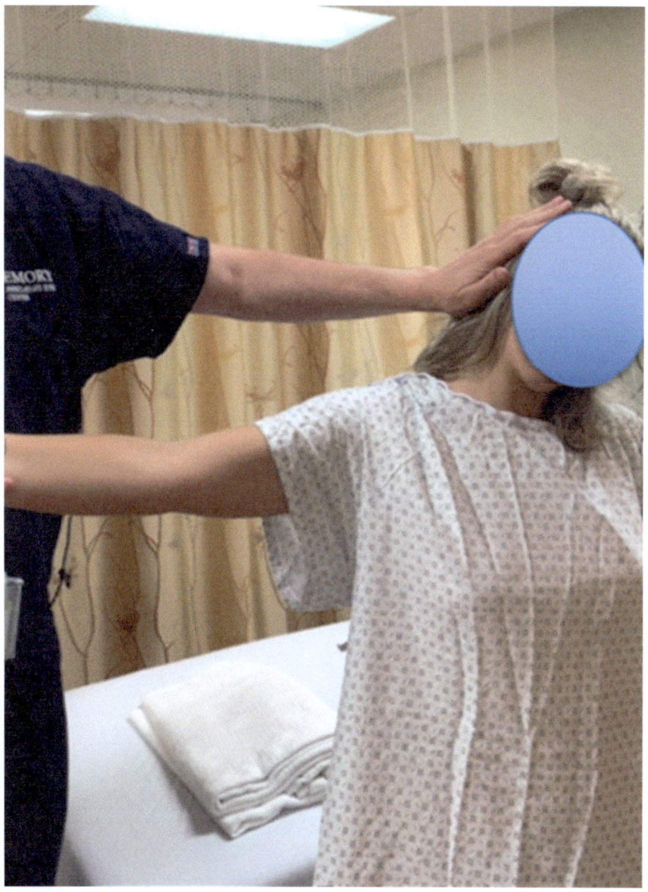

Fig. 22.3 Suprascapular nerve stretch test

22.4.5 Diagnostic Workup

- *Plain Radiographs*
  - In addition to standard shoulder X-ray views, the Stryker notch view should be included [37].
- *Ultrasound*
  - Ultrasound is not needed to make the diagnosis of suprascapular nerve entrapment but may be useful in challenging cases to examine the nerve for evidence of pathology in the form of enlargement/thickening or surrounding cyst/mass.
- *Magnetic Resonance Imaging*
  - MRI is recommended after a period of conservative treatment to rule out coinciding pathology such as supraspinatus and infraspinatus atrophy, labral or rotator cuff pathology, or anatomic lesions such as soft tissue masses or ganglion cysts around the shoulder. If no anatomic lesion is present, this may continue with non-operative treatment for 6–12 months [37, 38].
- *Nerve Conduction Study/Electromyography*
  - NCS/EMG is considered the gold standard in diagnosis of suspected suprascapular nerve entrapment and evaluated for denervation findings such as increased latency, fibrillations, and positive sharp waves. However, EMG is frequently normal [37].

22.4.6 Treatments

- *Medical Management*
- Initial management of suprascapular nerve injury is typically conservative with rest, protection, avoiding heavy lifting, and repetitive overhead activities [38].
- *Medications*
  - NSAIDs
  - Tricyclic antidepressants
  - Selective serotonin reuptake inhibitors
  - Anticonvulsants
- *Rehabilitation*
  - Shoulder range of motion
  - Strengthen compensatory muscles of the shoulder
  - Scapular stabilization
- *Procedures*
  - No therapeutic intervention is universally accepted as the most effective treatment for suprascapular nerve entrapment, but several options are available:
    - Suprascapular notch injection (Fig. 22.4)
    - Spinoglenoid notch injection
- *Surgery*
  - Surgeries listed below are reserved for refractory cases that do not respond to conservative measures outlined above [40–42]:
    - Surgical release of the transverse scapular ligament
    - Arthroscopic suprascapular nerve decompression
  - Surgical excision is indicated for cyst or tumor removal.

22.5 Quadrilateral Space Syndrome (S44.31, S44.32)

22.5.1 Synonyms

- Axillary nerve injury (S44.30XA)
- Axillary nerve palsy (G54.0)

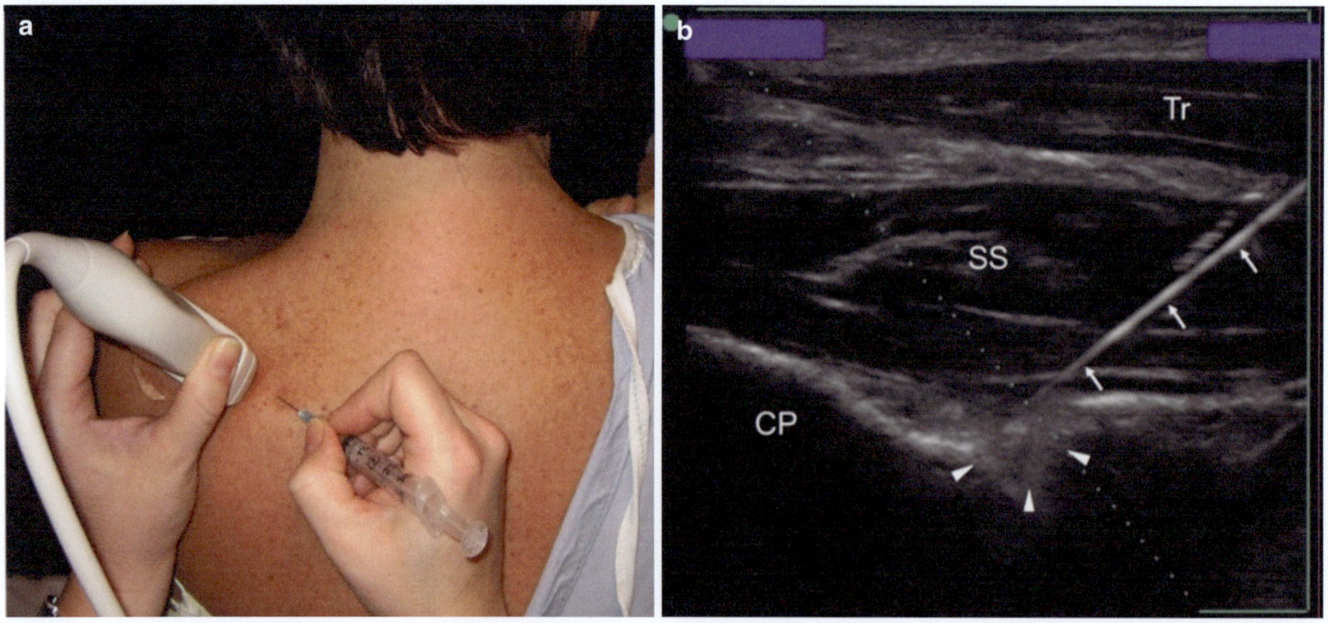

Fig. 22.4 Ultrasound-guided suprascapular nerve block. (**a**) Placement of probe and needle. (**b**) Ultrasound-guided in-plane approach injection of suprascapular notch. Tr trapezius, SS supraspinatus, CP coracoid process, arrows, needle, arrowheads, suprascapular nerve. (Courtesy of Malanga and Mautner [68])

- Axillary nerve compression (G54.0)
- Neuropathy, axillary nerve (G56.90)
- Disorder of axillary nerve (G54.0)
- Compression of axillary nerve (G54.0)

22.5.2 Definition

Often a diagnosis of exclusion and entrapment of the axillary nerve can occur as it travels through the quadrilateral space formed by the teres minor superiorly, humerus laterally, long head of triceps medially, and teres major inferiorly [43, 44].

22.5.3 Clinical Presentation

- Diffuse shoulder pain, fasciculations, weakness, and paresthesias in a non-dermatomal distribution.
- Point tenderness over the quadrilateral space.
- Vascular manifestations can include pain, pallor, absent pulses, cyanosis, digital ischemia, and cold intolerance [45].

22.5.4 Physical Exam

- Positioning the shoulder in flexion, abduction, and external rotation for several minutes reproduces symptoms [45].

22.5.5 Diagnostic Workup

- *Ultrasound*
  - Placing the probe slightly below the posterior glenohumeral joint and parallel to the long axis of the humeral shaft, visualization of the posterior circumflex humeral artery around the axillary nerve at the quadrilateral space can be achieved. This vessel may appear dilated, and the surrounding deltoid and teres minor muscle may demonstrate atrophic changes such as thinning and hyperechogenicity [46].
- *Magnetic Resonance Imaging*
  - Typically, MRI is the initial imaging choice but is often normal if it does not demonstrate focal fatty atrophy of teres minor and/or deltoid muscles [47] (Fig. 22.5).
  - May visualize associated mass displacing the neurovascular bundle.
- *Arteriography*
  - May reveal decreased outflow due to compression of posterior humeral circumflex artery with the arm in abduction and external rotation [45].
- *Nerve conduction study/electromyography*
  - Evaluate for denervation findings, such as increased latency, fibrillations, and positive sharp waves, of the teres minor and deltoid muscles which are supplied by the axillary nerve.

22.5.6 Treatments

- *Medical Management*
  - First-line treatment for quadrilateral space syndrome is nonoperative and may include activity modification, physical therapy, medications, and ultrasound-guided perineural steroid injections [46].
  - Recovery for patients with incomplete injury usually begins within 3–4 months [48, 49].
  - Medications: NSAIDs
- *Rehabilitation*
  - Therapeutic massage
  - Transverse friction
    - Active release soft tissue massage
    - Active shoulder range of motion
  - Scapular stabilization

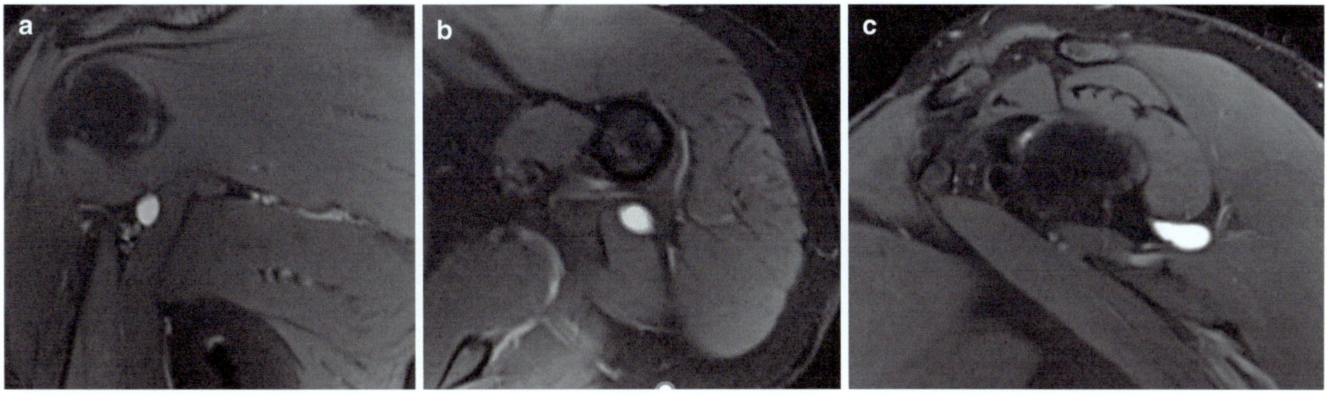

Fig. 22.5 Coronal (**a**), axial (**b**), and sagittal (**c**) T1-weighted magnetic resonance images of cyst in quadrilateral space

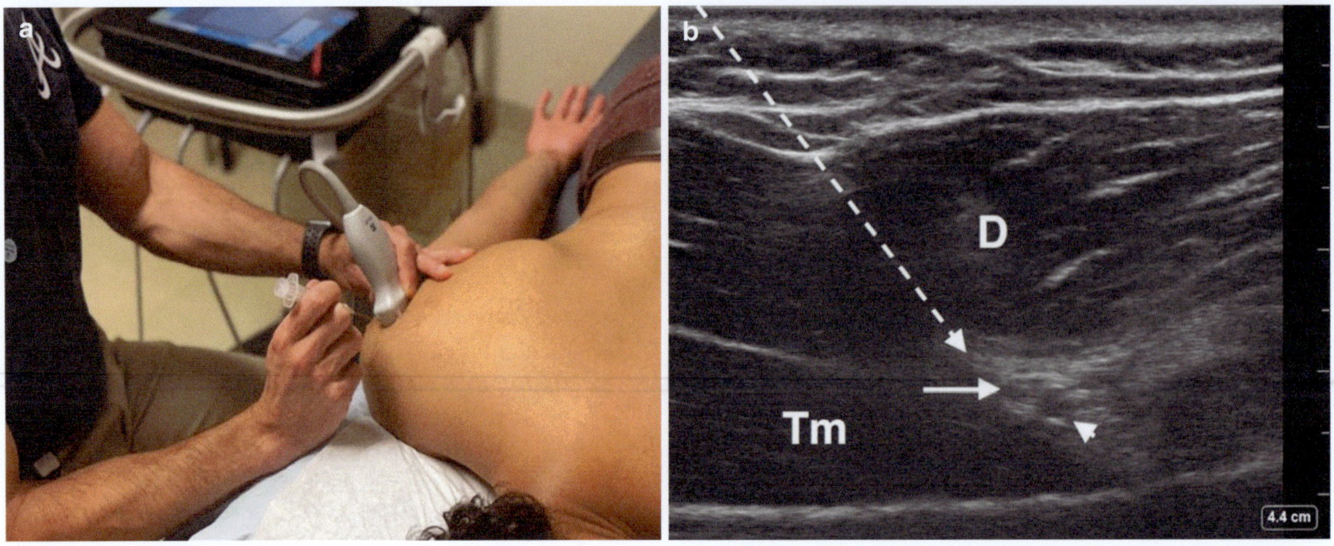

Fig. 22.6 Ultrasound-guided axillary nerve block approach. (**a**) Placement of probe and needle. (**b**) Ultrasound of quadrilateral space demonstrating in-plane injection approach. D deltoid, Tm teres minor, arrow, axillary nerve; dashed arrow, in-plane needle approach; arrowhead, posterior circumflex humeral artery

  - Posterior rotator cuff stretching
- *Procedures*
  - *Ultrasound-guided axillary nerve block* has been shown to decrease pain [46] (Fig. 22.6).
  - *Pulsed radiofrequency neuromodulation of the axillary nerve* [46].
- *Surgery*

  Surgical decompression: Surgery is reserved for refractory cases that do not respond to ≥6 months of conservative measures as outlined above or patients with recurrent shoulder dislocations [48, 49].

In surgical decompression, axillary nerve is dissected and palpated along with the posterior humeral circumflex artery with the arm in external rotation and abduction to confirm the nerve is decompressed and freely gliding and the artery maintains a strong pulse. Investigation for fibrous bands around neurovasculature is performed to identify any regions of structural compression. Postoperatively, the patient is placed in arm sling for comfort and immediately referred to physical therapy to prevent adhesions [45]. A case series suggests that four female athletes experienced return to full activity without pain or limitation in overhead function by 12 weeks postoperatively [50].

22.6 Winged Scapula (M95.8)

22.6.1 Synonyms

- Injury of unspecified nerve at the shoulder and upper arm level, unspecified arm, initial encounter (S44.90XA)
- Other specified acquired deformities of unspecified limb (M21.80)
- Other specified acquired deformities of musculoskeletal system (M95.8)

22.6.2 Definition

- The long thoracic nerve originates from the fifth, sixth, and seventh cervical nerve roots and carries motor fibers to the serratus anterior muscle. The main etiologies of long thoracic nerve injury are neuralgic amyotrophy; direct trauma to the shoulder or lateral chest wall seen in football players or invasive procedures such as first rib resections, mastectomies with axillary node dissections, scalenectomies, chest tube insertions, or infraclavicular plexus anesthesia; compression such as by heavy backpacks; traction seen postoperatively due to positioning during anesthesia; or stretch from repetitive activities while the arm is overhead and outstretched [31, 51–53]. Injury to the long thoracic nerve can lead to weakness of the serratus anterior, thereby producing a medially winged scapula (Fig. 22.7).
- The spinal accessory nerve is the tenth cranial nerve derived from the upper cervical nerve roots and carries motor fibers to the sternocleidomastoid and trapezius muscle. The main etiologies of isolated spinal accessory neuropathy include biopsy of the cervical lymph nodes in the posterior triangle, local surgery such as radical neck dissection, or blunt injuries due to sports or combat [54]. Injury to the spinal accessory nerve can lead to weakness of the trapezius, thereby producing a laterally winged scapula (Fig. 22.8).

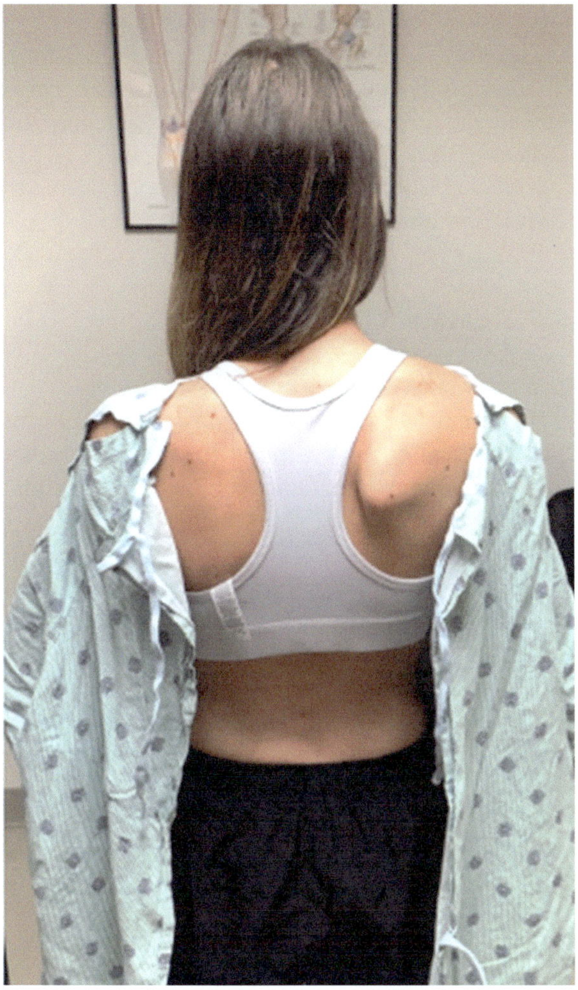

Fig. 22.7 Winged scapula medially due to serratus anterior weakness

- Winging of the scapula can also be seen due to dorsal scapular neuropathies causing rhomboid weakness, cervical radiculopathies, or primary muscle diseases.

22.6.3 Clinical Presentation

Classically, winged scapula as a result of neuralgic amyotrophy is characterized by prior onset of severe pain followed by patchy weakness in the distribution of a trunk or cord of the brachial plexus. However some cases demonstrate isolated long thoracic nerve involvement [31, 53].

Features of the winged scapula as a result of spinal accessory neuropathy include drooping or depression of the affected shoulder and weakness in abduction [54, 55]. Proximal lesions are associated with atrophy and weakness of the sternocleidomastoid, while distal lesions are associated with atrophy and weakness of the trapezius. Pain may also present due to traction on brachial plexus [54].

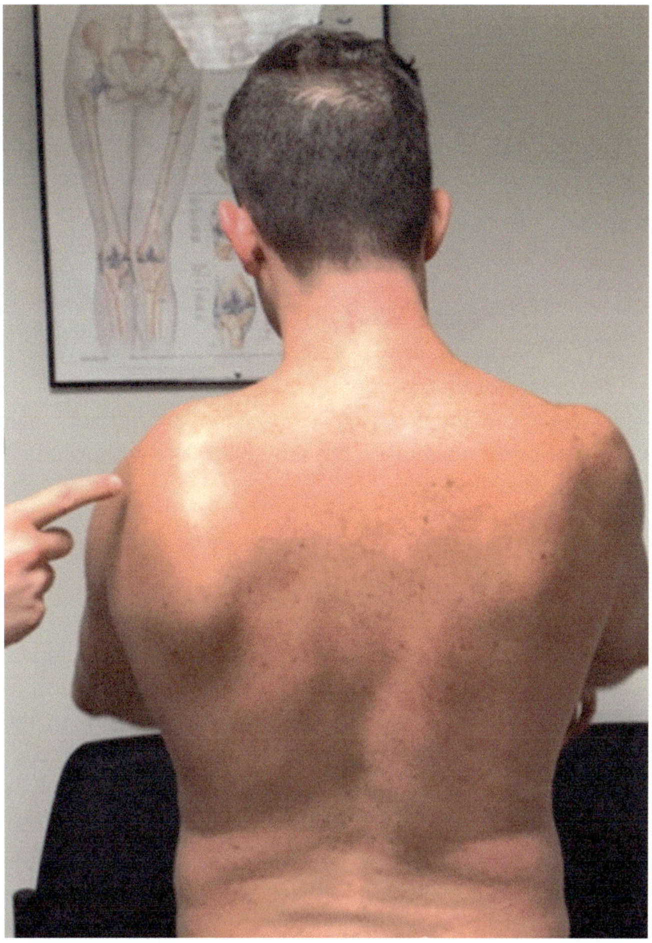

Fig. 22.8 Winged scapula laterally due to trapezius weakness

22.6.4 Physical Exam

- *Inspection* – Scapular winging may be observed posteriorly and can be accentuated by muscle activation in varied degrees of the affected shoulder flexion and abduction and scapular retraction and protraction [4].
- *Wall pushup* – The clinician observes the patient from behind as he/she presses his/her outstretched arms against a wall. This test is positive if the involved scapula projects medially or laterally from the thorax.
- *Lateral scapular slide test* – The patient relaxes arms at side (position 1) the examiner measures the distance between the nearest spinous process and the inferomedial border of the scapula. The patient then moves the hands onto the hips with fingers anterior and thumb posterior in approximately 10° of shoulder extension (position 2), and the examiner measures the same distance. The patient then abducts arms to about 90° with maximal internal rotation of the glenohumeral joint, and the examiner again measures the same distance. This is repeated for the unaffected side. The test is positive if there is at least 1–1.5 cm

difference between sides, depending on cited literature. The sensitivities and specificities of this test for pathology were low regardless of position measured [4].

- *Isometric pinch test* – The patient retracts the scapula pinching together posteriorly. This test is positive for scapular muscle weakness if burning pain is experienced after isometric hold for 15–20 s [4].
- *Nerve Conduction Study/Electromyography*
  - Currently the only definitive diagnostic test to determine specific muscle involvement indicated by resting denervation potentials, decreased motor unit recruitment, and polyphasic motor unit potentials during volitional activity in either the serratus anterior, trapezius, or rhomboid muscle [56].

22.6.5 Diagnostic Workup

- *Plain Radiographs*
  - X-rays of the neck, chest, shoulder, and thoracic inlet are rarely diagnostic but may help rule out structural abnormalities [56].
- *Ultrasound*
  - While the patient is seated upright, four views can be scanned to evaluate the scapula-stabilizing muscles for atrophy [57].
    - View 1 visualizes the serratus anterior and latissimus dorsi as the patient forward flexes their arm to 90° with support. To obtain a coronal view of the latissimus dorsi wedged between the serratus anterior and subcutaneous tissue, the transducer is placed on posterior-axillary line with the superior border positioned perpendicular to a horizontal line made with the inferior scapular angle [57].
    - View 2 visualizes the upper trapezius, levator scapulae, and supraspinatus. To obtain an oblique coronal view, the transducer is placed on the shoulder with the center positioned over the superior angle of the scapula which separates the levator scapula medially, supraspinatus laterally, and upper trapezius superficially [57].
    - View 3 visualizes the middle trapezius, rhomboids, and erector spinae. To obtain an axial view of the middle trapezius superficially, the rhomboids deep to it, and the erector spinae deeper still, the transducer is placed over the mid-back lateral to the midline and inferior to the spine of the scapula [57].
    - View 4 visualizes the infraspinatus and deltoid. To obtain this view, the sonographer may transition from View 3 by translating the probe laterally sliding over the medial edge of the scapula resting just inferior to the spine of the scapula at which point the trapezius will move out of view as the infraspinatus moves into view and further translation laterally will bring the deltoid into view superficially [57].
- *Magnetic Resonance Imaging*
  - MRI is rarely needed but may help rule out other diagnoses such as neurofibromatous-related injury, disk disease and radiculopathy, and mass lesions [56].

22.6.6 Treatment

- *Medical Management*
  - While management and prognosis vary according to mechanism of injury, initial treatment with conservative therapy including activity modifications to avoid precipitating factors and physical therapy is usually appropriate [56]. Neuralgic amyotrophy symptoms typically recover slowly over 1–3 years, while long thoracic nerve injuries caused by carrying or repetitive activity may recover within 6–24 months as they are usually incomplete injuries [56]. However, traumatic long thoracic nerve injuries are typically severe, and recovery may be limited or nonexistent [56]:
  - *Medications:* Muscle relaxants and NSAIDs
  - Winger's brace: Designed to manually press the scapula against the posterior thoracic wall and prevent stretching of paralyzed muscle [58].
- *Rehabilitation*
  - Range of motion exercises performed supine may prevent winging by compressing the scapula against the thorax [56].
  - Strengthening of adjacent muscle groups to compensate for cross-sectional area and direction of pull of the affected muscle [56].
- *Procedures*
  - *Perineural Corticosteroid Injection*: Injections around the affected nerves (e.g., long thoracic, spinal accessory, dorsal scapular) may decrease pain related to neuritis.
- *Surgery*
  - Surgery is reserved for refractory cases that do not respond to conservative measures outlined above as functional limitation resulting from isolated weakness of the serratus anterior can be reasonably mild and therefore not necessitate surgical management.
  - However, winged scapula due to spinal accessory nerve injury in comparison is not as responsive to conservative measures [56]:
    - Muscle transfers and fascial grafts – e.g., transfer of the sternal head of the pectoralis major muscle [31, 59, 60] or Eden-Lange muscle transfer procedure [56].

- Nerve transfer – e.g., thoracodorsal nerve or medial pectoral nerve [61, 62].

22.7 Scapulothoracic Bursopathy (M75.50)

22.7.1 Synonyms

- Scapulothoracic syndrome (G56.80)
- Other shoulder lesions, unspecified shoulder (M75.80)
- Bursitis of unspecified shoulder (M75.50)

22.7.2 Definition

Scapulothoracic bursitis arises from friction created by scapular range of motion between the scapula at the superior-medial angle and the anatomically adjacent ribs.

22.7.3 Clinical Presentation

Pain and popping aggravated by repetitive overhead movements associated with localized tenderness and palpable or audible crepitus.

22.7.4 Physical Exam [63]

Visual inspection of the scapula may demonstrate fullness, winging, or dyskinesis.

Palpation and auscultation while fully ranging the affected shoulder may demonstrate periscapular crepitus.

22.7.5 Diagnostic Workup [63]

- *Plain Radiographs*
  - X-rays including anteroposterior view and tangential view (Y view) may identify osseous abnormalities resulting in mechanical disruption of scapulothoracic range of motion.
- *Magnetic Resonance Imaging*
  - An effusion, soft tissue lesion, or hemorrhage into the area may be seen on MRI.
- *Computed Tomography*
  - May be helpful if radiographic studies are negative and the clinician suspects bony abnormality.
- *Nerve Conduction Study/Electromyography*
  - NCS/EMG of the shoulder girdle musculature should be considered as focal muscle weakness may contribute to idiopathic cases of scapulothoracic bursitis or crepitus.

22.7.6 Treatments

- *Medical Management*
  - As most cases spontaneously resolve, initial conservative management with physical therapy, medications (NSAIDS), and sometimes injections are indicated [64].
- *Rehabilitation* [63]
  - Postural training
  - Scapular strengthening
- *Procedures*
  - Scapulothoracic bursa ultrasound-guided corticosteroid injection
- *Surgery*
  - Surgery resection of the bursa and a portion of the scapula may provide relief but is reserved for refractory cases that do not respond to conservative measures outlined above [65, 66].

22.8 Snapping Scapula (M24.819)

22.8.1 Synonyms

- Other specified disorders of bone, shoulder (M89.8X1)
- Other specified acquired deformities of unspecified limb (M21.80)
- Other specified acquired deformities of musculoskeletal system (M95.8)

22.8.2 Definition

Snapping scapula results from a disruption of normal mechanics of the scapulothoracic articulation due to bursitis, muscle abnormality, and bony or soft tissue abnormalities such as excessive forward curvature of the superomedial border of the scapula and is especially common in the young, active patients [67].

22.8.3 Clinical Presentation

Audible and palpable crepitus near the superomedial border of the scapula is provoked by overhead and throwing activities.

22.8.4 Physical Exam [63]

- Visual inspection of the scapula may demonstrate fullness, winging, or dyskinesis.
- Palpation and auscultation while fully ranging the affected shoulder may demonstrate periscapular crepitus.

22.8.5 Diagnostic Workup

- *Plain Radiographs*
  - X-rays including anteroposterior view and tangential view (Y view) may identify osseous abnormalities resulting in mechanical disruption of scapulothoracic range of motion.
- *Magnetic Resonance Imaging*
  - An effusion, soft tissue lesion, or hemorrhage into the area may be seen on MRI.
- *Nerve Conduction Study/Electromyography*
  - NCS/EMG of the shoulder girdle musculature should be considered as focal muscle weakness may contribute to idiopathic cases of scapulothoracic bursitis or crepitus.

22.8.6 Treatments

- *Medical Management*
  - Conservative management with physical therapy and anti-inflammatory medications (NSAIDS) is considered first-line treatment and is curative in most cases.
- *Physical Therapy*
  - Scapular muscle strengthening
- *Procedures*
  - Scapulothoracic bursa ultrasound-guided corticosteroid injection
- *Surgery*
  - Surgery with both open and arthroscopic techniques is reserved for refractory cases that do not respond to conservative measures outlined above, especially if a soft tissue or bony mass is involved.

References

1. Lansdown DA, Feeley BT. Evaluation and treatment of rotator cuff tears. Phys Sportsmed. 2012;40(2):73–86. https://doi.org/10.3810/psm.2012.05.1967. PMID: 22759608.
2. Matthewson G, Beach CJ, Nelson AA, Woodmass JM, Ono Y, Boorman RS, Lo IK, Thornton GM. Partial thickness rotator cuff tears: current concepts. Adv Orthop. 2015;2015:458786. https://doi.org/10.1155/2015/458786. Epub 2015 Jun 11. PMID: 26171251; PMCID: PMC4480800.
3. American Academy of Orthopaedic Surgeons Management of Rotator Cuff Injuries Evidenced-Based Clinical Practice Guideline. https://www.aaos.org/globalassets/quality-and-practice-resources/rotator-cuff/rotator-cuff-cpg-final-12-20-19.pdf. Published 11 Mar 2019.
4. Malanga GA, Mautner KR. Musculoskeletal physical examination: an evidence-based approach. 2nd ed. Philadelphia: Elsevier; 2017. Print. ISBN: 978-0-323-39623-3.
5. Pribicevic M, Pollard H. Rotator cuff impingement. J Manip Physiol Ther. 2004;27(9):580–90. https://doi.org/10.1016/j.jmpt.2004.10.004. PMID: 15614246.
6. Lizzio VA, Meta F, Fidai M, Makhni EC. Clinical evaluation and physical exam findings in patients with anterior shoulder instability. Curr Rev Musculoskelet Med. 2017;10(4):434–41. https://doi.org/10.1007/s12178-017-9434-3. PMID: 29043566; PMCID: PMC5685956
7. Yocum LA. Assessing the shoulder. History, physical examination, differential diagnosis, and special tests used. Clin Sports Med. 1983;2(2):281–9. PMID: 9697638.
8. Burbank KM, Stevenson JH, Czarnecki GR, Dorfman J. Chronic shoulder pain: part I. Evaluation and diagnosis. Am Fam Physician. 2008;77(4):453–60. PMID: 18326164.
9. Greenberg DL. Evaluation and treatment of shoulder pain. Med Clin North Am. 2014;98(3):487–504. https://doi.org/10.1016/j.mcna.2014.01.016. Epub 2014 Mar 22. PMID: 24758957.
10. Challoumas D, Kirwan PD, Borysov D, Clifford C, McLean M, Millar NL. Topical glyceryl trinitrate for the treatment of tendinopathies: a systematic review. Br J Sports Med. 2019;53(4):251. Epub 2018 Oct 9
11. Page MJ, Green S, McBain B, Surace SJ, Deitch J, Lyttle N, Mrocki MA, Buchbinder R. Manual therapy and exercise for rotator cuff disease. Cochrane Database Syst Rev. 2016;6:CD012224. https://doi.org/10.1002/14651858.CD012224. PMID: 27283590.
12. Hurley ET, Lim Fat D, Moran CJ, Mullet H. The efficacy of platelet-rich plasma and platelet-rich fibrin in arthroscopic rotator cuff repair: a meta-analysis of randomized controlled trials. Am J Sports Med. 2019;47(3):753–61.
13. Chen X, Jones IA, Togashi R, Park C, Vangsness CT Jr. Use of platelet-rich plasma for the improvement of pain and function in rotator cuff tears: a systematic review and meta-analysis with bias assessment. Am J Sports Med. 2020;48(8):2028–41. https://doi.org/10.1177/0363545418771423. Epub 2019 Nov 19. PMID: 31743037; PMCID: PMC7234896.
14. Speed C. A systematic review of shockwave therapies in soft tissue conditions: focusing on the evidence. Br J Sports Med. 2014;48(21):1538. Epub 2013 Aug 5
15. van der Zwaal P, Thomassen BJ, Nieuwenhuijse MJ, Lindenburg R, Swen JW, van Arkel ER. Clinical outcome in all-arthroscopic versus mini-open rotator cuff repair in small to medium-sized tears: a randomized controlled trial in 100 patients with 1-year follow-up. Arthroscopy. 2013;29(2):266–73. https://doi.org/10.1016/j.arthro.2012.08.022. Epub 2012 Dec 1. PMID: 23206691.
16. Ketola S, Lehtinen JT, Arnala I. Arthroscopic decompression not recommended in the treatment of rotator cuff tendinopathy: a final review of a randomised controlled trial at a minimum follow-up of ten years. Bone Joint J. 2017;99-B(6):799.
17. Shah N, Lewis M. Shoulder adhesive capsulitis: systematic review of randomised trials using multiple corticosteroid injections. Br J Gen Pract. 2007;57(541):662–7. PMID: 17688763; PMCID: PMC2099674.
18. Bhatia M, Singh B, Nicolaou N, Ravikumar KJ. Correlation between rotator cuff tears and repeated subacromial steroid injections: a case-controlled study. Ann R Coll Surg Engl. 2009;91(5):414–6. https://doi.org/10.1308/003588409X428261. Epub 2009 Apr 30. PMID: 19409148; PMCID: PMC2758443.
19. Reilly P, Macleod I, Macfarlane R, Windley J, Emery RJ. Dead men and radiologists don't lie: a review of cadaveric and radiological studies of rotator cuff tear prevalence. Ann R Coll Surg Engl. 2006;88(2):116–21. https://doi.org/10.1308/003588406X94968. PMID: 16551396; PMCID: PMC1964063
20. Hsieh LF, Hsu WC, Lin YJ, Wu SH, Chang KC, Chang HL. Is ultrasound-guided injection more effective in chronic subacromial bursitis? Med Sci Sports Exerc. 2013;45(12):2205–13. https://doi.org/10.1249/MSS.0b013e31829b183c. PMID: 23698243.
21. Bloom JE, Rischin A, Johnston RV, Buchbinder R. Image-guided versus blind glucocorticoid injection for shoulder pain.

Cochrane Database Syst Rev. 2012;8:CD009147. https://doi.org/10.1002/14651858.CD009147.pub2. PMID: 22895984.

22. Henkus HE, de Witte PB, Nelissen RG, Brand R, van Arkel ER. Bursectomy compared with acromioplasty in the management of subacromial impingement syndrome: a prospective randomised study. J Bone Joint Surg Br. 2009;91(4):504–10. https://doi.org/10.1302/0301-620X.91B4.21442. PMID: 19336812.
23. Kolk A, Thomassen BJW, Hund H, de Witte PB, Henkus HE, Wassenaar WG, van Arkel ERA, Nelissen RGHH. Does acromioplasty result in favorable clinical and radiologic outcomes in the management of chronic subacromial pain syndrome? A double-blinded randomized clinical trial with 9 to 14 years' follow-up. J Shoulder Elb Surg. 2017;26(8):1407–15. https://doi.org/10.1016/j.jse.2017.03.021. Epub 2017 May 8. PMID: 28495574.
24. Cowderoy GA, Lisle DA, O'Connell PT. Overuse and impingement syndromes of the shoulder in the athlete. Magn Reson Imaging Clin N Am. 2009;17(4):577–93, v. https://doi.org/10.1016/j.mric.2009.06.003. PMID: 19887291.
25. Campbell RS, Dunn A. External impingement of the shoulder. Semin Musculoskelet Radiol. 2008;12(2):107–26. https://doi.org/10.1055/s-2008-1078699. PMID: 18509791.
26. Chang EY, Moses DA, Babb JS, Schweitzer ME. Shoulder impingement: objective 3D shape analysis of acromial morphologic features. Radiology. 2006;239(2):497–505. https://doi.org/10.1148/radiol.2392050324. Epub 2006 Mar 16. PMID: 16543591.
27. Hultenheim Klintberg I, Gunnarsson AC, Styf J, Karlsson J. Early activation or a more protective regime after arthroscopic subacromial decompression--a description of clinical changes with two different physiotherapy treatment protocols--a prospective, randomized pilot study with a two-year follow-up. Clin Rehabil. 2008;22(10–11):951–65. https://doi.org/10.1177/0269215508090771. PMID: 18955427.
28. Bishay V, Gallo RA. The evaluation and treatment of rotator cuff pathology. Prim Care. 2013;40(4):889–910, viii. https://doi.org/10.1016/j.pop.2013.08.006. PMID: 24209724.
29. Lähdeoja T, Karjalainen T, Jokihaara J, Salamh P, Kavaja L, Agarwal A, Winters M, Buchbinder R, Guyatt G, Vandvik PO, Ardern CL. Subacromial decompression surgery for adults with shoulder pain: a systematic review with meta-analysis. Br J Sports Med. 2020;54(11):665–73. https://doi.org/10.1136/bjsports-2018-100486. Epub 2019 Jan 15. PMID: 30647053.
30. Beard DJ, Rees JL, Cook JA, Rombach I, Cooper C, Merritt N, Shirkey BA, Donovan JL, Gwilym S, Savulescu J, Moser J, Gray A, Jepson M, Tracey I, Judge A, Wartolowska K, Carr AJ, CSAW Study Group. Arthroscopic subacromial decompression for subacromial shoulder pain (CSAW): a multicentre, pragmatic, parallel group, placebo-controlled, three-group, randomised surgical trial. Lancet. 2018;391(10118):329–38. https://doi.org/10.1016/S0140-6736(17)32457-1. Epub 2017 Nov 20. PMID: 29169668; PMCID: PMC5803129.
31. Goslin KL, Krivickas LS. Proximal neuropathies of the upper extremity. Neurol Clin. 1999;17(3):525–48, vii. https://doi.org/10.1016/s0733-8619(05)70151-1. PMID: 10393752.
32. Boykin RE, Friedman DJ, Higgins LD, Warner JJ. Suprascapular neuropathy. J Bone Joint Surg Am. 2010;92(13):2348–64. https://doi.org/10.2106/JBJS.I.01743. PMID: 20926731.
33. Cummins CA, Schneider DS. Peripheral nerve injuries in baseball players. Neurol Clin. 2008;26(1):195–215; x. https://doi.org/10.1016/j.ncl.2007.11.014. PMID: 18295091.
34. Dramis A, Pimpalnerkar A. Suprascapular neuropathy in volleyball players. Acta Orthop Belg. 2005;71(3):269–72. PMID: 16035699.
35. Romeo AA, Rotenberg DD, Bach BR Jr. Suprascapular neuropathy. J Am Acad Orthop Surg. 1999;7(6):358–67. https://doi.org/10.5435/00124635-199911000-00002. PMID: 11497489.
36. Fritz RC, Helms CA, Steinbach LS, Genant HK. Suprascapular nerve entrapment: evaluation with MR imaging. Radiology. 1992;182(2):437–44. https://doi.org/10.1148/radiology.182.2.1732962. PMID: 1732962.
37. Kostretzis L, Theodoroudis I, Boutsiadis A, Papadakis N, Papadopoulos P. Suprascapular nerve pathology: a review of the literature. Open Orthop J. 2017;28(11):140–53. https://doi.org/10.2174/1874325001711010140. PMID: 28400882; PMCID: PMC5366386
38. Neal S, Fields KB. Peripheral nerve entrapment and injury in the upper extremity. Am Fam Physician. 2010;81(2):147–55. PMID: 20082510.
39. Narakas A. Compression syndromes about the shoulder including brachial plexus. In: Szabo RM, editor. Nerve compression syndromes: diagnosis and treatment. Thorofare, NJ: Slack; 1989. p. 236–9.
40. Shah AA, Butler RB, Sung SY, Wells JH, Higgins LD, Warner JJ. Clinical outcomes of suprascapular nerve decompression. J Shoulder Elb Surg. 2011;20(6):975–82. https://doi.org/10.1016/j.jse.2010.10.032. Epub 2011 Feb 1. PMID: 21277808.
41. Lafosse L, Tomasi A, Corbett S, Baier G, Willems K, Gobezie R. Arthroscopic release of suprascapular nerve entrapment at the suprascapular notch: technique and preliminary results. Arthroscopy. 2007;23(1):34–42. https://doi.org/10.1016/j.arthro.2006.10.003. PMID: 17210425.
42. Piasecki DP, Romeo AA, Bach BR Jr, Nicholson GP. Suprascapular neuropathy. J Am Acad Orthop Surg. 2009;17(11):665–76. https://doi.org/10.5435/00124635-200911000-00001. PMID: 19880677.
43. Brown SA, Doolittle DA, Bohanon CJ, Jayaraj A, Naidu SG, Huettl EA, Renfree KJ, Oderich GS, Bjarnason H, Gloviczki P, Wysokinski WE, McPhail IR. Quadrilateral space syndrome: the Mayo Clinic experience with a new classification system and case series. Mayo Clin Proc. 2015;90(3):382–94. https://doi.org/10.1016/j.mayocp.2014.12.012. Epub 2015 Jan 31 PMID: 25649966.
44. Hoskins WT, Pollard HP, McDonald AJ. Quadrilateral space syndrome: a case study and review of the literature. Br J Sports Med. 2005;39(2):e9. https://doi.org/10.1136/bjsm.2004.013367. PMID: 15665194; PMCID: PMC1725134.
45. Hangge PT, Breen I, Albadawi H, Knuttinen MG, Naidu SG, Oklu R. Quadrilateral space syndrome: diagnosis and clinical management. J Clin Med. 2018;7(4):86. https://doi.org/10.3390/jcm7040086. PMID: 29690525; PMCID: PMC5920460.
46. Feng SH, Hsiao MY, Wu CH, Özçakar L. Ultrasound-guided diagnosis and management for quadrilateral space syndrome. Pain Med. 2017;18(1):184–6. https://doi.org/10.1093/pm/pnw256.
47. Palmer W, Bancroft L, Bonar F, et al. Glossary of terms for musculoskeletal radiology. Skelet Radiol. 2020;49:1–33. https://doi.org/10.1007/s00256-020-03465-1.
48. Steinmann SP, Moran EA. Axillary nerve injury: diagnosis and treatment. J Am Acad Orthop Surg. 2001;9(5):328–35. https://doi.org/10.5435/00124635-200109000-00006. PMID: 11575912.
49. Perlmutter GS. Axillary nerve injury. Clin Orthop Relat Res. 1999;368:28–36. PMID: 10613150.
50. McAdams TR, Dillingham MF. Surgical decompression of the quadrilateral space in overhead athletes. Am J Sports Med. 2008;36(3):528–32. https://doi.org/10.1177/0363546507309675. Epub 2007 Nov 30. PMID: 18055916.
51. Kauppila LI, Vastamäki M. Iatrogenic serratus anterior paralysis. Long-term outcome in 26 patients. Chest. 1996;109(1):31–4. https://doi.org/10.1378/chest.109.1.31. PMID: 8549212.
52. Krasna MJ, Forti G. Nerve injury: injury to the recurrent laryngeal, phrenic, vagus, long thoracic, and sympathetic nerves during thoracic surgery. Thorac Surg Clin. 2006;16(3):267–75, vi. https://doi.org/10.1016/j.thorsurg.2006.05.003. PMID: 17004555.
53. Seror P, Lenglet T, Nguyen C, Ouaknine M, Lefevre-Colau MM. Unilateral winged scapula: clinical and electrodiagnostic experience with 128 cases, with special attention to long thoracic nerve palsy. Muscle Nerve. 2018;57(6):913–20. https://doi.org/10.1002/mus.26059. Epub 2018 Feb 24. PMID: 29314072.

54. Wills AJ, Sawle GV. Accessory nerve palsies. Pract Neurol. 2010;10(4):191–4. https://doi.org/10.1136/jnnp.2010.217760. PMID: 20647524.
55. Kelley MJ, Kane TE, Leggin BG. Spinal accessory nerve palsy: associated signs and symptoms. J Orthop Sports Phys Ther. 2008;38(2):78–86. https://doi.org/10.2519/jospt.2008.2454. Epub 2007 Sep 7. PMID: 18560187.
56. Martin RM, Fish DE. Scapular winging: anatomical review, diagnosis, and treatments. Curr Rev Musculoskelet Med. 2008;1(1):1–11. https://doi.org/10.1007/s12178-007-9000-5. PMID: 19468892; PMCID: PMC2684151.
57. Krzesniak-Swinarska M, Caress JB, Cartwright MS. Neuromuscular ultrasound for evaluation of scapular winging. Muscle Nerve. 2017;56(1):7–14.
58. Marin R. Scapula winger's brace: a case series on the management of long thoracic nerve palsy. Arch Phys Med Rehabil. 1998;79(10):1226–30. https://doi.org/10.1016/s0003-9993(98)90266-0. PMID: 9779675.
59. Galano GJ, Bigliani LU, Ahmad CS, Levine WN. Surgical treatment of winged scapula. Clin Orthop Relat Res. 2008;466(3):652–60. https://doi.org/10.1007/s11999-007-0086-2. Epub 2008 Jan 8. PMID: 18196359; PMCID: PMC2505206.
60. Connor PM, Yamaguchi K, Manifold SG, Pollock RG, Flatow EL, Bigliani LU. Split pectoralis major transfer for serratus anterior palsy. Clin Orthop Relat Res. 1997;341:134–42. PMID: 9269166.
61. Novak CB, Mackinnon SE. Surgical treatment of a long thoracic nerve palsy. Ann Thorac Surg. 2002;73(5):1643–5. https://doi.org/10.1016/s0003-4975(01)03372-0. PMID: 12022573.
62. Tomaino MM. Neurophysiologic and clinical outcome following medial pectoral to long thoracic nerve transfer for scapular winging: a case report. Microsurgery. 2002;22:254–7.
63. Conduah AH, Baker CL 3rd, Baker CL Jr. Clinical management of scapulothoracic bursitis and the snapping scapula. Sports Health. 2010;2(2):147–55. https://doi.org/10.1177/1941738109338359. PMID: 23015932; PMCID: PMC3445084.
64. Higuchi T, Ogose A, Hotta T, Okamoto K, Kamura T, Sasai K, Hatano H, Morita T. Clinical and imaging features of distended scapulothoracic bursitis: spontaneously regressed pseudotumoral lesion. J Comput Assist Tomogr. 2004;28(2):223–8. https://doi.org/10.1097/00004728-200403000-00012. PMID: 15091127.
65. Lehtinen JT, Macy JC, Cassinelli E, Warner JJ. The painful scapulothoracic articulation: surgical management. Clin Orthop Relat Res. 2004;423:99–105. https://doi.org/10.1097/01.blo.0000128647.38363.8e.
66. Son SA, Lee DH, Lee YO, Lee SC, Kim KJ, Cho JY. Operative management in a patient with scapulothoracic bursitis. Korean J Thorac Cardiovasc Surg. 2013;46(6):486–9. https://doi.org/10.5090/kjtcs.2013.46.6.486. Epub 2013 Dec 6. PMID: 24368981; PMCID: PMC3868702.
67. Kuhne LT M, Boniquit N, Ghodadra N, Romeo AA, Provencher MT. The snapping scapula: diagnosis and treatment. Arthroscopy. 2009. https://doi.org/10.1016/j.arthro.2008.12.022.
68. Malanga G, Mautner K. Atlas of ultrasound-guided musculoskeletal injections. New York: McGraw-Hill Education; 2014.

Shoulder Dislocations and Fractures

23

Oluseun Olufade, Giorgio Negron, and Kenneth Mautner

23.1 Synonyms

- Shoulder anterior instability
- Shoulder posterior instability
- Shoulder subluxation
- Humeral shaft fracture
- Collar bone fracture

23.2 ICD-10 Codes

- Subluxation and dislocation of shoulder joint (S43.0)
- Anterior subluxation and dislocation of humerus (S43.01)
- Posterior subluxation and dislocation of humerus (S43.02)
- Fracture of clavicle (S42.0)
- Fracture of scapula (S42.1)
- Fracture of upper end of humerus (S42.2)
- Fracture of shoulder girdle (S42.9)

23.3 Description

There are four shoulder articulations that make up shoulder motion: sternoclavicular joint, glenohumeral joint, acromioclavicular joint, and scapulothoracic articulation. The glenohumeral joint is one of the most mobile joints in the body. With that said, the tradeoff for this freedom of movement is the lack of stability which makes this joint susceptible to injury. In this chapter, we will discuss shoulder dislocations and fractures.

O. Olufade (✉)
Orthopaedics and Physical Medicine & Rehabilitation, Emory University School of Medicine, Atlanta, GA, USA
e-mail: oolufad@emory.edu

G. Negron
Department of Orthopaedics and Physical Medicine and Rehabilitation, Emory University School of Medicine, Atlanta, GA, USA

K. Mautner
Primary Care Sports Medicine, Emory University, Atlanta, GA, USA

Anatomy The bony anatomy of the shoulder includes the scapula which forms the posterior aspect of the shoulder girdle with 17 muscular attachments and the glenoid that forms half of the primary shoulder joint [1, 2].

The clavicle connects the axial skeleton to the upper extremity skeleton, while the humeral proximal head articulates with the glenoid cavity. The proximal humerus can be divided into four parts: the lesser and greater tuberosities, the head, and the diaphyseal region.

Glenohumeral joint (GH) is a "ball-and-socket" joint with approximately 25% of the humeral head surface area interacting with the glenoid cavity [3, 4].

Labrum is a fibrocartilaginous structure that contributes to 50% of glenoid socket depth and is the attachment site of glenohumeral ligaments and bony glenoid [5]. In addition, the superior aspect of the labrum provides the origin site of the long head of the biceps attaching [6].

23.3.1 Shoulder Stabilizers

The shoulder stabilizers can be broken down to static and dynamic types:

Static Shoulder Stabilizers

1. The labrum provides a deep glenoid concavity that adds to stabilizing the humeral head [5].
2. Maintenance of negative intra-articular pressure that aids in translational stability [7].
3. Ligaments provide the most stability during end-range motion [8]:
   (a) Superior glenohumeral ligament (SGHL) prevents inferior translation of the humeral head and stabilizes the biceps tendons within the groove.
   (b) Inferior glenohumeral ligament (IGHL) is the thickest of all glenohumeral ligaments:
      - The anterior band prevents anterior translation of the humeral head when the arm is placed into abduction.

© The Author(s), under exclusive license to Springer Nature Switzerland AG 2022

S. A. Mostoufi et al. (eds.), *Clinical Guide to Musculoskeletal Medicine*, https://doi.org/10.1007/978-3-030-92042-5_23

- The posterior band prevents posterior translation of the humeral head when the arm is placed into abduction and external rotation.

(c) The coracohumeral ligament prevents posterior translation when the shoulder is flexed and internally rotated as well as prevents inferior translation when the arm is adducted and externally rotated.
(d) Coracoacromial ligament is responsible for restraint of superior humeral head displacement.

Dynamic Shoulder Stabilizers

1. Rotator cuff muscles provide dynamic stability that actively compresses the humeral head to the glenoid cavity [9]:
   (a) Subscapularis opposes inferior and anterior translation.
   (b) Infraspinatus opposes posterior and superior translation.
   (c) Teres minor opposes posterior and superior translation.
   (d) Supraspinatus has the least activity for dynamic stabilization.
2. Long head of the biceps tendon provides humeral head active depression and stability for anterior-posterior translation [5, 7, 10].

23.4 Shoulder Dislocations

Shoulder dislocations make up about 50% of all major joint dislocations. About 40% of acute shoulder dislocations include associated structural injury such as rotator cuff tears, neurological deficit (i.e., axillary nerve palsy), and greater tuberosity fracture [20]. Furthermore, shoulder dislocations may be associated with Bankart and Hill-Sachs lesions. A Bankart lesion is reported to be seen in 85% of anterior shoulder dislocations and defined as a subsequent disruption of the anterior labrum from the glenoid rim [21]. The Hill-Sachs lesion is a compression fracture of the posterolateral humeral head that is estimated to occur in 40–90% of dislocations [22]. Reverse Bankart and Hill-Sachs lesions are seen in posterior dislocations.

23.4.1 Anterior Shoulder Dislocation

This is the most common type of shoulder dislocation [11–13]. It is common in male, with bimodal distribution of 10–20 years of age being the most common and 50–60-year age group being the second most common [14, 15]. The mechanism of injury is classically from a forced abduction and external rotation of the upper extremity. Anterior shoulder dislocation may also be caused by posterior force to the shoulder or a fall on an outstretched arm.

23.4.2 Posterior Shoulder Dislocation

In a cast for approximately 3% of all shoulder dislocations, mechanism of injury usually involves an anterior force to the shoulder with axial loading of the flex-abducted internally rotated upper extremity [17, 18]. Seizures and electrocution may also cause posterior shoulder dislocation due to the imbalanced and substantial contractions of shoulder muscles [19].

23.4.3 Inferior Shoulder Dislocations

Also known as *luxatio erecta humeri*, inferior shoulder dislocation is a rare presentation (<1%) that is typically caused by shoulder hyperabduction or with axial loading on the abducted arm which presents as a fixed abducted position of the upper extremity following dislocation [16]. Connective tissue disease such as Ehlers-Danlos syndrome or bony abnormalities such as glenoid hypoplasia may contribute to non-traumatic dislocations.

Factors associated with a high risk of recurrent instability include [23]:

- Age <30 years old
- Male gender
- Hypermobility
- Glenoid cavity bone loss >20–25%
- Hill-Sachs lesion extending medially over the medial margin of the glenoid track or >5/8 of the humeral head
- Hill-Sachs defect >5/8 of the humeral head radius
- High level of activity/contact sport participation
- Bankart lesion plus another associated lesions
- Positive anterior apprehension test
- Anterior labral periosteal sleeve avulsion (ALPSA)

23.5 Shoulder Fractures

Fractures of the shoulders commonly involve the clavicle, proximal humerus, and scapula. Differential diagnosis of shoulder fracture and dislocation is outlined in Table 23.2.

23.5.1 Clavicle Fractures

The incidence of clavicle fractures is described as a bimodal distribution with the first peak under the age to 40 and the second peak above the age to 70 years [24]. Clavicle fractures in the youth usually are from a high-impact mechanism such as through contact sports or motor vehicle collision, while in the older population, they are sustained after a fall on an outstretched hand. It has been estimated

Table 23.1 Modified Neer classification

Type I	Fracture that is lateral to intact coracoclavicular (CC) ligaments Spares the acromioclavicular (AC) joint Stable
Type IIA	Fracture occurring medial to the CC ligaments Intact CC ligaments Unstable
Type IIB	Fracture occurring between the CC ligaments Conoid ligament is torn Trapezoid ligament is intact Unstable
Type III	Intra-articular fracture occurring lateral to the CC ligaments Involves the AC joint Stable
Type IV	Periosteal slippage of the proximal fragment at the epiphysis Seen in the pediatric population Intact CC ligaments Stable
Type V	Comminuted fracture pattern Inferior fragment attached to the intact CC ligaments Unstable

Table 23.2 Differential diagnosis of shoulder dislocations and fractures

Shoulder impingement syndrome	Glenoid labrum tear
AC joint sprain	Biceps tendon tear
Pseudo dislocation of the shoulder	Triceps tendon tear
Shoulder rotator cuff tear	Pectoralis major tear

that about 45% of sports-related clavicle fractures are non-displaced [25].

The modified Neer classification is used to label clavicle fractures in relation to the coracoclavicular ligaments (Table 23.1) [26].

23.5.2 Proximal Humeral Fractures

Proximal humeral fractures account for 5% of all fractures with high incidence in the elderly population especially in the setting of osteoporosis [27]. The most common mechanism of action is from a fall at an oblique angle onto an outstretched hand while in the younger population tends to be from a high-speed force to the lateral humerus of the shoulder [28].

Neer classification of proximal humeral fractures takes into account the involvement of the number and location of displaced fractures. A fracture is considered displaced if the angle of displacement was >45° or if there is a separation of >1 centimeter (cm).

Scapular fractures are typically uncommon which usually present after a high-velocity trauma involving the chest cavity and make up about 3–5% of upper extremity fractures [29]. The international scapula fracture classification system divides the scapular in four parts: glenoid fossa, coracoid, acromion, and body (Table 23.2) [30].

23.6 Clinical Presentation

23.6.1 Dislocations

Common patient presentations:

- Anterior dislocation: The arm is held flexed, internally rotated, and abducted.
- Posterior dislocation: The arm is in a fixed, internally rotated, and adducted position.
- Inferior dislocation: The arm is in a fixed, abducted position, and typically above their head.

23.6.2 Fractures

Individuals who sustained clavicle fractures usually hold the affected arm closely adducted to the body supporting it with the opposite hand as this limits the weight of the arm that is pulling on the fracture.

Proximal humeral head fractures often present with point tenderness at the upper arm with associated swelling and ecchymosis. The clinician should be wary on vascular compromise as fractures of the humeral head can place vascular structures including the axillary artery and anterior/posterior circumflex arteries are at risk of injury [31].

Scapular fractures are typically after a high-impact trauma directly to the scapula. At times, the patient is obtunded and unable to provide accurate history; therefore, there should be high suspicion when performing a secondary survey.

23.7 Physical Examination

The clinician should perform a thorough yet concise physical examination based on the medical history obtained.

Visual observation Bilateral shoulders should be exposed to compare symmetry. Evaluate for any muscular atrophy such as in the deltoid, supraspinatus, and infraspinatus. Atrophy of the deltoid may indicate axillary nerve involvement. Evaluate for swelling, erythema, open fractures, or tenting of the skin. A flattened shoulder silhouette with prominent acromion can be secondary to a shoulder dislocation. The clinician may also assess for scapular winging during static and provocative scapular motion.

Neurovascular exam Assess distal neurovascular in the setting of acute shoulder injuries (i.e., check for distal radial pulse). Assess for sensation around the lateral shoulder as there is risk of axillary nerve injury. Most of the shoulder girdle is innervated by the fifth and sixth cervical roots of the upper trunk of the brachial plexus.

Palpation The clinician should palpate all bony landmarks and superficial joints around the shoulder starting with the sternoclavicular joint, acromioclavicular joint, and glenohumeral joint. Evaluate for crepitus in the setting of trauma as this may be a sign of an underlying fracture. Along with the shoulder, assess the distal portion of the affected extremity.

Range of motion Active and passive range of motion of the bilateral shoulders should be assessed and compared.

Motor testing Strength testing should be performed on all rotator cuff muscles and compared them to the contralateral side:

- Supraspinatus (C5–C6): Assessed by having the arms abducted to 90° and internally rotated with thumbs pointing down. The clinician provides an inferior force with the patient providing resistance (Fig. 23.1).
- Infraspinatus (C5–C6)/teres minor (C6–C7): Assessed by resisting external rotation in 0 (infraspinatus) (Fig. 23.2) and 90° (teres minor) of shoulder abduction.
- Subscapularis (C5–C6): Assessed by belt press test where the patient is asked to have their hand on their abdomen with wrist neutral and resist the clinician's external rotation.

23.7.1 Special Tests

Apprehension Test Sensitivity 81%; specificity 90% [32]

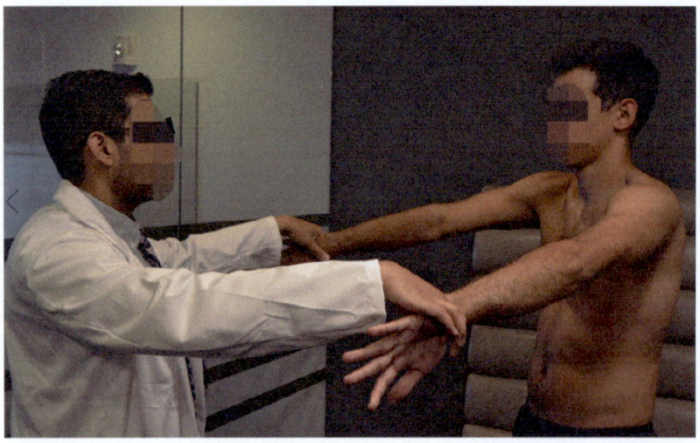

Fig. 23.1 Supraspinatus strength test: The patient has their arms abducted to 90° and internally rotated with thumbs pointing down. The clinician provides an inferior force with the patient providing resistance

Tests for anterior shoulder instability. The patient is standing or supine with the arm at 90° of abduction and elbow flexion. The clinical passively moves the shoulder to external rotation, and forward pressure is applied to the posterior shoulder. The test is positive if the patient becomes apprehensive about their shoulder dislocating (Fig. 23.3).

Jobe relocation (Fowler) test Sensitivity 68%; specificity 100% [33]

Tests for anterior shoulder instability. At the end of the apprehension test, the patient is asked where they feel discomfort, and the clinician provides a posteriorly directed force to the humeral head. If the sense of apprehension dissipates, then the test is positive (Fig. 23.4).

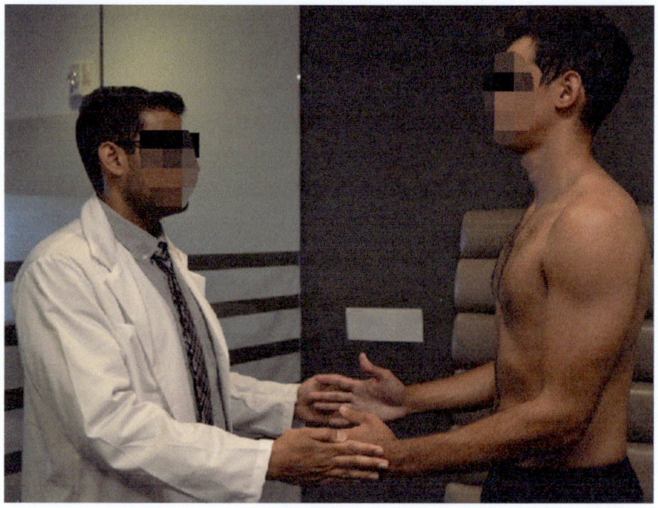

Fig. 23.2 Infraspinatus strength test: Assessed by resisting external rotation in 0° of shoulder abduction

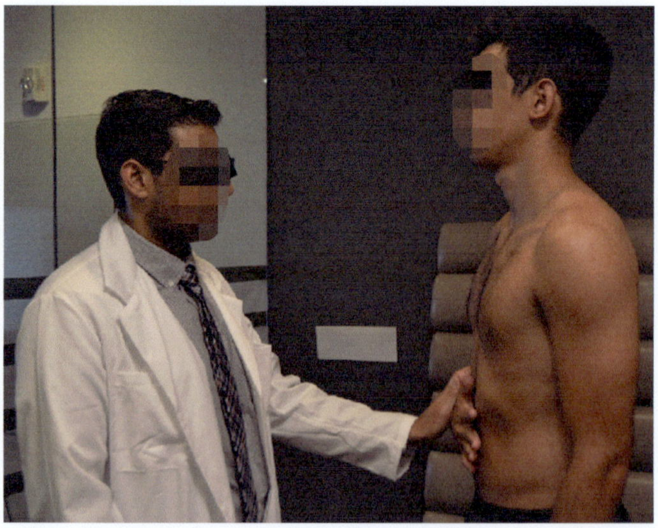

Fig. 23.3 Belt press test: The patient has their hand on their abdomen with the wrist neutral and resist the clinician's external rotation

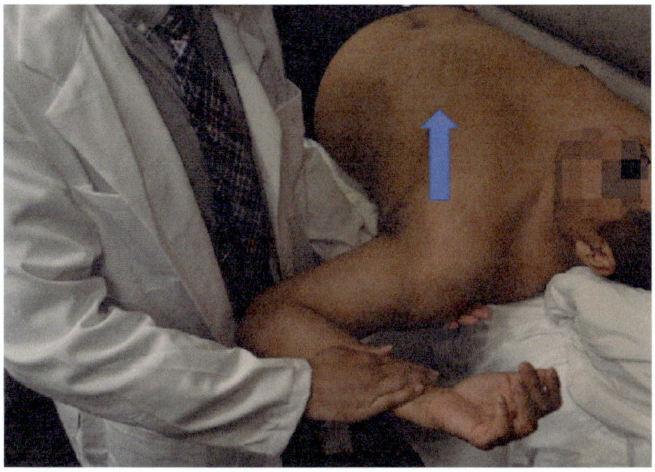

Fig. 23.4 Apprehension test: The patient has their arm at 90° of abduction and elbow flexion with the clinician passively moving the shoulder to external rotation and applying forward pressure to the posterior shoulder. The test is positive if the patient becomes apprehensive about their shoulder dislocating

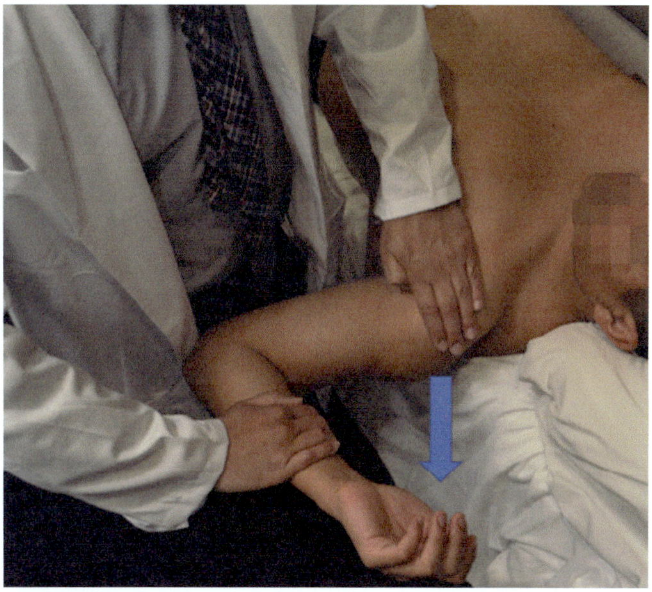

Fig. 23.5 Jobe relocation (Fowler) test: At the end of the apprehension test, the clinician provides a posteriorly directed force to the humeral head. If the sense of apprehension dissipates, then the test is positive

Anterior drawer test Sensitivity 53%; specificity 85% [32]

Tests for anterior shoulder instability. The patient is supine with the clinician stabilizing the scapula by firmly placing the scapular spine forward with the index and middle finger and thumb on the coracoid process. The clinician's other hand grasps the relaxed upper arm and gently translates it anteriorly. A positive test is a reproduction of instability symptoms (Fig. 23.5).

Posterior drawer test No sensitivity or specificity data available.

Tests for posterior shoulder instability. The patient is supine, and the clinician holds the arm in forward flexion and abduction at 45°. With the other hand, the clinician holds the scapular with the index and middle fingers on the scapular spine and thumb immediately lateral to the coracoid process. The clinician translates humeral head posterior with the thumb while lifting the arm forward. A positive test is a reproduction of instability symptoms (Fig. 23.6).

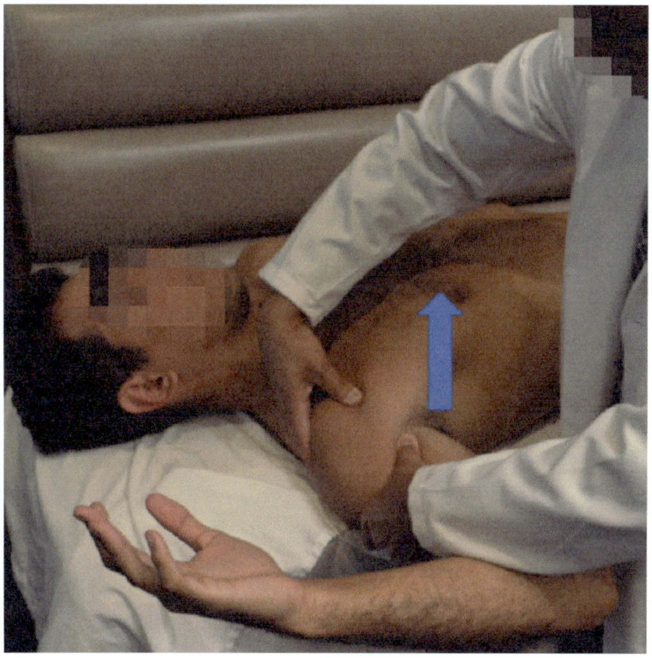

Fig. 23.6 Posterior drawer test. Firmly placing the scapular spine forward with the index and middle finger and the thumb on the coracoid process. The clinician's other hand grasps the relaxed upper arm and gently translates it anteriorly. A positive test is a reproduction of instability symptoms

Load and shift test Sensitivity 71.1%/Specificity 89.9%

Test for General Shoulder Instability. The patient is standing or supine with the clinician standing behind them and stabilizing the scapula over the acromion with one hand and the patient's upper arm with the other hand. The clinician applies a slight axial load, and the humeral head is then translated anteriorly and posteriorly (Fig. 23.7). Laxity can be graded with the modified Hawkins system [34], Grade I (no subluxation), and Grade II (subluxation over the glenoid rim).

Sulcus sign No sensitivity or specificity data available.

Tests for Inferior Shoulder Instability. The patient is standing or sitting upright with the shoulder in a relaxed neutral position. The clinician provides an inferior force onto the upper arm. A positive test is a reproduction of pain with humeral head subluxation (Fig. 23.8).

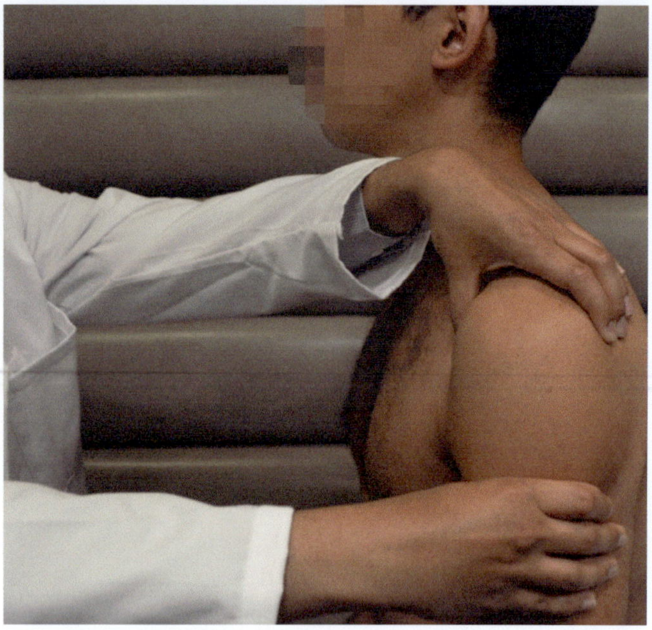

Fig. 23.7 Load and shift test: The clinician stabilizes the scapula over the acromion with one hand and the patient's upper arm with the other hand. A slight axial load is applied, and the humeral head is then translated anteriorly and posteriorly

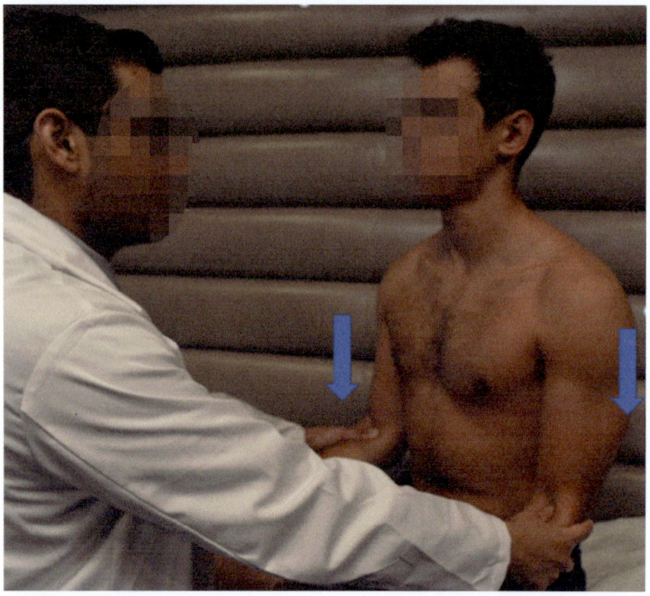

Fig. 23.8 Sulcus sign: With the shoulder in a relaxed neutral position, the clinician provides an inferior force onto the upper arm. A positive test is a reproduction of pain with humeral head subluxation

Specialized test for specific shoulder instability These tests are outlined in Table 23.3.

Table 23.3 Specialized test for specific shoulder instability

Type of instability	Test	Sensitivity/specificity
General instability	Load and shift test	Sensitivity 71.1%; specificity 89.9%
Anterior instability	*Apprehension test* *Jobe relocation (Fowler) test* *Anterior drawer test*	Sensitivity 81%; specificity 90% Sensitivity 68%; specificity 100% Sensitivity 53%; specificity 85%
Posterior instability	*Posterior drawer test*	No data available
Inferior instability	*Sulcus sign*	No data available

23.8 Diagnostic Workup

X-Ray A clinician should start with a plain radiograph including anterior posterior (AP), scapular Y, and axillary view to evaluate for bony abnormalities and alignment (Figs. 23.9 and 23.10). A serendipity view can be requested for suspicion of a clavicular fracture since this assesses bilateral clavicles, AC, and sternoclavicular joints. In the dislocated patient, radiographs should be taken before and after the reduction as there may be subsequent humeral head or glenoid involvement (Fig. 23.11).

Computer Tomography (CT) CT scan may be indicated to evaluate complex fractures and chronic fracture dislocations of the humeral head that are not caught by plain radiographs. Fractures of the proximal humerus and glenoid tubercle can be appreciated if suspicious for Hill-Sachs or bony Bankart lesions, respectively.

Magnetic Resonance Imaging (MRI) MRI of the shoulder is indicated when evaluating and/or concern for injuries to the rotator cuff, glenoid labrum, capsular and glenohumeral ligaments detachments, and neurovascular structures (Fig. 23.12).

Ultrasound Imaging A clinician trained in musculoskeletal ultrasound may use ultrasound as a point-of-care diagnostic method for acute shoulder injuries. This provides a non-invasive, dynamic, and radiation-free imaging modality. A systematic review investigating diagnostic accuracy for shoulder dislocation using ultrasound found specificity/sensitivity up to 100% when compared to X-ray imaging [35].

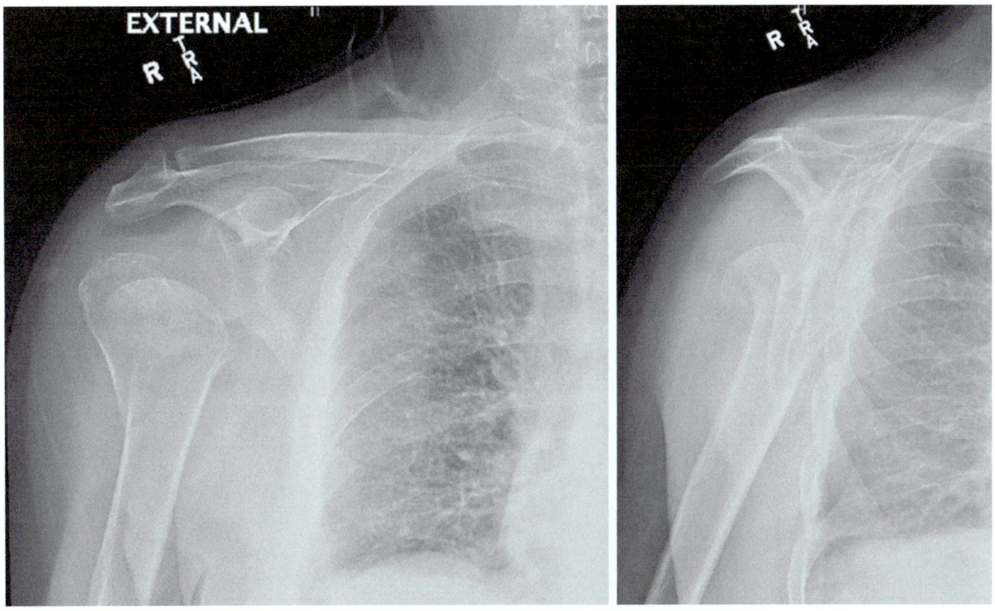

Fig. 23.9 AP and Y view of a comminuted intra-articular humeral head fracture with inferior subluxation of the humeral head

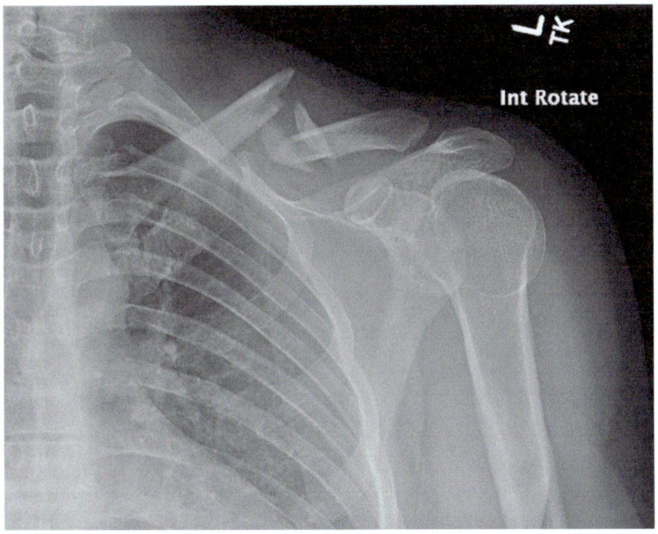

Fig. 23.10 AP view in internal rotation of a comminuted clavicular fracture

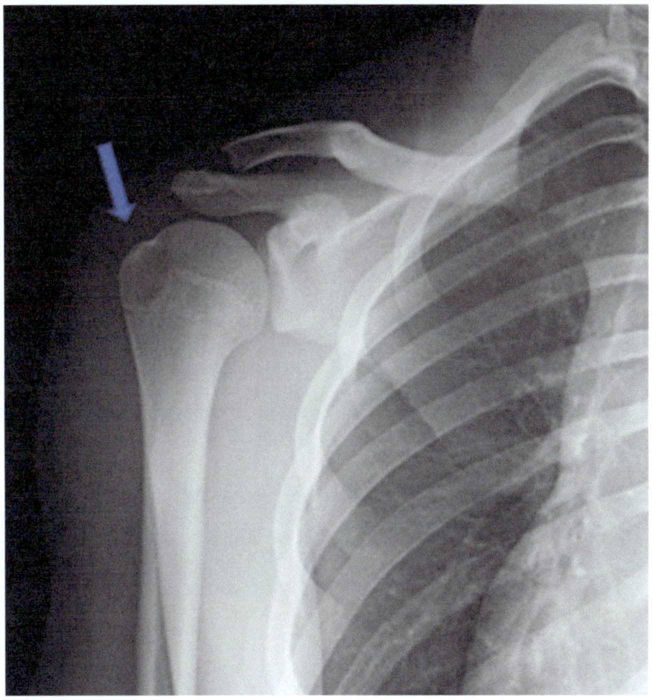

Fig. 23.11 AP view of the shoulder showing a small Hill-Sachs deformity post-reduction

23.9 Treatment

Different shoulder dislocations and shoulder fractures have different treatment algorithms. In this section we will go through them individually.

23.9.1 Shoulder Dislocation Treatment

23.9.1.1 Glenohumeral Reduction

Different methods of relocating the shoulder which has been dislocated. The technique depends on the direction in which the shoulder was dislocated. Table 23.4 outlines the different types of shoulder reduction techniques.

23.9.1.2 Anterior Glenohumeral Dislocations

There are multiple reduction techniques for the management of anterior shoulder dislocations. Here we will discuss four techniques [16]:

- *Kocher's Method* (Fig. 23.13)
  For Anterior Shoulder Dislocations
  This technique is noted to be painless and excludes traction using leverage alone.

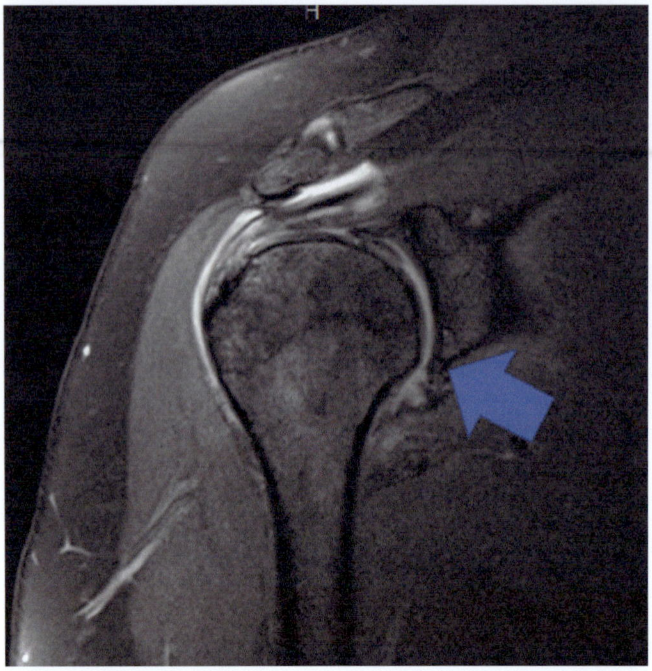

Fig. 23.12 Non-contrast T2 coronal MRI of the shoulder showing a mildly displaced subacute fracture of the anterior inferior glenoid (Bony Bankart)

Table 23.4 This table outlines the different techniques available for glenohumeral reduction relevant to the direction in which the shoulder has been dislocated

Type of glenohumeral dislocation	Reduction techniques
Anterior dislocation	Kocher's method Milch technique Scapular manipulation Chair technique
Posterior dislocation	Stimson technique Traction technique
Inferior dislocation	Two-step maneuver

  The clinician bends the affected arm at 90° adducted against the body.
  The arm is slowly externally rotated between 70° and 85° until resistance is felt.
  The arm is then forward flexed and reduction of the humeral head occurs.
  Success rates ranging from 81% to 100% have been reported.
- *Milch Technique* (Fig. 23.14)
  For Anterior Shoulder Dislocations
  Stand on the same side as the affected arm while the patient is seated or lies in a supine position.
  The clinician places fingers over the affected shoulder using the thumb to stabilize the humeral head.
  The arm is then gently abducted and externally rotated into an overhead position.
  Success rates ranging from 70% to 100% have been reported.
- *Scapular Manipulation* (Fig. 23.15)
  For Anterior Shoulder Dislocations
  Lie the patient on a prone position on an exam table.

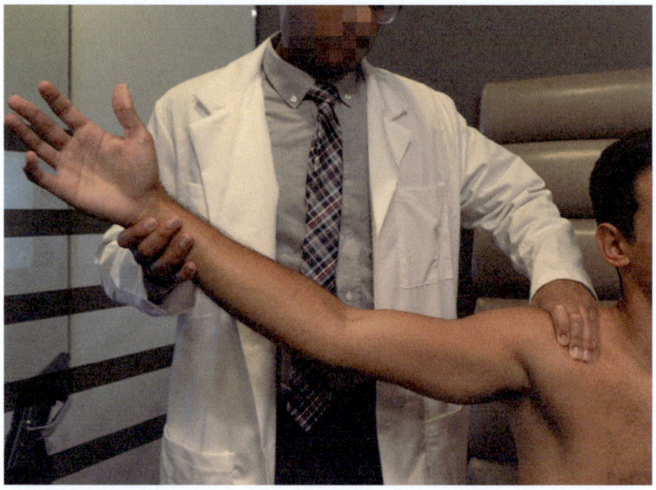

Fig. 23.14 Milch technique. The clinician places their fingers over the affected shoulder using the thumb to stabilize the humeral head. The arm is then gently abducted and externally rotated into an overhead position

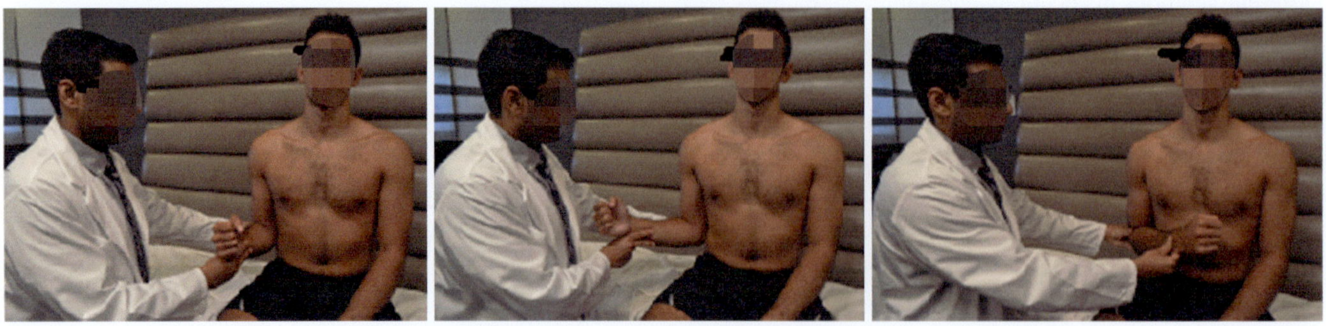

Fig. 23.13 Kocher's method: The clinician bends the affected arm at 90° adducted against the body, and the arm is slowly externally rotated between 70° and 85° until resistance is felt. The arm is then forward flexed, and reduction of the humeral head occurs

Allow the affected arm to hang vertically over the edge of the table with gentle traction being provided.
When patient begins to relax, reduction is then attempted by pushing on the tip of the scapula medially, with rotation of the superior aspect of the scapular laterally.
Success rates ranging from 79% to 96% have been reported.

- *Chair Technique* (Fig. 23.16)
  For Anterior Shoulder Dislocations
  The patient is seated sideways in a chair with the arm hanging over the backrest.
  The clinician holds the patient's arm, while the patient stands providing self-traction.
  Success rate of 73% has been reported.

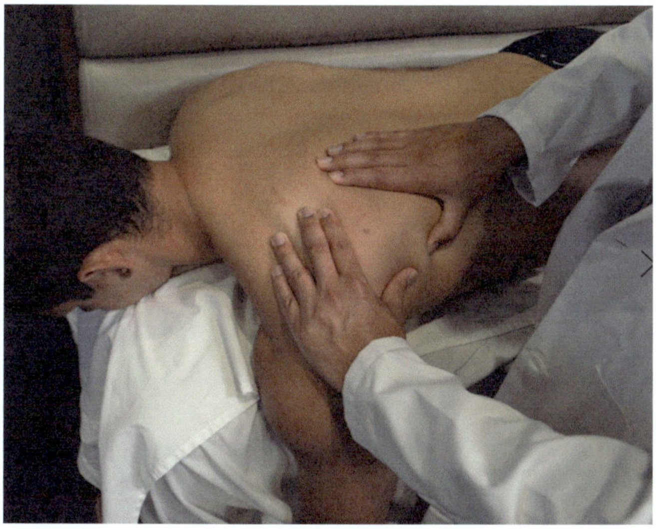

Fig. 23.15 Scapular manipulation: The patient lies on a prone position with the affected arm hanging vertically over the edge of the table. The clinician provides gentle traction, and reduction is attempted by pushing on the tip of the scapula medially, with rotation of the superior aspect of the scapula laterally

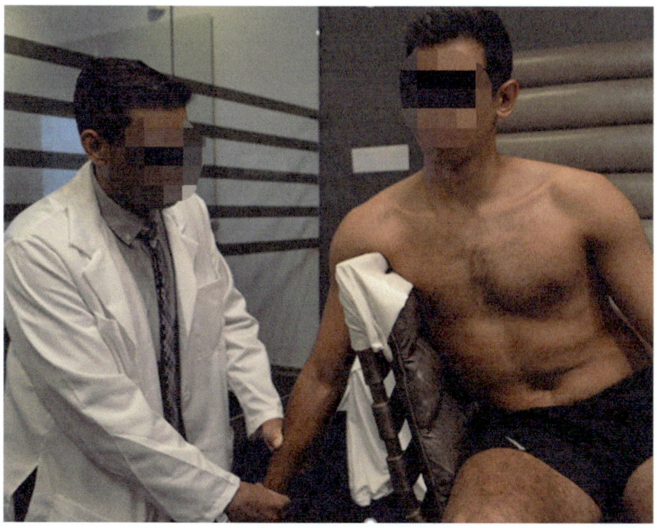

Fig. 23.16 Chair technique: The patient is seated sideways in a chair with the arm hanging over the backrest. The clinician then holds the patient's arm, while the patient stands providing self-traction

23.9.1.3 Posterior Glenohumeral Dislocations

Closed reduction of a posterior shoulder dislocation is recommended for those who have <20% of a reverse Hill-Sachs lesion [36].

- *Stimson Technique*
  For Posterior Shoulder Dislocations
  The patient is placed in a prone position on a table with the arm abducted and holding 5–10 LBS of weight in the hand.
- *Traction Technique*
  For Posterior Shoulder Dislocations
  The clinician forward flexes the shoulder to 90° then adducts and internally rotates the arm.
  An assistant provides longitudinal traction while the clinician provides anteriorly directed pressure on the humeral head.

23.9.1.4 Inferior Glenohumeral Dislocations

Since the humeral head separates inferiorly from the glenoid and lodges in the infra-glenoid region, the arm is in a fixed and abducted position. Two-step maneuver allows for conversion of an inferior shoulder dislocation to anterior dislocation. The clinical may then perform an anterior dislocation maneuver to complete reduction.

- *Two-step maneuver* [37]
  For Inferior Shoulder Dislocations
  The patient is lying supine, and the clinician is standing at the patient's head while placing one hand on the shaft of the humerus providing an anterior force with the other hand on the medial condyle. This will move the humeral head anteriorly converting the inferior dislocation to an anterior dislocation.

23.9.2 Rehabilitation

Post-glenohumeral reduction period may include a period of immobilization; however, there are conflicting evidence regarding the length of immobilization to patient outcomes as it is unclear if 3 weeks of immobilization is superior to 1 week [20, 38–42]. Generally, the patient may implement a *passive range of motion* (ROM) exercise program afterward as well as *isometric shoulder exercises* to maintain musculature. External rotation and internal rotation past neutral should be limited for anterior and posterior dislocations, respectively, for 4–6 weeks. Return to sports can be recommended after the patient has full strength and painless ROM.

23.9.3 Procedures

The clinician may inject 10–20 mL of lidocaine or bupivacaine into the glenohumeral joint for pain relief. Intra-articular lidocaine has been found as effective as using intravenous analgesia with or without sedation for pain relief prior to manual reduction [43]. For hospital-assisted glenohumeral dislocations, procedural sedation may be offered so the reduction could be tolerated by the patient.

23.9.4 Surgery

Patients with a high risk of recurrent glenohumeral dislocations may elect for surgical repair (arthroscopic versus open stabilization) which may also include anatomic repair of the Bankart lesion [23]. For more details please See Chap. 24: Shoulder surgeries.

23.10 Clavicle Fracture Treatments

23.10.1 Medical Management

A clinician must take in consideration hand dominance involvement which may be surrogate for functional outcomes as well as activity level for the treatment of clavicular fractures. Conservative management is preferred for almost all acute and nondisplaced (<5 mm) clavicle fracture (Neer I and III). Though a previous study by Rokito et al. [44] showed similar results with conservative and surgical management of Type II Neer fractures, other studies demonstrated rates ranging 28–44% of non-union outcomes after conservative management [45–48].

23.10.2 Rehabilitation

The patient should have a brief period of immobilization followed by range of motion exercises. Treatment with an arm sling is favored over a figure-of-eight dressing as it is better tolerated [49, 50]. The clinician may clear an athlete for initiation of non-contact sports after radiographic studies show healthy healing at 6 weeks after injury. In addition, it was found that most patients may return to contact sports after 16 weeks [51].

23.10.3 Surgery

Surgical consultation may be warranted if there is >5 mm displacement without any bony contact and if there is skin compromised by bony fragments [52, 53]. For a displaced distal clavicle fracture with intact CC ligaments (Type IIA, V), a pre-contoured locking plate or hook plate may be considered. For CC ligament disruption, other surgical options include intramedullary fixation or tension band wiring [53].

23.11 Proximal Humeral Fracture Treatments

23.11.1 Medical Management

It is estimated that around 80% of proximal humerus fractures are minimally displaced or nondisplaced. Conservative management is the preferred treatment [54]. A Cochrane review of 31 studies showed that compared with conservative management, surgery does not provide better outcomes at 1–2 years after sustaining a displaced proximal humeral fracture and may progress for a need of further surgery in the future [55].

23.11.2 Rehabilitation

Studies have shown that early ROM and physical therapy after 1 week may result in better functional and pain outcomes [56]. Early rehabilitation includes restoring early shoulder movement and prevention of pathological compensatory strategies for shoulder girdle movement. Intermediate and late stages include starting proprioceptive exercises to improve shoulder control and close-chain exercises to progressive resistance training. The clinician may recommend contact activities between 3 months and 5 months, depending on if radiographic studies show healthy healing [25].

23.11.3 Surgery

Young and active patients with two-, three-, and four-part fractures may be referred to an orthopedic surgeon. If surgery is considered, options included open reduction and internal fixation (ORIF), closed reduction and percutaneous pinning (CRPP), hemiarthroplasty (HA), and reverse total shoulder arthroplasty (RSA) [27].

23.12 Scapular Fracture Treatment

23.12.1 Medical Management

Most scapular fractures are managed conservatively.

23.12.2 Rehabilitation

There is a consensus of immobilization in a sling for 1–2 weeks with limiting weight-bearing restrictions following passive ROM with pendulum swings. Afterward, the patient may initiated active-assisted ROM at 4 weeks with progressive strengthening exercises at 8 weeks [57].

23.12.3 Surgery

Surgical intervention for internal fixation is generally considered during two occasions [25]:

- A fracture of scapular neck associated with a clavicle fracture creating an unstable floating shoulder
- A displaced fracture of the glenoid which can promote chronic shoulder dislocations

References

1. Cools AM, Dewitte V, Lanszweert F, Notebaert D, Roets A, Soetens B, et al. Rehabilitation of scapular muscle balance: which exercises to prescribe? Am J Sports Med. 2007;35(10):1744–51.
2. Kibler WB. The role of the scapula in athletic shoulder function. Am J Sports Med. 1998;26(2):325–37.
3. Adams CR, DeMartino AM, Rego G, Denard PJ, Burkhart SS. The rotator cuff and the superior capsule: why we need both. Arthroscopy. 2016;32(12):2628–37.
4. Turkel SJ, Panio MW, Marshall JL, Girgis FG. Stabilizing mechanisms preventing anterior dislocation of the glenohumeral joint. J Bone Joint Surg Am. 1981;63(8):1208–17.
5. Lugo R, Kung P, Ma CB. Shoulder biomechanics. Eur J Radiol. 2008;68(1):16–24.
6. Howell SM, Galinat BJ. The glenoid-labral socket. A constrained articular surface. Clin Orthop Relat Res. 1989;243:122–5.
7. Di Giacomo G, Piscitelli L, Pugliese M. The role of bone in glenohumeral stability. EFORT Open Rev. 2018;3(12):632–40.
8. Bakhsh W, Nicandri G. Anatomy and physical examination of the shoulder. Sports Med Arthrosc Rev. 2018;26(3):e10–22.
9. Halder AM, Itoi E, An KN. Anatomy and biomechanics of the shoulder. Orthop Clin North Am. 2000;31(2):159–76.
10. Abboud JA, Soslowsky LJ. Interplay of the static and dynamic restraints in glenohumeral instability. Clin Orthop Relat Res. 2002;400:48–57.
11. Wolfe JA, Christensen DL, Mauntel TC, Owens BD, LeClere LE, Dickens JF. A history of shoulder instability in the military: where we have been and what we have learned. Mil Med. 2018;183(5–6):e158–e65.
12. Enger M, Skjaker SA, Melhuus K, Nordsletten L, Pripp AH, Moosmayer S, et al. Shoulder injuries from birth to old age: a 1-year prospective study of 3031 shoulder injuries in an urban population. Injury. 2018;49(7):1324–9.
13. Lizzio VA, Meta F, Fidai M, Makhni EC. Clinical evaluation and physical exam findings in patients with anterior shoulder instability. Curr Rev Musculoskelet Med. 2017;10(4):434–41.
14. Rowe CR. Prognosis in dislocations of the shoulder. J Bone Joint Surg Am. 1956;38-A(5):957–77.
15. Leroux T, Wasserstein D, Veillette C, Khoshbin A, Henry P, Chahal J, et al. Epidemiology of primary anterior shoulder dislocation requiring closed reduction in Ontario, Canada. Am J Sports Med. 2014;42(2):442–50.
16. Youm T, Takemoto R, Park BK. Acute management of shoulder dislocations. J Am Acad Orthop Surg. 2014;22(12):761–71.
17. Kowalsky MS, Levine WN. Traumatic posterior glenohumeral dislocation: classification, pathoanatomy, diagnosis, and treatment. Orthop Clin North Am. 2008;39(4):519–33, viii.
18. Mc LH. Posterior dislocation of the shoulder. J Bone Joint Surg Am. 1952;24 A(3):584–90.
19. Goudie EB, Murray IR, Robinson CM. Instability of the shoulder following seizures. J Bone Joint Surg. 2012;94-B(6):721–8.
20. Robinson CM, Shur N, Sharpe T, Ray A, Murray IR. Injuries associated with traumatic anterior glenohumeral dislocations. J Bone Joint Surg Am. 2012;94(1):18–26.
21. Rowe CR, Patel D, Southmayd WW. The Bankart procedure: a long-term end-result study. J Bone Joint Surg Am. 1978;60(1):1–16.
22. Provencher MT, Frank RM, Leclere LE, Metzger PD, Ryu JJ, Bernhardson A, et al. The Hill-Sachs lesion: diagnosis, classification, and management. J Am Acad Orthop Surg. 2012;20(4):242–52.
23. Kane P, Bifano SM, Dodson CC, Freedman KB. Approach to the treatment of primary anterior shoulder dislocation: a review. Phys Sportsmed. 2015;43(1):54–64.
24. Kim W, McKee MD. Management of acute clavicle fractures. Orthop Clin North Am. 2008;39(4):491–505, vii.
25. Burnier M, Barlow JD, Sanchez-Sotelo J. Shoulder and elbow fractures in athletes. Curr Rev Musculoskelet Med. 2019;12(1):13–23.
26. Stenson J, Baker W. Classifications in brief: the modified NEER classification for distal-third clavicle fractures. Clin Orthop Relat Res. 2021;479(1):205–9.
27. Gupta AK, Harris JD, Erickson BJ, Abrams GD, Bruce B, McCormick F, et al. Surgical management of complex proximal humerus fractures-a systematic review of 92 studies including 4500 patients. J Orthop Trauma. 2015;29(1):54–9.
28. Court-Brown CM, Garg A, McQueen MM. The epidemiology of proximal humeral fractures. Acta Orthop Scand. 2001;72(4):365–71.
29. Goss TP. Scapular fractures and dislocations: diagnosis and treatment. J Am Acad Orthop Surg. 1995;3(1):22–33.
30. Harvey E, Audigé L, Herscovici DJ, Agel J, Madsen JE, Babst R, et al. Development and validation of the new international classification for scapula fractures. J Orthop Trauma. 2012;26(6):364–9.
31. Bahrs C, Rolauffs B, Dietz K, Eingartner C, Weise K. Clinical and radiological evaluation of minimally displaced proximal humeral fractures. Arch Orthop Trauma Surg. 2010;130(5):673–9.
32. Farber AJ, Castillo R, Clough M, Bahk M, McFarland EG. Clinical assessment of three common tests for traumatic anterior shoulder instability. J Bone Joint Surg Am. 2006;88(7):1467–74.
33. Speer KP, Hannafin JA, Altchek DW, Warren RF. An evaluation of the shoulder relocation test. Am J Sports Med. 1994;22(2):177–83.
34. McFarland EG. Examination of the shoulder: the complete guide. New York: Thieme; 2006.
35. Entezari P, Jalili M, Seyedhosseini J, Doosti-Irani A, Mirfazaelian H. Accuracy of ultrasonography in diagnosis of shoulder dislocation: a systematic review. Adv J Emerg Med. 2020;4(1):e9.
36. Rouleau DM, Hebert-Davies J, Robinson CM. Acute traumatic posterior shoulder dislocation. J Am Acad Orthop Surg. 2014;22(3):145–52.
37. Nho SJ, Dodson CC, Bardzik KF, Brophy RH, Domb BG, MacGillivray JD. The two-step maneuver for closed reduction of inferior glenohumeral dislocation (luxatio erecta to anterior dislocation to reduction). J Orthop Trauma. 2006;20(5):354–7.
38. Hovelius L, Olofsson A, Sandström B, Augustini BG, Krantz L, Fredin H, et al. Nonoperative treatment of primary anterior shoulder dislocation in patients forty years of age and younger. A prospective twenty-five-year follow-up. J Bone Joint Surg Am. 2008;90(5):945–52.

39. Hovelius L, Augustini BG, Fredin H, Johansson O, Norlin R, Thorling J. Primary anterior dislocation of the shoulder in young patients. A ten-year prospective study. J Bone Joint Surg Am. 1996;78(11):1677–84.
40. Hovelius L. Anterior dislocation of the shoulder in teen-agers and young adults. Five-year prognosis. J Bone Joint Surg Am. 1987;69(3):393–9.
41. Hovelius L, Eriksson K, Fredin H, Hagberg G, Hussenius A, Lind B, et al. Recurrences after initial dislocation of the shoulder. Results of a prospective study of treatment. J Bone Joint Surg Am. 1983;65(3):343–9.
42. Kiviluoto O, Pasila M, Jaroma H, Sundholm A. Immobilization after primary dislocation of the shoulder. Acta Orthop Scand. 1980;51(6):915–9.
43. Wakai A, O'Sullivan R, McCabe A. Intra-articular lignocaine versus intravenous analgesia with or without sedation for manual reduction of acute anterior shoulder dislocation in adults. Cochrane Database Syst Rev. 2011;(4):Cd004919.
44. Rokito AS, Zuckerman JD, Shaari JM, Eisenberg DP, Cuomo F, Gallagher MA. A comparison of nonoperative and operative treatment of type II distal clavicle fractures. Bull Hosp Jt Dis. 2002;61(1–2):32–9.
45. Robinson CM, Cairns DA. Primary nonoperative treatment of displaced lateral fractures of the clavicle. J Bone Joint Surg Am. 2004;86(4):778–82.
46. Robinson CM, Court-Brown CM, McQueen MM, Wakefield AE. Estimating the risk of nonunion following nonoperative treatment of a clavicular fracture. J Bone Joint Surg Am. 2004;86(7):1359–65.
47. Deafenbaugh MK, Dugdale TW, Staeheli JW, Nielsen R. Nonoperative treatment of Neer type II distal clavicle fractures: a prospective study. Contemp Orthop. 1990;20(4):405–13.
48. Neer CS 2nd. Fracture of the distal clavicle with detachment of the coracoclavicular ligaments in adults. J Trauma. 1963;3:99–110.
49. Andersen K, Jensen PO, Lauritzen J. Treatment of clavicular fractures. Figure-of-eight bandage versus a simple sling. Acta Orthop Scand. 1987;58(1):71–4.
50. Stanley D, Norris SH. Recovery following fractures of the clavicle treated conservatively. Injury. 1988;19(3):162–4.
51. Hebert-Davies J, Agel J. Return to elite-level sport after clavicle fractures. BMJ Open Sport Exerc Med. 2018;4(1):e000371.
52. Zlowodzki M, Zelle BA, Cole PA, Jeray K, McKee MD. Treatment of acute midshaft clavicle fractures: systematic review of 2144 fractures: on behalf of the Evidence-Based Orthopaedic Trauma Working Group. J Orthop Trauma. 2005;19(7):504–7.
53. Kim DW, Kim DH, Kim BS, Cho CH. Current concepts for classification and treatment of distal clavicle fractures. Clin Orthop Surg. 2020;12(2):135–44.
54. Skariah JM, Rasmussen C, Hollander-Rodriguez J, Carney PA, Dexter E, Waller E, et al. Rural curricular guidelines based on practice scope of recent residency graduates practicing in small communities. Fam Med. 2017;49(8):594–9.
55. Handoll HH, Ollivere BJ, Rollins KE. Interventions for treating proximal humeral fractures in adults. Cochrane Database Syst Rev. 2012;12:CD000434.
56. Hodgson S. Proximal humerus fracture rehabilitation. Clin Orthop Relat Res. 2006;442:131–8.
57. Seidl AJ, Joyce CD. Acute fractures of the glenoid. J Am Acad Orthop Surg. 2020;28(22):e978–e87.

Shoulder Surgeries

24

Alfred J. Tria Jr, Jeremy Silver, Casey Imbergamo, and Andrzej Brzezinski

24.1 Soft Tissue and Muscle Injuries

24.1.1 Rotator Cuff Injury

Injuries to the rotator cuff occur on a continuum ranging from impingement to full-thickness tendon tears. The supraspinatus is the most frequently damaged tendon; however, tears can occur in any of the four rotator cuff muscles [1]. Factors that impact the management of rotator cuff tears are vast and include patient age and activity level, etiology of the tear (degenerative vs. traumatic), size and location of the tear, and functional deficits. For patients that fail nonoperative management, several surgical options may be considered. In patients with partial tears, arthroscopic subacromial decompression or acromioplasty is indicated [2]. In full-thickness tears, arthroscopic or open rotator cuff repair is typically performed [3]. In select cases of massive or irreparable rotator cuff tears, pectoralis major or latissimus dorsi tendon transfer is the surgery of choice. Additionally, the use of allograft, xenograft, or synthetic patches to repair massive rotator cuff tears is a novel area of research [4].

Following rotator cuff repair, patients are immobilized in a sling for 4 weeks, removing it only for physical therapy. In the early postoperative period, it is imperative to protect the repair. At 3 weeks postoperatively, gentle passive range of motion (ROM) and pendulum exercises can be initiated. Limited active ROM can begin at 4 weeks with a gradual progression to full active ROM at approximately 10 weeks. By 4 months postoperatively, advanced strengthening exercises can be initiated with gradual return to full functional activities over the subsequent months. The rate-limiting step in rotator cuff repair is a biologic healing of the tendon to the humeral head, which may take approximately 8–12 weeks [5].

A. J. Tria Jr (✉) · J. Silver · C. Imbergamo · A. Brzezinski
Department of Orthopaedics, Rutgers-Robert Wood Johnson Medical School, New Brunswick, NJ, USA

24.1.2 Shoulder Labrum Injury

Shoulder labral injuries when associated with dislocations in younger individuals (<30 years of age) have varying injury patterns. The most prevalent are SLAP (superior labrum from anterior to posterior) and Bankart (anteroinferior labral tears with glenoid avulsion) lesions [6]. Labral tears that fail to respond to conservative management can be addressed surgically. Arthroscopic management of labral pathologies has been gaining popularity among orthopedic surgeons in recent years. Depending on the location and pattern of the tear, surgery can entail debridement of frayed tissue, repair of the labrum, capsulorrhaphy (tightening of the articular capsule), and additional tenotomy or tenodesis of the biceps tendon if needed [7, 8].

In the early rehabilitation stages, patients may remain in a sling throughout the day, coming out only for physical therapy. Isometric exercises and passive ROM are begun with limitations in order to protect the repair. Between 4 and 6 weeks postoperatively, patients may progress to active ROM with gradual advancement to strengthening and functional training by 12 weeks. Return to sport typically occurs at approximately 6 months but may be longer in throwing or overhead athletes [9].

24.1.3 Pectoralis Major Tendon Injury

Acute rupture of the pectoralis major muscle is typically observed in young athletes and is commonly associated with weightlifting. Primary repair is the treatment of choice for complete tears, and in rare cases of chronic tears that cannot be mobilized for primary repair, reconstruction with Achilles allograft can be considered [10, 11]. For patients who choose not to undergo surgical repair of a pectoralis rupture, a significant strength deficit is to be expected, specifically in shoulder adduction. Additionally, such patients may experience delayed recovery, unsatisfactory cosmetic outcomes, and for athletes, lower rates of return to competitive sports.

© The Author(s), under exclusive license to Springer Nature Switzerland AG 2022

S. A. Mostoufi et al. (eds.), *Clinical Guide to Musculoskeletal Medicine*, https://doi.org/10.1007/978-3-030-92042-5_24

Postoperatively, the arm is fully immobilized in a sling for 2 weeks to protect the repair. After 2 weeks, gentle passive ROM can be initiated with limitations on external rotation and abduction. Patients may discontinue the use of the sling at 4–6 weeks and begin progressing to active ROM. After 6 weeks, muscle strength and endurance are subsequently increased over the course of 3–4 months. By approximately 6 months, patients can gradually return to full activities as tolerated [12]. If non-surgical treatment is pursued, a short period of immobilization (2 weeks) followed by passive and active ROM exercises is recommended [10].

24.1.4 Proximal Biceps Tendon Injury

Proximal biceps tendon rupture is highly correlated with rotator cuff pathology, which must be considered when managing patients with this condition. Proximal biceps rupture is more common in elderly patients, and non-surgical management is often sufficient for this condition. However, in more active patients who opt for surgical intervention, biceps tenodesis can be performed with either interference screws or bio-absorbable suture anchors [13].

Postoperatively, the arm is immobilized in a sling with gentle passive ROM beginning at 1–2 weeks. Full passive ROM should be achieved by 4 weeks, with active ROM beginning at this point. At 6–8 weeks, progressive strengthening exercises can be implemented, and by approximately week 10, patients may return to full unrestricted activities as tolerated. More information on this topic can be found in the Elbow Chap. 25.

24.2 Shoulder Osteoarthritis

24.2.1 Glenohumeral Osteoarthritis (OA)

Glenohumeral arthritis is a common cause of shoulder pain, especially in the aging population. A multitude of etiologies contribute to glenohumeral arthritis including degenerative, post-traumatic, rotator cuff arthropathy, and inflammatory, among others. While there is no universal treatment algorithm, physical therapy and non-steroidal anti-inflammatory drugs (NSAIDS) are considered the first-line treatment, while intra-articular steroid injections are second line [14]. Patients that fail conservative management can be indicated for several surgeries ranging from arthroscopic debridement to arthroplasty [15]. Following arthroscopic debridement, patients may remain in a sling in the early postoperative period, typically weaning at 1–2 weeks. Gentle passive and active ROM can begin 1 week postoperatively, in addition to isometric rotator cuff exercises. Range of motion and progressive resistance exercises can be advanced from weeks 2–6, and full return to activity as tolerated can be expected at 6 weeks.

Arthroplasty can take the form of hemiarthroplasty, total shoulder arthroplasty (TSA), or reverse total shoulder arthroplasty (rTSA). While TSA maintains the anatomic alignment of having a convex humeral head and concave glenoid, a rTSA utilizes a convex glenoid and concave humeral head. Stability of the shoulder after TSA depends on the function of the rotator cuff muscles. rTSA is indicated in patients with rotator cuff damage, as it shifts the center of rotation inferiorly and medially, allowing the deltoid to raise the arm more effectively and stabilize the shoulder.

Following shoulder arthroplasty, patients should remain in a sling for 3 weeks to protect the repair. Gentle passive ROM can be initiated in the early postoperative period, and active ROM can be incorporated into rehabilitation at 4–6 weeks postoperatively. Following TSA, external rotation (ER) of the shoulder must be limited due to a risk of injury to the subscapularis tendon and further shoulder instability. In case of rTSA, stability and mobility of the shoulder joint depend upon the deltoid musculature. After rTSA, patients are at risk of dislocation with the arm in internal rotation and adduction in conjunction with extension. Thus, tucking in one's shirt or performing bathroom hygiene with the operative arm is particularly dangerous. These precautions should remain in effect for at least 12 weeks postoperatively.

24.2.2 Acromioclavicular Osteoarthritis (OA)

Another problem highly prevalent in the aging population is acromioclavicular (AC) joint arthritis. Treatment for AC arthritis also generally follows a stepwise approach with physical therapy, activity modification, use of NSAIDs, and occasionally joint injections. AC arthritis that is refractory to these conservative measures may be treated surgically with either arthroscopic or open distal clavicle resection [16].

Postoperatively, the patient should remain in the sling for a period of 4–6 weeks and avoid excessive arm abduction and rotation.

24.3 Shoulder Dislocation and Fractures

Fractures of the shoulder are managed based upon several anatomic and patient-specific variables. Anatomic factors include location, fracture pattern, and degree/direction of displacement, while patient factors include age, activity level, and mechanism of injury. Management of these injuries is frequently categorized based upon location.

24.3.1 Clavicle Fracture

Clavicle fractures are common in the young adult (mostly male <30 years of age) and generally are localized in the midshaft followed by lateral and medial end of the clavicle. Most clavicle fractures, regardless of location, can be treated with sling immobilization for a period of roughly 2 weeks followed by early ROM with weightbearing at around 6 weeks [17]. Surgical management should be considered in the case of open fractures, severely displaced (>100% displacing and >2 cm shortening), associated with disruption of the CC ligaments, neurovascular impairment, floating shoulder, or multitrauma [17]. Surgical treatment may also be considered for any displaced clavicle fracture in athletes to facilitate better postoperative mobility and earlier return to sport [18].

Rehabilitation protocol after surgery is similar to non-operative management.

24.3.2 Scapula Fracture

The scapula is a complex bone that can be fractured in multiple places. Non-operative management of scapular fractures consists of sling immobilization for 2–3 weeks followed by early motion. Indications for surgical management are ill-defined but include intra-articular glenoid fractures with significant displacement and floating shoulders. A floating shoulder is considered when there is a scapular neck fracture with associated AC joint injury or clavicle fractures. Open reduction and internal fixation (ORIF) is the preferred surgical management for these fractures.

Postoperatively, rehabilitation is generally performed similarly to non-surgical management [19].

24.3.3 Humerus Fracture

Management of humeral fractures depends on fracture morphology and location. Non-operative treatment is the mainstay for minimally displaced (<1 cm displacement or/and <45° angulation), extra-articular proximal humerus fractures and consists of 2 weeks of sling immobilization followed by early passive ROM [20]. Serial x-rays should accompany office evaluation of these fractures to ensure stability. Surgical intervention is recommended for displaced (>1 cm, >45°, or >0.5 cm for greater tuberosity) two or more-part proximal humerus fractures in active patients, head-splitting, open fractures, or fractures associated with shoulder dislocation. Most often fracture fixation is accomplished with ORIF or intramedullary nailing [20]. In older patients, arthroplasty should be considered [21].

Postoperative rehabilitation protocols depend on the surgical procedure; however, they generally include early passive ROM followed by active ROM with progressive resistance and strengthening.

24.3.4 Glenohumeral Dislocations

Dislocations of the shoulder most commonly occur in younger males but can occur at any age. Anterior shoulder dislocation is most common and results from forced abduction, external rotation, and extension of the shoulder. Posterior shoulder dislocations can occur with a fall onto an outstretched and internally rotated arm or might be associated with tetanic muscle contractions occurring during seizure or electric shock. Inferior shoulder dislocations are the least common and typically occur with sudden forceful arm hyperabduction. Closed reduction of shoulder dislocations should be attempted as early as possible. Following reduction of a shoulder dislocation, the arm is immobilized in a sling for 1–3 weeks [22]. After this period, the patient can advance to rotator cuff strengthening and ROM exercises, while avoiding activities that place the arm in a high-risk position (excessive IR for posterior dislocations, abduction/ER for anterior dislocations, and hyperabduction for inferior dislocations). Patients who suffer posterior shoulder dislocations are also immobilized in 10–20° of external rotation with the elbow at the patient's side.

Following anterior dislocations, placing the arm in ER may create a greater contact force between the glenoid and labrum [23]. However, the recent meta-analyses have failed to prove a difference in re-dislocation rates between immobilization in ER and IR, and most surgeons recommend immobilization in IR which is more tolerable by the patients [24, 25]. Surgical indications following shoulder dislocation aim at providing shoulder stability and preventing recurrent dislocations. There are multiple described techniques that vary from open vs. closed procedures and range from direct repair of the labrum to bone grafting and other techniques [24]. Postoperatively, patients are typically immobilized in a sling with the arm in a neutral position for 4–6 weeks, followed by gradual advancement of ROM and progressive resistance exercises. Full return to activities may occur at approximately 6 months postoperatively.

24.3.5 Acromioclavicular Separations/Dislocations

AC joint dislocation, commonly referred to as a "separated shoulder," generally occurs in younger patients. Rockwood classified these injuries into six types based on the degree and direction of displacement, as well as involvement of acromioclavicular (AC) and coracoclavicular (CC) ligaments. Management of AC injuries is generally based upon the integrity of the CC ligaments. Type I and II injuries (<100% displacement and intact CC ligament) are treated non-operatively. Treatment of type III injuries (AC and CC ligament is torn, <100% displacement) is individualized with the majority treated non-surgically with good functional results. Type IV–VI (AC and CC ligaments torn, >100% displacement posteriorly, superiorly, and inferiorly, respectively) injuries are treated with surgical management, which includes reduction of the AC joint with reconstruction of the CC ligaments. Technique for repair is surgeon-specific and may include ORIF of the AC joint with either direct repair or reconstruction of the CC ligaments with sutures, screws, autograft, or allograft.

Operative fixation is generally followed by a period of sling immobilization for roughly 6 weeks [26]. Shoulder ROM is prohibited for the first 6 weeks; however, gentle isometric rotator cuff exercises can be instituted at 2 weeks. Following 6 weeks of immobilization, patients may begin ROM and progressive resistance exercises with gradual progression over the subsequent months. Return to full activity can be expected at approximately 6 months.

References

1. Kim HM, Dahiya N, Teefey SA, Middleton WD, Stobbs G, Steger-May K, Yamaguchi K, Keener JD. Location and initiation of degenerative rotator cuff tears: an analysis of three hundred and sixty shoulders. J Bone Joint Surg Am. 2010;92(5):1088–96. https://doi.org/10.2106/JBJS.I.00686.
2. Khan M, Alolabi B, Horner N, Bedi A, Ayeni OR, Bhandari M. Surgery for shoulder impingement: a systematic review and meta-analysis of controlled clinical trials. CMAJ Open. 2019;7(1):E149–58. https://doi.org/10.9778/cmajo.20180179.
3. Huang R, Wang S, Wang Y, Qin X, Sun Y. Systematic review of all-arthroscopic versus mini-open repair of rotator cuff tears: a meta-analysis. Sci Rep. 2016;6:22857. https://doi.org/10.1038/srep22857.
4. Gillespie RJ, Knapik DM, Akkus O. Biologic and synthetic grafts in the reconstruction of large to massive rotator cuff tears. J Am Acad Orthop Surg. 2016;24(12):823–8. https://doi.org/10.5435/JAAOS-D-15-00229.
5. Lee BG, Cho NS, Rhee YG. Effect of two rehabilitation protocols on range of motion and healing rates after arthroscopic rotator cuff repair: aggressive versus limited early passive exercises. Arthroscopy. 2012;28(1):34–42. https://doi.org/10.1016/j.arthro.2011.07.012.
6. Sedeek SM, Bin Abd Razak HR, Ee GW, Tan AH. First-time anterior shoulder dislocations: should they be arthroscopically stabilised? Singap Med J. 2014;55(10):511–6. https://doi.org/10.11622/smedj.2014132.
7. Brockmeyer M, Tompkins M, Kohn DM, Lorbach O. SLAP lesions: a treatment algorithm. Knee Surg Sport Traumatol Arthrosc. 2016;24(2):447–55. https://doi.org/10.1007/s00167-015-3966-0.
8. Mair SD, Zarzour R, Speer KP. Posterior labral injury in contact athletes. Am J Sports Med. 1998;26(6):753–8. https://doi.org/10.1177/03635465980260060301.
9. Blackburn TA, Guido JA. Rehabilitation after ligamentous and labral surgery of the shoulder: guiding concepts. J Athl Train. 2000;35(3):373–81. PMID:16558650.
10. Durant EJ, De Cicco FL. Pectoralis major tear. StatPearls; 2020. PMID:31751065.
11. Lipman A, Strauss E. Treatment of pectoralis major muscle ruptures. Bull Hosp Jt Dis. 2016;74(1):63–72. PMID:26977551.
12. Manske RC, Prohaska D. Pectoralis major tendon repair post surgical rehabilitation. N Am J Sports Phys Ther. 2007;2(1):22–33. PMID21522200.
13. Scully WF, Wilson DJ, Grassbaugh JA, Branstetter JG, Marchant BG, Arrington ED. A simple surgical technique for subpectoral biceps tenodesis using a double-loaded suture anchor. Arthrosc Tech. 2013;2(2):e191–6. https://doi.org/10.1016/j.eats.2013.02.005.
14. Millett PJ, Gobezie R, Boykin RE. Shoulder osteoarthritis: diagnosis and management. Am Fam Physician. 2008;78(5):605–11. PMID: 18788237.
15. Izquierdo R, Voloshin I, Edwards S, Freehill MQ, Stanwood W, Wiater JM, Watters WC, Goldberg MJ, Keith M, Turkelson CM, Wies JL, Anderson S, Boyer K, Raymond L, Sluka P. Treatment of glenohumeral osteoarthritis. J Am Acad Orthop Surg. 2010;18(6):375–82. https://doi.org/10.5435/00124635-201006000-00010.
16. Menge TJ, Boykin RE, Bushnell BD, Byram IR. Acromioclavicular osteoarthritis: a common cause of shoulder pain. South Med J. 2014;107(5):324–9. https://doi.org/10.1097/SMJ.0000000000000101.
17. van der Meijden OA, Gaskill TR, Millett PJ. Treatment of clavicle fractures: current concepts review. J Shoulder Elb Surg. 2012;21(3):423–9. https://doi.org/10.1016/j.jse.2011.08.053.
18. Burnier M, Barlow JD, Sanchez-Sotelo J. Shoulder and elbow fractures in athletes. Curr Rev Musculoskelet Med. 2019;12(1):13–23. https://doi.org/10.1007/s12178-019-09530-0.
19. Cole PA, Gauger EM, Schroder LK. Management of scapular fractures. J Am Acad Orthop Surg. 2012;20(3):130–41. https://doi.org/10.5435/JAAOS-20-03-130.
20. Pencle FJ, Varacallo M. Proximal humerus fracture. [Updated 2020 Aug 16]. In: StatPearls [Internet]. Treasure Island (FL): StatPearls Publishing; 2021.
21. Khmelnitskaya E, Lamont LE, Taylor SA, Lorich DG, Dines DM, Dines JS. Evaluation and management of proximal humerus fractures. Adv Orthop. 2012:861598. https://doi.org/10.1155/2012/861598.
22. Paterson WH, Throckmorton TW, Koester M, Azar FM, Kuhn JE. Position and duration of immobilization after primary anterior shoulder dislocation: a systematic review and meta-analysis of the literature. J Bone Joint Surg Am. 2010;92(18):2924–33.
23. Gutkowska O, Martynkiewicz J, Gosk J. Position of immobilization after first-time traumatic anterior glenohumeral dislocation: a literature review. Med Sci Monit. 2017;23:3437–45.
24. Braun C, McRobert CJ. Conservative management following closed reduction of traumatic anterior dislocation of the shoulder. Cochrane Database Syst Rev. 2019;2019(5):CD004962. https://doi.org/10.1002/14651858.CD004962.pub4.
25. Kavaja L, Lähdeoja T, Malmivaara A, Paavola M. Treatment after traumatic shoulder dislocation: a systematic review with a network meta-analysis. Br J Sports Med. 2018;52(23):1498–506. https://doi.org/10.1136/bjsports-2017-098539.
26. Li X, Ma R, Bedi A, Dines DM, Altchek DW, Dines JS. Management of acromioclavicular joint injuries. J Bone Joint Surg Am. 2014;96(1):73–84. https://doi.org/10.2106/JBJS.L.00734.

Part V

Elbow

Section Editor
Jason L. Zaremski

Anterior Elbow Disorders

25

Julio A. Martinez-Silvestrini

25.1 Distal Biceps Tendinopathy at the Elbow

25.1.1 Synonyms

- Distal biceps tendonitis
- Distal biceps tendinosis
- Distal biceps enthesopathy
- Distal biceps paratenonitis
- Distal biceps peritendinitis

25.1.2 ICD-10 Codes

- S46.211 Strain of muscle, fascia and tendon of other parts of biceps, right arm
- S46.212 Strain of muscle, fascia and tendon of other parts of biceps, left arm
- M70.31 Other bursitis of elbow, right elbow
- M70.32 Other bursitis of elbow, left elbow

25.1.3 Description

Anterior elbow pain is uncommon, compared to medial or lateral elbow pain. The most common causes of anterior elbow pain involve the biceps brachii tendon. Biceps tendinopathy at the elbow presents with an insidious course of anterior elbow pain, particularly with repetitive or resisted flexion and resisted supination of the forearm. This injury is commonly seen in middle-aged men and related repetitive flexion, extension, pronation, and supination of the elbow, such as in the case of mechanics, construction workers, and carpenters [1, 2]. Further, exercises such as dumbbell curls can cause stress to the biceps distal tendon. The tendon may be primarily involved at the mid-substance (tendinosis), and its insertion (enthesopathy) or the sheath around it may be involved (paratenonitis) [3].

J. A. Martinez-Silvestrini (✉)
Baystate Physical Medicine and Rehabilitation, Baystate Medical Center, Springfield, MA, USA

Tufts University School of Medicine, Boston, MA, USA

University of Massachusetts Medical School – Baystate, Longmeadow, MA, USA
e-mail: Julio.martinez@bhs.org

25.1.3.1 Anatomy

The elbow joint is composed of three bones (humerus, radius, and ulna) and three joints (humeroulnar, proximal radioulnar, and radiocapitellar joint) (Fig. 25.1). The humeral trochlea articulates with the ulnar olecranon, while the radius head articulates with both the proximal ulna and the humeral capitellum. It is primarily a hinged joint which allows for shortening of the upper extremity to facilitate activities closer to the body (like buttoning a shirt) and lengthening of the limb to increase our reach and interactions with the environment [3]. Compared to other hinged joints like the knee, the elbow also allows for rotation of the terminal limb, the forearm, and the wrist, known as pronation and supination, allowing for increased range of motion and dexterity of the distal upper extremity. At the antecubital fossa, a neurovascular bundle including the radial and median nerves and the brachial artery is located. Due to the complexity of the anatomic structures at the elbow, multiple causes of pain should be considered in patients with anterior elbow pain (Table 25.1).

The biceps brachii muscle originates at the supraglenoid tubercle and the coracoid process of the scapula, crossing over the anterior humerus. The bicipital distal tendon inserts on the radial tuberosity, and the lacertus fibrosus (bicipital aponeurosis) inserts on the proximal ulna [4–6]. Also known as the "everyday supinator," the biceps brachii is the primary supinator of the forearm and flexes the elbow in concert with the brachioradialis and brachialis muscles [6].

© The Author(s), under exclusive license to Springer Nature Switzerland AG 2022
S. A. Mostoufi et al. (eds.), *Clinical Guide to Musculoskeletal Medicine*, https://doi.org/10.1007/978-3-030-92042-5_25

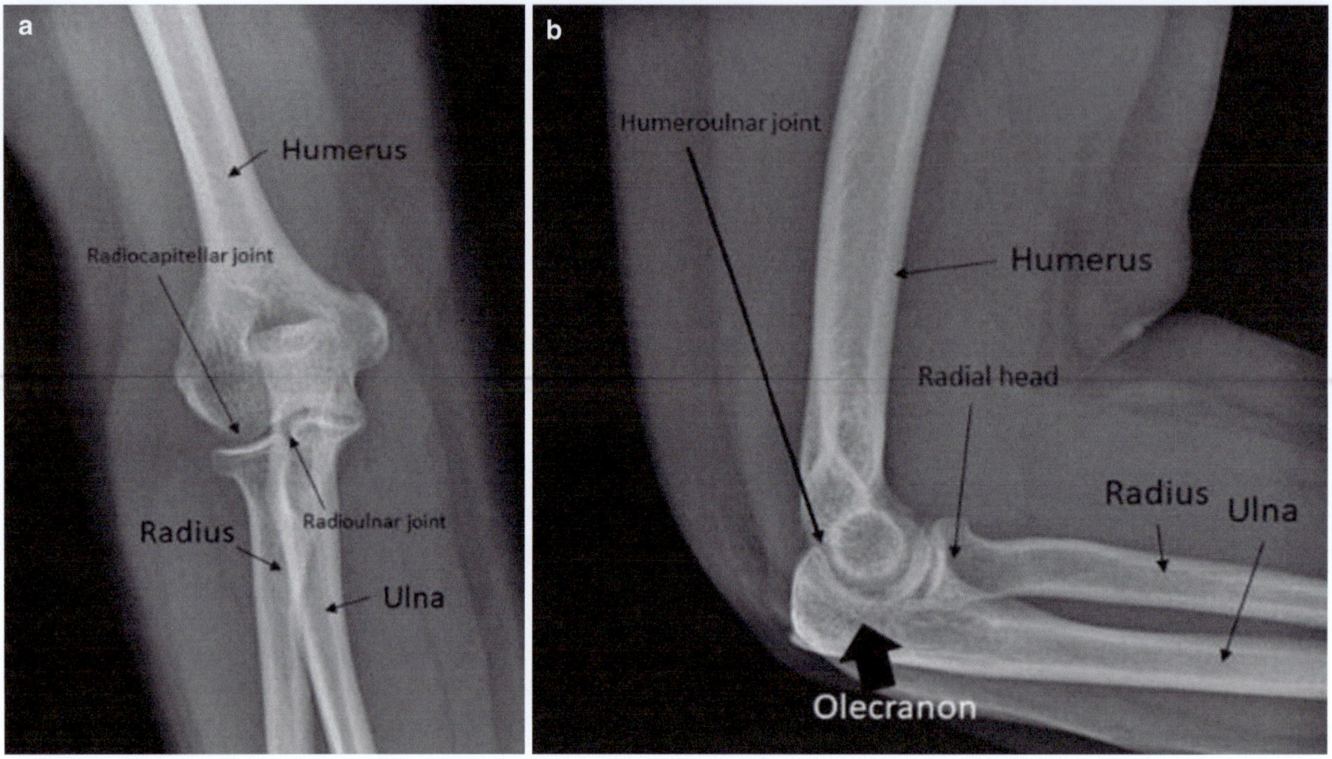

Fig. 25.1 Anteroposterior (**a**) and lateral (**b**) X-rays view of the right elbow demonstrating the three bones (humerus, radius, and ulna) and three joints (humeroulnar, proximal radio-ulnar, and radiocapitellar joint) of the elbow. The radial head and olecranon are also identified

Table 25.1 Differential diagnosis of anterior elbow pain

Anterior capsule strain	Osteoarthritis
Gout	Pronator syndrome
Intra-articular loose body	Rheumatoid arthritis
Muscular strain (biceps brachii, brachialis)	Tendon injury

25.1.4 Clinical Presentation

The patients commonly have personal or vocational history of repetitive elbow flexion or supination. The introduction of new exercises, like weighted biceps curls, may be related to the symptom origin. Patients state they usually do not have a specific single event associated with the onset of symptoms. They will complain of vague anterior elbow pain at the antecubital fossa with loss of elbow flexion strength. The symptoms are mostly chronic and a gradual decline in function if often observed.

25.1.5 Physical Examination

On inspection, swelling of the antecubital fossa may be observed. Ecchymosis in the area may be a sign of a partial or total biceps tendon rupture. Palpation of the tendon may show peritendinous swelling or crepitus, but the rope-like tendinous structure should be palpable and contiguous.

Passive supination and pronation of the forearm with the elbow flexed to 90° should reveal a normal piston-like movement of the biceps muscle belly. The absence of this motion indicates a complete tear. Resisted supination typically recreates pain deep in the antecubital fossa. No sensory loss is expected in patients with this condition. Sensory and motor examination of the proximal and distal upper extremity and cervical spine is recommended, as biceps tendinopathy at the elbow may occur as part of a repetitive stress injury syndrome or due to abnormal body mechanics at the elbow to compensate for other proximal or distal pathologies, as cervical radiculopathy, adhesive capsulitis of the shoulder, rotator cuff tendinopathy, or carpal tunnel syndrome.

25.1.6 Special Tests

(a) The hook test (Fig. 25.2): This test involves the examiner hooking the biceps tendon with his or her fingertip and will confirm an intact tendon and cause pain [3]. As this may be a naturally sensitive area, “hook test” comparison with the contralateral side is recommended. This test is also helpful to identify complete distal biceps tears, but not useful in identifying a partial tear [6, 7].
(b) The flexion initiation test (FIT): This test aims at improving diagnostic acuity of high-grade partial thickness tears, demonstrating a high sensitivity and specificity for both partial and complete biceps tendon tears. A positive FIT is when the patient cannot overcome the examiner’s counter force to initiate the first 10–15 of elbow flexion [6].

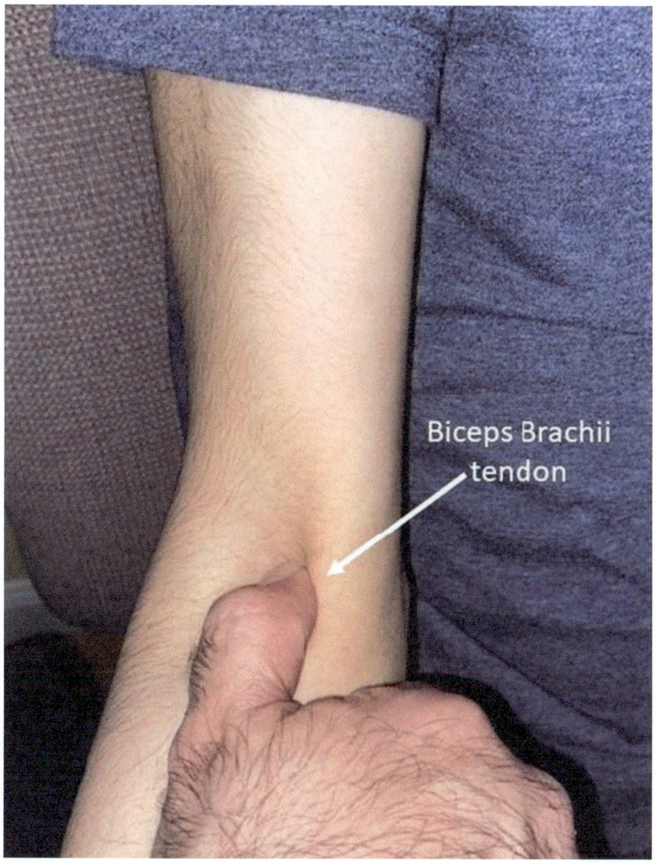

Fig. 25.2 The "hook test." The examiner hooking the biceps tendon with his or her fingertip will confirm an intact tendon and cause pain, in case of tendinopathy. If the examiner cannot hook the finger, it is suggestive of a tendon tear

25.1.7 Diagnostic Workup

X-rays of the elbow are usually normal but may be helpful to show osteophytes, loose bodies, or avulsion of the radial tuberosity. Magnetic resonance imaging (MRI) or musculoskeletal ultrasonography can be used to demonstrate continuity and changes in caliber of the tendon, yet ultrasonographic exam of the antecubital fossa is particularly difficult due to multiple anatomic structures in the region and the anatomy of the distal tendon [3]. These studies may help differentiate tendinopathy, enthesopathy (changes at the tendon insertion), or paratenonitis (inflammation of the tendon sheath) [4]. All these conditions are usually considered a continuum in the tendinopathy spectrum, and management may not change significantly from one to the other.

25.1.8 Treatments

25.1.8.1 Medical Management

Despite no significant evidence of inflammation on pathologic examination of tendinopathy, a course of simple analgesics or non-steroidal anti-inflammatories (NSAIDs) may be helpful to control pain and soft tissue swelling, specifically in patients with paratenonitis or inflammation of the tendon sheath.

25.1.8.2 Rehabilitation

The goals of rehabilitation are to decrease pain and improve range of motion, strength, and function.

To decrease pain modalities as cryotherapy, ultrasound and iontophoresis with dexamethasone may be utilized. Note that the median nerve is very close the distal biceps tendon and direct ice or heat modalities may cause irritation or even damage to the nerve. Close monitoring of sensory complaints while applying various modalities is advised.

Range of motion and stretching exercises of the shoulder capsule, elbow capsule, and wrist flexors and extensors are recommended, keeping in mind the versatility of movement at the elbow (flexion-extension and pronation-supination).

Isometric strengthening of the biceps in flexion and supination, followed by open and close kinetic chain, should be implemented, progressing to eccentric strengthening exercises. Clinically, it is reasonable to conclude that eccentric strengthening of the biceps will be helpful as it is a muscle that sustains significant eccentric forces, specifically during the throwing decelerations phase [2]. Yet, as of now, only two case reports of the use of eccentric strengthening in the rehabilitation of distal biceps tendinopathy were found [1, 2].

25.1.8.3 Procedure

Platelet-rich plasma (PRP) has been used in the treatment of distal biceps tendinopathy. Decreases in pain and improvements in strength and function have been reported. Unfortunately, due to the rarity of this diagnosis, there is minimal published data [8].

The distal tendon should not be injected with corticosteroids as this will traumatize the tendon by the needle insertion and alter the collagen matrix and decreased cellular viability by the corticosteroids [9]. Paratenonitis could potentially be injected safely with corticosteroids under ultrasound guidance, as the integrity of the tendon is maintained. Yet, considering the morbidity of a potential tendon tear, resulting in a significant loss of strength and cosmetic deformity, it is the author's opinion that corticosteroids should not be used, as other safer treatment options, as PRP are available.

25.1.8.4 Surgery

Surgical consultation for potential repair is usually recommended for patients with high-grade partial tears more of 50% of the tendon fibers, patients that fail conservative care or total tendon ruptures [10].

25.2 Distal Biceps Tendon Tear

25.2.1 Synonyms

Distal biceps tendon rupture

25.2.2 ICD-10 Codes

- S46.291A Biceps muscle/fascia/tendon injury – right arm, initial encounter
- S46.292A Biceps muscle/fascia/tendon injury – left arm, initial encounter

25.2.3 Description

Distal biceps tendon tears are rare, comprising 3–10% of all biceps brachii tendon ruptures, with an incidence of 2.6 per 100,000 patients and typically seen in middle-aged men [6, 10, 11].

25.2.4 Clinical Presentation

The typical patient is between the fourth and sixth decade with an average age of 50 years old [11]. The mechanism of injury is a sudden eccentric load that is applied to the flexed elbow, forcing it from flexion to extension. The dominant arm is usually affected by this injury [1, 6]. Most will experience a painful "pop" or "snap" and will complain of pain in the forearm, not the arm or anterior elbow [4]. Smoking, anabolic steroid use, and local corticosteroid injections are considered risk factors for distal biceps tendon tears [5]. Only about 30% of patients with distal biceps tendon tears are considered athletically active or have physical demanding vocational roles [10]. Patients present with acute pain and ecchymosis on the anterior elbow and weakness of elbow flexion and forearm supination, making some activities difficult for patients, like opening a jar.

25.2.5 Physical Examination

There will be ecchymosis and swelling on the antecubital fossa with tenderness to palpation. The distal biceps tendon will not be palpable, and there is pain with full elbow extension. As discussed above, resisted flexion of the elbow with the forearm supinated (Fig. 25.3) and supination of the forearm will be weak compared to the contralateral side. Due to the swelling close to the medial nerve in the anterior elbow, the patients may feel paresthesia in the sensory medial distribution without weakness on pronation of the forearm, flexion of the wrist, or median innervated musculature in the hand (thumb abduction). Muscle stretch reflexes will be normal except for the reflex biceps reflex, which as expected will be not only absent, but patients will experience pain with tapping on the anterior elbow.

25.2.6 Diagnostic Workup

Anteroposterior and lateral X-rays of the elbow and forearm will be helpful to look at a possible radial tuberosity avulsion fracture and other associated bony injuries. Due to the curved trajectory of the biceps brachii tendon, the musculoskeletal ultrasound evaluation of the distal biceps tendon is difficult [4]. MRI is rarely necessary for diagnosis of a complete tear,

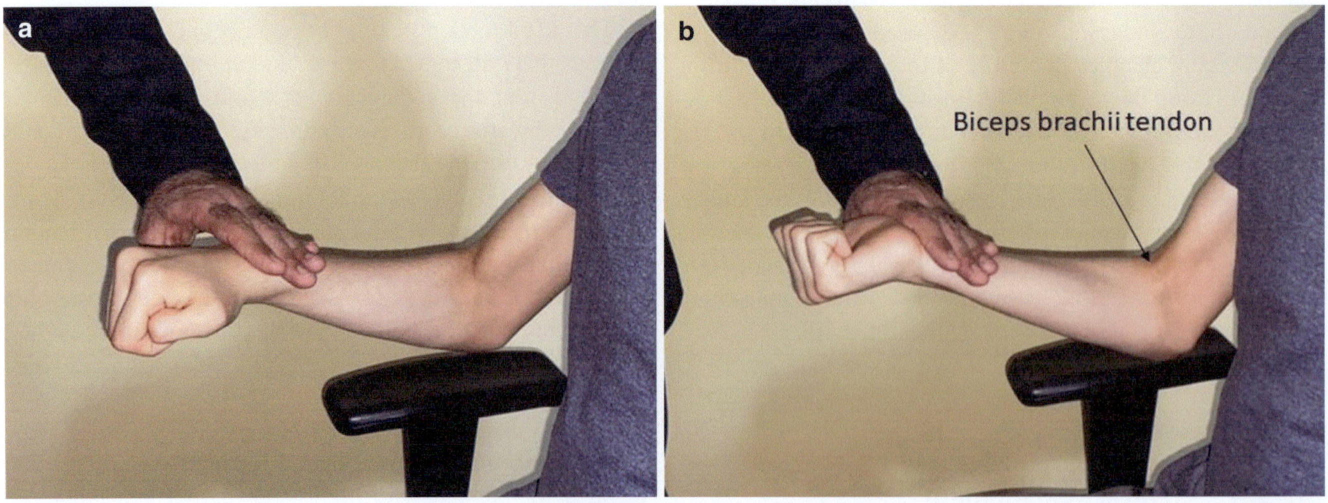

Fig. 25.3 Elbow flexion resistance with the forearm pronated and the hand dorsum up tests predominantly the brachialis muscle (**a**), while elbow flexion with the forearm supinated and the palm up will test the biceps brachii (**b**). Note that the biceps tendon is more visible with the forearm supinated, as this position provides better mechanical advantage to the biceps

although it can differentiate between complete tears, partial tears, and muscular strain. It is also helpful to quantify the degree of tendon retraction in cases of complete tears, which is necessary for surgical planning. MRI has high sensitivity and specificity, particularly for complete tears, and it is more accurate than ultrasound in detecting a tear [6].

25.2.7 Treatments

25.2.7.1 Medical Management

There may be a role of non-surgical treatment in patients with sedentary work or patients in which surgery is not possible due to complex medical conditions [10]. Compared with the contralateral arm, complete rupture of the distal biceps can produce a 40% loss of supination strength, a 47% loss of supination endurance, and up to 30% loss of flexion strength at the elbow, for which unless medically contraindicated, tendon repair is recommended [6]. Simple analgesics, such as acetaminophen and NSAIDs, if not contraindicated, can be used for pain control and control of soft tissue inflammation. In the acute setting, NSAIDS should be used carefully as they may result in excessive ecchymosis. Due to the magnitude of this injury, a short course of oral opioids may be considered initially after an acute injury.

25.2.7.2 Rehabilitation

Pain and swelling control are helpful for patients in the preamble of surgical repair or patients in which repair is not possible due to medical comorbidities. Protection with an elbow brace and/or sling for comfort can be used. Compression with an elbow or arm sleeve and elevation above the chest level will also help decrease swelling and excessive bruising. Stretching or elbow extension range of motion is not recommended if surgery is planned, but if conservative care is the only option, gentle passive range, progressing to active assistive and active range of motion, is recommended to prevent elbow capsulitis. Preservation of pronation and supination with range of motion exercises is also important. Lastly, for patients with non-surgical management, strengthening supplementary musculature as the brachialis, brachioradialis, and supinator muscles should be targeted, noting that even for fully rehabilitated non-surgical patients, they will persist with significant elbow weakness.

25.2.7.3 Procedures

Injections are not recommended for this diagnosis.

25.2.7.4 Surgery

Timely diagnosis of a complete distal biceps tendon rupture and primary repair to reestablish motion and strength is imperative. Early surgical repair is strongly recommended in athletes, patients with forceful supination vocational needs, and patients that consider arm deformity unacceptable, as non-surgical treatment will make the distal biceps tendon scar to the brachialis muscle, changing the arm contour [11]. The surgical technique results in reinserting the biceps tendon into the radial tubercle. Due to the risk of neurovascular injury of structures at the antecubital fossa, multiple surgical techniques have been developed [10]. Although normal strength is usually regained with surgery of the dominant arm, residual weakness has been observed in surgical repairs of the nondominant arm [12]. Common complications of surgical intervention include nerve injury, more commonly the lateral antebrachial cutaneous nerve, loss of motion, tendon re-rupture, and heterotopic ossification. In patients with chronic tendon injuries, surgery may not be possible. In patients with tears older than 6 weeks, repair may be difficult, and after 12 weeks, the tendon may not be repairable due to fiber retraction, atrophy, and scarring [10]. Elbow surgeries are further discussed in Chap. 30.

25.3 Brachialis Muscle Strain

25.3.1 Synonyms

Climber's elbow

25.3.2 ICD-10 Code

- S56.81 Strain of other muscles, fascia and tendons at forearm level
- S56.811 Strain of other muscles, fascia and tendons at the right forearm
- S56.812 Strain of other muscles, fascia and tendons at the left forearm

25.3.3 Description

Strains and tears of the brachialis muscle are uncommon compared to other muscle strains and other elbow injuries. The clinical presentation may be similar to other anterior elbow injuries, such as biceps tendon tears. As injuries to the brachialis muscle and tendon are rare, their incidence and prevalence are not well documented [13]. The information currently available in this type of injury are predominantly case reports [14]. The deep location of the brachialis muscle and scarcity of literature make diagnosis and treatment difficult.

25.3.3.1 Anatomy

Brachialis is composed of two heads, superficial and deep heads [14]. The origin of the superficial head is the deltoid tuberosity. It continues laterally on the attaching on anterior surface of the ulna at the ulnar tuberosity [15]. The deep head originates on the anterior surface of the humerus and inserts onto the ulna proximal to the superficial head, with some fibers penetrating the distal attachment of the superficial head. It is the primary elbow flexor, generating the greatest force, compared to the biceps brachii and brachioradialis. It has no role on elbow supination or pronation. While the forearm is held in full protonation, the biceps brachii is in a mechanical disadvantage, and the brachialis muscle performs most of the elbow flexion. High repetitive stress in this position, as in the case of rock climbers, can result in partial tears of the brachialis musculotendinous junction.

In contrast to brachialis, the biceps brachii is more commonly injured and usually involves the tendon. Brachialis muscle belly tears, while rare, are the most common injury observed in the brachialis muscle [14].

Due to the scarcity of medical evidence, adequate demographic and epidemiologic analysis reports are not available. This type of injury has been observed in both pediatric and adult patients [14, 16]. As the brachialis muscle tears are rare, and the muscle is deep in the arm and elbow, it is prone to misdiagnosis.

25.3.4 Clinical Presentation

The initial presentation of these patients is usually after repetitive elbow flexion with the arm pronated, as while doing pull-ups or rock climbing [17]. Another mechanism of injury may be the sudden hyperextension or forceful eccentric extension force to the elbow [14]. Brachialis muscle injury presents with pain and swelling in the anterior mid- and distal arm exacerbated by elbow flexion with the forearm pronated.

25.3.5 Physical Examination

Brachialis muscle injuries present with pain and swelling in the anterior mid- and distal arm exacerbated by elbow flexion with the forearm pronated. Unlike a biceps muscle injury, in which a palpable gap may be felt on physical examination, the brachialis muscle is difficult to palpate due to its position deep to the overlying biceps brachii. Resisted elbow flexion with the thumb up or palm up will not be painful (Fig. 25.3). Normal sensory examination and preserved biceps reflexes should be observed.

25.3.6 Diagnostic Workup

AP and lateral X-rays of the elbow may be obtained to rule out other more common bony causes of antecubital pain. Usually, muscular injury occurs where the brachialis crosses the elbow joint. Because of their close anatomical proximity to the radial nerve, median nerve, and brachial artery, ultrasound evaluation is recommended for the evaluation of brachialis injuries [15]. MRI is the gold standard to confirm the injury, unless an adequate musculoskeletal ultrasound can be obtained and performed by an experienced sonographer.

25.3.7 Treatments

25.3.7.1 Medical Management

Traumatic brachialis muscle injuries reported in the literature were treated non-operatively and responded well to conservative treatment. Treatment consists of resting the affected limb, ice, and non-steroidal anti-inflammatories if not contraindicated [16].

25.3.7.2 Rehabilitation

Swelling control followed by range of motion and strengthening exercises is imperative for recovery. Eccentric muscle strengthening is strongly recommended in the later stages of rehabilitation, due to the action of the brachialis muscle on elbow eccentric flexion [16].

25.3.7.3 Procedures

No procedures have been documented in the treatment of this injury.

25.3.7.4 Surgery

Brachialis muscle injury is a rare entity, and no surgical treatment has been documented for the treatment of this injury.

25.4 Elbow Capsular Strain

25.4.1 Synonyms

Elbow sprain

25.4.2 ICD-10 Code

- S53.401 Elbow sprain, right elbow
- S53.402 Elbow sprain, left elbow
- S59.901 Unspecified injury of right elbow
- S59.902 Unspecified injury of left elbow

25.4.3 Description

Activities requiring repetitive hyperextension of the elbow may strain the anterior capsule. The strain results in anterior elbow pain that becomes worse with passive extension or hyperextension stress testing [18]. Activities that should make one suspicious of a possible elbow capsular injury include weight-lifting with eccentric strain (such as decline dumbbell or barbell curls).

25.4.4 Clinical Presentation

Anterior elbow pain is specifically related to extension or a hyperextension injury to the joint. The patient may have a history of anterior elbow pain in the antecubital fossa after throwing a ball or overhead lifting, usually on the terminal phase of the action when the elbow is fully extended.

25.4.5 Physical Examination

Patients may have mild to no swelling in the anterior elbow. Severe swelling or ecchymosis may suggest a musculotendinous injury as described in previous sections of this chapter, as a biceps or brachialis injury. Patients will have pain with hyperextension of the elbow (bounce home test) or passive extension of the elbow. In cases of elbow capsulitis, an extensor lag at the elbow may be present. Generally, there is no significant pain with resisted elbow flexion or extension at midrange (90° of elbow flexion). A normal neurovascular exam is typically observed.

25.4.6 Diagnostic Workup

X-rays are commonly recommended to rule out other possible more serious injuries. Elbow radiographs are usually normal unless a bony avulsion injury, loose body, or a superimposed ruptured brachialis muscle with associated myositis ossificans is visible [18]. If there is suspicion of a more serious injury, imaging such as musculoskeletal ultrasound and/or MRI should be considered.

25.4.7 Treatments

25.4.7.1 Medical Management

Pain control with simple analgesics and NSAIDs may be needed in the initial phase of recovery. Activity modification, avoiding elbow hyperextension and activities that exacerbate symptoms, is encouraged. A shoulder sling may be used intermittently, keeping in mind that prolonged immobilization of the elbow in flexion and the shoulder in adduction may result in adhesive capsulitis of the elbow or shoulder. In the author's experience, therapeutic elbow taping may also be useful in preventing elbow hyperextension.

25.4.7.2 Rehabilitation

The elbow is known to react by a precipitous loss of motion even after minor injuries [19]. Preservation of the elbow's full range of motion including pronation and supination is vital. Modalities to decrease pain and/or inflammation such as cryotherapy and compression, followed by passive ROM, progressing to active ROM are advised. Once adequate ROM is achieved, strengthening of the elbow at all planes (flexion, extension, pronation, and supination) is recommended, progressing from isometrics to concentric exercises. As musculotendinous structures are not usually involved, the role of eccentric strengthening for this diagnosis is unknown. Follow-up physical examination during rehabilitation is important to determine other concomitant musculotendinous and/or osseous injuries that may have occurred and were missed.

25.4.7.3 Procedures

In patients with secondary adhesive capsulitis of the elbow, high-volume intra-articular injections may be considered. The author's preference is to use a mixture of normal saline solution, local anesthetics, and low dose corticosteroids (10–20 mg of triamcinolone acetate). A volume of 5 ml may be enough to cause significant capsular distention and improve range of motion if the limitation is secondary to capsular restrictions. Depending on the clinician's expertise, ultrasound or fluoroscopic guidance may be needed.

25.4.7.4 Surgery

No surgical intervention is recommended for capsular strains. In case of elbow adhesive capsulitis or stiff elbow, manipulation under anesthesia or arthroscopic debridement may be considered [19]. Elbow surgeries are further discussed in Chap. 30.

References

1. Jayaseelan DJ, Magrum EM. Eccentric training for the rehabilitation of a high level wrestler with distal biceps tendinosis: a case report. Int J Sports Phys Ther. 2012;7(4):413–24.
2. Holshouser C, Jayaseelan DJ. Multifaceted exercise prescription in the management of an overhead athlete with suspected distal biceps tendinopathy: a case report. J Funct Morphol Kinesiol. 2020;5(3):56.
3. Kane SF, Lynch JH, Taylor JC. Evaluation of elbow pain in adults. Am Fam Physician. 2014;89(8):649–57.
4. Brasseur JL. The biceps tendons: from the top and from the bottom. J Ultrasound. 2012;15(1):29–38.

5. Logan CA, Shahien A, Haber D, Foster Z, Farrington A, Provencher MT. Rehabilitation following distal biceps repair. Int J Sports Phys Ther. 2019;14(2):308–17.
6. Bono OJ, Shah SS, Peterson J, Golenbock SW, Ross G. The flexion initiation test and an evidence-based diagnostic algorithm for distal biceps tendon tears. Arthrosc Sports Med Rehabil [Internet]. 2021 [cited 2021 Apr 20]. Available from: https://www.sciencedirect.com/science/article/pii/S2666061X2100016X.
7. O'Driscoll SW, Goncalves LBJ, Dietz P. The hook test for distal biceps tendon avulsion. Am J Sports Med. 2007;35(11):1865–9.
8. Kwapisz A, Prabhakar S, Compagnoni R, Sibilska A, Randelli P. Platelet-rich plasma for elbow pathologies: a descriptive review of current literature. Curr Rev Musculoskelet Med. 2018;11(4):598–606.
9. Puzzitiello RN, Patel BH, Forlenza EM, Nwachukwu BU, Allen AA, Forsythe B, et al. Adverse impact of corticosteroids on rotator cuff tendon health and repair: a systematic review of basic science studies. Arthrosc Sports Med Rehabil. 2020;2(2):e161–9.
10. Sutton KM, Dodds SD, Ahmad CS, Sethi PM. Surgical treatment of distal biceps rupture. J Am Acad Orthop Surg. 2010;18(3):139–48.
11. Leighton MM, Bush-Joseph CA, Bach BR. Distal biceps brachii repair. Results in dominant and nondominant extremities. Clin Orthop. 1995;317:114–21.
12. Redmond CL, Morris T, Otto C, Zerella T, Semmler JG, Human T, et al. Functional outcomes after distal biceps brachii repair: a case series. Int J Sports Phys Ther. 2016;11(6):962–70.
13. Winblad JB, Escobedo E, Hunter JC. Brachialis muscle rupture and hematoma. Radiol Case Rep. 2008;3(4):251.
14. Forsythe CM, Burtis MT, Pfeiffer DC, Spurling GR, Ashby DB. Acute brachialis muscle tear in a pediatric patient. Radiol Case Rep. 2020;15(5):498–501.
15. Chang K-V, Wu W-T, Özçakar L. Ultrasound imaging and rehabilitation of muscle disorders: part 1. Traumatic injuries. Am J Phys Med Rehabil. 2019;98(12):1133–41.
16. Geiselman J, Gillespie R, Miller A. Brachialis strain in a collegiate Wrestler: a case report. Int J Athl Ther Train. 2020;25(4):181–4.
17. Cole KP, Uhl RL, Rosenbaum AJ. Comprehensive review of rock climbing injuries. J Am Acad Orthop Surg. 2020;28(12):e501–9.
18. Chumbley EM, O'Connor FG, Nirschl RP. Evaluation of overuse elbow injuries. Am Fam Physician. 2000;61(3):691–700.
19. Morrey BF. The posttraumatic stiff elbow. Clin Orthop. 2005;431:26–35.

Posterior Elbow Disorders

26

Eric W. Pettyjohn and Jason L. Zaremski

26.1 Olecranon Bursopathy (Bursitis)

26.1.1 Synonyms

- Baker's elbow
- Elbow bursitis
- Student's elbow

26.1.2 ICD-10 Codes

M70.20, M70.21, M70.22

26.1.3 Description

The olecranon bursa is a superficial synovial fluid membrane located just posterior to the olecranon. The bursa allows the olecranon to track smoothly across the surrounding tissues during elbow flexion and extension. Due to its superficial location, the bursa is susceptible to injury via multiple mechanisms. As an acute injury, olecranon bursitis can occur due to trauma, inflammation, or infection. When infection is suspected, this is usually due to direct spread, so typical skin flora is the common pathogen. Chronic inflammation can also be seen due to certain occupations, such as miners, plumbers, heating and air conditioning technicians, and even desk jobs with prolonged contact of the elbow on a hard surface. Systemic inflammatory conditions such as rheumatoid arthritis, psoriatic arthritis, gout, and chondrocalcinosis can also cause the condition. Whether the cause is noninfectious or infectious, the event causes an inflammatory cascade causing the release of protein and synovial type fluid into the bursa. This is manifested by swelling of the joint.

Olecranon bursitis typically affects men between the ages of 30 and 60 years old [1]. Two-thirds of the cases are nonseptic and occur with repeated trauma to the area resulting in a release of inflammatory mediators. There is no predisposition between sex and race. Differential diagnosis of olecranon bursitis is listed in Table 26.1.

26.1.4 Clinical Presentation

Clinical features can vary depending on whether the cause is acute or chronic and aseptic versus septic. Classic presentation of an acute injury includes symptoms of swelling and pain over the tip of the elbow in both aseptic and septic bursitis. Complaints of warmth overlying the elbow and fevers can favor a diagnosis of septic bursitis. In addition to this, septic cases tend to become symptomatic earlier than nonseptic forms, thus presenting earlier for evaluation [3]. In chronic cases patients may present with a remote history of significant swelling of the elbow that diminished in size, leading to small "lumps" when palpating their elbow. These lumps represent fibrotic scar tissue

Table 26.1 Differential diagnosis of olecranon bursopathy

Cause/category	Specific injury/process
Acute trauma	Olecranon process fracture
Autoimmune condition	Rheumatoid arthritis
Crystalline inflammatory arthropathy	Gout and pseudogout
Muscular	Triceps tendinitis or tear
Infectious	*Staphylococcus aureus* (MSSA most common) [2], *Streptococcus* (second most common)
Miscellaneous	Lipoma, synovial cyst

E. W. Pettyjohn
UF Health, University of Florida, Gainesville, FL, USA

J. L. Zaremski (✉)
Divisions of PM&R, Sports Medicine, & Research, Department of Orthopaedics and Rehabilitation, UF Health, University of Florida, Gainesville, FL, USA
e-mail: zaremjl@ufl.edu

© The Author(s), under exclusive license to Springer Nature Switzerland AG 2022

S. A. Mostoufi et al. (eds.), *Clinical Guide to Musculoskeletal Medicine*, https://doi.org/10.1007/978-3-030-92042-5_26

as a result of chronic inflammation and increased consistency of the bursal fluid [1].

26.1.5 Physical Examination

Initially, the clinician should inspect both elbows to assess for localized swelling. The normal appearance of the bursitis is round or "golf ball" in shape due to the fluid being confined within the bursa [4]. Patients may also experience tenderness to palpation over the posterior tip of the elbow. Erythema is present in 63–100% of patients with septic bursitis versus only 25% with nonseptic bursitis [1]. Fever is only present in approximately 70% of septic bursitis cases; therefore, infectious etiology cannot be ruled out in an afebrile patient [4].

26.1.6 Diagnostic Workup

The diagnosis is usually made by history and physical exam alone and does not require imaging to confirm. However, due to the overlapping of signs and symptoms of aseptic and septic bursitis, the clinician should highly consider the risk of septic bursitis in each patient. If septic bursitis is of concern, bursal aspiration and analysis are considered to be the gold standard in diagnosis [4]. Fluid should be sent for cell count, Gram stain, culture, and crystal examination. Radiographic evaluation is not recommended unless there is concern for an olecranon fracture in a setting of recent trauma [1].

26.1.7 Treatments

The treatment depends on whether it is infectious or noninfectious. Overall, nonsurgical management leads to better clinical resolution of aseptic bursitis compared to surgical management [5].

26.1.7.1 Medical Management

Acute, noninfectious bursitis is usually self-limiting and can be managed conservatively with rest, ice, and a course of NSAIDs. Infectious bursitis requires treatment with antibiotics targeted against streptococcal and staphylococcal organisms [4]. When the diagnosis between aseptic and septic bursitis is unknown and aspirated fluid results are pending, it is recommended to begin antibiotic therapy against the organisms noted above (including methicillin-resistant *Staphylococcus aureus*) until microbiological findings are available [6].

26.1.7.2 Rehabilitation

Application of a compressive, elastic bandage or sleeve has been shown to help with the treatment and further development of swelling [4].

26.1.7.3 Procedures

Nonseptic bursitis In a randomized trial by Kim et al., the likelihood of resolution of nonseptic olecranon bursitis and earliest resolution of symptoms were evaluated in three treatment groups: compression bandaging plus NSAID use, aspiration, and aspiration with steroid injection. At the end of 4 weeks, there were no differences in the proportion of patients whose bursitis resolved in the three groups. The steroid injection after aspiration group was associated with the earliest resolution (2.3 weeks), when compared to the aspiration alone group (3.1 weeks) and the compression bandaging and NSAID group (3.2 weeks) [7]. One systematic review found that CSI did not improve the rate of clinical resolution, but did increase overall complications and skin atrophy at the injection site [5].

Septic bursitis Traditionally, if there is concern for septic bursitis, the general recommendation in the literature is for bursal aspiration with fluid analysis. However, a study compared treatment outcomes of traditional bursal aspiration to empirical antibiotic management. They concluded that empiric management for uncomplicated septic bursitis was effective and may be considered [8].

26.1.7.4 Surgery

Surgical treatment options include aspiration and irrigation, incision and drainage, and total excision through either open or endoscopic approach [9]. When comparing endoscopic to an open approach, endoscopically treated patients tolerated local anesthesia (versus general anesthesia in an open approach), had decreased hospitalization time, and had superior treatment satisfaction scores [9]. When grouped together, clinical resolution was significantly more common after nonsurgical management than surgical management [5].

26.2 Posteromedial Elbow Impingement

26.2.1 Synonyms

- Posteromedial olecranon impingement (PMOI)
- Valgus extension overload syndrome (VEOS)

26.2.2 ICD-10 Codes

M19.029

26.2.3 Description

Posteromedial elbow impingement is classically seen in athletes who are involved in frequent and repetitive overhead athletes, such as swimmers, volleyball players, gymnasts, golfers, as well as baseball and softball players [10, 11]. While posteromedial elbow impingement is the most common elbow injury caused by overhead throwing in baseball players, it is an otherwise rare condition in the general population [12]. Pathophysiology involves repeated hyperextension, valgus stress, and supination of the elbow leading to progressive medial laxity. This causes abutment of the bony and soft tissue structures of the posteromedial elbow. As a result, osteoarthritic changes can be seen that include joint space narrowing, subchondral sclerosis, osteophyte formation, loose bodies, subchondral cyst formation, joint effusion, and secondary synovitis [13]. Differential diagnosis of posteromedial elbow impingement is given in Table 26.2.

26.2.4 Clinical Presentation

Patients typically report posteromedial elbow pain that is most pronounced during the extension or follow-through phase of throwing [14]. Patients may only present with complaints of decreased training capacity or performance due to premature fatigue, loss of velocity, or loss of control. There may also be reports of locking or catching (due to loose bodies) or an inability to fully extend the arm (due to olecranon osteophytes and/or loose bodies).

26.2.5 Physical Exam

Physical examination begins with visual inspection of the affected elbow in comparison to the unaffected side. The normal carrying angle in adults may vary from 5° to 15°; however it is not uncommon for throwers to have an increased carrying angle in their dominant elbow compared to their nondominant elbow [15]. Posteromedial elbow impingement does not typically cause a joint effusion or visible muscle atrophy of the triceps or forearm muscles. Tenderness to palpation along the posteromedial elbow is usually elicited. Range of motion testing may demonstrate a loss of terminal extension, as well as posterior elbow pain with pronation, valgus stress, and extension. Valgus stress can also induce pain or laxity of the ulnar collateral ligament (UCL).

Table 26.2 Differential diagnosis of posteromedial elbow impingement

Skeletal	Osteoarthritis, olecranon apophysitis, olecranon avulsion fracture, and olecranon stress fracture
Muscular/ ligamentous	Triceps tendinopathy/tear, ulnar collateral ligament insufficiency/injury
Nervous	Cubital tunnel syndrome

26.2.5.1 Special Tests

(a) *Arm bar test:* This maneuver has the patient standing with the shoulder in internal rotation with the elbow extended and index fingers resting on the examiner's shoulder. The examiner places their hand on the distal humerus and applies pressure on the distal humerus to the fully extended elbow. The test is positive if there is distinctive posteromedial pain [16].

(b) *Valgus overload test/posteromedial impingement test:* The patient is seated or standing with 20–30° of elbow flexion. The examiner stabilizes the upper arm while grasping the wrist. The examiner then forcibly extends the elbow while applying valgus stress. Posteromedial pain specifically indicates a positive test [11].

26.2.6 Diagnostic Workup

To definitively diagnose posteromedial elbow impingement, this requires the synthesis of a detailed history, thorough physical exam, and imaging evidence. One study found that less than half (14 out of 36) of their sample size of baseball players could be diagnosed with the condition confidently by clinical symptoms and physical examination alone [13]. The diagnosis can be further complicated by the presence of co-injuries, such as to the medial ulnar collateral ligament (UCL).

X-ray Can be useful to help aid in the diagnosis, as well as rule out other bony skeletal disorders that are within the differential. Anterior-posterior, lateral, and oblique views can detect posteromedial osteophytes, loose bodies, osteochondritis dissecans, and associated stress fracture of the olecranon seen in posteromedial impingement cases [13, 17]. X-ray has less utility when evaluating for joint space narrowing as well as associated soft tissue injuries.

Computer tomography (CT) One study concluded that characteristic imaging findings of posteromedial elbow impingement are more readily diagnosed by CT compared to MRI when it comes to joint space narrowing, medial olecranon subluxation, and the number of loose bodies [13]. This is because the joint spaces could be more definitively measured by CT.

Magnetic resonance imaging (MRI) MRI is considered the gold standard imaging modality for the entire aspect of the athlete's elbow, though utility of musculoskeletal ultrasound may be considered if one is an experienced ultrasonographer. When clinical suspicion is high for posteromedial impingement in baseball players, MRI should be considered necessary for a comprehensive evaluation of the affected elbow because associated bone marrow edema, secondary synovitis, and soft tissue and nerve-related injuries are more readily diagnosed. Common associated elbow injuries that would be more evident on MRI include UCL injury, distal medial triceps tendinosis, ulnar neuritis, and flexor-pronator tendinosis [13]. It should be noted that if there is a concern for concomitant UCL injury, MRI arthrogram has a higher sensitivity and specificity than MRI alone for partial UCL tears, but with stronger magnets (such as T3), MRI and MRA both have extremely high diagnostic accuracy, 100% in some studies [18].

26.2.7 Treatments

26.2.7.1 Medical Management

A conservative treatment approach lasting 6–10 weeks should be recommended first. Medical management includes a trial of relative rest, cryotherapy, restriction from throwing, and valgus stress-related activities and if needed may consider using non-steroidal anti-inflammatory drugs (NSAIDS).

26.2.7.2 Rehabilitation

Early implementation of specific rehabilitation exercises including rotator cuff strengthening as well as eccentric strengthening of the wrist flexors shoulder be initiated. After the initial physical therapy stage, a supervised throwing program with correction of flawed throwing mechanics is then recommended as long as there are no symptoms including pain when throwing.

26.2.7.3 Procedures

None

26.2.7.4 Surgery

Arthroscopy is a viable surgical option in patients who have failed a conservative approach and have characteristic findings on advanced imaging. In one study comparing MRI findings in overhead throwing athletes and results of arthroscopic treatment, patients that benefited subjectively and objectively (increased elbow extension range of motion) from surgery were found to have posteromedial synovitis, olecranon spurring, and loose bodies. Treatment consisted of arthroscopic debridement of the synovitis, loose body removal, and olecranon spur excision [17]. The presence of symptomatic loose bodies or impinging osteophytes typically has the greatest improvement after arthroscopic surgery, compared to patients with degenerative findings that seem to have less satisfactory results [19]. It is recommended that only osteophyte and not native olecranon be removed as a prior study revealed that 42% of baseball players who underwent partial olecranon excision for posteromedial impingement required a second surgery, several requiring UCL reconstruction [12]. Arthroscopy is also a viable surgical option in the teenage population for debridement, excision of olecranon spurs, and removal of any loose bodies [20]. All patients were able to return to their previous level of play in an average of 3.4 months, and no patient developed medial instability that required additional surgery at end follow-up of a mean of 26 months [20]. For more details, please see Chap. 30 "Surgeries in the Elbow."

26.3 Triceps Injury/Tendinopathy

26.3.1 Synonyms

Posterior tennis elbow

26.3.2 ICD-10 Codes

S46.311, S46.312, S46.319

26.3.3 Description

The term tendinopathy can be divided into two varying categories: tendinosis and tendinitis. Tendinosis is a more degenerative process characterized by fibroblastic changes, vascular hyperplasia, and immature/disorganized collagen that can be seen in histopathology, whereas tendinitis is an inflammatory process with the presence of neutrophils and lymphocytes seen on histopathology [21]. Triceps tendinopathy is the least common type of elbow tendinopathy [22]. Triceps tendinopathy is an enthesopathy due to damage to the triceps tendon from repetitive, resisted elbow extension [21]. The pathology most commonly occurs at the enthesis of the olecranon but can also occur within the tendon itself or the myotendinous junction. Differential diagnosis of triceps injury is listed in Table 26.3.

Table 26.3 Differential diagnosis of triceps injury

Posteromedial elbow impingement
Osteoarthritis
Olecranon bursitis
Snapping triceps
Olecranon stress fracture
Partial triceps tendon tear

26.3.4 Clinical Presentation

Patients will typically present with pain and swelling of the posterior elbow. For the majority of cases, the pain will develop progressively over time. Patients may report that the pain is elicited with resisted elbow extension, stretching of the triceps muscles, or even present at rest. They may also report limited mobility and reduced elbow extension strength due to pain inhibition. The clinician should focus on the mechanism of injury and chronicity and assess for any associated risk factors, including olecranon bursitis, injectable and/or oral steroid use, and type 1 diabetes when taking a history [23–25].

26.3.5 Physical Examination

Initial examination of the posterior elbow includes assessment signs of swelling, ecchymosis, direct trauma, or visible defects. Active range of motion with flexion and extension, as well as elbow extension strength, should be tested as both of these may be reduced. Patients with either tendinosis or tendinitis will have worsening of their pain with resisted elbow extension [21].

26.3.5.1 Special Tests

Triceps squeeze test The patient is positioned seated with the forearm hanging over the back of a chair to where their elbow is flexed at 90°. The examiner places one hand on the distal triceps tendon with the other around the muscle belly and squeezes both hands firmly. The lack of extension of the elbow indicated a total triceps rupture [26].

26.3.6 Diagnostic Workup

X-ray Plain radiographs have limited use as an imaging modality to aid in the diagnosis of triceps tendinopathy. Tendon-specific pathology will not be seen, but X-ray can show calcification within the tendon (usually at the osteotendinous junction), as well as an avulsion fragment proximal to the olecranon [27]. The utility of X-ray is to help rule out skeletal-specific pathologies that are within the differential.

Ultrasound The superficial location of the triceps tendon allows for a straightforward evaluation of the tendon. Tendinopathy will present as reduced echogenicity and possible calcification within the tendon [27]. Ultrasound is also able to visualize partial- and full-thickness tears.

Magnetic resonance imaging The advantage of MRI is that it can more readily assess for other causes of the patient's symptoms. Findings of tendinopathy show abnormal (increased) signal intensity on fluid-sensitive images. Further, the insertions of the superficial and deep tendons can be visualized separately, aiding in a more specific diagnosis [27].

26.3.7 Treatments

There is very limited data available reporting on the management of distal triceps tendinopathy. However, the general consensus is that it is a self-limiting condition that typically resolves with conservative management.

26.3.7.1 Medical Management

May include the use of cryotherapy, compression, and/or NSAIDs at first.

26.3.7.2 Rehabilitation

Rehabilitation management should follow the principles used to treat other types of tendinopathies [26]. Initially, activity modification and cessation of weight training and loading of the elbow is a general recommendation for most tendinopathies. Physical therapy can be utilized to address any strength or mobility deficits. A physical therapy routine incorporating stretching and strengthening exercises of the triceps and surrounding muscles, as well as specific eccentric strengthening exercises, should be attempted [28].

26.3.7.3 Procedures

Platelet-rich plasma (PRP) PRP does not have the potential complications that are associated with steroid injections such as skin atrophy, skin discoloration, and secondary tendon tear [29]. Evidence of PRP for triceps tendinopathy is lacking in the literature. There is one case report of a 47-year-old male with a partial distal triceps tendon rupture who was treated with PRP injection and a conservative therapy program [30]. A decrease in pain and increase in strength at 2 and 4 weeks, respectively, after injection were seen. However, the single report and lack of control group make PRP difficult to recommend as a treatment option for triceps tendinopathy.

Ultrasound-guided tenotomy (USGT) There is limited data in the literature in regard to USGT and triceps tendinopathy. In one case series, five patients that underwent USGT all reported moderate pain at baseline, which improved to no or mild pain at short-term follow-up (2, 6, and 12 weeks) [31].

26.3.7.4 Surgery

Surgical intervention should be reserved for refractory cases. Donaldson et al. propose that a minimum of 1 year should pass of attempted conservative treatment prior to surgical evaluation [27]. Surgical options include triceps debridement of degenerative tendinous tissue or excision of related olecranon osteophytes [32].

References

1. Del Buono A, Franceschi F, Palumbo A, Denaro V, Maffulli N. Diagnosis and management of olecranon bursitis. Surgeon. 2012;10(5):297–300.
2. Lormeau C, Cormier G, Sigaux J, Arvieux C, Semerano L. Management of septic bursitis. Joint Bone Spine. 2019;86(5):583–8.
3. Weinstein PS, Canoso JJ, Wohlgethan JR. Long-term follow-up of corticosteroid injection for traumatic olecranon bursitis. Ann Rheum Dis. 1984;43(1):44–6.
4. Pangia J, Rizvi TJ. Olecranon bursitis. In: StatPearls [Internet]. Treasure Island (FL): StatPearls Publishing; 2021 [cited 2021 Apr 7]. Available from: http://www.ncbi.nlm.nih.gov/books/NBK470291/.
5. Sayegh ET, Strauch RJ. Treatment of olecranon bursitis: a systematic review. Arch Orthop Trauma Surg. 2014;134(11):1517–36.
6. Shell D, Perkins R, Cosgarea A. Septic olecranon bursitis: recognition and treatment. J Am Board Fam Pract. 1995;8(3):217–20.
7. Kim JY, Chung SW, Kim JH, Jung JH, Sung GY, Oh K-S, et al. A randomized trial among compression plus nonsteroidal antiinflammatory drugs, aspiration, and aspiration with steroid injection for nonseptic olecranon bursitis. Clin Orthop. 2016;474(3):776–83.
8. Deal JB, Vaslow AS, Bickley RJ, Verwiebe EG, Ryan PM. Empirical treatment of uncomplicated septic olecranon bursitis without aspiration. J Hand Surg. 2020;45(1):20–5.
9. Meric G, Sargin S, Atik A, Budeyri A, Ulusal AE. Endoscopic versus open bursectomy for prepatellar and olecranon bursitis. Cureus. 2018;10(3):e2374.
10. Park J-Y, Yoo H-Y, Chung SW, Lee S-J, Kim NR, Ki S-Y, et al. Valgus extension overload syndrome in adolescent baseball players: clinical characteristics and surgical outcomes. J Shoulder Elb Surg. 2016;25(12):2048–56.
11. Dugas JR. Valgus extension overload: diagnosis and treatment. Clin Sports Med. 2010;29(4):645–54.
12. Andrews JR, Timmerman LA. Outcome of elbow surgery in professional baseball players. Am J Sports Med. 1995;23(4):407–13.
13. Ko CC, Tai MH, Lin CH, Tzeng WS, Chen JH, Shu G, et al. Posteromedial olecranon impingement of the pitching elbow: additional findings provided by CT. Eur J Radiol. 2016;85(1):211–7.
14. Loftice J, Fleisig GS, Zheng N, Andrews JR. Biomechanics of the elbow in sports. Clin Sports Med. 2004;23(4):519–30, vii–viii.
15. Erickson BJ, Chalmers PN, Zajac J, Sgroi T, Eno JJ, Altchek DW, et al. Do professional baseball players with a higher valgus carrying angle have an increased risk of shoulder and elbow injuries? Orthop J Sports Med. 2019;7(8):2325967119866734.
16. Zwerus EL, Somford MP, Maissan F, Heisen J, Eygendaal D, van den Bekerom MP. Physical examination of the elbow, what is the evidence? A systematic literature review. Br J Sports Med. 2018;52(19):1253–60.
17. Cohen SB, Valko C, Zoga A, Dodson CC, Ciccotti MG. Posteromedial elbow impingement: magnetic resonance imaging findings in overhead throwing athletes and results of arthroscopic treatment. Arthroscopy. 2011;27(10):1364–70.
18. Campbell RE, McGhee AN, Freedman KB, Tjoumakaris FP. Diagnostic imaging of ulnar collateral ligament injury: a systematic review. Am J Sports Med. 2020;48(11):2819–27.
19. Reddy AS, Kvitne RS, Yocum LA, Elattrache NS, Glousman RE, Jobe FW. Arthroscopy of the elbow: a long-term clinical review. Arthroscopy. 2000;16(6):588–94.
20. Matsuura T, Iwame T, Suzue N, Iwase J, Tamaki S, Yokoyama K, et al. Clinical outcome of arthroscopic treatment for posteromedial elbow impingement in adolescent baseball players. Arthroscopy. 2018;34(1):105–10.
21. Laratta J, Caldwell J-M, Lombardi J, Levine W, Ahmad C. Evaluation of common elbow pathologies: a focus on physical examination. Phys Sportsmed. 2017;45(2):184–90.
22. Anzel SH, Covey KW, Weiner AD, Lipscomb PR. Disruption of muscles and tendons; an analysis of 1, 014 cases. Surgery. 1959;45(3):406–14.
23. Sollender JL, Rayan GM, Barden GA. Triceps tendon rupture in weight lifters. J Shoulder Elb Surg. 1998;7(2):151–3.
24. Clayton ML, Thirupathi RG. Rupture of the triceps tendon with olecranon bursitis. A case report with a new method of repair. Clin Orthop. 1984;184:183–5.
25. Wagner JR, Cooney WP. Rupture of the triceps muscle at the musculotendinous junction: a case report. J Hand Surg. 1997;22(2):341–3.
26. Bracker MD, Achar SA, Pana AL, Taylor KS. The 5-minute sports medicine consult (5 minute consult series). 2nd ed. Philadelphia: Wolters Kluwer; Lippincott Williams & Wilkins; 2011. 721 p.
27. Donaldson O, Vannet N, Gosens T, Kulkarni R. Tendinopathies around the elbow part 2: medial elbow, distal biceps and triceps tendinopathies. Shoulder Elbow. 2014;6(1):47–56.
28. Hall MM, Woodroffe L. Ultrasonic percutaneous tenotomy for recalcitrant calcific triceps tendinosis in a competitive strongman: a case report. Curr Sports Med Rep. 2017;16(3):150–2.
29. Kwapisz A, Prabhakar S, Compagnoni R, Sibilska A, Randelli P. Platelet-rich plasma for elbow pathologies: a descriptive review of current literature. Curr Rev Musculoskelet Med. 2018;11(4):598–606.
30. Cheatham SW, Kolber MJ, Salamh PA, Hanney WJ. Rehabilitation of a partially torn distal triceps tendon after platelet rich plasma injection: a case report. Int J Sports Phys Ther. 2013;8(3):290–9.
31. Stover D, Fick B, Chimenti RL, Hall MM. Ultrasound-guided tenotomy improves physical function and decreases pain for tendinopathies of the elbow: a retrospective review. J Shoulder Elb Surg. 2019;28(12):2386–93.
32. van den Bekerom MPJ, Eygendaal D. Posterior elbow problems in the overhead athlete. Sports Med Arthrosc Rev. 2014;22(3):183–7.

27 Lateral Elbow Disorders

Julio A. Martinez-Silvestrini

27.1 Lateral Epicondylopathy

27.1.1 Synonyms

- Tennis elbow
- Lateral epicondylosis
- Lateral epicondylalgia
- Lateral elbow tendinopathy

27.1.2 ICD-10 Codes

- M77.11 Lateral epicondylitis, right elbow
- M77.12 Lateral epicondylitis, left elbow

27.1.3 Description

Lateral epicondylopathy (LE) is the most common cause of elbow pain. This overuse tendinopathy occurs in approximately 1–3% of the population annually, and although it is commonly called tennis elbow, only 5–10% of tennis players develop the condition. Most patients suffering this condition are in their 30s and 40s, affecting males and females equally, and affect predominantly the dominant upper extremity. Most patients develop elbow pain as a result of occupational rather than recreational activities [1]. The lateral elbow epicondyle is affected four to ten times more often than the medial side.

J. A. Martinez-Silvestrini (✉)
Baystate Rehabilitation Care, University of Massachusetts Medical School – Baystate, Longmeadow, MA, USA

Tufts University School of Medicine, Boston, MA, USA

University of Massachusetts Medical School – Baystate, Longmeadow, MA, USA
e-mail: Julio.martinez@bhs.org

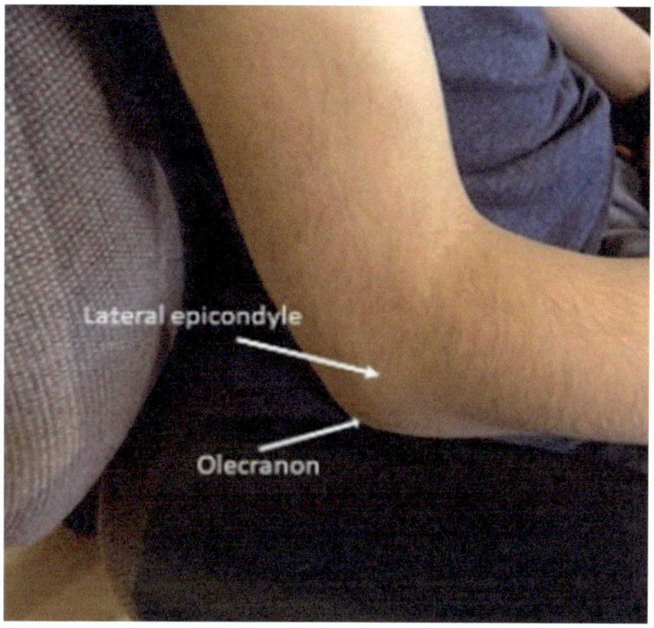

Fig. 27.1 Lateral elbow. Lateral epicondyle and olecranon process is identified

27.1.3.1 Anatomy of Lateral Epicondyle

The lateral epicondyle of humerus (Fig. 27.1) serves as the common origin for the anconeus muscle, supinator, extensor carpi radialis brevis, extensor digitorum, extensor digiti minimi, and extensor carpi ulnaris. As an overload or overuse syndrome, it is commonly associated with repetitive microtrauma from excessive gripping or wrist extension and/or forearm supination. The extensor carpi radialis brevis (ECRB) is the most frequently affected muscle, and the supinator and other extensor muscles are also commonly affected [1]. Lateral epicondylopathy was originally considered as an inflammatory process. However, the current evidence suggests a tendinosis, a degenerative process characterized by fibroblasts, vascular hyperplasia, and disorganized collagen, known as angiofibroblastic hyperplasia [1, 2]. Differential diagnosis of lateral elbow pain is given in Table 27.1.

© The Author(s), under exclusive license to Springer Nature Switzerland AG 2022
S. A. Mostoufi et al. (eds.), *Clinical Guide to Musculoskeletal Medicine*, https://doi.org/10.1007/978-3-030-92042-5_27

27.1.4 Clinical Presentation

A patient complains of lateral elbow pain with forceful grip or while lifting objects with the thumb up or the hand pronated. Limited range of motion of the wrist and elbow due to pain may be observed. Hand grip strength loss and/or swelling at the lateral epicondyle or surrounding tissue may also be a presenting complaint.

27.1.5 Physical Examination

On inspection, there is no swelling, although in chronic cases, soft tissue swelling at the lateral epicondylar region is observed. There is no discoloration or bruising. There will be exquisite tenderness at the lateral epicondyle. Extension of the wrist without resistance may reproduce some of the symptoms, but the pain is mainly reproduced with resisted extension of the wrist or fingers of the affected limb. In severe cases, pain may be reproduced with full elbow extension. Decreased grip strength secondary to pain may be present. Normal sensory exam and muscle stretch reflexes should be observed:

Special Tests

1. *Third digit extension*: The patient will forward flex the shoulder at 90° and keep the elbow extended, wrist at neutral position, and fingers extended. The examiner will apply downward pressure at the third digit, while the patient resists the force. Pain will be reproduced at the lateral epicondyle or dorsal forearm, not at the finger or wrist (Fig. 27.2).
2. *Chair lift test*: This maneuver requires the patient to lift a chair by the backrest with the shoulder at neutral position, forward flexed at 90°, the elbows extended, and forearm pronated (palm down) (Fig. 27.3).

Table 27.1 Differential diagnosis of lateral elbow pain [3]

Elbow synovitis or capsulitis	Posterolateral plica
Lateral epicondylitis	Posterolateral rotatory instability
Osteochondral defect	Radial tunnel syndrome
Posterior interosseous nerve syndrome	Radiocapitellar chondromalacia

27.1.6 Diagnostic Workup

1. *X-rays* are typically negative in patients with lateral epicondylitis, although in rare instances, calcifications of ECRB tendon (calcific tendinopathy) or spurring at the lateral epicondyle may be observed. X-rays are recom-

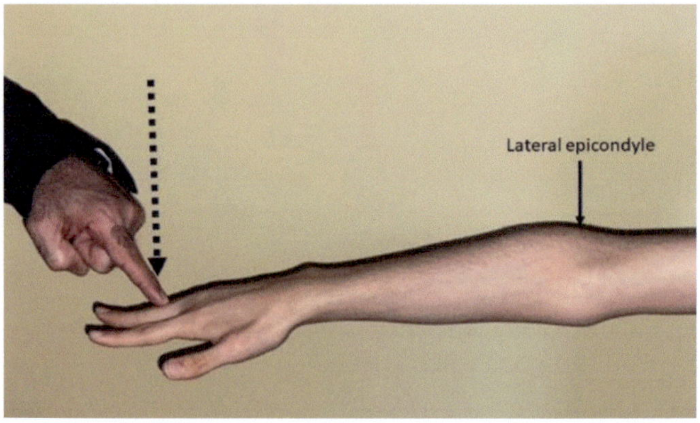

Fig. 27.2 Third digit extension test. The examiner will apply downward pressure at the third digit (dotted line), distal to the proximal interphalangeal joint (PIP), while the patient resists with the elbow and fingers extended. A positive test will reproduce the patient symptoms at the lateral elbow and extensor muscle mass

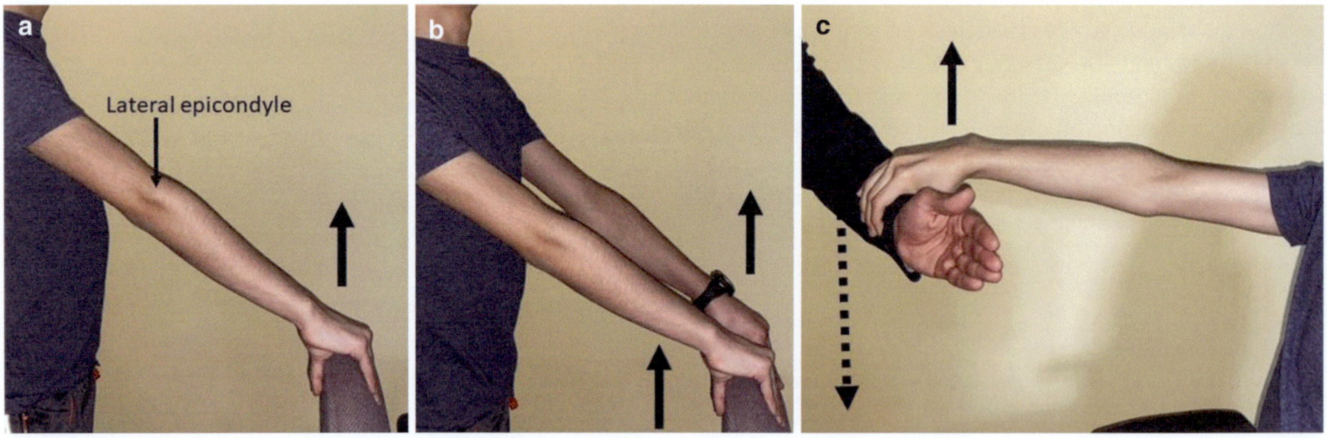

Fig. 27.3 Chair lift test. The patient will try to lift a chair straight up (solid arrow) while holding the back rest with a pinch grip (fingers and thumb in opposition), using one arm (**a**). The author recommends this variant of pulling with both arms (**b**). Alternatively, the examiners can use their own arm (**c**) to provide downward resistance (dotted line) to the upward motion. A positive test will reproduce the patient's symptoms at the lateral elbow

mended to rule-out other diagnosis with a similar clinical presentation (Table 27.1), such as arthropathy, osteochondral defects, or joint loose bodies [2].

2. *Ultrasound* is considered as an efficient, noninvasive, and relatively cost-effective imaging method for LE. Several findings may be observed on ultrasound to identify degenerative changes of the tendons, as bone irregularities, thickening, tears, or neovascularization [2, 4].
3. *MRI* can provide a better view of the complete anatomical structures of the lateral epicondyle. The findings observed in patients with LE include abnormal thickening tendon and increased signal intensity within the common extensor origin and epicondyle [1]. MRI can also identify partial- or full-thickness tears of the extensor muscle group, which can influence the need for surgical management and be helpful during preoperative planning. MRI is also considered to rule out intra-articular pathology. This imaging modality is not recommended routinely for concerns of LE, as it is costly and may not change the treatment [2].

27.1.7 Treatments

27.1.7.1 Medical Management

There is no consensus in the efficacy of oral non-steroidal anti-inflammatory drugs (NSAIDs), compared to topical NSAIDs. Due to the avascular nature of the ECRB and common extensor tendons, oral NSAIDs tend not to be as effective in controlling pain or inflammation and are normally contraindicated in patients with cardiovascular, renal, and severe hepatic disease or patients with gastrointestinal sensitivity to NSAIDS or history of gastrointestinal bleeding. Topical NSAIDs tend to be effective in controlling soft tissue swelling and minimizing pain with minimal systemic absorption. Placebo-controlled trials demonstrated topical NSAIDs are effective within 4 weeks in the treatment of LE [2]. Nitric oxide and topical glyceryl trinitrate patch is another modality that has been shown to be effective in the treatment of LE, as well [5–7].

Counterforce bracing or tennis elbow brace is often used in the treatment of LE. Using counterforce braces can decrease pain by pressing on the forearm extensor muscles, dispersing the stress on the lateral epicondyle. Stabilizing the wrist in neutral position with a cock-up wrist splint may also help reduce the insertional pull of forearm extensors and decrease symptoms. Biomechanical studies have shown that immobilizing the forearm with braces can significantly lessen the stress on the ECRB origin, decrease the frequency and severity of pain, and improve elbow function, compared with the placebo group [2].

27.1.7.2 Rehabilitation

Strengthening does not seem to have an overall effect on patient pain or function long term. The most important components of rehabilitation of lateral epicondylopathy are education, activity modifications, and regaining the tendon length to enable normal wrist extensor dynamics [8].

A rehabilitation program consisting of 4–6 visits, progressing to an independent home exercise regimen on education, stretches, activity modification, and pain management techniques, is possible and effective at reducing pain and increasing function in patients. Despite eccentric strengthening exercises that have been used successfully in the management of other tendinopathies, the addition of eccentric exercises failed to improve rehabilitation outcomes, as demonstrated by the author and confirmed by more recent studies [8, 9].

27.1.7.3 Procedures

Corticosteroid local injections may be considered in patients with subacute or chronic LE. They are not recommended for patients with acute onset of pain, as they have not proven to be effective in the acute setting. Corticosteroid injections are superior to NSAIDs at 4 weeks, without long-term benefits at 1 year. Despite its short-term pain relief, corticosteroid injections are inferior to a wait-and-see approach or physical therapy at 1-year follow-up. Multiple injections may result in iatrogenic tendon rupture and muscle atrophy [2].

The use of regenerative biologic products has become very popular recently in the management of chronic conditions as LE. Some of the treatments that have been studied include autologous blood injections (ABI) and platelet-rich plasma injections (PRP). ABI's work mechanism includes initiating the inflammatory response around the affected tendon, which may result in cellular and humoral mediators. ABI may also deliver growth factors promoting collagen formation and healing. The current evidence suggests that ABI can achieve good outcomes in the short term, but no benefit in long-term follow-up has been observed. PRP theoretically works by releasing high concentrations of platelet-derived growth factors enhancing wound, bone, and tendon healing. The current evidence yields conflicting results [2]. There is some evidence that PRP injection may reduce the need for surgical intervention in intractable lateral epicondylitis [10].

27.1.7.4 Surgery

Surgical intervention (open, percutaneous, or arthroscopic) can be an option for patients with persistent pain and disability that have failed appropriate nonoperative management. The current studies indicate fair to good results for these procedures and should be offered to patients that fail a course of conservative care including analgesics, rehabilitation, and possibly injections. The specific surgical techniques are discussed in the Chap. 30.

27.2 Osteochondritis Dissecans of the Capitellum

27.2.1 Synonyms

OCD

27.2.2 ICD-10 Codes

- M93.22 Osteochondritis dissecans of elbow
- M93.221 Osteochondritis dissecans, right elbow
- M93.222 Osteochondritis dissecans, left elbow

27.2.3 Description

Osteochondritis dissecans of the elbow (OCD) is often observed in the humeral capitellum in skeletally immature adolescent athletes. The etiology of capitellar OCD is still unclear, but genetic predisposition, microtrauma, and ischemia appear to play a critical role in the development of this condition. Repetitive valgus, hyperextension, and compression of the poorly vascularized capitellum [11] and radiocapitellar joint are postulated as the causes of capitellar OCD and are commonly observed in gymnasts and overhead-throwing athletes. In overhead-throwing athletes, the elbow is subjected to valgus overload with significant compression stress applied to the radiocapitellar joint, specifically during the late cocking and early acceleration phases of throwing [12]. This diagnosis is commonly confused with osteochondrosis or Panner's disease, which occurs in younger patients and will be discussed later in this chapter. Classification of the OCD is outlined in Table 27.2.

27.2.4 Clinical Presentation

The patients with this diagnosis are typically older than 11 years of age but still skeletally immature. They may complain of vague pain and stiffness deep at the lateral elbow, worsened with activity, and relieved by rest. The symptoms tend to start gradually and usually become chronic. It is not uncommon for athletes to be diagnosed over 1 year after the onset of symptoms [11].

Table 27.2 Minami classification of osteochondritis dissecans

Minami classification of osteochondritis dissecans [13]
Grade 1: A stable lesion with a translucent cystic shadow in the capitellum
Grade 2: Clear zone between the OCD and adjacent subchondral bone
Grade 3: The articular surface separates and forms a loose body

27.2.5 Physical Examination

Patients regularly present with swelling in the elbow. On inspection they hold their elbow in flexion, and they may have an elbow extension lag, in the later stages of the disease. An elbow effusion may be observed. A normal neurovascular examination is expected. Locking of the elbow may be suggestive of an intra-articular loose body.

27.2.5.1 Diagnostic Workup

Radiography of the elbow is commonly performed as the first diagnostic study. As typical OCD lesions are in the anterior aspect of the capitellum, the anteroposterior (AP) view with the elbow in 45° of flexion is recommended for throwing athletes. In the case of gymnasts, AP views with the elbows at 30° of flexion may be more accurate. Ultrasonography is effective in detecting early-stage capitellar OCD and may be helpful for athletes that do not participate in overhead-throwing sports with suspicion of this diagnosis. Computer tomography (CT) scan is usually reserved for patients with advanced OCD. CT appears to be more sensitive and superior to MRI in the classification of OCD, with a sensitivity of 100% (CT) vs 96% (MRI) [11–13]. Some investigators do not recommend CT for patients that will be treated conservatively. As the patients are not exposed to radiation during MRI, it may be a superior imaging tool in the pediatric population.

27.2.6 Treatments

27.2.6.1 Medical Management

Short courses of immobilization and NSAIDs may be considered.

27.2.6.2 Rehabilitation

1. The first step to determine the adequate treatment of OCD is to classify the lesion to determine whether it is stable or unstable. This will determine the type of treatment and is closely related to the prognosis (Table 27.2). A stable lesion will most likely heal naturally with rest of the elbow, but when a lesion has become unstable or fragmented, surgery provides significantly better results [11]. Stable lesions are characterized by an immature capitellum with an open growth plate, and flattening or radiolucency of the subchondral bone, in a patient with (almost) normal elbow motion. Unstable lesions have at

least one of the following findings: a capitellum with a closed growth plate, fragmentation, restriction of elbow motion 20°, or more [13]. The mainstay of care for non-operative management of this condition is rest. Patients with a stable lesion should not be participating in activities that aggravate the elbow pain and symptoms, including conditioning exercises, weight-bearing on the upper extremities, or weightlifting. Throwing should be avoided. General conditioning exercises as running, lower extremity strengthening and stretching, and core stability work without upper extremity stress is advised.
2. Suboptimal throwing mechanics may result in this condition as poor throwing mechanics can result in increased valgus stress to the elbow. For which, adequate throwing technical training is recommended.
3. Mechanical stress to the elbow during upper extremity weight-bearing may contribute to development of the capitellar OCD in gymnasts. Gymnasts who develop capitellar OCD tend to demonstrate scapular dyskinesis like baseball players. Elbow "locking" or hyperextension can also cause excessive stress to the radiocapitellar joint. Scapular stabilizer exercises and avoiding elbow hyperextension are recommended during their return to sports participation training.
4. Both proper technique training and periscapular conditioning may have a role in prevention of OCD.

27.2.6.3 Procedures

Regenerative biologic products have been used in combination with surgical care. At this time, there is no evidence of orthobiologics use independent of surgical interventions [14].

27.2.6.4 Surgery

It is estimated that more than 50% of OCD can be treated conservatively. Surgical treatment is recommended for those that fail conservative management and patients with unstable (as described above in the rehabilitation section), displaced, or fragmented lesions [13]. Surgical procedures include arthrotomy with loose body removal, curettage of the residual osteochondral defect, and arthroscopic debridement and microfracture procedures. Elbow arthroscopy is considered the standard of care and allows for a minimally invasive detailed lesion assessment and treatment. Even with surgical care, the prognosis of advanced osteochondral lesions is guarded [13, 15]. Open procedures are commonly recommended for patients that fail arthroscopic surgery. Good clinical results were observed in patients with open growth plates and shorter duration of symptoms. However, only about 2/3 of patients returned to high-level sports participation [16].

27.3 Osteochondrosis of the Capitellum

27.3.1 Synonyms

Panner's disease

27.3.2 ICD-10 Codes

M92.0 Juvenile osteochondrosis of humerus

27.3.3 Description

Osteochondrosis of the capitellum (Panner's disease) is a rare medical condition associated with irregularity of the humeral capitellum on plain radiographs. Panner's disease (PD) occurs after the appearance of the ossification nucleus of the capitellum, in patients typically younger than 11 years of age [17]. It has been reported more commonly in males, and the dominant arm tends to be more commonly involved. As this is an uncommon condition, good-quality demographic studies are not available [17]. The author observed most initial studies on this diagnosis were done between 1927 and 1970, according to a recent review bibliography, when boys were more likely to participate in sports. It is unclear to the author if the reason for males to be more commonly seen with this diagnosis is secondary to selection bias or delayed ossification compared to females [17]. It has been associated with direct trauma and repetitive microtrauma, as well as increased valgus stress and compression to the lateral elbow, specifically in sports like baseball and gymnastics. This diagnosis is commonly confused with osteochondritis dissecans (OCD), described above.

27.3.4 Clinical Presentation

Patients with Panner's disease complain of limited range of motion, pain, and/or swelling. Stiffness and increased elbow temperature have also been observed. Regularly the symptoms worsen by activity and relieved with rest. Duration of symptoms may vary from a few weeks to years.

27.3.5 Physical Examination

On inspection, there is objective evidence of inflammation with swelling, small elbow effusion, redness, and/or increased temperature. Limited range of motion of approximately 20° is the most common feature and seen in 77% of patients. An extension lag is more common, although cases with limited elbow flexion have also been reported [17]. No elbow locking and sensorimotor deficits are expected in this diagnosis. Ligamentous examination of the elbow is normal, yet patients may feel lateral elbow pain on valgus stress (Fig. 27.4).

27.3.6 Diagnostic Workup

X-rays of the elbow reveal the following changes in the capitellum: irregularity of the epiphysis, irregularity of the capitellum contour, sclerosis, and/or flattening of the capitellum. Destruction of the epiphysis or lytic lesions has been reported in rare instances. MRI of the elbow reveals joint effusion with decreased T1 signal of the capitellum. Bone scan will show increased radionuclide capitellar uptake.

27.3.7 Treatments

27.3.7.1 Medical Management

PD is considered a self-limiting disease, in which immobilization and relative rest are the mainstays of care. Avoidance of activities that worsen the elbow symptoms as throwing and lifting heavy objects are recommended. Some investigators suggest immobilizing the elbow and use of NSAIDs. There is no consensus on the length of immobilization and the degree of flexion in immobilization. As the elbow is a joint that is known to react by a precipitous loss of motion [18] even after minor injuries, it is the recommendation of the author to minimize the use of plaster immobilizers and instead consider the use of shoulder sling, progressing to a soft elbow brace or hinged elbow braces.

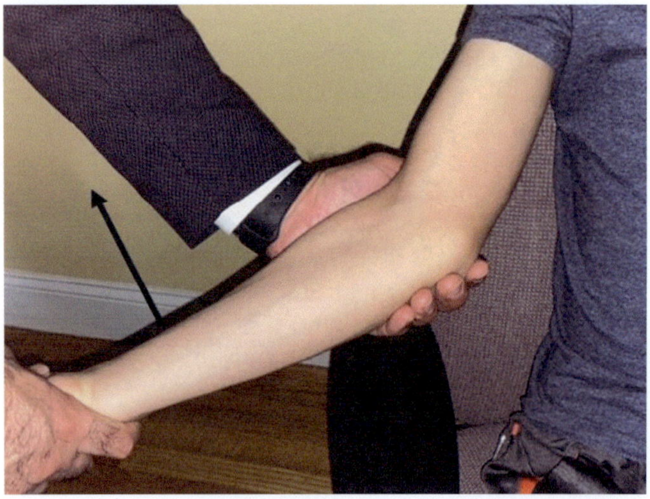

Fig. 27.4 Elbow valgus stress. The examiner will provide medial elbow stress, applying a lateral force to the distal forearm (arrow) while stabilizing the distal humerus with the opposite hand. Positioning the shoulder of the limb to be examined in full external rotation makes this test easier while the patient is sitting, as the shoulder capsule will provide stability to the humerus. This test is usually performed to test the medial collateral ligament and other medial structures of the elbow, but lateral elbow pain may be observed in patients with PD

27.3.7.2 Rehabilitation

Gradual pain-free return to activities is recommended with an emphasis in regaining ROM. Follow-up X-rays are recommended. Most patients will have a full recovery and bony healing, although in some cases, persistent flattening or sclerosis of the capitellum with reduced ROM may be observed.

27.3.7.3 Procedures

None

27.3.7.4 Surgery

Failure to respond to treatment may require arthroscopic surgical debridement. Surgeries in elbows are discussed in Chap. 30.

27.4 Lateral Collateral Ligament Complex Injury

27.4.1 Synonyms

Radial collateral ligament sprain

27.4.2 ICD-10 Codes

- S53.43 Radial collateral ligament sprain
- S53.431 Radial collateral ligament sprain of right elbow
- S53.432 Radial collateral ligament sprain of left elbow

27.4.3 Description

The lateral collateral ligamentous complex is composed of the lateral ulnar collateral ligament (LUCL), annular ligament (AL), and radial collateral ligament (RCL). Injuries to the lateral ligamentous complex (LLC) are considered the primary lesion associated with elbow dislocations. The mechanism of injury of the LLC includes trauma, previous elbow surgery, corticosteroid injections, severe LE, and cubitus varus deformities [19].

27.4.4 Clinical Presentation

Injury to the LLC typically occurs after elbow dislocations. This type of injury typically occurs secondary to a fall on an outstretched hand, generating an axial load, and valgus stress to the elbow. This causes the radial head and proximal ulna to subluxate posterolaterally, detaching or tearing the lateral collateral ligament [19]. Patients may present primarily with vague, lateral-sided pain rather than complaining of symptoms of instability. Clicking and popping at the elbow may be present. Transient elbow deformity may be a sign of episodic subluxations.

Some patients with elbow dislocations will develop chronic laxity of the LLC, resulting in posterolateral rotatory instability of the elbow, which can result in pain and functional limitation. This rotary instability may range from elbows subluxation to gross, recurrent elbow instability [20].

27.4.5 Physical Examination

On inspection, when the radial head is subluxed, an indentation may be observed in the lateral aspect of the forearm. There may be tenderness to palpation at the radial head and proximally at the lateral elbow. Range of motion is generally normal, but patients may feel instability with active or resisted elbow extension. Neurovascular examination of the upper extremity is typically normal.

Special Tests

1. *Posterolateral rotatory drawer test:* It is the most sensitive maneuver for posterolateral elbow instability, but it may be difficult if the patient is not fully relaxed [20]. The arm is stabilized between the trunk and arm of the examiner. To examine the right upper extremity, it is recommended that the examiner secures the right limb of the patient by the examiner's left side of the trunk and the left upper extremity. The humerus is held securely, while a posterolateral rotatory force is applied to the proximal radius (Fig. 27.5).
2. *Push-up tests*: The patient will start with the elbows fully flexed and do a push-up on a table or while holding a chair arm rest (chair push-up test). The test is positive if the patient feels instability (apprehension) moving from elbow flexion to extension (Fig. 27.6). Symptoms improve if the test is repeated with the forearm in the pronated position [21].

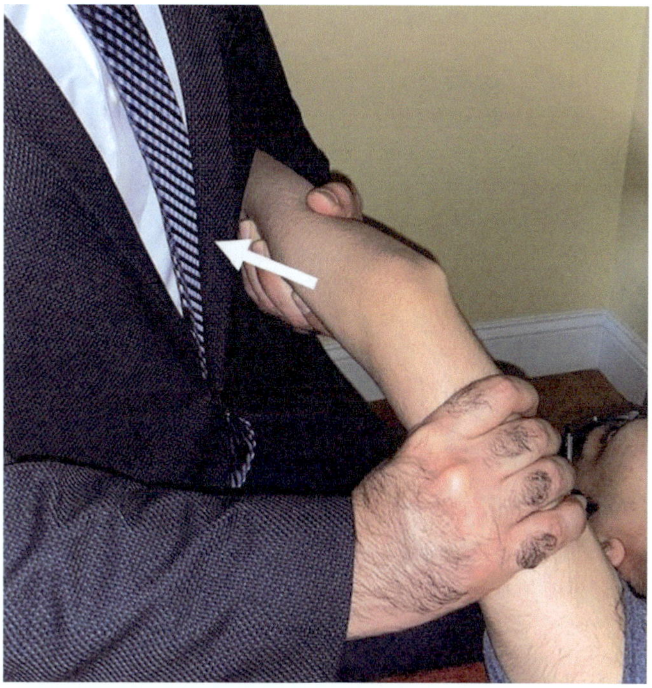

Fig. 27.5 Posterolateral rotatory drawer test: The distal upper extremity is secured between the trunk and arm of the examiner. The humerus is held securely with one hand, while a posterolateral rotatory force is applied to the proximal radius (arrow) with the opposite hand. Maximal instability generally occurs between 20° and 40° of elbow flexion

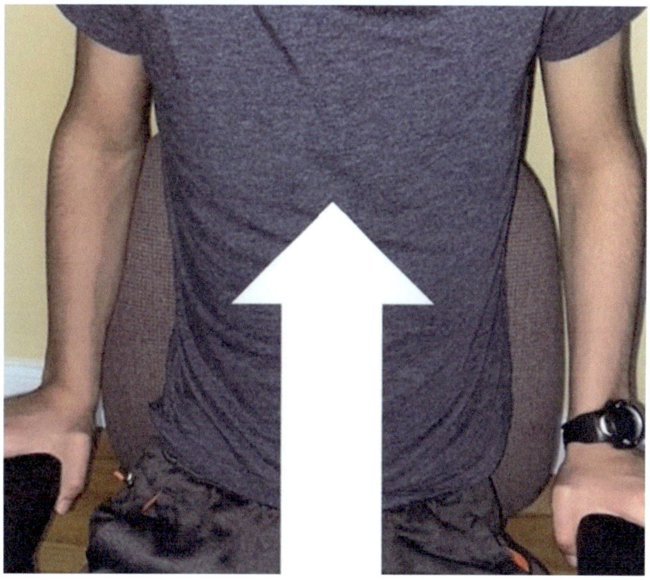

Fig. 27.6 Push-up tests: The patient will start with the elbows fully flexed and do a push-up and extend both elbows while holding a chair arm rest. The test is positive if the patient feels instability moving from elbow from flexion to extension

27.4.6 Diagnostic Workup

AP, lateral, and oblique radiographic views of the elbow are routinely negative, but occasionally posterolateral subluxation of the radial head may be observed. CT should be considered in skeletally immature patients with elbow instability, specifically looking for dysplasia of the coronoid, radial head, or trochlea. CT with 3D reconstruction is normally preferred to see these deformities. Impaction injuries of the capitellum may also be seen in CT scan. MRI may reveal disruption in the lateral ligamentous complex. Examination under fluoroscopy or ultrasound guidance may be helpful making the diagnosis of dynamic instability [21].

27.4.7 Treatments

27.4.7.1 Medical Management

If there is a complex injury to the lateral collateral ligament, there is usually no role for conservative care. Immobilization in a position of stability (based on physical exam) is recommended. Plaster or locked hinged braces limiting the range of motion to the range in which the elbow is stable can be used until definite surgical treatment. Prolonged immobilization for more than 3 weeks often results in elbow stiffness [18].

27.4.7.2 Rehabilitation

A rehabilitation trial may be considered for patients with mild elbow instability symptoms and no bony abnormalities. The common extensor tendon originates at the lateral aspect of the distal humerus, with the ECRB attachment extending distal to the radiocapitellar joint line and can provide dynamic elbow stability [19]. For which strengthening of wrist extensors, elbow supination and finger extensors may result in increased lateral elbow stability. Ergonomic evaluation and education on avoiding activities that promote instability is recommended.

27.4.7.3 Procedures

Regenerative biologics (such as PRP) have been extensively used in the treatment of medial elbow pain and medial ulnar collateral ligament injuries, as well as for the treatment of LE, but no evidence of its use on LLC injuries was found.

27.4.7.4 Surgery

Surgery is generally recommended in patients with traumatic lateral ligamentous complex injury and patients with symptomatic elbow instability. Surgical procedures include acute ligament repair or reconstruction in patients with severe or chronic instability. Surgeries in elbows are discussed in Chap. 30.

References

1. Cutts S, Gangoo S, Modi N, Pasapula C. Tennis elbow: a clinical review article. J Orthop. 2020;17:203–7.
2. Ma K-L, Wang H-Q. Management of lateral epicondylitis: a narrative literature review. Pain Res Manag. 2020;2020:6965381.
3. Kane SF, Lynch JH, Taylor JC. Evaluation of elbow pain in adults. Am Fam Physician. 2014;89(8):649–57.
4. Ricci V, Schroeder A, Özçakar L. Ultrasound imaging for lateral elbow pain: pinpointing the epicondylosis. Am J Phys Med Rehabil. 2020;99(6):560–1.
5. Ozden R, Uruç V, Doğramaci Y, Kalaci A, Yengil E. Management of tennis elbow with topical glyceryl trinitrate. Acta Orthop Traumatol Turc. 2014;48(2):175–80.
6. Bokhari AR, Murrell GAC. The role of nitric oxide in tendon healing. J Shoulder Elb Surg. 2012;21(2):238–44.
7. McCallum SDA, Paoloni JA, Murrell GAC. Five-year prospective comparison study of topical glyceryl trinitrate treatment of chronic lateral epicondylosis at the elbow. Br J Sports Med. 2011;45(5):416–20.
8. McQueen KS, Powell RK, Keener T, Whalley R, Calfee RP. Role of strengthening during nonoperative treatment of lateral epicondyle tendinopathy. J Hand Ther. 2021;34(4):619–26.
9. Martinez-Silvestrini JA, Newcomer KL, Gay RE, Schaefer MP, Kortebein P, Arendt KW. Chronic lateral epicondylitis: comparative effectiveness of a home exercise program including stretching alone versus stretching supplemented with eccentric or concentric strengthening. J Hand Ther. 2005;18(4):411–9, quiz 420.
10. Haasti G, Soufi M, Wilson J. Platelet rich plasma injections for lateral epicondylitis of the elbow reduce the need for surgical intervention. J Orthop. 2018;15(1):239–41.
11. van den Ende KIM, Keijsers R, van den Bekerom MPJ, Eygendaal D. Imaging and classification of osteochondritis dissecans of the capitellum: X-ray, magnetic resonance imaging or computed tomography? Shoulder Elbow. 2019;11(2):129–36.
12. Kajiyama S, Muroi S, Sugaya H, Takahashi N, Matsuki K, Kawai N, et al. Osteochondritis dissecans of the humeral capitellum in young athletes: comparison between baseball players and gymnasts. Orthop J Sports Med. 2017;5(3):2325967117692513.
13. van Bergen CJ, van den Ende KI, Ten Brinke B, Eygendaal D. Osteochondritis dissecans of the capitellum in adolescents. World J Orthop. 2016;7(2):102–8.
14. Guerra E, Fabbri D, Cavallo M, Marinelli A, Rotini R. Treatment of capitellar osteochondritis dissecans with a novel regenerative technique: case report of 3 patients after 4 years. Orthop J Sports Med. 2018;6(9):2325967118795831.
15. Baker CL, Romeo AA, Baker CL. Osteochondritis dissecans of the capitellum. Am J Sports Med. 2010;38(9):1917–28.
16. Bexkens R, van den Ende KIM, Ogink PT, van Bergen CJA, van den Bekerom MPJ, Eygendaal D. Clinical outcome after arthroscopic debridement and microfracture for osteochondritis dissecans of the capitellum. Am J Sports Med. 2017;45(10):2312–8.
17. Claessen FMAP, Louwerens JKG, Doornberg JN, van Dijk CN, Eygendaal D, van den Bekerom MPJ. Panner's disease: literature review and treatment recommendations. J Child Orthop. 2015;9(1):9–17.
18. Morrey BF. The posttraumatic stiff elbow. Clin Orthop Relat Res. 2005;431:26–35.
19. Bernholt DL, Rosenberg SI, Brady AW, Storaci HW, Viola RW, Hackett TR. Quantitative and qualitative analyses of the lateral ligamentous complex and extensor tendon origins of the elbow: an anatomic study. Orthop J Sports Med. 2020;8(10):2325967120961373.
20. Camp CL, Smith J, O'Driscoll SW. Posterolateral rotatory instability of the elbow: part I. Mechanism of injury and the posterolateral rotatory drawer test. Arthrosc Tech. 2017;6(2):e401–5.
21. Camp CL, Smith J, O'Driscoll SW. Posterolateral rotatory instability of the elbow: part II. Supplementary examination and dynamic imaging techniques. Arthrosc Tech. 2017;6(2):e407–11.

28 Medial Elbow Disorders

Eric W. Pettyjohn and Jason L. Zaremski

28.1 Medial Epicondylopathy (Epicondylosis)

28.1.1 Synonyms

- Golfer's elbow
- Baseball elbow
- Little league elbow

28.1.2 ICD-10 Codes

M77, M77.00, M77.01, M77.02

28.1.3 Description

Medial epicondylopathy (ME) is a relatively common injury that may affect as many as 3.8–8.2% of patients with occupational settings requiring repetitive forceful grip, manual handling of loads over 20 kg, or exposure to constant vibratory forces at the elbow [1, 2]. The injury occurs primarily due to repetitive eccentric loading of the forearm flexor-pronator tendon group, a common flexor tendon (CFT), that conducts wrist flexion and forearm pronation, as well as valgus strain of the elbow [3]. The flexor-pronator tendon is made up of five muscles: the pronator teres, flexor carpi radialis, palmaris longus, flexor carpi ulnaris, and flexor digitorum superficialis [4]. This injury is common in overhead athletes due to the valgus strain that occurs with stabilization of the elbow joint from eccentric contraction of the CFT [4]. The action of wrist flexion and forearm pronation during ball release places additional stress on the CFT. This supraphysiologic stress eventually results in peritendinous inflammation that, if continued, will result in angiofibroblastic hyperplasia [4]. This hyperplasia replaces normal tendon with fibroblastic, calcific tissue [4].

An important alternative diagnosis that can be a sequela of ME in a patient with medial elbow pain, especially one that participates in an overhead sport, is an avulsion fracture of the medial epicondyle. This type of injury is typically seen in between the ages of 9 and 14 years of age [5]. Mechanisms of injury that have been proposed include direct trauma, increased sudden tension of the flexor-pronator tendon group on the epicondyle itself, elbow dislocation in which the UCL provides the avulsion force, and a chronic, stress-related injury. Chronic injuries are most often seen in childhood or adolescent baseball pitchers who either have high pitch counts or limited rest in between pitching episodes [6]. Differential diagnosis of medial epicondylopathy is presented in Table 28.1.

28.1.3.1 Clinical Presentation

It is important to inquire about a patient's job or take into account an athlete's sports when they present to the clinic with medial elbow pain. In the athlete, this condition is primarily associated with overhead-throwing sports and/or sports with grip, such as golf and/or tennis; however, other sports including football, weightlifting, and bowling have been documented in the literature [2]. Patients present with

Table 28.1 Differential diagnosis of medial epicondylopathy

Ulnar collateral ligament (UCL) injury
Ulnar neuritis
Intra-articular pathology
Osteochondritis dissecans lesion

E. W. Pettyjohn
UF Health, University of Florida, Gainesville, FL, USA

J. L. Zaremski (✉)
Divisions of PM&R, Sports Medicine, & Research, Department of Orthopaedics and Rehabilitation, UF Health, University of Florida, Gainesville, FL, USA
e-mail: zaremjl@ufl.edu

© The Author(s), under exclusive license to Springer Nature Switzerland AG 2022

S. A. Mostoufi et al. (eds.), *Clinical Guide to Musculoskeletal Medicine*, https://doi.org/10.1007/978-3-030-92042-5_28

medial elbow pain that can be localized to a location of maximal pain at the medial epicondyle, with radiation into the proximal forearm. The pain is commonly insidious in onset and does not necessarily resolve with rest. In athletes specifically, they may note that the pain is at its worst during the late cocking phase in overhead throwing or early acceleration phase in the tennis player or golfer [7].

28.1.3.2 Physical Examination

Patients with ME typically do not show any abnormalities of the elbow on inspection; however, some may present with a flexion contracture due to pain and guarding. Most patients have full active and passive range of motion at the elbow and wrist. Physical examination is significant for tenderness to palpation approximately 5–10 mm distal and anterior to the medial epicondyle with soft tissue swelling [3]. Strength testing with resisted wrist flexion, forearm pronation, and grip strength may elicit medial elbow pain, as well as weakness in these maneuvers when compared to the contralateral side. Patients should be neurovascularly intact in the affected extremity.

However, it should be noted that an avulsion fracture may present with soft tissue swelling on inspection, with crepitus of the medial epicondyle on palpation, and decreased range of motion if the fracture fragment is entrapped within the joint [5].

28.1.3.3 Diagnostic Work-up

1. *X-ray*: X-ray is not the imaging modality of choice for diagnosing ME, but radiographs may reveal up to 25% may show signs of calcification of the CFT [3]. In regard to an avulsion fracture, X-ray is the imaging modality of choice for diagnosis and includes AP, lateral, and oblique views to help with assessing fracture displacement [5].
2. *Ultrasound*: Diagnostic accuracy is highly dependent on the operator but can be a cost-effective option to visualize pathology in the CFT. Park et al. showed that an ultrasound performed by a trained radiologist had sensitivity, specificity, and positive and negative predictive values greater than 90% for the diagnosis of ME in patients who had been diagnosed with the condition based on their symptoms and clinical signs on physical examination [8]. The most commonly discovered finding was hypoechoic or anechoic areas of tendon degeneration. Ultrasound also allows for dynamic examination of the tendon through range of motion and strength testing.
3. *Magnetic resonance imaging*: MRI is the standard of care for radiologic detection of ME. Advanced imaging with MRI is chosen when either there is high concern for concomitant pathology or the clinical picture is unclear when deciding the source of the medial elbow pain. When reviewing the image sequences, increased signal intensity at the CFT, especially with associated peritendinous edema on T2-weighted images, is the most specific finding of ME [9].

28.1.4 Treatments

28.1.4.1 Medical Management

Non-steroidal anti-inflammatory drugs (NSAIDs) may provide pain relief and can be used for 1–2 weeks as tolerated by the patient. The clinician should be sure to take into account the patient's medical history, including a history of hypertension, coronary artery disease, chronic kidney disease, history of gastrointestinal bleed, and/or gastric ulcer prior to initiating NSAID therapy. NSAIDs are particularly effective in reducing the synovitis accompanied with CFT degeneration [3].

28.1.4.2 Rehabilitation

In ME, patients should initially refrain from activities that exacerbate their symptoms, especially activities that require repetitive wrist flexion, forearm pronation, and valgus stress of the elbow [4]. Once acute symptoms improve, the focus is on flexor-pronator mass stretching and strengthening. Initially, the return of full, painless range of motion is the goal with implementing open-chain exercises and self-directed passive stretching techniques [4]. Once there is no pain with functional motion, tendon strengthening is focused on with concentric exercises to increase flexor-pronator strength. Finally, eccentric strengthening exercises are added [4]. Return to sport is generally recommended in a stepwise manner once the patient can tolerate sprint repetitions of concentric and eccentric resistance exercises [3].

Regarding avulsion fractures, nondisplaced and minimally displaced (5 mm or less) fractures can be treated nonoperative with cast or hinge brace immobilization for a period of 4 weeks. Then, a progressive physical therapy is routine focused on initially regaining full range of motion and then establishing full strength of the affected extremity [5, 10].

28.1.4.3 Procedures

Extracorporeal shockwave therapy (ESWT) It provides electrical stimulation to the diseased tendon to help promote angiogenesis, tendon healing, and pain relief [11]. Long-term outcomes were not promising in one study. Only 7 of 30 patients reported either excellent or good results at 1 year follow-up after ESWT sessions were completed on a weekly basis [12].

Platelet-rich plasma (PRP) In a study by Halpern et al., the utilization of PRP was significantly effective in treating ME from a clinical and structural standpoint. Further, PRP was linked to reduced needs for narcotic medication, improved sleep, and reduction in perception of pain [13]. However, the study noted unanswered questions in regard to the optimal concentration of platelets, what cell types should be present, and ideal application frequency that still need to be explored [13].

Percutaneous ultrasonic tenotomy (PCU) Limited data is available but is promising in highlighting its use in patients with tendinopathy refractory to conservative measures. In a systematic review by Vajapey et al., percutaneous ultrasonic tenotomy resulted in decreased pain/disability scores and improved functional outcome scores for chronic elbow tendinopathy [14]. When comparing PCU to PRP, both were successful in producing clinically and statistically significant improvements in pain, function, and quality of life; however, there was no statistical significance found between the two [15].

Bone marrow aspirate concentrate (BMAC) To date, no research studies are available evaluating BMAC therapy for ME. However, stem cell therapy was beneficial from a pain, function, and improving the structural defect seen on ultrasound in patients with lateral epicondylitis consistently from 2 to 52 weeks post-injection [16].

28.1.4.4 Surgery

Surgery for ME is typically reserved for patients with recurrent and/or persistent symptoms despite nonsurgical management for at least 4–6 months [4]. However, an elite athlete with definitive tendon disruption on MRI may return to pre-injury performance levels with early surgical intervention, compared to initial nonsurgical treatment [3]. Common surgical management involves an open procedure with debridement of injured tissue of the CFT and tendon repair [3].

The decision for surgical intervention of an avulsion fracture includes absolute and relative indications. Absolute indications include open fractures and fracture fragments that are within the joint [17]. Relative indications are controversial in the literature but can include valgus instability, athletes with high-demand elbow function in their sport, and associated ulnar nerve dysfunction [5]. Typically, if the displacement is greater than 5 mm, this is an indication for a surgical consultation. Multiple studies have shown either good to excellent results with open reduction and internal fixation or continued radiographic findings of nonunion with non-operative treatment with fractures having a displacement of greater than 5 mm [18–20]. Surgeries in the elbow are further discussed in Chap. 30.

28.2 Ulnar (Medial) Collateral Ligament Injury

28.2.1 Synonyms

Tommy John injury

28.2.2 ICD-10 Codes

S53.441, S53.442, S53.449, S53.31

28.2.3 Description

The elbow is a hinged joint that is composed of three articulations: the radiocapitellar joint, the ulnohumeral joint, and the proximal radioulnar joint. All three joints are enclosed by a single fibrous and synovial capsule that thickens and create the medial and lateral ligaments of the elbow [21]. The configuration of the joint itself provides stability of the elbow against varus and valgus stress at less than 20 degrees and more than 120 degrees of flexion; however, between these angles, stability is heavily provided by the medial and lateral ligaments of the elbow [22]. The ulnar collateral ligament (UCL) is composed of three parts: an anterior oblique ligament, a fan-shaped posterior oblique ligament, and a transverse oblique ligament. The transverse oblique is relatively nonfunctional in terms of stability [22]. It has been shown that the anterior oblique ligament is the primary stabilizer to valgus stress.

UCL injury occurs due to repetitive extremes of high force valgus stress of the ligament. This injury can be seen in any overhead-throwing athlete or any athlete that performs high-velocity overhead rotation motions such as baseball, softball, American football quarterbacks, Javlineers, gymnastics, tennis, golf, wresting, hand ball, and water polo [23]. The ligament is specifically vulnerable during the late cocking and early acceleration phases of the throwing motion with the arm abducted to 90 degrees, externally rotated at the shoulder, and flexed 90 degrees or greater at the elbow [24]. This portion of the throwing motion places maximum valgus stress on the elbow, which can lead to chronic microtrauma or eventual complete rupture of the ligament. There has been a rising incidence of UCL injury across age groups and skill levels over the past couple of decades. The incidence of UCL rupture in baseball players in 15- to 19-year-olds increased by more than 9% between 2007 and 2011 [25]. In Major League Baseball, 24.1% of all elbow injuries from 2011 to 2014 were due to UCL-related injury [26]. Further, the prevalence of UCL reconstruction (UCL-R) in all professional pitchers was 13% with major league pitchers reporting 26% prevalence of UCL-R [27].

28.2.4 Clinical Presentation

Given this injury is prevalent in overhead-throwing sports, it is important to determine the patient's athletic participation and level of competition. Injuries to the UCL can be acute or chronic, and they present in slightly different ways. Acute injuries make up approximately two-thirds of injuries and present with intense pain during throwing followed by an inability to continue [28]. Some athletes may feel a "pop" in their elbow after a specific pitch without having prior elbow pain [29]. Chronic injuries have an insidious onset and present over a longer period of time with symptoms of medial elbow pain while throwing combined with decreased throwing velocity and accuracy as well as decreased sport performance as listed in Table 28.2 [24].

28.2.5 Physical Examination

Physical examination should include inspection, palpation, range of motion, and neurological examination of both the affected and unaffected sides. Inspection should be used to rule out other pathologies as UCL injury does not typically cause a joint effusion or overlying skin changes. Patients typically have tenderness to palpation at the medial epicondyle and/or at the sublime tubercle, where the ligament inserts [24]. Passive and active range of motion (ROM) is typically preserved in isolated UCL injuries, but loss of extension or pain with terminal extension can indicate an associated posteromedial impingement. Shoulder ROM should be evaluated, including a patient's total arc of motion. Total arc of motion is evaluated by placing the patient in 90 degrees of shoulder abduction and combining the measurements of maximal internal and external rotation [30]. In a study by Ruotolo et al., college-level baseball players with shoulder pain had a significant decrease in total arch of motion and internal rotation when compared to their nondominant shoulder and with pain-free athletes [30]. This loss of motion has been associated with conditions such as scapular dyskinesis and glenohumeral internal rotation deficit (GIRD) [31].

Table 28.2 Differential diagnosis of ulnar collateral ligament injury

Ulnar neuritis
Ulnar nerve subluxation
Subluxation of medial head of triceps
Medial epicondylopathy
Osseous fragmentation or avulsion or loose body
Valgus extension overload syndrome
Stress reaction/fracture of bone

28.2.5.1 Special Tests

1. *Milking maneuver*: The patient should be placed in 90 degrees of shoulder abduction and elbow flexion and forearm sully supinated while pulling the patients thumb posteriorly to apply a valgus load. The presence of pain, instability, or apprehension is a positive test [29] (see Fig. 28.1).
2. *Moving valgus stress test*: The patient should be placed in 90 degrees of shoulder abduction with maximal external rotation and full flexion of the elbow. Then a valgus stress is applied to the elbow while quickly extending the elbow to 30 degrees. Eliciting pain indicates a positive test [32].

28.2.5.2 Diagnostic Workup

1. *X-ray*: Radiographs can be used to evaluate for any associated osseous abnormalities of the elbow; this could include olecranon osteophytes, loose bodies, ligament avulsions, and calcification of the UCL. Utilizing non-stressed and stressed radiographs to determine ligament insufficiency has shown conflicting results; therefore, a negative stress radiograph should not be used to rule out UCL pathology [24].

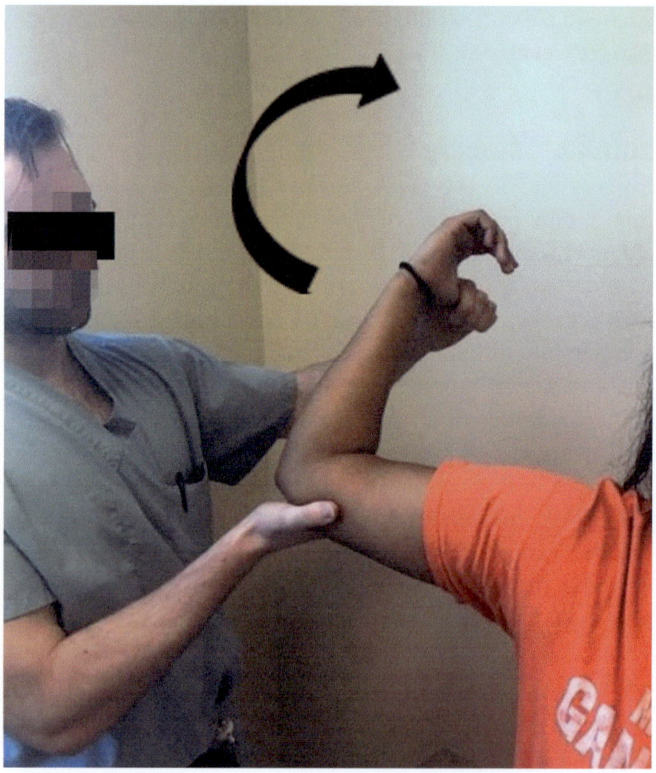

Fig. 28.1 Milking maneuver. While the affected limb's elbow is flexed to approximately 90 degrees, the examiner grabs the patient's thumb and applies a valgus load with a posterior strain (arrow). Pain, instability, or apprehension is considered a positive test

2. *Ultrasound*: Stress ultrasonography can be an accurate, cost-effective, and timely imaging modality to detect medial elbow gapping seen in UCL injury as well as ligamentous changes. One recent study compared the distance in joint space gapping with stress ultrasonography of cadaveric elbows with different anatomical locations of partial UCL tears: distal anterior/posterior, midsubstance anterior/posterior, and proximal anterior/posterior. Both distal partial tear groups had mean gapping distance similar to intact UCLs [33]. Midsubstance partial tears had the largest distance, similar to those of complete tears [34]. These findings suggest that whether non-operative treatment or early reconstruction is recommended could depend on where the partial tear occurs. UCL ruptures can present as discontinuity of the ligament with anechoic fluid of a heterogeneous echogenicity [35].
3. *MRI or MRI arthrography:* Advanced imaging with MRI or MRI arthrography (MRA) is the best way to visualize both full- and partial-thickness tears of the UCL along with other concomitant elbow pathologies. Specifically, MRA has been shown to be more accurate than MRI for the diagnosis of UCL tears (sensitivity and specificity, 92% and 100%, respectively, compared to 57% and 100%, respectively) [36]. Abnormal appearance on MRI depends on the acuity and severity of the injury. Sprains are demonstrated by ligament thickening and signal hyperintensity with no area of discontinuity. Acute, complete tears show increased T2 signal within and around the ligament [35]. Partial tears present as focal areas of disruption of the ligament with increased signal [35].

28.2.6 Treatments

Tailoring treatment options for each patient will require taking into account the age, athletic level, desire to return to competitive play, and potentially location of the tear. Unless there is evidence of a complete tear, pediatric athletes should be managed initially non-operatively due to injury in this age group which is typically a result of poor throwing technique and overuse [37]. However, location of injury is important to note as research indicated that distal partial tears more likely to fail non-operative treatment compared to proximal partial tears [38].

28.2.6.1 Medical Management

When beginning non-operative treatment, all patients should be initially managed with a period of rest, ice, and potentially anti-inflammatory medications if pain control is needed. Patients should also be counseled to avoid valgus stress to the elbow to help with decreasing inflammation and to avoid any further stress on the ligament [39].

28.2.6.2 Rehabilitation

When taking an initial conservative approach, a gradually progressive physical therapy program beginning after the initial rest period is recommended. Strengthening and stretching exercises of the wrist extensors and flexors, improving shoulder motion, and periscapular strengthening should be focused on at first [40]. Further, proprioceptive training, lower body strength, and core training should be implemented to help strengthen the entire kinetic chain to help prevent future injuries [40]. Once a patient has pain-free full range of motion, pain-free with valgus stress, and full strength of shoulder and elbow, sports-specific related activities and an interval throwing program can be started [39, 40]. If the patient experiences pain at any point during the rehabilitation process, the elbow should be rested. Once symptoms resolve, rehabilitation can be started again either from the beginning or an earlier phase of the protocol [40].

If surgery is indicated, the rehabilitation process varies compared to the conservative approach. During the initial month of therapy, goals are to protect healing tissue, decrease pain and inflammation, and begin the process of restoring range of motion. During the initial postoperative week, the elbow is fixed in 90 degrees of flexion and allowed to rest. At week 2, a functional brace is applied, and the patient is allowed limited ROM with a goal of achieving a ROM of roughly 30–100 degrees. Initiating wrist ROM and gripping exercises, as well as scapular and shoulder isometrics, is important. During the second month of rehabilitation, full ROM with flexion and extension should be achieved. Initiating light resistance exercises (one pound) of wrist curls, extension, pronation/supination, and elbow flexion/extension is begun, as well as incorporating a strengthening program for the rotator cuff. Elbow bracing is typically discontinued once full range of motion is achieved, usually by 8 weeks. During the third month, the major goal is to obtain full strength in the entire upper extremity. Typically, throwers will begin a throwing program at 4 months with a gradual return to competitive throwing at around 6 months (Ellenbecker) [41]. It is important to emphasize the continued need for incorporating flexibility and strengthening exercises for the elbow and shoulder into their training program to help prevent reinjury.

28.2.6.3 Procedures

1. *Platelet-rich plasma (PRP) injection* is a sample of autologous blood that contains an increased concentration of platelets. These platelets release growth factors such as platelet-derived growth factor, transforming growth factor beta, and vascular endothelial growth factor that potentially stimulate endothelial growth and angiogenesis [42]. PRP has shown promising results in studies and may be useful in initiating a healing response, but the lack

of randomized controlled trials as well as variability in preparation and dosing limits any definitive treatment recommendations. In a study by Rettig et al., there was a 42% return-to-play rate of throwing athletes who were treated non-operatively with anti-inflammatory drugs, icing, night-time bracing, graduated physical therapy, and a throwing program. The average time to return to play was 24.5 weeks [43]. In contrast, studies with protocols including PRP have shown return-to-play rates of 66% to 88% [42, 44]. More recent data has suggested that low-grade injuries have successful outcomes after PRP when combined with physical therapy and rehabilitation compared with higher-grade UCL injuries [45].

2. *Corticosteroid injection*: Corticosteroid injections are not recommended due to the potential risk of damage to articular cartilage and/or further tendon injury or rupture [46].

28.2.6.4 Surgery

Indications for surgical evaluation include failure of non-operative treatment, continued medial elbow pain/instability, and/or full-thickness UCL rupture [25]. There are multiple commonly used surgical techniques for UCL-R as well as, more recently, UCL repair using internal bracing. The most common graft option is the palmaris longus tendon [25]. Surgeries in the elbow are further discussed in Chap. 30.

References

1. Descatha A, Leclerc A, Chastang JF, Roquelaure Y, Study Group on Repetitive Work. Medial epicondylitis in occupational settings: prevalence, incidence and associated risk factors. J Occup Environ Med. 2003;45(9):993–1001.
2. Vangsness CT, Jobe FW. Surgical treatment of medial epicondylitis. Results in 35 elbows. J Bone Joint Surg Br. 1991;73(3):409–11.
3. Ciccotti MG, Ramani MN. Medial epicondylitis. Tech Hand Up Extrem Surg. 2003;7(4):190–6.
4. Amin NH, Kumar NS, Schickendantz MS. Medial epicondylitis: evaluation and management. J Am Acad Orthop Surg. 2015;23(6):348–55.
5. Gottschalk HP, Eisner E, Hosalkar HS. Medial epicondyle fractures in the pediatric population. J Am Acad Orthop Surg. 2012;20(4):223–32.
6. Wilkins KE. Fractures involving the medial epicondylar apophysis. In: Rockwood Jr CA, Wilkins KE, King RE, editors. Fractures in children. 3rd ed. Philadelphia: JB Lippincott; 1991. p. 509–828.
7. Cain EL, Dugas JR, Wolf RS, Andrews JR. Elbow injuries in throwing athletes: a current concepts review. Am J Sports Med. 2003;31(4):621–35.
8. Park G-Y, Lee S-M, Lee MY. Diagnostic value of ultrasonography for clinical medial epicondylitis. Arch Phys Med Rehabil. 2008;89(4):738–42.
9. Kijowski R, De Smet AA. Magnetic resonance imaging findings in patients with medial epicondylitis. Skelet Radiol. 2005;34(4):196–202.
10. Ostrander JD, O'Connell M, Dolch HJ. Open reduction internal fixation of a medial epicondyle avulsion fracture with incarcerated fragment. J Orthop Trauma. 2019;33(Suppl 1):S9–10.
11. Sems A, Dimeff R, Iannotti JP. Extracorporeal shock wave therapy in the treatment of chronic tendinopathies. J Am Acad Orthop Surg. 2006;14(4):195–204.
12. Krischek O, Pompe JD, Hopf C, Vogel J, Herbsthofer B, Nafe B, et al. [Extracorporeal shockwave therapy in epicondylitis humeri ulnaris or radialis--a prospective, controlled, comparative study]. Z Orthop Ihre Grenzgeb. 1998;136(1):3–7.
13. Halpern BC, Chaudhury S, Rodeo SA. The role of platelet-rich plasma in inducing musculoskeletal tissue healing. HSS J Musculoskelet J Hosp Spec Surg. 2012;8(2):137–45.
14. Vajapey S, Ghenbot S, Baria MR, Magnussen RA, Vasileff WK. Utility of percutaneous ultrasonic tenotomy for tendinopathies: a systematic review. Sports Health. 2020;30:1941738120951764.
15. Boden AL, Scott MT, Dalwadi PP, Mautner K, Mason RA, Gottschalk MB. Platelet-rich plasma versus Tenex in the treatment of medial and lateral epicondylitis. J Shoulder Elb Surg. 2019;28(1):112–9.
16. Lee SY, Kim W, Lim C, Chung SG. Treatment of lateral epicondylosis by using allogeneic adipose-derived mesenchymal stem cells: a pilot study. Stem Cells Dayt Ohio. 2015;33(10):2995–3005.
17. Fowles JV, Kassab MT, Moula T. Untreated intra-articular entrapment of the medial humeral epicondyle. J Bone Joint Surg Br. 1984;66(4):562–5.
18. Louahem DM, Bourelle S, Buscayret F, Mazeau P, Kelly P, Dimeglio A, et al. Displaced medial epicondyle fractures of the humerus: surgical treatment and results. A report of 139 cases. Arch Orthop Trauma Surg. 2010;130(5):649–55.
19. Josefsson PO, Danielsson LG. Epicondylar elbow fracture in children. 35-year follow-up of 56 unreduced cases. Acta Orthop Scand. 1986;57(4):313–5.
20. Lee H-H, Shen H-C, Chang J-H, Lee C-H, Wu S-S. Operative treatment of displaced medial epicondyle fractures in children and adolescents. J Shoulder Elb Surg. 2005;14(2):178–85.
21. Miller null, Savoie null. Valgus extension injuries of the elbow in the throwing athlete. J Am Acad Orthop Surg. 1994;2(5):261–9.
22. Schwab GH, Bennett JB, Woods GW, Tullos HS. Biomechanics of elbow instability: the role of the medial collateral ligament. Clin Orthop. 1980;146:42–52.
23. Dugas J, Chronister J, Cain EL, Andrews JR. Ulnar collateral ligament in the overhead athlete: a current review. Sports Med Arthrosc Rev. 2014;22(3):169–82.
24. Raducha JE, Gil JA, Harris AP, Owens BD. Ulnar collateral ligament injuries of the elbow in the throwing athlete. JBJS Rev. 2018;6(2):e1.
25. Erickson BJ, Nwachukwu BU, Rosas S, Schairer WW, McCormick FM, Bach BR, et al. Trends in medial ulnar collateral ligament reconstruction in the United States: a retrospective review of a large private-payer database from 2007 to 2011. Am J Sports Med. 2015;43(7):1770–4.
26. Ciccotti MG, Pollack KM, Ciccotti MC, D'Angelo J, Ahmad CS, Altchek D, et al. Elbow injuries in professional baseball: epidemiological findings from the major league baseball injury surveillance system. Am J Sports Med. 2017;45(10):2319–28.
27. Leland DP, Conte S, Flynn N, Conte N, Crenshaw K, Wilk KE, et al. Prevalence of medial ulnar collateral ligament surgery in 6135 current professional baseball players: a 2018 update. Orthop J Sports Med. 2019;7(9):2325967119871442.
28. Nassab PF, Schickendantz MS. Evaluation and treatment of medial ulnar collateral ligament injuries in the throwing athlete. Sports Med Arthrosc Rev. 2006;14(4):221–31.
29. Jang S-H. Management of ulnar collateral ligament injuries in overhead athletes. Clin Shoulder Elb. 2019;22(4):235–40.

30. Ruotolo C, Price E, Panchal A. Loss of total arc of motion in collegiate baseball players. J Shoulder Elb Surg. 2006;15(1):67–71.
31. Wilk KE, Macrina LC, Fleisig GS, Aune KT, Porterfield RA, Harker P, et al. Deficits in glenohumeral passive range of motion increase risk of shoulder injury in professional baseball pitchers: a prospective study. Am J Sports Med. 2015;43(10):2379–85.
32. Madden C, Putukian M, McCarty E, Young C. Netter's sports medicine. Elsevier; 2017. p. 816.
33. Ciccotti MG, Atanda A, Nazarian LN, Dodson CC, Holmes L, Cohen SB. Stress sonography of the ulnar collateral ligament of the elbow in professional baseball pitchers: a 10-year study. Am J Sports Med. 2014;42(3):544–51.
34. Ciccotti MC, Hammoud S, Dodson CC, Cohen SB, Nazarian LN, Ciccotti MG. Medial elbow instability resulting from partial tears of the ulnar collateral ligament: stress ultrasound in a cadaveric model. Am J Sports Med. 2020;48(11):2613–20.
35. Ford GM, Genuario J, Kinkartz J, Githens T, Noonan T. Return-to-play outcomes in professional baseball players after medial ulnar collateral ligament injuries: comparison of operative versus nonoperative treatment based on magnetic resonance imaging findings. Am J Sports Med. 2016;44(3):723–8.
36. Magee T. Accuracy of 3-T MR arthrography versus conventional 3-T MRI of elbow tendons and ligaments compared with surgery. AJR Am J Roentgenol. 2015;204(1):W70–5.
37. Greiwe RM, Saifi C, Ahmad CS. Pediatric sports elbow injuries. Clin Sports Med. 2010;29(4):677–703.
38. Frangiamore SJ, Lynch TS, Vaughn MD, Soloff L, Forney M, Styron JF, et al. Magnetic resonance imaging predictors of failure in the nonoperative management of ulnar collateral ligament injuries in professional baseball pitchers. Am J Sports Med. 2017;45(8):1783–9.
39. Zaremski JL, Vincent KR, Vincent HK. Elbow ulnar collateral ligament: injury, treatment options, and recovery in overhead throwing athletes. Curr Sports Med Rep. 2019;18(9):338–45.
40. Kadri OM, Okoroha KR, Patel RB, Berguson J, Makhni EC, Moutzouros V. Nonoperative treatment of medial ulnar collateral ligament injuries in the throwing athlete: indications, evaluation, and management. JBJS Rev. 2019;7(1):e6.
41. Ellenbecker TS, Wilk KE, Altchek DW, Andrews JR. Current concepts in rehabilitation following ulnar collateral ligament reconstruction. Sports Health. 2009;1(4):301–13.
42. Podesta L, Crow SA, Volkmer D, Bert T, Yocum LA. Treatment of partial ulnar collateral ligament tears in the elbow with platelet-rich plasma. Am J Sports Med. 2013;41(7):1689–94.
43. Rettig AC, Sherrill C, Snead DS, Mendler JC, Mieling P. Nonoperative treatment of ulnar collateral ligament injuries in throwing athletes. Am J Sports Med. 2001;29(1):15–7.
44. Dines JS, Williams PN, ElAttrache N, Conte S, Tomczyk T, Osbahr DC, et al. Platelet-rich plasma can be used to successfully treat elbow ulnar collateral ligament insufficiency in high-level throwers. Am J Orthop Belle Mead NJ. 2016;45(5):296–300.
45. Mills FB, Misra AK, Goyeneche N, Hackel JG, Andrews JR, Joyner PW. Return to play after platelet-rich plasma injection for elbow UCL injury: outcomes based on injury severity. Orthop J Sports Med. 2021;9(3):2325967121991135.
46. Freire V, Bureau NJ. Injectable corticosteroids: take precautions and use caution. Semin Musculoskelet Radiol. 2016;20(5):401–8.

29 Elbow Joint Dislocations and Fractures

Jason L. Zaremski, Julio A. Martinez-Silvestrini, and Eric W. Pettyjohn

29.1 Elbow Dislocation

29.1.1 ICD-10 Codes

M24.429, M24.421, M24.422, M24.321, M24.322, M24.329 S53.1, S53.104A, S53.105A, S53.194A, S53.195A

29.1.2 Synonyms

None

29.1.3 Definition

When the proximal radius and/or ulna become malaligned with respect to the distal humerus.

29.1.4 Symptoms

Elbow dislocations, which are the most commonly dislocated joint in children and second most common overall (the shoulder is the first), are typically due to a traumatic forceful impact [1]. Specifically, axial loading with supination or external rotation of the forearm combined with a valgus posterolateral force may result in this injury. The most common ages for this injury are typically 10–20 years old. The most common direction of an elbow dislocation is posterolateral (about 80%) [2]. For a posteromedial dislocation, the force is due to a varus posteromedial mechanism.

As with nearly all dislocations, these injuries are acute in nature. Patients will have gross deformities of their elbow joint with immediate pain and associated swelling. Sports that have the greatest number of injuries are reported to be American football, wrestling, and gymnastics.

29.1.5 Physical Exam

Given the severity of the injury, the immediate focus should be to first assess the skin and confirm there are no signs of an open injury. Next, neurovascular status should be assessed at the wrist, elbow, and upper arm due to the risk of neurovascular injury or compromise in upward of 20% of cases [3]. Further, injuries to the wrist or shoulder occur with elbow dislocations in about 10–15% of cases, and these joints should be initially assessed, as well [3].

Finally, checking for the presence of compartment syndrome by assessing compartments in the upper arm and forearm is paramount. With posterior elbow dislocations, the upper extremity may be shortened, and the elbow minimally flexed with a prominent olecranon. Any crepitus with active range of motion (AROM) or passive range of motion (PROM) is an indicator of a potential fracture, and radiograph prior to attempted reduction is recommended [3].

J. L. Zaremski (✉)
Divisions of PM&R, Sports Medicine, & Research, Department of Orthopaedics and Rehabilitation, UF Health, University of Florida, Gainesville, FL, USA
e-mail: zaremjl@ufl.edu

J. A. Martinez-Silvestrini
Baystate Rehabilitation Care, University of Massachusetts Medical School – Baystate, Longmeadow, MA, USA

Tufts University School of Medicine, Boston, MA, USA

University of Massachusetts Medical School – Baystate, Longmeadow, MA, USA
e-mail: Julio.martinez@bhs.org

E. W. Pettyjohn
UF Health, University of Florida, Gainesville, FL, USA

© The Author(s), under exclusive license to Springer Nature Switzerland AG 2022
S. A. Mostoufi et al. (eds.), *Clinical Guide to Musculoskeletal Medicine*, https://doi.org/10.1007/978-3-030-92042-5_29

29.1.6 Diagnostic Workup

Imaging workup includes elbow radiographs that include anterior-posterior and lateral views, though one may consider oblique views as well. After an attempted reduction follow-up, immediate repeat radiographs are recommended to assess for joint congruency as well as potential secondary fractures [1]. A computed tomography (CT) scan may be indicated once reduction is achieved to identify occult fractures not present on radiographs [4].

The treating provider should be aware of the "terrible triad" of the elbow. This is when there is a traumatic elbow dislocation, radial head fracture, and associated coronoid fracture. This injury pattern may lead to poorer outcomes and has been associated with recurrent and/or chronic instability and posttraumatic arthritis. Early referral to surgical specialists are indicated in this scenario [4, 5].

29.1.7 Treatments

For any dislocation, immediate reduction is the primary treatment [1]. Once this has been achieved, the patient should be splinted at 90 degrees for 5–10 days. Repeated neurovascular and compartment checks after injury are recommended, as well [1, 4].

29.1.7.1 Elbow Reduction Maneuvers

For patients that are not in a hospital or emergency room setting, while immediate reduction is recommended, reductions should only be performed with a healthcare provider that is experienced in evaluating and treating the injury. For sporting events, it has been recommended by the National Athletic Trainers' Association that "onsite elbow reductions should not be attempted by athletic trainers in most cases given that elbow dislocations typically involve fracture(s) and significant potential for neurovascular compromise." However, the consensus recommendations state that "If emergency transport will be delayed, an AT, under the direction of a physician, may attempt a reduction provided no signs and symptoms of fracture or neurovascular damage are present. Multiple attempts at reduction are not recommended " [6].

There are different techniques for elbow reduction in supine and prone planes using traction and countertraction. After any elbow reduction, always repeat neurovascular status and compartment checks [1]:

1. Elbow reduction technique 1: [4, 7, 8]

The patient will lay supine with the elbow and forearm supinated. Traction should be applied to the forearm with countertraction to the upper arm. Then, force should be applied to the olecranon distally in order to reduce into the olecranon fossa (Fig. 29.1).

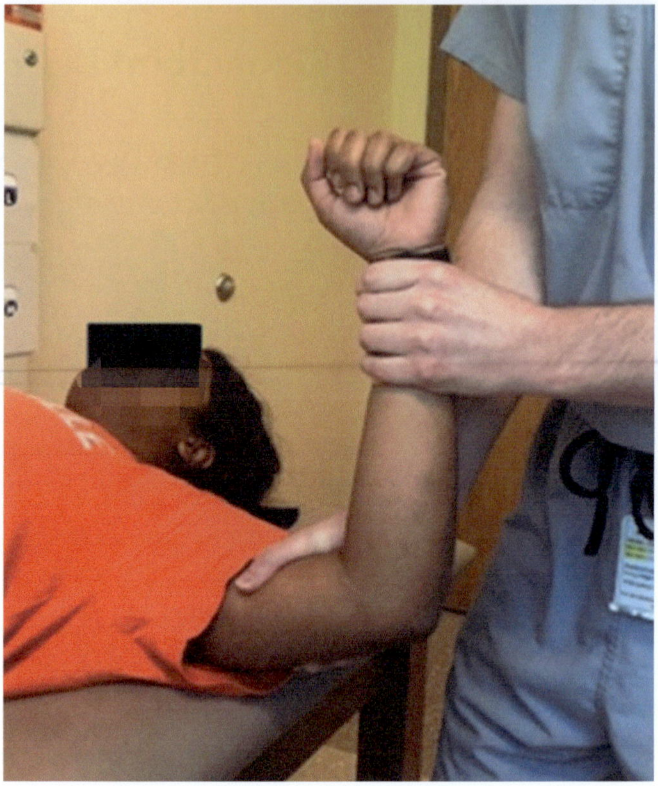

Fig. 29.1 Technique 1 elbow reduction maneuver

2. Elbow reduction technique 2: [9]

With the patient in a prone position, and the affected arm/forearm laying off of the examination table, traction is applied via a downward force on the forearm with one hand while there is countertraction to the humerus. Then, olecranon is pushed into the olecranon fossa to achieve reduction (Fig. 29.2).

3. Elbow reduction: technique 3: [10]

The patient is supine with the affected arm across the chest. The elbow is flexed to 90 degrees with the forearm in supination. Traction is applied to the forearm with one hand, while the other hand pulls the arm in the opposite direction. The elbow is then flexed, and the thumb pushes the olecranon into the olecranon fossa. As noted in previous literature, it is important that the forearm is supinated during reduction so the coronoid can clear the trochlea (Fig. 29.3) [4].

29.1.7.2 Splinting

Splinting should then take place as elbow stability evaluation is not recommended as the elbow is likely unstable, in particular in valgus and with extension. The splint should be placed with the elbow in at least 90° of elbow flexion. Of note if there is suspicion of radial collateral ligament rupture, splint with the elbow in pronation is recommended. However, if there is concern of an ulnar collateral

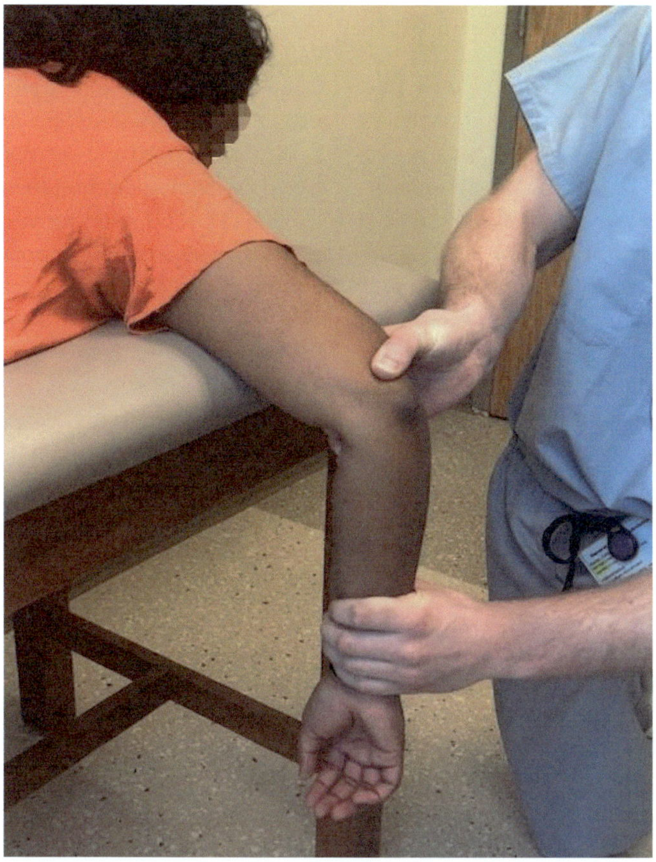

Fig. 29.2 Technique 2: elbow reduction maneuver

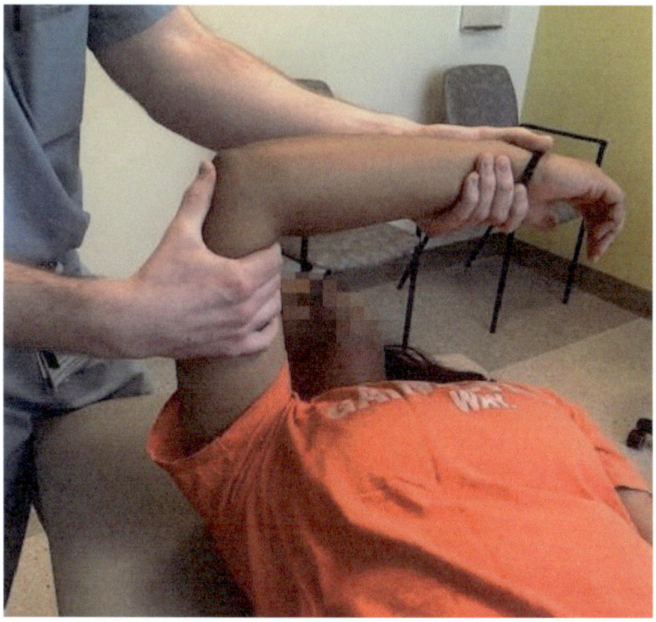

Fig. 29.3 Technique 3: elbow reduction maneuver

ligament rupture, then splinting in supination is recommended. Once splinting has occurred, obtain post-reduction radiographs.

Elbow dislocations are divided into simple and complex. Simple indicates no fracture, whereas a complex elbow dislocation is associated with a fracture,

For dislocations that result in more significant associated injuries (i.e., fractures of the coronoid, radial head, olecranon, as well as radial collateral ligament, and/or ulnar collateral ligament ruptures), surgical referral is indicated. Persistent post-reduction instability or inability to perform a reduction also requires a surgical referral.

29.1.7.3 Medical Management

The goals of treatment include a stable elbow joint with ability to achieve early active ROM [1]. For closed reduction and non-operative management, typically patients are immobilized for only about 5–10 days. Further, research has indicated that immobilization for more than 1–3 weeks results in poor ROM and possible elbow contracture [4, 11, 12]. As patients progress after the first 5–10 days, early active assisted ROM (AAROM) with a physical therapist is strongly recommended with a limited ROM arc. Extension blocks may be used for up to 3–4 weeks. Gradually the extension block is removed such that approximately 6–8 weeks post injury a patient has full AROM [4]. A hinged elbow brace that has ROM locking capability is typically very helpful once the initial splint is removed.

29.1.7.4 Rehabilitation

Clearance for return to sport without restriction will be allowed once the patient has full AROM without pain as well as no signs of instability with valgus, varus, and posterolateral rotational testing without the use of a stabilization brace [1].

29.1.7.5 Procedures

Once reduced, no additional intervention needed.

29.1.7.6 Surgery

For further details of surgical interventions and postoperative rehabilitation, please refer to Chap. 30.

29.2 Elbow Fractures

29.2.1 Synonyms

- Intercondylar fracture
- Olecranon fracture
- Radial head fracture
- Supracondylar fracture

29.2.2 ICD-10 Code

- S42.4: Fracture of distal end of humerus
- S42.41: Simple supracondylar fracture

- S52.90XA: Unspecified fracture of forearm
- S52.02: Fracture of olecranon process
- S52.12: Fracture of head of radius

29.2.3 Description

Elbow fractures are one of the most common upper extremity fractures. They are the most common type of fractures in the pediatric population with acute supracondylar fractures as the most frequent type [13, 14]. The adult population includes a large variety of acute fractures, with radial head and olecranon fractures as the most common [14]. At the distal humerus, intercondylar fractures are the most common surgery requiring internal fixation [15]. The overall incidence of elbow fractures in pediatric patients is reported at approximately 30/10,000 per year, a fraction of elbow fractures in adults, 4/10,000. Supracondylar fractures have an incidence of 177/100,000 children [13]. Acutely they may be seen in combination with neurovascular injuries. And if left untreated, they may also result in non-union, valgus or varus elbow deformities, and chronic nerve injuries [13]. Due to the heterogeneity of pathologic fractures, this entity will be excluded from this chapter.

29.2.4 Clinical Presentation

Most pediatric elbow fractures have a peak between 6 and 10 years old and occur after a fall from a play structure as trampoline or monkey bars [13, 14]. Skateboard and scooter (caster-boarding) injuries are five times more common than after a fall while riding a bicycle [13]. The male:female ratio of elbow fractures is 1.6:1. The non-dominant upper extremity is mostly involved, as it is postulated that the dominant arm is in use, while the non-dominant arm assumes a protective role [13]. The elbow joint is the most common joint dislocation in pediatric patients and is the second most common in adults [14]. One-third to half of all elbow dislocation may be complex dislocation-fracture injuries, requiring surgical care. Multiple elbow fractures can coexist and are common in adults suffering dislocation-fractures, with the radial head and coronoid fractures mostly involved [14].

29.2.5 Physical Examination

On inspection, findings may range from mild swelling to obvious deformity of the elbow. Patients guard the injured elbow in flexion with the shoulder internally rotated. The

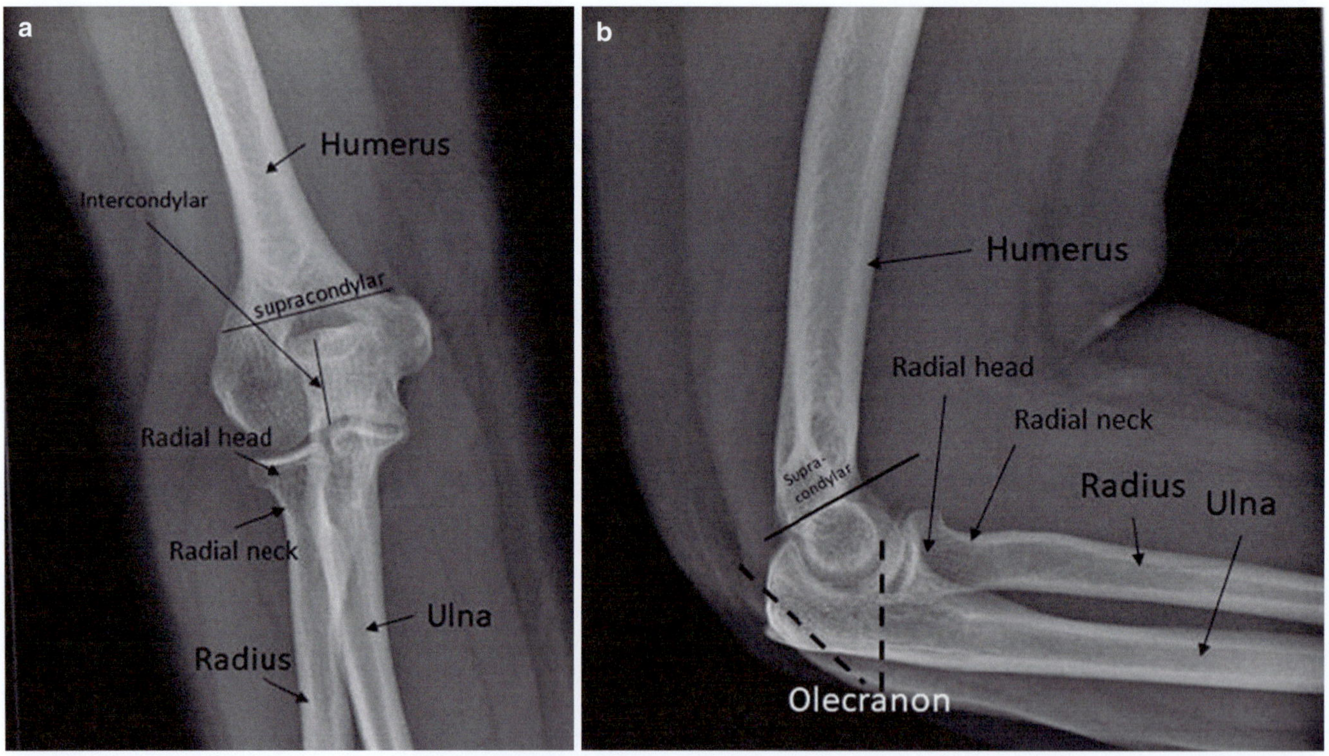

Fig. 29.4 Anteroposterior (**a**) and lateral (**b**) views of the elbow illustrating common areas of elbow fractures. The solid lines in anteroposterior and lateral views mark common areas of supracondylar and intercondylar fractures, while the dotted lines in the lateral views mark common sites of olecranon fractures. The arrows mark the humerus, radius, and ulnar bones, as well as the radial head and radial neck and common fracture sites of the proximal radius

olecranon, medial epicondyle, lateral epicondyle, and radial head should be palpated looking for exquisite local tenderness (Fig. 29.4). It is not uncommon for the patient to "jump" when the fracture site is palpated (known by one of the authors as the "jack in the box" sign). ROM is usually limited on extension. Pronation and supination may be painful or limited in cases of radial head fractures [16].

The elbow extension test can be used as an examination screening tool to determine the presence of elbow fractures in adults. The test is done with the patient seated, shoulders flexed forward at 90°, and forearms supinated (palms up). The patient can rest the arms on an examination table if needed for comfort. Then the patient is asked to fully extend and lock both elbows. Injured and uninjured elbows' range of motion is compared. Patients who cannot fully extend their affected elbow after injury should be referred for imaging. X-rays can be deferred if the patient has full elbow extension, there is no concern for an olecranon fracture and the patient can return for a 7–10 days of follow-up. This test has a sensitivity of 97% but has a low specificity of 50%. This test should be used with caution in the pediatric population [17].

Neurovascular injuries by traction, compression (by hematoma formation or compartment syndrome), or laceration by sharp bone fragments may occur acutely [13, 16]. Injuries involving the median nerve and brachial artery at the antecubital fossa, the ulnar nerve medially, or radial nerve, specifically posterior interosseous nerve, in cases of radial head fractures may be observed [16]. After elbow trauma and suspected fracture or dislocation, a detailed neurovascular physical examination of the wrist and hand is imperative. Active range of motion and strength examination as tolerated as well as palpation of the upper extremity compartments, sensory examination, pulses, and capillary refill should be performed.

29.2.6 Diagnostic Workup

At least two perpendicular X-ray views of the elbow (Fig. 29.4), full-length humerus and full-length radius and ulna, are a standard practice in patients after acute trauma. Imaging of the joint above and below the fracture site is also commonly obtained. The lateral radiograph is helpful for the identification of the "posterior fat pad sign" [16], which may represent an elbow effusion in patients with a fracture difficult to visualize. In addition, a raised anterior fat pad (a.k.a. "the sail sign") may also be present in an intra-articular fracture such as in an occult radial head fracture [18]. Contralateral X-rays are recommended in pediatric patients for detailed comparison of ossification centers [16]. Proximal radial fractures are associated with other fractures or elbow dislocations in 30–50% of cases, for which once a proximal radial fracture is identified, the examiner should look for another possible fracture [16]. Elbow arthrogram and computer tomography (CT) are particularly helpful for elbow injuries due to the anatomic complexity of the joint and bony overlap on X-rays AP and lateral images.

29.2.7 Treatments

29.2.7.1 Medical Management

To prevent elbow fractures in the pediatric population, the use of protective elbow pads is recommended while riding skateboards and bicycles [13]. Most radial fractures and minimally displaced radial neck fractures can be treated conservatively resulting in excellent results in most patients [14, 16]. Some displaced proximal radial fractures can be treated with close reduction. Pronation and supination ROM loss is common in pediatric patients with radial head fractures [16], and proactive warning and education should be given to the patient and family members. Recommendation of 2–3 weeks of immobilization in a long arm cast with the forearm in neutral rotation or slight pronation after reduction is indicated. Ninety to ninety-five percent of excellent to good outcomes are seen in patients treated conservatively for proximal radial fractures [16]. If a patient has a non-displaced or minimally displaced radial head or neck fracture, recommendations include the use of a sling with early ROM in flexion and extension planes only (no supination or pronation), but non-weight-bearing is recommended for the first 2–4 weeks.

29.2.7.2 Rehabilitation

Early rehabilitation is recommended to prevent function loss after elbow fractures. The best interventions of a comprehensive rehabilitation program are exercise, education, and functional activities. The optimal rehabilitation after elbow fractures is unknown due to the lack of medical evidence and clarity defining rehabilitation interventions. The current expert consensus is that elbow fracture rehabilitation can begin within days of the initial injury and continue throughout the recovery process [19]. Direct input of ROM limitations, splinting, and weight-bearing status should be obtained from the orthopedic surgeon or sports physician treating the fracture.

The rehabilitation program post-elbow fracture can be divided in two phases:

1. *Acute phase*: Posture, ergonomic, and precautions education is considered an important part of this phase of the rehabilitation program. AROM and AAROM are more commonly used, compared to passive ROM (PROM) and stretching. Static or dynamic splinting is commonly used to protect the joint and promote healing. Modalities to control pain and inflammation as rest, ice compression,

elevation, and heat are also used in this phase by most practitioners.

2. *Rehabilitation phase*: This phase focuses more on the restoration of function and less on pain and edema management. AROM, stretching, strengthening, and functional exercises are the most common treatments prescribed [19]. The goal is to maintain adequate range of motion, prevent a "stiff elbow," and then restore strength and function.

29.2.7.3 Procedures

No other procedures are recommended for this diagnosis.

29.2.7.4 Surgery

Surgery is recommended in patients with open fractures, non-reducible fracture fragments, joint instability, or neurovascular dysfunction [13]. Less than 50% of pediatric fracture will require surgical care, with medial epicondyle fracture accounting for close to 80% of all cases requiring surgery [13]. Numerous methods of percutaneous reduction have been described for pediatric displaced radial head fractures, and surgical care should be considered in patients failing closed reduction. Open reduction should be avoided if possible, as they are associated with poor outcomes [16]. Close to 80% of adult patients report their post-surgical outcome from excellent to good [15]. Olecranon fractures are the most common adult fracture requiring hospital admission and subsequent surgical care [14]. Tension band wiring, K-wires, screw fixation, and plate fixation are some of the procedures done for the treatment of olecranon and other adult elbow fractures [14]. Radial head arthroplasty may be required in rare instances for adult patients with proximal radial fractures. In cases with open fractures and complex comminuted fractures, external fixation may be needed.

Possible post-surgical complications include non-union, neurovascular injury, elbow stiffness, permanent loss of ROM, hardware fracture, myositis ossificans, and infection [15].

Contractures and elbow stiffness after surgery are considered problematic and are observed in patients with the following risk factors: elbow dislocation, specifically those involving the humeroulnar joint, complex or comminuted fractures, other fractures not involving the elbow, limited elbow ROM, and presence of radiographic heterotopic ossification at 6 weeks postoperatively. Patients with these risk factors should receive aggressive physical therapy and be counseled as to the possible development of elbow stiffness and needing subsequent surgery [20].

In the pediatric population, bony overgrowth, osteonecrosis, and premature physeal closure are possible complications. Elbow stiffness is also seen in the pediatric population and has poor functional outcomes. Other factors associated with poor outcome include greater initial bony angulation and displacement, associated injuries, age more than 10 years, articular involvement, and the need for open reduction [16]. For more details, please see the Chap. 30.

References

1. McGuire DT, Bain GI. Management of dislocations of the elbow in the athlete. Sports Med Arthrosc Rev. 2014;22(3):188–93.
2. Grazette AJ, Aquilina A. The assessment and management of simple elbow dislocations. Open Orthop J. 2017;11:1373–9.
3. Hodge DK, Safran MR. Sideline management of common dislocations. Curr Sports Med Rep. 2002;1(3):149–55.
4. Rezaie N, Gupta S, Service BC, Osbahr DC. Elbow dislocation. Clin Sports Med. 2020;39(3):637–55.
5. Hotchkiss RN. Fractures and dislocations of the elbow. In: Rockwood CA, Green DP, Bucholz RW, et al., editors. Rockwood and Green's fractures in adults. 4th ed. Philadelphia: Lippincott-Raven; 1996. p. 929–1024.
6. Rozzi SL, Anderson JM, Doberstein ST, Godek JJ, Hartsock LA, McFarland EG. National Athletic Trainers' Association position statement: immediate management of appendicular joint dislocations. J Athl Train. 2018;53(12):1117–28.
7. O'Driscoll SW, Jupiter JB, King GJ, Hotchkiss RN, Morrey BF. The unstable elbow. Instr Course Lect. 2001;50:89–102.
8. Schreiber JJ, Warren RF, Hotchkiss RN, Daluiski A. An online video investigation into the mechanism of elbow dislocation. J Hand Surg. 2013;38(3):488–94.
9. Parvin RW. Closed reduction of common shoulder and elbow dislocations without anesthesia. AMA Arch Surg. 1957;75(6):972–5.
10. Kumar A, Ahmed M. Closed reduction of posterior dislocation of the elbow: a simple technique. J Orthop Trauma. 1999;13(1):58–9.
11. Mehlhoff TL, Noble PC, Bennett JB, Tullos HS. Simple dislocation of the elbow in the adult. Results after closed treatment. J Bone Joint Surg Am. 1988;70(2):244–9.
12. McCabe MP, Savoie FH. Simple elbow dislocations: evaluation, management, and outcomes. Phys Sportsmed. 2012;40(1):62–71.
13. Okubo H, Nakasone M, Kinjo M, Onaka K, Futenma C, Kanaya F. Epidemiology of paediatric elbow fractures: a retrospective multicentre study of 488 fractures. J Child Orthop. 2019;13(5):516–21.
14. Bolt A, Govilkar S, Dover C, Blackwell J, Hay S. A 7-year prospective epidemiological study of acute elbow admissions to a trauma unit. J Surg. 2020;8(6):190.
15. Holdsworth BJ, Mossad MM. Fractures of the adult distal humerus. Elbow function after internal fixation. J Bone Joint Surg Br. 1990;72(3):362–5.
16. Nicholson LT, Skaggs DL. Proximal radius fractures in children. J Am Acad Orthop Surg. 2019;27(19):e876–86.
17. Appelboam A, Reuben AD, Benger JR, Beech F, Dutson J, Haig S, et al. Elbow extension test to rule out elbow fracture: multicentre, prospective validation and observational study of diagnostic accuracy in adults and children. BMJ. 2008;337:a2428.
18. Saeed W, Waseem M. Elbow Fractures Overview. In: StatPearls [Internet]. Treasure Island (FL): StatPearls Publishing; 2021 [cited 2021 May 11]. Available from: http://www.ncbi.nlm.nih.gov/books/NBK441976/.
19. Macdermid JC, Vincent JI, Kieffer L, Kieffer A, Demaiter J, Macintosh S. A survey of practice patterns for rehabilitation post elbow fracture. Open Orthop J. 2012;6:429–39.
20. Carlock KD, Bianco IR, Kugelman DN, Konda SR, Egol KA. Risk factors for elbow joint contracture after surgical repair of traumatic elbow fracture. J Am Acad Orthop Surg. 2021;29(4):e178–87.

30 Elbow Surgeries

Anna H. Green, Andrew J. Butler, Matthew H. Nasra, and Alfred J. Tria Jr

30.1 Distal Biceps Tendon Rupture

Distal biceps tendon ruptures most often occur when a flexed elbow is eccentrically loaded and is best diagnosed on magnetic resonance imaging (MRI). Risk factors for rupture include a history of anabolic steroid use, smoking, and impingement of the tendon during motion. Both nonoperative and operative treatment options are available. Nonoperative treatment may leave the patient with reduced strength in forearm supination and elbow flexion and can be considered in patients who are low-demand, elderly, or willing to sacrifice function and potential limitations to activities of daily living (ADL). Surgical fixation is indicated in young patients with complete tendon ruptures who do not want to sacrifice function and patients with partial tears who fail nonoperative treatment. Early operative fixation within 2–3 weeks is favorable, as delayed repair leads to adhesions, loss of elasticity, and retraction of the tendon which may necessitate a more extensile approach, and is associated with a higher complication rate [1].

There are multiple methods of surgical treatment for distal biceps tendon ruptures, including suture button, suture anchor, bone tunnel, and interference screw fixation. Biomechanical studies have shown the Endobutton (Smith & Nephew, Andover, MA, USA) (Fig. 30.1), a type of suture button, to be superior [2]. Dual fixation involving the use of an interference screw in conjunction with suture button or anchor has also been described. The repair may use a single- or dual-incision approach. The single-incision technique carries a higher risk of neurological injury, primarily to the lateral antebrachial cutaneous nerve. The two-incision technique is associated with a greater risk of radio-ulnar synostosis.

After surgery, the elbow is initially placed in a splint or brace at 90 degrees of flexion for 1–2 weeks until suture removal. Then, active elbow extension with passive elbow flexion is initiated, with the goal to reach full range of motion by 6 weeks postoperatively. Resistance training may begin at 10–12 weeks postoperatively. Dual fixation using both suture buttons with an interference screw may allow more aggressive early therapy, where splinting is discontinued after 3–5 days and the patient is transitioned to a compression sleeve by 1 week to allow gentle range of motion [3]. Strengthening begins 1-week postoperatively with 1 pound (lb) weights, with return to daily activities at 2–3 weeks.

30.2 Lateral Epicondylitis

Surgery for lateral epicondylitis can be performed with an open, arthroscopic, or percutaneous approach. Studies have shown all three methods to be highly effective [4, 5] with the reported success rate of operative intervention approximating 80% good to excellent results in most studies, regardless of the surgical technique used [6].

The surgery includes open or arthroscopic release of the common extensor tendon with resection of degenerative extensor carpi radialis brevis tissue and tendon repair:

- Arthroscopic debridement enables examination of the intra-articular structures, provides greater ligament stability, and can treat concomitant elbow pathologies, such as plica, loose bodies, or chondral lesions [4]. An arthroscopic approach offers a faster recovery time and a quicker return

A. H. Green
Robert Wood Johnson University School of Medicine, Department of Orthopaedic Surgery, New Brunswick, NJ, USA

A. J. Butler
Department of Orthopaedic Surgery, Robert Wood Johnson University School of Medicine, New Brunswick, NJ, USA

Department of Orthopaedic Surgery, Rutgers-Robert Wood Johnson Medical School, New Brunswick, NJ, USA

M. H. Nasra
Robert Wood Johnson University School of Medicine, New Brunswick, NJ, USA

Department of Orthopaedic Surgery, Rutgers-Robert Wood Johnson Medical School, New Brunswick, NJ, USA

A. J. Tria Jr (✉)
Department of Orthopaedics, Rutgers-Robert Wood Johnson Medical School, New Brunswick, NJ, USA

© The Author(s), under exclusive license to Springer Nature Switzerland AG 2022

S. A. Mostoufi et al. (eds.), *Clinical Guide to Musculoskeletal Medicine*, https://doi.org/10.1007/978-3-030-92042-5_30

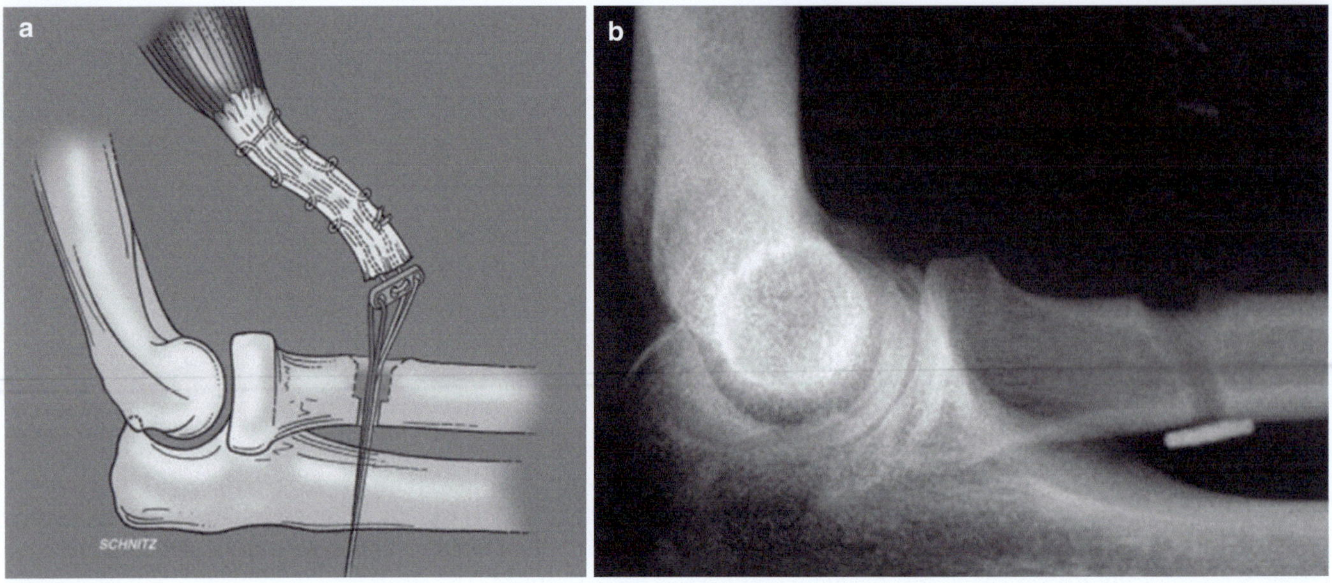

Fig. 30.1 (**a**) Illustration of the Endobutton (Smith & Nephew, Andover, MA, USA) fixation of a distal biceps tendon rupture. (**b**) Lateral radiograph showing Endobutton fixation. (With permission from Greenberg et al. [2])

to activities compared to an open procedure. Active and passive range of motion (ROM) exercises can begin immediately, followed by stretching and progressive strengthening exercises, with return to light activities at 2 weeks postoperatively [7].

- Open release allows for complete removal of the pathologic tissue and improved vascularity to the region but can result in higher postoperative morbidity due to ligament damage [5]. The rehabilitation after open procedures generally requires a longer recovery course postoperatively to allow for adequate healing. The upper extremity is splinted with the elbow in 90 degrees of flexion for 1–2 weeks. After this time, active ROM exercises begin, followed by strengthening exercises 6 weeks postoperatively or once painless ROM is achieved [4].

Radial tunnel syndrome and posterior interosseous nerve (PIN) syndrome can be associated with lateral epicondylitis. Concurrent PIN entrapment has been reported in up to 5% of patients [7]. For these patients, surgical decompression of the radial nerve or PIN is necessary. If there is associated lateral collateral ligament complex instability, ligamentous repair and reconstruction are performed as well.

30.3 Medial Epicondylitis

Surgical treatment for medial epicondylitis is indicated after 6 months of failed conservative measures or the elite athlete with indications of tendon disruption [8]. The open release is the standard of care for the treatment of medial epicondylitis [9]. This technique involves epicondylar debridement and repair of the common flexor tendon. An open approach affords the surgeon the ability to visualize and protect the ulnar collateral ligament (UCL) and ulnar nerve posterior to the medial epicondyle [9]. Studies have reported ulnar nerve involvement in 23–60% of patients requiring operative treatment for medial epicondylitis [7]. When ulnar neuropathy is present, surgical decompression, submuscular transposition, or subcutaneous transposition of the ulnar nerve is necessary. Patients with concurrent ulnar neuritis experience less favorable outcomes.

Rehabilitation protocols are similar to that of lateral epicondylitis. Postoperatively, the upper extremity is splinted with the elbow in 90 degrees of flexion for 1–2 weeks. This is followed by passive and active ROM exercises of the upper extremity. Isometric exercises begin 3–4 weeks postoperatively, while wrist flexion and forearm pronation exercises begin 6 weeks postoperatively [8]. Strengthening exercises of the hand, wrist, and forearm can begin at 6–8 weeks with return to regular activities 3–6 months postoperatively [9].

30.4 Medial Ulnar Collateral Ligament Injury

Injury to the medial ulnar collateral ligament (MUCL) leads to valgus instability of the elbow and is more common in throwing athletes due to repetitive stress. UCL reconstruction (UCL-R) is indicated for intractable pain and dysfunction when all nonoperative measures have failed or the athlete desires to return to pre-injury performance levels. Operative treatment involves ligamentous reconstruction with tendon autograft via the Jobe or modified Jobe technique. Alternatively, UCL repair with collagen-treated internal brace is another viable treatment option, which involves the use of a suture tape to reinforce the repair of the native ligament [10].

UCL-R requires a rigorous recovery course. Erickson et al. [11] describe a standard rehabilitation program. Postoperatively, the elbow is placed in 90 degrees of flexion for 1 week and then transitioned to a hinged elbow brace. Gentle progressive ROM exercises begin, increasing by 5 degrees of extension and 10 degrees of flexion per week until full ROM is established. Progressive strengthening exercises of the elbow, shoulder, and scapular stabilizers can commence at 4–8 weeks, followed by isotonic and manual resistance exercises, proprioception, and dynamic stabilization drills at 9–13 weeks. Throwing progression is initiated at weeks 14–26, and patients can return to competitive throwing at 7–9 months [11].

UCL repair with internal brace allows for faster rehabilitation and a quicker return to sports and activities compared to traditional UCL-R, which makes it an appealing procedure for high-level throwing athletes [10]. The rehabilitation protocol proceeds similarly to UCL-R except when patients generally progress more rapidly through the stages and can expect to return to competitive throwing at 5 months postoperatively [10].

30.5 Olecranon Bursitis

Olecranon bursitis may be classified as acute versus chronic and aseptic versus septic. Acute olecranon bursitis is typically secondary to direct pressure or trauma to the bursa. Chronic olecranon bursitis may develop after prolonged stress is inflicted on the bursa or from systemic illnesses such as rheumatoid arthritis. A septic bursitis may develop from a skin opening where microbes can enter or via local spread from cellulitis and requires antibiotics to treat the infection. As noted in the posterior elbow chapter, needle aspiration is helpful to determine the organism and antibiotic susceptibility. Incision and drainage may be necessary in cases that fail isolated antibiotic therapy.

Overall, surgical treatments for olecranon bursitis are associated with higher complication rates compared to nonsurgical treatments and should therefore only be pursued when nonsurgical treatments have failed [12]. Olecranon bursectomy, open or arthroscopic, is an option for unrelenting cases of olecranon bursitis:

- Open bursectomy is often associated with wound healing complications, where up to 27% of patients develop postoperative hematoma, exudate, or skin necrosis [12]. Physicians should take care when considering open bursectomy in patients with rheumatoid arthritis, as these patients tend to have significantly lower rates (40% versus 94%) of success following this procedure [13]. After open bursectomy, patients are often placed into a well-padded posterior splint in approximately 90 degrees of flexion, which reduces the dead space available for fluid accumulation. After adequate skin healing in 1–2 weeks, the splint may be removed and replaced with a light compressive wrap to reduce swelling.
- Gentle ROM at the elbow may begin, as well as at the shoulder and wrist to prevent stiffness. A pad or cushion may be applied for several weeks postoperatively to prevent irritation to the area.
- Arthroscopic bursectomy was developed to combat the wound complications associated with an open procedure. Offending osteophytes can be removed at the same time, and recovery is usually quicker. Some studies show equivalent success rates between arthroscopic and open olecranon bursectomy but with less soft tissue compromise, faster healing, and fewer complications [14]. Patients may initially be splinted or placed in a sling for a few days postoperatively and ROM advanced as tolerated to preserve motion.

30.6 Elbow Dislocation

The treatment of elbow dislocations is variable depending on associated fracture and ligamentous structures injured. The majority of elbow dislocations (up to 74%) are simple dislocations without bony fracture [15]. These can primarily be treated with closed reduction and posterior splint with the elbow in 90 degrees of flexion [15]. Stability of the elbow should be assessed through ROM and stressing the ligaments. ROM exercises for simple dislocations should begin approximately a week after initial injury. Immobilization for longer periods has been associated with worse outcomes, usually related to stiffness [15]. An extension block brace is often used for 3–4 weeks. ROM should be instituted within the stable arc as determined by physical exam.

Open reduction internal fixation (ORIF) is indicated in complex elbow dislocations or a persistently unstable elbow. The "terrible triad" injury describes the constellation of injuring the lateral ulnar collateral ligament (LUCL), radial head fracture, and coronoid fracture and is so named for its association with poor outcomes (Fig. 30.2) [15]. Coronoid fractures may be treated with internal fixation if the fragment is large enough but are often too small for hardware. The radial head may be addressed with plate and screw construct (Fig. 30.3) or radial head arthroplasty (Fig. 30.3) if the fragments are irreparable.

The rehabilitation following internal fixation of elbow dislocations depends on the stability at the conclusion of the surgical procedure. Patients are often initially splinted for 1–2 weeks after the procedure. The timing of initiating ROM exercises should be correlated with the surgical stability with the knowledge that stiffness is the most common complication.

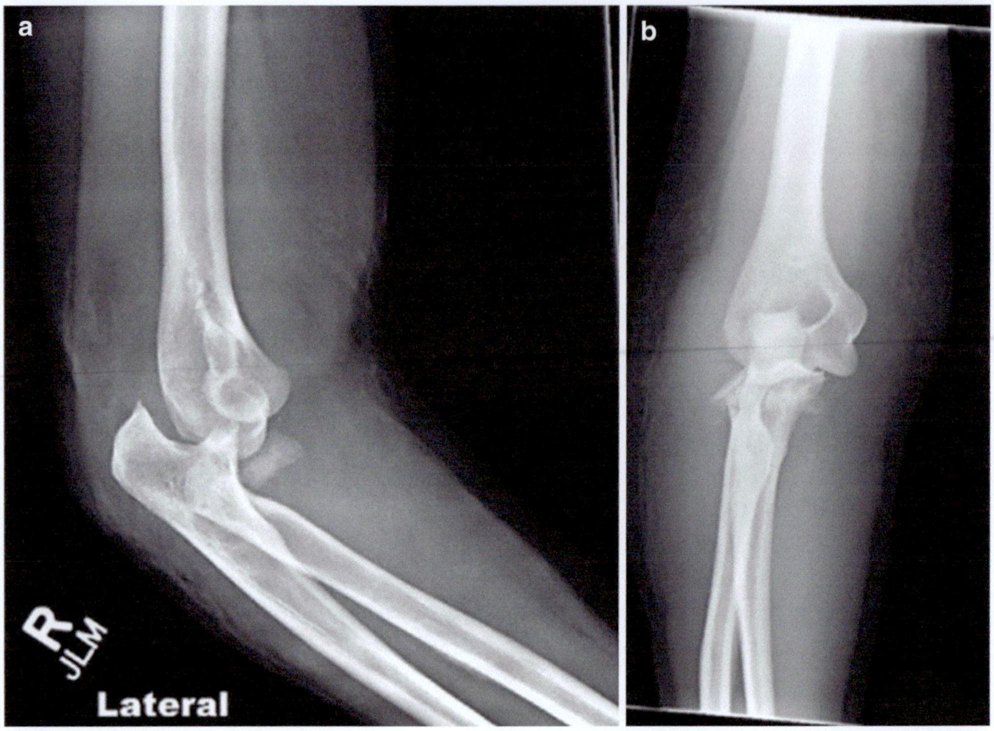

Fig. 30.2 Lateral (**a**) and AP (**b**) radiographs of a terrible triad elbow dislocation. (With permission from Rezaie et al. [15], p. 646. Fig. 9)

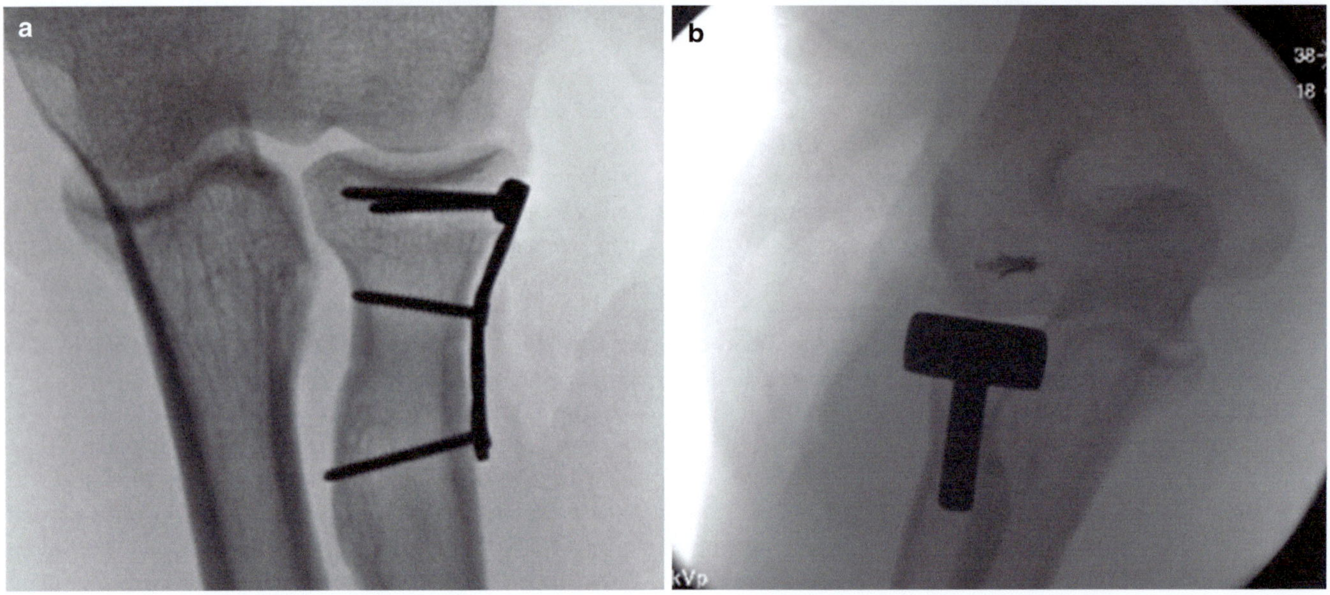

Fig. 30.3 (**a**) Operative fixation of the radial head with plate and screw construct. (**b**) Radial head fracture replacement with LUCL repair. (With permission from Rezaie et al. [15], p. 649)

30.7 Elbow Osteoarthritis

Surgical management of primary osteoarthritis of the elbow consists of either arthroscopic or open arthrotomy procedures, as well as total elbow arthroplasty (TEA), depending on the severity of symptoms and joint degeneration. Ulnar nerve transposition may be done concomitantly with any of these procedures, especially if cubital tunnel symptoms are present:

- In younger patients or those with milder symptoms, arthroscopic debridement may help remove inflamed synovium, loose bodies, and osteophytes that may contribute to pain and loss of motion [16]. Such a minimally invasive procedure allows immediate ROM exercises to restore motion.
- The Outerbridge-Kashiwagi procedure, also known as the OK procedure or ulnohumeral arthroplasty, entails osteophyte removal through a burr hole in the olecranon fossa

[16]. This may be done open or arthroscopically and is indicated in younger patients with limited range of motion secondary to impinging osteophytes as their primary complaint [16]. Postoperatively, heavy lifting should be avoided for 2–3 weeks, but ROM exercises at the elbow may begin immediately.

- In cases of severe osteoarthritis that is unresponsive to conservative treatment, the primary surgical consideration is age and level of function of the patient. In younger patients (less than 60 years of age), interposition arthroplasty involving placement of graft tissue (tensor fascia lata, Achilles tendon, etc.) between the ulnohumeral articulating surfaces may be considered [17]. A hinged external fixator is often applied intra-operatively to allow early stable range of motion while protecting the graft and soft tissue repair. The external fixator is removed after 6–8 weeks [17].
- In older, low-demand patients with inflammatory, primary, or post-traumatic arthritis with painful arc of motion, TEA is indicated [16]. Patients who undergo this procedure must understand the lifelong limitations of this procedure, which often include restriction not to lift more than 5 lb. Rehabilitation following TEA is dependent on whether or not the triceps was detached during surgery and the strength of the repair. If the triceps was detached, then active flexion may be limited for the first 6 weeks in order to protect the repair. Otherwise, full active and passive ROM is encouraged in order to prevent stiffness.

References

1. Cain RA, Nydick JA, Stein MI, Williams BD, Polikandriotis JA, Hess AV. Complications following distal biceps repair. J Hand Surg Am. 2012;37(10):2112–7. https://doi.org/10.1016/j.jhsa.2012.06.022. Epub 2012 Aug 30. PMID: 22938802.
2. Greenberg JA, Fernandez JJ, Wang T, Turner C. EndoButton-assisted repair of distal biceps tendon ruptures. J Shoulder Elb Surg. 2003;12:484–90.
3. Heinzelmann AD, Savoie FH 3rd, Ramsey JR, Field LD, Mazzocca AD. A combined technique for distal biceps repair using a soft tissue button and biotenodesis interference screw. Am J Sports Med. 2009;37:989–94.
4. Brummel J, Baker CL 3rd, Hopkins R, Baker CL Jr. Epicondylitis: lateral. Sports Med Arthrosc Rev. 2014;22(3):e1–6.
5. Szabo SJ, Savoie FH 3rd, Field LD, Ramsey JR, Hosemann CD. Tendinosis of the extensor carpi radialis brevis: an evaluation of three methods of operative treatment. J Shoulder Elb Surg. 2006;15(6):721–7.
6. Lo MY, Safran MR. Surgical treatment of lateral epicondylitis: a systematic review. Clin Orthop Relat Res. 2007;463:98–106.
7. Van Hofwegen C, Baker CL 3rd, Baker CL Jr. Epicondylitis in the athlete's elbow. Clin Sports Med. 2010;29(4):577–97.
8. Ciccotti MC, Schwartz MA, Ciccotti MG. Diagnosis and treatment of medial epicondylitis of the elbow. Clin Sports Med. 2004;23(4):693–705, xi.
9. Amin NH, Kumar NS, Schickendantz MS. Medial epicondylitis: evaluation and management. J Am Acad Orthop Surg. 2015;23(6):348–55.
10. Wilk KE, Arrigo CA, Bagwell MS, Rothermich MA, Dugas JR. Repair of the ulnar collateral ligament of the elbow: rehabilitation following internal brace surgery. J Orthop Sports Phys Ther. 2019;49(4):253–61.
11. Erickson BJ, Harris JD, Chalmers PN, Bach BR Jr, Verma NN, Bush-Joseph CA, Romeo AA. Ulnar collateral ligament reconstruction: anatomy, indications, techniques, and outcomes. Sports Health. 2015;7(6):511–7.
12. De Degreef L, Smet. Complications following resection of the olecranon bursa. Acta Orthop Belg. 2006;72:400–3.
13. Stewart NJ, Manzanares JB, Morrey BF. Surgical treatment of aseptic olecranon bursitis. J Shoulder Elb Surg. 1997;6:49–54.
14. Sayegh S. Treatment of olecranon bursitis: a systematic review. Arch Orthop Trauma Surg. 2014;134(11):1517–36. https://doi.org/10.1007/s00402-014-2088-3.
15. Rezaie N, Gupta S, Service BC, Osbahr DC. Elbow dislocation. Clin Sports Med. 2020;39(3):637–55. https://doi.org/10.1016/j.csm.2020.02.009.
16. Gallo RA, Payatakes A, Sotereanos DG. Surgical options for the arthritic elbow. J Hand Surg Am. 2008;33(5):746–59.
17. Blaine TA, Wiseman SP, Kovacevic D, Morrey BF. Interposition arthroplasty for posttraumatic ulnohumeral arthritis. J Shoulder Elb Arthrop. 2019; https://doi.org/10.1177/2471549219836390.

Part VI

Wrist-Hand

Section Editor
Jason L. Zaremski

31 Dorsal Wrist Disorders

Nadia N. Zaman, Alexandra St Clair, Cara Rodriguez, and Charles Cassidy

31.1 Ganglion Cysts

31.1.1 Synonyms

- Synovial cyst
- Gideon's disease

31.1.2 ICD-10 Codes

M67.431, M67.432, M67.439

31.1.3 Description

Ganglion cysts are the most common soft tissue masses seen amongst hand and wrist pathologies; they are more commonly seen on the dorsal aspect of the wrist and measure approximately 1–2 centimeters in size [1, 2] (Fig. 31.1). They are thought to occur due to repetitive irritation and microtrauma, leading to the accumulation of a highly viscous fluid within a ganglion; this fluid contains a large amount of hyaluronic acid, as well as glucosamine, globulins, and albumin [2]. The exact mechanism of where the fluid comes from, as well as how the cyst walls form, is not fully understood, though multiple theories exist regarding both extra-articular and intra-articular origins [2]. Differential diagnosis for wrist ganglion cysts is in Table 31.1.

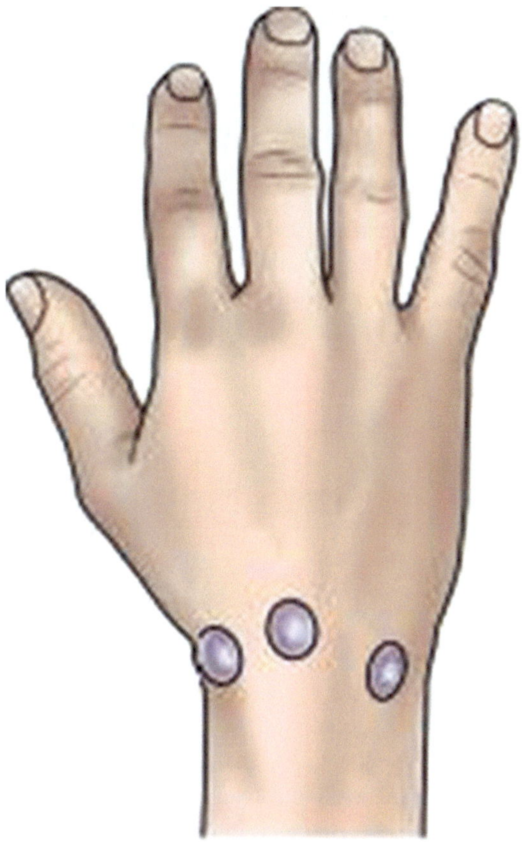

Fig. 31.1 Common locations for a ganglion cyst on the dorsal wrist. (From: Schnur and Keith [4]; with permission)

N. N. Zaman (✉)
Department of Orthopedics & Rehabilitation Medicine, Tufts University School of Medicine, Boston, MA, USA
e-mail: nzaman1@tuftsmedicalcenter.org

A. St Clair
Department of Occupational Therapy, Tufts Medical Center, Boston, MA, USA
e-mail: astclair@tuftsmedicalcenter.org

C. Rodriguez
Department of Physical and Occupational Therapy, Tufts Medical Center, Boston, MA, USA
e-mail: crodriguez@tuftsmedicalcenter.org

C. Cassidy
Department of Orthopedic & Rehabilitation Medicine, Tufts University School of Medicine, Tufts Medical Center, Boston, MA, USA

© The Author(s), under exclusive license to Springer Nature Switzerland AG 2022

S. A. Mostoufi et al. (eds.), *Clinical Guide to Musculoskeletal Medicine*, https://doi.org/10.1007/978-3-030-92042-5_31

Table 31.1 Differential diagnosis for wrist ganglion cysts [4]

Neuroma
Lipoma
Tenosynovitis
Gouty tophus
Giant cell tumor of tendon sheath
Soft tissue sarcoma

31.1.4 Clinical Presentation

Patients will often present with pain located at the dorsal or volar aspect of the wrist, with concern regarding the growth that has developed. For some patients, there may be no pain at all, but concern regarding a new growth that was not present before. If pain is present, they will report increased pain with activities, as well as decreased range of motion in flexion/extension. If the ganglion cyst is located on the volar aspect of the wrist, patients may report paresthesia due to compression of the median or ulnar nerves [2].

31.1.5 Physical Examination

A firm, well-circumscribed lesion is seen on inspection of the wrist. On palpation, it may be painful and will be immobile as most of these cysts are tethered to underlying tissues, as opposed to a lipoma, which is more likely to be mobile [2]. There will not be any erythema or warmth. Ganglion cysts will also transilluminate versus solid masses. If the ganglion cyst is causing compression of a nerve or is large, there may be findings of decreased range of motion or reduced grip strength on physical examination.

31.1.6 Diagnostic Workup

A diagnosis of ganglion cyst can often be made based on the history and physical examination alone. Plain radiographs will reveal a normal wrist; magnetic resonance imaging (MRI) is usually not necessary but would show a well-circumscribed mass with homogenous fluid signal intensity. You may consider the above imaging if there is concern for a more malignant process. The best imaging modality to confirm the presence of a ganglion cyst is ultrasound, where a well-marginated hypoechogenic mass would be seen [3]. The differential diagnosis to consider is in Table 31.1 [4].

31.1.7 Treatment

31.1.7.1 Medical Management

First and foremost, patients should be reassured of the benign nature of a ganglion cyst. The management is largely conservative, focusing on observation or immobilization when painful. Some, especially smaller-sized, cysts may even resolve on their own if patients modify their activities to decrease repetitive microtrauma for a period of time [1].

31.1.7.2 Rehabilitation

The timeline for hand therapy varies in nonoperative management of a ganglion cyst, depending on symptoms and functional impairment. Therapeutic interventions may include fitting the patient with a wrist immobilization orthosis to address discomfort, issuing a home exercise program (HEP) consisting of gentle range of motion (ROM) to address joint stiffness and function, and educating the patient on heat and cold modalities to address pain and swelling [5]. It is important to educate the patient that therapy will not resolve the ganglion. Education on activity modification, adaptation, and ergonomics is beneficial in preventing repetitive microtrauma. Postoperative treatment of a ganglion excision should focus on early ROM (active and passive) of the wrist and digits to prevent postoperative stiffness. For dorsal wrist ganglion excisions, wrist flexion should be emphasized to avoid development of extrinsic tightness [6]. The therapist should monitor the patient's symptoms with progression of motion, strengthening, and activity. The therapist should additionally educate the postoperative patient on scar management techniques to reduce scar formation and adherence to underlying structures [5]. Moist heat, transcutaneous electrical nerve stimulation (TENS), and orthotic fabrication may be beneficial to patients experiencing significant postoperative pain [5, 6].

31.1.7.3 Procedures

Aspiration of a ganglion cyst can be performed and has been considered the mainstay of nonsurgical treatment for many years; however, it has been found in recent studies that the recurrence rate is very high [1, 2]. Some studies have compared aspiration with reassurance alone and found no significant difference with respect to outcomes [1]. Blind aspiration of volar wrist ganglion cysts should be avoided due to the neurovascular structures in its proximity [2].

31.1.7.4 Surgery

Surgical excision is considered when there are recurrent cysts or if there are neurologic deficits present. On meta-analysis, recurrence was found to be less common in those who have surgical incision than aspiration [1]. For more details on surgery for dorsal wrist disorders, refer to Chap. 37.

31.2 Posterior Interosseous Nerve (PIN) Entrapment Syndrome

31.2.1 Synonyms

- Posterior interosseous nerve syndrome (PINS)
- Posterior interosseous neuropathy
- Posterior interosseous nerve palsy
- Dorsal interosseous nerve syndrome

31.2.2 ICD-10 Codes

G56.3

31.2.3 Description

The posterior interosseous nerve syndrome (PINS) is a motor nerve that branches off the radial nerve and supplies the muscles of the extensor compartment of the wrist and hand [Table 31.2]. PIN palsy can occur due to both compressive and non-compressive etiologies. The most common sites of compression include the Arcade of Frohse, a fibrous connection between the two heads of the supinator muscle, and at the supinator muscle itself; it can also be compressed by extrinsic factors, such as fibrous bands at the radial tunnel, as well as masses, such as ganglion cysts or tumors [7]. Non-compressive etiologies are often due to disruption of the nerve from a medical diagnosis like neuralgic amyotrophy, rheumatoid arthritis, and hourglass-like fascicular constriction [7]. PINS is often confused with radial tunnel syndrome (RTS); however, the major difference lies in the clinical presentation of these two pathologies. Differential diagnosis for PIN entrapment syndrome is given in Table 31.3 [8]. Table 31.2 lists the muscles innervated by posterior interosseous nerve.

31.2.4 Clinical Presentation

Patients with posterior interosseous nerve syndrome (PINS) will usually present with weakness of finger and thumb extensors without any associated pain; the wrist extensors and forearm supinators are generally spared because their innervations are more proximal to the area of compression [8]. The dorsal part of the forearm and wrist receives their sensory innervation from the superficial radial nerve; therefore, the PIN is a purely motor nerve with no sensory component. This is one of the main distinctions between PINS and RTS, as the latter will usually have pain as the primary presenting symptom.

Table 31.2 Muscles innervated by posterior interosseous nerve

Extensor carpi radialis brevis (*deep branch of radial nerve*)	Supinator muscle (*deep branch of radial nerve*)
Extensor indicis	Abductor pollicis longus
Extensor digiti minimi	Extensor pollicis longus
Extensor carpi ulnaris	Extensor digitorum
Extensor pollicis brevis	

Table 31.3 Differential diagnosis for ganglion cysts [7, 8]

Differential diagnosis for PIN entrapment syndrome
Radial tunnel syndrome
Neuralgic amyotrophy
Radial nerve injury/palsy
Brachial plexopathy
Cervical radiculopathy
Extensor tendon rupture

31.2.5 Physical Examination

The forearm should be inspected and palpated to identify any mass that may be present. A thorough neurologic examination is important to rule out more proximal causes of the weakness that may be present, such as cervical radiculopathy or brachial plexopathy. Whenever possible, muscles should be isolated and tested with their specific innervations in mind [8]. Elbow joint ROM is not affected.

31.2.6 Diagnostic Workup

Posterior interosseous nerve syndrome (PINS) can be diagnosed based on history and physical examination findings; imaging can be helpful in looking for space-occupying masses that may be extra-neural [8]. Plain radiographs can be obtained to look for fractures or soft tissue swelling but should be accompanied by MRI and ultrasound imaging to look more closely at the anatomy of the forearm and explore the common sites of compression [7]. Additionally, electrodiagnostic studies can be considered to determine both the severity of muscle denervation and the site of compression [7]. Timing of the electrophysiologic studies can affect their usefulness in the management of PINS; a study that is performed too early will be negative regardless of the clinical presentation. The ideal time to perform a needle electromyography is at least 3–4 weeks after symptom onset [8]. The differential diagnosis to consider is in Table 31.3 [7, 8].

31.2.7 Treatment

31.2.7.1 Medical Management

A significant component of the medical management of PINS is focused on nonoperative care, emphasizing rest, anti-inflammatory medications, splinting, and activity modifications. One study found 73% of those with PINS due to a non-compressive etiology like neuralgic amyotrophy will recover in 1 year and 80–90% will recover in 2 years; PINS due to hourglass-like fascicular constriction should have some improvement in pain and weakness in 3 months, after which surgical consultation should be considered [8].

31.2.7.2 Rehabilitation

Given the low occurrence of PINS in the population, high-level evidence for current clinical treatments is lacking. Current best practice in this area is derived from the study of anatomy, clinical data on radial tunnel, and research of treatment techniques in other nerve entrapments [9]. Conservative rehabilitation for PINS should focus on decreasing pressure to the radial nerve through activity modification, splinting, taping, and incorporation of exercises aimed at increasing free gliding of the nerve and lengthening of surrounding muscles (Fig. 31.2). Stretching of cervical and scapular muscles can also be beneficial to relieve proximal pressure to the radial nerve [9]. Patients should be taught to avoid activities that require combined forearm rotation, elbow extension, and repetitive grasp or pinch. The use of an orthosis with the wrist positioned in extension may also be helpful for relieving tension on the nerve. The use of counterforce bracing for lateral epicondylitis can be a causative factor for PINS and should be avoided [9]. As the patient awaits motor return to wrist and finger extensors, they may benefit from adapted equipment and use of a low-profile wrist and digit extension splint to maintain the wrist and metacarpal joints in extension during functional tasks [10] (Fig. 31.3). Postoperatively, gentle AROM of the wrist and forearm is encouraged to improve nerve gliding and to prevent scar adhesions. A wrist immobilization orthosis is often used to provide support and decrease inflammation during functional tasks [10]. Other areas of postoperative rehabilitation include scar management, desensitization, edema management, and modalities for pain relief [10].

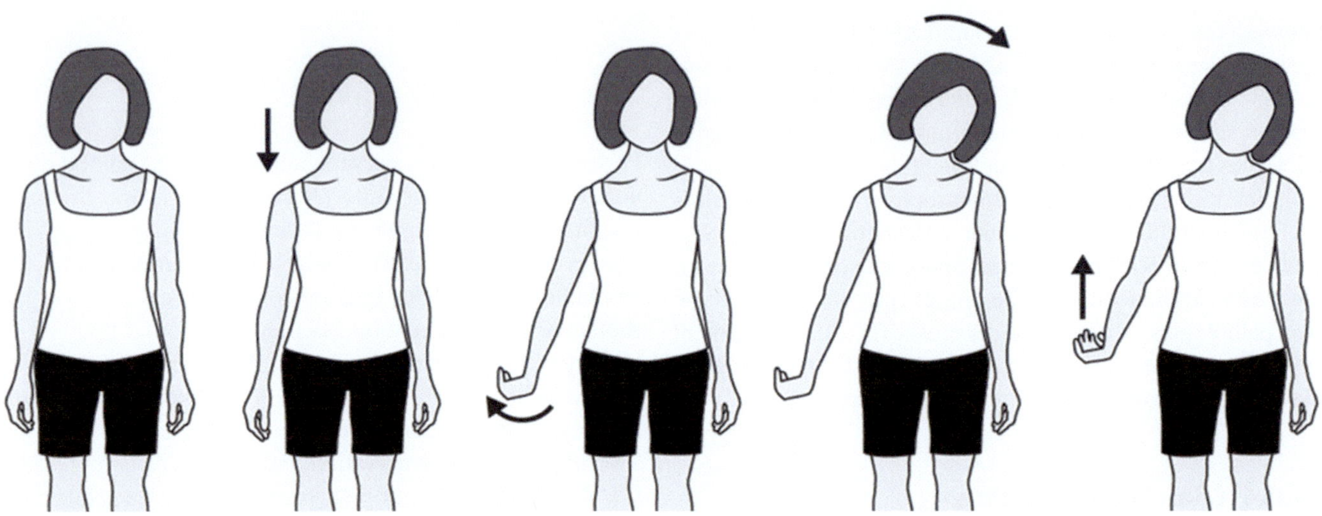

Fig. 31.2 Radial nerve glides are a series of motions aimed at providing a gentle stretch and gliding to the affected nerve. To complete: (1) Stand with your body in a relaxed position. (2) Lower your affected shoulder. (3) Internally rotate your shoulder and flex your wrist. (4) Tilt your head away from the affected arm. (5) Bring your shoulder back while maintaining your head tilted and wrist bent. (Reproduced with permission from OrthoInfo. © American Academy of Orthopaedic Surgeons. https://orthoinfo.org/)

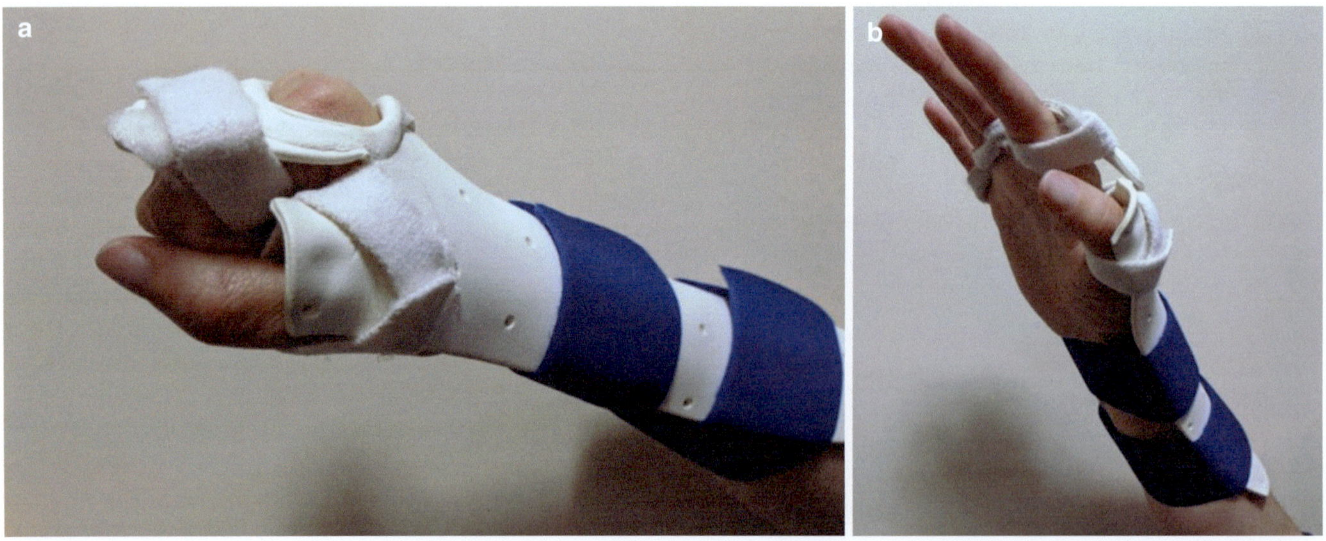

Fig. 31.3 (**a**) Patients with weakness of paralysis of the wrist and finger extensors may benefit from the use of a low-profile digit and wrist extension splint. (**b**) This splint has elastics that hold the fingers and thumb in extension. This will provide the extension force to straighten the fingers after the patient has actively flexed. (Photos by Cara Rodriguez)

31.2.7.3 Procedures

There are no particular injections that assist in the recovery of PINS. One can, however, consider a local anesthetic injection as a part of the diagnostic workup, especially if trying to determine if a radial tunnel syndrome or lateral epicondylitis is present [8].

31.2.7.4 Surgery

For PINS that results from a space-occupying lesion seen on imaging, surgery is often the preferred treatment [7]. This will often lead to better and faster recovery once the offending mass is removed. PINS that presents as paralysis often requires surgery as well. Additionally, PINS that has not responded to nonoperative management for 3 months should have surgical consultation [8]. For more details on surgery for dorsal wrist disorders, refer to Chap. 37.

31.3 Triangular Fibrocartilage Complex Injuries

31.3.1 ICD-10 Codes

M24.131, M24.132

31.3.2 Description

The triangular fibrocartilage complex (TFCC) is a ligamentous complex that is considered one of the main stabilizers on the ulnar side of the wrist. Located between the carpus and the ulna, it not only serves as a load-bearing structure but also stabilizes the distal radioulnar joint (DRUJ). The relevant anatomy is highlighted in Fig. 31.4 [11]. When a wrist

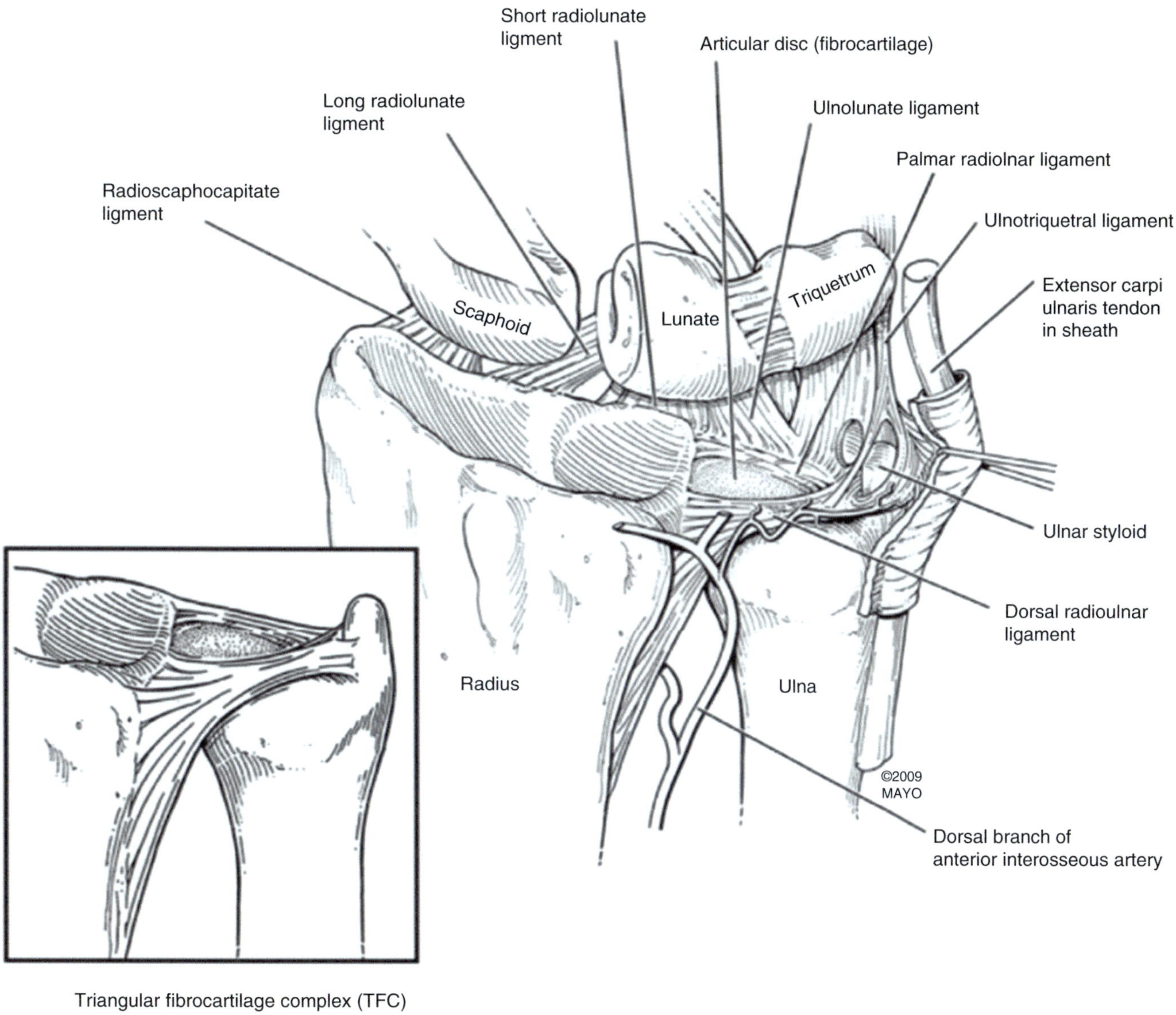

Fig. 31.4 TFCC and its relevant anatomy. (From: Kovachevich and Elhassan [26]; with permission)

Table 31.4 Palmer classification for TFCC tears

The Palmer classification for TFCC injuries			
I	Traumatic	**II**	Degenerative
IA	Central perforation of the articular disk	**IIA**	Central wear of TFCC
IB	Foveal insertional tear, with or without ulnar styloid fracture	**IIB**	Wear with chondromalacia of the lunate or ulnar head
IC	Tear of ulnocarpal ligaments (ulnolunate and ulnotriquetral)	**IIC**	TFCC perforation with chondromalacia
ID	Radial-sided insertional tear	**IID**	TFCC perforation with chondromalacia and wear or tear of the LT ligament
		IIE	TFCC perforation with chondromalacia and wear or tear of the LT ligament, with ulnocarpal arthritis

From: Adams [13]; with permission

has neutral ulnar variance, the TFCC transmits and absorbs approximately 20% of the forces that cross the wrist [11, 12]. This force is increased in positive ulnar variance, where the thickness of the TFCC is decreased, while the force is decreased in negative ulnar variance where the thickness of the TFCC is increased [12].

Blood supply to the TFCC comes from the terminal branches of the anterior and posterior interosseous arteries. While the peripheral 10–30% of the TFCC has adequate blood supply for healing, the central and radial aspects are more poorly vascularized [13]. The Palmer classification is widely recognized as one of the best classifications for TFCC injuries [Table 31.4] [14].

31.3.3 Clinical Presentation

Injuries to the TFCC can result both from a traumatic incident and from degenerative changes to the structures above over time. Patients will usually present with ulnar-sided wrist pain with or without DRUJ instability that is aggravated by repetitive axial loading or activities that require pronation/supination or ulnar deviation [12]. With more degenerative tears, patients may report a clicking or clunking with forearm rotation, which may signify DRUJ instability [13]. Because ulnar-sided wrist pain can result from a wide assortment of pathologies, care must be taken in gathering a thorough history from the patient to rule out other etiologies.

31.3.4 Physical Examination

A thorough musculoskeletal and neurologic physical examination is required to determine the best course of action. Inspection of the skin over the dorsal and volar wrist should be performed to look for any lesions, trophic changes, ecchymosis, or edema. Palpation of the bony prominences along the dorsal and ulnar wrist will assist in determining if there is suspicion for a fracture. Patients with TFCC injury will often have tenderness over the ulnar fovea, lunotriquetral interval, ECU tendon, or DRUJ [13]. Range of motion should be checked in flexion-extension, radial-ulnar deviation, and pronation/supination planes and compared bilaterally. Functional testing includes asking patients to turn a doorknob or having them push up from a chair, which leads to axially loading of the wrist in pronation [13].

Special maneuvers are often used to rule out other injuries in the ulnar wrist:

- Piano key test: Performed by holding the patient's arm in pronation with the wrist in a neutral position. A force is applied to the ulna dorsally and ventrally to look for instability at the DRUJ.
- TFCC stress test: Performed by axially loading the wrist while in ulnar deviation and then applying pronation-supination force. The test is positive if it reproduces the patient's pain but is nonspecific.
- Fovea sign: Performed by placing the patient's elbow at 90° of flexion with the forearm and wrist in neutral position. The examiner places their thumb in the soft space between the ulnar styloid and the flexor carpi ulnaris tendon, the location of the ulnar fovea. The test is positive if applying pressure in this area causes pain and may indicate ulnotriquetral or distal radioulnar ligaments disruption [12].

31.3.5 Diagnostic Workup

Initial workup for TFCC injuries includes plain radiographs to identify any underlying fractures, arthritic changes, bony malalignment, or gapping of the radius and ulna that would denote DRUJ instability [12]. These should include posteroanterior (PA), lateral and oblique films, as well as posteroanterior grip views [13]. Radiographs will also allow for the measurement of ulnar variance, as a majority of TFCC injuries are thought to occur in positive or neutral ulnar variance [11]. More advanced imaging can include computed tomographic arthrography (CTA) or MRI. MRI sensitivity and specificity are 67–100% and 71–100%, respectively; magnetic resonance arthrography (MRA) has also been used and found to be superior to MRI alone in some studies, while others note that a 3.0T scanner has excellent resolution to diagnose TFCC tears, and an arthrogram is not necessary [12, 13]. CTA is an alternative modality and found to be 100% sensitive and specific for accuracy in the diagnosis of TFCC tears, especially for those who cannot undergo MRI [13, 15]. The differential diagnosis to consider is in Table 31.5 [16].

31.3.6 Treatment

31.3.6.1 Medical Management

If there is no DRUJ instability present, the initial management of TFCC injuries is conservative. Symptom management is the focus of care, with the concepts of RICE applied. This may include bracing of the wrist for immobilization and comfort [12]. It also includes activity modifications, as well as anti-inflammatory medications as needed in the acute phase.

31.3.6.2 Rehabilitation

The primary goal of rehabilitation after TFCC injury is to restore the normal joint mechanics and anatomy of the DRUJ [17]. In conservative management of TFCC injuries, initial therapy will focus on techniques to decrease inflammation including rest, use of modalities, taping, and supportive splinting. Splinting needs will vary depending on the patient's pain level and the stability of the DRUJ. The use of a wrist immobilization splint, a long arm orthosis that immobilizes the wrist and forearm, or use of a wrist strap, such as a WristWidget®, are all common forms of support after this injury [17, 18] (Fig. 31.5). Patients should be instructed to avoid activities that require forearm pronation, ulnar deviation, weight-bearing, or gripping. As pain allows, occupational therapy and physical therapy will incorporate pain-free active ROM exercises of the wrist and forearm into the therapy program. This would be followed by progressive strengthening with a focus on wrist stabilization [18] (Fig. 31.6). Postoperative therapy for TFCC injuries will vary depending on the surgery that was performed. Open or arthroscopic TFCC repairs will require a period of immobilization to the wrist and forearm to minimize tension to the repair site. The patient's status post-TFCC debridement does not require as extensive protection and are advanced through the rehab stages above as post-surgical inflammation resolves. It is important with all TFCC surgeries to respect pain during the healing process. Increases in pain, edema, and inflammation are indications that therapy is progressing too rapidly [17, 19].

Table 31.5 Differential diagnosis for TFCC tears [16]

ECU tendinopathy
DRUJ sprain or instability
Triquetral fracture
Ulnar neuropathy at Guyon's canal
Lunotriquetral tear
Ulnar impaction syndrome

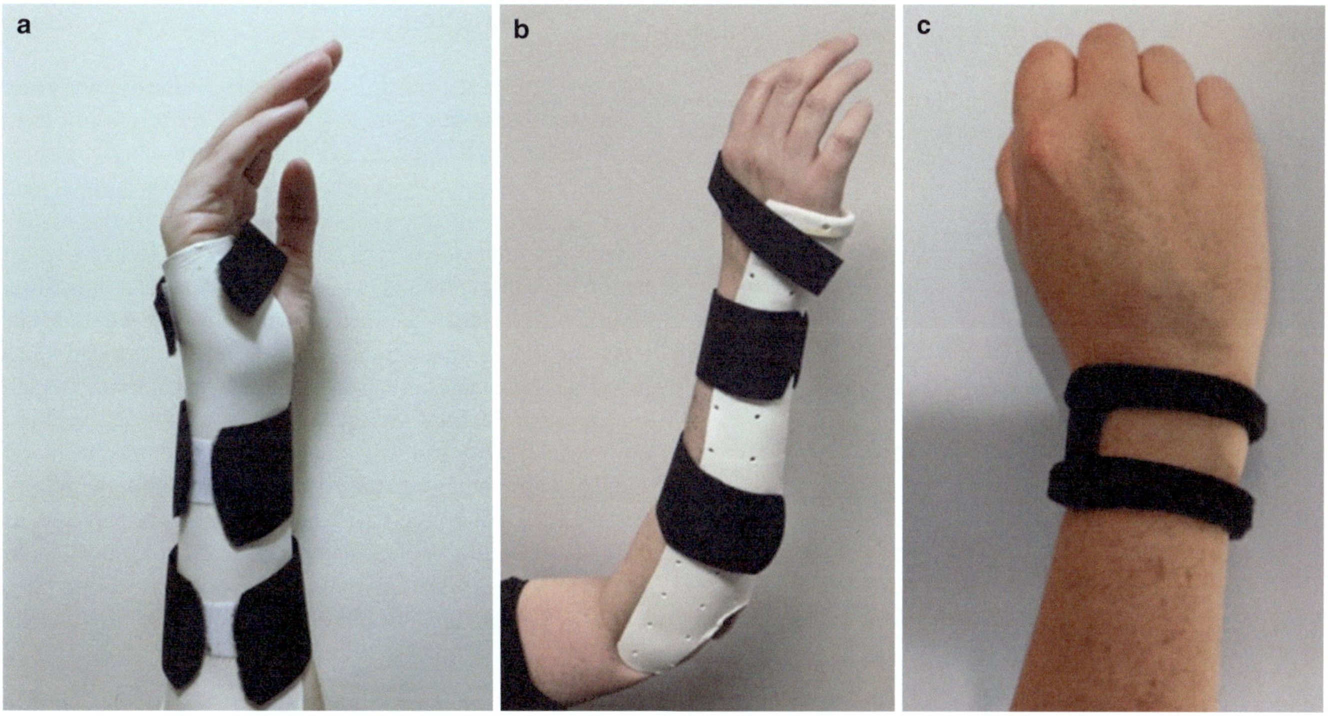

Fig. 31.5 (**a**) An ulnar gutter splint. (**b**). A long arm orthosis that immobilizes the wrist and forearm. (**c**) A wrist strap such as a WristWidget®. (Photos by Cara Rodriguez)

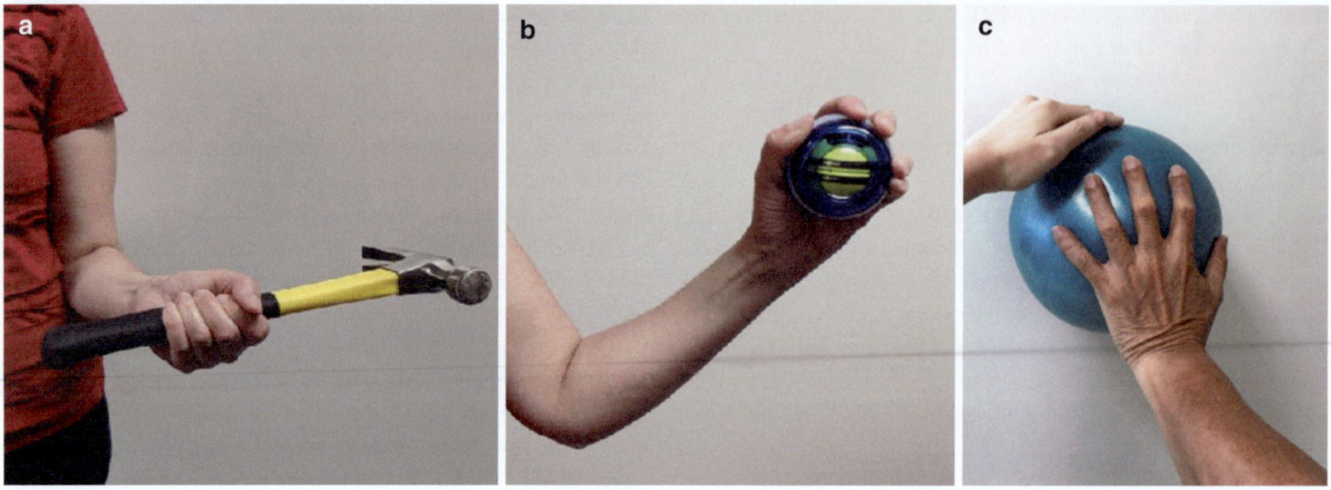

Fig. 31.6 (**a**) Activities that might be included in a progressive strengthening program after TFCC injury include (**a**) rotation of a hammer for forearm strengthening, (**b**) use of a gyroscope for wrist stability, and (**c**) incorporation of progressive weight-bearing activities. (Photos by Cara Rodriguez)

31.3.6.3 Procedures

Management begins with bracing, activity modification, anti-inflammatory medications, and hand therapy as mentioned above. In those who cannot tolerate rehabilitation due to severe pain, corticosteroid injections can be considered.

31.3.6.4 Surgery

Most patients will improve with conservative management as listed above. Surgery may be indicated in those with central tears of the TFCC, due to the poor vascularity for healing, or in those with concomitant fractures [13, 16]. Those with DRUJ instability may not improve with conservative management alone and require surgery. For more details on surgery for dorsal wrist disorders, refer to Chap. 37.

31.4 Kienböck's Disease

31.4.1 Synonyms

- Avascular necrosis of the lunate
- Osteonecrosis of the lunate
- Osteomalacia of the lunate

31.4.2 ICD-10 Codes

M92.21, M93.1

Table 31.6 Differential diagnosis for Kienböck's disease [21, 22]

Perilunate dislocation
Ulnar impaction syndrome
Lunate contusion/acute fracture
Arthritis (early rheumatoid arthritis, gout, osteoarthritis)
Intraosseous ganglion cyst
Osteoid osteoma

31.4.3 Description

The first known description of Kienböck's disease was from a cadaveric case study in 1843, but the term was not used until Dr. Robert Kienböck, a radiologist, presented the clinical and radiographic evidence for osteonecrosis of the lunate in 1910 [20]. While the exact mechanism of why this occurs is not fully understood, it is thought to result from a combination of multiple factors, such as altered vascular perfusion, repetitive microtrauma, variable anatomy, and altered biomechanics and kinematics [21]. The lunate typically has blood supply from both palmar and dorsal arteries, which serves as protection should there be vascular disruption; however, 20–26% of lunates may only have a palmar blood supply, which increases the risk for developing Kienböck's disease [21]. Anatomic variations in lunate morphology, as well as ulnar variance, has also been thought to contribute to abnormal load distribution through the radiolunate joint [20]. Table 31.6 lists the differential diagnosis for Kienböck's disease.

31.4.4 Clinical Presentation

Kienböck's disease is often seen in males 20–40 years of age, who may have a history of trauma to the wrist or those who do repetitive wrist loading. Because the osteonecrosis of the lunate may be slow to develop, patients will usually present with generalized wrist pain, altered range of motion, decreased grip strength, or pain with grip and edema, depending on the stage at initial presentation [20, 21]. Symptoms are usually seen in the dominant wrist and are rarely bilateral. Because of the insidious onset of usually low-grade pain, most patients will report continuing work duties or other activities despite having symptoms.

31.4.5 Physical Examination

Physical examination will reveal tenderness over the dorsal lunate and radiolunate facet, with an effusion or fullness palpated over the radiocarpal joint [20]. Range of motion testing will usually reveal limitations in flexion/extension arc with pain. Testing grip strength with a dynamometer and comparing to the contralateral, asymptomatic side will show up to 50% decrease in strength [20].

31.4.6 Diagnostic Workup

Imaging starts with posterior-anterior (PA) and lateral radiographs with the affected wrist in neutral rotation. While initial stages of Kienböck's disease may produce negative plain films, later stages of the disease may show increased lunate density, which signifies osteonecrosis, as well as progressive collapse and fragmentation of the lunate [20] (Fig. 31.7). Measurements should be taken for ulnar variance, as well as to look for dorsal intercalary segmental instability (DISI). Suspicion of Kienböck's disease should prompt more advanced imaging, such as CT or MRI, despite negative plain radiographs. MRI can detect early stages of osteonecrosis that are not seen in other imaging modalities and aids in developing the best management plan [21]. The differential diagnosis to consider is in Table 31.6 [21, 22].

31.4.7 Treatment

31.4.7.1 Medical Management

The proper management is determined based on the stage of the disease. The most commonly known and frequently used classification scheme was developed by Lichtman and col-

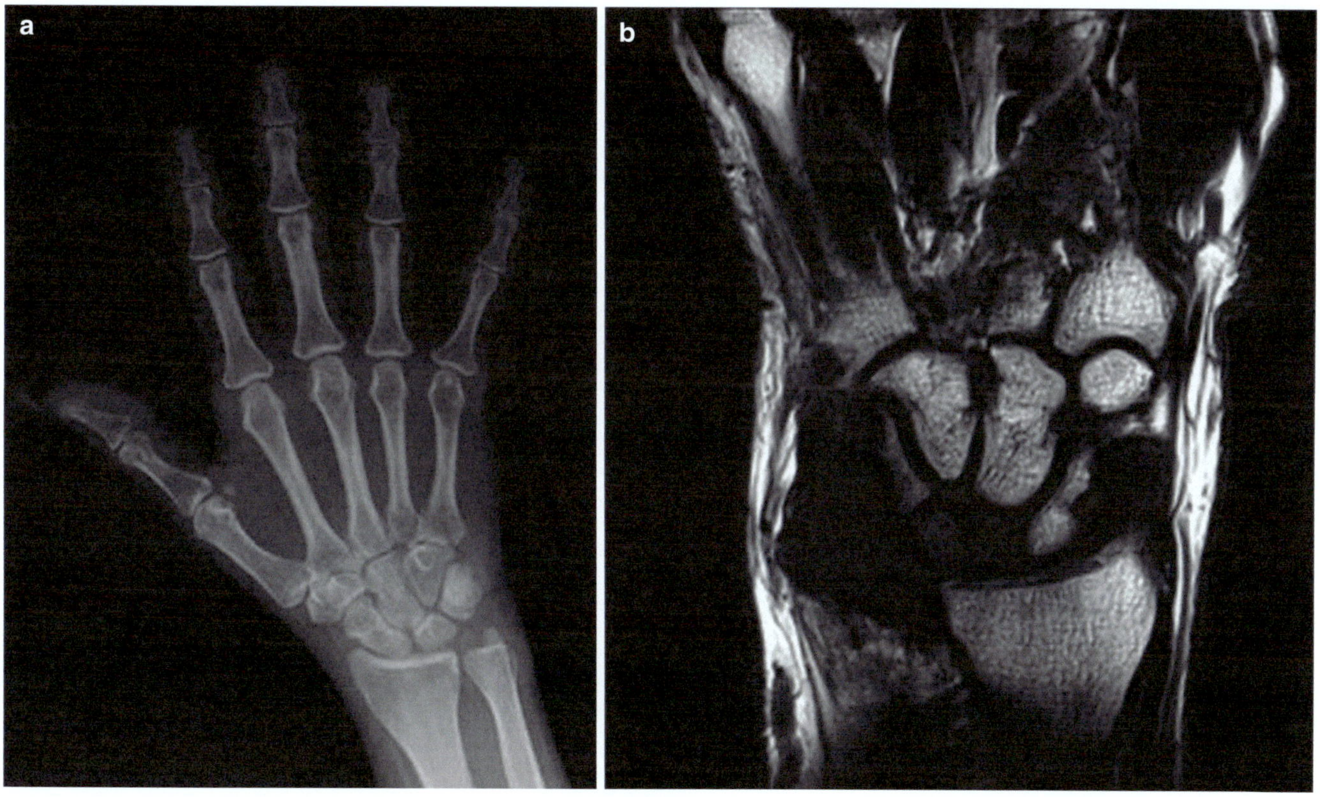

Fig. 31.7 (**a**) AP radiograph of a wrist with known stage I disease, showing no acute changes. (**b**) Coronal T1-weighted MRI showing decreased signal intensity in the lunate. (From: Pientka et al. [27]; with permission)

Table 31.7 Lichtman classification for Kienböck's disease

Stage I	Radiographs are normal, and MRI will show signal decrease in T1-weighted images
Stage II	Radiographs: lunate sclerosis without collapse, +/− fracture lines
Stage IIIA	Lunate collapse, but no change in carpal height and alignment
Stage IIIB	Lunate collapse, as well as carpal height loss, capitate migration proximally, and/or flexed and rotated scaphoid
Stage IV	Stage IIIB + radiocarpal or midcarpal degenerative changes

From: Cross and Matullo [20]; with permission

leagues [23] [Table 31.7]. Conservative management including the use of anti-inflammatory medications and immobilization has shown to be successful in early stage I disease [21]. However, a large number of those with stage I will likely progress, so close monitoring is paramount to ensuring healing or need for surgical management.

31.4.7.2 Rehabilitation

While a patient with early Kienböck's disease may benefit from a wrist immobilization orthosis in providing short-term relief, there is little research supporting effective long-term success in addressing progressed stages of the disease with conservative management [24]. Therefore, a patient with Kienböck's disease is generally treated by hand therapy as a post-surgical intervention. While casted, the patient should begin digit and elbow ROM immediately following surgery to avoid stiffness. Active and gentle passive ROM is initiated upon cast removal and the patient provided a HEP. A wrist immobilization orthosis may be fitted for comfort and protection as indicated. Scar management techniques may be included in treatment as well as the HEP in order to reduce scar formation. Progressive strengthening is initiated in accordance with the surgeon's postoperative protocol. It is important to note that the primary goal of surgery is to provide a stable, pain-free wrist [6]. With this in mind, the therapist should set clear, realistic expectations with the patient regarding long-term wrist ROM and grip strength and should not attempt to achieve motion beyond the expected range. Education on activity adaptation and modifications may be necessary given post-surgical biomechanical changes.

31.4.7.3 Procedures

Because localized corticosteroid injections have been known to worsen osteonecrosis, these should be avoided in Kienböck's disease. There is no evidence for the use of orthobiologics for this condition [25].

31.4.7.4 Surgery

Any evidence of sclerotic changes in the lunate or lunate collapse will require surgical management to prevent further worsening. For more details on surgery for dorsal wrist disorders, refer to Chap. 37.

References

1. Head L, Gencarelli JR, Allen M, Boyd KU. Wrist ganglion treatment: systematic review and meta-analysis. J Hand Surg Am. 2015;40(3):546–53.e8.
2. Gude W, Morelli V. Ganglion cysts of the wrist: pathophysiology, clinical picture, and management. Curr Rev Musculoskelet Med. 2008;1(3–4):205–11.
3. Zhang A, Falkowski AL, Jacobson JA, Kim SM, Koh SH, Gaetke-Udager K. Sonography of wrist ganglion cysts: which location is Most common? J Ultrasound Med. 2019;38(8):2155–60.
4. Schnur D, Keith J. Ganglion cysts. In: Miller M, editor. Essential Orthopaedics. 2nd ed. Philadelphia: Elsevier, Inc; 2020. p. 305–7.
5. Pal J, Wallman J. Ganglions and tumors of the hand and wrist. In: Cooper C, editor. Fundamentals of hand therapy. 2nd ed. St. Louis: Elsevier, Inc.; 2014. p. 500–7.
6. Cannon NM. Diagnosis and treatment manual for physicians and therapists: upper extremity rehabilitation. 4th ed. Indianapolis, IN: The hand rehabilitation center of Indiana; 2001. p. 287.
7. McGraw I. Isolated spontaneous posterior interosseous nerve palsy: a review of aetiology and management. J Hand Surg Eur. 2019;44(3):310–6.
8. Knutsen EJ, Calfee RP. Uncommon upper extremity compression neuropathies. Hand Clin. 2013;29(3):443–53.
9. Cleary C. Management of radial tunnel syndrome: a therapist's clinical perspective. J Hand Ther. 2006;19(2):186–91.
10. Porretto-loehrke A, Soika E. Therapist's management of other nerve compression syndromes of the wrist and elbow. In: Skirven™. Osterman AL. Fedorcczyk JM, Amadio PC, editors. Rehabilitation of the hand and upper extremity. 6th ed. St. Louis: Mosby; 2011, p. 845–57.
11. Skalski MR, White EA, Patel DB, Schein AJ, RiveraMelo H, Matcuk GR. The traumatized TFCC: an illustrated review of the anatomy and injury patterns of the triangular fibrocartilage complex. Curr Probl Diagn Radiol. 2016;45(1):39–50.
12. Pang EQ, Yao J. Ulnar-sided wrist pain in the athlete (TFCC/DRUJ/ECU). Curr Rev Musculoskelet Med. 2017;10(1):53–61.
13. Adams JE. Disorders of the distal radioulnar joint. In: Miller MD, Thompson SR, editors. DeLee & Drez's orthopaedic sports medicine. 5th ed. Philadelphia: Elsevier, Inc; 2020. p. 865–72.
14. Palmer AK. Triangular fibrocartilage complex lesions: a classification. J Hand Surg Am. 1989;14:594–606.
15. Lee RKL, Ng AWH, Tong CSL, Griffith JF, Tse WL, Wong C, et al. Intrinsic ligament and triangular fibrocartilage complex tears of the wrist: comparison of MDCT arthrography, conventional 3-T MRI, and MR arthrography. Skelet Radiol. 2013;42(9):1277–85.
16. Boatright JD. Triangular fibrocartilage complex injuries. In: Miller M, editor. Essential orthopaedics. 2nd ed. Philadelphia: Elsevier, Inc; 2020. p. 294–8.
17. Dell, P. Ulnar wrist pain and impairment: a therapist's algorithmic approach to the triangular fibrocartilage complex. In: Skirven™. Osterman AL. Fedorcczyk JM, Amadio PC, editors. Rehabilitation of the hand and upper extremity. 6th ed. St. Louis: Mosby; 2011, p. 974–87.
18. Chen Z. A novel staged wrist sensorimotor rehabilitation program for a patient with triangular fibrocartilage complex injury: a case report. J Hand Ther. 2019;32(4):525–34.

19. Altman E. The ulnar side of the wrist: clinically relevant anatomy and biomechanics. J Hand Ther. 2016;29(2):111–22.
20. Cross D, Matullo KS. Kienböck disease. Orthop Clin North Am. 2014;45(1):141–52.
21. Rioux-Forker D, Shin AY. Osteonecrosis of the lunate: Kienböck's disease. J Am Acad Orthop Surg. 2020;28(14):570–84.
22. Thaller JB, Iaculli MC. Kienböck's disease. In: Miller M, editor. Essential orthopaedics. 2nd ed. Philadelphia: Elsevier, Inc; 2020. p. 290–3.
23. Lichtman DM, Mack GR, MacDonald RI, Gunther SF, Wilson JN. Kienböck's disease: the role of silicone replacement arthroplasty. J Bone Joint Surg Am. 1977;59(7):899–908.
24. Divelbiss B, Baratz ME. Kienböck disease. J Am Soc Surg Hand. 2001;1(1):61–72.
25. Steiner MM, Calandruccio JH. Biologic approaches to problems of the hand and wrist. Orthop Clin North Am. 2017;48(3):343–9.
26. Kovachevich R, Elhassan BT. Arthroscopic and open repair of the TFCC. Hand Clin. 2010;26(4):485–94.
27. Pientka WF, Hanalla B, Barber RB, Niacaris T, Lichtman DM. Clinical presentation, natural history, and classification of Kienböck's disease. In: Lichtman D, Bain G, editors. Kienböck's disease. Springer: Cham; 2016. p. 97–109. Available from: https://doi-org.ezproxy.library.tufts.edu/10.1007/978-3-319-34226-9_9.

32 Ventral Wrist Disorders

Christopher Elmore, Walter I. Sussman, Riley Rousakis, William A. Berrigan, Kenneth Mautner, and Charles Cassidy

32.1 Carpal Tunnel Syndrome

32.1.1 Synonyms

- CTS
- Median nerve entrapment
- Repetitive motion injury

32.1.2 ICD 10 Code

G56.00

C. Elmore (✉)
Department of Physical Medicine and Rehabilitation, Tufts Medical Center, Boston, MA, USA

W. I. Sussman
Department of Orthopedics & Rehabilitation Medicine, Tufts University School of Medicine, Boston, MA, USA

Boston Sports & Biologics PC, Wellesley, MA, USA

R. Rousakis
Boston Sports & Biologics PC, Private Practice, Wellesley, MA, USA

Department of Physical Medicine and Rehabilitation, Veterans Administration Medical Center, Boston, MA, USA

W. A. Berrigan
Clinical Sports Medicine Fellow, Department of Physical Medicine and Rehabilitation, Emory University School of Medicine, Atlanta, GA, USA

K. Mautner
Primary Care Sports Medicine Fellowship, Emory University, Atlanta, GA, USA

Department of Orthopaedics and Physical Medicine and Rehabilitation, Emory University School of Medicine, Atlanta, GA, USA

C. Cassidy
Department of Orthopedic & Rehabilitation Medicine, Tufts University School of Medicine, Tufts Medical Center, Boston, MA, USA

32.1.3 Description

Carpal tunnel syndrome (CTS) is a symptomatic focal median mononeuropathy at the wrist. It is caused by compression of the median nerve as it passes through the osteofibrous carpal tunnel in the volar wrist between the transverse carpal ligament (TCL; flexor retinaculum) and carpal bones. CTS is the most common focal entrapment mononeuropathy representing about 90% of all entrapment mononeuropathies and has a lifetime risk around 10% [1]. CTS typically presents with a characteristic pattern of abnormal sensation and pain in the ventral palm, thumb, index, middle, and radial half of the ring fingers and is bilateral in about 65% of patients at first presentation [2].

Etiology and pathophysiology CTS is caused by ischemia of the median nerve due to elevated pressure within the confined carpal tunnel. Risk factors for the development of CTS include elevated body mass index (BMI), female gender (3:1 ratio), diabetes, hypothyroidism, rheumatoid arthritis, and occupational risk factors, which predispose to repetitive wrist flexion and extension [2]. The increased pressure can be a result of wrist position, flexor tenosynovitis (e.g., rheumatoid arthritis), wrist trauma, fibrosis of the surrounding connective tissue, congenitally small tunnel, or idiopathic. CTS is also fairly common during pregnancy, especially during the third trimester and may persist after delivery if the mother is breastfeeding.

Normal CT pressure is less than 5 mm Hg in a neutral position but can be elevated to 20–30 mm Hg when using a computer mouse. At these elevated pressures, there is a decrease in median nerve blood flow [1]. An increased pressure can result in demyelination and, in more advanced cases, axonal loss. Sensory nerves are typically affected first and undergo demyelination followed later by axonal loss. Motor fibers are affected later and muscle atrophy is often considered an absolute indication for surgery.

Anatomy The median nerve is formed by the convergence of the medial and lateral cord of the brachial plexus and has contributions from the ventral roots of C5 to T1. The nerve

© The Author(s), under exclusive license to Springer Nature Switzerland AG 2022
S. A. Mostoufi et al. (eds.), *Clinical Guide to Musculoskeletal Medicine*, https://doi.org/10.1007/978-3-030-92042-5_32

descends lateral to the brachial artery in the arm until the nerve crosses over the brachial artery at the elbow and under the bicipital aponeurosis between the pronator teres and the biceps tendon. The nerve then passes between the two heads of the pronator teres. Compression at these points can lead to pronator syndrome. The nerve then innervates the flexor–pronator muscles, including the superficial layer (pronator teres, flexor carpi radialis, and palmaris longus) and the intermediate layer (flexor digitorum superficialis) before the takeoff of the anterior interosseous nerve, which innervates the deep layer (the flexor digitorum profundus of the index and middle fingers, flexor pollicis longus, and pronator quadratus). Approximately 5 cm proximal to the wrist, the palmar cutaneous branch of the median nerve arises from the main trunk and travels superficial to the carpal tunnel to innervate the skin in the radial palm; this area is spared in CTS. The median nerve then passes into the carpal tunnel and divides into the recurrent motor branch supplying the thenar muscles (opponens pollicis, abductor pollicis brevis, superficial head flexor pollicis brevis) and the palmar digital branches innervating the ulnar two lumbricals and the median-innervated skin. Table 32.1 outlines differential diagnosis of carpal tunnel syndrome.

32.1.4 Clinical Presentation

Patients commonly endorse a nighttime sensation of burning, tingling, or numbness primarily in the median nerve distribution of the affected hand. In some instances, the discomfort will radiate proximally as well. The symptoms may be aggravated during the day by activities such as driving, reading, or computer use. They may "shake out" their hands to relieve the numbness. As the condition progresses, the irritability symptoms may subside and be replaced by constant numbness. Over time, the numbness may become constant, and patients may have difficulty with activities such as fastening buttons or picking up small objects. In the physical examination and diagnostic workup sections, we will address differentiating CTS from some other pathologies that can mimic symptoms of CTS (Table 32.1).

32.1.5 Physical Examination

Evaluation of the median nerve should include both sensory and motor examination. Sensation should be assessed proximal and distal to the carpal tunnel, as proximal sensory changes may be indicative of other diagnoses. Muscle bulk and strength should be evaluated and one should also consider the patient's comorbidities. Thenar atrophy in numerous studies is considered an absolute indication for operative release.

Table 32.1 Differential diagnosis of carpal tunnel syndrome

Cervical radiculopathy (particularly C6, C7)	Brachial plexopathy
Cervical spondylotic myelopathy	Proximal median neuropathy
Motor neuron disease (e.g., ALS)	Fibromyalgia
Ligament disruption	Forearm or hand compartment syndrome

32.1.5.1 Provocative Maneuvers

Tinel test: Firm percussion just proximal to or over the transverse carpal ligament (Fig. 32.1). A positive test elicits tingling or electric shock–like sensations in the median nerve distribution. It is estimated to be about 50% sensitive and 77% specific [2]. It may be negative in advanced cases.

Phalen maneuver Patient fully flexes the wrist with the elbow extended or, alternatively, presses the dorsum of the hands together causing hyperflexion of both wrists (Fig. 32.2). It is estimated to be about 68% sensitive and 73% specific [2].

Carpal compression test Examiner applies manual pressure over the transverse carpal ligament recreating the pain or paresthesias in the median dermatome (Fig. 32.3). It is estimated to be about 64% sensitive and 83% specific [2].

The hand elevation test The patient holds their hand above their head for 1 minute and is positive if their symptoms are recreated. It is estimated to have similar sensitivity and specificity to the Phalen maneuver and Tinel test [2].

32.1.6 Diagnostic Workup

32.1.6.1 Electrodiagnostic Testing (EDX)

Nerve conduction studies (NCS) can localize the lesion, assess the degree of injury, and rule out other pathology. Needle electromyography (EMG) is frequently used to augment the NCS and can help rule out plexopathy, polyneuropathy, and radiculopathy. The NCS and EMG combined provide a high degree of sensitivity and specificity, and studies should be conducted bilaterally.

Nerve compression initially causes demyelination, which will cause delayed distal latencies in the NCS. With progression, there can be axonal loss, which manifests as decreased amplitude of the compound motor action potential (CMAP) and sensory nerve action potentials (SNAP). The degree of severity is important in deciding the appropriate course of treatment and the likelihood of improvement versus progression of disease. More advanced cases are unlikely to resolve with conservative management and should be referred for operative release.

32.1.6.2 Neuromuscular Ultrasound

In patients with CTS, there is an increase in the cross-sectional area of the median nerve at the distal wrist crease.

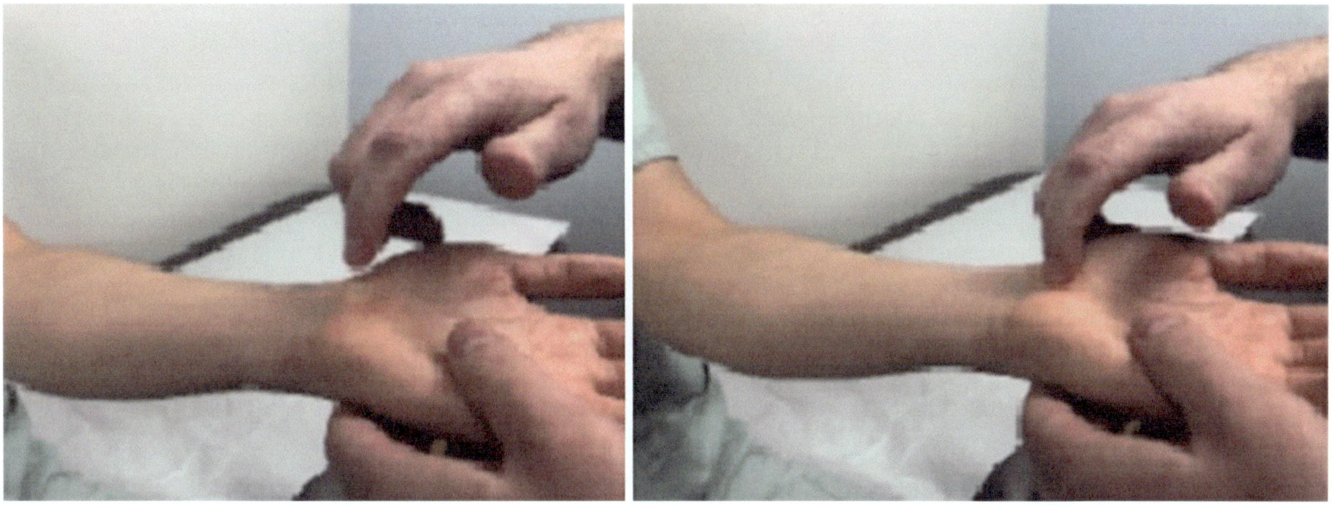

Fig. 32.1 Tinel test

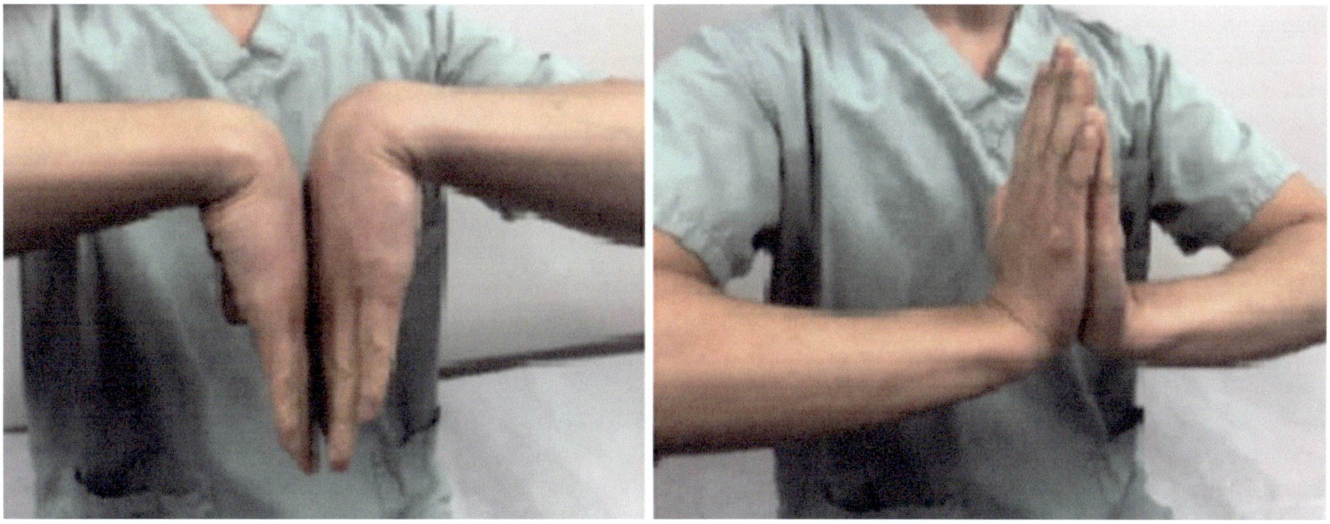

Fig. 32.2 Phalen maneuver

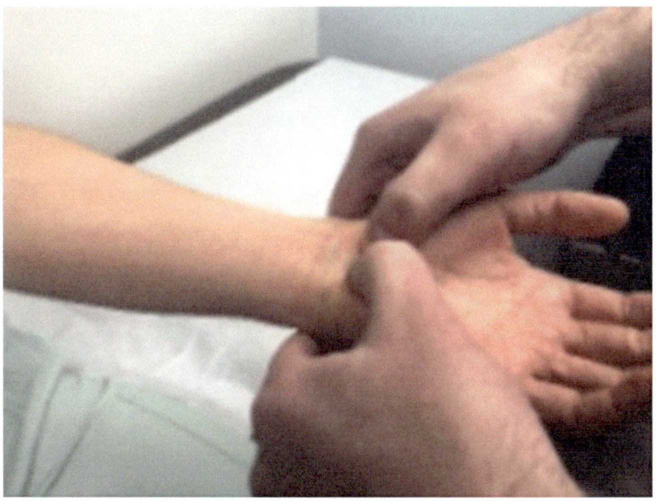

Fig. 32.3 Carpal compression test

Multiple high-quality studies use a cutoff of 8.5–10 mm for diagnosis, though the optimal cutoff has varied [2]. Some recent studies using cross-sectional area cutoffs have demonstrated good interrater reliability and sensitivity and specificity approaching or surpassing electrodiagnostic studies. Additionally, ultrasound can shed light on anatomic abnormalities that may be causing injury such as ganglion cysts. It is also helpful to compare the cross-sectional area of the affected versus contralateral nerve at the distal wrist crease. One such study used a cross-sectional area difference of $2.5 mm^2$ and was 97% sensitive and 100% specific [3].

32.1.6.3 Magnetic Resonance Imaging

Magnetic resonance imaging (MRI) is typically reserved for unusual cases or to rule out other pathology such as a mass. It can provide information on abnormal nerve, tendon, vascular structures, or other soft tissue anomalies.

32.1.7 Treatments

32.1.7.1 Medical Management

Splinting is a commonly used and widely available non-surgical treatment for CTS. It is most effective in mild cases and has less evidence of support in moderate to severe cases [1]. In addition to providing pain relief and improving duration or quality of sleep, splints help patients become more aware of hand positioning and those activities that exacerbate their symptoms. Although NSAIDs are commonly prescribed, there is little evidence to support its effectiveness in treating CTS. Oral corticosteroids can also be used but may be more limited by comorbidities, patient tolerance, and duration due to their systemic effects.

32.1.7.2 Rehabilitation

Occupational and physical therapy can be beneficial in both conservative and surgical management of CTS. Conservative management focuses on symptom reduction and typically includes splinting, tendon gliding exercises, and patient education. Education includes activity modifications, ergonomics, and adaptive equipment to reduce symptoms and improve the client's ability to participate in daily activities. Physical agent modalities such as ultrasound and iontophoresis have been used in the conservative treatment of CTS but are not strongly supported by evidence.

If conservative treatment is unsuccessful, patients may be referred for surgical intervention. Rehabilitation after carpal tunnel release surgery begins with wound care, splinting, edema control, and ROM exercises. This is followed by scar mobility, desensitization, tendon gliding exercises, and progression of strengthening exercises as appropriate. The therapist will also educate the client on postoperative precautions, adaptive equipment, and activity modifications to promote healing of the surgical site and maximize independence with daily activities.

32.1.7.3 Procedures

CTS Corticosteroid Injection (CPT Code 20526)

Corticosteroid is a widely accepted treatment for relief of symptoms in CTS. The INSTINCTS trial showed that when compared to night splinting alone, patients undergoing carpal tunnel injection had less pain and better hand function at 6 weeks and no adverse events were reported. Additionally, the treatment was found to be cost-effective because of the low cost of a single dose of methylprednisolone and the earlier onset of relief that was sustained over 6 months [4]. Injections are commonly performed under landmark or imaging guidance (Fig. 32.4).

Median Nerve Hydrodissection

This is another treatment for nerve entrapment via injection of anesthetic, saline, or 5% dextrose and is sometimes accompanied by a small volume of steroid. The goal is to provide separation of the nerve from the surrounding tissue, fascia, or adjacent structures relieving compressive forces that may cause relative ischemia. Hydrodissection (HD) with normal saline (NS) has been shown to outperform an injection of NS subcutaneously placed above the carpal tunnel (control) by a greater decrease in Boston Carpal Tunnel Syndrome Questionnaire (BCTSQ) score, better functional status, and decreased nerve cross-sectional area at 6 months. Studies have also demonstrated an even greater improvement in pain, functional status, and edema in a group comparing dextrose 5% in water HD with NS HD at 6 months [5].

CTS PRP Injection (CPT: 0232T)

Several RCTs have compared platelet-rich plasma (PRP) injections to various conservative treatments, and multiple systematic reviews and meta-analyses have evaluated the efficacy of PRP in carpal tunnel syndrome (CTS) [6–8].

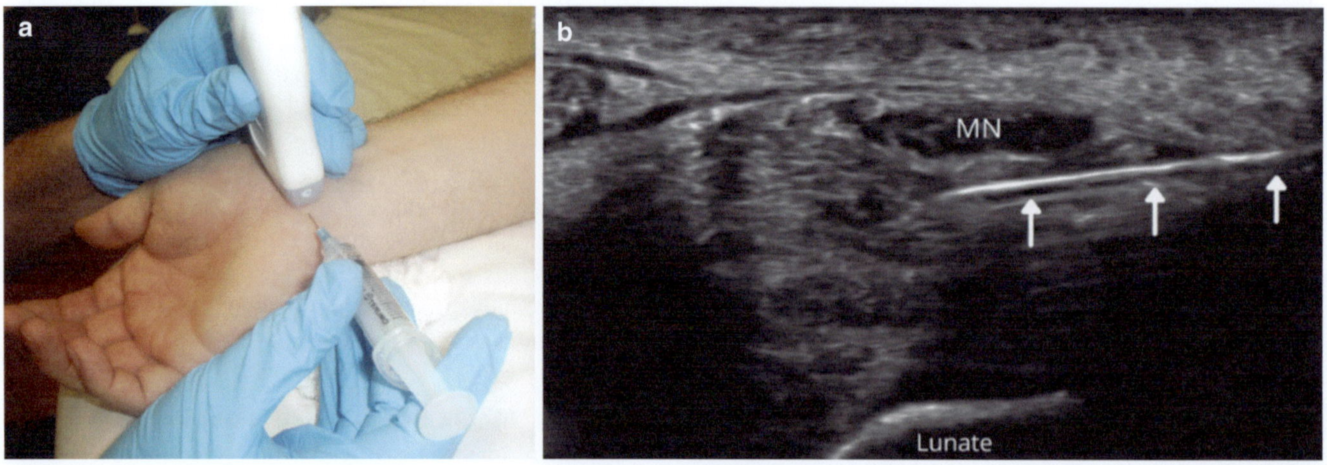

Fig. 32.4 Ultrasound-guided carpal tunnel injection. (**a**) Transducer position for transverse imaging of the carpal tunnel and in-plane needle approach. (**b**) Transverse sonogram of the carpal tunnel with a 25 gauge needle (arrows) passing a shallow oblique angle deep to the median nerve (MN)

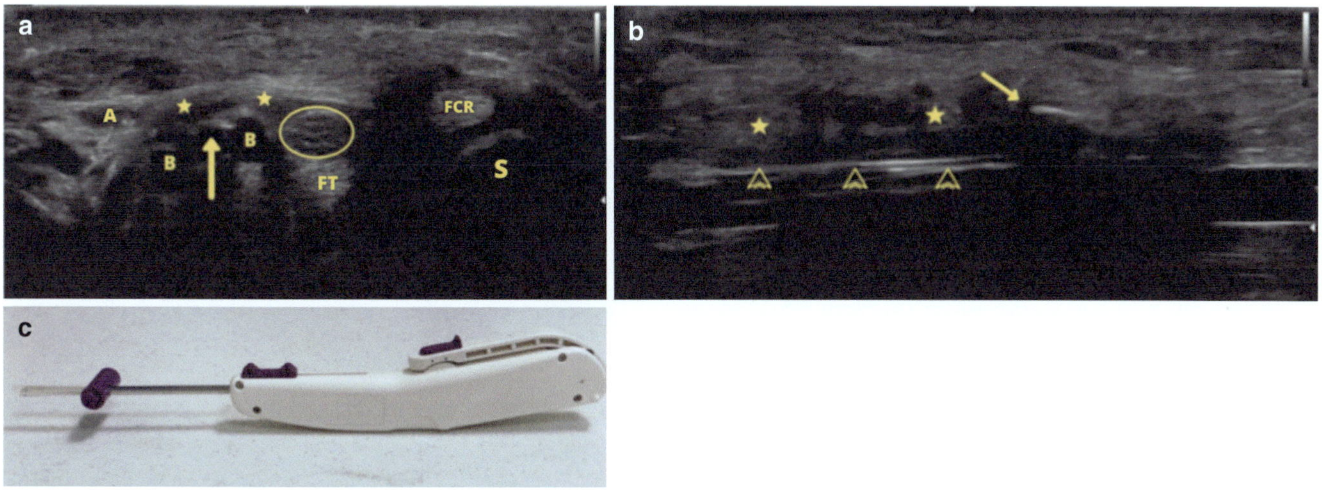

Fig. 32.5 Ultrasound-guided carpal tunnel release. (**a**) Intraprocedural ultrasound images during transverse carpal ligament transection demonstrate a short-axis image of the carpal tunnel following insertion of the device (arrow) and inflation of the balloon (**b**). The device is positioned within the transverse safe zone ulnar to the median nerve (circle). S scaphoid, FCR flexor carpi radialis, FT flexor tendons, A ulnar artery. (**b**) Longitudinal image (distal to the right, proximal to the left) shows the device (arrowheads) cutting the transverse carpal ligament (star) with the hook of the device deployed (arrow). (**c**) The SX-One MicroKnife device (Sonex Health) used to transect the transverse carpal ligament

While corticosteroids consistently had short-term benefit over PRP injections, the 3–6 months data suggest better symptom relief with PRP treatment compared with corticosteroids and other conservative treatments [6–8]. The studies are limited due to the variability in PRP preparations and the definition of the control group (splint, steroid, or saline injection, no treatment.) PRP may also be effective as an adjuvant treatment with carpal tunnel release, facilitating earlier recovery of grip strength [9]. Studies including median nerve cross-sectional area by ultrasound and NCS have not conclusively demonstrated a clear benefit of PRP over traditional treatment [8, 10, 11].

Percutaneous CTS Release (CPT: 64721+ 76342 US Guidance)

Ultrasound-guided carpal tunnel release is a minimally invasive procedure performed under local anesthesia to release the median nerve by transecting the transverse carpal ligament (TCL). It combines a small incision with real-time ultrasound visualization of at-risk structures including the median nerve, recurrent motor branch, ulnar vessels, and superficial palmar arch. Several methods for release have been described ranging from the use of a spinal needle and surgical dissecting thread to single-use disposable devices with a retractable cutting blade (Fig. 32.5) [12–17]. These various techniques have proven clinical success of greater than 95% with a reduced post-procedure recovery time compared to traditional surgical approaches and without any significant complications reported to date [12, 13, 18, 19].

32.1.7.4 Surgery

Open surgical treatments are discussed in Chap. 37.

References

1. Wang L. Guiding treatment for carpal tunnel syndrome. Phys Med Rehabil Clin N Am. 2018;29(4):751–60.
2. Kothari M. Carpal tunnel syndrome: clinical manifestations and diagnosis. UpToDate. UpToDate, Waltham, MA. Accessed 1 Apr 2021.
3. Elnady B, Rageh EM, Ekhouly T, Fathy SM, Alshaar M, Fouda ES, et al. Diagnostic potential of ultrasound in carpal tunnel syndrome with different etiologies: correlation of sonographic median nerve measures with electrodiagnostic severity. BMC Musculoskelet Disord. 2019;20(1):634.
4. Chesterton LS, Blagojevic-Bucknall M, Burton C, Dziedzic KS, Davenport G, Jowett SM, et al. The clinical and cost-effectiveness of corticosteroid injection versus night splints for carpal tunnel syndrome (INSTINCTS trial): an open-label, parallel group, randomised controlled trial. Lancet. 2018;392(10156):1423–33.
5. Lam KHS, Hung CY, Chiang YP, Onishi K, Su DCJ, Clark TB, et al. Ultrasound-guided nerve hydrodissection for pain management: rationale, methods, current literature, and theoretical mechanisms. J Pain Res. 2020;13:1957–68.
6. Catapano M, Catapano J, Borschel G, Alavinia SM, Robinson LR, Mittal N. Effectiveness of platelet-rich plasma injections for nonsurgical management of carpal tunnel syndrome: a systematic review and meta-analysis of randomized controlled trials. Arch Phys Med Rehabil. 2020;101(5):897–906.
7. Dong C, Sun Y, Qi Y, Zhu Y, Wei H, Wu D, et al. Effect of platelet-rich plasma injection on mild or moderate carpal tunnel syndrome: an updated systematic review and meta-analysis of randomized controlled trials. Biomed Res Int. 2020;2020:5089378.

8. Malahias MA, Chytas D, Mavrogenis AF, Nikolaou VS, Johnson EO, Babis GC. Platelet-rich plasma injections for carpal tunnel syndrome: a systematic and comprehensive review. Eur J Orthop Surg Traumatol. 2019;29(1):1–8.
9. Trull-Ahuir C, Sala D, Chismol-Abad J, Vila-Caballer M, Lison JF. Efficacy of platelet-rich plasma as an adjuvant to surgical carpal ligament release: a prospective, randomized controlled clinical trial. Sci Rep. 2020;10(1):2085.
10. Amini D. Occupational therapy interventions for work-related injuries and conditions of the forearm, wrist, and hand: a systematic review. Am J Occup Ther. 2011;65(1):29–36.
11. Wu YT, Ho TY, Chou YC, Ke MJ, Li TY, Huang GS, et al. Six-month efficacy of platelet-rich plasma for carpal tunnel syndrome: a prospective randomized, single-blind controlled trial. Sci Rep. 2017;7(1):94.
12. Henning PT, Yang L, Awan T, Lueders D, Pourcho AM. Minimally invasive ultrasound-guided carpal tunnel release: preliminary clinical results. J Ultrasound Med. 2018;37(11):2699–706.
13. Rojo-Manaute JM, Capa-Grasa A, Chana-Rodriguez F, Perez-Mananes R, Rodriguez-Maruri G, Sanz-Ruiz P, et al. Ultra-minimally invasive ultrasound-guided carpal tunnel release: a randomized clinical trial. J Ultrasound Med. 2016;35(6):1149–57.
14. Chappell CD, Beckman JP, Baird BC, Takke AV. Ultrasound (US) changes in the median nerve cross-sectional area after micro-invasive US-guided carpal tunnel release. J Ultrasound Med. 2020;39(4):693–702.
15. Hebbard PD, Hebbard AIT, Tomka J, Appleyard R. Ultrasound-guided microinvasive carpal tunnel release using a novel retractable needle-mounted blade: a cadaveric study. J Ultrasound Med. 2018;37(8):2075–81.
16. Joseph AE, Leiby BM, Beckman JP. Clinical results of ultrasound-guided carpal tunnel release performed by a primary care sports medicine physician. J Ultrasound Med. 2020;39(3):441–52.
17. Guo D, Guo D, Guo J, Schmidt SC, Lytie RM. A clinical study of the modified thread carpal tunnel release. Hand (N Y). 2017;12(5):453–60.
18. Kamel SI, Freid B, Pomeranz C, Halpern EJ, Nazarian LN. Minimally invasive ultrasound-guided carpal tunnel release improves long-term clinical outcomes in carpal tunnel syndrome. AJR Am J Roentgenol. 2021;217(2):460–8.
19. Leiby BM, Beckman JP, Joseph AE. Long-term clinical results of carpal tunnel release using ultrasound guidance. Hand (N Y) 2021:1558944720988080. https://doi.org/10.1177/1558944720988080

Radial-Side Wrist Disorders

33

Christopher Elmore, Walter I. Sussman, Riley Rousakis, and Charles Cassidy

33.1 De Quervain's Tenosynovitis

33.1.1 Synonyms

- Radial styloid tenosynovitis
- Stenosing tenosynovitis
- De Quervain's tendinosis
- Washerwoman's sprain

33.1.2 ICD 10 Code

M65.4

33.1.3 Description

De Quervain's tenosynovitis is a painful condition involving the abductor pollicis longus (APL) and the extensor pollicis brevis (EPB) in the first dorsal wrist compartment. It is an overuse injury resulting in thickening of the APL and/or EPB tendon and extensor retinaculum. Local trauma and scar tissue can restrict tendon movement and precipitate pain. The APL and EPB tendons pass through the first wrist compartment, in a fibro-osseous tunnel, and inflammation of the tendon or thickening of the extensor retinaculum can restrict gliding of the tendons resulting in a local stenosing effect. Chronic de Quervain's tenosynovitis has also been attributed to myxoid degeneration and increased vascularity rather than acute inflammation [1]. Differential diagnosis of de Quervain's tenosynovitis is given in Table 33.1.

C. Elmore (✉)
Department of Physical Medicine and Rehabilitation, Tufts Medical Center, Boston, MA, USA

W. I. Sussman
Department of Orthopedics & Rehabilitation Medicine, Tufts University School of Medicine, Boston, MA, USA

Boston Sports & Biologics PC, Wellesley, MA, USA

R. Rousakis
Boston Sports & Biologics PC, Private Practice, Wellesley, MA, USA

Department of Physical Medicine and Rehabilitation, Veterans Administration Medical Center, Boston, MA, USA

C. Cassidy
Department of Orthopedic & Rehabilitation Medicine, Tufts University School of Medicine, Tufts Medical Center, Boston, MA, USA

Table 33.1 Differential diagnosis of de Quervain's tenosynovitis

Differential diagnosis	Key elements
Osteoarthritis of the first carpometacarpal joint (base of the thumb)	Radiographs will show the first CMC OA typical progressive.
Intersection syndrome	Pain is more proximal than de Quervain's tenosynovitis.
Gamekeeper or skier's thumb	Due to radial deviation of the thumb and pain is focal over the medial thumb. Typically traumatic.
Flexor tenosynovitis	Pain is volar to the first compartment. Can be acute or chronic presentation. Pyogenic cases are surgical emergencies.

33.1.3.1 Anatomy

Extensor pollicis brevis EPB originates from the dorsal radius and inserts on the proximal phalanx of the thumb. Functionally, it is involved in radial abduction of the wrist and thumb extension. Innervation is by the radial nerve.

Abductor pollicis longus APL originates from the dorsal radius and ulna. The APL may have multiple tendon slips and inserts onto the trapezium with the abductor pollicis brevis, opponens pollicis, and anterior oblique ligament. It is one of the deep extensor muscles of the forearm and lies deep to the supinator. Functionally, the APL is involved in abduction of the thumb and extension of the first carpometacarpal (CMC) joint. Innervation is by a terminal branch of the radial nerve.

© The Author(s), under exclusive license to Springer Nature Switzerland AG 2022

S. A. Mostoufi et al. (eds.), *Clinical Guide to Musculoskeletal Medicine*, https://doi.org/10.1007/978-3-030-92042-5_33

33.1.4 Clinical Presentation

Patients typically present with pain over the radial styloid joint, which worsens with activities that cause ulnar deviation such as clenching a fist. Activities associated with this type of pain include golfing, lifting children, and hammering. The patient may also endorse paresthesias and/or weakness in the affected hand. A thorough history should include trauma, evolution of symptoms, work or daily activities, and current or recent pregnancy. History can help eliminate some of the differentials noted above (Table 33.1).

33.1.5 Physical Examination

There is tenderness over the base of the radial thumb. A "catching" or "snapping" sensation may be palpable over the first dorsal compartment of the wrist when performing range of motion (ROM) testing.

33.1.5.1 Special Test

Finkelstein's test Patient thumb is flexed and held inside a closed fist and the wrist is then ulnarly deviated. Test is positive if it reproduces pain over the first dorsal compartment. Eichhoff's test is similar, but the patient performs the movements themselves (Fig. 33.1).

33.1.6 Diagnostic Workup

X-rays These are non-diagnostic for de Quervain's tenosynovitis but can be used to rule out osteoarthritis (OA) of the first carpometacarpal joint or radiostyloid joint and other bony abnormalities that may cause radial wrist pain.

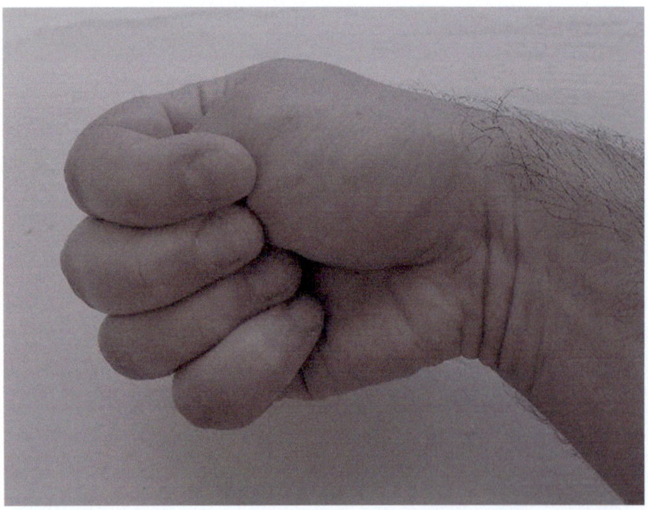

Fig. 33.1 Eichhoff's test with thumb clinched within grip and ulnar deviation. Finkelstein's test is similar, but the ulnar deviation is performed actively by the examiner

Ultrasound (US) Findings can include hypoechoic thickening of the APL and EPB tendons (Fig. 33.2), tenosynovitis of the tendon sheath, split tear of the tendon, thickening of the overlying retinaculum (Fig. 33.3), and neovascularization on power Doppler imaging. An inter-tendinous septum between the APL and EPB tendons can usually be identified and may have implications for management when injection of the tendon sheath is considered [2].

Magnetic resonance imaging (MRI) Findings can include tenosynovitis or tendinosis of the APL and EPB, thickening of the retinaculum, and linear split tear. MRI has a high sensitivity and specificity for de Quervain's tenosynovitis [3].

33.1.7 Treatments

33.1.7.1 Medical Management

Nonsteroidal anti-inflammatory drugs (NSAIDs) NSAIDs can be administered in oral, topical, or injectable formulations. Iontophoresis has also been used in delivery of anti-inflammatory medications (typically dexamethasone).

Thumb spica splints Splinting has been shown to decrease pain by immobilizing thumb and wrist joint tendons and decreasing thumb metacarpal phalangeal (MP) joint flexion and wrist ulnar deviation. A forearm-based thumb spica splint should position the wrist joint in neutral, carpometacarpal joint in 30° of flexion and abduction, while leaving the thumb interphalangeal joint free [4].

33.1.7.2 Rehabilitation

Physical or occupational therapy for de Quervain's tenosynovitis therapy focuses on splinting, therapeutic ultrasound, iontophoresis, eccentric therapeutic exercise to assist in soft tissue mobilization, and education. The goal of therapeutic exercises is to enhance gliding of the APL and EPB tendons in the first dorsal compartment. Pain-free active range of motion (AROM) exercise is initiated to the patient's tolerance, focusing on the wrist and thumb joints. Tendon gliding of the APL and EPB tendons is gently incorporated into thumb MP flexion combined with wrist ulnar deviation [5]. Strengthening exercises are then initiated to assist in return to functional activity. Activity modifications and adaptive equipment can improve an individual's function and decrease symptoms during daily activities.

In post-surgical cases after a first dorsal compartment release, rehabilitation will start with splinting, gentle range of motion exercise, scar management, and desensitization. The therapist will then progress the patient through strengthening exercises and returning to daily activities as appropriate.

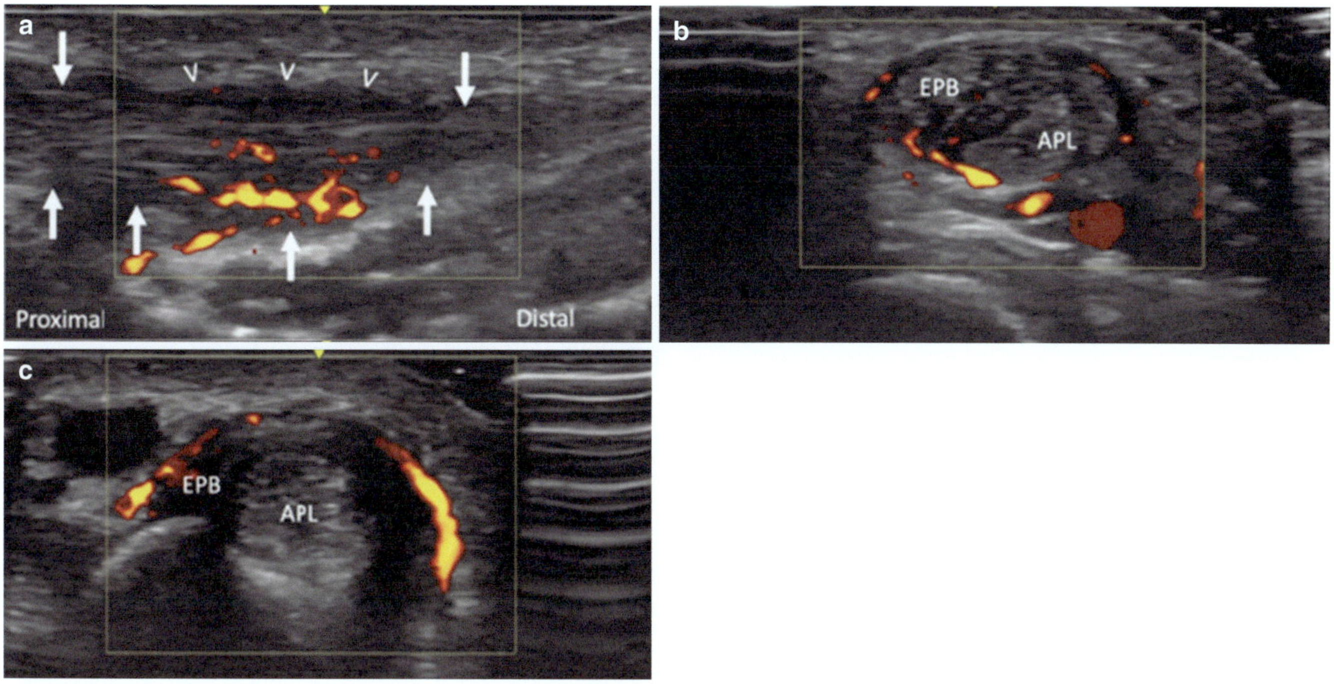

Fig. 33.2 (**a**) Sonogram of the first dorsal compartment in a postpartum wrist, showing neovascularization of the tendon (arrows) in the long axis and thickening of the retinaculum (arrowheads). (**b**) Short-axis views of the tendons demonstrate neovascularization of the extensor pollicis brevis (EPB) and abductor pollicis longus (APL). The APL tendon appears thickened with degenerative changes. (**c**) There is a hypoechoic halo with neovascularization surrounding the EPA and APL tendons with thickening of the APL. (Image courtesy of Ali Mostoufi, MD, Boston Regenerative Medicine)

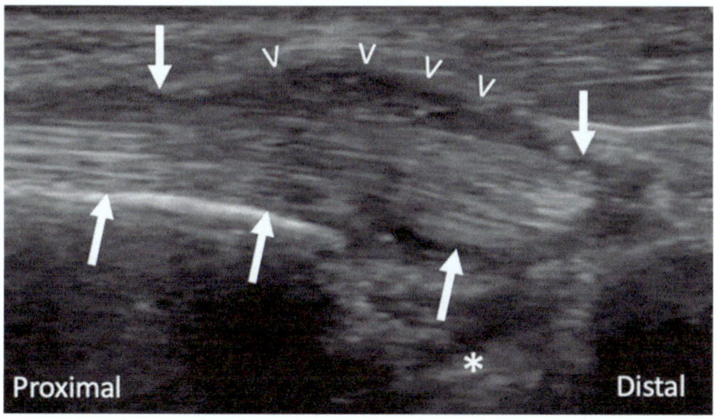

Fig. 33.3 Ultrasound of the radial wrist joint (*) in the long axis demonstrating thickened retinaculum (open arrows) causing stenosing tenosynovitis of APL/EPB (arrows). (Image from authors library)

33.1.7.3 Procedures

Corticosteroid Injection (CSI)
Corticosteroids have been shown to be effective, with patients remaining symptom free at 6 months in up to 80–82% of cases [1, 6]. In another study, 70% of patients responded to 1 or 2 *injections* [1].

Platelet-Rich Plasma (PRP)
The literature on PRP's role in treatment is still being evaluated, but one case study combined US-guided percutaneous needle tenotomy with PRP injection and found that at 6 months, visual analog scale (VAS) pain scale had decreased by 63% [7].

Prolotherapy
Another option for failed conservative management is prolotherapy with a mix of local anesthetic and dextrose. One case study showed that a 4 mL combination of 1% lidocaine with 12.5% dextrose provided complete pain relief for 2 months, equivalent to steroid injection, without any adverse effects [8].

33.1.8 Surgery

33.1.8.1 Ultrasound-Guided Percutaneous Release

Ultrasound (US) is highly effective in visualizing superficial structures of the forearm, wrist, and hand. Emerging techniques such as US-guided percutaneous release of the reti-

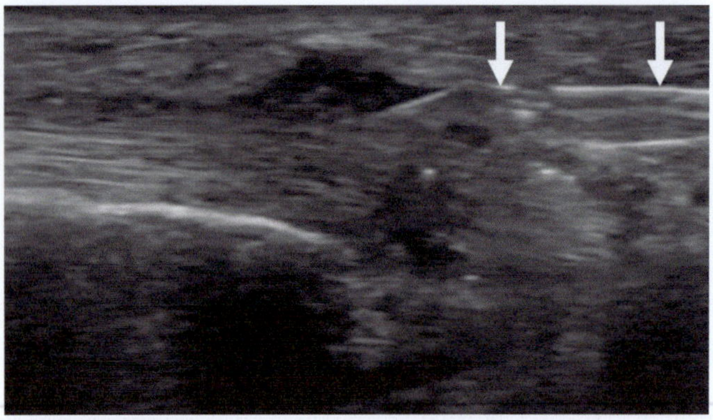

Fig. 33.4 Percutaneous release for de Quervain's tenosynovitis with a Nokor (arrows). (Image from authors' library)

naculum overlying the first dorsal extensor compartment have shown promising results (Fig. 33.4). In one study, 91.4% of patients had a negative Finkelstein test at the 1 month follow-up and decreased pain within 7 days of the procedure [6].

33.1.8.2 Open Surgical Release

In recalcitrant cases, surgical intervention can be considered. An incision through the extensor retinaculum is made over the first dorsal extensor compartment followed by the release of any sub-compartments such as the one frequently found with EPB, and return to activity is typically 2–3 weeks after surgery [1]. Surgical treatment of wrist and hand is discussed in Chap. 37.

33.2 Thumb Carpometacarpal Osteoarthritis

33.2.1 Synonyms

- First CMC OA
- Thumb arthritis
- Basal joint arthritis
- CMC osteoarthritis
- Trapeziometacarpal arthritis

33.2.2 ICD 10 Code

M18.9

33.2.3 Description

Degenerative osteoarthritis of the carpometacarpal (CMC) joint is a common, progressive, and painful condition, eventually causing weakness and decreased range of motion of the joint. Differential diagnosis of thumb carpometacarpal osteoarthritis is presented in Table 33.2.

Table 33.2 Differential diagnosis of thumb carpometacarpal osteoarthritis

De Quervain's tenosynovitis
Carpal tunnel syndrome
Gamekeeper's thumb
Rheumatoid arthritis
Arthritis of the radial styloid
Arthritis of scaphotrapezial trapezoidal (STT) joint
Trigger thumb

Etiology The first CMC joint is the most affected single joint involved in hand OA [9]. The risk factors include age and female sex, white ethnic groups, high body mass index (BMI), history of traumatic radial subluxation [10], and Ehlers–Danlos syndrome or hereditary ligament laxity [9]. The lifetime prevalence has varied in the literature. A 2020 meta-analysis found the prevalence of radiographic CMC osteoarthritis to be 5.8% in males and 7.3% in females at age 50. At age 80, the prevalence was 33.1% in males and 39% in females [9].

Pathophysiology Osteoarthritis is a chronic degenerative disease of the cartilage. Progression of the first CMC osteoarthritis can eventually result in instability and subluxation of the first metacarpal on the trapezium. Studies also suggest a role for the peptide hormone relaxin, which may help explain an elevated female predilection [11]. Instability contributes to progressive deterioration of the cartilage and pain, altered thumb mechanics, and hyperextension of the metacarpophalangeal joint.

Anatomy The first CMC joint is a synovial saddle joint between the trapezium and first metacarpal. Movement includes flexion, extension, abduction, adduction, opposition, retroposition, and circumduction (Table 33.3). Multiple ligaments may be implicated in the progressive instability, including the dorsal deltoid ligament complex of the thumb, anterior and posterior oblique carpometacarpal ligaments, lateral ligament, and fibrous capsule. Blood supply comes from the first dorsal metacarpal branch of the radial artery. The joint is innervated by a combination of the lateral antebrachial cutaneous nerve, palmar cutaneous branch of the median nerve, and the superficial radial nerve.

33.2.4 Clinical Presentation

History typically involves the insidious onset of progressive pain at the base of the thumb. The first CMC osteoarthritis can greatly impact an individual's ability to participate in

Table 33.3 Movement of the thumb and corresponding muscle activation

Flexion	Opponens pollicis, flexor pollicis brevis, flexor pollicis longus
Extension	Abductor pollicis longus, extensor pollicis longus, extensor pollicis brevis
Abduction	Abductor pollicis longus, abductor pollicis brevis
Adduction	Adductor pollicis, extensor pollicis longus
Opposition	Simultaneous activation of muscles of abduction, flexion, and pronation
Retroposition	Extensor pollicis longus
Circumduction	Sequential extension, abduction, flexion, and abduction

Opposition is a motion in which thumb pulp contacting the fifth digit pulp. Retroposition is elevation of pulp of the thumb into extension and ulnar adduction

daily activities, and activity may worsen symptoms, including turning of door knobs, pinching and gripping maneuvers, and wringing out washcloths. As noted above (Table 33.2), a variety of pathology can present similarly so the special tests noted below can help narrow the differential.

33.2.5 Physical Examination

Grip strength should be tested to assess for weakness or recreation of symptoms. The provider should assess for tenderness over the first CMC joint as well as range of motion.

33.2.5.1 Special Test

1. Axial grind test assesses the integrity of the thumb CMC joint and a positive test is indicative of arthrosis and/or synovitis. The test is performed by gripping the thumb metacarpal, applying axial force and rotating in a circle. Reproduction of pain and crepitus is a positive test. The sensitivity and specificity are estimated to be 30% and 97%, respectively [11].
2. Traction-shift test: In this test, the metacarpal is passively subluxed and relocated. Reproduction of pain is considered a positive test. Sensitivity and specificity have been estimated at 67% and 100%, respectively [11].

33.2.6 Diagnostic Workup

33.2.6.1 X-Rays

Imaging typically includes posteroanterior, lateral, and oblique views. These may be supplemented with a basal joint stress view, which is obtained in the posterior–anterior (PA) projection with the patient firmly pressing the thumbs together, and provides an increased visualization of the basal joint articulations, and allows assessment of trapeziometacarpal joint subluxation, which may not be apparent on routine radiographs [12]. These images can then be applied to the Eaton–Littler classification system for staging (Table 33.4).

Table 33.4 Eaton–Littler classification of thumb carpometacarpal (CMC) osteoarthritis [4]

Stage I	Subtle carpometacarpal (CMC) joint space widening
Stage II	Slight (CMC) joint space narrowing, sclerosis, cystic changes with osteophytes or loose bodies <2 mm
Stage III	Advanced CMC joint space narrowing, sclerosis, and cystic changes with osteophytes or loose bodies >2 mm
Stage IV	Stage III changes + scaphotrapezial OA

- *The Robert view*, with thumb positioned with the dorsal side of the hand flat on the plate with pronation of the wrist, allows visualization of all four trapezial articulations
- *The Lewis modification* is similar to the Robert view but angles 15^0 proximally and is preferred by some.

33.2.6.2 Ultrasound

It can be used to evaluate thickness and integrity of ligaments, including the anterior oblique ligament, joint effusions, synovitis, and osteophytes.

33.2.6.3 MRI and MR Arthrography

They both can be used to provide an in-depth ligamentous information to delineate between superficial and deep AOL and 3D reconstruction for operative planning.

33.2.6.4 CT Scan

It also can be used in perioperative planning in addition to plain films due to a higher inter-observer reliability and OA detection [12].

33.2.7 Treatment

33.2.7.1 Medical Management

Conservative management in mild to moderate cases typically includes activity modification, oral and topical nonsteroidal anti-inflammatory (NSAID) and analgesic medications, orthoses, and strengthening and flexibility exercises. At least one randomized controlled trial (RCT) trial showed oral analgesics supplemented with a topical NSAID showed an improvement in pain of 40% in hand osteoarthritis, though it does not alter the natural history [12]. Renal function should be monitored when prolonged NSAID use is considered.

33.2.7.2 Rehabilitation

Occupational and physical therapy may include splinting, therapeutic exercises, and education. Education includes joint protection strategies, activity modifications, and the use of adaptive equipment to increase independence with daily activities. Thermal modalities such as paraffin and hot packs are commonly used for pain management and have been shown to decrease pain in some cases; however, they are not strongly supported by evidence [13, 14].

33.2.7.3 Procedures

Corticosteroid injection (CSI), with or without local anesthetic, has shown short-term benefit [11, 15]. Hyaluronic acid and platelet-rich plasma (PRP) injections have also been studied for the first CMC osteoarthritis. A systematic review suggested that hyaluronic acid and CSI both provided pain relief with hyaluronic acid shown to be more effective and longer lasting [11].

A RCT published in 2021 comparing intra-articular PRP to CSI found that in mild to moderate disease, PRP was effective and yielded significantly better results in VAS pain scores, functional scores using Q-DASH, and patient satisfaction when compared to CSI [15].

33.2.7.4 Surgery

Failing other treatment modalities, a number of surgical approaches exist. These include extension osteotomy, CMC arthroscopy and debridement, trapeziectomy with or without ligament reconstruction, trapeziectomy with tightrope suspension, CMC arthrodesis, and implant arthroplasty. Surgical treatment of the wrist and hand is discussed in Chap. 37.

33.3 Intersection Syndromes

33.3.1 Synonyms

- Oarsmen's wrist
- Crossover syndrome
- Squeaker's wrist
- Abductor pollicis longus bursitis
- Abductor pollicis longus syndrome
- Subcutaneous polymyositis
- Peritendinitis crepitans

33.3.2 ICD 10 Code

- M65.841, other synovitis and tenosynovitis, right hand
- M65.842, other synovitis and tenosynovitis, left hand
- M65.849, other synovitis and tenosynovitis, unspecified hand

33.3.3 Description

Intersection syndrome is a painful condition of the forearm that has been described in two locations. Proximal intersection syndrome is a tenosynovitis involving the first and second dorsal compartments of the wrist extensors about 4–6 cm proximal to Lister's tubercle. Distal intersection syndrome is a tenosynovitis involving the second and third extensor compartments.

Anatomy The dorsal wrist extensor tendons are split into six compartments, and each is occupied by one or two extensor tendons (Table 33.5).

Etiology In the forearm, the extensor tendons cross over each other predisposing them to friction-type forces, and similar to other tendinopathies, overuse can predispose to inflammation and pain. The risk factors are similar to those of other tendinopathies of the hand and wrist and include activities such as rowing, weightlifting, cycling, skiing, and repetitive flexion/extension activities. Incidence and prevalence among males and females are equal. The overall incidence of proximal intersection syndrome is 0.2–0.37% [16]. Distal intersection syndrome is rare compared to the more common proximal intersection syndrome [17].

Pathophysiology Repetitive flexion and compressive forces can irritate and damage the tendon sheath leading to inflammation, tenosynovitis, swelling, pain, and decreased functional ability.

- *Proximal intersection syndrome* is defined anatomically as where the abductor pollicis longus (APL) and extensor pollicis brevis (EPB) cross over the extensor carpi radialis brevis (ECRB) and extensor carpi radialis longus (ECRL). This point of intersection between the first and second extensor compartment typically occurs 4–6 cm proximal to the radial styloid, just proximal to the extensor retinaculum and Lister's tubercle.
- *Distal intersection syndrome* is defined anatomically as where the extensor pollicis longus (EPL) tendon crosses over the extensor carpi radialis tendons (ECRB and

Table 33.5 Dorsal wrist extensor compartments and its tendons (radial to ulnar)

Compartment 1 (most radial)	Abductor pollicis brevis Extensor pollicis brevis
Compartment 2	Extensor carpi radialis brevis (ECRB) Extensor carpi radialis longus (ECRL)
Compartment 3	Extensor pollicis longus
Compartment 4	Extensor indices Extensor digitorum communis
Compartment 5	Extensor digiti minimi
Compartment 6	Extensor carpi ulnaris

ECRL), and pathology occurs at the intersection of the second and third extensor compartment. Lister's tubercle acts as a pully for the EPL, mechanically predisposing the tendon to injury due to the mechanical disadvantage placed on the tendon. Progression to EPL tendon rupture has been reported [17].

33.3.4 Clinical Presentation

History typically includes focal dull aching pain in the dorsoradial distal forearm over the area of intersection. Patients are likely to deny any known history of trauma or falls. The pain may be exacerbated by wrist extension or ulnar deviation. History, exam, and imaging can all be used to help narrow the differential (Table 33.6).

33.3.5 Physical Examination

Examination usually reveals tenderness to palpation at the sites of intersection. Localized swelling and crepitus may be felt with passive ranging and palpation. Pain and crepitus can also be elicited with resisted wrist and thumb extension. Resisted pronation can recreate the symptoms and is specific to intersection syndrome. This test can help differentiate the condition from de Quervain's tenosynovitis [16, 18]. Tenderness in de Quervain's tenosynovitis is near the radial styloid, whereas tenderness in intersection syndrome is found 4–6 cm proximal to the radial styloid and Lister's tubercle.

33.3.6 Diagnostic Workup

Clinical exams are usually sufficient, but imaging, in particular the US, may assist with accurate diagnosis.

Radiographs Plain films have minimal utility in diagnosing intersection syndrome but can be used to rule out other pathology.

Ultrasound US is the imaging of choice for intersection syndrome. The structures are superficial and easily imaged with a linear probe. Images consistent with the syndrome may show areas of hypoechoic inflammatory fluid between the two compartments. The US may also visualize tendon thickening or damage. US can also be used in interventional treatment [16].

Table 33.6 Differential diagnosis of intersection syndrome

De Quervain's tenosynovitis	Ganglion cyst
Myofascial pain or muscle strain	Osteoarthritis of the wrist first CMC joint
Metacarpophalangeal ligament tear	Radial nerve entrapment (Wartenberg's syndrome)
Scaphoid fracture	Cervical radiculopathy

MRI MRI can provide high fidelity images of the soft tissues and compartments but is usually not necessary as the US is more accessible, faster, and more cost-effective. In distal intersection syndrome, the anatomy of the EPL is difficult to examine with MRI as the tendon is flat and the tendon's course results in false positives [17].

33.3.7 Treatment

33.3.7.1 Medical Management

Initial management is conservative, including activity modification, oral and topical nonsteroidal anti-inflammatory medications, cryotherapy, and short-term splinting.

33.3.7.2 Rehabilitation

After an initial rest phase, therapy consists of progressive stretching exercises and joint mobilization techniques. Progressive strength training should be initiated carefully to avoid relapse of symptoms and gradual return to daily activities.

33.3.7.3 Procedures

Corticosteroid injection, PRP, or prolotherapy may be effective options if conservative management has failed, although high-quality data is still lacking.

33.3.7.4 Surgery

In recalcitrant cases, surgical decompression has been reported. Return to full activities is suggested to be about 4–6 weeks [1]. Surgical treatment of the wrist and hand is discussed in Chap. 37.

33.4 Scapholunate Ligament Injury

33.4.1 ICD 10 Code

S63, dislocation and sprain of joints and ligaments at wrist and hand level

33.4.2 Description

Scapholunate ligament (SLL) injury is a source of dorsoradial wrist pain, and chronic injuries are the most common cause of carpal instability [19].

Etiology Most scapholunate ligament injuries are traumatic due to sudden force on the wrist with an extended and ulnarly deviated wrist [20]. In one study, 13.4% of distal radius fractures were associated with scapholunate ligament dissociation [21]. The position a hand assumes when holding a steering wheel has also been described as a mechanism of injury to the ligament [20]. Individuals with chronic inflammatory conditions such as gout can have gradual breakdown of the scapholunate ligament as well as other carpal ligaments [22].

Pathophysiology The stability of the wrist is dependent on the anatomy and biomechanics of the wrist with the SLL playing a critical role in carpal stability. Disruption of the ligament results in altered carpal alignment and biomechanics. Axial loads through the distal carpal row are evenly distributed, while 50% of the load through the proximal role is transmitted through the radioscaphoid joint and 35% across the radiolunate joint [20]. The SLL is between these load-sustaining bones and predisposes the ligament to injury. There are four stages of injury based on imaging classification (Table 33.8), which range from stage I (occult), stage II (dynamic), stage III (SLL dissociation), and stage IV (dorsal intercalated segment instability [DISI]). Patients with stage I injuries may not initially seek out evaluation and only complain of symptoms during certain activities involving mechanical loading. This stage has been termed pre-dynamic instability because of the implied progression for some but not all [19]. Higher-energy impacts are likely to lead to higher-grade injuries. Once the SLL is incompetent, there are altered kinematics and progressive deterioration of other ligaments and abnormal pressure on the cartilage of the wrist. This can lead to a pattern of wrist arthritis, namely, scapholunate advanced collapse (SLAC).

Anatomy The carpal bones are generally organized into two rows. The proximal row from radial to ulnar is made up of scaphoid, lunate, triquetrum, and pisiform. The distal row from radial to ulnar includes trapezium, trapezoid, capitate, and hamate. There is no direct tendinous insertion to the scaphoid, lunate, or triquetrum, and their movement is dependent on mechanical forces of the surrounding tissues.

The scaphoid and lunate are bound by the SLL, which is composed of three histologically distinct regions [19]. The scapholunate interosseous ligament (SLIL) is the primary stabilizer of this joint, and this joint is the most frequently injured of the ligaments [19]. The SLIL attaches on the dorsal, proximal, and volar margins with the dorsal being the thickest and strongest [19]. The dorsal component resists distraction, torsion and translation. The palmar component contributes to rotational stability. Disruption of the SLIL can lead to progressive wear of the secondary stabilizers (scapho-capitate, scapho-trapezio-trapezoid, radio-scapho-capitate, and dorsal intercarpal ligaments) leading to further disruption and instability.

33.4.3 Clinical Presentation

Patients may describe a fall onto an outstretched hand followed by progressive pain, decreased ability to bear weight with the wrist, and/or a feeling of instability. In the acute phase, there may be swelling and acute tenderness with pain potentially limiting provocative testing. In the subacute phase, patients may complain of continued pain, painful clunking or clicking sensation in the wrist, decreased grip strength, and localized pain over the dorsoradial wrist. Differential diagnosis of scapholunate ligament injury is presented in Table 33.7.

33.4.4 Physical Examination

Palpation of anatomic landmarks may elicit tenderness. The range of motion of the wrist and grip strength should be compared to the contralateral wrist.

Scaphoid shift test The examiner's thumb applies pressure to the scaphoid tubercle, while the subject's hand is moved from ulnar deviation and slight extension to radial deviation and slight flexion. Pain should be recreated in a positive test, and if instability is present, there may be an audible or palpable click as pressure is released and the scaphoid is allowed to spontaneously reduce. False positives occur in up to one-third of patients due to ligament hyperlaxity allowing for capito-lunate translation with similar findings [19].

33.4.5 Diagnostic Workup

X-rays Radiographs can help determine if there is malalignment of the carpal bones. Four views should be obtained: posteroanterior (PA), lateral, scaphoid projection, and oblique view. Clenched fist views will load the carpal bones and widen the diastasis in cases of dynamic instability (Table 33.8).

Table 33.7 Differential diagnosis of scapholunate ligament injury

Pseudogout	Scaphoid nonunion advanced collapse
Scaphotrapezial trapezoidal arthritis	Idiopathic osteonecrosis (Keinbock's disease)
Infection	

Table 33.8 Stages of scapholunate instability

	I. Occult	II. Dynamic	III. SL dissociation	IV. DISI
Ligament(s)	Partial SLIL	Incomplete or complete SLIL; partial volar extrinsics	Complete SLIL; dorsal or volar extrinsics	Complete SLIL, volar extrinsics, changes in RL, ST and DIC ligaments
Static XR	Normal	Usually normal	SL gap ≥3 mm; RS angle ≥60⁰	SL angle ≥70°, SL gap ≥3 mm; RL angle ≥15°, CL angle ≥15°
Stress XR	Normal–abnormal fluoroscopy	Abnormal	Grossly abnormal	Unnecessary
Treatment	Pinning or capsulodesis	SLIL repair with capsulodesis	SLIL repair with capsulodesis vs triligament reconstruction	Reducible: triligament reconstruction Fixed: intercarpal arthrodesis

Adapted from reference [19]

CT arthrography Has improved upon traditional arthroscopy and has been noted to be as sensitive as 85% and specific as 86% in detecting SLIL tears, although still rarely performed today [19].

MRI MRI depends on the strength of the magnet with some studies reporting as high as 89% sensitivity and 100% specificity with a 3-T magnet [19]. This is notably dependent on the radiologist and clinical provider. Results are improved with new wrist specific protocols and more powerful magnets [19, 23].

33.4.6 Treatment

33.4.6.1 Medical Management

Nonsurgical management involves symptomatic treatment including activity modification, splinting, NSAIDs, and intra-articular corticosteroid injection (CSI). As in other wrist pathology, surgery is indicated in more severe cases or those poorly controlled with conservative management [24].

33.4.6.2 Rehabilitation

Rehabilitation of a scapho-lunate ligament injury will vary depending on the severity of the injury. For mild injuries, the first step is typically to immobilize the wrist in a neutral position with a splint and allow the ligament to heal. After the immobilization period, the patient can begin progressive stretching and strengthening exercises under the supervision of an occupational or physical therapist. In addition, wrist stabilization exercises focused on the surrounding musculature are key to regaining carpal stability.

In more severe injuries, surgical intervention may be required to repair the ligament. Postoperative rehabilitation will begin with splinting, edema management, scar mobilization, and active range of motion (AROM) of uninvolved joints to preserve joint mobility. In the next phase, the patient can begin AROM of the wrist in certain planes under the guidance of an occupational therapist (OT) or physical therapist (PT). Modalities such as moist heat and ultrasound are often used during this phase but are not strongly supported by evidence. Finally, the patient can initiate weight bearing of the surgical hand and begin progressive strengthening exercises with the supervision of a therapist. Emerging research is exploring the role of dart thrower's motion (DTM) and proprioception activities in the rehabilitation of these particular injuries [25].

33.4.6.3 Procedures

Wrist arthroscopy can be used in the acute phase for diagnosis and treatment decision-making by visualizing the involved ligaments.

33.4.6.4 Surgery

Early surgical intervention is considered the mainstay of treatment and should be repaired within 4–6 weeks as failure to intervene early can lead to deterioration of function, instability, pain, loss of grip strength, and articular damage [26], although stage 1 occult injuries may be amenable to conservative management [19]. Acute or partial tears may involve arthroscopic debridement with or without capsulodesis. Complete tears can be repaired via direct repair of the SLL and dorsal radioscaphoid capsulodesis. Chronic or severe tears may require reconstruction of which there are numerous options available [27]. Surgical treatment of the wrist and hand is discussed in Chap. 37.

33.5 Thumb Sprain

33.5.1 Synonyms

- Skier's thumb
- Gamekeeper's thumb

33.5.2 ICD 10 Code

- S63.642A, sprain of metacarpophalangeal joint of left thumb, initial encounter
- S63.621A, sprain of interphalangeal joint of right thumb, initial encounter

Table 33.9 Differential diagnosis of thumb sprain

De Quervain's tenosynovitis	MCP dislocation
Distal metacarpal fracture	Proximal phalanx fracture

33.5.3 Description

Injury to the ulnar collateral ligament (UCL) of the thumb along the medial metacarpophalangeal (MCP) joint can result in disruption of the UCL complex with or without an avulsion fracture. This is often called gamekeeper's thumb in chronic valgus strain injuries and skier's thumb for the acute counterpart prevalent among skiers where poles can cause a forced radial deviation of the thumb [28]. Differential diagnosis of thumb sprain is presented in Table 33.9.

Etiology Disruption of the UCL of the thumb MCP joint was first reported as laxity in Scottish gamekeepers due to chronic repetitive valgus strain. The same injury can also occur acutely. The most frequent mechanism of injury involves skiers falling on an outstretched hand holding a ski pole [28] and is the second most common skiing injury [29], accounting for up to one-third of all skiing injuries of the upper extremity [28]. It can also occur in sports where there are falls on the outstretched hand or those with direct ball impact on the thumb, as seen in volleyball and handball.

Pathophysiology Acute injury to the UCL is typically caused by forceful radial deviation of the thumb or a twisting injury to the thumb, causing a range of injuries from simple sprains to complete rupture of the ulnar ligamento-capsular complex and/or avulsion fracture of the ulnar-volar base of the proximal phalanx [28]. Even if the UCL is not completely torn, the aponeurosis can become interposed between a distally damaged UCL and metacarpal head causing disrupted healing, known as a Stener lesion [28].

Anatomy The thumb MCP joint is a hinge joint, which moves mainly in flexion and extension and to a lesser-degree adduction, abduction, and rotation [30]. The joint involves a proximal convex surface and distal concave surface. The soft-tissue structures that provide static restraint of the CP joint include the dorsal capsule, volar plate, radial collateral ligament (RCL), and UCL [30]. The collateral ligaments resist varus–valgus stress in varying degrees of flexion [30].

33.5.4 Clinical Presentation

Patients typically present with a history of trauma and complain of pain in the MCP area, which is worsened by thumb extension or abduction. Swelling and hematoma may be present in the acute phase. In the subacute and acute phase, patients may report instability, [31] weakness, and difficulty holding large objects [28]. As with other pathology, history and physical exams are important in narrowing the differential (Table 33.9).

33.5.5 Physical Examination

A high degree of suspicion based on the history of the injury and localization of pain should lead to a detailed examination of the thumb, including observation for any anatomic abnormalities, swelling, and ecchymosis. Palpation may reveal localized tenderness to the MCP joint and UCL [28]. A Stener lesion (Fig. 33.5) may have a palpable and tender mass proximal to the adductor aponeurosis [28]. Valgus stress testing with the MCP joint in both neutral and flexed (about 45 degrees) can reveal laxity and pain. When tested in the flexed position, the UCL is isolated from other stabilizers [31]. This should be compared to the uninjured side, and a relative increase of 15–20^0 in laxity may indicate a UCL rupture [31]. Pinch strength may also be decreased. Median and radial nerve block with local anesthesia can be used to augment the exam if stress testing cannot be assessed due to pain [28, 31].

33.5.6 Diagnostic Workup

X-rays Standard posteroanterior, lateral, and oblique radiographs are used to identify bony lesions and avulsion fracture of the metacarpal or proximal phalanx. Stress films can also be obtained to determine the degree of UCL laxity.

Ultrasound (US) US is cost-effective and lends itself to dynamic evaluations where the MCP joint can undergo a valgus stress to further elucidate any defect. Sensitivity and specificity of ultrasound in detecting injuries of the UCL varied from 76% to 100% and 81% to 100%, respectively, across the literature [32].

MRI MRI is more accurate and is the standard test in detecting UCL injuries of the thumb with sensitivity and specificity of 96–100% and 100%, respectively [32].

33.5.7 Treatment

33.5.7.1 Medical Management

Conservative treatments are based on symptomatic management and early immobilization of the thumb MCP joint. The interphalangeal joint is not immobilized and ROM is encouraged. Many patients with partial injuries, or even tears with

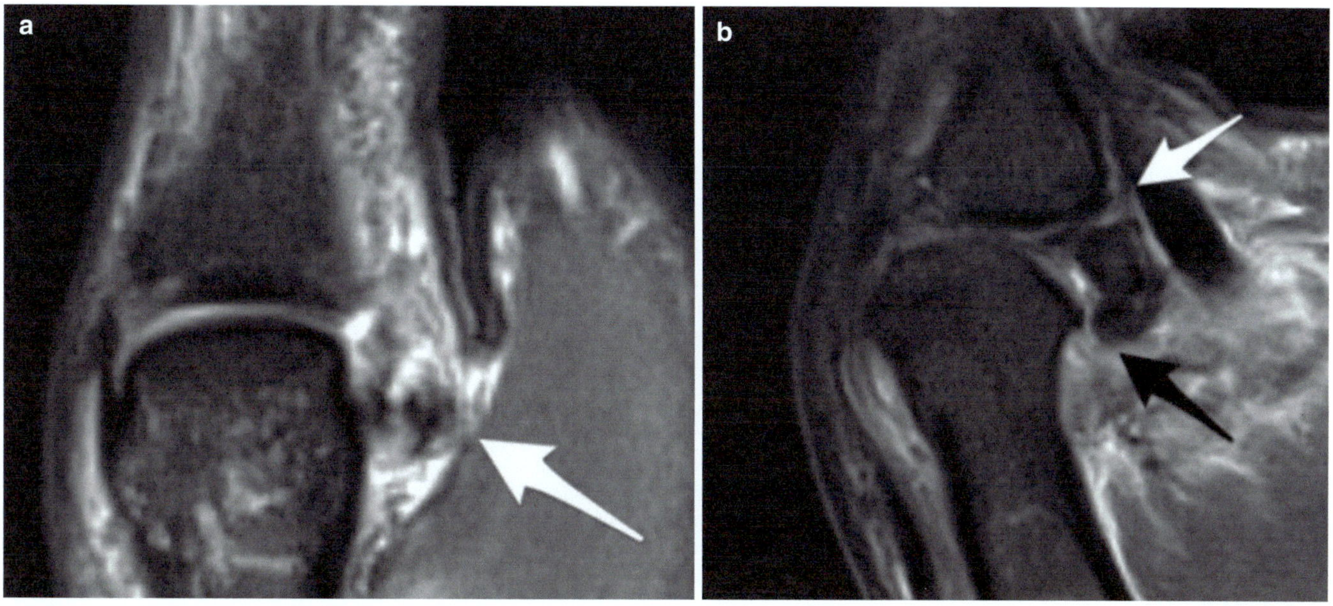

Fig. 33.5 Coronal intermediate-weighted fat-saturated image (**a**) demonstrates a Stener lesion (white arrow). The dislocated distal stump is retracted proximally and wrapped around the adductor pollicis aponeurosis (yo-yo on a string appearance). Sagittal intermediate-weighted fat-saturated image (**b**) demonstrates a concomitant complete disruption of the volar ligaments, the checkrein (black arrow), and phalangoglenoidal ligaments (white arrow)

avulsion injuries, do well with splinting. Some studies suggest that up to 85% heal without residual instability, pain, or stiffness [31]. They can eventually move into a supervised therapy program 3–4 weeks after the injury [28].

33.5.7.2 Rehabilitation

Following a period of immobilization, rehabilitation includes progressive ROM exercises and a transition to strengthening exercises. Following surgical repair, the patient may require a rehabilitation program to regain full function of the hand. Postoperative therapy will begin with splinting, wound management, and edema management. After a period of immobilization, patients can begin ROM exercises and progression to grip and pinch strengthening exercises as appropriate, with a gradual return to daily activities.

33.5.7.3 Procedure

PRP or prolotherapy may be an effective next treatment option if conservative options have failed, but clinical trials are lacking to this point.

33.5.7.4 Surgery

Surgical referral is indicated in patients with radiographs showing a bony avulsion fragment >2 mm displaced or fracture involving >10–20% of the articular surface. Surgery is also indicated if there is evidence of a complete UCL tear [31] or if a Stener lesion is present (Fig. 33.5) [31]. Surgical treatment of the wrist and hand is discussed in Chap. 37.

References

1. Patrick NC, Hammert WC. Hand and wrist tendinopathies. Clin Sports Med. 2020;39(2):247–58.
2. Diop AN, Ba-Diop S, Sane JC, Tomolet Alfidja A, Sy MH, Boyer L, et al. Role of US in the management of de Quervain’s tenosynovitis: review of 22 cases. J Radiol. 2008;89(9 Pt 1):1081–4.
3. Glajchen N, Schweitzer M. MRI features in de Quervain's tenosynovitis of the wrist. Skelet Radiol. 1996;25(1):63–5.
4. Goel R, Abzug JM. de Quervain’s tenosynovitis: a review of the rehabilitative options. Hand (N Y). 2015;10(1):1–5.
5. Jaworski CA, Krause M, Brown J. Rehabilitation of the wrist and hand following sports injury. Clin Sports Med. 2010;29(1):61–80, table of contents.
6. Lapegue F, Andre A, Pasquier Bernachot E, Akakpo EJ, Laumonerie P, Chiavassa-Gandois H, et al. US-guided percutaneous release of the first extensor tendon compartment using a 21-gauge needle in de Quervain's disease: a prospective study of 35 cases. Eur Radiol. 2018;28(9):3977–85.
7. Peck E, Ely E. Successful treatment of De Quervain’s tenosynovitis with ultrasound-guided percutaneous needle tenotomy and platelet-rich plasma injection: a case presentation. PM R. 2013;5(5):438–41.
8. Chen H, Yuan A. Prolotherapy treatment for Dequervain's tenosynovitis and intersection syndrome. J Pain. 2015;16(4):S113.
9. van der Oest MJW, Duraku LS, Andrinopoulou ER, Wouters RM, Bierma-Zeinstra SMA, Selles RW, et al. The prevalence of radiographic thumb base osteoarthritis: a meta-analysis. Osteoarthr Cartil. 2021;29(6):785–92.
10. Hunter DJ, Zhang Y, Sokolove J, Niu J, Aliabadi P, Felson DT. Trapeziometacarpal subluxation predisposes to incident trapeziometacarpal osteoarthritis (OA): the Framingham Study. Osteoarthr Cartil. 2005;13(11):953–7.
11. Pickrell BB, Eberlin KR. Thumb basal joint arthritis. Clin Plast Surg. 2019;46(3):407–13.

12. Melville DM, Taljanovic MS, Scalcione LR, Eble JM, Gimber LH, DeSilva GL, et al. Imaging and management of thumb carpometacarpal joint osteoarthritis. Skelet Radiol. 2015;44(2):165–77.
13. Beasley J. Osteoarthritis and rheumatoid arthritis: conservative therapeutic management. J Hand Ther. 2012;25(2):163–71; quiz 72.
14. Neumann DA, Bielefeld T. The carpometacarpal joint of the thumb: stability, deformity, and therapeutic intervention. J Orthop Sports Phys Ther. 2003;33(7):386–99.
15. Malahias MA, Roumeliotis L, Nikolaou VS, Chronopoulos E, Sourlas I, Babis GC. Platelet-rich plasma versus corticosteroid intra-articular injections for the treatment of trapeziometacarpal arthritis: a prospective randomized controlled clinical trial. Cartilage. 2021;12(1):51–61.
16. Balakatounis K, Angoules AG, Angoules NA, Panagiotopoulou K. Synthesis of evidence for the treatment of intersection syndrome. World J Orthop. 2017;8(8):619–23.
17. Mattox R, Battaglia PJ, Scali F, Ottolini K, Kettner NW. Distal intersection syndrome progressing to extensor pollicis longus tendon rupture: a case report with sonographic findings. J Ultrasound. 2017;20(3):237–41.
18. Michols NJ, Kiel J. Intersection syndrome. Treasure Island: StatPearls; 2021.
19. Kitay A, Wolfe SW. Scapholunate instability: current concepts in diagnosis and management. J Hand Surg Am. 2012;37(10):2175–96.
20. Konopka G, Chim H. Optimal management of scapholunate ligament injuries. Orthop Res Rev. 2018;10:41–54.
21. Gunal I, Ozaksoy D, Altay T, Satoglu IS, Kazimoglu C, Sener M. Scapholunate dissociation associated with distal radius fractures. Eur J Orthop Surg Traumatol. 2013;23(8):877–81.
22. Beck JD, Deegan JH, Riehl JT, Klena JC. Incidence of scapholunate ligament dissociation in patients with aspiration-confirmed gout. J Hand Surg Am. 2010;35(12):1938–42.
23. Shahabpour M, Staelens B, Van Overstraeten L, De Maeseneer M, Boulet C, De Mey J, et al. Advanced imaging of the scapholunate ligamentous complex. Skelet Radiol. 2015;44(12):1709–25.
24. Wahed K, Deore S, Bhan K, Vinay S, Jayasinghe G, Dutta A, et al. Management of chronic scapholunate ligament injury. J Clin Orthop Trauma. 2020;11(4):529–36.
25. Wolff AL, Wolfe SW. Rehabilitation for scapholunate injury: application of scientific and clinical evidence to practice. J Hand Ther. 2016;29(2):146–53.
26. Andersson JK. Treatment of scapholunate ligament injury: current concepts. EFORT Open Rev. 2017;2(9):382–93.
27. Pulos N, Kakar S. Hand and wrist injuries: common problems and solutions. Clin Sports Med. 2018;37(2):217–43.
28. Fricker R, Hintermann B. Skier's thumb. Treatment, prevention and recommendations. Sports Med. 1995;19(1):73–9.
29. Tsiouri C, Hayton MJ, Baratz M. Injury to the ulnar collateral ligament of the thumb. Hand (N Y). 2009;4(1):12–8.
30. Earp B, Cefalu C, Blazar P. Thumb metacarpophalangeal joint arthritis. J Am Acad Orthop Surg. 2019;27(23):e1029–e39.
31. Gammons M. Ulnar collateral ligament injury (gamekeeper's or skier's thumb). In: Grayzel J, editor. UpToDate. Waltham. (Accessed 9 June 2021): UpToDate; 2021.
32. Shekarchi B, Mokhdanzadeh Dashti M, Shahrezaei M, Karimi E. The accuracy of ultrasonography in detection of ulnar collateral ligament of thumb injuries; a cross-sectional study. Emerg (Tehran). 2018;6(1):e15.

34 Ulnar-Sided Wrist Disorders

Eileen M. Colliton, Ashleigh Gibula, Cara Rodriguez, Nadia Zaman, and Charles Cassidy

34.1 Triangular Fibrocartilage Complex Injuries

34.1.1 Synonyms

None

34.1.2 ICD-10 Codes

- M24.131
- M24.132

34.1.3 Description

The triangular fibrocartilage complex (TFCC) is a ligamentous complex that is one of the main stabilizers on the ulnar side of the wrist. Located between the carpus and the ulna, it not only serves as a load-bearing structure but also stabilizes the distal radioulnar joint (DRUJ). It is composed of the triangular fibrocartilage disc proper (or central articular disc), dorsal and volar distal radioulnar ligaments, meniscal homolog, ulnocarpal collateral ligament, ulnotriquetral ligament, ulnolunate ligament, and extensor carpi ulnaris (ECU) tendon subsheath [1] (Fig. 34.1). When a wrist has neutral ulnar variance, the TFCC transmits and absorbs approximately 20% of the forces that cross the wrist [1, 2]. Blood supply to the TFCC comes from the terminal branches of the anterior and posterior interosseous arteries. While the peripheral 10–30% of the TFCC has adequate blood supply for healing, the central and radial aspects are more poorly vascularized [3]. The Palmer classification is widely recognized as one of the best classifications for TFCC injuries [4] (Table 34.2). The differential diagnosis of TFCC injury is broad (Table 34.1).

34.1.4 Clinical Presentation

Injuries to the TFCC can result from both a traumatic incident and degenerative changes over time. Patients will usually present with ulnar-sided wrist pain with or without DRUJ instability that is aggravated by repetitive axial loading, activities that require pronosupination, or ulnar deviation [2]. Patients may report a clicking or clunking with forearm pronosupination, which may signify DRUJ instability [3]. Because ulnar-sided wrist pain can result from a wide assortment of pathologies, care must be taken in gathering a thorough history from the patient to rule out other etiologies.

34.1.5 Physical Examination

A thorough musculoskeletal and neurologic physical examination is required in order to determine the best course of action. Inspection of the skin over the dorsal and volar wrist should be performed to look for any lesions, trophic changes, ecchymosis, or edema. Palpation of the bony prominences along the dorsal and ulnar wrist will assist in determining if there is suspicion for a fracture. Patients with TFCC injury will often have tenderness over the ulnar fovea, lunotriquetral interval, ECU tendon, or DRUJ [3]. The range of motion

E. M. Colliton · C. Cassidy (✉)
Department of Orthopedic & Rehabilitation Medicine, Tufts Medical Center, Boston, MA, USA
e-mail: ecolliton@tuftsmedicalcenter.org; ccassidy@tuftsmedicalcenter.org

A. Gibula
Tufts University School of Medicine, Boston, MA, USA
e-mail: Ashleigh.Gibula@tufts.edu

C. Rodriguez
Department of Occupational Therapy, Tufts Medical Center, Boston, MA, USA
e-mail: crodriguez@tuftsmedicalcenter.org

N. Zaman
Department of Orthopedics & Rehabilitation Medicine, Tufts University School of Medicine, Boston, MA, USA
e-mail: Nzaman1@tuftsmedicalcenter.org

© The Author(s), under exclusive license to Springer Nature Switzerland AG 2022
S. A. Mostoufi et al. (eds.), *Clinical Guide to Musculoskeletal Medicine*, https://doi.org/10.1007/978-3-030-92042-5_34

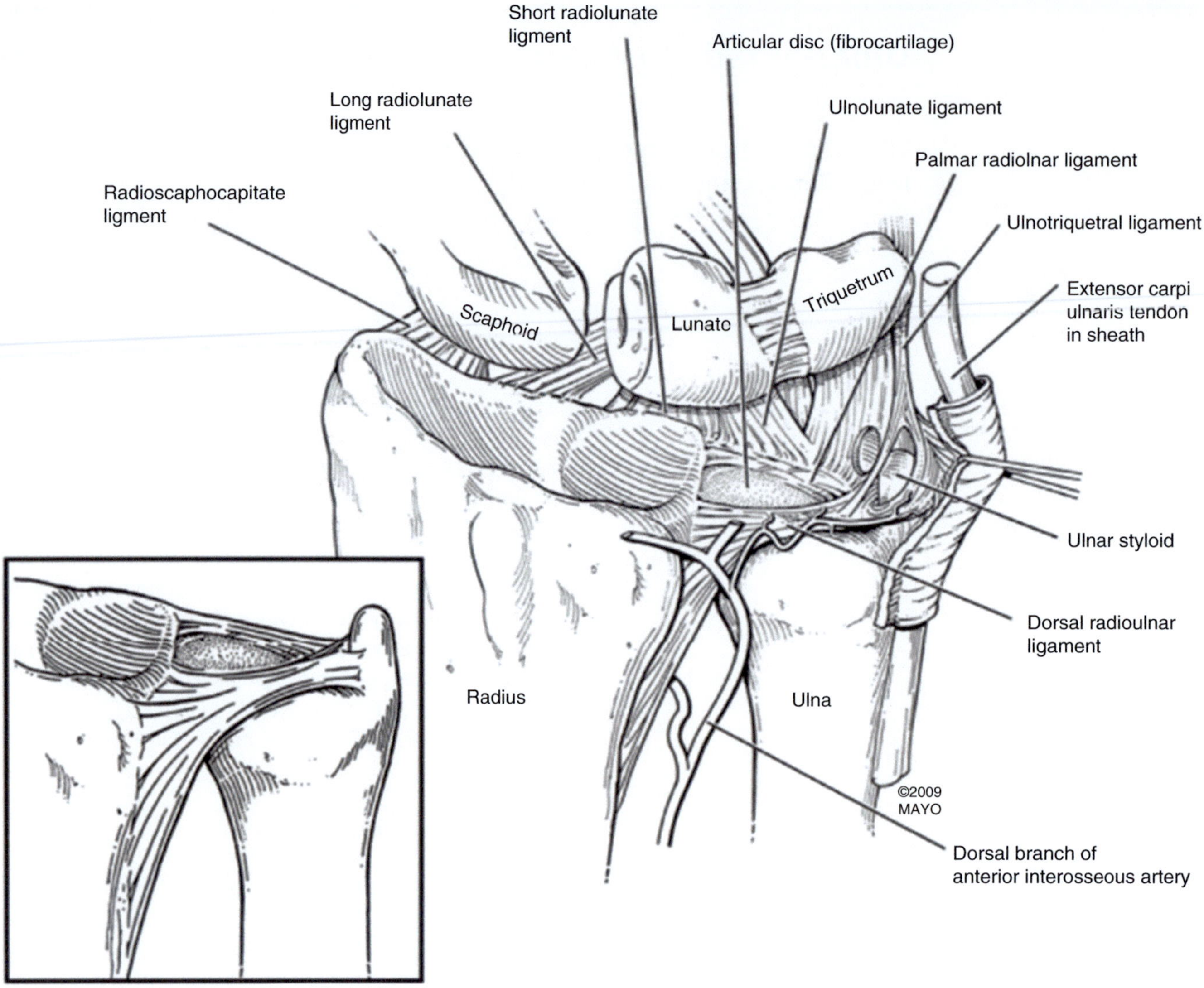

Fig. 34.1 TFCC and its relevant anatomy. (From: Kovachevich and Elhassan [41]; with permission)

Table 34.1 Differential diagnosis for TFCC tears

ECU tendinopathy
DRUJ arthritis
Triquetral fracture
Ulnar neuropathy at Guyon's canal
Lunotriquetral tear
Ulnar impaction syndrome

Table 34.2 Palmer classification of TFCC injury

Type 1 traumatic	Type 2 degenerative
A. Central perforation	**A.** TFCC wear
B. Ulnar avulsion, with or without distal ulna fracture	**B.** TFCC wear and lunate or ulnar chondromalacia
C. Distal avulsion	**C.** TFCC perforation and lunate or ulnar chondromalacia
D. Radial avulsion, with or without sigmoid notch fracture	**D.** Type 2C injury plus lunotriquetral ligament perforation
	E. Type 2D injury plus ulnocarpal arthritis

should be checked in flexion–extension, radial–ulnar deviation, and pronation–supination planes and compared bilaterally. Functional testing includes asking patients to turn a doorknob or having them push up from a chair, which leads to axial loading of the wrist in pronation [4].

Special Tests

It is important to note that these examination maneuvers are applicable in the assessment of suspected TFCC tears, ulnocarpal impaction, and ulnar collateral ligament injuries but may not be specific enough to localize the exact structure(s) involved.

- *Piano key/ballottement test*: The examiner uses one hand to stabilize the patient's wrist/hand in pronation while, with the other hand, applying dorsal-volar translation force to the ulnar head. Increased laxity (compared to the uninjured side) is suggestive of DRUJ instability [5].
- *Fovea sign*: The flexor carpi ulnaris (FCU)–ECU interval is a "window" into the region of the ulnar fovea. Tenderness in the soft space immediately volar to the ulnar styloid between the ulnar head and the pisiform (Fig. 34.2) is suggestive of a foveal TFCC lesion, with a sensitivity of 95.2% and specificity of 86.5% [2, 6].
- *Ulnocarpal stress test*: The patient's wrist is placed in maximal ulnar deviation, and an axial load is applied while passively rotating the forearm from supination to pronation [3, 7] (Fig. 34.3). Pronation makes the ulna relatively longer, impinging on the lunate and exacerbating the pain [8]. This test is sensitive for ulnar-sided wrist pain but not specific as it may be positive in ulnar impaction syndrome, ulnocarpal arthritis, and lunotriquetral ligamentous injury [9].
- Ulnar grinding test: Pain with an axial force applied to an ulnar-deviated wrist while passively directing the wrist through flexion, extension, pronation, and supination.
- Pisiform boost: Pain with dorsal elevation of the pisiform with volar-directed depression of the ulnar head. Examiner may elicit crepitus while rotating the forearm during this maneuver [7].

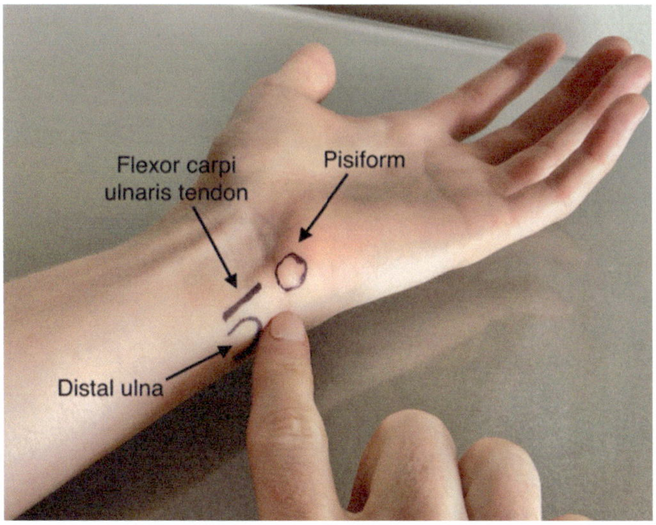

Fig. 34.2 Ulnar fovea sign, with examiner indicating site of ulnar fovea

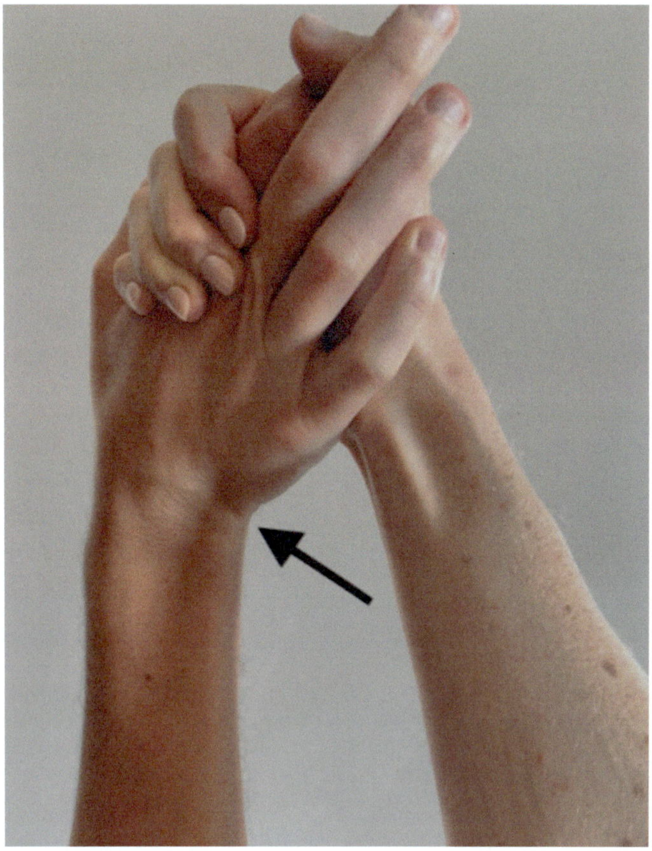

Fig. 34.3 Ulnocarpal stress test with arrow indicating site of pain

34.1.6 Diagnostic Workup

Initial workup for suspected TFCC injuries should include neutral rotation posteroanterior (PA), lateral, and oblique radiographs [2, 3]. Radiographs will also allow for the measurement of ulnar variance, as a majority of TFCC injuries are associated with positive (Fig. 34.4) or neutral ulnar variance [1]. Pronated PA grip views accentuate positive ulnar variance by making the radius relatively shorter than the fixed ulna (Fig. 34.5) [9, 11, 12]. A more advanced imaging can include computed tomographic arthrography (CTA) or

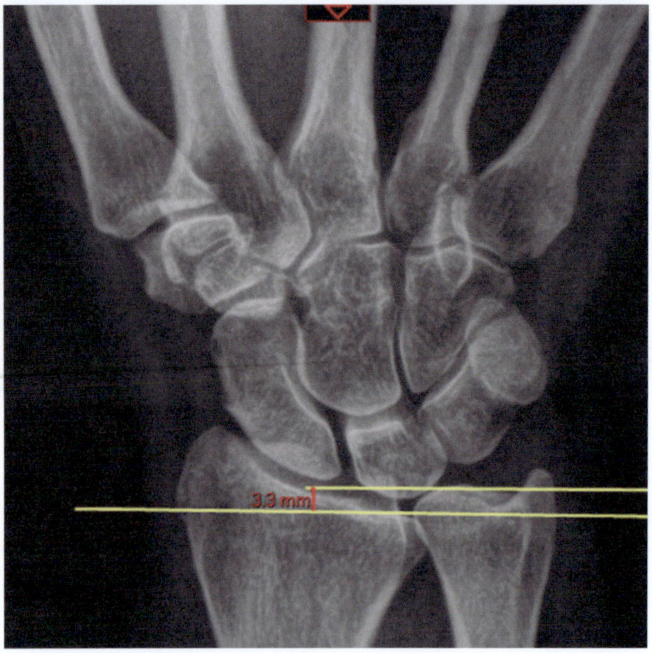

Fig. 34.4 PA wrist radiograph demonstrating a positive ulnar variance of 3.3 mm. A line is drawn tangential to the articular surface of the ulnar and perpendicular to the ulnar shaft. A second line is drawn tangential to the articular surface of the distal radius lunate facet and perpendicular to the shaft of the radius. The distance between these two lines is the ulnar variance

magnetic resonance imaging (MRI). MRI sensitivity and specificity are 67–100% and 71–100%, respectively. Magnetic resonance arthrography (MRA) has also been used and found to be superior to MRI alone in some studies, while others note that a 3.0 T MRI scanner has excellent resolution to diagnose TFCC tears, and an arthrogram is not necessary [2, 3]. CTA is an alternative modality and found to be 100% sensitive and specific for accuracy in the diagnosis of TFCC tears, especially for those who cannot undergo MRI [13].

34.1.7 Treatment

(a) *Medical Management*

If no DRUJ instability is present, the initial management of TFCC injuries is conservative. Symptom management is the focus of care, with the concepts of RICE applied. This may include bracing of the wrist for immobilization and comfort [2]. It also includes activity modifications and anti-inflammatory medications as needed in the acute phase.

(b) *Rehabilitation*

The primary goal of rehabilitation after TFCC injury is to restore the normal joint mechanics and anatomy of the DRUJ [14]. In conservative management of TFCC

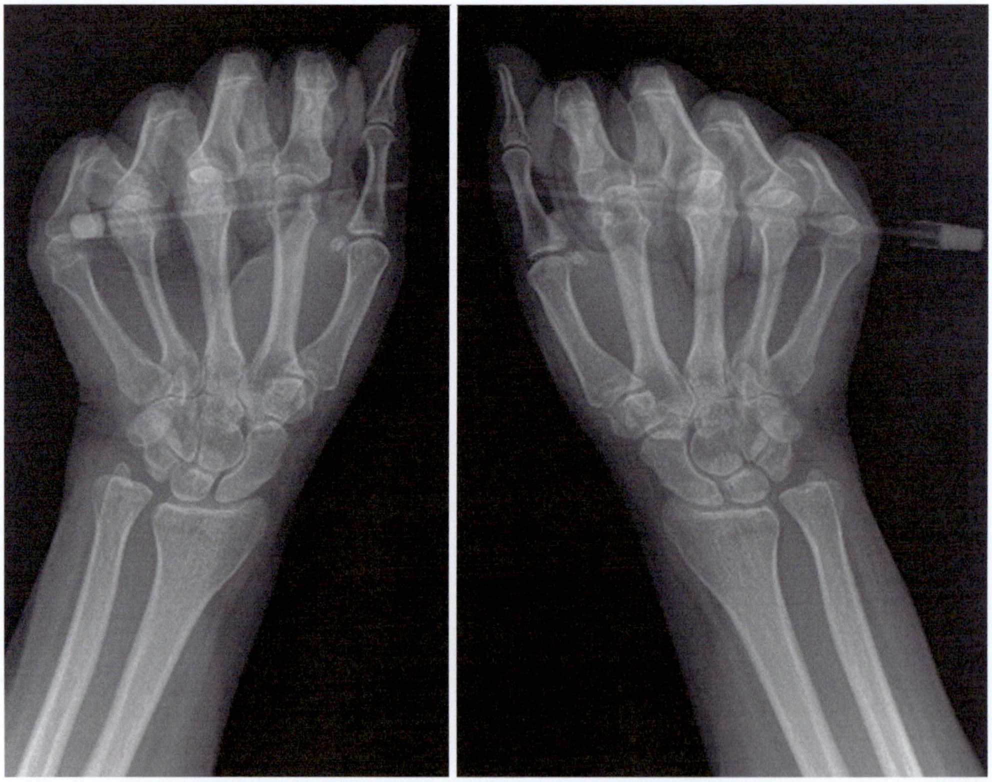

Fig. 34.5 A pronated grip PA wrist radiograph demonstrating bilateral positive ulnar variance

injuries, initial therapy will focus on techniques to decrease inflammation including rest, use of modalities, taping, and supportive splinting. Splinting needs will vary depending on the patient's pain level and the stability of the DRUJ. The use of a wrist immobilization splint, a long arm orthosis that immobilizes the wrist and forearm, and the use of a wrist strap, such as a wrist widget, are all common forms of support after this injury [14, 15] (Fig. 34.6). Patients should be instructed to avoid activities that require forearm pronation, ulnar deviation, weight-bearing, or gripping. As pain allows, therapy will incorporate active range of motion (AROM) exercises of the wrist and forearm into the therapy program. This would be followed by progressive strengthening with a focus on wrist stabilization [15] (Fig. 34.7). Postoperative therapy for TFCC injuries will vary depending on the surgery that was performed. Open or arthroscopic TFCC repairs will require a period of immobilization to the wrist and forearm to minimize tension on the repair site. Patients who have undergone TFCC debridement do not require an extensive protection and are advanced through the rehabilitation stages above as postsurgical inflammation resolves. It is important with all TFCC surgeries to respect pain during the healing process. Increases in pain, edema, and inflammation are indications that therapy is progressing too rapidly [16].

(c) *Procedures*

Management begins with bracing, activity modification, anti-inflammatory medications, and hand therapy as mentioned above. For ulnar-sided wrist pain without instability, intra-articular corticosteroid injections can be helpful. Ultrasound guidance facilitates accurate placement and minimizes pain.

(d) *Surgery*

Surgery is reserved for refractory ulnar-sided wrist pain and/or DRUJ instability. For more details on surgery for dorsal wrist disorders, refer to Chap. 50.

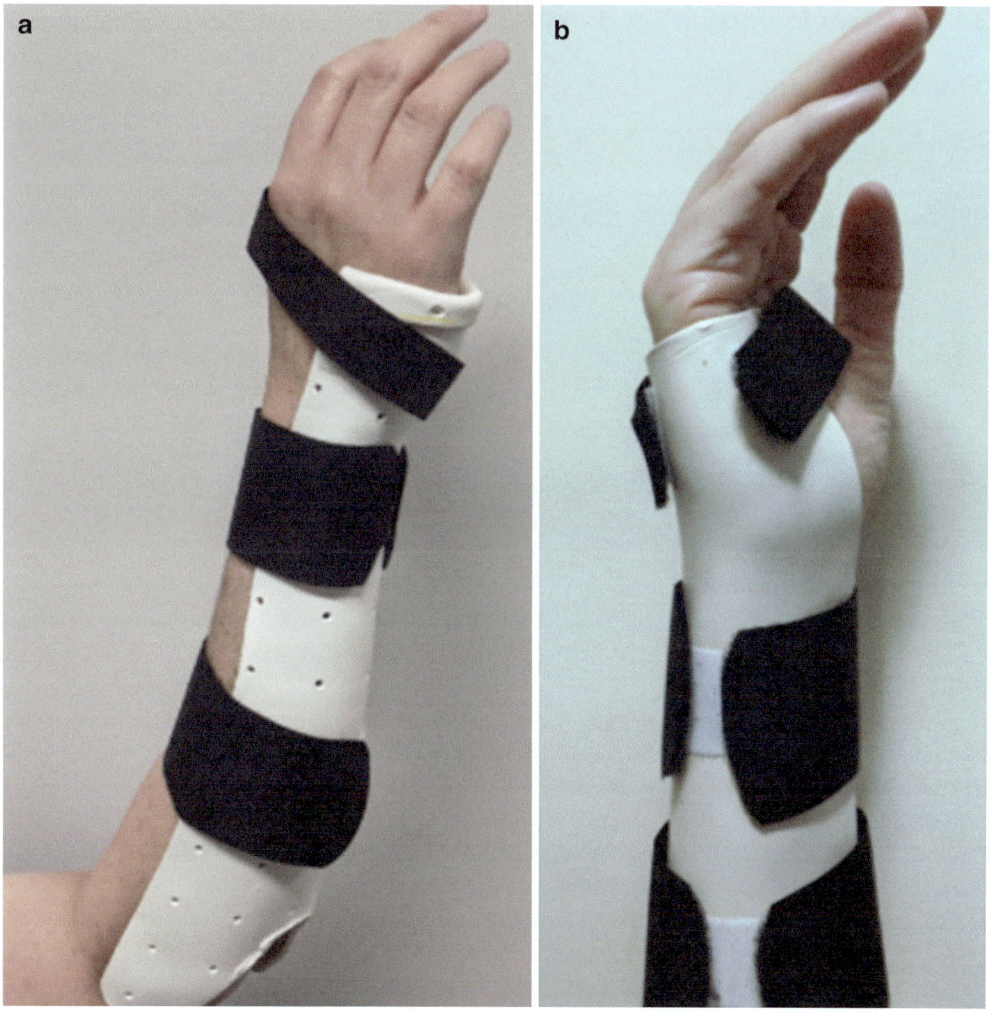

Fig. 34.6 An ulnar gutter splint (A), a long arm orthosis that immobilizes the wrist and forearm (center), or a wrist strap such as a wrist widget (B) are all common forms of support used after a TFCC tear. (Photos by Cara Rodriguez)

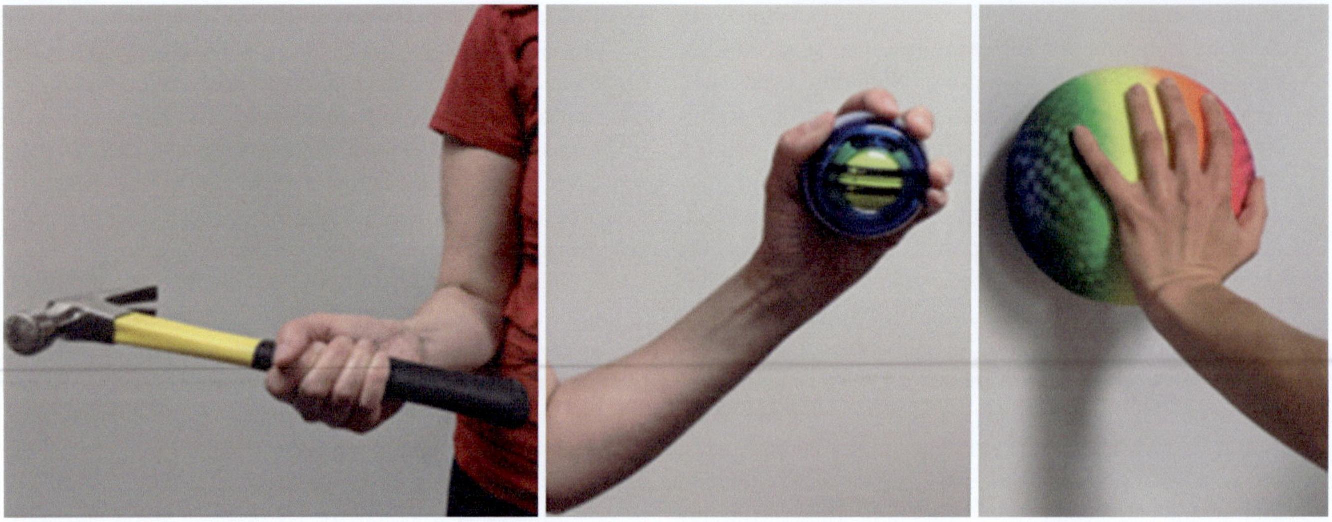

Fig. 34.7 Activities that might be included in a progressive strengthening program after TFCC injury include rotation of a hammer for forearm strengthening, the use of a gyroscope for wrist stability (center), and incorporation of progressive weight-bearing activities (right). (Photos by Cara Rodriguez)

34.2 Ulnar Impaction Syndrome

34.2.1 Synonyms

- Ulnar abutment syndrome
- Ulnocarpal impaction
- Ulnocarpal abutment
- Ulnocarpal impingement

34.2.2 ICD-10 Codes

- M24.831, other specific joint derangements of right wrist, not elsewhere classified
- M24.832, other specific joint derangements of left wrist, not elsewhere classified
- M24.839, other specific joint derangements of unspecified wrist, not elsewhere classified

34.2.3 Description

Not surprisingly, there is considerable overlap between TFCC injuries and ulnar impaction syndrome. Ulnar impaction syndrome is caused by excessive, repetitive stress through the ulnocarpal joint, leading to degenerative changes [17]. The triangular fibrocartilage complex (TFCC), or the load-bearing structure between the ulnar head and the carpus, plays a key role in load transfer. In a normal wrist, 18–20% of the load is transmitted through the ulna [17]. Positive ulnar variance, congenital or acquired, is a significant risk factor for ulnar impaction syndrome due to the resulting increase in loading of the ulnocarpal joint [11]. Small changes in ulnar variance can have a significant impact on the force transmitted through the ulnocarpal joint.

A cadaveric study by Palmer et al. [17] demonstrated that a decrease in ulnar variance of 2.5 mm resulted in a decrease of ulnocarpal joint load to 4% and an increase in ulnar variance of 2.5 mm resulted in an increase of ulnocarpal joint load to 42%. Positive ulnar variance can be acquired in multiple conditions, including distal radius physeal injury, Madelung's deformity, radius malunion, and Essex-Lopresti injury [11, 13]. Additionally, developmentally positive ulnar variance is more common in Asian populations, possibly making idiopathic ulnar impaction more prevalent in this racial group [13].

The thickness of the TFCC is inversely related to ulnar variance [11, 13, 18]. Patients with positive ulnar variance have been shown to have thinner TFCC discs that are therefore more susceptible to injury [17]. Ulnar variance can also change with forearm position, as pronation and grip result in relative shortening of the radius, causing a physiologic, dynamic increase in ulnar variance [11, 13].

Persistent stress between the distal ulna and the carpus results in the spectrum of findings in ulnar impaction, including TFCC tears, chondromalacia of the ulnar aspect of the lunate and ulnar head, and lunotriquetral ligament tears [11, 13]. The differential diagnosis of ulnar impaction syndrome is broad (Table 34.3).

34.2.4 Clinical Presentation

Patients with ulnar impaction syndrome generally present with ulnar-sided wrist pain that is insidious, is onset, and

Table 34.3 Differential diagnosis for ulnar impaction syndrome

Distal radial ulnar joint (DRUJ) arthritis or instability
Triangular fibrocartilage complex (TFCC) tear
Extensor carpi ulnaris (ECU) instability or tendonitis
Pisotriquetral arthritis
Dorsal cutaneous ulnar nerve branch neuritis
Lunotriquetral interosseous ligament (LTIL) injury
Hypothenar hammer syndrome
Carpal fracture or instability

worsens over time [13]. Patients may experience associated swelling and loss of wrist or forearm motion. Any activities that involve forearm pronation, hand grip, and ulnar deviation of the wrist will exacerbate symptoms [13]. Patient may or may not have a history of wrist trauma prior to symptom onset.

34.2.5 Physical Examination

Ulnar impaction syndrome can be diagnosed based on clinical exam with the support of radiographic findings. Patients may have swelling in the affected area with tenderness to palpation around the ulnar head: just distal to the ulnar head dorsally and just volar to the ulnar styloid ulnarly [11, 13]. Ulnar deviation of the wrist, both passive and active, will produce pain, which can be intensified by providing a dorsal force on the pisiform and a volar force on the ulnar head to better replicate the ulnocarpal joint forces during grip activities [11]. The distal radioulnar joint (DRUJ) should be evaluated to assess for pain and stability since this can impact treatment decisions, and the contralateral wrist should be examined for comparison purposes [13].

Special tests: Please refer to the previous section on TFCC injuries, with specific attention to ulnocarpal stress test and pisiform boost.

34.2.6 Diagnostic Workup

Radiographs Please refer to the previous section on TFCC injuries [9, 10]. It is important to look for distal radius physeal growth arrest, distal radius malunion, or other pathology that may result in ulnar positive variance. With distal radius malunions, it is beneficial to compare X-rays to the contralateral side. Additionally, bony changes may be evident on radiographs secondary to ulnar impaction syndrome, including subchondral sclerosis and cysts of the ulnar head, radial triquetrum, and ulnar proximal lunate, which can progress to ulnocarpal arthritis [10]. Radiographs should also be examined for DRUJ arthritis and stability.

Magnetic resonance imaging MRI can detect early disease or other pathology that can present similarly [10]. MRI in ulnar impaction syndrome will often show early articular cartilage wear and bony edema in the involved areas [17].

34.2.7 Treatment

Conservative Care

For medical, rehabilitation, and procedural treatments, please refer to the TFCC injuries.

Surgery

Surgery is considered in patients with symptoms refractory to a 6- to 12-week course of non-operative treatment. Arthroscopy alone is less effective in patients who are ulnar positive, and consideration should be made for ulnar shortening osteotomy (Fig. 34.8.) Please refer to Chap. 50 for more details.

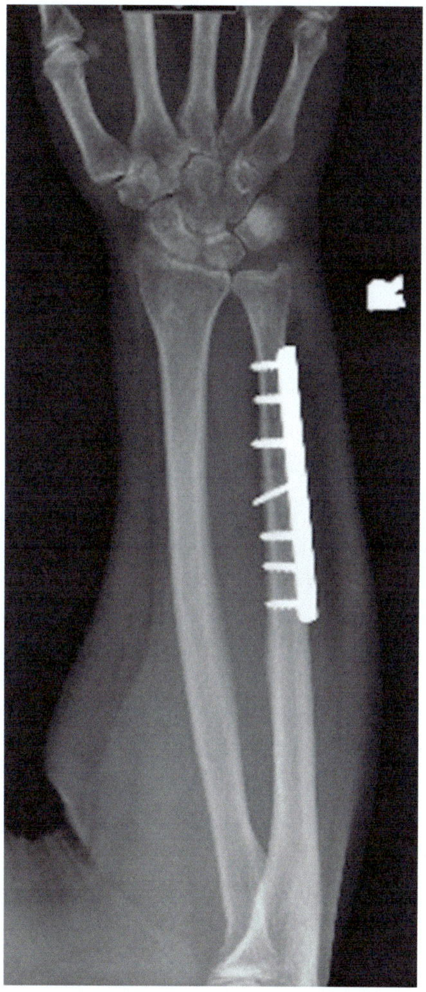

Fig. 34.8 Postoperative anterior–posterior (AP) forearm radiograph demonstrating an ulnar shortening osteotomy with a resulting negative ulnar variance

34.3 Extensor Carpi Ulnaris (ECU) Tendinopathy

34.3.1 Synonyms

- ECU tendinosis
- ECU tenosynovitis
- ECU tendon instability
- ECU tendon subluxation
- ECU tendon dislocation

34.3.2 ICD-10 Codes

- M65.849, other synovitis and tenosynovitis, unspecified hand
- M65.841, other synovitis and tenosynovitis, right hand
- M65.842, other synovitis and tenosynovitis, left hand
- S63.509, unspecified sprain of unspecified wrist
- S63.501, unspecified sprain of right wrist
- S63.502, unspecified sprain of left wrist

34.3.3 Description

Extensor carpi ulnaris (ECU) tendinopathy includes a spectrum of tendon pathology, ranging from tenosynovitis to tendon instability, and is a common cause of ulnar-sided wrist pain. The ECU tendon occupies the sixth dorsal compartment, passing along a bony groove in the ulnar before inserting on the fifth metacarpal base. The ECU tendon is held in the osseous groove by deep antebrachial fascia duplication, which forms the tendon subsheath, acting as a tunnel that inserts on the ulna [18]. The dorsal wrist retinaculum also helps to stabilize the ECU tendon, running like a bridge over the sixth dorsal compartment [18]. With forearm rotation, the relative position of the tendon changes due to the rotation of the hand around the stable ulna. With full forearm pronation, the ECU tendon travels in a linear path, and with full supination, the tendon travels around the ulnar styloid at an angle to insert on the base of the fifth metacarpal. The floor of the ECU tendon sheath is an important stabilizer for the TFCC, making ECU tendon pathology difficult to distinguish from TFCC pathology [19].

Instability of the ECU tendon can coexist with tenosynovitis or exist in isolation. ECU tendon instability can occur when there is disruption to the stable osseofibrous sheath through which the ECU tendon travels [18]. The ECU tendon can completely dislocate out of the sheath, or it can subluxate during supination and reduce during pronation [18]. There are three reported types of ECU tendon instability (Fig. 34.9) [18]:

1. Type A ulnar-sided subsheath tear
2. Type B radial-sided subsheath tear
3. Type C detachment of the subsheath from the ulna resulting in sheath attenuation and a false pouch

Due to differences in treatment, it is important to differentiate between an acute injury resulting in instability and instability secondary to chronic tendonitis [19]. Acute ECU instability is more commonly seen in athletes, often after a forceful forearm supination activity, such as playing tennis, baseball, hockey, or golf [18]. The differential diagnosis of ECU tendinopathy is presented in Table 34.4.

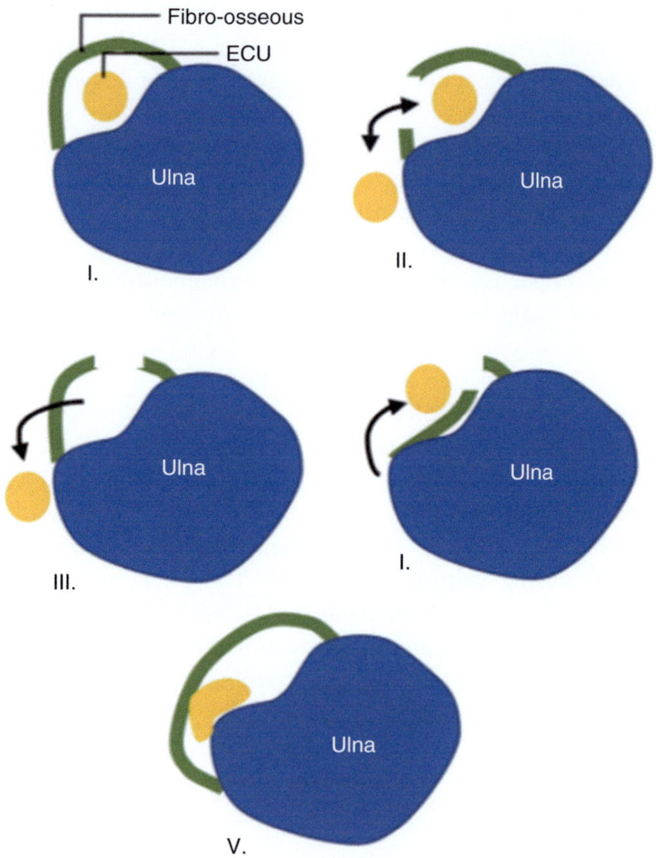

Fig. 34.9 Types of ECU tendon instability. I demonstrates normal anatomic relationship of ECU tendon in the ulnar groove, stabilized by the fibro-osseous sheath. II demonstrates type A tendon instability with an ulnar-sided subsheath tear. III and IV demonstrate type B tendon instability with a radial-sided subsheath tear, which can result in the torn fibro-osseous sheath underlying the ECU tendon with reduction into the groove, preventing healing. V demonstrates detachment of the subsheath from the ulna, resulting in subsheath attenuation and a false pouch

Table 34.4 Differential diagnosis for ECU tendinopathy

Triangular fibrocartilage complex (TFCC) tear
Ulnar impaction syndrome
DRUJ instability or arthritis
Lunotriquetral interosseous ligament (LTIL) injury
Flexor carpi ulnaris (FCU) tendonitis
Dorsal cutaneous ulnar nerve branch neuritis

34.3.4 Clinical Presentation

Patients with ECU tendinopathy commonly present with ulnar-sided wrist pain after an overuse or a twisting injury. Pain is exacerbated with any wrist range of motion and generally is difficult to localize and may radiate up the forearm [19]. Nocturnal pain that interferes with sleep is common. Patients may report dysesthesias along the dorsal ulnar wrist, in the distribution of the dorsal sensory branch of the ulnar nerve [19]. If patients are experiencing ECU tendon instability, they may report a painful snapping sensation with certain wrist movements.

34.3.5 Physical Examination

On examination of patients with ECU tendinopathy, there may be notable swelling overlying the dorsal ulnar wrist. The ECU sheath swelling is often tender with palpation in the ulnar groove, and sometimes crepitus can be felt by the examiner [18, 19]. Pain is elicited with any wrist motion, and active wrist extension with ulnar deviation against resistance will exacerbate the patient's symptoms [19].

Special Tests

ECU tendon stability: Tendon instability may be elicited on exam by palpating the tendon sheath while having the patient hold their wrist in extension and actively rotate the forearm through full pronosupination [19]. The ECU tendon should reduce with forearm pronation. The examiner may also feel the tendon subluxation or snap as the wrist is held in supination and brought from extension to flexion with ulnar deviation [19].

Extensor carpi ulnaris synergy test: In this test for ECU tendinitis, the patient's elbow is flexed at 90 degrees with the wrist in full supination and fingers extended and abducted. The examiner squeezes the patient's thumb and middle finger with one hand, while the other hand palpates the ECU tendon. (Fig. 34.10). The test is positive if pain is reproduced along the ECU tendon [22].

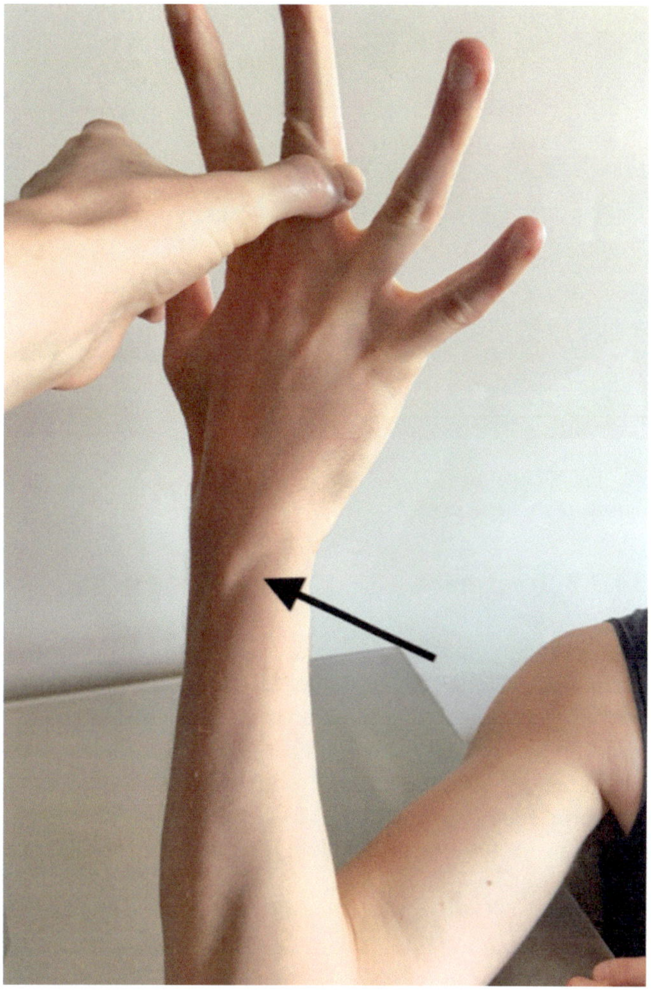

Fig. 34.10 Extensor carpi ulnaris synergy test with arrow indicating location of ECU tendon

34.3.6 Diagnostic Workup

Radiographs A standard wrist radiographic series should be obtained in all patients presenting with ulnar-sided wrist pain; however, radiographs should show no acute pathology in patients with ECU tendinopathy.

Magnetic resonance imaging Magnetic resonance imaging (MRI) is often helpful for diagnosis and will commonly show tenosynovitis surrounding the ECU tendon. Other ECU tendon or ulnar wrist pathology can also be seen on MRI, such as a shallow ECU tendon groove, TFCC injury, degenerative tendon tears or rupture, and accessory anomalous tendon slips [19]. If there is concern for possible tendon instability, obtaining an MRI with the forearm in full pronation and full supination can be helpful for diagnosis [19] (Fig. 34.11).

Ultrasound Ultrasound is a beneficial diagnostic and real-time imaging modality, which can reveal tenosynovitis surrounding the ECU tendon, as well as tendon instability with forearm rotation [19].

Injection To confirm the diagnosis of ECU tendonitis, lidocaine can be injected in the ECU tendon sheath and should provide complete but transient pain relief [11].

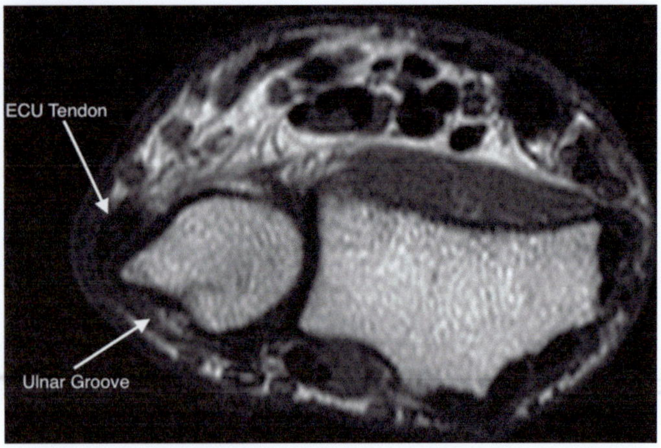

Fig. 34.11 MRI of the wrist demonstrating ECU tendon dislocation outside of the ulnar groove

34.3.7 Treatment

Medical Management
Prior to considering surgical intervention, conservative non-operative treatment should be provided. This includes rest, ice, splint, or cast immobilization, nonsteroidal anti-inflammatory medication, and activity modification [19]. The arm should be immobilized in pronation with radial deviation to allow appropriate rest of the soft tissues and keep the ECU within the ulnar groove [20].

Rehabilitation
After a period of immobilization, patients can begin physical therapy with active and active-assistive range of motion exercises as tolerated [21]. Once motion is greater than 75% of normal, patients can begin a strengthening program. If patients experience mechanical symptoms of ECU tendon subluxation or dislocation during physical therapy, circumferential taping proximal and distal to the ulnar styloid can be considered to add to stability [21]. Once strength is greater than 75% of normal, patients can begin sport-specific training if indicated [21].

Procedures
If splinting and anti-inflammatory medications fail to provide adequate treatment, corticosteroid injection (CPT 20550) can be considered in conjunction with physical therapy; however, corticosteroids should be administered with caution as there is an increased risk of tendon rupture following corticosteroid injection [19]. Patients may be immobilized for 3–5 days following corticosteroid injection prior to resuming therapy, and injections can be performed under ultrasound guidance [21, 22].

Surgery
If non-operative conservative treatment modalities fail to provide adequate symptom relief, operative intervention can be considered. Please refer to Chap. 50 for details.

34.4 Ulnar Tunnel Syndrome

34.4.1 Synonyms

- Ulnar nerve entrapment at the wrist
- Guyon's canal syndrome
- Handlebar palsy

34.4.2 ICD-10 Codes

- G56.20, lesion of ulnar nerve, unspecified upper limb
- G56.21, lesion of ulnar nerve, right upper limb
- G56.22, lesion of ulnar nerve, left upper limb
- S64.00XA, injury of ulnar nerve at wrist and hand level of unspecified arm, initial encounter
- S64.01XA, injury of ulnar nerve at wrist and hand level of right arm, initial encounter
- S64.02XA, injury of ulnar nerve at wrist and hand level of left arm, initial encounter

34.4.3 Description

Ulnar tunnel syndrome refers to the motor and/or sensory impairment caused by compression of the ulnar nerve at the wrist. In contrast to cubital tunnel syndrome, ulnar tunnel syndrome is relatively rare [23, 24]. This condition is most commonly caused by ganglia arising from the triquetrohamate, pisotriquetral, ulnocarpal, or other midcarpal joints, but it may be the result of acute or chronic repetitive trauma to the hand, as seen in cyclists or those who operate machinery like jackhammers [25, 26]. Other etiologies include vascular aneurysms, abnormal musculature, nerve sheath lesions, rheumatoid arthritis, osteoarthritis, and iatrogenic injury from prior surgery [27].

Arising from the C8 and T1 nerve roots, the ulnar nerve is often compressed in the cubital tunnel [23]. In differentiating ulnar tunnel syndrome from cubital tunnel syndrome, it is important to recognize that the ulnar nerve innervates the FCU and FDP to the ring and small fingers proximal to the wrist [23, 25]. In addition, the dorsal sensory branch of the ulnar nerve arises from the main trunk six to eight centimeters proximal to the wrist to provide sensation to the dorsal ulnar aspect of the hand. Since this branch does not enter Guyon's canal, sensation of the dorsal ulnar aspect of the hand is preserved in ulnar tunnel syndrome, whereas it is affected in cubital tunnel syndrome [23, 27].

The floor of the ulnar tunnel is the transverse carpal ligament, the roof is the palmar carpal ligament, and the pisiform and hamate hook are the ulnar and radial borders, respectively [26]. The ulnar nerve enters the tunnel as a mixed sensory and motor nerve (zone 1) before it bifurcates into the motor-predominant deep ulnar nerve (zone 2) and the superficial sensory branch (zone 3). This separation divides the ulnar tunnel into three zones (Fig. 34.12). Presenting symptoms can help guide clinicians as to which zone is involved and the potential etiology of nerve compression (Table 34.6) [23, 25–27]. The differential diagnosis of ulnar tunnel syndrome is broad (Table 34.5).

34.4.4 Clinical Presentation

Ulnar tunnel syndrome is most frequently a clinical diagnosis [23]. Depending on the location of compression, patients most commonly present with numbness and tingling, burning, or loss of sensation over the palmar aspect of the ring and small fingers. Motor complaints may include reports of weakness with grip, inability to adduct the small finger, or

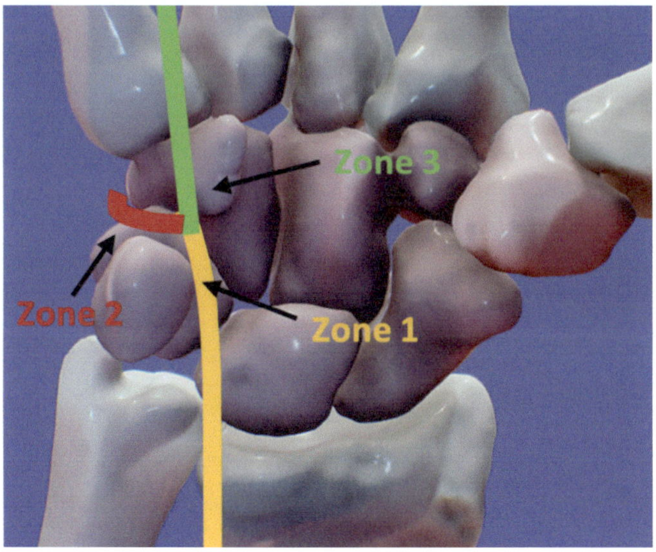

Fig. 34.12 Zones of the ulnar nerve in Guyon's canal. Zone 1 contains mixed motor and sensory fibers, zone 2 contains only motor fibers, and zone 3 contains mainly sensory fibers. (Modified from "Wrist bones anatomy" from MDCT/STL, created by Chair Digital Anatomy at Paris University; Licensed under Creative Commons Attribution. https://skfb.ly/6UpB8 To view a copy of this license, visit https://creativecommons.org/licenses/by/4.0/)

Table 34.5 Differential diagnosis of ulnar tunnel syndrome

Cubital tunnel syndrome	Malignant peripheral nerve sheath tumor
Carpal tunnel syndrome	Guillain–Barre syndrome
Cervical nerve root compression	Rheumatoid or osteoarthritis
CNS lesions	Diabetic neuropathy
Motor neuron disease (ALS)	ETOH neuropathy, B12 deficiency

Table 34.6 Ulnar tunnel zones

Zones	Ulnar nerve branch	Causes of compression	Symptoms
Zone 1	Mixed motor and sensory ulnar nerve from entrance to tunnel to just proximal to the bifurcation	Ganglia, hook of hamate fracture	Mixed motor and sensory impairment
Zone 2	Deep motor branch of ulnar nerve	Ganglia, hook of hamate fracture, repetitive trauma	Impaired innervation of the hypothenar muscles (flexor digiti minimi, opponens digiti minimi, adductor digiti minimi), third and fourth lumbricals, palmar and dorsal interosseous muscles, adductor pollicis, and deep head of the flexor pollicis brevis
Zone 3	Superficial sensory branch of ulnar nerve, with motor fibers to palmaris brevis	Ulnar artery thrombosis, ulnar artery aneurysm, abnormal musculature	Impaired innervation of the palmaris brevis, loss of sensation, paresthesia, or burning of palmar aspect of ulnar half of fourth digit, fifth digit

clawing of the ring and small fingers due to loss of ulnar lumbrical innervation leading to imbalance. In advanced cases, wasting of the hypothenar muscles and first dorsal interosseous muscle may be seen.

A comprehensive history should be gathered to rule out proximal compression. Assessment of symptom duration and severity, occupational and recreational history, repetitive palmar stress (construction work, cyclists, tennis players), surgical history, and medical history should be reviewed for causes of peripheral neuropathy that may influence management and prognosis [24, 27].

34.4.5 Physical Examination

The principal differential diagnosis is cubital tunnel syndrome. The entire path of the ulnar nerve should be examined, looking for any signs of trauma, tenderness, masses, deformity, cyanosis, or edema. Symmetry of both hands should be assessed, looking for ulnar digit clawing or intrinsic atrophy. The radial and ulnar arteries should be palpated for any thrill or pulsatile mass.

Sensation of the cervical dermatomes should be assessed to rule out cervical root compression. Special attention should be paid to both the ulnar and median nerve sensory distributions of the hand to rule out concurrent carpal tunnel syndrome [23]. Loss of only palmar sensation of the ulnar half of the ring and entire small finger is suggestive of ulnar tunnel syndrome. If the lesion is isolated to zone 3, only sensation should be affected with preservation of motor function; however, zone 1 lesions will have mixed motor and sensory loss. If there is loss of both palmar and dorsal ulnar sensation, it suggests compression proximally in extremity.

Motor involvement in the ulnar tunnel may result in weakness of thumb adduction, clawing of the ring and small fingers, and the inability to adduct the small finger. Grip strength and pinch strength may be impaired in the affected hand [18]. Isolated motor loss with preservation of sensation is suggestive of a zone 2 lesion; zone 1 lesions will have mixed motor and sensory impairment.

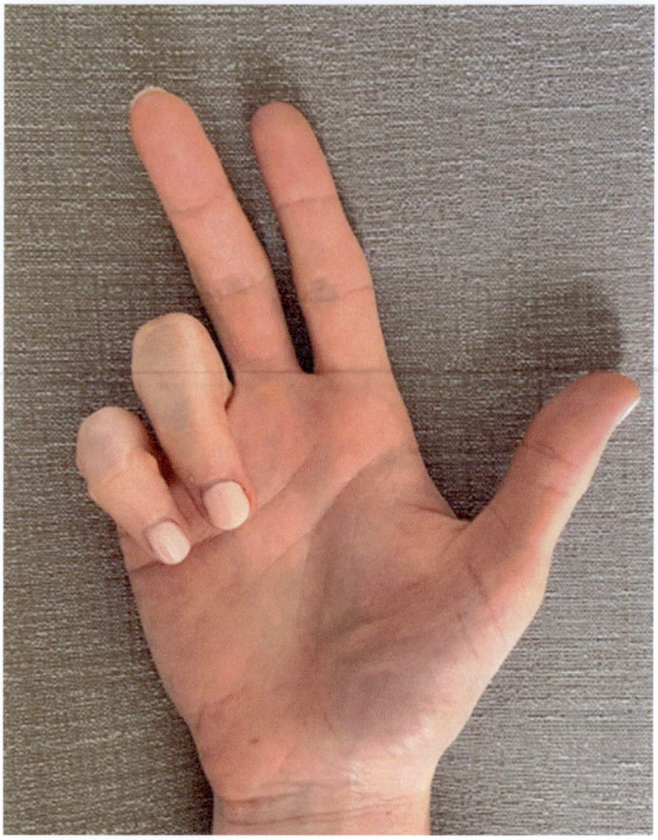

Fig. 34.13 Hand of benediction sign

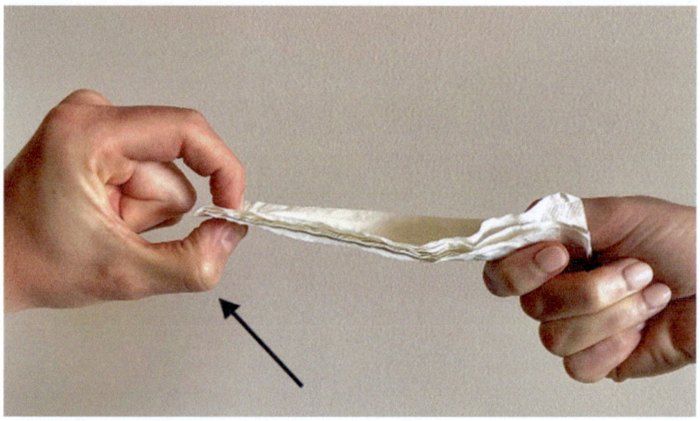

Fig. 34.14 Froment sign with arrow indicating compensatory thumb interphalangeal joint flexion during pinch grip

Special Signs and Tests

- *Ulnar claw hand*: Clawing of the ring and small fingers (metacarpophalangeal hyperextension with proximal and distal interphalangeal flexion) due to loss of the third and fourth lumbrical innervation leading to digital imbalance (Fig. 34.13).
- *Palmaris brevis sign*: Contraction of the palmaris brevis muscle (evidenced by wrinkling of the skin over the proximal ulnar-sided palm) with abduction of the fifth digit. This sign suggests preserved innervation via the superficial sensory branch of the ulnar nerve. This finding would be absent in zone 1, zone 3, and ulnar nerve compression proximal to the ulnar tunnel.
- *Froment sign*: Interphalangeal joint hyperflexion of the thumb during pinch grip to compensate for loss of adductor pollicis function. This may be seen in conjunction with the first dorsal interosseous atrophy (Fig. 34.14).
- *Wartenberg sign*: Inability to adduct the small finger resulting from the unopposed ulnar moment of the extensor digiti minimi.
- *Finger cross test*: Inability to cross the first and second digits, suggestive of paralysis of the first palmar and the second dorsal interosseous paralysis. If this sign is positive with preservation of hypothenar motor innervation, this is suggestive of a distal deep ulnar nerve lesion [24].
- *Tinel's sign*: Percussion over the entire distribution of the ulnar nerve especially over the elbow and wrist. The sign is positive if symptoms of numbness, tingling, or a shock are reproduced. This sign may be positive in multiple locations, suggestive of multiple areas of ulnar nerve compression.
- *Allen test*: Simultaneous compression of the ulnar and radial arteries while the patient rapidly contracts the hand. Pressure on one artery is then released to assess for return

of blood flow before repeating the test on the opposite side. Capillary refill should be <2 seconds; ≥5 seconds is abnormal and is suggestive of some arterial compromise.
- *Elbow flexion test*: Patient maximally flexes elbow for 1 minute; the presence of pain or paresthesias in the ulnar nerve distribution suggests compression of the ulnar nerve at the elbow.

34.4.6 Diagnostic Workup

Radiographs Conventional radiographs, including carpal tunnel and hamate views, should be obtained to evaluate for a hook of hamate fracture.

Ultrasound Ultrasound is limited in the assessment of osseous pathology but is useful for assessment of soft tissue lesions and inflammatory changes of the tendons and ligaments, which may be causing ulnar nerve compression [29]. Ultrasound, however, is limited by operator dependence and the thick, fibrous structures within the palm, which may limit views and lead to false-negative diagnoses [30].

Magnetic resonance imaging MRI is considered to be the gold standard for examination.[1] It has been used in the identification of soft tissue pathology, nerve and vessel anatomy, and anatomical variations. In addition, cross-sectional area and compartment space may also be assessed [23]. MRI is frequently used to assess ganglion anatomy, origin, and relationship to other structures, which is critical for preoperative planning [29, 30].

Electromyography and nerve conduction studies (EMG/NCS) Electromyography and nerve conduction studies are performed to localize focal nerve compression, acuity, and severity of the nerve impairment [28] and differentiate focal versus more systemic or radicular cause of neuropathic complaint. EMG/NCS also provide useful information regarding prognosis [23] and are considered an extension to our physical exam and not a replacement for it. Other limitations include patient tolerance, technical skills, and confounding effects of other pathologies and age-related changes impacting study results [23].

Arteriography Arteriography may be beneficial in the case of suspected ulnar arterial pathology, including thrombosis, aneurysm, and pseudoaneurysm [23, 24].

[1] Text

34.4.7 Treatment

Medical Management

Discontinuation of the offending activity is indicated in some cases. If diagnostic studies demonstrate compression from a mass, such as a ganglion, surgery is the next step. Aspiration is not recommended due to limited success, risk of recurrence, and potential damage to numerous vulnerable anatomic structures within the area [24]. In other circumstances, the decision between conservative and operative management depends on symptom severity and duration. In the case of mild to moderate symptoms lasting less than 3 months, conservative management involves activity modification and splint immobilization [28]. Nonsteroidal anti-inflammatory drugs (NSAIDs) are not beneficial for the treatment of ulnar tunnel syndrome due to the lack of a significant contribution from inflammation worsening compression [23–25].

Rehabilitation

As part of the conservative non-operative management, immobilization in a wrist splint may be beneficial. Physical therapy is not typically utilized in the treatment of ulnar tunnel syndrome; however, occupational therapy can be helpful in educating patients on activity modification, including avoiding aggravating motions.

Procedures

There is a consensus agreement that corticosteroid injections are not beneficial for the treatment of ulnar tunnel syndrome due to the lack of a significant contribution from inflammation worsening compression [23–25, 29–31].

Surgery

Decompression of Guyon's canal and removal of any compressive structures are the major components of any surgical interventions. Please refer to Chap. 50 for more details.

34.5 Ulnar Collateral Ligament of the Wrist Injury (UCL)

34.5.1 Synonyms

- Ulnocarpal collateral ligament (UCCL)
- Distal peripheral TFCC injury

34.5.2 ICD-10 Codes

- S63.31, traumatic rupture of collateral ligament of wrist

- S63.311, traumatic rupture of collateral ligament of right wrist
- S63.312, traumatic rupture of collateral ligament of left wrist
- S63.319, traumatic rupture of collateral ligament of unspecified wrist

34.5.3 Description

Injury of the ulnar collateral ligament (UCL) of the wrist usually results from a fall on an outstretched hand but may also be seen after a forceful ulnar deviation, pronation, or supination of the wrist [6, 32, 33]. Isolated injury to the UCL of the wrist is rare due to its location and anatomy and thus is frequently associated with lesions of the ECU tendinous subsheath, other structures within the TFCC, and lunotriquetral carpal ligaments [5, 6, 33, 34].

The UCL is an extrinsic wrist ligament that serves an important role in stabilization of the ulnocarpal joint during pronation and supination of the wrist [35–37].

The UCL is found at the floor of the sixth extensor compartment, just deep to the ECU tendon [36, 37]. Proximally, the UCL is attached to the ulnar styloid and extends distally to attach to the medial aspect of the triquetrum. The ulnar styloid also serves as a site of attachment to the superficial fibers of the dorsal and palmar distal radioulnar ligaments and the tendinous sheath of the ECU. The attachment of the UCL may be at the tip (type 1) or medial base (type 2) of the ulnar styloid, and type 2 attachments are found more frequently in symptomatic wrists, which suggests that a type 2 UCL may predispose patients to ulnar-sided wrist injury [38]. The differential diagnosis for ulnar collateral ligament injury of the wrist is broad (Table 34.7).

34.5.4 Clinical Presentation

Patients most commonly present with complaints of ulnar-sided wrist pain, localized swelling, and restricted range of motion. Injury to the ulnar attachment of the TFCC has been demonstrated to be more reliably symptomatic than central or radial lesions [39]. Patients may report a history of either a fall on a hyperextended wrist, lifting a heavy object, or a forceful rotation of the wrist resulting in injury. There may be associated weakness of grip, which tends to exacerbate the pain. Rotation of the wrist, such as twisting a doorknob, using a screwdriver, or wringing a cloth, is also often painful [6, 33]. Assessment of DRUJ instability is critical as it influences management of the injury. In such cases, patients may report a history of the wrist giving out during rotation, a sensation of grinding within the wrist, or crepitus with pronation and supination [32, 40]. Hand dominance, previous injury and response to treatment, and repetitive movements related to occupation should be assessed as this may impact treatment and prognosis [40].

Table 34.7 Differential diagnosis of ulnar collateral ligament injury

Distal radioulnar joint arthritis/ instability	Kienböck's disease (osteonecrosis of lunate)
Pisotriquetral arthritis	Ulnar styloid impaction syndrome
Extensor carpi ulnaris tendonitis/ tendinopathy	Ulnar impingement syndrome
Triangular fibrocartilage complex tear	Lunotriquetral ligament tear
Ulnar impaction syndrome	Ulnar carpal or styloid fracture

34.5.5 Physical Examination

A thorough wrist exam is indicated to differentiate UCL injury from the broad differential of ulnar-sided wrist pain.

The wrist should first be inspected, looking for any swelling, bruising, deformity, or other signs of trauma. Point tenderness over the ulnar styloid is common, and palpable prominence of the ulnar head dorsally may be present, which would suggest DRUJ instability. Limitation of ulnar deviation, pronation, and supination is most common, but flexion and extension of the wrist may be limited depending on the severity of disease. Passive and active ulnar deviation commonly elicits pain, and pain with active pronation is often greater than pain with supination. Resisted rotation of the affected wrist is frequently weak, and grip strength may be decreased as well.

Special Tests

Please refer to the section on TFCC injuries. There are no specific physical exam maneuvers that differentiate UCL of the wrist from TFCC given their close anatomic relationship and the fact that they are commonly injured together.

34.5.6 Diagnostic Workup

Radiographs Standard wrist radiographs have limited utility in the diagnosis of UCL injury; however, they may be useful for assessment of associated fracture, arthritic changes, or measurement of ulnar variance, which may predispose patients to ulnar-sided injury [38].

Magnetic resonance imaging MR arthrography (MRA) is emerging as the favored imaging modality for assessment of TFCC pathology (Fig. 34.15). Some studies have concluded that MRA is of equal diagnostic value when compared to arthroscopy in the diagnosis of ligamentous wrist injury [5,

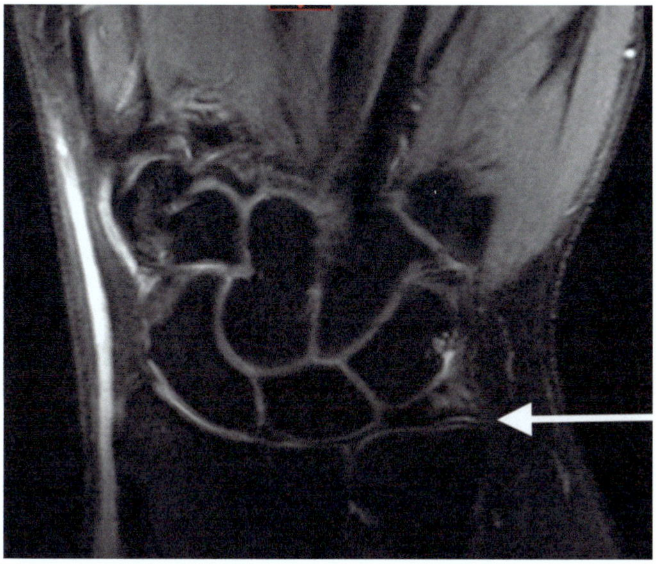

Fig. 34.15 MRI of the wrist demonstrating a complex tear of the TFCC at its ulnar attachment

37, 38]. MRA is especially useful in the diagnosis of peripheral, extrinsic wrist injury when utilizing injection of contrast into the radiocarpal joint and DRUJ.

34.5.7 Treatment

Medical Management

Treatment of UCL injury is dependent on multiple factors including the size of the tear, the presence or absence of concomitant TFCC injury, and the condition of the cartilage of the DRUJ. In general, most acute traumatic injuries and degenerative injuries can be first managed with a trial of non-operative treatment, including splinting and NSAIDs [38, 39]. If symptoms persist, further diagnostic workup and imaging are recommended.

Rehabilitation

Please refer to the section on TFCC injuries.

Procedures

Corticosteroid injection can be considered in conjunction with immobilization followed by therapy. Ultrasound guidance can be utilized to ensure appropriate placement of steroid injection. Again, corticosteroids should be administered with caution as there is an increased risk of tendon rupture following corticosteroid injection [19].

Surgery

Wrist arthroscopy may be considered for treatment of ulnar-sided wrist pain refractory to conservative measures. Please refer to Chap. 50 for more details.

References

1. Skalski MR, White EA, Patel DB, Schein AJ, RiveraMelo H, Matcuk GR. The Traumatized TFCC: an illustrated review of the anatomy and injury patterns of the triangular fibrocartilage complex. Curr Probl Diagn Radiol. 2016;45(1):39–50.
2. Pang EQ, Yao J. Ulnar-sided wrist pain in the athlete (TFCC/DRUJ/ECU). Curr Rev Musculoskelet Med. 2017;10(1):53–61.
3. Adams JE. Disorders of the distal radioulnar joint. In: Miller MD, Thompson SR, editors. DeLee & Drez's orthopaedic sports medicine. 5th ed. Philadelphia: Elsevier, Inc; 2020. p. 865–72.
4. Palmer AK. Triangular fibrocartilage complex lesions: a classification. J Hand Surg Am. 1989;14:594–606.
5. Atzei A, Luchetti R. Foveal TFCC tear classification and treatment. Hand Clin. 2011;27(3):263–72.
6. Vezeridis PS, Yoshioka H, Han R, Blazar P. Ulnar-sided wrist pain. Part I: anatomy and physical examination. Skelet Radiol. 2010;39(8):733–45.
7. Nakamura R, Horii E, Imaeda T, et al. The ulnocarpal stress test in the diagnosis of ulnar-sided wrist pain. J Hand Surg Br. 1997;22(6):719–23.
8. Michelotti B, Chung KC. Ulnar shortening osteotomy for ulnar impaction syndrome. In: Chung KC, editor. Hand and wrist surgery. 3rd ed. Philadelphia: Elsevier; 2018. p. 251–8.
9. Tomaino MM. The importance of the pronated grip x-ray view in evaluating ulnar variance. J Hand Surg Am. 2000;25(2):352–7.
10. Cerezal L, del Pinal F, Abascal F, et al. Imaging findings in ulnar-sided wrist impaction syndromes. Radiographics. 2002;22(1):105–21.
11. Adams BD, Leversedge FJ. Distal radioulnar joint. In: Wolfe SW, Hotchkiss RN, Kozin SH, Pederson WC, Cohen MS, editors. Green's operative hand surgery. 7th ed. Philadelphia: Elsevier; 2017. p. 479–515.
12. Palmer AK, Werner FW. Biomechanics of the distal radioulnar joint. Clin Orthop Relat Res. 1984;187:26–35.
13. Sammer DM, Rizzo M. Ulnar impaction. Hand Clin. 2010;26:549–57.
14. Dell P. Ulnar wrist pain and impairment: a therapist's algorithmic approach to the triangular fibrocartilage complex. In: Skirven TM, Osterman AL, Fedorcczyk JM, Amadio PC, editors. Rehabilitation of the hand and upper extremity. 6th ed. St. Louis: Mosby; 2011. p. 974–87.
15. Chen Z. A novel staged wrist sensorimotor rehabilitation program for a patient with triangular fibrocartilage complex injury: a case report. J Hand Ther. 2019;32(4):525–34.
16. Altman E. The ulnar side of the wrist: clinically relevant anatomy and biomechanics. J Hand Ther. 2016;29(2):111–22.
17. Palmer AK, Glisson RR, et al. Relationship between ulnar variance and triangular fibrocartilage complex thickness. J Hand Surg [Am]. 1984;9:681–2.
18. Montalvan B, Parier J, Brasseur JL, et al. Extensor carpi ulnaris injuries in tennis players: a study of 28 cases. Br J Sports Med. 2006;40(5):424–9.
19. Wolfe S. Tendinopathy. In: Wolfe SW, Hotchkiss RN, Kozin SH, Pederson WC, Cohen MS, editors. Green's operative hand surgery. 7th ed. Elsevier; 2017. p. 1904–25.
20. Inoue G, Tamura Y. Recurrent dislocation of the extensor carpi ulnaris tendon. Br J Sports Med. 1998;32:172–4.
21. Graham T. Pathologies of the extensor carpi ulnaris (ECU) tendon and its investments in the athlete. Hand Clin. 2012;28:345–56.
22. Adams JE, Habbu R. Tendinopathies of the hand and wrist. JAAOS. 2015;23(12):741–50.
23. Aleksenko D, Varacallo M. Guyon canal syndrome. In: StatPearls. Treasure Island (FL): StatPearls Publishing; 2020.

24. Bachoura A, Jacoby SM. Ulnar tunnel syndrome. Orthop Clin North Am. 2012;43(4):467–74.
25. Earp BE, Floyd WE, Louie D, Koris M, Protomastro P. Ulnar nerve entrapment at the wrist. J Am Acad Orthop Surg. 2014;22(11):699–706.
26. Ramage JL, Varacallo M. Anatomy, shoulder and upper limb, hand Guyon canal. In: StatPearls. Treasure Island (FL): StatPearls Publishing; 2020.
27. Sharrak S, M Das J. Hand nerve compression syndromes. In: StatPearls. Treasure Island (FL): StatPearls Publishing; 2020.
28. Ginanneschi F, Mondelli M, Cioncoloni D, Rossi A. Impact of carpal tunnel syndrome on ulnar nerve at wrist: systematic review. J Electromyogr Kinesiol. 2018;40:32–8.
29. Wang B, Zhao Y, Lu A, Chen C. Ulnar nerve deep branch compression by a ganglion: a review of nine cases. Injury. 2014;45(7):1126–30.
30. Tottas S, Kougioumtzis I, Titsi Z, Ververidis A, Tilkeridis K, Drosos GI. Correction to: ulnar nerve entrapment in Guyon's canal caused by a ganglion cyst: two case reports and review of the literature. Eur J Orthop Surg Traumatol. 2019;29(7):1575–8.
31. Hoogvliet P, Coert JH, Fridén J, Huisstede BMA, European HANDGUIDE group. How to treat Guyon's canal syndrome? Results from the European HANDGUIDE study: a multidisciplinary treatment guideline. Br J Sports Med. 2013;47(17):1063–70.
32. Malshikare VA. Perthes-like lesion in wrist joint: stripping of ulnar collateral ligament. J Wrist Surg. 2019;8(2):152–6.
33. Kirchberger MC, Unglaub F, Muhldorfer-Fodor M, et al. Update TFCC: histology and pathology, classification, examination, and diagnostics. Arch Orthop Trauma Surg. 2015;135(3):263–72.
34. Maizlin ZV, Brown JA, Clement JJ, Grebenyuk J, Fenton DM, Smith DE, et al. MR arthrography of the wrist: controversies and concepts. Hand (N Y). 2009;4(1):66–73.
35. Türker T, Sheppard JE, Klauser AS, Johnston SS, Amerongen H, Taljanovic MS. The radial and ulnar collateral ligaments of the wrist are true ligaments. Diagn Interv Radiol. 2019;25(6):473–9.
36. DiTano O, Trumble TE, Tencer AF. Biomechanical function of the distal radioulnar and ulnocarpal wrist ligaments. J Hand Surg Am. 2003;28(4):622–7.
37. Nozaki T, Wu WD, Kaneko Y, Rafijah G, Yang L, Hitt D, et al. High-resolution MRI of the ulnar and radial collateral ligaments of the wrist. Acta Radiol. 2017;58(12):1493–9.
38. Watanabe A, Souza F, Vezeridis PS, Blazar P, Yoshioka H. Ulnar-sided wrist pain. II. Clinical imaging and treatment. Skelet Radiol. 2010;39(9):837–57.
39. Atzei A, Luchetti R, Garagnani L. Classification of ulnar triangular fibrocartilage complex tears. A treatment algorithm for Palmer type IB tears. J Hand Surg Eur. 2017;42(4):405–14.
40. Henderson CJ, Kobayashi KM. Ulnar-sided wrist pain in the athlete. Orthop Clin North Am. 2016;47(4):789–98.
41. Kovachevich R, Elhassan BT. Arthroscopic and open repair of the TFCC. Hand Clin. 2010;26(4):485–94.

Disorders of the Fingers

35

Margaret Shields, Andrew Felber, and Charles Cassidy

35.1 Boutonnière and Swan Neck Deformity

35.1.1 Synonyms and ICD 10 Code

- Boutonnière deformity, M20.02
- Swan neck deformity, M20.03

35.1.2 Description

Anatomy: Distal interphalangeal (DIP) and proximal interphalangeal (PIP) joint extension is a complex interplay between the extensor digitorum communis (EDC) tendon and the interosseous and lumbrical tendons [1]. Over the metacarpophalangeal (MCP) joint, the EDC is stabilized by the sagittal bands. There is no direct attachment to the proximal phalanx; MCP extension occurs via the sling of the lateral bands lifting up the proximal phalanx. Over the proximal phalanx, the extensor tendon trifurcates into the central slip and lateral slips (Figs. 35.1, 35.2, and 35.3). On the sides of the digit, the interossei and lumbrical tendons merge as lateral bands, bifurcating to blend with the central slip and to the lateral slips of the EDC, forming conjoined lateral bands. The central slip inserts at the dorsal base of the middle phalanx, applying an extension force at the PIP joint. The conjoined lateral bands proceed on the radial and ulnar sides of the PIP joint and then combine over the middle phalanx to form the terminal extensor tendon that inserts at the dorsal base of the distal phalanx, extending the DIP joint. The conjoint lateral bands are stabilized by the triangular ligament on the dorsal side of the middle phalanx, limiting volar migration, and by the transverse retinacular ligament on the volar side, limiting dorsal migration.

Boutonnière deformity is a condition in which the central slip (Figs. 35.2 and 35.3) of the extensor tendon and the triangular ligament are disrupted. The injury causes flexion at the proximal interphalangeal (PIP) joint in combination with volar migration of the lateral bands, resulting in hyperextension at the distal interphalangeal (DIP) joint [2].

Boutonnière deformities can be caused by attenuation of the central slip from chronic PIP synovitis (e.g., rheumatoid arthritis) or from trauma, including forced flexion of the digit, open laceration, or volar dislocation of the PIP joint. These mechanisms cause disruption to the central slip and triangular ligament [2]. The extent of deformity is classified into four Burton stages:

- Stage I is a supple, passively correctable deformity.
- Stage II is a fixed contracture with contracted lateral bands and no joint involvement.
- Stage III involves volar plate and collateral ligament contractures with intra-articular fibrosis.
- Stage IV involves volar plate and collateral ligament contractures, intra-articular fibrosis, and PIP joint arthritis.

Swan neck deformity is a condition in which a disruption to the volar plate of the PIP joint leads to the classic appearance of hyperextension at the PIP joint and flexion at the DIP joint (Fig. 35.2) [2]. There are three general categories of swan neck deformities: extrinsic, intrinsic, and articular. Extrinsic causes include mallet finger or flexor digitorum superficialis (FDS) tendon disruption in patients with volar plate laxity or posttraumatic MCP joint flexion contractures that increase tension on the extensor tendons. Intrinsic causes include intrinsic muscle contracture related to chronic MCP joint volar ulnar subluxation (e.g., rheumatoid arthritis). Articular causes include volar plate disruption or arthritis.

M. Shields
Department of Orthopaedics and Rehabilitation Medicine, Tufts Medical Center, Boston, MA, USA
e-mail: mshields@tuftsmedicalcenter.org

A. Felber
Tufts University School of Medicine, Boston, MA, USA

C. Cassidy (✉)
Department of Orthopedic & Rehabilitation Medicine, Tufts University School of Medicine, Tufts Medical Center, Boston, MA, USA
e-mail: ccassidy@tuftsmedicalcenter.org

© The Author(s), under exclusive license to Springer Nature Switzerland AG 2022
S. A. Mostoufi et al. (eds.), *Clinical Guide to Musculoskeletal Medicine*, https://doi.org/10.1007/978-3-030-92042-5_35

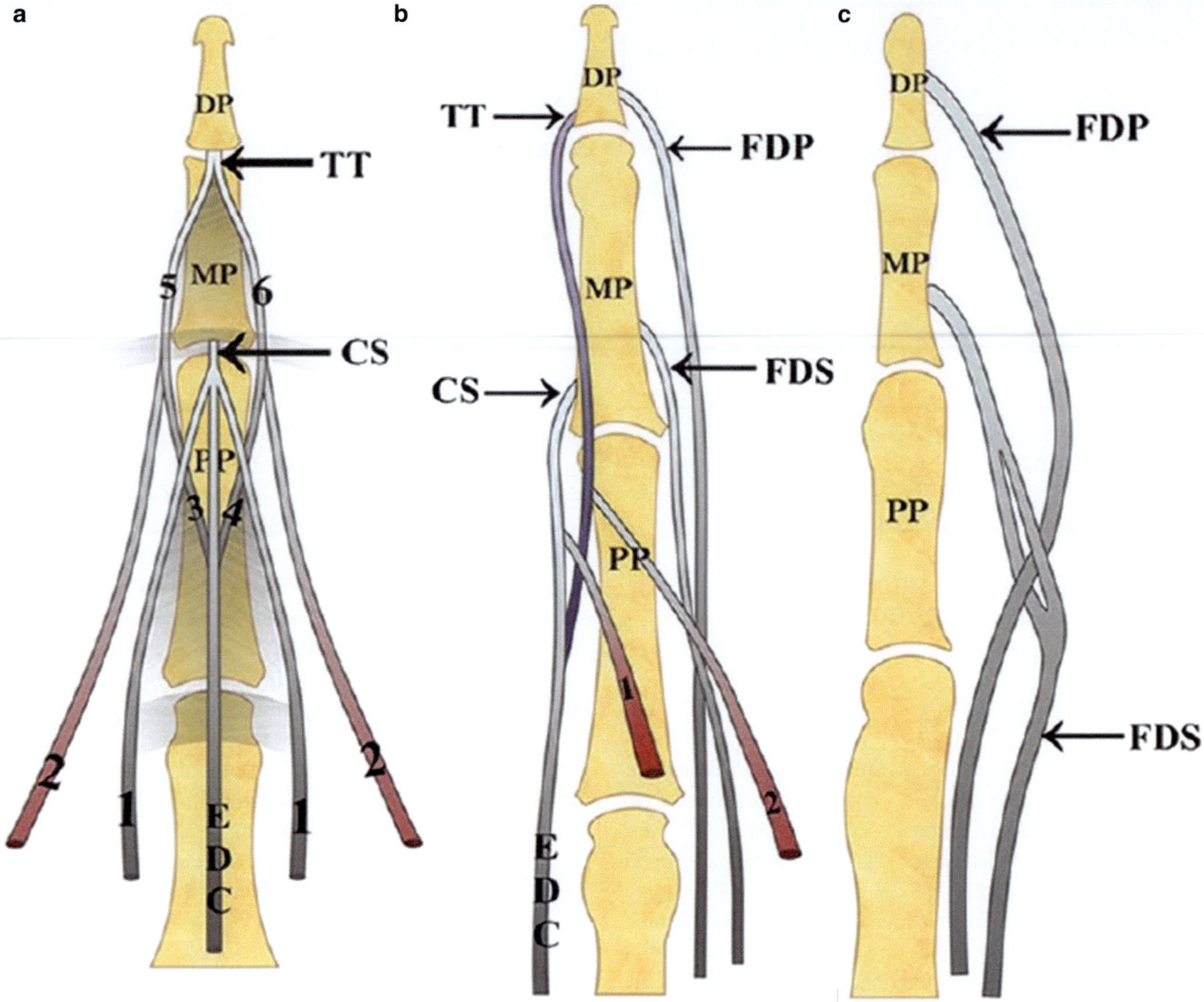

Fig. 35.1 This illustration depicts the complex anatomy of the extensor mechanism of the digits of the hand mechanism. (**a**) Diagrammatic representation of the dorsal aspect and (**b**) the lateral aspect of the finger to show the flexor and extensor tendons of the finger including the CS and the TT. (**c**) Schematic drawing of the finger showing the FDS and FDP. EDC, extensor digitorum communis; PP, proximal phalanx; MP, middle phalanx; DP, distal phalanx; 1, interosseous muscle; 2, lumbrical muscle; 3, lateral slip; 4, medial slip; 5, lateral conjoined tendon; 6, medial conjoined tendon; FDS, flexor digitorum superficialis; FDP, flexor digitorum profundus; CS, central slip; TT, terminal tendon. (Open access image Chin Med J (Engl). 2018 May 5; 131(9): 1051–1058)

35.1.3 Clinical Presentation

- *Boutonnière deformity*: The classic presentation of a boutonnière deformity is a patient with recent trauma who reports a painful finger deformity with flexion at the PIP joint and hyperextension at the DIP joint.
- *Swan neck deformity*: The typical presentation of a swan neck deformity is a patient with a history of inflammatory arthritis or previous trauma with hyperextension of the PIP joint and flexion of the DIP joint. They often report a locking sensation of the finger as it is flexed from a fully extended position and occasionally report pain (for the differential diagnosis, see Table 35.1).

35.1.4 Physical Examination

Inspect the fingers for abrasions, lacerations, swelling, or deformity. Look for signs of inflammatory arthritis such as involvement of multiple joints. Palpate along the length of the finger assessing for tenderness or warmth. Assess active (with and without resistance) and passive range of motion (ROM) at the DIP, PIP, and MCP joints. Normal ROM includes DIP from 0 to 90° flexion, PIP from 0 to 100° flexion, and MCP from +30° to −90° flexion. A snapping sensation may occur during flexion with a swan neck deformity. Always do a thorough neurovascular exam.

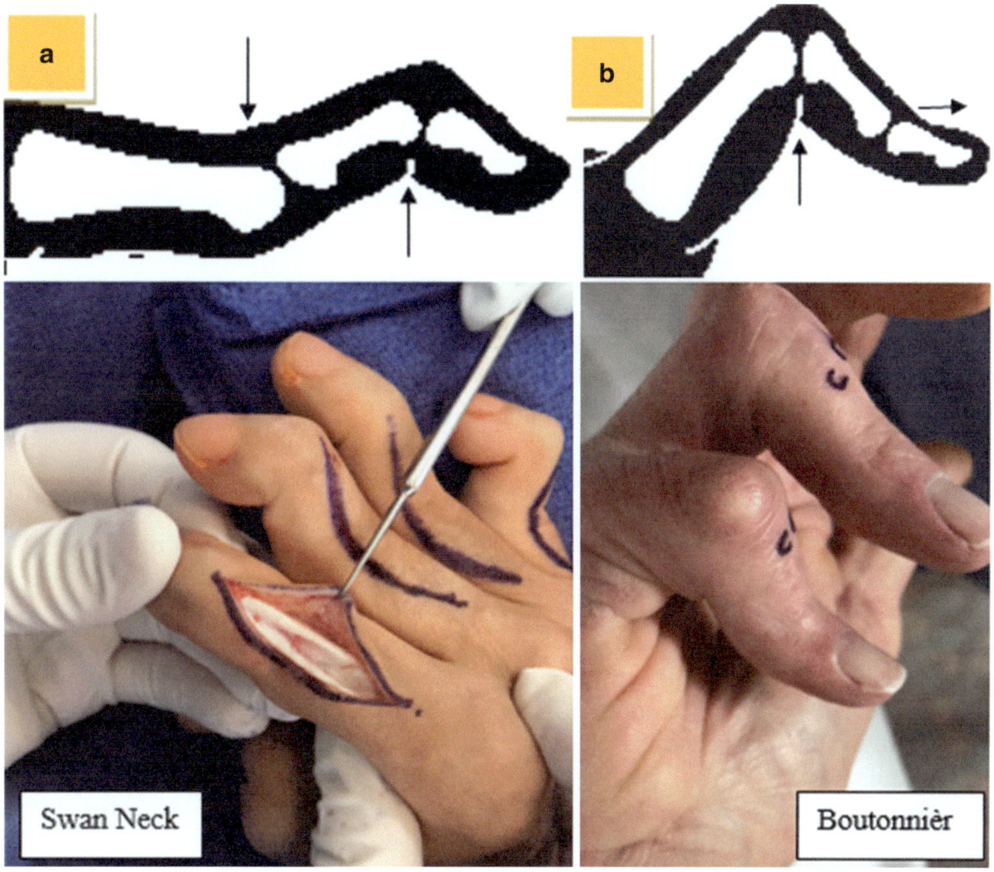

Fig. 35.2 Swan neck deformity (**a**) and boutonnière deformity (**b**)

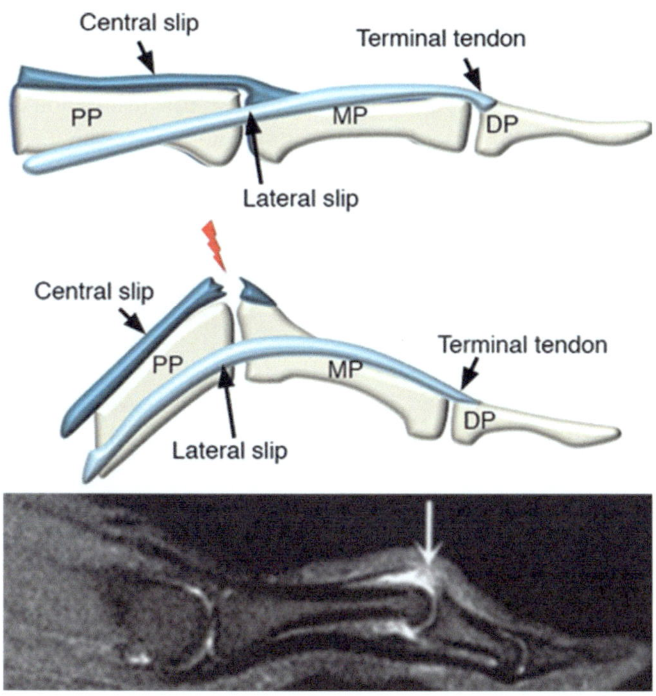

Fig. 35.3 Boutonnière deformity illustration and MR. Boutonnière deformity is an injury involving the central slip of the extensor tendon over the proximal interphalangeal joint. DP, distal phalanx; MP, middle phalanx; PP, proximal phalanx. (Open access image Chin Med J (Engl). 2018; 131(9): 1051–1058. and www.e-ultrasonography.org)

35.1.4.1 Special Test

- *Elson's test*: This test is the most reliable in assessing for boutonnière deformity [3]. The physician holds the PIP joint in 90° flexion and the patient actively extends the PIP joint against resistance. If a central slip injury is present, there will be weak PIP extension and a rigid DIP joint. If no injury is present, the PIP extension is strong and the DIP joint is passively flexible.
- *Bunnel test*: This test assesses intrinsic muscle tightness in the setting of swan neck deformities. The MCP joint is held in extension while passively flexing the PIP joint, noting the ROM. The test is then repeated with the MCP joint in the flexed position. If passive PIP joint flexion is limited with the MCP extended, but full with the MCP flexed, then intrinsic tightness is present.

35.1.5 Diagnostic Workup

For both swan neck and boutonnière deformities, plain radiographs of the injured finger should be obtained. Treatment plans may be altered by the presence of arthritis or fractures on radiographs. Occasionally, central slip injuries can involve a bony avulsion fracture and swan neck deformities can be

Table 35.1 Differential diagnoses for the common finger disorders

Boutonnière deformity	Swan neck deformity	Dupuytren's contracture	Mallet finger	Skier's thumb	Trigger finger
Rheumatoid arthritis Pseudo boutonnière deformity	Mallet finger Rheumatoid arthritis Flexor digitorum superficialis injury	Trigger finger Skin callus Soft tissue tumor Ulnar nerve palsy	Swan neck deformity Rheumatoid arthritis	Dislocation of the thumb MCP joint Wrist sprain or fracture Fracture of the thumb proximal phalanx or metacarpal	Dupuytren's contracture Sagittal band rupture Inflammatory arthritis Soft tissue tumor

associated with a bony mallet or an avulsion of the PIP volar plate [1]. Advanced studies such as ultrasound or magnetic resonance imaging (MRI) are rarely required.

35.1.6 Treatments

35.1.6.1 Medical Management

Conservative management is the preferred first line of treatment for patients who present with an acute, closed boutonnière injury (Burton stage I) and is often preferred for chronic, fixed boutonnière deformities (Burton stage II) as well. Conservative management includes specific splinting and rehabilitation protocols (see the next section).

Conservative management is also indicated in patients with mild swan neck deformities that have full active flexion of the PIP joint. These patients frequently report pain when initiating PIP flexion due to the hyperextension deformity and occasionally report snapping with PIP flexion due to lateral band subluxation. These patients typically benefit from splinting and rehabilitation.

35.1.6.2 Rehabilitation

Rehabilitation management for acute boutonnière deformity (Burton stage I) includes relative motion flexion splint or splinting of the PIP in extension for 4–12 weeks [2, 4]. The purpose of these splinting techniques is to decrease tension across the central slip to allow for healing, to allow the lateral bands to migrate dorsally, and to prevent progression to a boutonnière deformity. To prevent lateral band volar subluxation, active DIP flexion exercises should be initiated during the splinting phase. McKeon et al. advocate for full-time extension splinting for 4–8 weeks, followed by nighttime splinting for 4–6 additional weeks while beginning active PIP flexion exercises.

For a fixed flexion contracture, serial PIP extension casting is performed until the patient can comfortably be placed into a dynamic PIP extension splint for daytime use and a static extension splint at night. Splinting must be continued for at least 8–12 weeks. Focus should still be maintained on active DIP flexion exercises to prevent volar migration of the lateral bands.

For swan neck deformities due to an acute mallet finger, the DIP joint should be immobilized in full extension for 8 weeks. For supple swan neck due to other causes, rehabilitation includes splinting (e.g., oval 8 splints), which limit PIP hyperextension while allowing PIP flexion.

35.1.6.3 Procedures

For chronic, supple boutonnière deformities, ultrasound-guided percutaneous extensor tenotomy over the middle phalanx level can rebalance the finger, relaxing the extensor force over the DIP joint and transferring the force to the PIP joint. Iatrogenic mallet finger is a complication of this method of treatment.

35.1.6.4 Surgery

Operative indications for acute boutonnière deformity include open injuries, especially those associated with large avulsion fragments. Irrigation and debridement are followed by surgical repair of the central slip or bone fragment. This repair is followed by pinning of the PIP joint in extension for 4–6 weeks. In chronic boutonnière deformity, restoration of full passive PIP extension is required before performing any tendon procedure and is achieved via serial casting, dynamic extension splinting, dynamic external fixation, or joint contracture release. Tendon rebalancing procedures range from a simple extensor tenotomy to complex central slip reconstructions. It is important to counsel patients that the results are somewhat unpredictable. PIP arthrodesis is recommended for concomitant PIP arthritis.

Surgery is indicated for treatment of swan neck deformity in patients who are not amenable to splint wear or those with severe deformity. Options include soft tissue procedures to limit PIP hyperextension with or without arthrodesis of the DIP joint. Postoperatively, the PIP is splinted in 30° of flexion for 3 weeks with gradual restoration of extension. In the setting of intrinsic tightness, release of the intrinsic tendon at the MCP joint level can rebalance the digit. Associated PIP joint stiffness must be corrected before or during the tendon rebalancing procedure. Associated arthritis is best treated with PIP arthroplasty or arthrodesis.

35.2 Dupuytren's Contracture

35.2.1 Synonyms and ICD 10 Code

- Dupuytren's disease
- ICD10, M72.0

35.2.2 Description

Dupuytren's contracture is a benign fibroproliferative disorder of the palmar fascia complex characterized by collagen deposition in the form of nodules and cords within the fascia (Fig. 35.3). The disease is often progressive, as evidenced by cords shortening with time, which leads to contractures and fixed flexion at the MCP and PIP joints [3].

Anatomy The palmar fascia complex of the hand is divided into three zones; the palmar fascia (includes the radial, ulnar, and central aponeuroses), the palmodigital fascia, and the digital fascia. The central aponeurosis (CA) is where most of Dupuytren's pathology occurs. It is triangular in shape with a proximal apex and fibers running longitudinally, transversely, and vertically [5]. Normal fascial structures are called bands, whereas the pathologic changes are termed cords. The longitudinal fibers of the CA are the pretendinous bands, which bifurcate distally before inserting at the three layers of the central digits. The superficial layer inserts into the dermis, the middle layer encircles the MCP joint forming the spiral band and then travels distally as the lateral digital sheet, and the deep layer inserts into the flexor and extensor mechanism. The CA transverse fibers are parallel and include the more distal natatory ligament located in the palmodigital region and the more proximal transverse ligament of the palmar aponeurosis (TLPA). The TLPA gives origin to the vertical fibers septa of Legueu and Juvara [5]. Continuing distally, the digital fascia encompasses the neurovascular structures with Grayson's ligament palmarly, Cleland's ligament dorsally, the lateral digital sheet laterally, and a retrovascular fascia medially.

The risk factors for Dupuytren's disease include genetic predisposition, alcohol abuse, smoking, manual labor, and vibrational exposure [3]. The pathophysiology of Dupuytren's contracture involves increased fibroblast proliferation leading to disordered type III collagen deposition. Fibroblasts differentiate into myofibroblasts, which are pathologic cells that produce excess collagen and also have a smooth muscle component that contributes to contracture formation [3, 5].

35.2.3 Clinical Presentation

Dupuytren's contracture first presents with slowly progressing palmar skin thickening, pitting, or well-defined, raised palmar nodules. It may be painful at first. In 50% of patients, the disease progresses with nodule regression and cord formation. Cord involvement usually starts in the palm and continues to the palmodigital area or digits (Fig. 35.4a).

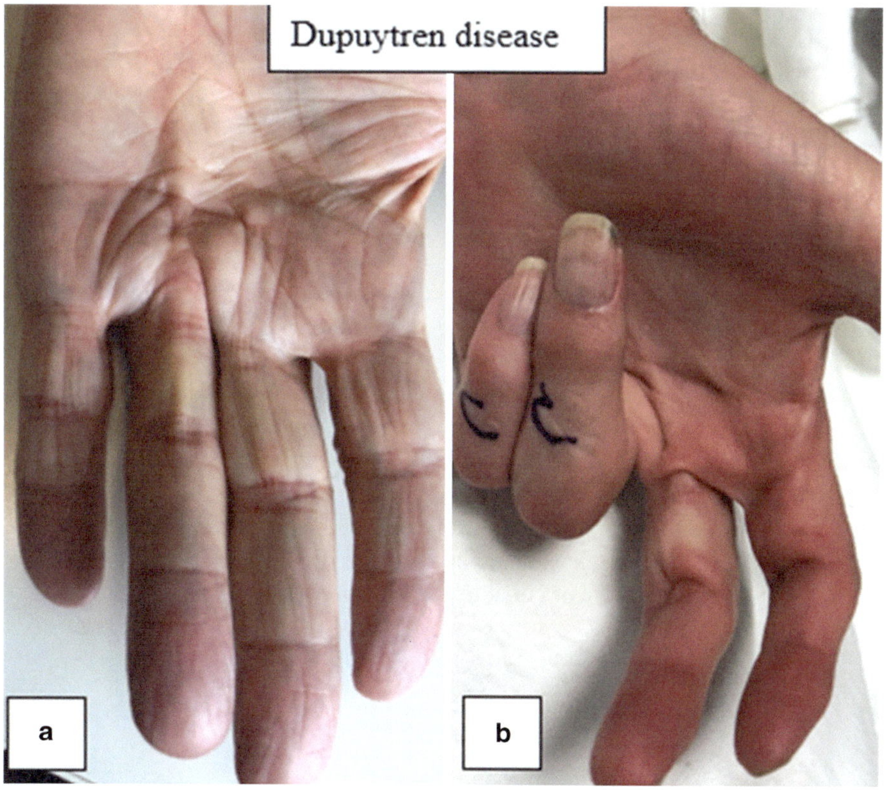

Fig. 35.4 (**a**) Early Dupuytren's disease involves the ring finger, with a nodule and cord in the palm in line with the ring finger, resulting in a mild MCP contracture. (**b**) Advanced Dupuytren's disease, with severe contractures of all digits, worst in the MCP and PIP of the ring and small fingers. (Photos courtesy of Charles Cassidy, MD)

Advanced disease presents with contractures at the MCP and PIP joints, most commonly on the ring finger (Fig. 35.4b).

35.2.4 Physical Examination

Inspect the hand for any dorsal skin changes including dorsal Dupuytren's nodules (Garrod's knuckle pads) or palmar skin changes such as skin rippling or dimpling caused by skin thickening and adherence. Palpate the palmar hand and digits for nodules, which are firm, well-defined masses that are fixed to the fascia. Simultaneously, feel for tight, tendon-like cords. Assess active and passive ROM at the PIP and MCP joints with and without resistance. Always do a thorough neurovascular exam (for the differential diagnosis, see Table 35.1).

35.2.4.1 Special Test

Hueston's tabletop test Place the palm of the hand on a flat surface. The test is positive if MCP or PIP contracture prevents the patient from completely flattening the hand against the surface.

35.2.5 Diagnostic Workup

No diagnostic workup is necessary in the evaluation of Dupuytren's disease.

35.2.6 Treatments

35.2.6.1 Medical Management

The most common form of noninvasive management of Dupuytren's disease is observation alone, as isolated nodules and isolated cord contractures do not always progress [6]. While many pharmacologic and radiation therapy interventions have been tested, they are not currently the mainstay of treatments.

35.2.6.2 Rehabilitation

Immobilization with splinting or casting and occupational therapy have not been proven to be successful in the preoperative period for patients with Dupuytren's disease.

35.2.6.3 Procedures

While many nonsurgical treatment options have been proposed for the management of Dupuytren's disease, the two most commonly performed are percutaneous needle aponeurotomy (PNA) and injection of collagenase *Clostridium histolyticum* (CCH).

- PNA is a technique involving the use of a needle to incrementally transect the contracted cord until the release has been achieved. It is attractive due to its minimal invasiveness, quick healing time, and rapid recovery. While short-term effectiveness has been shown to be comparable to surgical release [3], Pess et al. reviewed PNA in over 1000 fingers and demonstrated significant recurrence with patients maintaining 72% of correction at the MP joint and 31% at the PIP joints [7]. They found that correction was more likely to be maintained in older patients (>55 years old) and patients with MP joint contractures rather than PIP joint contractures.
- CCH is a technique that involves injection of an enzyme that lyses cord tissue, allowing the physician to manually rupture the cord on the following day [3]. Hurst et al. paved the way for CCH injections in their 2009 study where they performed as many as three CCH injections and manipulations at monthly intervals [8]. One month after the last injection, they found that 64% of patients had reduction of their contracture to <5° and range of motion of the involved joint improved from 44 to 80 degrees. However, as with PNA, long-term relief was not as reliable [8].

35.2.6.4 Surgery

Surgical management of Dupuytren's disease is generally indicated if a patient has >30° MCP contracture or any of PIP contracture [6]. Surgical options include fasciotomy, limited or radical fasciectomy, and dermatofasciectomy. Fasciotomy is minimally invasive, but the recurrence rate is high. Limited fasciectomy involves removal of the pathologic tissue alone. Dermatofasciectomy involves removal of the overlying skin in addition to the cord and placement of a skin graft. This is reserved primarily for revision surgery. Given the similar results of the latter three procedures, limited fasciectomy is generally the preferred treatment [3]. Leafblad et al. found significantly lower rates of re-intervention at 2 and 5 years post intervention for patients treated surgically (4% at 2 years, 4% at 5 years) versus PNA (24% at 2 years, 61% at 5 years) and CCH (41% at 2 years, 55% at 5 years) [9].

35.3 Mallet Finger

35.3.1 Synonyms and ICD 10 Code

- Mallet finger
- M20.012

35.3.2 Description

Mallet finger is the result of disruption of the terminal extensor tendon insertion on the base on the distal phalanx. This alters the balance of flexion and extension forces on the DIP joint, resulting in the inability to extend the joint (Fig. 35.5). For anatomy of mallet finger, please review the section Boutonnière and Swan Neck Deformity and its figures.

Mallet finger injury may occur from minor trauma such as pulling up stockings or from sports participation or workplace trauma [1]. In sports, the mechanism of injury is forced flexion or an axial–hyperextension load to the DIP joint. This force leads to tendon disruption or to a bony avulsion at the base of the distal phalanx. A laceration, crush injury, or deep abrasion may also cause open mallet finger injury [1, 10]. Mallet injuries are divided into four types based on Doyle's classification:

Type I is closed injuries either with or without an avulsion fracture.

Type II is open tendon injuries resulting from a laceration.

Type III is open injuries with soft tissue abrasions that cause loss of skin or tendon substance.

Type IV is mallet fractures subdivided into three sub-types:

- Sub-type IV: Distal phalanx physeal injuries (in pediatrics)
- Sub-type IVB: Fractures involving 20–50% of the articular surface
- Sub-type IVC: Fractures involve >50% of the articular surface

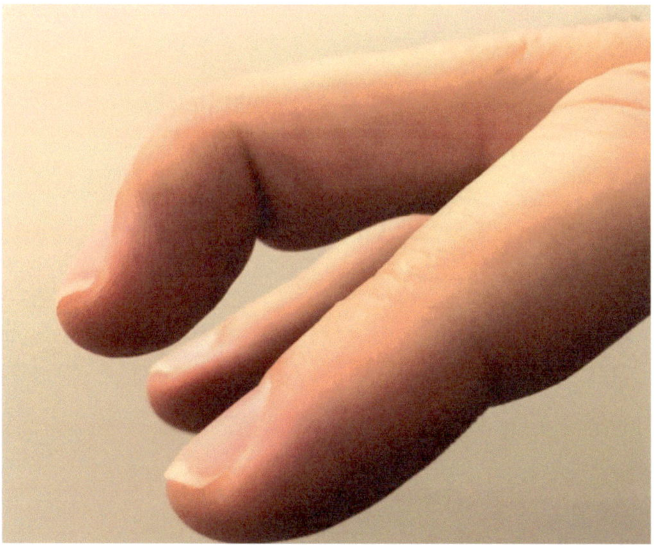

Fig. 35.5 Mallet finger

35.3.3 Clinical Presentation

Mallet finger classically presents as a flexed DIP joint of the affected digit. The long, ring, or small fingers of the dominant hand are most frequently injured [10].

35.3.4 Physical Examination

Inspect the finger for any abrasions, lacerations, swelling, and resting finger position. There may be local tenderness and swelling over the DIP joint. Assess active and passive ROM at the DIP joint bilaterally to look for symmetry. Patients with mallet finger will not be able to actively extend at the DIP, but the digit can usually be extended passively. Radiographs should be reviewed before performing stress testing. Patients with underlying ligamentous laxity may present with an acute swan neck deformity. The clinician should be aware that an extensor lag at the DIP joint does not always present immediately after injury and may be delayed hours to days (for the differential diagnosis, see Table 35.1) [1].

35.3.5 Diagnostic Workup

Radiographs are an important part of the evaluation for any patient with a suspected mallet finger. Clinicians should assess for bony avulsion fractures and joint congruence using the standard AP and lateral X-ray views.

35.3.6 Treatments

35.3.6.1 Medical Management

Splinting is the mainstay of treatment of mallet finger injuries. While the agreement on acceptable outcomes is variable, the general goal of treatment is to end up with minimal pain, less than 20° of residual DIP extension lag, and greater than 50° of DIP flexion arc [1].

35.3.6.2 Rehabilitation

The vast majority of mallet fingers are amenable to splinting as a primary treatment. Splinting is also indicated for closed mallet fingers with less than one-third articular surface fracture involvement and no joint subluxation. Studies have shown that extension or slight hyperextension splinting of the DIP joint alone provides sufficient decrease in tension to allow healing [1]. Splints should be used for 8 weeks full time and then at nighttime for an additional 2 weeks. Outcomes are excellent with appropriate splint wear, as many studies have shown high patient satisfaction and extensor lag of the DIP joint <10° at five-year follow-up. Casting is rare but can be utilized in patients who are noncompliant with splinting and in children.

35.3.6.3 Procedures

Manipulation and percutaneous DIP joint Kirschner wire fixation is an option for patients who are unable to work with splints, such as healthcare workers.

35.3.6.4 Surgery

Please refer to chapter "Surgical Management of Mallet Finger Injuries."

35.4 Thumb Sprain (Skier's Thumb)

35.4.1 Synonyms

Thumb collateral ligament injury, Ulnar collateral ligament (UCL) injury, UCL avulsion fracture, Gamekeeper's thumb

35.4.2 ICD 10 Code

S63.642

35.4.3 Description

Skier's thumb is a condition in which the ulnar collateral ligament (UCL) of the thumb MCP joint is injured by a radial stress on the joint, resulting in pain, disability, and joint instability.

Anatomy The thumb MCP joint is a condyloid joint that achieves static stability from a flattened metacarpal head coupled with the UCL, radial collateral ligament (RCL), volar plate, and dorsal capsule [11]. The UCL and RCL are comprised of proper and accessory components (Fig. 35.6). The proper UCL attaches to the side of the metacarpal head and the proximal volar aspect of the proximal phalanx, whereas the accessory UCL attaches to the volar plate. The proper ligament resists lateral force when the thumb is flexed, while the accessory ligament resists load when the thumb is in extension. There are also intrinsic and extrinsic muscles and tendons that provide dynamic support to the thumb MCP joint.

Acute injury to the UCL most often occurs during skiing, sports, or falls on the thumb due to a radially directed force on the thumb resulting in hyperabduction. In 90% of the cases, the force causes the UCL to avulse with or without a bony attachment from the proximal phalanx. The distal end of the avulsed ligament may become entrapped proximal to the aponeurosis of the adductor pollicis muscle, causing a Stener lesion. The extent of joint instability is classified into three grades:

- Grade 1 injury: incomplete ligament tear with no joint instability
- Grade 2 injury: incomplete tear with asymmetric joint laxity with an endpoint
- Grade 3 injury: complete tear with joint instability that lacks a firm end point

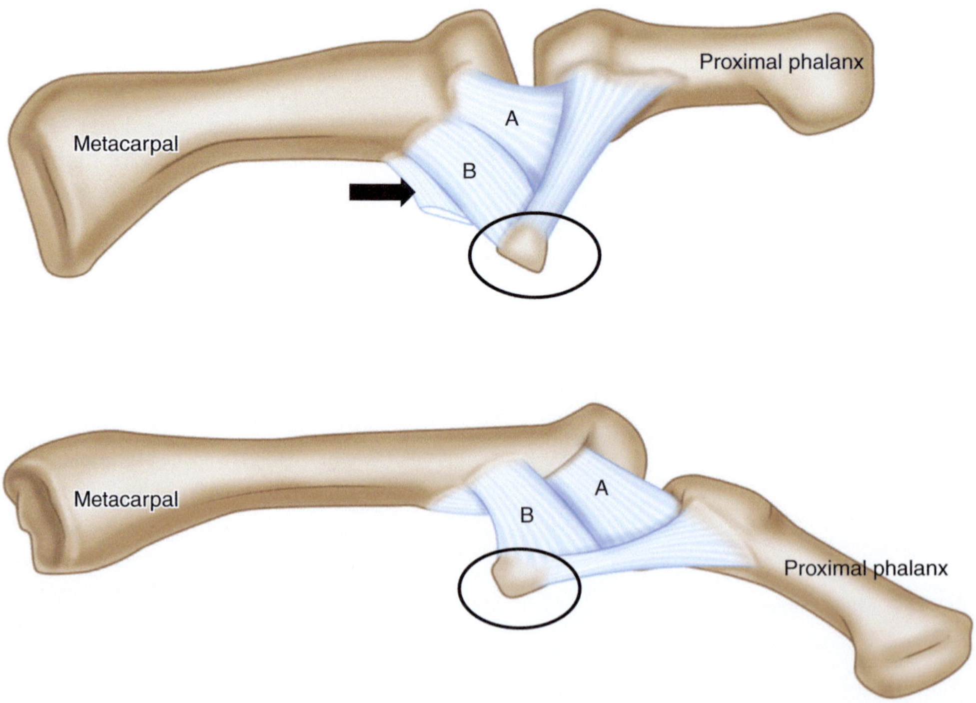

Fig. 35.6 This figure shows UCL ligaments. (**a**) is the proper collateral (PC) ligament and (**b**) is accessory collateral (AC) ligament. The volar plate is pointed out by an arrow. The sesamoid bone is highlighted by a circle. The volar plate and AC ligament are taught in interphalangeal joint extension, while the PC ligament is taught in flexion (Illustration reproduced by Yamine Mostoufi)

35.4.4 Clinical Presentation

Skier's thumb can present with acute thumb pain localized around the MCP joint that is exacerbated with pinch or grasp movement such as writing or turning a key. The patient often reports acute hyperabduction of the thumb leading to associated swelling, ecchymosis, and decreased ROM.

35.4.5 Physical Examination

Inspect the hands for any swelling, ecchymosis, and static deformity of the MCP. Palpate the ulnar aspect of the MCP joint and dorsal capsule to assess for tenderness. Occasionally, Stener lesions can present with a tender mass on the ulnar side of the metacarpal head from the avulsed UCL. Assess active and passive ROM at the thumb interphalangeal (IP) and MCP joints. Normal IP ROM is +1–80° flexion and MCP joint is +0–55° flexion [12]. Assess muscle strength with pinching and gripping activities (for the differential diagnosis, see Table 35.1).

35.4.5.1 Special Tests

Radial stress test Apply a radial stress to the proximal phalanx while holding the metacarpal stable. Evaluate stability with the thumb MCP joint in 0° extension and 30° flexion. Joint instability is defined as radial deviation of the proximal phalanx of greater than 30°. With partial tears, the joint is typically lax in flexion and stable in extension. Patient guarding may interfere with an accurate evaluation requiring intra-articular block or local anesthesia.

35.4.6 Diagnostic Workup

Radiographs should be a routine part of a complete examination for a patient with a suspected thumb UCL injury. Specific attention should be made to evaluate for fractures and joint subluxation or dislocation. Instability can be tested using stress radiographs. While the diagnosis typically is made based on physical exam and radiographs, if the diagnosis is unclear, either ultrasonography (specificity 81% and sensitivity 76%) or MRI (specificity and sensitivity 100%) can be utilized to confirm a complete tear in the UCL.

35.4.7 Treatment

35.4.7.1 Medical Management

There is no indication for medical management of UCL tears. However, splinting in the acute phase can be used for localized pain control.

35.4.7.2 Rehabilitation

Thumb spica cast or splint (without incorporation of the IP joint) immobilization for 4 weeks is indicated for incomplete (grade 1 and 2) UCL tears and complete (grade 3) tears that are not associated with a Stener lesion. Active and passive motion should be initiated at 4 weeks or sooner if the splint is removable, being cautious to avoid radial/ulnar stress at the MP joint. This is followed by grip and pinch strength at 6 weeks. Restrictions for return to sports are different for the dominant versus non-dominant extremity. The non-dominant thumb should be protected for sports activities for at least 3 months. For the throwing athlete, the dominant thumb should be protected for a longer period of time and the protection may interfere with performance. The protection is these cases must be determined on a case-by-case basis.

35.4.7.3 Procedures

There are no procedures indicated for treatment of skier's thumb.

35.4.7.4 Surgery

Please refer to chapter "Surgical Management of Mallet Finger Injuries."

35.5 Trigger Finger

35.5.1 Synonyms and ICD 10 Code

- Trigger thumb, M65.312
- Trigger finger index, M65.322
- Trigger finger middle, M65.332
- Trigger finger ring, M65.342
- Trigger finger little, M65.352

35.5.2 Description

Trigger finger (TF) is a condition in which fibrous thickening of either the flexor tendon or A1 pulley impedes smooth flexor tendon gliding. The mechanical impingement can present with progressive palmar pain, along with clicking, catching, and locking of the digit [13].

Anatomy The flexor tendon sheath is a complex system of retinacular structures also known as pulleys (see Fig. 35.7). The flexor pulley system consists of the palmar aponeurosis pulley, three cruciform pulleys, and five annular pulleys. The pulleys maintain proper alignment of the flexor digitorum profundus (FDP) and FDS tendons and translate flexion force efficiently. TF is associated with pathology in the first annular pulley (A1 pulley). The A1 pulley originates in the region of the palmar plate of the MCP joint and travels dis-

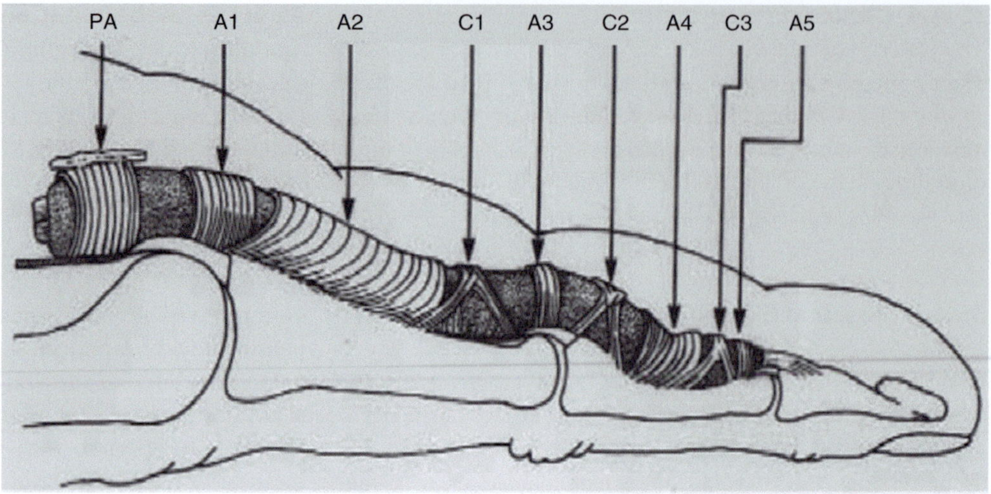

Fig. 35.7 This illustration displays the flexor pulley system in the digits of the hand, including the palmar aponeurosis (PA) pulley, the five annular pulleys (A1–5), and the three cruciate pulleys (C1–3). (Reprinted with permission from Doyle [14])

tally to the proximal portion of the proximal phalanx, encompassing the flexor tendons throughout its course [15].

Although the etiology of TF is likely multifactorial and not well understood, it is more commonly seen in females, patients who perform repetitive tasks with their fingers, and patients with inflammatory arthritis and systemic conditions such as diabetes mellitus and hypothyroidism [13]. The impairment in smooth tendon gliding is caused by hypertrophy of either the A1 pulley or flexor tendon, often at the proximal end of the interface. The disease severity is classified by Green [16]:

- Grade I (pre-triggering) is palm pain and tenderness over the A1 pulley.
- Grade II (active) demonstrates catching with preserved active extension at the PIP joint.
- Grade III (passive) demonstrates catching of the digit requiring passive extension to release.
- Grade IV (contracture) is a fixed flexion contracture at the PIP joint.

35.5.3 Clinical Presentation

The typical presentation of TF is painful clicking or locking of the affected digit, most commonly involving the middle and ring fingers and the thumb. There may be swelling and tenderness in the palm.

35.5.4 Physical Examination

Inspect the fingers and hands for any swelling or finger locking in the flexed position. Palpate the A1 pulley on the palmar surface of the hand at the head of the metacarpals. Assess for tenderness to palpation or warmth. Passively flex and extend the digit fully while palpating for a nodule. Assess active and passive ROM at the PIP and MCP joints, with and without resistance. Observe for any locking of the PIP joint in the flexed position with active ROM. Pain and impaired ability to grasp and hold objects may be observed with TF (for the differential diagnosis, see Table 35.1).

35.5.5 Diagnostic Workup

The diagnosis of trigger finger is primarily made through the patient's history and physical examination. Although rarely utilized, ultrasonography can visualize pathology at the tendon pulley interface if confirmation of diagnosis is needed [13]. There is no utility for radiographs or advanced imaging.

35.5.6 Treatment

35.5.6.1 Medical Management

NSAIDs can help reduce inflammation and pain. NSAIDS are often utilized in conjunction with either immobilization or cortisone injections to provide adequate symptomatic relief.

35.5.6.2 Rehabilitation

Full-time splint immobilization for 6–12 weeks can be performed to decrease the amount of tendon excursion, thereby decreasing pain and improving function [13, 17]. Only one joint (DIP, PIP, or MCP) needs to be immobilized to decrease tendon gliding. Studies have shown that PIP joint blocking orthoses have superior compliance and functional outcomes over MCP joint blocking orthoses, and MCP orthoses provides better pain relief than DIP orthoses [13, 17]. The success rate of splinting for management of trigger finger ranges from 47% to 93% [17].

35.5.6.3 Procedures

Flexor tendon sheath steroid injection is an effective option for TF. The response rates range from 45% to 80% [13]. The success rate of steroid injection is lower for patients of a younger age, diabetic patients, long-standing triggering (>6 months), and patients with multiple trigger fingers. Steroids can be repeated up to three times before the cost-effectiveness of surgical release outweighs another injection.

35.5.6.4 Surgery

Surgical treatment for trigger finger includes either percutaneous or open A1 pulley release. Open release is currently the gold standard; however, recent studies have shown that percutaneous release is a safe and effective alternative to open release. The success rates of open TF release range from 90% to 100% [13]. If open TF surgery does not provide symptomatic relief, additional procedures may be indicated, including release of the palmar aponeurosis pulley, the proximal A2 pulley, and the FDS tendon slip excision.

References

1. Bendre AA, Hartigan BJ, Kalainov DM. Mallet finger. J Am Acad Orthop Surg. 2005;13(5):336–44.
2. McKeon KE, Lee DH. Posttraumatic boutonnière and swan neck deformities. J Am Acad Orthop Surg. 2015;23(10):623–32.
3. Gil JA, Akelman MR, Hresko AM, Akelman E. Current concepts in the management of Dupuytren disease of the hand. J Am Acad Orthop Surg. 2021;29(11):462–9.
4. Merritt WH, Wong AL, Lalonde DH. Recent developments are changing extensor tendon management. Plast Reconstr Surg. 2020;145(3)
5. Rayan GM. Dupuytren's disease: anatomy, pathology, and presentation. In: Eaton C, Seegenschmiedt M, Bayat A, Gabbiani G, Werker P, Wach W, editors. Dupuytren's disease and related hyperproliferative disorders. Berlin, Heidelberg: Springer; 2012.
6. Black EM, Blazar PE. Dupuytren disease: an evolving understanding of an age-old disease. Am Acad Orthop Surg. 2011;19(12):746–57.
7. Pess GM, Pess RM, Pess RA. Results of needle aponeurotomy for Dupuytren contracture in over 1,000 fingers. J Hand Surg Am. 2012;37(4):651–6.
8. Hurst LC, Badalamente MA, Hentz VR, Hotchkiss RN, Kaplan FT, Meals RA, Smith TM, Rodzvilla J, CORD I Study Group. Injectable collagenase clostridium histolyticum for Dupuytren's contracture. N Engl J Med. 2009;361(10):968–79.
9. Leafblad ND, Wagner E, Wanderman NR, et al. Outcomes and direct costs of needle aponeurotomy, collagenase injection, and fasciectomy in the treatment of Dupuytren contracture. J Hand Surg Am. 2019;44(11):919–27.
10. Lamaris GA, Matthew MK. The diagnosis and management of mallet finger injuries. Hand. 2016;12(3):223–8.
11. Tang P. Collateral ligament injuries of the thumb metacarpophalangeal joint. J Am Acad Orthop Surg. 2011;19(5):287–96.
12. Normal range of motion reference values. http://www.eatonhand.com/nor/nor002.htm. Accessed 19 Apr 2021.
13. Gil JA, Hresko AM, Weiss A-PC. Current concepts in the management of trigger finger in adults. J Am Acad Orthop Surg. 2020;28(15):642–50.
14. Doyle JR. Anatomy of the finger flexor tendon sheath and pulley system. J Hand Surg. 1988;13A:473–84.
15. Doyle JR. Palmar and digital flexor tendon pulleys. Clin Orthop Relat Res. 2001;383:84–96.
16. Green D, Green D, Hotchkisss R, Pederson W, Wolfe S. Green's operative hand surgery. 5th ed. Philadelphia: Livingston; 2005.
17. Lunsford D, Valdes K, Hengy S. Conservative management of trigger finger: a systematic review. J Hand Ther. 2019;32(2):212–21.

Wrist and Hand Dislocations and Fractures

36

Gabriel S. Perrone, Nicholas J. Coccoluto, Jennifer Hoffman, and Charles Cassidy

36.1 Distal Radius Fracture

36.1.1 Synonyms

- Colles' fracture
- Smith's fracture
- Barton's fracture
- Fracture of the forearm

36.1.2 ICD 10 Code

S52.50–S52.59

36.1.3 Description

Anatomy The distal radius has two articulations, the distal articular surface, which articulates with the scaphoid and lunate, and the sigmoid notch, which articulates with the head of the ulna [1, 2, 10]. These joints are stabilized, respectively, by the volar extrinsic and distal radioulnar ligaments (Fig. 36.1), permitting axial load transmission. The metaphyseal cortex is relatively thin and susceptible to fracture, particularly in the setting of osteoporosis.

Distal radius fractures are among the most common orthopedic injuries, accounting for 20% of all fractures seen in the emergency department [1]. The injury is equally likely to occur in both males and females, with the vast majority being the result of a traumatic incident in which the patient falls onto an outstretched hand [1–4]. There is a bimodal age distribution, with fractures in younger patients typically the result of high-energy injuries and geriatric fractures the result of low-energy falls. The Colles' fracture, an extra-articular, dorsally angulated, shortened fracture, is the most common type [1]. Fractures can also involve the articular surface (intra-articular fractures), which can predispose to arthritis if displaced [1, 5]. Of note, over 50% of distal radius fractures are associated with fracture of the ulnar styloid, with possible disruption of the radioulnar ligaments [2, 6–9]. Closed reduction and cast treatment are usually adequate for simple fracture patterns in younger patients. Comminuted (multi-fragmentary), displaced, intra-articular fractures are often best treated surgically. The most common long-term complication of this injury is malunion, which may result in chronic pain, wrist stiffness, and arthritis. Differential diagnosis for distal radius fracture is presented in Table 36.1.

36.1.4 Clinical Presentation

Patients sustaining distal radius fractures commonly report having fallen onto an outstretched hand. In the elderly, such fractures raise the suspicion of osteoporosis. Patients usually describe an acute onset of wrist pain and may have numbness and tingling in the median nerve distribution. They often will have difficulty moving the wrist and fingers.

36.1.5 Physical Examination

In addition to ruling out other associated trauma, physical examination of a patient with a suspected distal radius fracture involves a focused musculoskeletal examination.

Inspection The affected wrist may be grossly deformed, with swelling and ecchymosis. Examination for any lacerations or open wounds should be done circumferentially to exclude an open fracture.

G. S. Perrone · C. Cassidy (✉)
Department of Orthopedic Surgery, Tufts University School of Medicine, Boston, MA, USA
e-mail: ccassidy@tuftsmedicalcenter.org

J. Hoffman
Department of Orthopaedics & Rehabilitation Medicine, Tufts University School of Medicine, Boston, MA, USA

N. J. Coccoluto
Tufts University School of Medicine, Boston, MA, USA

© The Author(s), under exclusive license to Springer Nature Switzerland AG 2022

S. A. Mostoufi et al. (eds.), *Clinical Guide to Musculoskeletal Medicine*, https://doi.org/10.1007/978-3-030-92042-5_36

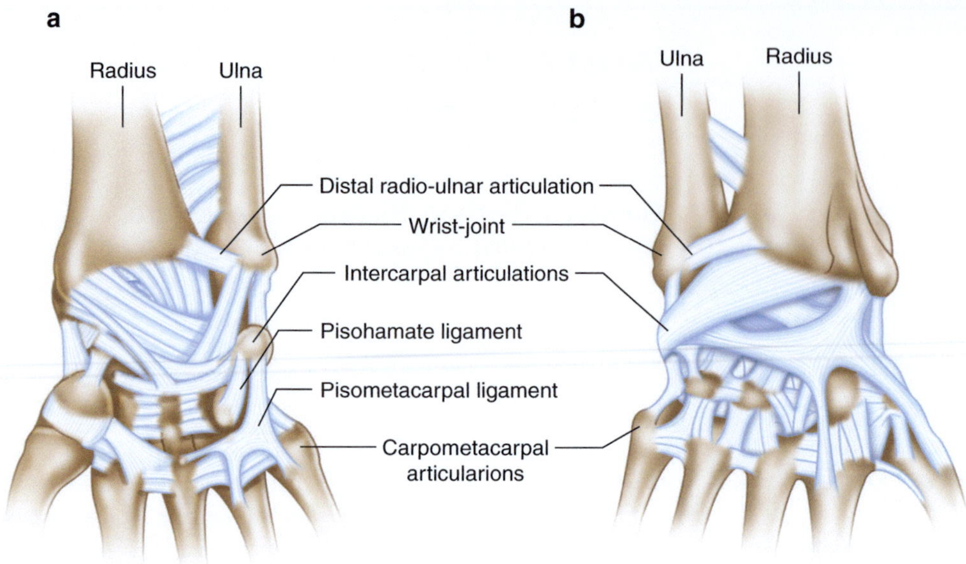

Fig. 36.1 Volar (**a**) and dorsal (**b**) views of the wrist with associated ligamentous attachments. (Courtesy of Williams et al. 2020)

Table 36.1 Differential diagnosis for distal radius fracture

Scapholunate ligament tear
Scaphoid fracture
Kienbock's disease
Extensor tenosynovitis
Lunotriquetral tear

Palpation Tenderness is present, particularly over Lister's tubercle. Patients typically have intact distal pulses and capillary refill.

Neurovascular Sensation to the hand is normally intact, although numbness in median nerve distribution can occur due to contusion of the median nerve or compression due to swelling in the carpal tunnel. The hand should be warm and well perfused, but checking the radial and ulnar pulses is a must with any wrist fracture.

Strength Strength is likely to be diminished due to pain and fracture instability.

Range of motion Wrist motion is often limited due to pain. Patients usually retain the ability to manipulate their fingers although many will endorse pain due to finger flexor and extensor tendons crossing near the fracture site.

36.1.6 Diagnostic Workup

Radiographs

Routine X-ray evaluation of a suspected distal radius fracture includes posteroanterior (PA), lateral, and oblique views (Fig. 36.2) [1, 11]. The images are scrutinized for displacement, including angulation, translation, comminution, shortening, and intra-articular extension. If a reduction maneuver is performed, repeat radiographs are obtained to evaluate the adequacy of the reduction [1].

Computed Tomography

Computed tomography (CT) provides an enhanced level of detail over plain radiographs and may be useful in complex cases, occult fractures (Fig. 36.3), or those with significant articular involvement and displacement [1]. The CT scan can inform the surgeon as to the best approach and method of fixation for a given fracture.

Magnetic Resonance Imaging

Magnetic resonance imaging (MRI) is not typically used in evaluating acute distal radius fractures. However, this modality may be of benefit in evaluating concomitant soft tissue injuries, such as scapholunate ligament or triangular fibrocartilage tears, or occult fractures. [1, 11]

36.1.7 Treatment

The goal in treating distal radius fractures is to achieve appropriate alignment to preserve wrist and hand function. This can be achieved through both operative and nonoperative means depending on the fracture pattern, bone quality, adequacy of reduction, and articular involvement.

Medical Management

Immobilization is the mainstay of treatment for distal radius fractures. Nondisplaced fractures can be treated with immobilization alone, typically with a plaster splint acutely and subsequently transitioned to a cast after a few days once the swelling has subsided. For displaced fractures, closed reduc-

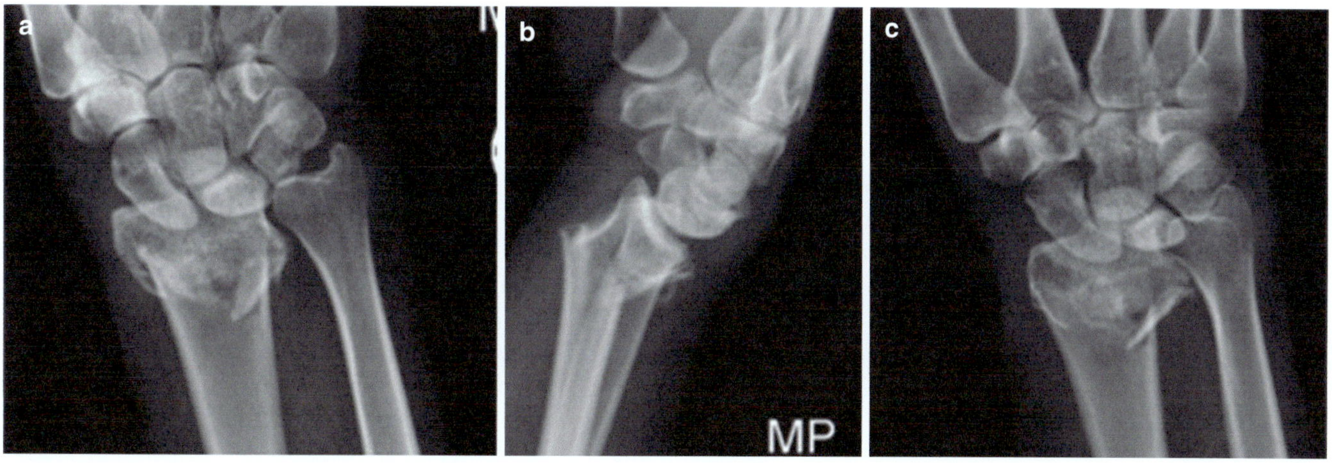

Fig. 36.2 PA (**a**), lateral (**b**), and oblique (**c**) radiographs demonstrating a comminuted, dorsally displaced distal radius fracture. (Figures from author's library)

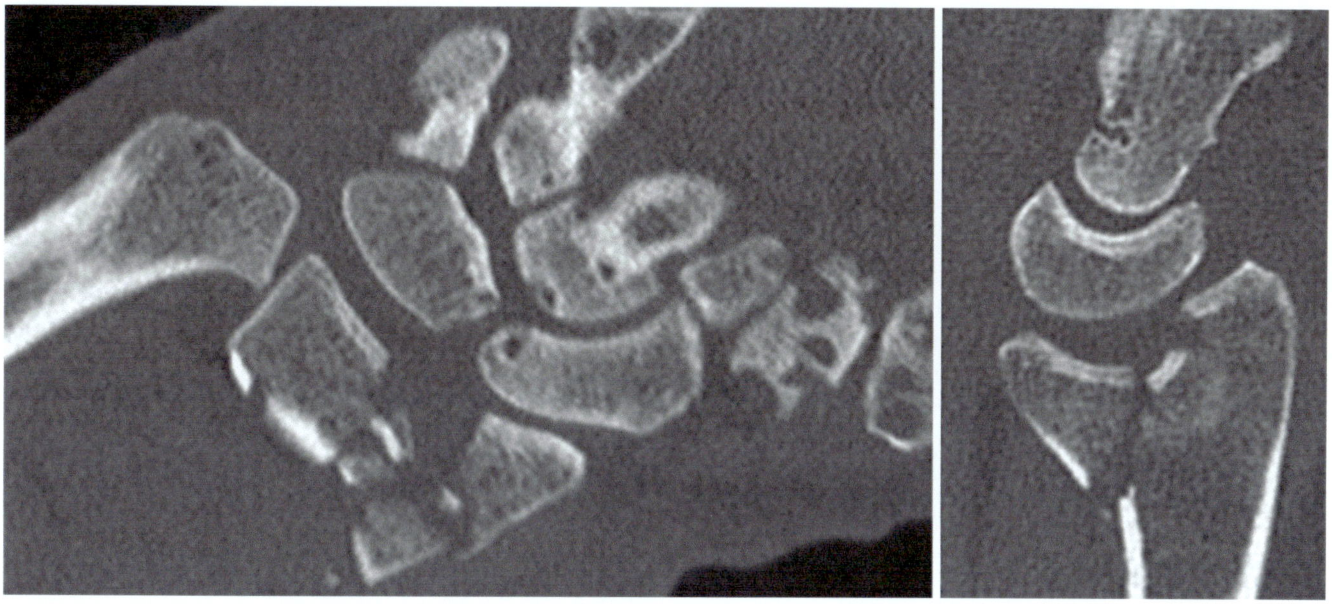

Fig. 36.3 Coronal (left) and sagittal (right) CT images of a comminuted intra-articular distal radius fracture. (Figures from author's library)

tion and splinting are performed acutely. It is important to monitor these patients with weekly serial radiographs for the first 3 weeks to evaluate for loss of reduction that may require surgical intervention. If reduction is maintained, the patient is transitioned to a short arm cast for an additional 3 weeks. The important parameters to evaluate include maintenance of radial height, volar tilt, and radial inclination; radiographs of the non-injured side can be obtained to gauge the patient's normal anatomy [12, 13].

Rehabilitation

There is much debate regarding the utility of formal therapy in the period following distal radius fractures [14]. The vast majority of studies on the subject have been of low quality, with limited participants and a high potential bias. Though physicians may favor a course of therapy to reduce pain and improve range of motion, there is not a clear benefit of formal therapy over a home exercise program. Formal therapy is usually reserved for patients who have delayed recovery of motion and function after a course of home exercises. The initial treatment is directed to edema control and restoration of digital motion. This is followed by strengthening, active-assisted, and passive motion of the wrist and forearm.

Procedure

In patients undergoing closed reduction of distal radius fracture, 32.2% patients developed complex regional pain (CRP) syndrome. Procedures to treat CRP may become relevant including sympathetic blocks and neuromodulation [55].

Surgery
Surgical options are described in the Chap. 37. Indications include persistent displacement after attempted closed reduction, open fractures, significant articular involvement, and acute carpal tunnel syndrome. Volar plate fixation is the most common surgical intervention, usually permitting earlier return to function and reducing the risk of post-traumatic osteoarthritis compared to nonoperative treatment [15–17].

36.2 Ulnar Styloid Fracture

36.2.1 Synonyms

Fracture of the distal ulna

36.2.2 ICD 10 Code

S52.611–S52.616

36.2.3 Description

Anatomy The most distal portion of the ulna, known as the styloid, is a protrusion that serves as an attachment point for the triangular fibrocartilage complex (TFCC), including the palmar and dorsal radioulnar ligaments (Fig. 36.4), which is responsible for providing stability to the distal radioulnar joint (DRUJ) [21, 22]. The ulnocarpal ligaments also originate from this area. The ulnar styloid serves as an attachment point for the ligamentous stabilizers of the distal radioulnar joint and ulnar wrist.

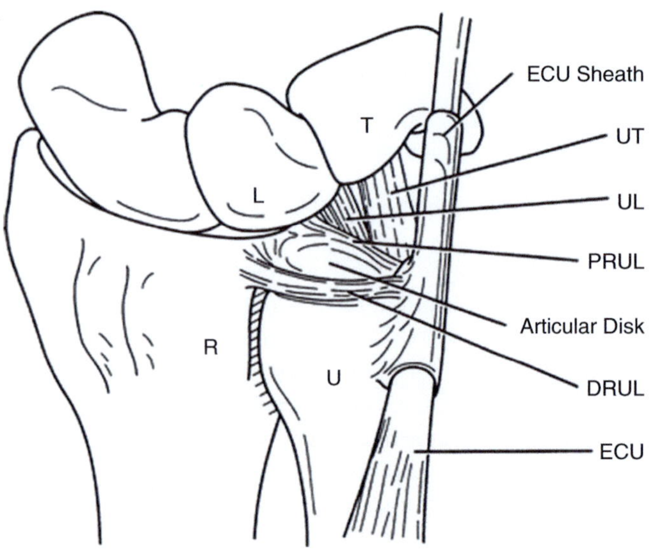

Fig. 36.4 Illustration of the wrist with the TFCC. R radius, U ulna, ECU extensor carpi ulnaris, DRUL dorsal radioulnar ligament, PRUL palmar radioulnar ligament, L lunate, T triquetrum, UL ulnolunate ligament, UT ulnotriquetral ligament

Table 36.2 Differential diagnosis for ulnar styloid fracture

TFCC tear
ECU subluxation/dislocation
Triquetral fracture
Lunotriquetral tear

The deep portion of the distal radioulnar ligament (DRUL) attaches to the fovea of the ulna. The superficial portion of the DRUL surrounds the articular disc at its apex and is integrated into the meniscus homologue. The attachment of the superficial ligament is poorly defined. The superficial ligament lies distal to the deep ligament. The tissue between and peripherally integrated into the ulnar aspect of the superficial ligament and the ulnar capsule is the meniscus homologue. The ligamentum subcruentum is between the deep portion of the DRUL and the meniscus homologue.

Ulnar styloid fractures are usually associated with distal radius fractures and are the result of a fall onto an outstretched hand [6, 8, 9, 18, 19]. Isolated styloid fractures are rare but can be the result of direct trauma to the ulnar portion of the wrist [20]. Diagnosis is made with traditional radiographs. These fractures are usually treated nonoperatively. Fibrous unions are relatively common and are often asymptomatic. Surgery is reserved for ulnar styloid fractures associated with distal radioulnar joint instability [19, 20]. Differential diagnosis for ulnar styloid fracture is presented in Table 36.2.

36.2.4 Clinical Presentation

Many patients with ulnar styloid fractures present with wrist pain in the hours after a fall onto an outstretched hand [1, 3, 18, 23]. A majority of these patients have an associated distal radius fracture [6, 8, 9, 18, 19]. Individuals with acute isolated ulnar styloid fractures will describe a recent direct blow to the ulnar portion of the wrist or a forced radial deviation injury [20]. In cases of nonunion, the patient may report a history of a prior distal radius fracture.

36.2.5 Physical Examination

In addition to ruling out other associated trauma, including distal radius fractures, physical examination of a patient with a suspected ulnar styloid fracture involves a focused musculoskeletal examination.

Inspection Obvious deformity may be seen as a result of an associated distal radius fracture, including swelling and ecchymosis. In cases of chronic ulnar styloid fractures, the wrist may appear normal or there may be a prominence of the ulnar head.

Palpation Tenderness is present over the region of the ulnar styloid. Laxity may be present with stress of the radioulnar joint.

Neurovascular Sensation to the hand is normally intact, though numbness in the median nerve distribution may be present due to compression from swelling in the carpal tunnel. Patients may report vague numbness in the ulnar nerve distribution from an isolated ulnar styloid fracture. As noted, checking pulses and warmth of the hand and wrist, and comparison to contralateral side, is imperative if someone has sustained an injury such as a fracture.

Strength Strength may be decreased due to pain.

Range of motion Wrist motion, including forearm rotation, may be decreased due to pain. Patients usually retain the ability to manipulate their fingers without issue.

36.2.6 Diagnostic Workup

Radiographs
Routine evaluation of a suspected fracture of the ulnar styloid includes plain radiographs of the wrist with posteroanterior (PA), lateral, and oblique views [20] (Fig. 36.5).

Computed Tomography
CT provides an enhanced level of detail over plain radiographs and may be useful in more complex cases of ulnar styloid fractures where the plan radiographs are inconclusive or in cases where the physician may require a greater level of detail [20].

Magnetic Resonance Imaging
MRI may be useful in diagnosing concomitant soft tissue injuries that may be in the differential for ulnar-sided wrist pain. These include but are not limited to TFCC tears or extensor carpi ulnaris (ECU) tears or subluxation.

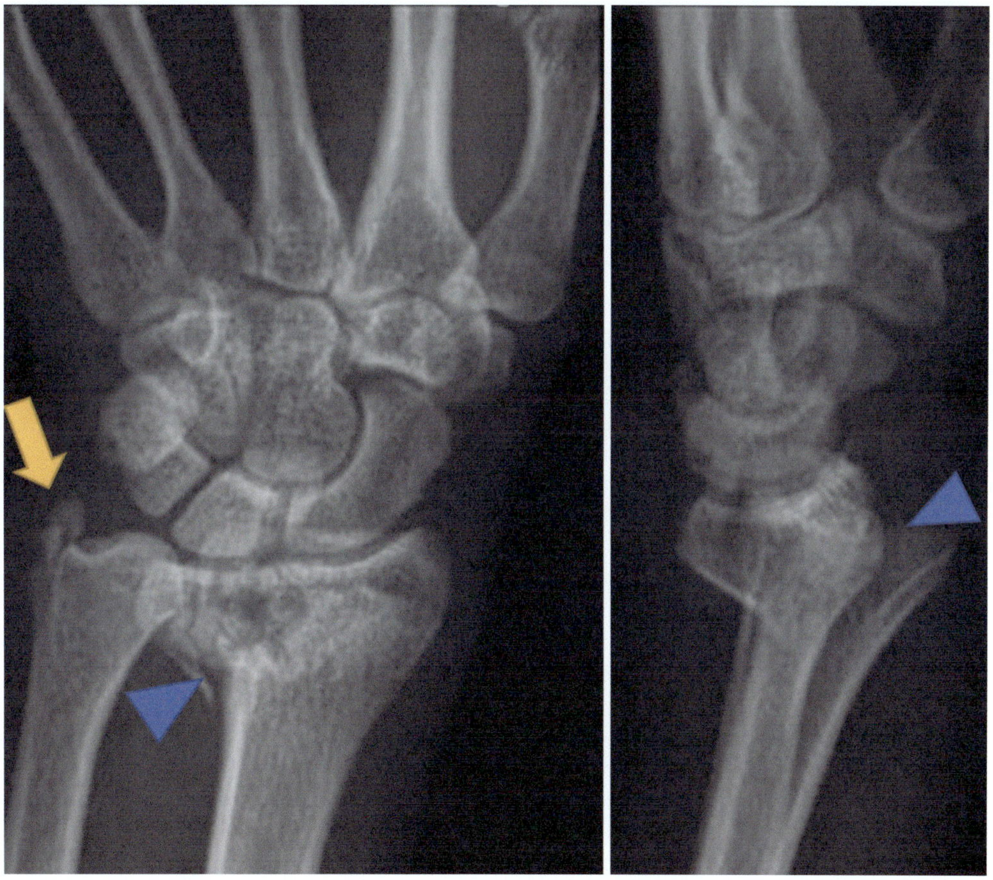

Fig. 36.5 PA and lateral radiographs of distal radius fracture (triangle) with dorsal displacement with associated ulnar styloid fracture (arrow). (Used with permission from Springer publication, Chen AC et al., Indian J Orthop. 2017;51 (1):93–98)

36.2.7 Treatment

For the majority of ulnar styloid fractures associated with distal radius fractures, the major focus of attention is on the distal radius. [9, 18, 19] In many instances, reducing the radius will simultaneously reduce the ulnar styloid, though nonunion is still possible [17, 20]. The ulnar side of the wrist tends to be painful for several months after the distal radius is healed [17, 23, 25–31].

Medical Management
Splint or cast treatment is typically below the elbow (e.g., a short arm cast), unless the injury is associated with distal radioulnar joint instability in which case a long arm or above the elbow cast is indicated [7, 27].

Surgery
Surgical options are described in the Chap. 37. Indications include concomitant distal radioulnar joint instability, which is more common with fractures at the base of the styloid rather than the tip [32]. Surgery may also be indicated in the treatment of symptomatic nonunion [20, 27].

36.3 Scaphoid Fractures

36.3.1 ICD-10 Codes

S62.00–03

36.3.2 Description

Anatomy The scaphoid has a complex three-dimensional anatomy that has been described as a "twisted peanut." The term is derived from the Greek word "skaphe," meaning boat or skiff [36]. It is considered to be the most important carpal bone due to its function in bridging the proximal and distal carpal rows. Due to its complex shape, scaphoid fractures are difficult to diagnose and treat.

Scaphoid fractures account for 50–80% of all carpal fractures [33, 35] and typically result from a fall on an outstretched hand with hyperextension of the wrist. They commonly occur in young, active adult males [35]. Diagnosis can be difficult as initial radiographs may be negative and many patients do not present immediately. CT or MRI may be necessary to confirm a suspected fracture. Untreated scaphoid fractures may result in wrist arthritis later in life. Treatment options range from cast immobilization for non-displaced fractures to open reduction internal fixation with or without bone grafting for displaced fractures and nonunions.

The scaphoid is predominantly covered with articular cartilage (80%) due to its numerous articulations with the distal radius, lunate, capitate, trapezium, and trapezoid [34, 36]. As a result, there are very few points of entry for the blood supply, mainly through the non-articular dorsal ridge and the distal tubercle (Fig. 36.6). Consequently, proximal pole fractures are more prone to osteonecrosis and nonunion due to the retrograde blood supply. The stability of the wrist is dependent on the integrity of the scaphoid. An unstable scaphoid fracture results in the typical "humpback deformity" (apex dorsal and radial), due to the ligamentous attachments of the proximal row. This results in extension of the lunate and subsequent dorsal intercalated segment instability (DISI). Differential diagnosis for scaphoid fracture is presented in Table 36.3.

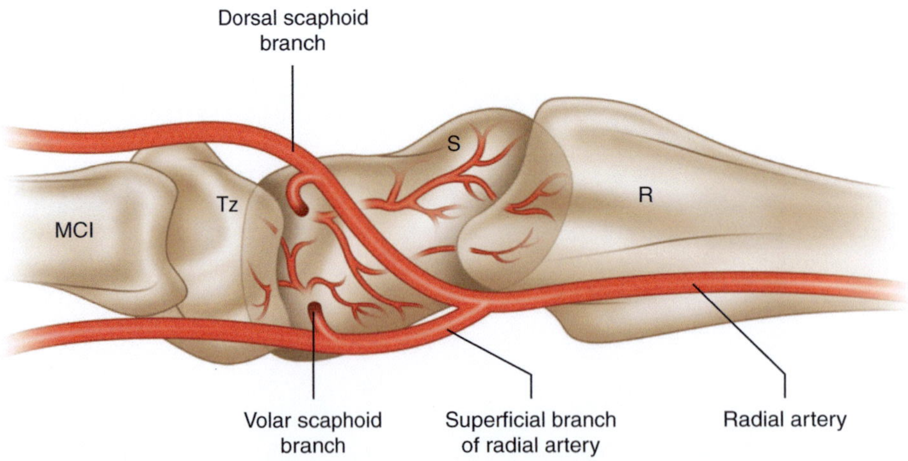

Fig. 36.6 Scaphoid blood supply. Most of the blood flow enters the scaphoid distally at the level of the dorsal ridge and through the proximal tubercle. Hence, fractures of the proximal pole may leave a segment of proximal bone with poor intrinsic blood supply and at risk of nonunion and avascular necrosis [34]. (Image adopted and modified by Yasmine from open access article by Jamie Corcoran et al. Surgical angiogenesis for scaphoid non-union: a literature review Vascular Cell. 2020; 12 (1):1)

Table 36.3 Differential diagnosis for scaphoid fracture

Distal radius fracture
Scapholunate ligament tear
De Quervain's tenosynovitis
First carpometacarpal dislocation

36.3.3 Clinical Presentation

Patients are typically young, active individuals. As with patient's age, the distal radial metaphysis is more likely to be the point of failure rather than the scaphoid for falls on an outstretched hand. Concomitant injuries are commonly seen, including distal radius fractures, fractures of other carpal bones, and associated perilunate injuries in cases of high-energy trauma. In the case of scaphoid nonunion, it is not uncommon for patients to present with wrist pain following a minor injury and report having had wrist trauma years earlier that was felt to be a "sprain."

36.3.4 Physical Examination

Evaluation of a patient with a suspected scaphoid fracture should involve the entire carpus and hand. Given the difficulty of diagnosis on a physical exam alone, any patient with a concern for occult scaphoid fracture should be immobilized until further imaging is obtained.

Inspection The affected wrist usually has deceptively little swelling. In the setting of a more severe trauma such as a trans-scaphoid perilunate injury, the wrist may be grossly deformed with swelling and ecchymosis.

Palpation Patients will have tenderness in the "anatomic snuff box," which is located between the tendons of the first and third extensor compartments, the abductor policis longus (APL)/extensor policis brevis (EPB) and extensor policis longus (EPL), respectively. Patients may also have tenderness on the volar aspect of the hand along the scaphoid tubercle.

Sensation Sensation to the hand is normally intact.

Strength Strength can be decreased due to pain.

Range of motion Wrist motion may be limited due to pain, particularly at the wrist and base of the thumb. Patients usually retain the ability to manipulate their fingers without issue.

Special Test

Special maneuvers include the compression test and pinching of the thumb and index finger in pronation. *Compression test*: Axial compression of the thumb or palpation of the scaphoid tubercle on the volar aspect of the wrist will elicit pain. Pinching of the thumb and index finger with the forearm in pronation may elicit pain [37].

36.3.5 Diagnostic Workup

Radiograph

X-rays should be obtained that include PA (Fig. 36.7) and lateral radiographs with the wrist in neutral position, oblique radiographs at 45–60° of pronation, and a posteroanterior radiograph with the wrist in 45° of ulnar deviation and pronation. X-rays tend to underestimate the true displacement of the fracture and will often miss nondisplaced fractures, with a false-negative rate as high as 25% [2]. If there is an obvious fracture line present on plain radiographs, the fracture is considered displaced. If no fracture line is evident, but there is clinical concern for a scaphoid fracture, there are two options. First, the patient can be placed in a short arm thumb spica cast for 10–14 days prior to repeat imaging. Second, advanced imaging such as CT or MRI can be obtained.

Magnetic Resonance Imaging (MRI)

MRI has been found to have a pooled estimate for sensitivity of 96% and specificity of 99% in many studies. [53] It prevents unnecessary radiation and prolonged immobilization in individuals that require their hands for work or sport. However, MRI can also "over diagnose" fractures as bone bruises can be difficult to distinguish from fractures. MRI is typically reserved for evaluation of concomitant ligament tears. It can also be used to assess vascularity of the proximal pole of the scaphoid.

Ultrasound (US)

US is becoming popular as an alternative for diagnosis as it is available in most emergency departments and clinics. Further, it can be quickly and safely performed while avoiding radiation exposure. US can diagnose scaphoid fracture with sensitivity of 85.6% and specificity of 83.3% based on a systematically review by Kwee et al [54].

36.3.6 Treatment

Treatment is dictated by the location of the fracture, degree of displacement, associated injuries, and patient-specific factors such as occupation or activity level. [39]

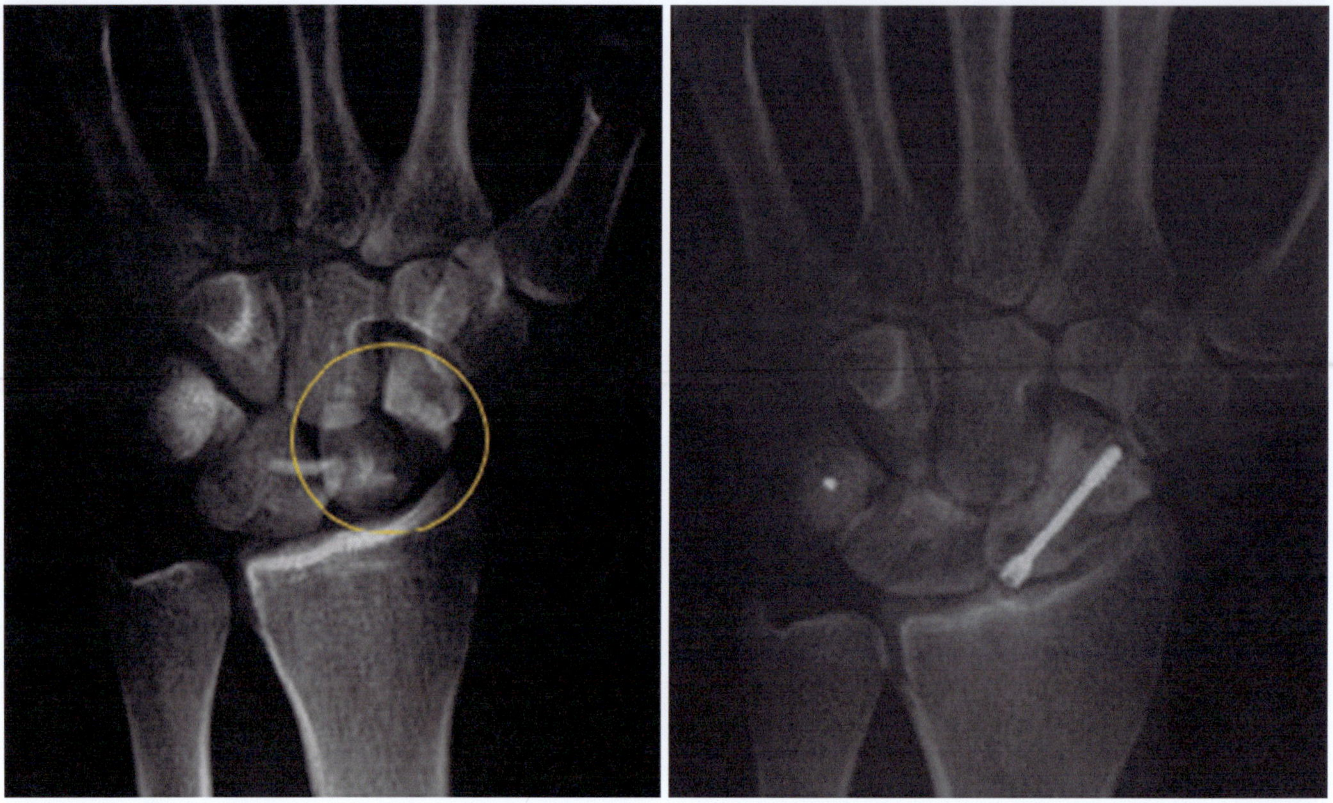

Fig. 36.7 Wrist PA X-ray at presentation showing a displaced scaphoid fracture with disruption of Gilula's arcs. A 20-month postoperative PA films suggesting scaphoid fracture union. (Used with permission, Springer publication, Orthop Traumatol. 2011;12 (3):159–162)

Medical Management

In addition to immobilization as described below, multiple adjunctive therapies have been described, including low-intensity pulsed ultrasound (LIPUS) and pulsed electromagnetic fields (PEMF), which have been used to stimulate bone growth. [35]

Immobilization

Nondisplaced, distal, and middle one-third scaphoid fractures can be managed with immobilization for 6–12 weeks in a short arm thumb spica cast. X-rays are taken at 3-week intervals until union is assured. CT may be helpful in equivocal cases. Approximately 95% of nondisplaced scaphoid waist and distal pole scaphoid fractures will heal with this form of treatment. Short-term complications related to cast treatment include stiffness, muscle atrophy, weakness, and pain.

Rehabilitation

After discontinuation of immobilization, therapy is first directed at restoration of range of motion in the wrist. The "dart thrower's" motion from wrist extension and radial deviation to wrist flexion and ulnar deviation appears to result in low stress across the proximal row of carpal bones. Once motion is reestablished, the next phase includes wrist and forearm strengthening prior to resumption of unrestricted activity.

Surgery

Surgery is reserved for displaced scaphoid fractures and proximal pole fractures and for patients that require skilled use of their hand and earlier return to function. [39] Athletes typically undergo surgery more commonly than non-athletes as operative fixation results in decreased immobilization time and quicker return to play [37]. Surgery results in faster union rate and approximately 1 month earlier return to full activity. Complications, while uncommon, include infection and hardware prominence.

36.4 Hook of Hamate Fractures

36.4.1 ICD-10 Codes

S62.141–156

36.4.2 Description

Anatomy As the name implies, there is a slight curvature in the hook, with the arc traveling from ulnar to radial as the bone progresses more volarly. This creates a smooth concave radial surface that allows for smooth gliding of the ulnar-sided finger flexors as they pass through the carpal tunnel. The hook is an ulnar attachment point for the transverse carpal ligament and the piso-hamate ligament. Similar to the scaphoid, the blood supply of the hook places it at risk for avascular necrosis. The more prominent vessels are at the radial base of the hook.

Hamate fractures are subdivided into body and hook fractures. In this section, we will detail the hook of hamate fractures (Figs. 36.8 and 36.9). The hook of the hamate is a bony prominence that projects volarly from the body of the hamate. These are uncommon carpal bone fractures, accounting for 2–4% of all carpal fractures [40, 41], and are difficult to diagnose given the often-delayed presentation and the lack of sensitivity of conventional wrist X-rays. Due to the vascular supply and biomechanical factors, complications include avascular necrosis, nonunion, ulnar-sided finger flexor tendonitis, and tendon rupture. Treatment options include immobilization alone, which rarely results in union, surgical excision, and open reduction and internal fixation [41, 42]. Differential diagnosis for the hook of hamate fracture is presented in Table 36.4.

36.4.3 Clinical Presentation

Acute fractures of the hook of the hamate result from either direct or indirect trauma. Direct injuries result from a fall, crush injury, or direct blow to the hook. Patients will describe vague pain in the hypothenar area of the palm or occasionally dorsally, aggravated by finger flexion or grip. In athletic activities that require the use of a handled object such as a racket, bat, or golf club, the butt of the handle can result in a fracture during a swing as a single event or from repetitive microtrauma [44]. Indirect injuries result from force transmission through its muscular and ligamentous attachments during a fall or from sudden wrist extension and ulnar deviation. Finally, forceful contraction of the ulnar finger flexors (small and ring finger) can cause a shear force at the base of the hook, thereby resulting in a fracture. Failure of healing is related to the tenuous blood supply and the repetitive stress of the ring and small finger flexor tendons against the radial side of the hamate hook.

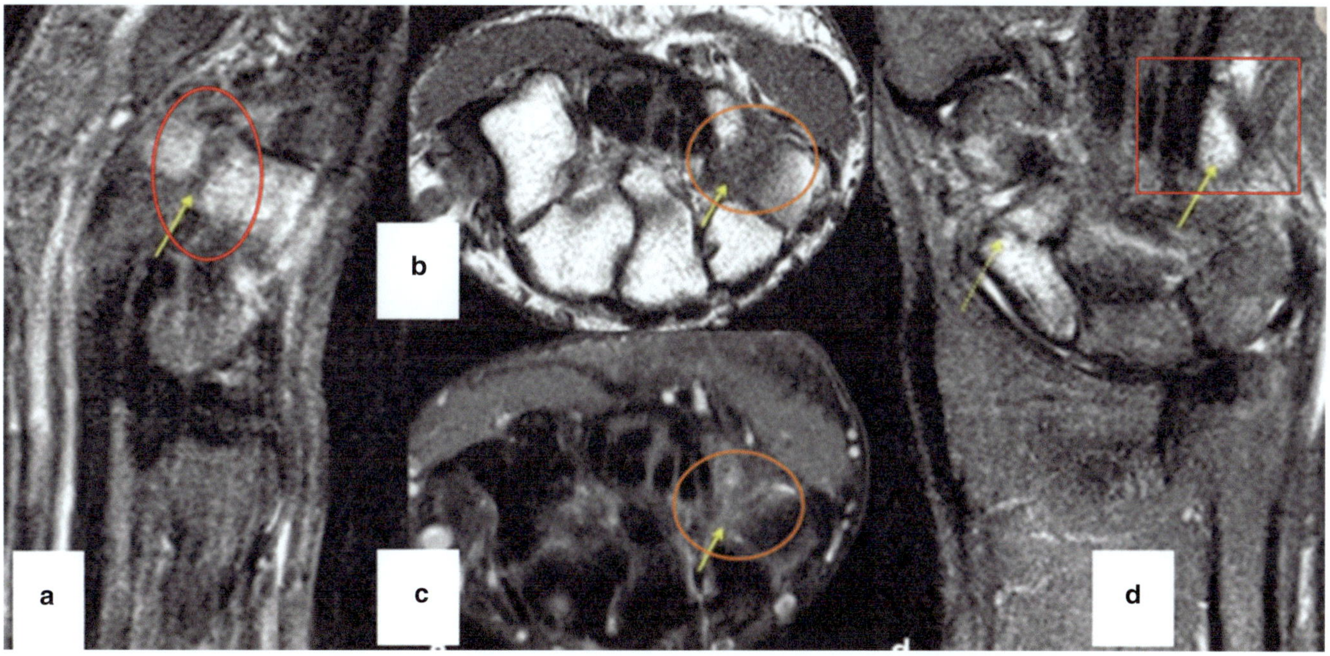

Fig. 36.8 MRI images of hook of hamate fracture and concomitant left scaphoid fracture. (**a**) Sagittal STIR shows significant marrow edema involving the hook and body of the hamate. (**b**) Hook of hamate fracture on axial T1. (**c**) Corresponding axial STIR sequences. (**d**) Coronal STIR sequences demonstrate marked edema with angulated fracture of the distal scaphoid pole (star) and marrow edema of the hook of hamate. (Image adopted and modified. Used with permission from Springer publication, Skeletal Radiology, 2018.47 (4) 505–510)

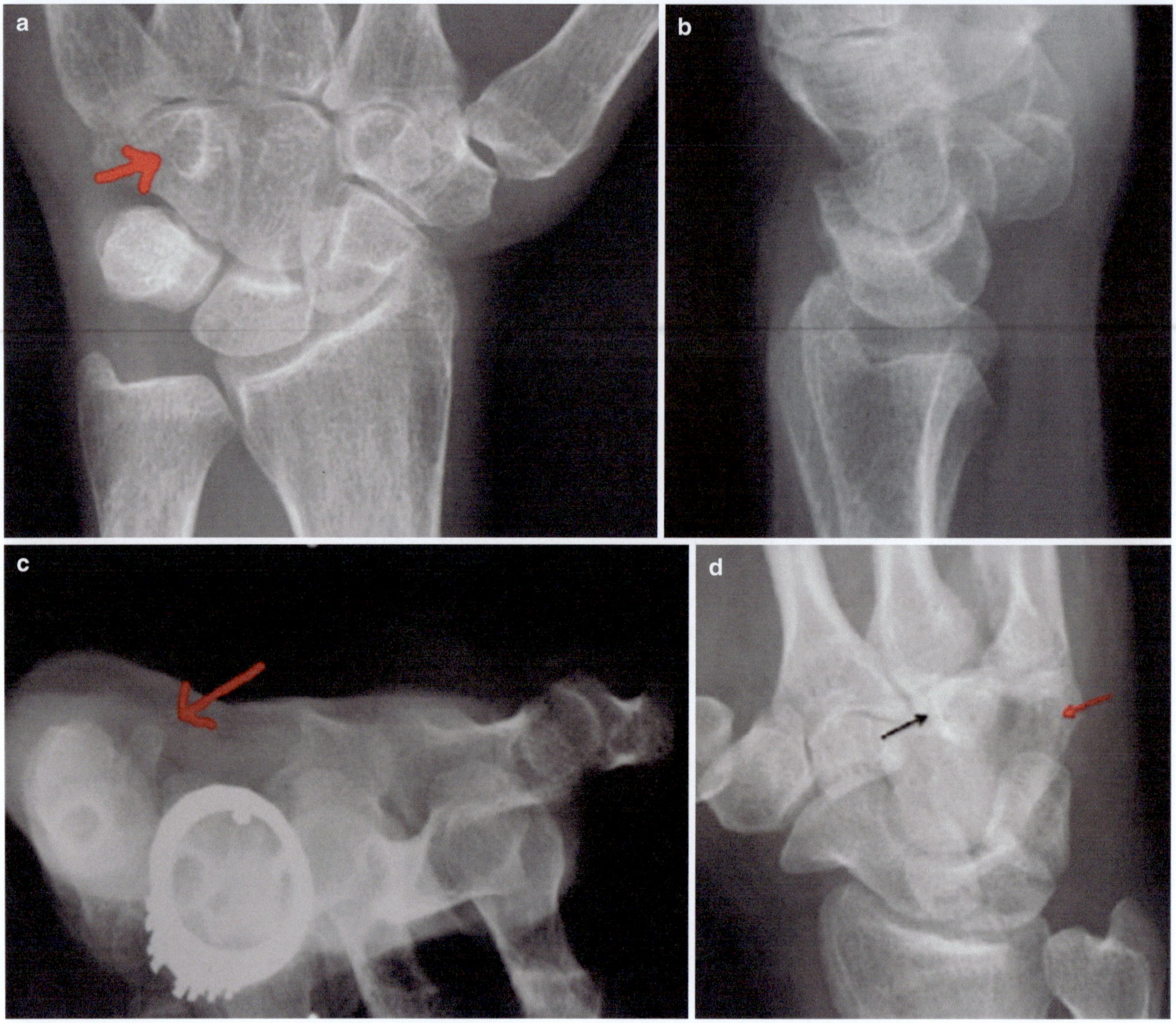

Fig. 36.9 (**a**) Shows posteroanterior (PA) view and (**b**) shows lateral wrist and carpal tunnel radiographs of a subtle hook of hamate fracture. The red arrow on the PA view demonstrates a "ring sign" or discontinuity of the cortical ring of the hook of hamate. The hook of hamate is difficult to visualize on the lateral radiograph. Although the hamate hook (arrow) is seen on the carpal tunnel view (**c**) the fracture is not apparent. (**d**) demonstrates a lucency projecting over the hamate in the expected location of the hook of hamate, i.e., "ghostly shadow" (red arrow). The black arrow in **d** shows the displaced hook of hamate. (Figures from author's library.)

Table 36.4 Differential diagnosis for the hook of hamate fracture

Pisiform fracture
Lunotriquetral tear
Triquetral fracture
Ulnar artery thrombosis
FCU tendinitis
Ulnar neuropathy

36.4.4 Physical Examination

Hamate hook fractures are usually isolated injuries. In the setting of crush injuries, however, there may be multiple fractures that deserve attention.

Inspection In athletes, there may be a callous in the palm directly overlying the hamate hook, the result of chronic pressure from the handle of a baseball or softball bat or hand-held racket. With acute trauma, there may be swelling, ecchymosis, and possibly damage to the overlying skin.

Palpation The location of the hamate hook in the palm is at the intersection between a line drawn along the fully abducted thumb and a line along the ring finger ray. Palpation in this area may demonstrate tenderness.

Sensation Patient may report paresthesias in the ulnar nerve distribution and, less commonly, the median nerve distribution.

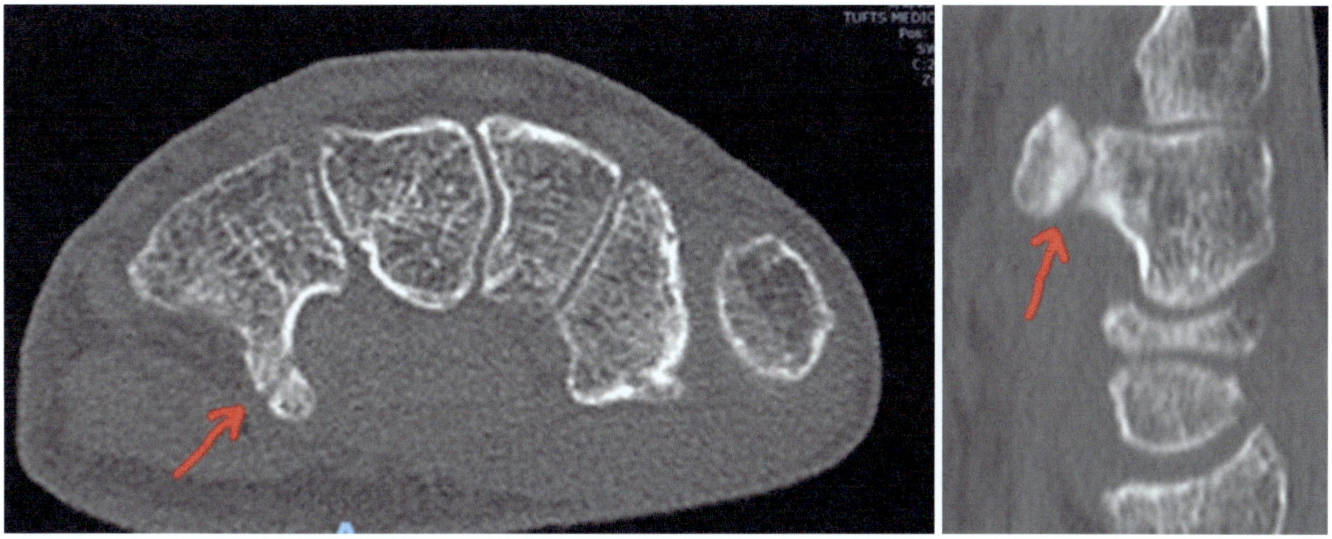

Fig. 36.10 Axial and sagittal CT images of a patient with subacute fracture of the tip of the hamate hook. (Figures from author's library)

Strength Strength can be decreased due to pain, especially in the ulnar-sided finger flexors. On rare occasions, the deep motor branch of the ulnar nerve can be injured, resulting in intrinsic weakness.

Range of motion Wrist motion is usually preserved, except in cases of acute severe trauma. Chronic injuries can result in rupture of the flexor tendons to the small and ring fingers.

Special Test

Hook of hamate pull test: With the hand in an ulnarly deviated position and the wrist supinated, the patient is asked to flex the ulnar two digits against resistance. Since the hook of the hamate acts as a pulley for the ulnar digital flexors, this maneuver may gap the fracture site, resulting in pain [40, 42, 45].

36.4.5 Diagnostic Workup

Radiographs

Fracture of the hook of the hamate is often missed on standard radiographs [41]. If there is a strong suspicion for a hook of hamate fracture, a carpal tunnel view should also be obtained. There are many radiographic signs on X-ray that may suggest a hook of hamate fracture. These include the "ring sign" and "ghostly shadow," which refer to discontinuity of the hook of hamate cortical ring and non-visualization of the hook of hamate with a lucency in its expected location (Fig. 36.1), respectively. [2] "Diffuse sclerosis" can be seen in chronic hook of hamate fractures (Fig. 36.9).

Computed Tomography

CT scans are obtained in cases where there is a high suspicion of hook of hamate fractures, as plain radiographs may miss the fracture initially. Further, CT scan can give more details to the location and displacement of the fracture (Fig. 36.10).

Magnetic Resonance Imaging

MRI allows for definitive diagnosis and for the determination of any complications such as avascular necrosis. Further, MRI can be useful in diagnosis of stress fractures that may occur in swinging athletes. [41] Despite its limited utilization, MRI has the highest imaging detection rate (100%) compared to CT (92%), carpal tunnel view (43%), and plain radiographs (10%) [42].

36.4.6 Treatment

Management of hook of hamate fractures is controversial, and treatment options range from immobilization alone to fragment excision, open reduction, and internal fixation. Acute fractures resulting from severe trauma are usually treated initially with immobilization, and in contrast, chronic injuries in athletes are usually treated with hamate hook excision.

Medical Management

Unless there are associated flexor tendon ruptures, a trial of immobilization is appropriate for most of the hook of hamate fractures. Complications include persistent pain, nonunion, stiffness, delayed return to sport, and flexor tendon rupture. [46]

Surgery

Early surgery, usually involving hamate hook excision, is indicated for competitive athletes and chronic fractures associated with flexor tendon rupture [42]. Surgical options are described in the Chap. 37.

Rehabilitation

Following hamate hook excision, patients are generally able to return to competitive athletics at about 6 weeks postoperatively. The surgical site may be tender, and a silicone gel pad and alteration in grip of the racket or bat may be necessary in the short term.

36.5 Metacarpal and Phalangeal Fractures

36.5.1 Synonyms

Hand fractures, finger fractures, boxer's fracture

36.5.2 ICD-10 Codes

S62, multiple codes depending on which finger and/or phalanx

36.5.3 Description

Anatomy The five metacarpals articulate proximally with the distal row of the carpus and distally with the proximal phalanges of the digits. These bones are tubular and have a dorsal convexity. The second and third carpometacarpal joints have significantly less mobility than the fourth and fifth [1]. The wrist extensors insert into the bases of the second, third, and fifth metacarpals. These attachment points produce deforming forces in certain metacarpal fractures. Distally, the metacarpals serve as attachment points for a portion of the pulley system on the volar aspect that keeps the flexor tendons from bowstringing. The extensor tendons run dorsally along the metacarpal. The deep transverse metacarpal ligaments connect the volar plates of the metacarpophalangeal joints, forming a thick fibrous transverse arch linking the metacarpal heads.

The index, middle, ring, and small fingers each have three phalanges that form three articulations: the metacarpophalangeal (MCP) joint, proximal interphalangeal (PIP) joint, and distal interphalangeal (DIP) joint. The thumb has two phalanges that form two articulations: MCP and interphalangeal (IP) joint. There are numerous muscles, ligaments, and tendons that attach to the phalanges in the hand. The extensor tendons continue dorsally along the phalanges to their terminal insertion at the base of the distal phalanx of the index through the small fingers. The flexor digitorum superficialis and profundus tendons insert at base of the middle phalanx and distal phalanx, respectively.

Table 36.5 Differential diagnosis for metacarpal and phalangeal fracture

CMC, MCP, or PIP dislocation
Collateral ligament tear
Volar plate injury
Finger pulley rupture

Metacarpal and phalangeal fractures are common, accounting for 40% of upper extremity fractures [46, 47]. The proximal phalanx is the most common phalanx fracture, while the fifth metacarpal is the most common metacarpal fracture. [48] They result from direct or indirect trauma to the hand such as sports, industrial accidents, or falls from standing height. Management options include immobilization and surgical repair. Complications are common and include residual stiffness, malunion, nonunion, contracture, malrotation, loss of knuckle prominence, arthritis, and extensor lag. Differential diagnosis for metacarpal and phalangeal fracture is presented in Table 36.5.

36.5.4 Clinical Presentation

Clinical presentations for metacarpal or phalangeal fractures are variable but involve direct or indirect trauma. Patients may present after a fall on an outstretched hand, a direct blow from an object, or a punch to another object/individual. It is important to obtain an accurate history and mechanism of injury in the case of open wounds near the metacarpal head as these can reflect wounds from another person's tooth and change management as discussed below.

36.5.5 Physical Examination

Depending on the mechanism of the injury, there could be multiple hand fractures or associated ligament injuries. Therefore, a thorough assessment of the entire injured hand is imperative.

Inspection Swelling, ecchymosis, and skin damage may be present. The loss of knuckle contour, malrotation, or gross deformity may be present with angulated or rotated (Fig. 36.11). Nail bed injuries may disguise an open distal phalanx fracture. A break in the skin overlying the metacarpal head is suggestive of a "fight bite." [50]

Palpation Tenderness will be present in the area of the fracture or dislocation and bony crepitus may be palpable.

Sensation Sensation to the hand is normally intact although patients may report vague numbness or paresthesias in the affected finger. In penetrating, open, or crush injuries, there may be numbness indicating digital nerve injury.

Vascular Capillary refill should be assessed, and if there is a concern for decreased perfusion, the digital arteries should be assessed via Doppler. This is especially important in penetrating, open or crush fractures.

Strength Strength is decreased due to pain.

Range of motion Both passive and active range of motion can be decreased due to pain particularly in the affected finger although neighboring digits may also be affected. Cascade of the fingers should be examined. Rotational deformity can be assessed by asking the patient to make a fist or passively extending the wrist and observing for any abnormal finger overlap, non-parallel nails among the fingers, or any flexion and angulation not seen on the uninjured side [4]. Malalignment is poorly tolerated in these fractures [51]. Extension and flexion of each finger and individual joint should be assessed to determine any concomitant ligamentous injury.

36.5.6 Diagnostic Workup

Radiographs
Standard radiographs include PA, oblique, and lateral views (Figs. 36.11 and 36.12). When there is a concern for a fracture or dislocation of a phalanx, dedicated views of that finger alone can help better determine the degree of displacement or presence of any joint dislocation or subluxation.

Computed Tomography (CT)
CT scans are reserved for intra-articular fractures to better characterize the degree and location of joint involvement. Also, CT of severely comminuted fractures may help dictate management and surgical approach [51].

Magnetic Resonance Imaging (MRI)
MRI is rarely utilized in metacarpal or phalanx fractures except in cases where this is suspected ligamentous or tendinous injury such as in the base of the thumb ulnar collateral ligament (UCL) injuries. Plain radiographs are oftentimes unable to differentiate a purely bony avulsion fracture versus an associated ligamentous injury in these cases.

36.5.7 Treatment

Medical Management
Metacarpal fractures that have no rotational deformity and are extra-articular are amenable to non-surgical management with immobilization. Generally, metacarpal fractures that are more ulnar and distal can tolerate more degrees of angulation and are, thus, more amenable to immobilization. For example, metacarpal shaft fractures of the ring and small fingers can tolerate 30 and 40 degrees of angulation, respectively, while the index and middle fingers can tolerate 20 degrees of angulation [52]. In general, immobilization includes the fractured metacarpal and the neighboring digits to provide further stability. However, the literature varies drastically on the need to immobilize the wrist and the recommended degree of flexion of the metacarpophalangeal joint. Studies have shown equivalent outcomes regardless of the immobilization technique. [52]

If the fracture is displaced (typically apex dorsal), a reduction is performed using the Jahss technique, whereby the metacarpophalangeal joint and proximal interphalangeal joint are held in 90° degrees flexion while applying a dorsally directed pressure. Similarly, phalangeal fractures that have no rotational deformity and do not have significant articular involvement can be managed with immobilization. Depending on the finger and phalanx injured, immobilization can range from a finger splint to the neighboring digits or an intrinsic plus splint including the wrist/hand. For any dislocation, a reduction should be performed followed by immobilization and repeat imaging to determine the adequacy of the reduction.

Rehabilitation
Loss of digital motion can significantly impair function following hand fractures. Consequently, it is imperative to encourage the patient to move all joints that are not included in the splint or cast. The safe position for PIP immobilization is in full extension, whereas the safe position for the MCP joint is in full flexion, or the "intrinsic plus" position tendon gliding exercises are important in combined injuries. Supplemental splints, such as static progressive or dynamic finger extension splints, are often prescribed to restore PIP joint extension.

Surgery
The indications for operative treatment of metacarpal fractures include any rotational deformity, greater than 5 mm of metacarpal shortening, greater than 1 mm of articular step-

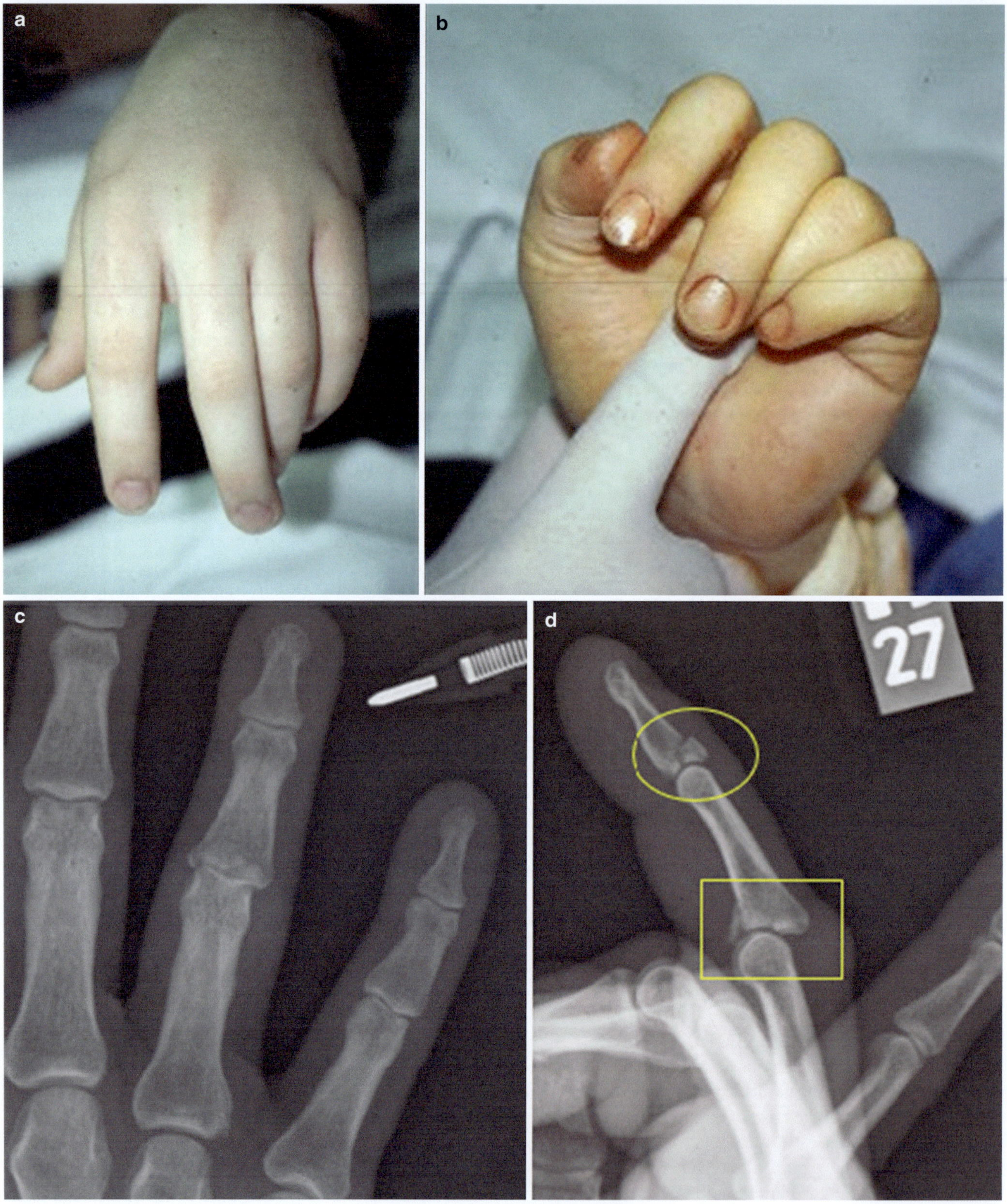

Fig. 36.11 Hand pain following a twisting injury to the middle finger. Inspection (**a**) demonstrates subtle ulnar deviation and pronation of the digit, which is magnified by tenodesis or passive extension of the wrist (**b**). (**c**) PA radiograph of the right hand demonstrates a spiral fracture of the third metacarpal. (**d**) Oblique radiograph of the patient demonstrates both a fracture-subluxation of the proximal interphalangeal joint and a distal phalanx "bony mallet" fracture

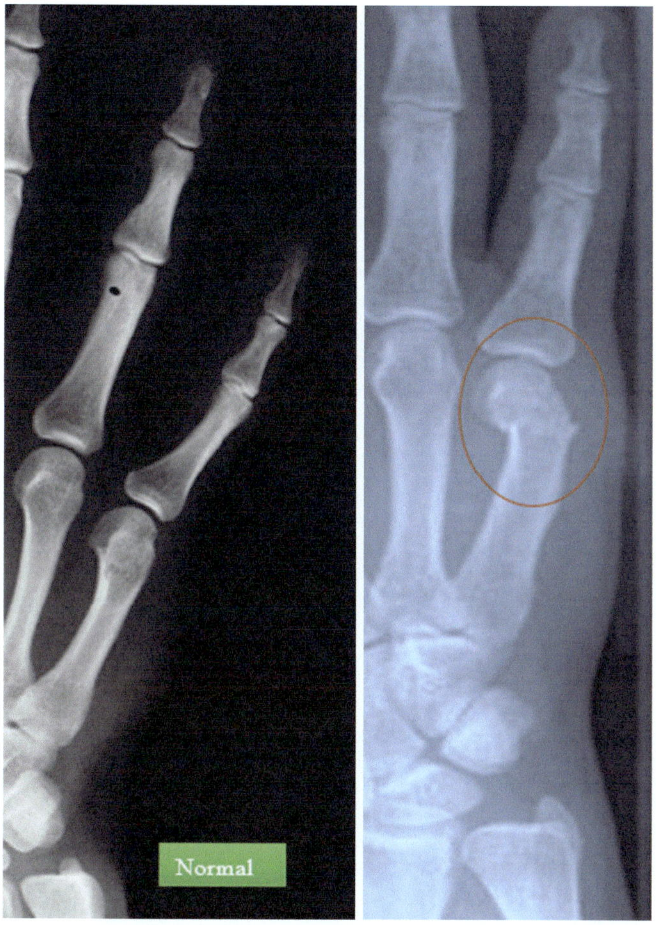

Fig. 36.12 Radiographs of a normal fifth metacarpal bone as compared to a fifth metacarpal fracture with angulation. (Images courtesy of Ali Mostoufi, MD)

off, or greater than 25% of articular involvement. Additionally, patient-specific factors are considered. Surgical options are described in the Chap. 37.

References

1. Meena S, Sharma P, Sambharia AK, Dawar A. Fractures of distal radius: an overview. J Family Med Primary Care. 2014;3(4):325. https://doi.org/10.4103/2249-4863.148101.
2. Frykman G. Fracture of the distal radius including sequelae-shoulder–handfinger syndrome, disturbance in the distal radio-ulnar joint and impairment of nerve function: a clinical and experimental study. Acta Orthopaed Scand. 1967;38(sup108):1–61. https://doi.org/10.3109/ort.1967.38.suppl-108.01.
3. Lindau TR, Aspenberg P, Arner M, Redlundh-Johnell I, Hagberg L. Fractures of the distal forearm in young adults: an epidemiologic description of 341 patients. Acta Orthop Scand. 1999;70(2):124–8. https://doi.org/10.3109/17453679909011248.
4. Pogue DJ, Viegas SF, Patterson RM, Peterson PD, Jenkins DK, Sweo TD, Hokanson JA. Effects of distal radius fracture malunion on wrist joint mechanics. J Hand Surg Am. 1990;15(5):721–7. https://doi.org/10.1016/0363-5023(90)90143-f. PMID: 2229966.
5. Solomon L, Warwick D, Nayagam S. Apley's system of orthopaedics and fractures. Boca Raton: CRC Press; 2010.
6. Ekenstam FA, Jakobsson OP, Wadin K. Repair of the triangular ligament in Colles' fracture: no effect in a prospective randomized study. Acta Orthop Scand. 1989;60(4):393–6. https://doi.org/10.3109/17453678909149304.
7. Hollingsworth R, Morris J. The importance of the ulnar side of the wrist in fractures of the distal end of the radius. Injury. 1975;7(4):263–6. https://doi.org/10.1016/s0020-1383(75)80004-0.
8. Lindau T, Arner M, Hagberg L. Intraarticular lesions in distal fractures of the radius in young adults: a descriptive arthroscopic study in 50 patients. J Hand Surg. 1997;22(5):638–43. https://doi.org/10.1016/s0266-7681(97)80364-6.
9. Sammer DM, Shah HM, Shauver MJ, Chung KC. The effect of ulnar styloid fractures on patient-rated outcomes after volar locking plating of distal radius fractures. J Hand Surg Am. 2009;34(9):1595–602. https://doi.org/10.1016/j.jhsa.2009.05.017.
10. Mehta JA, Bain GI. An overview of distal radial fractures. Aust J Rural Health. 1999;7(2):121–6. https://doi.org/10.1046/j.1440-1584.1999.00226.x.
11. Metz VM, Gilula LA. Imaging techniques for distal radius fractures and related injuries. Orthop Clin N Am. 1993;24(2):217–28. PMID: 8479720.
12. Tsukazaki T, Iwasaki K. Ulnar wrist pain after Colles' fracture: 109 fractures followed for 4 years. Acta Orthop Scand. 1993;64(4):462–4. https://doi.org/10.3109/17453679308993668.
13. Villar RN, Marsh D, Rushton N, Greatorex RA. Three years after Colles' fracture. A prospective review. J Bone Joint Surg Br. 1987; 69(4):635–8. https://doi.org/10.1302/0301-620X.69B4.3611172.
14. Ziebart C, Nazari G, MacDermid JC. Therapeutic exercise for adults post-distal radius fracture: an overview of systematic reviews of randomized controlled trials. Hand Ther. 2019;24(3):69–81. https://doi.org/10.1177/1758998319865751.
15. Bartl C, Stengel D, Gülke J, Gebhard F. Clinical results following conservative and surgical treatment of osteoporotic distal radius fractures in the elderly: overview of best available evidence. Unfallchirurg. 2016;119(9):723–31. https://doi.org/10.1007/s00113-016-0216-y.
16. Trumble TE, Culp RW, Hanel DP, Geissler WB, Berger RA. Intra-articular fractures of the distal aspect of the radius. Instr Course Lect. 1999;48:465–80. https://doi.org/10.4103/2249-4863.148101.
17. Ikpeze TC, Smith HC, Lee DJ, Elfar JC. Distal radius fracture outcomes and rehabilitation. Geriatr Orthop Surg Rehabil. 2016;7(4):202–5. https://doi.org/10.1177/2151458516669202.
18. Frykman G. Fracture of the distal radius including sequelae-shoulder–handfinger syndrome, disturbance in the distal radio-ulnar joint and impairment of nerve function: a clinical and experimental study. Acta Orthop Scand. 1967;38(sup108):1–61. https://doi.org/10.3109/ort.1967.38.suppl-108.01.
19. Logan AJ, Lindau TR. The management of distal ulnar fractures in adults: a review of the literature and recommendations for treatment. Strat Trauma Limb Recon. 2008;3(2):49–56. https://doi.org/10.1007/s11751-008-0040-1.
20. Hauck RM, Skahen J III, Palmer AK. Classification and treatment of ulnar styloid nonunion. J Hand Surg Am. 1996;21(3):418–22. https://doi.org/10.1016/S0363-5023(96)80355-8.
21. Ekenstam FA. Osseous anatomy and articular relationships about the distal ulna. Hand Clin. 1998;14(2):161–4. PMID: 9604150.
22. Garcia-Elias M. Soft-tissue anatomy and relationships about the distal ulna. Hand Clin. 1998;14(2):165–76. PMID: 9604151.
23. Niver GE, Ilyas AM. Carpal tunnel syndrome after distal radius fracture. Orthop Clin North Am. 2012;43(4):521–7. https://doi.org/10.1016/j.ocl.2012.07.021.
24. Ishii S, Palmer AK, Werner FW, Short WH, Fortino MD. An anatomic study of the ligamentous structure of the triangular fibrocartilage complex. J Hand Surg Am. 1998;23(6):977–85. https://doi.org/10.1016/S0363-5023(98)80003-8.
25. May MM, Lawton JN, Blazar PE. Ulnar styloid fractures associated with distal radius fractures: incidence and implications for distal

radioulnar joint instability. J Hand Surg Am. 2002;27(6):965–71. https://doi.org/10.1053/jhsu.2002.36525.
26. Chen AC, Chiu CH, Weng CJ, Chang SS, Cheng CY. Early and late fixation of ulnar styloid base fractures yields different outcomes. J Orthop Surg Res. 2018;13(1):1–5. https://doi.org/10.1186/s13018-018-0899-6.
27. Shaw JA, Bruno A, Paul EM. Ulnar styloid fixation in the treatment of posttraumatic instability of the radioulnar joint: a biomechanical study with clinical correlation. J Hand Surg Am. 1990;15(5):712–20. https://doi.org/10.1016/0363-5023(90)90142-e. PMID: 2229965.
28. Wijffels M, Ring D. The influence of non-union of the ulnar styloid on pain, wrist function and instability after distal radius fracture. J Hand Microsurg. 2011;3(1):11–4. https://doi.org/10.1007/s12593-011-0033-z.
29. Catalano LW III, Cole RJ, Gelberman RH, Evanoff BA, Gilula LA, Borrelli J Jr. Displaced intra-articular fractures of the distal aspect of the radius. Long-term results in young adults after open reduction and internal fixation. JBJS. 1997;79(9):1290–302. https://doi.org/10.2106/00004623-199709000-00003. PMID: 9314391.
30. Knirk JL, Jupiter JB. Intra-articular fractures of the distal end of the radius in young adults. J Bone Joint Surg Am. 1986;68(5):647–59. PMID: 3722221.
31. Mansat M, Gay R, Mansat C, Martinez C. Vicious callus of the lower end of the radius and" disturbances" of the inferior radio-ulnar joint (author's transl). InAnnales de chirurgie 1977;31(4):297–301. PMID: 879690.
32. Reeves B. Excision of the ulnar styloid fragment after Colles' fracture. Int Surg. 1966;45(1):46–52. PMID: 5905484.
33. Pinder RM, Brkljac M, Rix L, Muir L, Brewster M. Treatment of scaphoid nonunion: a systematic review of the existing evidence. J Hand Surg Am. 2015;40(9):1797–1805.e3. https://doi.org/10.1016/j.jhsa.2015.05.003. Epub 2015 Jun 24. PMID: 26116095.
34. Sabbagh MD, Morsy M, Moran SL. Diagnosis and management of acute scaphoid fractures. Hand Clin. 2019;35(3):259–69. https://doi.org/10.1016/j.hcl.2019.03.002. Epub 2019 May 11. PMID: 31178084.
35. Tada K, Ikeda K, Okamoto S, Hachinota A, Yamamoto D, Tsuchiya H. Scaphoid fracture–overview and conservative treatment. Hand Surg. 2015;20(2):204–9. https://doi.org/10.1142/S0218810415400018. PMID: 26051761.
36. Ring D, Jupiter JB, Herndon JH. Acute fractures of the scaphoid. J Am Acad Orthop Surg. 2000;8(4):225–31. https://doi.org/10.5435/00124635-200007000-00003. PMID: 10951111.
37. Fowler JR, Hughes TB. Scaphoid fractures. Clin Sports Med. 2015;34(1):37–50. https://doi.org/10.1016/j.csm.2014.09.011. Epub 2014 Nov 25. PMID: 25455395.
38. Cheung GC, Lever CJ, Morris AD. X-ray diagnosis of acute scaphoid fractures. J Hand Surg Br. 2006;31(1):104–9. https://doi.org/10.1016/j.jhsb.2005.09.001. Epub 2005 Oct 28. PMID: 16257481.
39. Jernigan EW, Morse KW, Carlson MG. Managing the athlete with a scaphoid fracture. Hand Clin. 2019;35(3):365–371. https://doi.org/10.1016/j.hcl.2019.03.011. PMID: 31178093. 1. O'Shea K, Weiland AJ. Fractures of the hamate and pisiform bones. Hand Clin 2012;28(3):287–300, viii. https://doi.org/10.1016/j.hcl.2012.05.010. PMID: 22883867.
40. O'Shea K, Weiland AJ. Fractures of the hamate and pisiform bones. Hand Clin. 2012;28(3):287–300, viii. https://doi.org/10.1016/j.hcl.2012.05.010. PMID: 22883867.
41. Spencer J, Hunt SL, Zhang C, Walter C, Everist B. Radiographic signs of hook of hamate fracture: evaluation of diagnostic utility. Skelet Radiol. 2019;48(12):1891–8. https://doi.org/10.1007/s00256-019-03221-0. Epub 2019 May 27. PMID: 31134315.
42. Kadar A, Bishop AT, Suchyta MA, Moran SL. Diagnosis and management of hook of hamate fractures. J Hand Surg Eur Vol. 2018;43(5):539–45. https://doi.org/10.1177/1753193417729603. Epub 2017 Sep 11. PMID: 28893146.
43. Davis DL. Hook of the Hamate: the spectrum of often missed pathologic findings. AJR Am J Roentgenol. 2017;209(5):1110–8. https://doi.org/10.2214/AJR.17.18043. Epub 2017 Aug 23. PMID: 28834449; PMCID: PMC5892414.
44. Sochacki KR, Liberman SR, Mehlhoff TL, Jones JM, Lintner DM, McCulloch PC. Progression of Hamate Hook stress reactions in elite baseball players. Orthop J Sports Med. 2020;8(5):2325967120919389. https://doi.org/10.1177/2325967120919389. PMID: 32537475; PMCID: PMC7268571.
45. Klausmeyer MA, Mudgal CS. Hook of hamate fractures. J Hand Surg Am 2013;38(12):2457–2460; quiz 2460. https://doi.org/10.1016/j.jhsa.2013.06.004. Epub 2013 Jul 26. PMID: 23891177.
46. Yamazaki H, Kato H, Nakatsuchi Y, Murakami N, Hata Y. Closed rupture of the flexor tendons of the little finger secondary to non-union of fractures of the hook of the hamate. J Hand Surg Br. 2006;31(3):337–41. https://doi.org/10.1016/j.jhsb.2005.12.015. Epub 2006 Mar 30. PMID: 16580104.
47. Kollitz KM, Hammert WC, Vedder NB, Huang JI. Metacarpal fractures: treatment and complications. Hand (N Y). 2014;9(1):16–23. https://doi.org/10.1007/s11552-013-9562-1. PMID: 24570632; PMCID: PMC3928373.
48. Neumeister MW, Webb K, McKenna K. Non-surgical management of metacarpal fractures. Clin Plast Surg. 2014;41(3):451–61. https://doi.org/10.1016/j.cps.2014.03.008. PMID: 24996464.
49. Henry MH. Fractures of the proximal phalanx and metacarpals in the hand: preferred methods of stabilization. J Am Acad Orthop Surg. 2008;16(10):586–95. https://doi.org/10.5435/00124635-200810000-00004. PMID: 18832602.
50. Haughton D, Jordan D, Malahias M, Hindocha S, Khan W. Principles of hand fracture management. Open Orthop J. 2012;6:43–53. https://doi.org/10.2174/1874325001206010043. Epub 2012 Feb 23. PMID: 22423303; PMCID: PMC3296112.
51. Taghinia AH, Talbot SG. Phalangeal and metacarpal fractures. Clin Plast Surg. 2019;46(3):415–23. https://doi.org/10.1016/j.cps.2019.02.011. Epub 2019 Apr 13. PMID: 31103086.
52. Wong VW, Higgins JP. Evidence-based medicine: management of metacarpal fractures. Plast Reconstr Surg. 2017;140(1):140e–51e. https://doi.org/10.1097/PRS.0000000000003470. PMID: 28654615.
53. Yin ZG, Zhang JB, Kan SL, et al. Diagnosing suspected scaphoid fractures: a systematic review and meta-analysis. 2010. In: Database of Abstracts of Reviews of Effects (DARE): quality-assessed Reviews [Internet]. York (UK): Centre for Reviews and Dissemination (UK); 1995. Available from: https://www.ncbi.nlm.nih.gov/books/NBK80083/.
54. Kwee RM, Kwee TC. Ultrasound for diagnosing radiographically occult scaphoid fracture. Skelet Radiol. 2018;47(9):1205–12. https://doi.org/10.1007/s00256-018-2931-7. Epub 2018 Apr 4. PMID: 29619506.
55. Jellad A, Salah S. Ben Salah Frih Z. Complex regional pain syndrome type I: incidence and risk factors in patients with fracture of the distal radius. Arch Phys Med Rehabil. 2014;95(3):487–92.

Wrist and Hand Surgeries

37

Todd Alter, Matthew H. Nasra, Andrew J. Butler, and Alfred J. Tria Jr

37.1 Surgery for Tendons and Ligament in the Wrist and Hand

37.1.1 Description

In this section, we discuss surgical intervention for the following injuries to tendons and ligaments in the wrist and hand: intersection syndrome, carpal tunnel syndrome, triangular fibrocartilage complex (TFCC) tears, trigger finger, de Quervain's syndrome, and thumb ulnar collateral ligament (UCL) injuries.

37.1.1.1 Intersection Syndrome

Operation

Intersection syndrome is an inflammatory condition that results from repetitive gliding between the first and second dorsal compartment extensor tendons during wrist flexion and extension movements. Surgery for this entity is reserved for the most recalcitrant cases. Operative treatment involves fasciotomy and synovectomy of the abductor pollicis longus (APL) and extensor pollicis brevis (EPB) tendons, decompression of the second dorsal compartment tendons, and debridement of the inflamed tissue [5].

Rehabilitation

Postoperatively, the patient is placed in a dressing/splint for 1–7 days. Active range of motion (ROM) and progressive resistive exercises follow, with a return to full activities at 10 days [6].

T. Alter · M. H. Nasra · A. J. Butler
Robert Wood Johnson University School of Medicine, New Brunswick, NJ, USA

A. J. Tria Jr (✉)
Department of Orthopaedics, Rutgers-Robert Wood Johnson Medical School, New Brunswick, NJ, USA

37.1.1.2 Carpal Tunnel Syndrome

Operation

When conservative measures fail, surgical decompression of the transverse carpal ligament by endoscopic, open release, or percutaneous approach can effectively alleviate carpal tunnel symptoms. Studies have compared endoscopic and open approaches with only a week faster return to work with the endoscopic technique [7]. In the past few years, office-based ultrasound-guided percutaneous approach has become an additional option for the release of transverse carpal ligament.

Rehabilitation

The goals of postoperative rehabilitation include reducing pain and swelling, promoting scar desensitization, and improving functional recovery. Active ROM and passive ROM (PROM) exercises can be initiated within the first week after surgery and return to full activities within eight weeks [8].

37.1.1.3 Triangular Fibrocartilage Complex (TFCC) Tears

Operation

Numerous surgical interventions can be implemented depending on the type of TFCC injury. For acute type 1A tears (central), arthroscopic debridement is indicated due to inadequate blood supply for healing. Arthroscopic or open repair may be performed for acute type 1B (ulnar), 1C (distal), and 1D (radial) injuries. Chronic (type 2) TFCC tears can be managed based on the amount of ulnar variance. For chronic tears with ulnar positive variance <2 mm, a wafer procedure (debridement with partial distal ulna resection), limited ulnar head resection, or ulnar shortening can be performed. For chronic tears with ulnar positive variance >2 mm, ulnar shortening osteotomy can be performed. Other less frequent options include a Darrach ulnar head resection, which is mainly used as a salvage procedure for recalcitrant

© The Author(s), under exclusive license to Springer Nature Switzerland AG 2022

S. A. Mostoufi et al. (eds.), *Clinical Guide to Musculoskeletal Medicine*, https://doi.org/10.1007/978-3-030-92042-5_37

pain [9]. After an isolated debridement without repair, the patient can be placed in a soft dressing or short arm cast/splint for 1–2 weeks to allow for surgical site healing. Strengthening can begin when near normal active ROM (AROM) is achieved and full activity at 4–6 weeks. If the TFCC tear has been repaired, the patient is placed in a long arm cast in supination for 4–6 weeks.

Rehabilitation
After cast removal, active and passive therapy is begun, followed by progressive strengthening, but full activity is not allowed until 3–4 months [4]. For ulnar shortening osteotomy, the short arm cast/splint is removed at 2 weeks, followed by ROM as tolerated and unrestricted activity after union at around 3 months.

37.1.1.4 Trigger Finger

Operation
The release of the A1 pulley can effectively alleviate triggering symptoms in >90% of patients. While surgical release via a mini-open approach remains the gold standard, many clinicians prefer percutaneous A1 pulley release with a needle or hook blade. On occasion, persistent triggering may exist after A1 pulley release, necessitating the release of additional structures (e.g., flexor digitorum superficialis slip, A2 pulley) [1].

Rehabilitation
Postoperatively, patients are placed into a non-restrictive soft dressing and allowed full use of the operative hand [2]. Dedicated hand therapy is typically not needed except in cases with residual symptoms or significant preoperative contractures.

37.1.1.5 De Quervain's Syndrome

Operation
The operative technique involves surgical release of the sheath of the first dorsal compartment with decompression of the abductor pollicis longus (APL) and extensor pollicis brevis (EPB) tendons [3]. Following surgery, a thumb spica splint is used for the first 1–2 weeks.

Rehabilitation
Early range of motion (ROM) exercises for the hand may begin right after the procedure with return to unrestricted activities after removal of the sutures and splint. For athletes and more severe cases, progressive strengthening with attention to the status of the radial sensory nerve and accessory branches [4] may require up to 6–8 weeks prior to unrestricted activity.

37.1.1.6 Thumb Ulnar Collateral Ligament (UCL) Injuries

Operation
Early surgical intervention is indicated for the acute thumb UCL tear with an indistinct endpoint to valgus stress examination. Oftentimes, the adductor aponeurosis can become caught between the torn ends of the UCL (Stener lesion) [14]. The surgery includes direct ligamentous repair with occasional K-wire protection. The hand is immobilized in a thumb spica splint for 4–6 weeks, followed by ROM exercises and progressive strengthening. Unrestricted use of the hand is allowed at about 3 months [15].

Rehabilitation
Rehab after surgical treatment of chronic tears is similar but with a slower progression.

37.2 Surgery for Fractures and Dislocations in the Wrist and Hand

37.2.1 Description

In this section, we will discuss surgical intervention for the following fracture and dislocations in the wrist and hand: scaphoid fractures, perilunate dislocation (PLD), distal radius fractures, mallet finger, and digital fractures.

37.2.1.1 Scaphoid Fractures

Operation
Operative intervention is indicated for scaphoid fractures that are displaced, unstable, or located at the proximal pole as these have a higher risk of non-union and osteonecrosis. Open reduction and internal fixation (ORIF) with cannulated headless compression screws are the most frequently utilized techniques and can be performed by multiple approaches [16]. A short arm or thumb spica splint is applied postoperatively and remains for 1–2 weeks, followed by a cast or thermoplastic splint for 6–10 weeks (duration depends on evidence of healing).

Rehabilitation
After cast removal, active and passive ROM exercises are initiated for 1–2 weeks, followed by progressive strengthening. A removable splint is used for protection with athletic activities for at least 3 months after cast removal. Athletes will have variations in rehab depending on their sport.

37.2.1.2 Perilunate Dislocation

Operation

All perilunate dislocations (PLD) and perilunate fracture-dislocations (PFLD) should be treated surgically. Closed reduction of the injury is performed acutely, followed by open reduction, ligamentous repair, and internal fixation when the swelling has improved [17]. This procedure can be performed with a dorsal, volar, or combined approach. Median nerve injury is frequently associated with these injuries, and the release of the carpal tunnel is recommended if symptoms are present. Chronic PLD or perilunate fracture dislocation (PLFD) can be treated with open reduction and internal fixation (ORIF), proximal row carpectomy, or total wrist arthrodesis.

Rehabilitation

Postoperative rehabilitation begins with splint immobilization for 1–2 weeks followed by casting for 6–8 weeks total. After cast removal, active and passive ROM exercises of the wrist, forearm, and thumb are initiated, followed by progressive strengthening protocols with hardware removal at approximately 12 weeks [17].

37.2.1.3 Distal Radius Fractures

Operation

Closed reduction and immobilization are the preferred treatments for non-displaced and stable distal radius fractures. ORIF is most often indicated for unstable, displaced, or comminuted distal radius fractures [18]. Distal radius ORIF can be accomplished with a dorsal-, volar-, or fragment-specific approach based on the fracture and patient characteristics.

Rehabilitation

Postoperatively, active and passive ROM of the fingers, elbow, and shoulders can begin immediately. Postoperative splints are removed at about 2 weeks, and active ROM of the wrist is initiated, followed by passive ROM 1–2 weeks later. A removable splint is to be worn at all times when not exercising or bathing. From 6–12 weeks, the patient can begin progressive strengthening and weaning of the splint until unrestricted activity at about 12 weeks [4].

37.2.1.4 Mallet Finger

Operation

Surgical management is indicated for specific injuries, noncompliance, and in professions where splinting would not be feasible. Doyle [10] classified these injuries into four types. Type I mallet fingers are closed injuries with or without small avulsion fractures, type II are open injuries, type III have skin and tendon tissue loss, and type IV have a fracture fragment >20% of the articular surface or involving the physis. Surgical treatment of type I injuries involves immobilization of the distal interphalangeal (DIP) joint in extension with a K-wire. Type II injuries may be treated with direct open tendon repair. Type III injuries require reconstruction and tendon grafting. Type IV injuries are treated operatively if the fractures involve >50% of the articular surface or DIP joint subluxation exists.

Rehabilitation

After surgery, the DIP joint is immobilized in extension with or without a K-wire for 6–8 weeks followed by a period of nighttime splinting [11] with progressive ROM for an additional 6 weeks. Following these strict DIP extension protocols is essential for healing, but PIP flexion should still be encouraged while the DIP joint is immobilized [4].

37.2.1.5 Other Digital Fractures

Operation

Surgical intervention may be indicated for injuries with displaced articular fragments, rotational malalignment, or significant angulation/shortening. Distal phalangeal fractures rarely require surgical fixation, but closed reduction and percutaneous pinning (CRPP) is preferred when indicated. CRPP remains the treatment of choice for unstable proximal and middle phalanx fractures and metacarpal fractures that can be reduced by closed means. When open reduction is required, fixation can be achieved with pins, interfragmentary screws, or a plate and screws depending on the fracture pattern. Other dislocations, such as at the metacarpophalangeal joint, may also require open reduction due to interposition of the surrounding soft tissues [12].

Rehabilitation

Postoperative rehabilitation is as variable as the treatment modalities used for these injuries. For less rigid constructs (i.e., Kirschner wires), immobilization is required for about 4 weeks until fracture healing and pin removal. For more rigid constructs (screws or plates), early active finger motion should be encouraged to promote tendon gliding and decrease adhesions and contractures. Fabricated static splints can be made for these patients to be used between exercise sessions. After open reduction of dislocations, the affected joint is generally splinted in flexion for 2–4 weeks, followed by progressive protected motion [13].

37.3 Surgery for Wrist and Hand Osteoarthritis (OA)

37.3.1 Wrist OA

Arthritis affecting the wrist is not one condition, but rather a spectrum of arthritides with varying etiologies, presentations, and treatments. Etiology aside, these can be broadly categorized by the affected joints into pan-carpal arthritis, radiolunate arthritis, radioscaphoid arthritis, and radioscapholunate arthritis.

37.3.1.1 Operation

The overall goal in surgical management of these conditions is to produce a pain free and stable wrist while preserving as much strength and motion as possible. Surgical treatment of pan-carpal arthritis is most commonly radiocarpal fusion, especially in young and higher-demand patients. However, total wrist arthroplasty can be utilized in lower-demand patients who will not be placing high levels of stress across the implant. Isolated radiolunate arthritis with a preserved midcarpal joint can be treated with radiolunate fusion. Arthritis affecting the radioscaphoid articulation is differentially treated depending on capitate and lunate involvement. If the capitate and lunate are involved, four-corner fusion is the preferred surgical intervention. However, if the capitate and lunate are preserved, the surgeon has the option of four-corner fusion or proximal row carpectomy. For arthritis affecting the radius, scaphoid, and lunate with preservation of the midcarpal joint, radioscapholunate fusion is indicated [22].

37.3.1.2 Rehabilitation

Postoperative rehabilitation protocols differ depending on the procedure performed. In general, rehab progresses less aggressively in fusion patients, as excessive early motion can prevent or delay adequate fusion [23]. For the first 2 weeks after total wrist fusion, the patient is left in the postoperative splint. After 2 weeks, a short or long arm splint is applied. A fitted, moveable splint in the neutral position can also be used if it is worn at all times. Active and passive ROM for the fingers and elbow can be started immediately but without wrist motion. At 6 weeks, gentle hand strengthening is incorporated, and a removable splint can be used when not in therapy. After 10 weeks, the splint can gradually be removed with no restrictions after 12 weeks. The postoperative management for the limited arthrodesis is similar, but some ROM of the wrist is preserved. Once rigid, immobilization is discontinued at 6 weeks.

ROM can be started earlier after proximal row carpectomy because fusion is not necessary. AROM of the wrist can start at 4 weeks with a removable orthosis at all other times, and by 6 weeks, the splint can gradually be removed and full PROM instituted. Strengthening can commence at 8 weeks with a goal to be done with therapy at 12 weeks. Similarly, patients undergoing total wrist arthroplasty can begin gentle wrist AROM and active-assisted range of motion (AAROM) in therapy as early as a few days after surgery, with a wrist splint at all other times [24]. At two weeks, therapy can begin to focus on functional tasks, with strengthening starting at 4 weeks and a gradual weaning of the splint until week 6. The remainder of the therapy focuses predominantly on ROM and activities of daily living (ADLs), as these implants are not designed for significant weighted exercises.

37.3.2 Thumb Metacarpophalangeal (Basal Joint) Arthritis

One of the most common complaints in elderly is painful first metacarpophalangeal joint (trapeziometacarpal). It interferes with ADLs and work and at times requires surgical intervention for improvement in function and pain.

37.3.2.1 Operation

Trapeziectomy is the most common surgical treatment when conservative measures fail. Simple trapeziectomy may be modified to include ligament reconstruction, tendon interposition with temporary Kirschner wires, or suture button constructs [19]. Rehab consists of 3–6 weeks of immobilization [20] followed by active and passive ROM and subsequent progressive strengthening and a return to full function at 3 months [21]. In some cases, mobilization may be started as soon as 3 days after surgery.

37.3.2.2 Rehabilitation

The rehab protocols for other procedures that include thumb metacarpal extension osteotomies, carpometacarpal arthrodesis, and implants (e.g., spacers, resurfacing, prostheses) are tailored individually for each procedure.

37.3.3 Interphalangeal Joint Arthritis

Surgical intervention for arthritis of the interphalangeal (IP) joint is indicated for functional impairment or intractable pain after a failed conservative management. Arthrodesis is the most commonly utilized method and is the treatment of choice for both distal interphalangeal (DIP) joint and proximal interphalangeal (PIP) joint arthritis.

37.3.3.1 Operation

PIP joint arthroplasty with silicone or metal implant prosthesis is a viable treatment option in the appropriate patient that desires motion of the joint. The recovery course following arthroplasty is longer compared to arthrodesis. Postoperatively, the patient is placed in a finger gutter or volar/dorsal splint.

Fusion of the DIP joint involves internal fixation with either crossed K-wires, interosseous wiring, a combination of K-wire and wire loop, or intramedullary screw [25]. For the PIP joint, internal fixation can be achieved with K-wires, interosseous wire loops, and tension band wiring. Following arthrodesis, the patient is placed in a finger gutter or volar/dorsal splint.

37.3.3.2 Rehabilitation

Postoperatively DIP Splinting of the DIP joint with a focus on ROM exercises of the other fingers and joints is initiated early. Patients typically return to full activity by 6–8 weeks [25]. Gentle active ROM of joints proximal and distal to the fused joint is begun with solid union by six to eight weeks [25].

Postoperatively PIP Active ROM and PROM exercises can begin within a few days and buddy taping; dynamic or static flexion splint can be added. ROM exercises are increased at week 3, followed by gentle progressive strengthening at week 8 and discontinuation of the splint by 12–14 weeks [25].

37.3.4 Metacarpophalangeal Joint Arthritis

Arthrodesis is generally reserved for the index finger MCP joint, especially in the younger patient or manual laborer [25].

37.3.4.1 Operation

Fixation can be achieved with tension band wiring, K-wires, or plate fixation. Postoperatively, static forearm splinting of the involved MCP joint with active ROM of the uninvolved joints can be initiated, and patients can discontinue the splint by 6–8 weeks depending upon the evidence of union [25].

37.3.4.2 Rehabilitation

Arthroplasty with silicone or metal implant prosthesis is the most widely accepted technique. Postoperatively, the patient is placed in a forearm dynamic outrigger splint to be worn during the day for 6–8 weeks and a forearm MCP and IP extension splint to be worn at rest or sleeping for three months until the joint is stable [25]. Alternatively, buddy taping with active ROM exercises or compressive isotoner glove with composite flexion and extension exercises can be utilized instead of the outrigger split [25].

References

1. Gil JA, Hresko AM, Weiss AC. Current concepts in the management of trigger finger in adults. J Am Acad Orthop Surg. 2020;28(15):e642–50.
2. Fiorini HJ, Tamaoki MJ, Lenza M, Gomes Dos Santos JB, Faloppa F, Belloti JC. Surgery for trigger finger. Cochrane Database Syst Rev. 2018;2(2):CD009860.
3. Ilyas AM, Ast M, Schaffer AA, Thoder J. De quervain tenosynovitis of the wrist. J Am Acad Orthop Surg. 2007;15(12):757–64.
4. Jaworski CA, Krause M, Brown J. Rehabilitation of the wrist and hand following sports injury. Clin Sports Med. 2010;29(1):61–80.
5. Balakatounis K, Angoules AG, Angoules NA, Panagiotopoulou K. Synthesis of evidence for the treatment of intersection syndrome. World J Orthop. 2017;8(8):619–23.
6. Williams JG. Surgical management of traumatic non-infective tenosynovitis of the wrist extensors. J Bone Joint Surg Br. 1977;59-B(4):408–10.
7. Scholten RJ, Mink van der Molen A, Uitdehaag BM, Bouter LM, de Vet HC. Surgical treatment options for carpal tunnel syndrome. Cochrane Database Syst Rev. 2007;2007(4):CD003905.
8. Peters S, Page MJ, Coppieters MW, Ross M, Johnston V. Rehabilitation following carpal tunnel release. Cochrane Database Syst Rev. 2016;2:CD004158.
9. Minami A. Triangular fibrocartilage complex tears. Hand Surg. 2015;20(1):1–9.
10. Doyle JR. Extensor tendons-acute injuries. In: Green DP, Hotchkiss RN, Pederson WC, editors. Green's operative hand surgery. 4th ed. New York: Churchill Livingstone; 1999. p. 1962–87.
11. Bendre AA, Hartigan BJ, Kalainov DM. Mallet finger. J Am Acad Orthop Surg. 2005;13(5):336–44.
12. Kozin SH, Thoder JJ, Lieberman G. Operative treatment of metacarpal and phalangeal shaft fractures. J Am Acad Orthop Surg. 2000;8(2):111–21.
13. Prucz RB, Friedrich JB. Finger joint injuries. Clin Sports Med. 2015;34(1):99–116.
14. Daley D, Geary M, Gaston RG. Thumb metacarpophalangeal ulnar and radial collateral ligament injuries. Clin Sports Med. 2020;39(2):443–55.
15. Ritting AW, Baldwin PC, Rodner CM. Ulnar collateral ligament injury of the thumb metacarpophalangeal joint. Clin J Sport Med. 2010;20(2):106–12.
16. Tait MA, Bracey JW, Gaston RG. Acute scaphoid fractures: a critical analysis review. JBJS Rev. 2016;4(9):01874474-201609000-00004.
17. Stanbury SJ, Elfar JC. Perilunate dislocation and perilunate fracture-dislocation. J Am Acad Orthop Surg. 2011;19(9):554–62.
18. Mauck BM, Swigler CW. Evidence-based review of distal radius fractures. Orthop Clin North Am. 2018;49(2):211–22.
19. Weiss AC, Goodman AD. Thumb basal joint arthritis. J Am Acad Orthop Surg. 2018;26(16):562–71.
20. Yuan F, Aliu O, Chung KC, Mahmoudi E. Evidence-based practice in the surgical treatment of thumb carpometacarpal joint arthritis. J Hand Surg Am. 2017;42(2):104–112.e1.
21. Baker RHJ, Al-Shukri J, Davis TRC. Evidence-based medicine: thumb basal joint arthritis. Plast Reconstr Surg. 2017;139(1):256e–66e.
22. Logan JS, Warwick D. The treatment of arthritis of the wrist. Bone Joint J. 2015;97-B(10):1303–8.
23. Hayden RJ, Jebson PJL. Wrist arthrodesis. Hand Clin. 2005;21:631–40.
24. Lin E, Paksima N. Total wrist arthroplasty. Bull Hosp Jt Dis (2013). 2017;75(1):9–14.
25. Estes JP, Bochenek C, Fassler P. Osteoarthritis of the fingers. J Hand Ther. 2000;13(2):108–23.

Part VII

Hip

Section Editor
Timothy Tiu

Anterior Hip Disorders

38

Kristian Von Rickenbach, Joanne Borg-Stein, and Haylee Borgstrom

38.1 Femoroacetabular Impingement

38.1.1 Synonyms

- Cam impingement
- Pincer impingement

38.1.2 ICD 10 Code

M25.85

38.1.3 Description

Anatomy The hip joint is a multidirectional ball-and-socket joint with the femoral head articulating with the concave acetabulum. The most inferior aspect of the acetabulum is incomplete, known as the acetabular notch. A fibrocartilaginous labrum adheres to the acetabular edge and thickens inferiorly to bridge the acetabular notch as the transverse acetabular ligament.

K. Von Rickenbach
Department of Physical Medicine & Rehabilitation, Spaulding Rehabilitation Hospital, Harvard Medical School, Charlestown, MA, USA

J. Borg-Stein
Department of Physical Medicine & Rehabilitation, Spaulding Rehabilitation Hospital, Massachusetts General Hospital, Harvard Medical School, Boston, MA, USA

Physical Medicine and Rehabilitation, Newton Wellesley Hospital Spine Center at Newton Wellesley Hospital, Boston, MA, USA
e-mail: borgstein@partners.org

H. Borgstrom (✉)
Department of Physical Medicine & Rehabilitation, Spaulding Rehabilitation Hospital, Massachusetts General Hospital, Harvard Medical School, Boston, MA, USA
e-mail: hborgstrom@partners.org

The proximal portion of the femur includes the articulating spherical femoral head and the narrowed femoral neck. A 125–130° inclination angle exists between the femoral neck and the femoral body, also known as the femoral neck–shaft angle. A fibrous joint capsule including the iliofemoral, ischiofemoral, and pubofemoral ligaments provides stability to the joint. Normal hip range of motion (ROM) is approximately 120° of flexion, 10° of extension, 45° of abduction, 25° of adduction, 45° of external rotation, and 35° of internal rotation, though normal ranges vary and symmetry is an important consideration.

Femoroacetabular impingement (FAI) is a common source of hip pain in the young- and middle-aged population, occurring secondary to abnormal abutment of the acetabulum and the proximal femur with associated soft tissue impingement. Accordingly, FAI is a mechanical and often multifactorial process with both static and dynamic risk factors. Congenital or acquired bony morphologic characteristics that result in approximation of the proximal femur on the acetabular rim, often in extreme ranges of flexion and internal rotation, may predispose to FAI. These morphologic changes may be idiopathic or secondary to repetitive stress during adolescence [1]. Dynamically, weak hip abductors, particularly gluteus medius, may result in increased hip adduction and exacerbation of impingement symptoms.

Based on bony morphology, FAI is commonly described as cam type, pincer type, or combined, with combined being the most common:

- A *cam lesion* is defined by a non-spherical enlargement of the femoral head at the femoral head–neck junction, also described as a pistol grip deformity (Fig. 38.1).
- A *pincer lesion* results from acetabular over-coverage of the femoral head [1]. Cam lesions are generally more prevalent in young males, while pincer lesions are more prevalent in middle-aged women [1]. Among athletes, however, cam lesions have been described to occur more commonly in both females and males [2].

© The Author(s), under exclusive license to Springer Nature Switzerland AG 2022
S. A. Mostoufi et al. (eds.), *Clinical Guide to Musculoskeletal Medicine*, https://doi.org/10.1007/978-3-030-92042-5_38

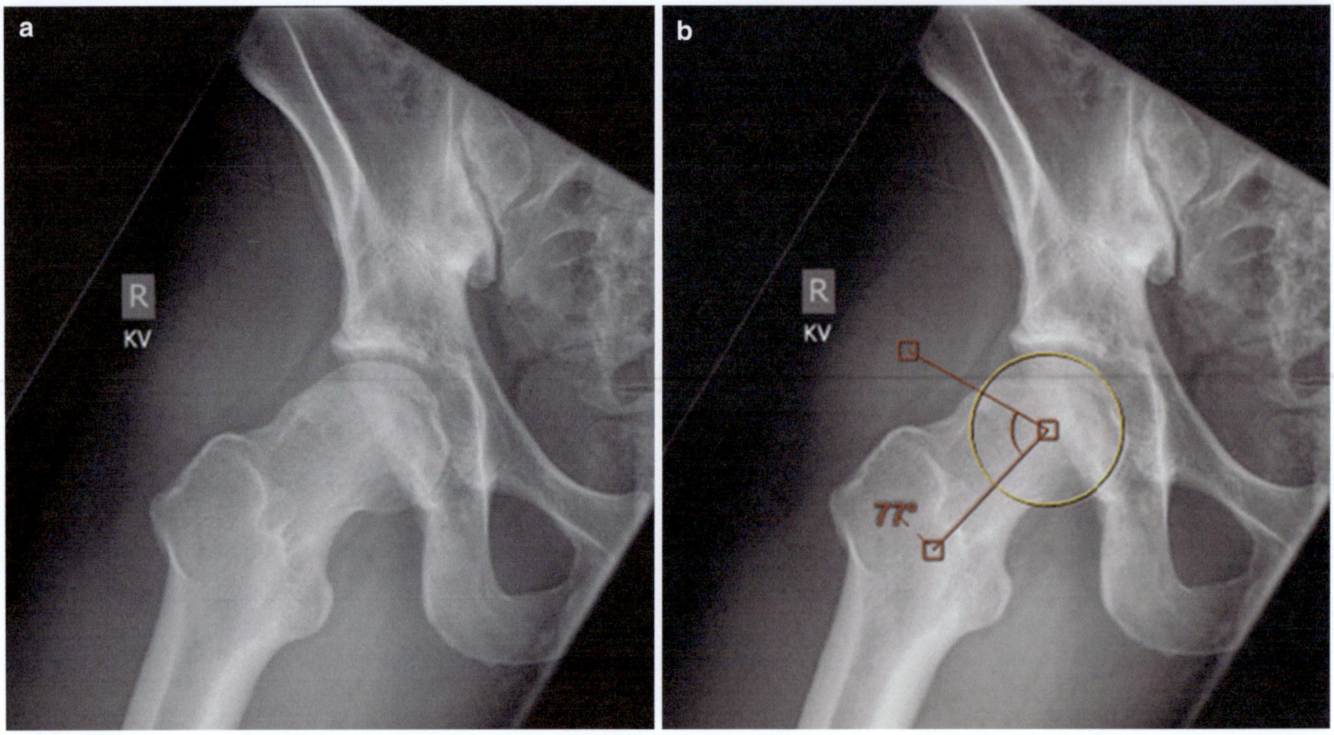

Fig. 38.1 Cam-type morphology with prominence of the femoral head–neck junction on elongated femoral neck radiograph (**a**). Alpha angle (normal <55 degrees) is measured by the angle between two intersecting lines: one along the femoral neck axis, the other from the center of the femoral head to the point where femoral head sphericity is lost (**b**)

It is important to note that radiographic FAI does not imply symptomatology as these findings are often present in asymptomatic individuals [3]. FAI is an important risk factor for the development of labral tears and early hip osteoarthritis. Among those undergoing surgery for FAI, 55% were found to have labral pathology, which is associated with early joint degenerative changes [4].

38.1.4 Clinical Presentation

Classically, FAI presents as anterior hip or groin pain, which is often described as sharp, pinching, or deep in nature and is typically insidious in onset. Patients may demonstrate the "C" sign with cupping of the fingers anteriorly and the thumb posteriorly demonstrating location of hip pain common with intra-articular hip pathology (Fig. 38.2). Given frequent concomitant intra-articular hip pathology such as chondral injuries or labral tears, pain may refer in complex and variable patterns, most commonly to the anterolateral thigh and buttock region. Radiation below the knee has been described in nearly 25% of cases [5]. Commonly, pain is worse with movements that result in hip flexion, adduction, and/or internal rotation, such as prolonged sitting, squatting, or pivoting, as well as impact activity and transitional movements. Mechanical symptoms such as locking, clicking, or popping may be present.

38.1.5 Physical Examination

The differential diagnosis for anterior hip pain is broad (Table 38.1). Physical examination must include a thorough bilateral hip evaluation with special attention to asymmetries. In addition, a comprehensive spine, bony pelvis, soft tissue, sacroiliac, and neurologic assessment must be performed. Depending on history, additional examination for intra-abdominal or intrapelvic pathology can be included.

Gait evaluation Gait is typically non-antalgic, but Trendelenburg gait may be present due to weak hip abductors further contributing to dynamic hip adduction and impingement positioning. Patients may endorse reproduction of pain with stance phase on the affected leg. Gait speed may be reduced.

Observation Inspection for posture, pelvic tilt, leg length discrepancy, and deformity should be completed, noting significant asymmetries. Often inspection is normal in FAI with or without labral tear, though the affected hip may be held in external rotation to avoid impingement position.

Palpation Palpatory examination is often normal, though hip flexor tendon pain/dysfunction, gluteal and iliotibial band tendinopathy, and regional myofascial pain may also coexist, which should prompt further evaluation.

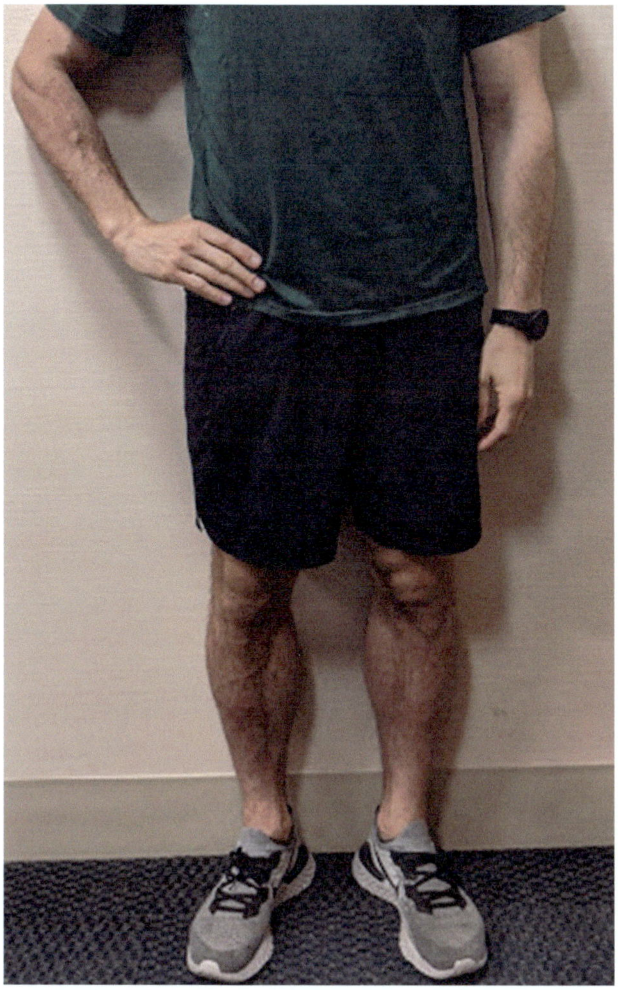

Fig. 38.2 Classic "C" sign with cupping of the fingers anteriorly and the thumb posteriorly demonstrating location of hip pain common with intra-articular hip pathology

Table 38.1 Differential diagnosis for anterior hip pain

Intra-articular pathology	
Femoroacetabular impingement	Cartilage defect
Labral tear	Osteoarthritis
Hip dysplasia	Joint arthropathies
Hip fracture/bone stress injury	Avascular necrosis
Ligamentum teres tear	Septic arthritis
Peri-articular pathology	
Anterior snapping hip	Athletic pubalgia
Iliopsoas tendinopathy/bursopathy	Osteitis pubis
Adductor or hip flexor strain	Hernia
Referred pain	
Lumbar spine pathology including radiculopathy	Intra-abdominal referred pain
Peripheral nerve impingement	Intrapelvic referred pain

Range of motion (ROM) Both passive and active ROM should be examined in all planes. Reproduction of index anterior hip or groin pain, particularly in flexion, adduction, and internal rotation, is suggestive of FAI. Unilateral limitations in end ROM indicate intra-articular hip pathology and possibly associated labral tear or osteoarthritis, which may be asymmetric compared to contralateral hip.

Sensory testing Upper lumbar/lower thoracic radiculopathy may mimic the classic groin pain distribution of FAI. Bilateral sensory examination should be normal in FAI (T12-S1). If deficits are present, further workup for radiculopathy is warranted.

Deep tendon reflexes Lower extremity reflexes should be tested, including patellar (L4 predominant), medial hamstring (L5), and Achilles (S1) tendons. Reflexes should be normal 2+ and symmetric in FAI. If changes or asymmetries are present, neurologic etiology should be considered.

Motor testing Pain-limited weakness may be noted with manual muscle testing in supine and/or seated hip flexion, adduction, abduction, side-lying hip abduction, and/or prone extension in FAI. Strength assessment including L2-S1 myotomes should also be completed to evaluate for possible neurologic etiology.

Joint testing Careful assessment of the lumbar spine including pubic symphysis, facet joints, and sacroiliac joints should be performed.

38.1.6 Special Maneuvers

FADIR (anterior impingement) test With the patient in a supine position, the affected hip is passively moved into *Flexion, ADduction, and Internal Rotation* (Fig. 38.3a). A positive test reproduces index hip pain in FAI as this position results in approximation of the proximal femur and acetabulum. This is the most sensitive clinical test for FAI and labral tears with sensitivity reported over 90% though with low specificity [6, 7].

FABER (Patrick's) test Also with the patient in supine position, the affected hip is passively moved in *Flexion, ABduction, and External Rotation* (Fig. 38.3b). Reproduction of index anterior hip pain suggests intra-articular hip pathology with sensitivity of approximately 80%, but is not specific for FAI alone [7]. Posterior pain with this maneuver may suggest sacroiliac joint disease.

Single-leg squat may demonstrate gluteal weakness with increased dynamic hip adduction contributing to impingement positioning. Other maneuvers that are commonly utilized to evaluate for intra-articular hip pathology include the *log roll* (Fig. 38.3c), *Stinchfield's test* (or resisted straight leg raise) (Fig. 38.3d), *hop test*, and *scour test* (all with lower sensitivities and specificities for FAI and labral tears) [6, 7].

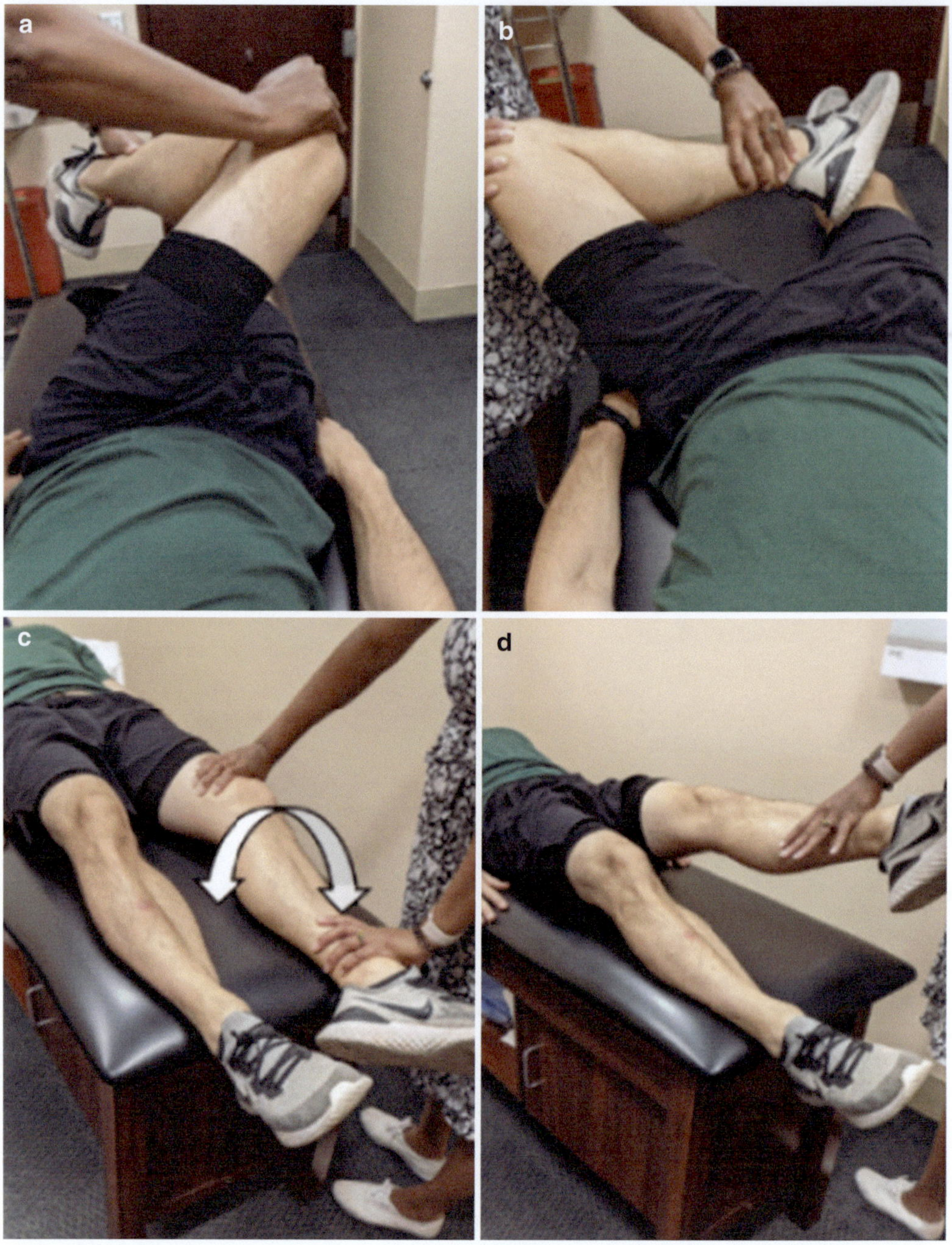

Fig. 38.3 Common clinical examination maneuvers to evaluate for intra-articular hip pathology: FADIR (**a**), FABER (**b**), logroll (**c**), and Stinchfield's test (**d**)

38.1.7 Diagnostic Workup

FAI is a clinical diagnosis. Imaging is often utilized to further characterize contributing bony morphology; evaluate for concomitant labral, chondral, or soft tissue pathology; or rule out other differential diagnoses.

X-ray Plain radiographs are typically the main imaging modality in patients with suspected FAI and should include anteroposterior (AP) and lateral views of the hip. Weight-bearing AP pelvis is recommended as this allows for evaluation of concomitant joint degenerative change. The elongated femoral neck (or Dunn) view, which is obtained with 45 degrees of hip flexion, better reveals the anterior femoral head–neck junction where cam-type lesions are most commonly located [8]. Though with limited clinical utility, an alpha angle greater than 55 degrees on Dunn radiograph and a lateral center-edge angle (LCEA) greater than 40 degrees on AP radiograph are suggestive of cam and pincer deformities, respectively [8] (Figs. 38.1 and 38.4). The presence of os acetabuli, or a small ossicle at the superolateral acetabular margin, has been associated with FAI and underlying labral tear.

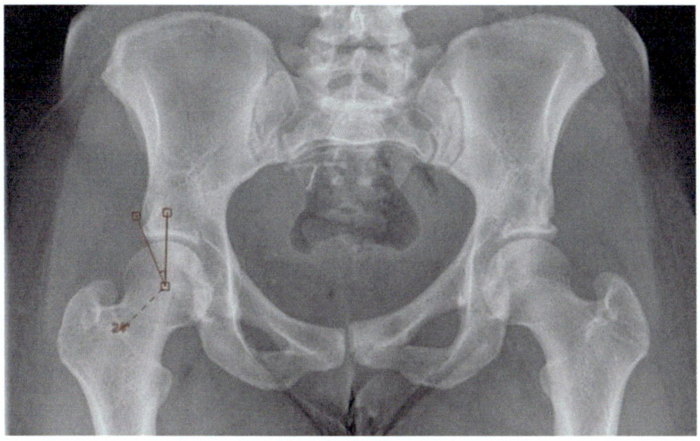

Fig. 38.4 AP pelvic radiograph demonstrating borderline hip dysplasia with under-coverage of the femoral heads bilaterally. Lateral center-edge angle (LCEA, normal >25 degrees) is measured by the angle between a vertical line and a line extending to the lateral acetabular rim, both originating from the center of the femoral head

Computed tomography (CT) CT is typically reserved for preoperative assessment and surgical planning to better understand its structural anatomy.

Magnetic resonance images Magnetic resonance imaging (MRI) with or without arthrography is often utilized to assess for concurrent articular cartilage or labral defects, both of which are associated with FAI.

Musculoskeletal ultrasound Both cam and pincer lesions can be seen on ultrasound by an experienced sonographer. Dynamic hip range of motion may demonstrate impingement.

Diagnostic intra-articular hip injection In cases where diagnosis remains ambiguous, a single ultrasound- or fluoroscopy-guided intra-articular hip injection with local anesthesia can be performed.

38.1.8 Treatment

38.1.8.1 Medical Management

Conservative treatment for FAI typically consists of patient education, activity modification including avoidance of impingement positioning, ice, and nonsteroidal anti-inflammatory drugs (NSAIDs) for pain management.

38.1.8.2 Rehabilitation

A 6- to 8-week course of physical therapy is often successful for the treatment of FAI and labral tears and should focus on core and gluteal strengthening, correction of dynamic malalignment contributing to hip adduction/impingement positioning, postural optimization to address lumbar hyperlordosis or anterior pelvic tilt, and manual therapy as indicated [1, 9]. Common rehabilitation exercises for FAI and labral tears are depicted in Fig. 38.5. Forced stretching, especially at the end range of motion, should be avoided.

38.1.8.3 Procedures

Intra-articular hip injection A single ultrasound- or fluoroscopy-guided intra-articular hip injection with local anesthetic with or without corticosteroids may be used for diagnostic and/or therapeutic purposes (Fig. 38.6). Pain relief has a high sensitivity for intra-articular pathology [1]. Alternative injectates including platelet-rich plasma, hyaluronic acid, and other orthobiologics may be considered, though limited high-quality evidence exists for their therapeutic benefit.

38.1.8.4 Surgery

Surgical interventions including arthroscopic debridement and osteoplasty may be considered for refractory cases and are discussed in detail in a subsequent chapter. If present, labral pathology is often addressed simultaneously. Surgical outcomes are typically positive with most patients returning to their previous level of activity. Poorer outcomes are associated with increased age, obesity, and pre-existing osteoarthritis [1]. Surgical risks include neurovascular injury, heterotopic ossification, deep venous thrombosis, and infection. See Chapter 42 for more details on hip surgeries.

38.2 Acetabular Labral Tear

38.2.1 Synonyms

Hip labral tear

38.2.2 ICD 10 Code

S73.1, M24.159

38.2.3 Description

Anatomy The horseshoe-shaped labrum contributes to joint stability and acetabular depth, force absorption and distribution, and maintenance of joint hydrostatic pressure. It is a fibrocartilaginous structure with a dense connective tissue capsular component that is inferiorly contiguous with the transverse acetabular ligament [1]. Vascular supply is via superior and inferior gluteal and obturator arteries [10] and sensory innervation from branches of the nerve to the quadratus femoris and the obturator nerve.

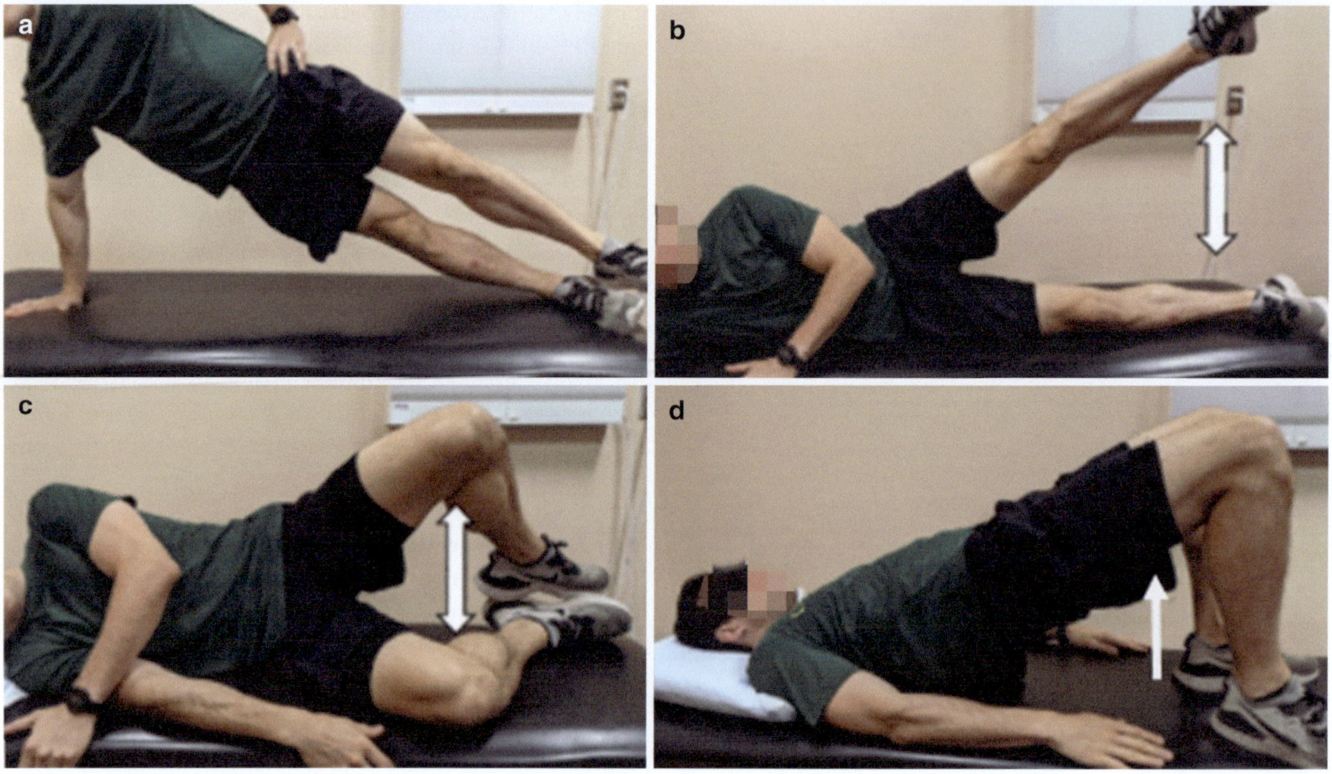

Fig. 38.5 Common hip rehabilitation exercises focused on core and gluteal strengthening: side plank (**a**, can be performed on flexed elbow as well to decrease force through the wrist), side-lying straight leg raises (**b**, hip in neutral to slight extension), clamshells (**c**), and gluteal bridges (**d**, may be performed on single leg)

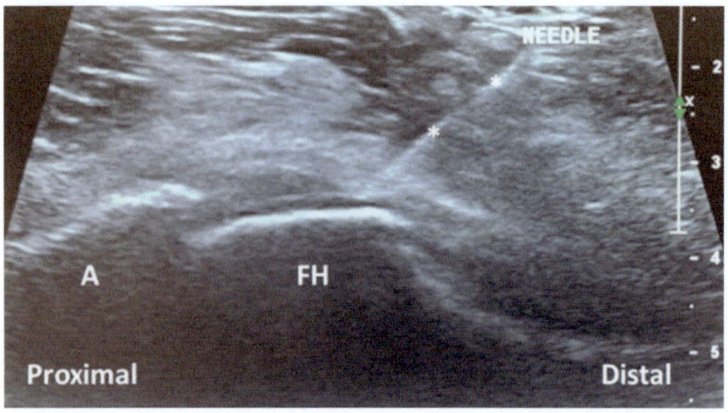

Fig. 38.6 Ultrasound-guided intra-articular hip injection performed with patient in supine position with distal-to-proximal in-plane approach (asterisks indicate needle) targeting just superior to typical femoral head–neck junction given small osseous bump/irregularity at this level (A acetabulum, FH femoral head)

Acetabular labral tears can occur in isolation or concurrently with other intra-articular hip pathology. Tears can be classified as traumatic, degenerative, dysplastic, or idiopathic [10]. Acute labral tears are less common and often occur in the setting of trauma, including during hip dislocation or with sudden high-velocity twisting or pivoting motions. Chronic degenerative tears are much more common and occur in the setting of repetitive stress and chronic inflammatory change. The risk factors for the development of labral tears include FAI, capsular laxity/hypermobility, hip dysplasia, and joint degenerative disease [10]. Labral tears are more common in females, likely due to increased frequency of associated risk factors [11].

The most common location for labral tears is the anterosuperior chondrolabral junction, which corresponds to a region of relatively low vascularization and high innervation that is prone to repetitive injury with hip impingement [11]. Posterior tears can occur secondary to posterior hip dislocation or dysplasia. Of note, labral tears have been demonstrated to increase risk for joint degenerative change by at least two-fold with chondral damage occurring in the same zone as labral injury in over 90% of cases [10]. Thus, early diagnosis and appropriate management are key for optimizing long-term joint health.

38.2.4 Clinical Presentation

Acetabular labral tears typically present with vague anterior hip or groin pain, often described as dull with episodes of sharp pain. They are commonly seen in the active, young female population, though they occur in both sexes and all age groups. Distribution of pain is similar to that of FAI as discussed in this chapter. Pain is more often insidious in onset but may be secondary to a specific traumatic event. Aggravating factors are also similar to those in FAI, but with increased occurrence of night pain. Mechanical symptoms and antalgic gait are reported more frequently than with isolated FAI.

38.2.5 Physical Examination

Physical exam components for labral tears is nearly identical to that of FAI with notable clinical differences in gait and ROM.

Gait evaluation Gait may more commonly be antalgic when compared to isolated FAI. In an older population, antalgic gait often correlates with hip osteoarthritis.

Range of motion (ROM) Clicking or limitation in motion is more commonly elicited with passive and active ROM in the setting of labral tear compared to isolated FAI. Additionally, active hip flexion and passive extension may provoke pain given close proximity of the hip flexor tendons, specifically the iliopsoas tendon, to the anterosuperior capsulolabral complex, which is the most common location for labral tears.

38.2.6 Diagnostic Workup

X-ray Plain radiographs may demonstrate associated bony abnormalities including os acetabuli, cam or pincer lesions, hip dysplasia, or osteoarthritis.

Computer tomography CT is typically not needed except in the case of surgical planning or suspected fracture.

MRI MR arthrogram is the preferred imaging modality for diagnosis of labral pathology with increased sensitivity and specificity compared to MRI alone (Fig. 38.7). Labral tears may be partial thickness, full thickness (detached), or complex. Adjacent chondral injury or paralabral cyst may be identified [8].

Musculoskeletal ultrasound Some labral tears and paralabral cysts can be visualized on ultrasound by an experienced sonographer. However, MR is the preferred modality to diagnose and characterize labral tears.

Diagnostic intra-articular hip injection In cases where diagnosis remains ambiguous, a single ultrasound- or fluoroscopy-guided intra-articular hip injection with local anesthesia can be performed.

38.2.7 Treatment

38.2.7.1 Medical Management, Rehabilitation, and Procedures

Conservative treatment for labral tears is similar to that for FAI as previously detailed. Repeat intra-articular steroid and anesthetic injections are generally avoided, especially in the younger population without underlying joint degenerative change, given concern for potential cumulative chondrotoxicity. Orthobiologic injections can be considered, though they are lacking in high-quality supportive evidence [1].

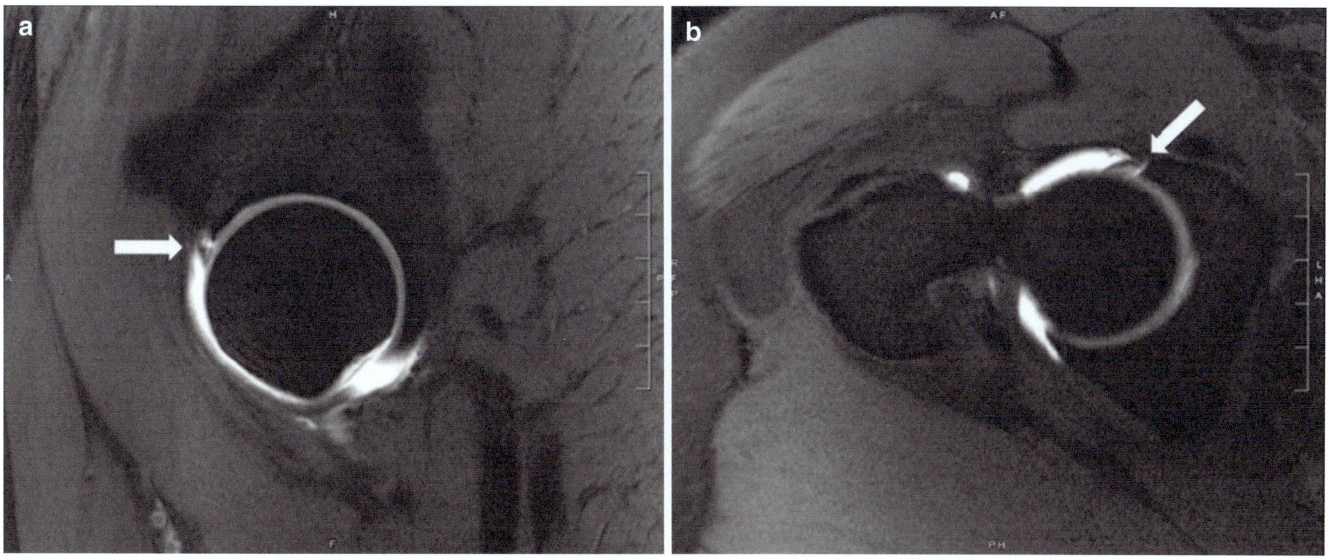

Fig. 38.7 MR arthrogram of the hip demonstrating complex detached tear of the anterosuperior labrum (arrows) on sagittal (**a**) and oblique axial (**b**) T1-weighted imaging with fat suppression

38.2.7.2 Surgery

In cases of symptomatic labral tears refractory to conservative treatment, surgical referral for consideration of arthroscopy with debridement of labral repair should be made. Particularly in the absence of significant underlying joint degenerative change, surgical management has been demonstrated to have good outcomes related to pain, functional improvement, and overall joint preservation. Concomitant bony FAI morphology or chondral injury is often addressed concurrently. See Chapter 42 for more details on hip surgeries.

38.3 Hip Dysplasia

38.3.1 Synonyms

- Developmental dysplasia of the hip (DDH)
- Acetabular dysplasia
- Congenital dysplasia of the hip

38.3.2 ICD 10 Code

Q65.89

38.3.3 Description

Anatomy The acetabulum is the concave socket of the hip joint formed by the coalescence of the pubic, ilium, and ischium bones with ossification occurring at 14–16 years. The acetabulum is oriented to face anteriorly and caudally. The superior dome is the weight-bearing portion of the acetabulum. In a normal hip, the labrum supports 1–2% of the loading force. In a dysplastic hip, the labrum bears up to 4–11% of this total load [12]. Labral or acetabular hypertrophy may occur as a physiologic attempt to increase femoral head coverage in dysplastic hips [13].

Hip dysplasia is a condition in which structural acetabular osseous deficits, or a shallow socket, lead to under-coverage of the femoral head (Fig. 38.4), resulting in reduced inherent joint stability [14]. Developmental dysplasia of the hip is a congenital condition that persists into adulthood in 40% of cases [11]. Hip dysplasia can occur in isolation or with concurrent pathology related to repetitive microtrauma/overload of the surrounding soft tissue structures, including labral tears; capsular injury; tendinopathies affecting hip flexor tendons, gluteal tendons, and the iliotibial band; and early osteoarthritis [14].

38.3.4 Clinical Presentation

Hip dysplasia typically presents as atraumatic, insidious onset of groin or lateral hip pain. It is commonly diagnosed in the young, skeletally mature, active adult. It is more common in females, and symptoms are often present for months to years prior to diagnosis. Pain is described as deep and aching, also commonly with the presence of the "C" sign (Fig. 38.2). Aggravating factors include prolonged sitting, weight-bearing, and activities involving hip flexion, external rotation, and rotational movement, particularly under load [14]. Given frequent association with labral pathology and osteoarthritis, mechanical symptoms may be described, and sensation of instability or subjective weakness is not uncommon [12].

38.3.5 Physical Examination

Hip dysplasia can be difficult to differentiate from labral injury or FAI by physical exam alone given overlapping constellations of findings and their frequent concurrent presentation [14]. Thus, physical examination should include all of the previously discussed components related to FAI and labral pathology with the following notable clinical differences.

Gait evaluation Gait may more commonly be antalgic compared to FAI occurring in nearly 50% of cases [14]. Additionally, the patient may describe apprehension with end-range hip extension during terminal stance phase related to loading of the edge of the femoral head on the acetabular rim. Trendelenburg gait may be present due to chronically weak hip abductors.

Range of motion (ROM) Active and passive ROM are often increased in the setting of hip dysplasia due to decreased joint stability and are often accompanied by pain at end range and other findings related to concomitant joint disease as previously discussed. Increased femoral anteversion associated with hip dysplasia may result in a pattern of increased internal rotation and decreased external rotation [14], which is typically in contrast to FAI, labral pathology, and hip osteoarthritis.

Beighton score Testing for generalized hypermobility may be accomplished with the use of the Beighton score (Table 38.2). A score of 4 or greater out of 9 suggests joint laxity, which is important to consider during treatment and rehabilitation and may prompt further specialty referral for evaluation of underlying connective tissue disease in certain clinical contexts.

Table 38.2 Components of the Beighton score for assessing generalized joint hypermobility

Passive extension of the fifth metacarpal-phalangeal joint beyond 90 degrees	1 point for each side
Passive thumb apposition to the forearm	1 point for each side
Passive hyperextension of the elbow beyond 10 degrees	1 point for each side
Passive hyperextension of the knees beyond 10 degrees	1 point for each side
Active trunk forward flexion with palms able to rest flat on the floor	1 point
TOTAL	9

38.3.6 Diagnostic Workup

X-ray Weight-bearing AP pelvic and lateral hip radiographs are often diagnostic for hip dysplasia in the correct clinical setting. LCEA less than 25 degrees on AP pelvic radiographs suggests hip dysplasia [8, 14] (Fig. 38.4). There are a variety of other imaging measurements to characterize dysplasia on radiographs, CT, and MRI. As previously discussed, radiographs may also demonstrate associated bony abnormalities including os acetabuli, cam or pincer lesions, or osteoarthritis.

CT CT represents the best imaging modality to assess acetabular coverage and version, though it is typically only required for surgical planning.

MRI MRI with or without arthrography is useful in evaluating for concurrent soft tissue pathology that is common in hip dysplasia, including chondral, labral, capsular, or tendon disorders.

Diagnostic intra-articular hip injection A single image-guided intra-articular hip injection with local anesthesia can be performed if diagnosis and symptomatology are unclear and may be particularly helpful in the setting of comorbid spine disease.

38.3.7 Treatments

38.3.7.1 Medical Management, Rehabilitation, and Procedures

In general, it is similar to FAI and labral tears with addition of focused core and gluteal strengthening programs. Overstretching and strengthening through supra-physiologic ranges of motion should be avoided, particularly in the case of generalized hypermobility. Intra-articular corticosteroid injection therapy may be therapeutic in milder cases of dysplasia but is unlikely to be beneficial in more advanced cases.

38.3.7.2 Surgery

Surgical consultation should be considered early in the management of hip dysplasia, especially in young patients (less than 40 years old) without significant joint degenerative change. These patients may be candidates for hip preservation surgery with periacetabular osteotomy (PAO) even in the case of only mild symptoms refractory to conservative care in an effort to avoid or delay the need for early total hip arthroplasty, which is more frequent in those with hip dysplasia compared to FAI or normal hips due to earlier degenerative change [13, 14]. See Chapter 42 for more details on hip surgeries.

38.4 Iliopsoas Tendon Dysfunction and Related Disorders

38.4.1 Synonyms

- Anterior/internal snapping hip
- Anterior/internal coxa saltans
- Iliopsoas impingement
- Iliopsoas tendinopathy
- Iliopsoas bursopathy

38.4.2 ICD 10 Code

M76.1

38.4.3 Description

Anatomy The iliopsoas muscle is a dynamic hip flexor and stabilizer composed of three muscles: the psoas major, minor, and iliacus. The psoas major and minor originate from T12-L5 vertebral bodies, transverse processes, and intervertebral discs, while the iliacus originates from the anterior iliac crest and fossa and sacral ala [15]. Innervation is by the ventral rami of L1-L3 for the psoas and the femoral nerve for the iliacus. The muscles converge at the L5-S2 vertebral level, forming the iliopsoas muscle–tendon unit. The iliopsoas tendon travels just anterior to the anterosuperior capsulolabral complex and inserts onto the lesser trochanter. The iliopsoas bursa lies deep to the tendon, superficial to the iliopectineal eminence, and may communicate with the hip joint in up to 15% of patients [15].

Iliopsoas tendon dysfunction is a common cause for anterior hip pain and may result in variable pathophysiology, including internal snapping hip, iliopsoas impingement, tendinopathy, and/or bursopathy. Iliopsoas tendon dysfunction may occur primarily or secondarily as a result of compensatory overuse in the setting of intra-articular hip pathology. As these disorders frequently occur concomitantly, clinical evaluation and treatment recommendations are similar. The risk factors may include tight hip flexors, weak core and posterior chain, anterior pelvic tilt, and joint hypermobility, among others.

38.4.3.1 Internal Snapping Hip, or Internal Coxa Saltans

It refers to snapping of the iliopsoas tendon during dynamic movement, most frequently from flexion, abduction, and external rotation back into a neutral position. Internal snapping hip may not be symptomatic and is more commonly painful in an athletic population, especially females, compared to the general population [11, 15]. Dynamic ultrasound has demonstrated that internal snapping hip results from a rotatory movement of the tendon within the muscle belly before snapping back into place again the superior pubic ramus [16] rather than translation over the iliopectineal eminence as often purported. Persistent snapping can lead to iliopsoas tendinopathy or bursopathy, though occurrence is rare [11, 17].

38.4.3.2 Iliopsoas Impingement

This may occur with or without concurrent internal snapping hip. Given the anatomic proximity of the iliopsoas tendon to the anterosuperior labrum (Fig. 38.8), specifically in the region where most labral pathology occurs, a dysfunctional tendon may impinge upon the capsulolabral complex increasing the risk for underlying labral injury.

38.4.4 Clinical Presentation

Iliopsoas tendon dysfunction most often presents with insidious onset anterior hip or groin pain. If present, the patient may be able to reproduce audible or palpable snapping, which may be painful or associated with a sensation of joint instability. Aggravating factors include active hip flexion, hip extension, weight-bearing or impact exercise, and transitional movements [15]. Symptomatic internal snapping hip is most commonly seen in athletes, especially in sports with increased hip range of motion such as dance, soccer, and hockey [15].

38.4.5 Physical Examination

Previously described principles related to comprehensive hip, spine, pelvis/SI joint, and neurologic assessment should be applied during evaluation of iliopsoas tendon dysfunction.

Gait evaluation Gait is typically non-antalgic. Patients may describe pain during terminal stance and pre-swing phase on the affected side.

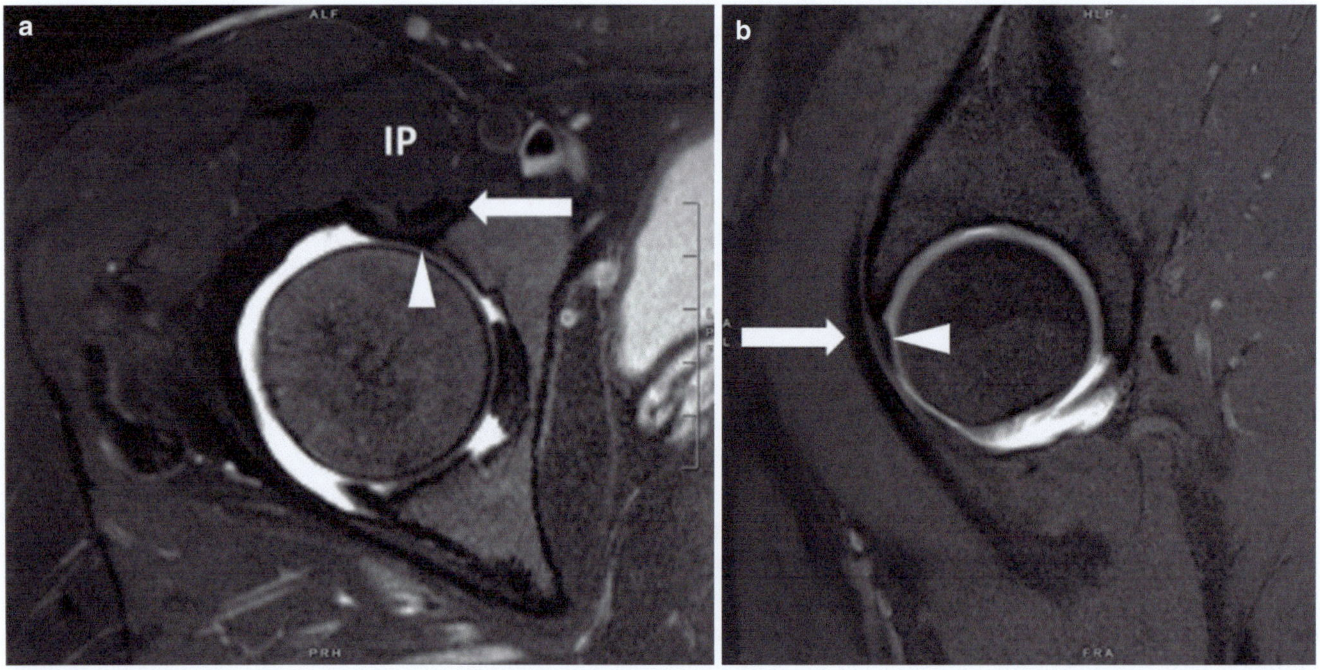

Fig. 38.8 MR arthrogram of the right hip demonstrating the proximity of the hypointense iliopsoas tendon (arrow) and labrum (arrowhead) on axial T2-weighted (**a**) and sagittal T1-weighted (**b**) sequences with fat suppression. IP iliopsoas muscle

Observation Inspection for risk factors associated with iliopsoas tendon dysfunction including anterior pelvic tilt should be completed. If the patient is able to reproduce snapping, provocative movement should be observed.

Palpation Palpatory exam often demonstrates tenderness directly over the iliopsoas tendon, which should be differentiated from the nearby direct head of the rectus femoris, which lies just lateral. If present, palpation of snapping during provocative movement should be completed.

Range of motion (ROM) Both passive and active ROM are often preserved in isolated iliopsoas tendon dysfunction, though index groin pain may be reproduced with active hip flexion and passive extension resulting in iliopsoas stretch. Limitation in ROM suggests intra-articular hip pathology. Passive reproduction of snapping is most commonly accomplished with movement of the hip from FABER position into neutral or into extension, adduction, and internal rotation [11, 15].

Motor testing, joint Testing Isolation of the iliopsoas from other hip flexors can be achieved with strength testing at 90 degrees of hip flexion or greater. Resisted hip flexion can be tested in seated or supine position, both of which may reproduce pain in the setting of iliopsoas tendon dysfunction, though strength should be maintained [15, 17]. Concomitant intra-articular hip pathology may be present; thus, previously described special maneuvers should be conducted as well.

38.4.5.1 Special Maneuvers

Thomas test In supine position, the patient pulls bilateral knees to the chest wall into maximal hip and knee flexion. The patient then releases one leg, extending it back toward the table. A positive test occurs when the patient is unable to extend the hip to neutral or if lumbar lordosis occurs, indicating a tight or shortened iliopsoas.

Active iliopsoas snapping test Similar to previously described passive ROM maneuver to reproduce snapping, in this case, the patient actively moves from FABER position to neutral while the examiner palpates the iliopsoas tendon. An audible or palpable snap typically occurs between 30 and 45 degrees of hip flexion [15].

38.4.6 Diagnostic Workup

X-ray AP pelvic and lateral hip radiographs are typically normal as with other soft tissue pathology, though they are useful to evaluate for concurrent bony abnormalities.

MRI MRI may demonstrate iliopsoas tendinopathy or bursopathy, though these findings are rare. Iliopsoas bursopathy may appear as a hyperintense fluid collection posteromedial to the myotendinous unit on T2-weighted sequences [17]. MRI or MR arthrography may also evaluate for common concurrent intra-articular pathology, including underlying labral tear.

Musculoskeletal ultrasound Ultrasound may demonstrate asymmetric tendon thickening or heterogeneity consistent with tendinopathy and bursitis, though again this is a rare finding. Dynamic testing for visualization of the snapping iliopsoas tendon may be performed.

Diagnostic injection Under direct ultrasound visualization, injection of local anesthesia into the iliopsoas tendon sheath can be performed for diagnostic purposes. This may be particularly useful in the setting of concomitant intra-articular hip pathology.

38.4.7 Treatments

38.4.7.1 Medical Management

Conservative treatment for iliopsoas tendon dysfunction is similar to that of aforementioned diagnoses in this chapter given frequent concurrent nature. Patient education, activity modification, ice, and nonsteroidal anti-inflammatory drugs (NSAIDs) can be utilized. Reassurance and education should be provided in the case of non-painful internal snapping hip.

38.4.7.2 Rehabilitation

Physical therapy should focus on stretching/lengthening of the iliopsoas and hip flexors, core and gluteal strengthening, and postural optimization to correct lumbar hyperlordosis and anterior pelvic tilt.

38.4.7.3 Procedures

Trigger point injections (TPIs) Targeting the iliopsoas musculature and other hip flexor musculature with TPI can be utilized to address myofascial pain limiting rehabilitation efforts. Often this is performed with ultrasound guidance given nearby neurovascular structures.

Corticosteroid injection Under direct ultrasound or fluoroscopic visualization, injection of corticosteroid into the iliopsoas tendon sheath can be performed. If bursopathy is present, this can also be targeted, keeping in mind that the bursa communicates with the hip joint in 15% of people [15]. Symptomatic relief may allow for enhanced participation in physical therapy.

38.4.7.4 Surgery

In the vast majority of cases, iliopsoas tendon dysfunction is managed successfully with non-operative care. For refractory cases, arthroscopic iliopsoas tendon release may be considered, along with additional surgical management of concurrent intra-articular hip pathology [15]. Failure to recognize iliopsoas tendon dysfunction and impingement prior to hip arthroscopy for other primary indications may result in poorer outcomes with nearly a third of patients undergoing revision arthroscopy found to have symptoms of iliopsoas impingement [18]. See Chapter 42 for more details on hip surgeries.

References

1. Hankins DA, Korcek L, Richter DL. Femoroacetabular impingement and management of labral tears in the athlete. Clin Sports Med. 2021;40(2):259–70.
2. Gerhardt MB, Romero AA, Silvers HJ, Harris DJ, Watanabe D, Mandelbaum BR. The prevalence of radiographic hip abnormalities in elite soccer players. Am J Sports Med. 2012;40(3):584–8.
3. Frank JM, Harris JD, Erickson BJ, Slikker W 3rd, Bush-Joseph CA, Salata MJ, et al. Prevalence of femoroacetabular impingement imaging findings in asymptomatic volunteers: a systematic review. Arthroscopy. 2015;31(6):1199–204.
4. Kuhlman GS, Domb BG. Hip impingement: identifying and treating a common cause of hip pain. Am Fam Physician. 2009;80(12):1429–34.
5. Lesher JM, Dreyfuss P, Hager N, Kaplan M, Furman M. Hip joint pain referral patterns: a descriptive study. Pain Med. 2008;9(1):22–5.
6. Reiman MP, Goode AP, Cook CE, Holmich P, Thorborg K. Diagnostic accuracy of clinical tests for the diagnosis of hip femoroacetabular impingement/labral tear: a systematic review with meta-analysis. Br J Sports Med. 2015;49(12):811.
7. Maslowski E, Sullivan W, Forster Harwood J, Gonzalez P, Kaufman M, Vidal A, et al. The diagnostic validity of hip provocation maneuvers to detect intra-articular hip pathology. PM R. 2010;2(3):174–81.
8. Hegazi TM, Belair JA, McCarthy EJ, Roedl JB, Morrison WB. Sports injuries about the hip: what the radiologist should know. Radiographics. 2016;36(6):1717–45.
9. Terrell SL, Olson GE, Lynch J. Therapeutic exercise approaches to nonoperative and postoperative management of femoroacetabular impingement syndrome. J Athl Train. 2021;56(1):31–45.
10. Groh MM, Herrera J. A comprehensive review of hip labral tears. Curr Rev Musculoskelet Med. 2009;2(2):105–17.
11. Borgstrom H, McInnis KC. Female athlete hip injuries: a narrative review. Clin J Sport Med. 2020. https://doi.org/10.1097/JSM.0000000000000857.
12. Kraeutler MJ, Safran MR, Scillia AJ, Ayeni OR, Garabekyan T, Mei-Dan O. A contemporary look at the evaluation and treatment of adult borderline and Frank hip dysplasia. Am J Sports Med. 2020;48(9):2314–23.
13. Hartig-Andreasen C, Soballe K, Troelsen A. The role of the acetabular labrum in hip dysplasia. A literature overview. Acta Orthop. 2013;84(1):60–4.
14. Harris JD, Lewis BD, Park KJ. Hip dysplasia. Clin Sports Med. 2021;40(2):271–88.
15. Anderson CN. Iliopsoas: pathology, diagnosis, and treatment. Clin Sports Med. 2016;35(3):419–33.
16. Deslandes M, Guillin R, Cardinal E, Hobden R, Bureau NJ. The snapping iliopsoas tendon: new mechanisms using dynamic sonography. AJR Am J Roentgenol. 2008;190(3):576–81.
17. Christopher ZK, Hassebrock JD, Anastasi MB, Economopoulos KJ. Hip flexor injuries in the athlete. Clin Sports Med. 2021;40(2):301–10.
18. Heyworth BE, Shindle MK, Voos JE, Rudzki JR, Kelly BT. Radiologic and intraoperative findings in revision hip arthroscopy. Arthroscopy. 2007;23(12):1295–302.

39 Posterior Hip Disorders

Stephanie DeLuca, Haylee Borgstrom, and Kelly C. McInnis

39.1 Proximal Hamstring Tendinopathy/ Tear

39.1.1 Synonyms

- Hamstring tendonitis
- Hamstring tendinosis
- High hamstring tendinopathy

39.1.2 ICD-10 Codes

M76.899, S76.311, S76.309

39.1.3 Description

Anatomy The hamstring myotendinous unit is frequently injured due to a bi-articular anatomic course across the hip and knee joints and the composition of mostly type II fast-twitch fibers. The proximal hamstring consists of two tendons, the semimembranosus and conjoint tendon (formed by the long head of the biceps femoris and semitendinosus). The proximal hamstring muscles originate on the lateral ischial tuberosity (IT) with the semimembranosus tendon origin lateral and anterior to the conjoint tendon. The sciatic nerve traverses in close proximity, 1–1.4 cm lateral to this origin [5]. In proximal hamstring tendinopathy, the semimembranosus tendon is most affected [4]. The paucity of blood flow at the enthesis is responsible for morbidity and delayed healing in many cases [6].

Proximal hamstring tendinopathy (PHT) is a chronic overuse injury due to repetitive microtrauma from mechanical overload and repetitive stretch on the hamstring origin at the ischial tuberosity (IT), with resultant tendon thickening, disorganization, and degeneration. It is commonly associated with enthesopathy or degenerative tears. While the onset of proximal hamstring tendinopathy is typically gradual and occurs without a traumatic event, it can be stressed acutely during eccentric contraction with the hip flexed and knee extended or an extreme stretch of the hamstring muscle–tendon unit [1]. There is maximum tension of the hamstring tendon origin at the ischial tuberosity during the terminal swing and early stance phases of the running cycle [2].

Potential risk factors for proximal hamstring tendinopathy include impact exercise overuse, muscular imbalance (particularly weakness at the hamstring and core), and lumbopelvic instability [3, 4]. Proximal hamstring tendinopathy most commonly affects runners, including sprinters, mid-distance, and long-distance runners, and athletes who participate in running sports with frequent directional changes.

Proximal hamstring tendon rupture/avulsion should be distinguished from proximal hamstring tendinopathy as acute tears that occur after forceful eccentric contraction of the hamstrings with sudden hip flexion and concurrent knee extension. Such injuries occur most frequently in high-ballistic sports such as weightlifting, water skiing, and gymnastics. Athletes may recall a pop or sensation of tearing with immediate onset of pain [3].

39.1.4 Clinical Presentation

Contrary to hamstring strain, proximal hamstring tendinopathy classically presents with a more insidious onset. Patients typically report gradually progressive pain at the deep buttock near the ischial tuberosity with occasional radiation of

S. DeLuca
Department of Physical Medicine & Rehabilitation, Spaulding Rehabilitation Hospital, Harvard Medical School, Charlestown, MA, USA
e-mail: sdeluca3@partners.org

H. Borgstrom
Department of Physical Medicine & Rehabilitation, Spaulding Rehabilitation Hospital, Massachusetts General Hospital, Harvard Medical School, Boston, MA, USA
e-mail: hborgstrom@partners.org

K. C. McInnis (✉)
Harvard–Spaulding PM&R Sports Medicine, Physical Medicine and Rehabilitation, Harvard Medical School, Boston, MA, USA
e-mail: kcmcinnis@partners.org

© The Author(s), under exclusive license to Springer Nature Switzerland AG 2022

S. A. Mostoufi et al. (eds.), *Clinical Guide to Musculoskeletal Medicine*, https://doi.org/10.1007/978-3-030-92042-5_39

pain to the posterior thigh. Symptoms may heighten with static stretching in end range of hip flexion. Sciatic neuralgia can be present in some cases. Sitting intolerance is often present and can be quite limiting. Provocative factors include running, particularly uphill as the proximal hamstring is subjected to higher energy storage, repetitive eccentric hamstring contraction, acceleration, forward trunk flexion, deep hip flexion, and direct pressure to the ischial tuberosity [4].

39.1.5 Physical Examination

Full musculoskeletal (MSK) examination of the lumbar spine and hip is needed to differentiate proximal hamstring tendinopathy from other causes of posterior hip pain (Table 39.1). Lower extremity neurologic assessment is indicated to rule out a neurologic component. Depending on findings, the examination may need to expand to assess for other potential sources of pain.

Gait Gait is typically unaffected in proximal hamstring tendinopathy. Assessment is useful to rule out other potential diagnoses. In the case of acute avulsion, patients usually have difficulty bearing weight.

Visual observation It is important to inspect the affected area and the bulk and tone of the hamstring muscles. In acute rupture, ecchymosis may be seen at the posterior thigh.

Palpation Direct palpation of the ischial tuberosity, gluteal muscles (including the piriformis), and hamstring muscle belly should be performed assessing for pain provocation. There may be focal tenderness at the ischial tuberosity. Taut bands and trigger points are commonly identified in the piriformis and hamstring muscles. In avulsion injuries, a palpable deformity may be appreciated on passive knee flexion in the prone position.

Table 39.1 Differential diagnosis of posterior hip pain

Hamstring strain	L5-S1 radiculopathy, lumbar facet pain lumbar plexopathy, lumbar stenosis
Proximal hamstring tendinopathy	Sacroiliac joint dysfunction, sacroiliitis
Ischiofemoral impingement	Pelvic floor dysfunction
Ischial bursitis	Sacrotuberous ligament pain
Intra-articular hip pathology	Gluteal tendinopathy
Adductor magnus enthesopathy	Piriformis myofascial pain
Obturator internus dysfunction	Pudendal neuralgia or posterior femoral cutaneous neuralgia

Range of motion (ROM) Hip and lumbar spine ROM should be examined in all planes. ROM is preserved in proximal hamstring tendinopathy. Normal measurements for hip and lumbar spine ROM are discussed in the anterior hip chapter and spine disorders section.

Sensory testing Light touch should be tested in bilateral lower extremities throughout the L1-S1 dermatomes. Sensory deficit warrants further investigation, as this is not expected in proximal hamstring tendinopathy.

Deep tendon reflexes The following lower extremity reflexes should be tested bilaterally to assess for radiculopathy: patellar tendon (L2-L4, L4 primary), Achilles tendon (S1), and hamstring tendon (L5). Reflexes should be normal and symmetric in proximal hamstring tendinopathy.

Motor testing It is important to test L2-S2 myotomes, specifically hip flexion (L2/L3), knee extension (L2/L3/L4), ankle dorsiflexion (L4/L5), great toe extension (L5), ankle planar flexion (S1/S2), knee flexion (S1/S2), and gluteus medius strength (L4/L5/S1), to exclude other pathology. In the prone position, resisted knee flexion should be tested at 30 degrees and 90 degrees while looking for pain provocation. Resisted hip extension can elicit pain. In the case of an avulsion injury, weakness can be seen with resisted hip extension and knee flexion.

Joint testing Careful assessment of the hip joint with special provocative tests is important to differentiate proximal hamstring tendinopathy from intra-articular hip sources of posterior hip pain. It is also important to assess the lumbar facet and sacroiliac joints. Specifics of such testing are highlighted in the spine disorders section and anterior hip disorders chapter.

39.1.5.1 Special Maneuvers

Several provocative maneuvers have been shown to have high validity and reliability for proximal hamstring tendinopathy [2, 4]. These are not indicated for acute proximal hamstring ruptures.

- *Puranen-Orava test*: The patient's foot rests on an elevated support about 90 degrees to their body with the hip flexed and knee extended while they reach with their ipsilateral arm toward the foot to stretch the hamstring. Provocation of pain is associated with proximal hamstring tendinopathy.
- *Bent-knee test/modified bent-knee stretch test*: With the patient supine, the examiner puts the affected side into maximum hip and knee flexion and then slowly passively

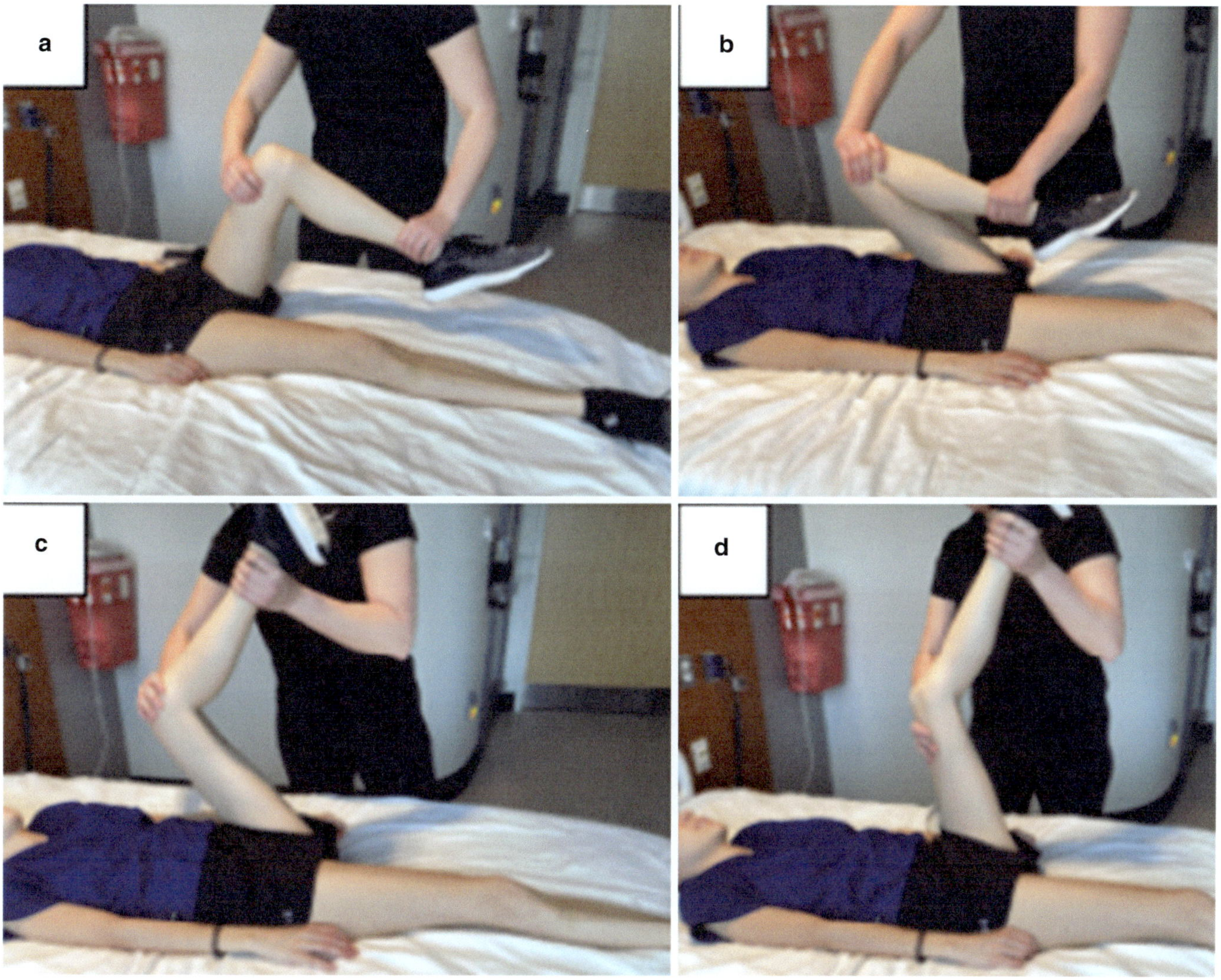

Fig. 39.1 Modified bent-knee stretch test performed stepwise fashion progressing from **a** through **d**

extends the knee. The modified bent-knee stretch test is similar, but with rapid passive knee extension instead (Fig. 39.1). In both tests, knee extension commonly elicits pain at the proximal hamstring.

- *Single-leg deadlift*: With knee slightly flexed, the patient stands on the affected leg while gradually bending forward at the hip, lifting the contralateral hip into extension to load the affected hamstring. This provokes pain.
- *Supine plank*: During this loading maneuver, the patient is supine with heels and elbows resting on the table. The patient rises up on their elbows while keeping their knees in extension and raising the unaffected leg while keeping the injured side on the table to elevate the pelvis (Fig. 39.2). A positive test reproduces the patient's index pain. Examiners may need to modify this test depending on the patient's ability to perform the maneuver. For instance, the examiner can hold the heel of the unaffected side off the table while the patient extends the hip on the affected side and elevates the pelvis. A single-leg bridge can also substitute; however, it is important to keep in mind that this places reduced load on the hamstring.

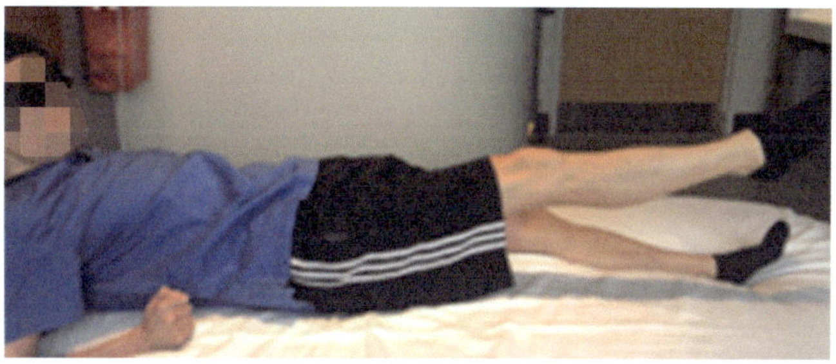

Fig. 39.2 Supine plank with single leg raise

- *Nordic hamstring exercise*: The patient kneels on a flat surface with their knees flexed at 90 degrees while the examiner holds their heels. While maintaining a straight spine, the patient gradually leans forward in a controlled

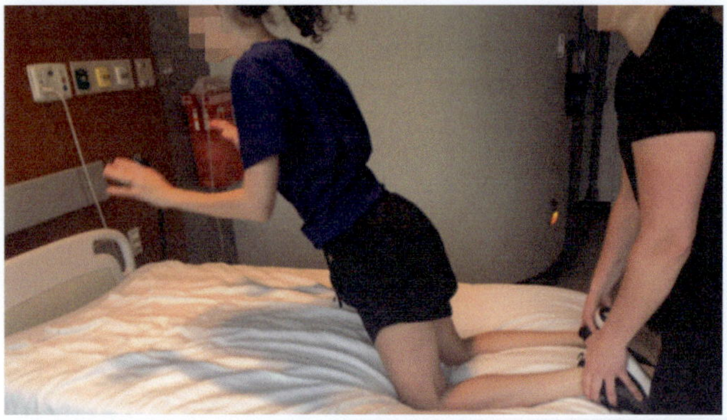

Fig. 39.3 Nordic hamstring exercise

fashion until they have to put their hands out to catch themselves (Fig. 39.3). The patient then performs a hamstring curl to return to the starting position. In cases of proximal hamstring tendinopathy, the eccentric load on the hamstring provokes pain.

39.1.6 Diagnostic Workup

For most cases, proximal hamstring tendinopathy is a clinical diagnosis. When the diagnosis is unclear, magnetic resonance imaging (MRI) and musculoskeletal ultrasound are the preferred imaging studies as they not only identify tendinosis but also characterize the severity of the injury.

X-ray Plain radiographs of the hips and pelvis are typically inconclusive. In chronic cases, they can identify enthesopathy or intra-tendinous calcifications at the ischial tuberosity.

MRI MRI has a higher sensitivity than musculoskeletal ultrasound. MRI findings of proximal hamstring tendinopathy may include bone edema at the ischial tuberosity, tendon thickening, intra-substance heterogeneity of the tendon, and tendinous/peritendinous edema with a distal feathery appearance (Fig. 39.4). Partial- and full-thickness tears can be identified and characterized. The degree of retraction can be important for surgical decision-making in the case of acute rupture.

Musculoskeletal ultrasound Ultrasound evaluation for proximal hamstring tendinopathy commonly demonstrates tendon thickening and degenerative changes along with peritendinous fluid at the site of the proximal hamstring. There may be cortical irregularity at the ischial tuberosity attachment site.

39.1.7 Treatment

Proximal hamstring tendinopathy can be challenging to manage. In most cases, nonoperative management can successfully return patients to activity within 3–6 months.

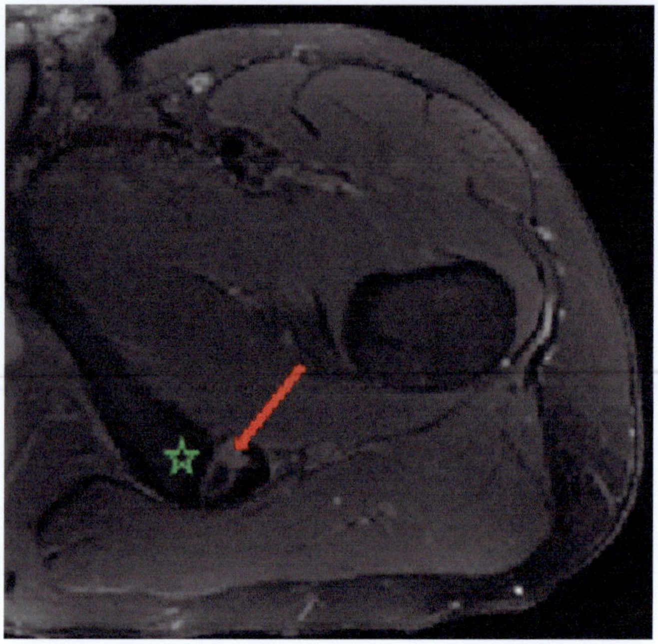

Fig. 39.4 MRI hip demonstrating proximal hamstring tendinopathy with increased signal intensity at the semimembranosus tendon (red arrow) near the ischial tuberosity (green star) on axial proton density fat suppression sequence

39.1.7.1 Medical Management

Pain control can be achieved with topical or oral anti-inflammatories such as nonsteroidal anti-inflammatory drugs (NSAIDs). If the patient is unable to tolerate NSAIDs, they may take acetaminophen for analgesia. In the acute phase of proximal hamstring tendinopathy, ice may be beneficial.

39.1.7.2 Rehabilitation

Postural modifications include seat cushions to offload compression at the tendon attachment site. Standing workstations are often helpful. Patients should avoid impact exercise and focus on non-impact activities as tolerated, such as cycling in the standing position, elliptical, and swimming. Soft tissue mobilization to the proximal hamstring may also be beneficial. Early engagement in physical therapy should focus on core and lumbosacral stabilization with activation of the gluteal musculature. As in other lower extremity enthesopathies, stretching of the hamstrings is not recommended for proximal hamstring tendinopathy; however, patients should focus on stretching the piriformis and hip flexors to optimize pelvic position and encourage posterior pelvic tilt. Guided by the patient's pain, a progressive hamstring strengthening protocol should be implemented with gradual progression from isometric to isotonic exercises. Once the tendon is less reactive, eccentric exercises should be incorporated and advanced as tolerated.

39.1.7.3 Procedures

For refractory cases, more invasive procedures can be tried.

Trigger point injections If myofascial pain limits rehabilitation progress, trigger point injections can target the proximal hamstring or gluteal musculature.

Ultrasound-guided percutaneous needle tenotomy with or without platelet-rich plasma (PRP) In an attempt to incite a proinflammatory response and promote tendon healing, an ultrasound-guided percutaneous needle tenotomy can be performed with or without PRP [7].

Extracorporeal shockwave therapy (ESWT) An alternative and effective treatment is ESWT. While treatment protocols vary, the following has been successfully utilized in a population of professional athletes—weekly radial shockwave sessions with 2500–3000 impulses per session at pressure of 4 bars and frequency of 10 shocks/second (0.18 mJ/mm^2 energy flux density) for 3–4 weeks [1]. Combined therapy consisting of radial and focused shockwave can also be considered.

Ultrasound-guided corticosteroid injection If patients are unable to fully participate in a progressive loading program, a one-time ultrasound-guided corticosteroid injection to the proximal hamstring complex tendon sheath can be performed, provided there is no evidence of a partial tear. More than one peritendinous corticosteroid injection is not recommended given potential for tenotoxicity [8].

39.1.7.4 Surgery

Operative management is reserved for recalcitrant cases or in patients where proximal hamstring tendinopathy progresses to high-grade partial- or full-thickness tear. In contrast, for acute proximal hamstring tendon injuries, surgical referral is indicated for complete avulsion or two-tendon injuries with >2 cm tendon retraction [2]. Early surgical repair leads to more favorable outcomes. Surgical interventions may consist of open tendon debridement and primary tendon repair. See Chap. 42 for more details on hip surgeries.

39.2 Ischial Bursitis

39.2.1 Synonyms

- Ischial bursopathy
- Ischiogluteal bursitis

39.2.2 ICD-10 Codes

M70.70

39.2.3 Description

Anatomy The ischial bursa is an adventitial bursa that lies between the proximal hamstring tendon origin at the ischial tuberosity and the overlying gluteus maximus muscle, in close proximity to the sciatic nerve, posterior femoral cutaneous nerve, and pelvic vasculature. As an adventitial bursa, it is not formed during normal embryologic development but develops in response to friction and pressure between the ischial tuberosity and overlying soft tissue. Chronic irritation results in an inflammatory response with increased vascular permeability and vasodilation at the bursa [10].

The bursa is rather dynamic in that load exposure changes depending on the patient's position. In the standing position, the gluteus maximus muscle covers the bursa. In the seated position, the gluteus maximus moves superiorly leaving only the subcutaneous tissue to protect the ischial bursa and heightening the risk for irritation.

Ischial bursitis is an infrequent cause of posterior hip pain. It is most commonly a noninfectious inflammatory process due to chronic, direct bursal irritation in the setting of prolonged sitting. It can also be reactive to chronic loading of the proximal hamstring and systemic inflammatory diseases such as rheumatoid arthritis and crystal arthropathy. Acute ischial bursitis is rare and classically occurs in the setting of trauma. Ischial bursitis most commonly affects individuals with sedentary lifestyles. Interestingly, it was previously referred to as "weaver's" or "tailor's bottom," as such professions put a great amount of pressure on the ischial bursa resulting in irritation and inflammation [9]. Ischial bursitis may also affect cyclists due to repetitive irritation on the saddle. Due to reduced subcutaneous tissue in patients with cachexia or severe weight loss, the ischial bursa may be under increased pressure, raising the risk for ischial bursitis [10].

39.2.4 Clinical Presentation

Patients with ischial bursitis classically present with insidious onset of dull, aching pain localized to the inferior gluteal region with or without radiation down the posterior leg. Provocative maneuvers include prolonged sitting and increased hip flexion commonly seen in cycling, rowing, horseback riding, sprinting, and running uphill [9]. Sleep may be interrupted due to pain.

39.2.5 Physical Examination

In many ways, physical examination of a patient with suspected ischial bursitis is similar to proximal hamstring tendinopathy.

Gait In the case of ischial bursitis, gait is rarely altered.

Visual observation Overlying erythema is a rare finding in ischial bursitis. This finding warrants further investigation for an infectious process.

Palpation Direct palpation of the ischial tuberosity will generally reproduce index pain in ischial bursitis. If swelling or a mass is detected, further studies should be initiated to rule out malignancy, abscess, and hematoma [9]. Clinicians should also include palpation at the following landmarks: origin, muscle belly, and insertion points of the gluteal, piriformis, and hamstring muscles.

Range of motion Hip and lumbar spine ROM should be examined in all planes.

Sensory testing A complete lower extremity sensory exam should be performed as part of the neurologic assessment. Sensory deficits are not detected in isolated ischial bursitis.

Deep tendon reflexes The following lower extremity reflexes should be performed—patellar tendon (L2-L4, L4 primary), Achilles tendon (S1), and hamstring tendon (L5). Reflexes are preserved in ischial bursitis.

Motor testing Strength assessment of the L2-S1 myotomes should be performed.

Joint testing Careful examination of the hip joint, sacroiliac joint, and lumbar facets is important to differentiate ischial bursitis from other causes of posterior hip pain.

Special Maneuvers

There are no specific physical examination maneuvers for ischial bursitis. It is important to perform the special maneuvers for proximal hamstring tear (discussed above) to differentiate ischial bursitis from proximal hamstring tendinopathy. These maneuvers are less likely to produce pain in isolated ischial bursitis.

39.2.6 Diagnostic Workup

X-ray Plain radiographs of the pelvis are generally normal in ischial bursitis. Occasionally, there may be nonspecific findings of cortical irregularity or calcifications at the ischial tuberosity.

MRI MRI of the hip or pelvis is the gold standard imaging study for cases of ischial bursitis associated with a palpable mass in order to rule out malignancy, abscess, cyst, or hematoma. Ischial bursitis presents similarly to other forms of bursitis on MRI with high signal intensity and bursal distention on fluid-sensitive sequences. Unique to ischial bursitis is the cystic appearance of the bursa, with frequent internal hemorrhage due to shearing, irritative forces placed on the ischial tuberosity (Fig. 39.5) [9]. Ischial bursitis can be dif-

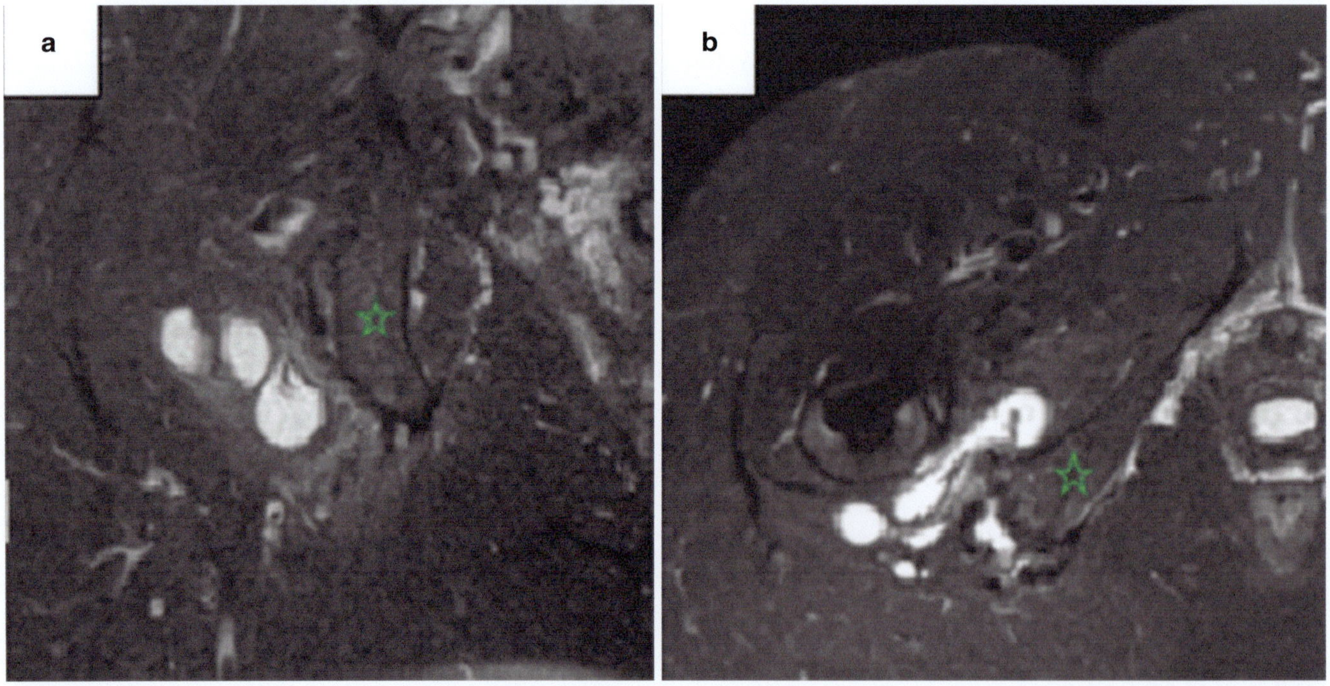

Fig. 39.5 MRI hip demonstrating ischial bursitis with high signal intensity and distention of the ischial bursa (outlined in red) in relation to the ischium (green star) on coronal (**a**) and axial (**b**) STIR sequences

ferentiated from neoplasm based on bursal contents. The bursa in ischial bursitis contains only fluid with soft tissue components confined to the bursal wall. On the contrary, neoplasms are predominantly composed of solid tissue [11].

Musculoskeletal ultrasound Point-of-care ultrasound can be useful for real-time evaluation of the compressible and cystic nature of the ischial bursitis [11].

Diagnostic ultrasound-guided local anesthetic injection In cases where the diagnosis is unclear, a diagnostic ultrasound-guided intra-bursal anesthetic injection can be helpful [12].

39.2.7 Treatment

39.2.7.1 Medical Management

Ischial bursitis is typically managed conservatively with a course of either topical or oral anti-inflammatories and cold compresses.

39.2.7.2 Rehabilitation

The rehabilitation course for ischial bursitis is very similar to proximal hamstring tendinopathy. Activity modifications include avoidance of impact exercise and provocative positions such as prolonged sitting. Patients are encouraged to resume non-impact exercises as tolerated for cardiovascular fitness. Soft tissue mobilization to the proximal hamstrings and gluteal muscles may alleviate reactive myofascial pain. Stretching of the piriformis, gluteal muscles, and hamstrings is recommended as well as core and lumbosacral stabilization with implementation of a progressive gluteal and hamstring strengthening protocol.

39.2.7.3 Procedures

Ultrasound-guided corticosteroid injection For refractory cases, ultrasound-guided procedures may be helpful for therapeutic purposes. Ultrasound-guided corticosteroid injection to the ischial bursa can be performed with the patient lying in the lateral decubitus position with their hips flexed to 90 degrees to increase the distance between the ischial bursa and sciatic nerve [12].

39.2.7.4 Surgery

Surgery is generally not indicated for this diagnosis. In cases of refractory symptoms affecting quality of life, ischial bursectomy has been described.

39.3 Ischiofemoral Impingement

39.3.1 Synonyms

- Quadratus femoris (QF) impingement
- Extra-articular hip impingement

39.3.2 ICD-10 Codes

M25.859, M24.859

39.3.3 Description

Anatomy It is important to note the boundaries of the ischiofemoral space (IFS) and quadratus femoris space (QFS). As mentioned, the ischiofemoral space is the distance between the ischium and lesser trochanter. The quadratus femoris space is the area between the superolateral aspect of the hamstring tendons and the posteromedial aspect of the iliopsoas tendon; the functional space for the quadratus femoris muscle originates from the anterior ischial tuberosity and inserts on the posteromedial proximal femur. The primary function of the quadratus femoris is hip adduction and external rotation. The sciatic nerve lies just superficial to the quadratus femoris within the ischiofemoral space.

Ischiofemoral impingement (IFI) is an extra-articular impingement of the soft tissues, namely, the quadratus femoris (QF) muscle, between the lesser trochanter of the femur and the ischial tuberosity. There are several factors, including congenital, positional, and acquired, which contribute to narrowing of the ischiofemoral space (IFS). Congenital factors consist of hip dysplasia and alignment abnormalities, specifically coxa valga. The ischiofemoral space is narrowed with hip extension, external rotation, and adduction [13]. Hip abductor weakness contributes to dynamic adduction and ischiofemoral space narrowing. Acquired anatomic changes, specifically hypertrophy of the superomedial aspect of the femur seen in hip osteoarthritis, total hip arthroplasty, lesser trochanter fractures/avulsions, proximal hamstring tendinopathy and enthesopathy, and regional osteochondromas, may also contribute to ischiofemoral space narrowing and impingement [14].

39.3.4 Clinical Presentation

Patients often present with insidious onset of deep gluteal and/or groin pain with occasional radiation down the posterior leg due to the close proximity of the quadratus femoris muscle to the sciatic nerve. Pain may be exacerbated with weight-bearing activity and hip adduction, extension, and external rotation [13]. Mechanical impingement symptoms may occur during exaggerated hip extension as seen in running or long-stride walking [14]. Ischiofemoral impingement may affect individuals of any age but most commonly affects adult females [14]. This predilection may be attributed to the frequency of hip abduction weakness in women. Approximately 25–40% of cases have bilateral involvement [14].

39.3.5 Physical Examination

Gait Patients may report pain and/or a snapping/locking sensation of the posterior hip region during the long-stride walking test, which has a sensitivity of 92% and specificity of 82% [14]. Patients may also demonstrate compensatory hip abduction to increase the ischiofemoral space.

Visual observation Inspection of the affected area should be normal.

Palpation Clinicians should palpate the ischial tuberosity, quadratus femoris, gluteal muscles, piriformis muscle, and hamstring muscle belly for tenderness. Typically, the palpatory exam is normal in ischiofemoral impingement. In cases of concurrent proximal hamstring tendinopathy, there may be tenderness of the ischial tuberosity.

Range of motion It is important to assess ROM for the lumbar spine and hip joint. Patients with ischiofemoral impingement classically report pain in hip extension, adduction, and external rotation.

Sensory testing Due to similar pain patterns between ischiofemoral impingement and lumbar radiculopathy, it is important to perform a sensory examination including L1-S1 dermatomes. Sensory deficits should not be present in ischiofemoral impingement. Rare sciatic neuropathy has been described.

Deep tendon reflexes Reflexes should be normal and symmetric in ischiofemoral impingement.

Motor testing Lower extremity motor strength testing should be carried out for L2-S1 myotomes to rule out a neurologic component. Strength should be preserved in ischiofemoral impingement with the rare exception of associated sciatic neuropathy, where hamstring and/or calf weakness may be seen.

Joint testing Assessment of the hip joint, lumbar facets, and sacroiliac joint should be performed to rule out other causes of posterior hip pain.

Special maneuvers Pain may be elicited with a combination of passive hip extension, adduction, and external rotation and generally alleviated with hip abduction as this widens the ischiofemoral space. This maneuver is occasionally referred to as the "ischiofemoral impingement test" and is performed in a lateral decubitus position. However, it is common to not find pain provocation on examination.

39.3.6 Diagnostic Workup

X-ray Plain radiographs of the pelvis and hip can assess intra-articular hip pathology. Plain radiographs are used to identify bony morphologic changes that may contribute to ischiofemoral impingement (discussed above).

MRI MRI of the hip/pelvis may demonstrate characteristic findings including ischiofemoral space and quadratus femoris narrowing with adjacent quadratus femoris muscle edema, suggestive of acute or chronic inflammation due to impingement (Fig. 39.6). Proximal hamstring tendinopathy with tendon thickening contributing to ischiofemoral space narrowing may also be seen [15]. An ischiofemoral space of <15 mm is the radiographic criteria utilized for ischiofemoral impingement [14, 16, 17]. It may not correlate with symptomatology.

Musculoskeletal ultrasound Dynamic ultrasound evaluation can be useful to demonstrate soft tissue impingement between the ischial tuberosity and lesser trochanter during hip external rotation. While MRI is the gold standard, ultrasound can be considered to measure the ischiofemoral space in the hands of an advanced ultrasonographer. It is helpful to perform side-by-side evaluations to determine if such impingement is a normal variant or the primary pain generator.

39.3.7 Treatment

39.3.7.1 Medical Management

NSAIDs or acetaminophen can be utilized for pain management. Aggravating factors such as long-stride walking should be avoided.

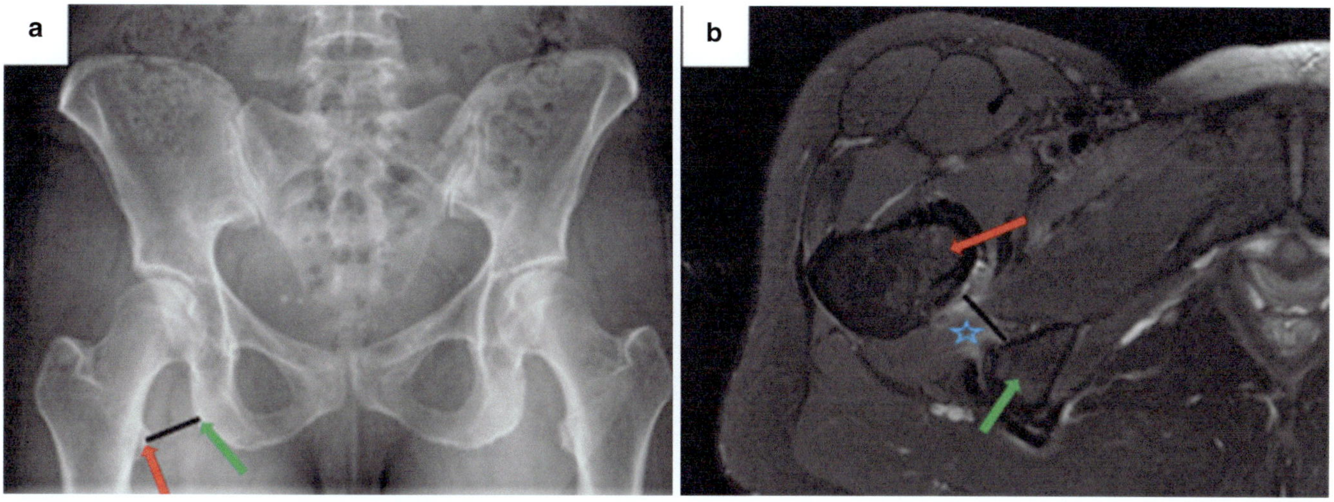

Fig. 39.6 Plain AP pelvic radiograph demonstrating ischiofemoral space (black line) between the lesser trochanter (red arrow) and ischial tuberosity (green arrow) (**a**). Axial T2-weighted MRI hip with narrowed ischiofemoral space (black line) with quadratus femoris muscle edema (blue star), which can be seen in ischiofemoral impingement (**b**). MRI is used to diagnose ischiofemoral impingement while radiograph is not

39.3.7.2 Rehabilitation

Patients should avoid movements that narrow the ischiofemoral space, including hip extension, adduction, and external rotation. While it is recommended to restrict weight-bearing exercise, patients may continue with non-impact exercise. Manual therapy to the gluteal muscles, including the piriformis and quadratus femoris, can mitigate reactive myofascial pain. A progressive core and lumbopelvic stabilization program with an emphasis on strengthening the hip abductors and external rotators and optimizing hip biomechanics should be started once pain is controlled.

39.3.7.3 Procedures

Ultrasound-guided injection For refractory cases, more invasive ultrasound-guided procedures can be trialed for diagnostic and therapeutic purposes. For cases where the diagnosis is unclear or patients are unable to fully participate in a course of physical therapy due to pain, an ultrasound-guided trigger point injection targeting the quadratus femoris with local anesthesia alone or in combination with corticosteroid can be performed, with careful attention to avoid the sciatic nerve.

39.3.7.4 Surgery

Ischiofemoral impingement is treated almost entirely with conservative measures. Surgical referral is recommended only when pain is severe and persistent despite rehabilitation and injection therapy and limits quality of life. The goal of surgical intervention for ischiofemoral impingement is to increase the ischiofemoral space through resection of the lesser trochanter [18, 19]. See Chap. 42 for more details on hip surgeries.

39.4 Piriformis Myofascial Pain

39.4.1 Synonyms

- Piriformis syndrome
- Deep gluteal syndrome
- Extra-spinal sciatica

39.4.2 ICD-10 Codes

G57.00

39.4.3 Description

Anatomy The piriformis muscle is pyramidal shaped and originates from the anterior aspect of the sacrum (S2-S4), courses through the greater sciatic notch, and inserts on the greater trochanter. The function of the piriformis muscle varies with hip position. In hip extension, it functions as a hip external rotator; in hip flexion, it predominantly serves as a hip abductor. The anatomic relationship between the sciatic nerve and piriformis muscle is variable. Traditionally, the sciatic nerve travels inferior to the piriformis muscle. Anatomic variants of the nerve course with relation to the piriformis muscle can further predispose it to entrapment [22].

Piriformis myofascial pain (PMP) is a common cause of posterior hip pain. It can be a source of extra-spinal sciatic neuralgia, referred to as "non-discogenic sciatica," due to compression of the sciatic nerve under the spastic piriformis muscle [20]. Piriformis myofascial pain typically results from repetitive hip flexion, internal rotation, and adduction, which is theorized to cause cumulative microtrauma to the piriformis muscle leading to myofascial pain. Such biomechanics are seen in cyclists, dancers, gymnasts, and skiers [21]. Though the pathophysiology is largely unknown, it is theorized that gluteal weakness/fatigue leads to compensatory piriformis overuse [20]. Piriformis myofascial pain may also present in the setting of acute traumatic fall or penetrating injury. Individuals with leg length discrepancy, pelvic obliquity, or scoliosis may demonstrate compensatory gait mechanics that heighten the risk for piriformis myofascial pain [21]. Additionally, piriformis myofascial pain may be more common in women due to biomechanics associated with a larger quadriceps angle (Q angle) [22]. Piriformis myofascial pain is frequently seen in association with spine (scoliosis) and hip joint pathology and proximal hamstring tendinopathy. The exact prevalence is unknown, due in part to variable diagnostic criteria.

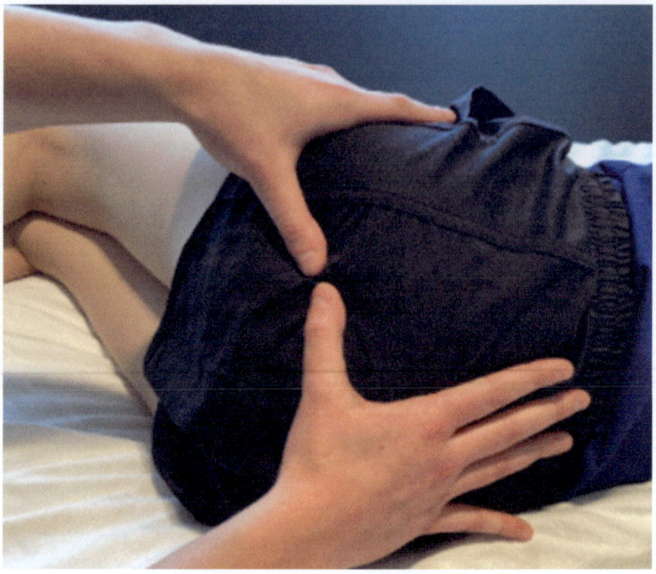

Fig. 39.7 Side-lying palpatory examination of the piriformis muscle. The examiner's left hand is on the greater trochanter, while the medial portion of the examiner's right hand is on the sacral sulcus. The examiner's thumbs overlie the fibers of the piriformis muscle

39.4.4 Clinical Presentation

Piriformis myofascial pain typically presents with gradual onset of deep gluteal pain and may be associated with radiating pain down the posterior limb and paresthesias in the distribution of the sciatic nerve. Patients may describe pain provocation with sitting or maneuvers that strain the piriformis muscle such as hip flexion, internal rotation, and adduction.

39.4.5 Physical Examination

Gait Generally, gait is unaffected in piriformis myofascial pain; however, in cases attributed to a leg length discrepancy, there can be increased internal rotation or adduction [21].

Visual observation The affected area will appear normal in most cases of piriformis pain. Static and dynamic knee valgus should be noted as a greater degree of valgus angulation may be associated with piriformis pain.

Palpation Patient can be examined in side-lying or prone position. In most cases, pain is reproduced with deep palpation of the piriformis muscle, with one hand over the greater trochanter and the other hand on the sacral sulcus with the thumbs overlying over the piriformis muscle fibers (in particular with simultaneous dynamic hip internal external rotation in prone examination). Taut bands and/or trigger points may be palpated along the gluteal and piriformis muscles (Fig. 39.7). While palpating this muscle, one should examine the distal sacroiliac joint, which is the closest axial structure to the piriformis muscle. It is important to palpate the contralateral piriformis muscle as it may be normally tender and not necessarily pathologic.

Range of motion ROM is generally preserved in piriformis myofascial pain.

Sensory testing Lower extremity sensory examination of L4-S1 dermatomes should be performed to exclude more common lumbar spine pathologies as sensation is preserved in piriformis myofascial pain.

Deep tendon reflexes Reflexes are normal and symmetric in piriformis myofascial pain.

Motor testing Motor strength testing of bilateral lower extremities is carried out to exclude other causes of posterior hip pain.

Joint testing Assessment of the hip, sacroiliac joint, and lumbar facets is warranted.

39.4.5.1 Special Maneuvers

There are several special maneuvers that passively stretch the piriformis muscle and may reproduce symptoms:

- *Pace test or passive seated piriformis test*: During this test, the patient is seated with hips flexed to 90 degrees followed by resisted hip abduction. Pain may be elicited. This test has a sensitivity of 0.53 and specificity of 0.90 [22].
- *Freiberg maneuver*: This maneuver can reproduce symptoms as the hip is extended and then passively internally rotated to stretch the piriformis (sensitivity and specificity unknown).
- *Beatty test*: With the patient side-lying on the unaffected side, the affected hip is flexed to 90 degrees with resisted hip abduction (sensitivity and specificity unknown).
- *FAIR test*: The details of this maneuver are highlighted in the anterior hip chapter. In many instances of piriformis myofascial pain, pain in the gluteal region may be elicited with the FAIR test with a sensitivity of 0.88 and specificity of 0.83 [22].
- *Straight leg raise (Lasegue sign), seated slump*: Such tests place neural tension along the sciatic nerve and commonly reproduce symptoms in patients with PMP. At 90 degrees of hip flexion with the knee extended, the patient may report buttock and posterior thigh pain [22]. The straight leg raise has a sensitivity of 0.15 and a specificity of 0.95 [22].

39.4.6 Diagnostic Workup

Piriformis myofascial pain is a clinical diagnosis. Referred pain from the lumbar spine should be excluded. Imaging studies are obtained to rule out other causes of posterior hip pain.

X-ray Plain radiographs of the lumbar spine, pelvis, and hip are considered to look for other sources of pain.

MRI MRI of the lumbar spine may rule out sources of referred pain from the L5-S1 disc as S1 radiculopathy may have a gluteal pain component. MRI of the pelvis may demonstrate anatomic variants associated with a predisposition for piriformis pain. Some studies have proposed that the piriformis muscle may appear enlarged in cases of piriformis myofascial pain, but this is not pathognomonic, and most MRI studies are unremarkable [21, 22]. MR neurography may have a role in this diagnosis, but availability may be limited.

MSK ultrasound Ultrasound evaluation of the sciatic nerve (with comparison to contralateral side) including cross-sectional area and sono-palpation of the piriformis muscle can be useful in making a diagnosis of piriformis myofascial pain and less-frequent coexisting sciatic neuralgia.

Diagnostic ultrasound-guided local anesthetic injection A diagnostic anesthetic injection can be considered to guide further management.

Electrodiagnostic testing (EMG/NCS) Electrodiagnostic testing is done primarily to exclude lumbosacral radiculopathy. Interestingly, studies have demonstrated a prolonged H-reflex in some cases of piriformis myofascial pain with sciatic neuralgia. However, electrodiagnostic sciatic neuropathy is generally not seen and studies are most often normal [22, 24].

39.4.7 Treatment

39.4.7.1 Medical Management

Pain control may be accomplished with NSAIDs and neuropathic agents including gabapentin and pregabalin.

39.4.7.2 Rehabilitation

It is recommended to avoid aggravating positions including prolonged sitting and frequent hip flexion, internal rotation, and adduction. Non-impact exercise is encouraged. Manual treatment for myofascial pain includes osteopathic manipulative treatment (OMT), proprioceptive neuromuscular facilitation (PNF), and soft tissue mobilization with deep tissue or self-massage of the piriformis and gluteal musculature. Dry needling of the piriformis and gluteal muscles can be utilized for pain management. Piriformis stretching can also be beneficial. Piriformis myofascial pain is often compensatory to deficiencies in gluteal strength and core control; therefore, a strengthening protocol should focus on lumbosacral and core stability with strengthening of the gluteal muscles and hip, particularly the hip extensors and abductors.

39.4.7.3 Procedures

Piriformis muscle trigger point injections Palpation-guided trigger point injections to the gluteal and piriformis muscles with local anesthesia can provide a longer duration of relief compared to dry needling [23]. Such injections can facilitate rehabilitation. If done under ultrasound, twitch response may be visualized in either the gluteus maximums or piriformis muscle.

Ultrasound-guided corticosteroid injection A corticosteroid injection to the piriformis muscle and/or muscle sheath can be performed for diagnostic and therapeutic measures.

Botulinum toxin If there is reduction in pain from an ultrasound-guided diagnostic injection, a botulinum toxin injection to the piriformis muscle can be considered for refractory cases [22]. Cost and side effects usually prohibit this as a first-line treatment.

39.4.7.4 Surgery

In very rare instances of chronic, recalcitrant pain, surgical release of the piriformis with decompression of the sciatic nerve can be considered. Diagnostic tools for piriformis syndrome remain obscure, and careful selection of patients for surgery is necessary to obtain good outcomes. Current surgical methods include open or endoscopic decompression of the sciatic nerve by release of the piriformis muscle [21, 24]. In a study of surgical resection of the piriformis muscle in 64 patients, it has obtained 82% initial and 76% long-term good or excellent outcomes [25].

References

1. Cacchio A, Rompe JD, Furia JP, Susi P, Santilli V, De Paulis F. Shockwave therapy for the treatment of chronic proximal hamstring tendinopathy in professional athletes. Am J Sports Med. 2011;39(1):146–53.
2. Arner JW, McClincy MP, Bradley JP. Hamstring injuries in athletes: evidence-based treatment. J Am Acad Orthop Surg. 2019;27(23):868–77.
3. Degen RM. Proximal hamstring injuries: management of tendinopathy and avulsion injuries. Curr Rev Musculoskelet Med. 2019;12(2):138–46.
4. Chu SK, Rho ME. Hamstring injuries in the athlete: diagnosis, treatment, and return to play: diagnosis, treatment, and return to play. Curr Sports Med Rep. 2016;15(3):184–90.
5. Miller SL, Gill J, Webb GR. The proximal origin of the hamstrings and surrounding anatomy encountered during repair: a cadaveric study. J Bone Joint Surg Am. 2007;89(1):44–8.
6. Sharma P, Maffulli N. Biology of tendon injury: healing, modeling and remodeling. J Musculoskelet Neuronal Interact. 2006;6(2):181–90.
7. Fader RR, Mitchell JJ, Traub S, Nichols R, Roper M, Mei Dan O, et al. Platelet-rich plasma treatment improves outcomes for chronic proximal hamstring injuries in an athletic population. Muscles Ligaments Tendons J. 2014;4(4):461–6.
8. Auriemma MJ, Tenforde AS, Harris A, McInnis KC. Platelet-rich plasma for treatment of chronic proximal hamstring tendinopathy. Regen Med. 2020;15(4):1509–18.
9. Cho KH, Lee SM, Lee YH, Suh KJ, Kim SM, Shin MJ, et al. Non-infectious ischiogluteal bursitis: MRI findings. Korean J Radiol. 2004;5(4):280–6.
10. Van Mieghem IM, Boets A, Sciot R, Van Breuseghem I. Ischiogluteal bursitis: an uncommon type of bursitis. Skelet Radiol. 2004;33(7):413–6.
11. Kim SM, Shin MJ, Kim KS, Ahn JM, Cho KH, Chang JS, et al. Imaging features of ischial bursitis with an emphasis on ultrasonography. Skelet Radiol. 2002;31(11):631–6.
12. Wisniewski SJ, Hurdle M, Erickson JM, Finnoff JT, Smith J. Ultrasound-guided ischial bursa injection: technique and positioning considerations. PM R. 2014;6(1):56–60.
13. Finnoff JT, Johnson AC, Hollman JH. Can ultrasound accurately assess ischiofemoral space dimensions? A validation study. PM R. 2017;9(4):392–7.
14. Gollwitzer H, Banke IJ, Schauwecker J, Gerdesmeyer L, Suren C. How to address ischiofemoral impingement? Treatment algorithm and review of the literature. J Hip Preserv Surg. 2017;4(4):289–98.
15. Torriani M, Souto SCL, Thomas BJ, Ouellette H, Bredella MA. Ischiofemoral impingement syndrome: an entity with hip pain and abnormalities of the quadratus femoris muscle. AJR Am J Roentgenol. 2009;193(1):186–90.
16. Singer AD, Subhawong TK, Jose J, Tresley J, Clifford PD. Ischiofemoral impingement syndrome: a meta-analysis. Skelet Radiol. 2015;44(6):831–7.
17. Finnoff JT, Johnson AC, Hollman JH. Can ultrasound accurately assess Ischiofemoral space dimensions? A validation study. PM&R. 2016;9(4):392–7.
18. de Sa D, Alradwan H, Cargnelli S, Thawer Z, Simunovic N, Cadet E, et al. Extra-articular hip impingement: a systematic review examining operative treatment of psoas, subspine, ischiofemoral, and greater trochanteric/pelvic impingement. Arthroscopy. 2014;30(8):1026–41.
19. Wilson MD, Keene JS. Treatment of ischiofemoral impingement: results of diagnostic injections and arthroscopic resection of the lesser trochanter. J Hip Preserv Surg. 2016;3(2):146–53.
20. Cassidy L, Walters A, Bubb K, Shoja MM, Shane Tubbs R, Loukas M. Piriformis syndrome: implications of anatomical variations, diagnostic techniques, and treatment options. Surg Radiol Anat. 2012;34(6):479–86.
21. Byrd JWT. Piriformis syndrome. Oper Tech Sports Med. 2005;13(1):71–9.
22. Probst D, Stout A, Hunt D. Piriformis syndrome: a narrative review of the anatomy, diagnosis, and treatment. PM&R. 2019;11(S1):S54–63.
23. Hong CZ. Lidocaine injection versus dry needling to myofascial trigger point: the importance of the local twitch response. Am J Phys Med Rehabil. 1994;73(4):256–63.
24. Hopayian K, Song F, Riera R, Sambandan S. The clinical features of the piriformis syndrome: a systematic review. Eur Spine J. 2010;19(12):2095–109.
25. Filler AG, Haynes J, Jordan SE, Prager J, Villablanca JP, Farahani K, McBride DQ, Tsuruda JS, Morisoli B, Batzdorf U, Johnson JP. Sciatica of nondisc origin and piriformis syndrome: diagnosis by magnetic resonance neurography and interventional magnetic resonance imaging with outcome study of resulting treatment. J Neurosurg Spine. 2005;2(2):99–115. https://doi.org/10.3171/spi.2005.2.2.0099. PMID: 15739520.

Lateral Hip Disorders

40

Sean Schowalter, Joanne Borg-Stein,
and Haylee Borgstrom

40.1 Gluteal Tendinopathy and Bursopathy

40.1.1 Synonyms

Gluteal tendinopathy

- Gluteus medius tendinopathy
- Gluteus minimus tendinopathy
- Gluteal tendinitis
- Greater trochanteric enthesopathy
- Greater trochanteric pain syndrome
- Dead butt syndrome

Greater trochanteric bursopathy

- Trochanteric bursitis
- Subgluteus maximus bursitis
- Greater trochanteric pain syndrome (GTPS)

Calcific tendinitis of the hip

- Calcific gluteal tendinopathy

40.1.2 ICD-10 Codes

- Gluteal tendinopathy (M76.0–M76.02)
- Greater trochanteric bursopathy (M70.6–M70.62)
- Calcific tendinitis of the hip (M65.25–M65.252)

40.1.3 Description

Anatomy Gluteal tendinopathy or tendinosis (GT) most often occurs at the distal tendinous insertions onto the greater trochanter, with the gluteus medius tendon affected much more frequently than the gluteus minimus tendon. The gluteus minimus tendon inserts at the anterior facet, while the gluteus medius tendon inserts at the lateral and posterosuperior facets of the greater trochanter (Figs. 40.1 and 40.2). Intra-substance degenerative tears, partial-thickness tears (typically on the undersurface of tendon), or full-thickness tears may occur [1]. The primary action of both muscles is hip abduction with

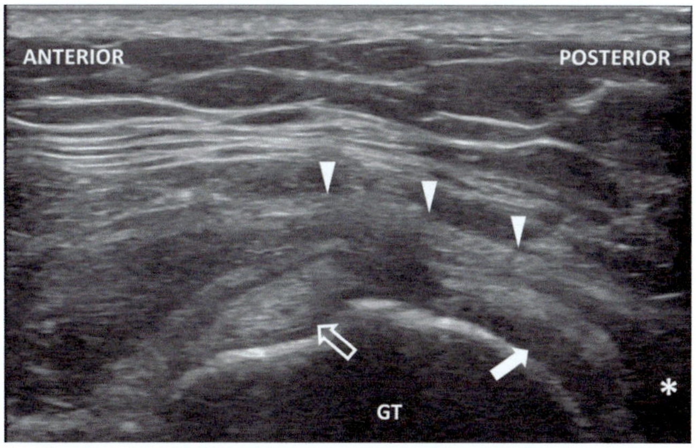

Fig. 40.1 Short-axis ultrasound image at the greater trochanter (GT) depicting the ITB (arrowheads), gluteus minimus tendon (open arrow), gluteus medius tendon (closed arrow), and anterior gluteus maximus fibers (asterisk). Respective bursae are not typically visible and lie deep to their respective tendons

S. Schowalter
Department of Physical Medicine & Rehabilitation, Spaulding Rehabilitation Hospital, Harvard Medical School, Charlestown, MA, USA
e-mail: sschowalter@partners.org

J. Borg-Stein
Associate Professor, Department of Physical Medicine & Rehabilitation, Spaulding Rehabilitation Hospital, Massachusetts General Hospital, Harvard Medical School, Boston, MA, USA

Chief of Physical Medicine and Rehabilitation, Newton Wellesley Hospital, Medical Director: Spine Center at Newton Wellesley Hospital, Newton, MA, USA
e-mail: jborgstein@partners.org

H. Borgstrom (✉)
Clinical Instructor, Department of Physical Medicine & Rehabilitation, Spaulding Rehabilitation Hospital, Massachusetts General Hospital, Harvard Medical School, Boston, MA, USA
e-mail: hborgstrom@partners.org

© The Author(s), under exclusive license to Springer Nature Switzerland AG 2022

S. A. Mostoufi et al. (eds.), *Clinical Guide to Musculoskeletal Medicine*, https://doi.org/10.1007/978-3-030-92042-5_40

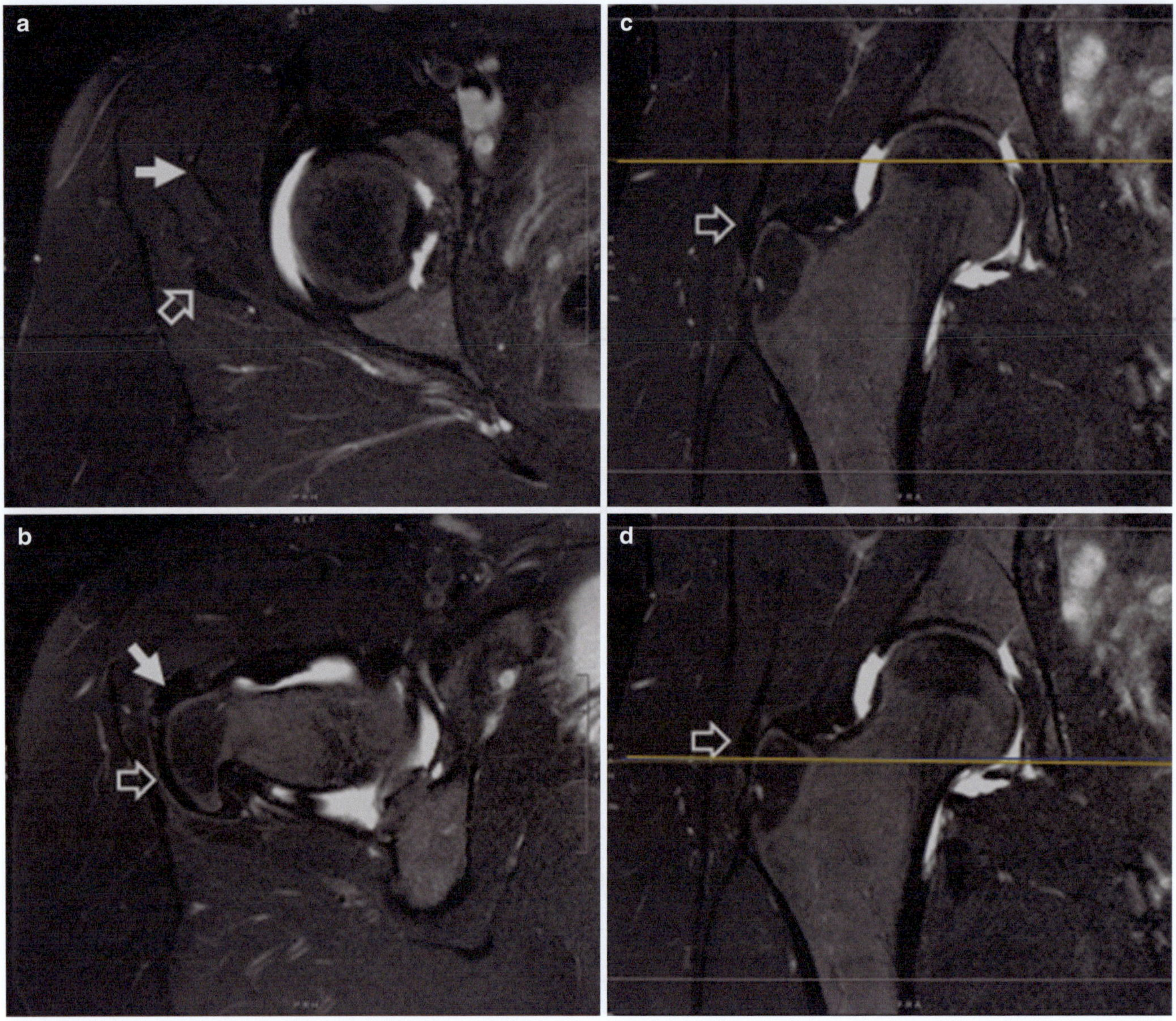

Fig. 40.2 Normal appearance of gluteus minimus (closed arrowhead) and medius (open arrowhead) tendons on fat-suppressed T2-weighted axial MRI, both superior to insertion (**a**) and at insertion (**b**) on the anterior and lateral facets, respectively. Corresponding level of axial cuts are demonstrated on coronal sequences (**c**, **d**) identified by the yellow line

secondary actions including internal rotation (gluteus minimus, anterior gluteus medius fibers) and external rotation (posterior gluteus medius fibers). The sub-gluteus maximus bursa, or trochanteric bursa, lies superior to the posterior facet of the greater trochanter. The sub-gluteus medius and minimus bursae lie deep to their respective tendons (Fig. 40.1).

Gluteal tendinopathy or tendinosis (GT) is a chronic, degenerative, non-inflammatory condition and is the most common cause of lateral hip or peri-trochanteric pain. In fact, gluteus medius and/or minimus tendinopathies are the most prevalent lower extremity tendinopathies, estimated to affect 10–25% of the general population [1]. While GT can occur in any age group, it is most prevalent in those aged 40–60 years old and attributed to overuse, repetitive loading, and cumulative microtrauma. Additionally, it displays a 2.5- to 4-fold greater predilection for females compared to males, likely due to several sex-specific anatomic and biomechanical differences, including increased acetabular anteversion, decreased gluteus medius insertional area, shorter gluteal abductor moment arm, and increased peripheral adiposity in females [2]. Dynamically, female athletes more often exhibit increased hip adduction during single-leg stance as a result of relative gluteus medius weakness, which has been demonstrated to increase tensile load on the hip abductors and further contribute to the risk of GT [3]. Decreased femoral neck–shaft angle (coxa vara) and leg length discrepancy have also been associated with increased risk for GT.

Calcific gluteal tendinopathy, or the deposition of calcium hydroxyapatite within the tendons, may also occur. The pathogenesis of calcific gluteal tendinopathy remains unclear but has been associated with diabetes, altered estrogen metabolism, and hypothyroidism.

Trochanteric bursopathy may affect one or more of the three major bursae in the lateral hip region. Once thought to be a distinct entity, trochanteric bursopathy is now generally accepted as a relatively rare sequela of underlying gluteal tendinosis, similar to bursopathies in the shoulder. If present, the overwhelming majority of cases involve the sub-gluteus maximus bursa with sub-gluteus minimus and sub-gluteus medius bursae accounting for less than 5% of cases [4]. In rarer cases, however, trochanteric bursitis can occur due to traumatic compression of the bursa or inflammation secondary to rheumatologic diseases such as gout, rheumatoid arthritis, or psoriasis.

40.1.4 Clinical Presentation

Patients with GT, with or without accompanying trochanteric bursopathy, typically present with chronic, insidious, dull pain at the posterolateral hip region. Far less commonly, pain can occur acutely and may be related to traumatic or inflammatory bursitis or calcific tendinitis. Radiation into the groin, posterior hip, and/or down the lateral thigh mimicking radicular symptoms has also been reported. Often patients will describe worsening of pain when laying on the affected side. Other exacerbating factors may include prolonged standing, transitional movements, sitting with the affected leg crossed, climbing stairs, running, or other high-impact or single-leg support activities.

40.1.5 Physical Examination

A comprehensive musculoskeletal examination should be performed, including both the affected and unaffected hip. It is imperative that the patient be examined in shorts to allow for appropriate access to the hip and observation of the entire kinetic chain. Thorough lumbar spine, sacroiliac joint, and neurologic examinations must be conducted as well given the broad differential diagnosis for lateral hip pain (Table 40.1).

Table 40.1 Differential diagnosis for lateral hip pain

Gluteal tendinopathy	Hip dysplasia
Calcific tendinitis	Avascular necrosis
Lateral snapping hip syndrome	Labral tear
Femoral neck fracture (stress or trauma)	Septic joint
Femoroacetabular impingement	Nerve entrapment (meralgia paresthetica, superior/inferior gluteal nerves)
Osteoarthritis of the hip	Referred pain (SI joint, spine, disc disease)
Inflammatory arthritides (RA, spondyloarthritis)	Tumors/neoplasm

Gait evaluation Gait is typically normal; however, patients may complain of reproduction of lateral hip pain during stance phase on the affected leg. In more severe cases, patients may have an antalgic gait or a Trendelenburg gait (Fig. 40.3a), indicating a significant gluteus medius weakness or even tear.

Observation Inspection for swelling, erythema, or deformity should be completed, noting asymmetries compared to the contralateral side. In cases of gluteal tendinopathy, there will typically be no obvious abnormalities. However, factors that may contribute to a higher risk can be observed, such as leg length discrepancy, peripheral adiposity, or a prominent greater trochanter, which can be a sign of coxa vara.

Palpation Palpatory examination is best performed with the patient in lateral decubitus position with hip and knee flexion. Tenderness to palpation at or near the greater trochanter is suggestive of GT if reproductive of index hip pain. Focal palpation of the individual trochanteric facets can better define specific tendon involvement.

Range of motion (ROM) Both passive and active ROM should be tested in all planes. In patients with isolated GT, ROM should remain full, though maneuvers should be performed slowly and with reassurance as it is not uncommon to elicit pain. True restriction with passive ROM generally indicates primary or concomitant intra-articular hip pathology.

Sensory testing Sensory examination should be performed in T12-S1 dermatomes and should be normal in the case of GT.

Deep tendon reflexes Lower extremity deep tendon reflexes (DTRs) including patellar, Achilles, and medial hamstring tendons should be tested and should be normal in GT.

Motor testing Reproduction of lateral hip pain with resisted hip abduction is suggestive of gluteal tendinopathy. Given that the tensor fascia latae (TFL) is a frequently overutilized hip abductor in the setting of gluteal weakness, specific effort should be made to isolate the gluteal musculature by testing hip abduction in the side-lying position with 10–15 degrees of hip extension.

Joint testing Careful assessment of the hip, sacroiliac, and facet joints should be performed to differentiate GT from other conditions that may mimic symptoms.

40.1.5.1 Special Maneuvers

FABER (Patrick's) test While non-specific, this test may elicit lateral hip pain in the setting of GT by stretching the portions of the gluteus medius/minimus involved with hip internal rotation (Fig. 40.3b). It is important to ask where the patient experiences pain during this maneuver as pain can be

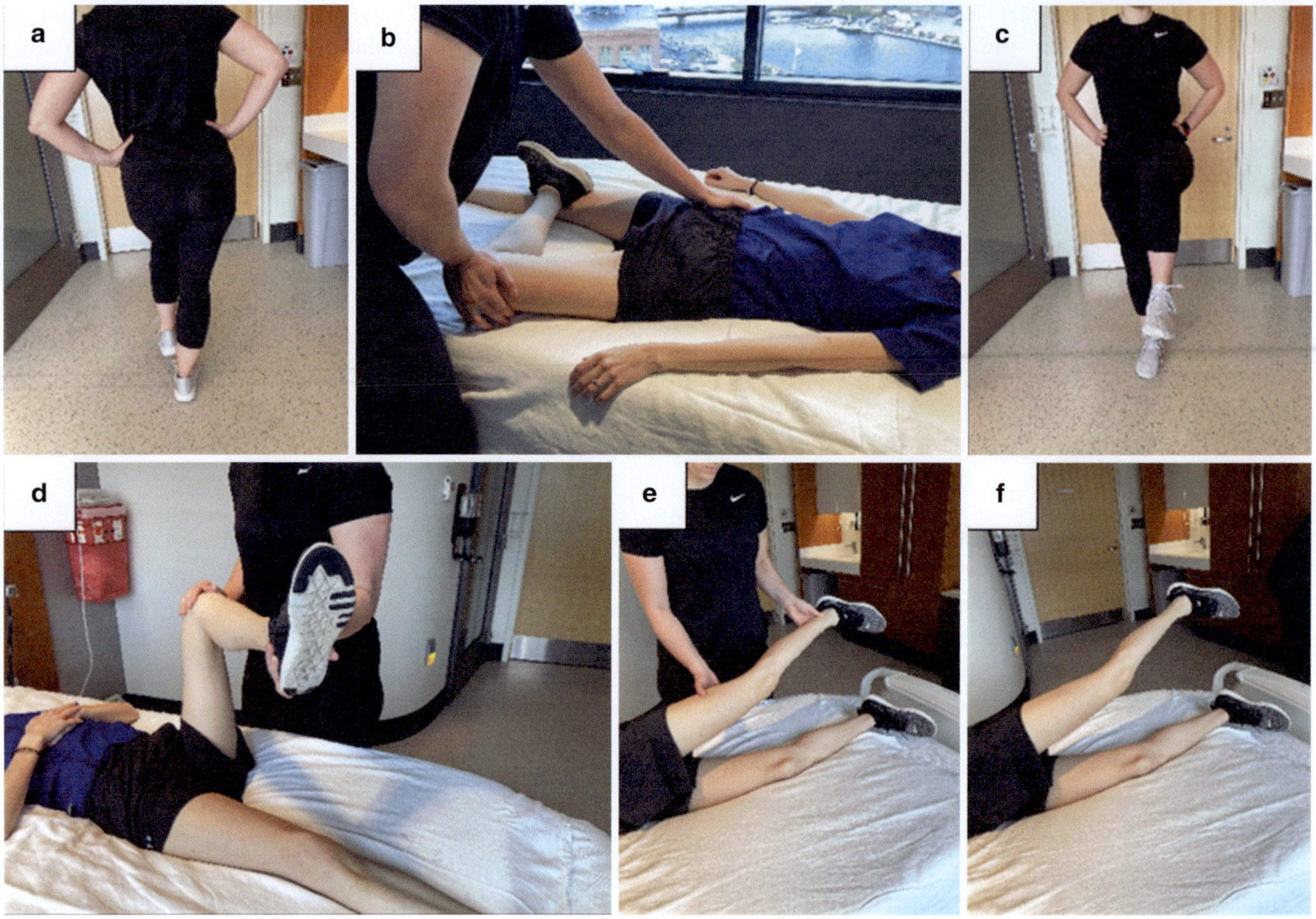

Fig. 40.3 Physical exam maneuvers for gluteal tendinopathy: Trendelenburg gait (**a**), FABER test (**b**), single-leg stance test (**c**), resisted internal rotation test (**d**), positioning patient for hip lag sign (**e**), and a negative hip lag sign (**f**)

elicited in many locations depending on pathology. Groin pain can suggest intra-articular hip process, whereas posterior pain can suggest sacroiliac joint disease.

Single-leg stance The patient is asked to stand on the painful leg for 30 seconds with the unaffected leg at 90 degrees of hip and knee flexion (Fig. 40.3c). Lateral hip pain during this period suggests GT with reported sensitivity of 100% and specificity of 97% in patients with at least 4 months of lateral hip pain [5].

Resisted internal rotation (resisted external derotation) While in the supine position, the symptomatic leg is brought to 90 degrees of hip and knee flexion, followed by 15 to 20 degrees of external rotation. Next, resisted internal rotation is tested using one hand to stabilize the knee and the other to apply a rotational force at the ankle (Fig. 40.3d). Pain or weakness with this maneuver has a reported sensitivity of 90%, specificity of 85%, and positive predictive value (PPV) of 85% for GT when correlated with MRI [6].

Hip lag sign While in the side-lying position with the affected hip upward, the hip is passively moved into 10 degrees of extension and 20 degrees of abduction and then internally rotated as far as possible. The examiner then releases the leg (Fig. 40.3e, f). An inability of the patient to maintain this position is considered a positive test with 89% sensitivity, 97% specificity, and 94% PPV for gluteus medius and/or minimus pathology [7].

40.1.6 Diagnostic Evaluation

GT is generally a clinical diagnosis; however, imaging may evaluate for secondary or concomitant pathologies or assess the integrity of the gluteal tendons or guide further interventions in the case of refractory disease.

X-ray Radiographs are frequently obtained to evaluate for other potential etiologies of hip pain, such as arthritis, fractures, avascular necrosis, or bony morphologies associated with femoroacetabular impingement. Radiographs have low sensitivity for detecting gluteal tendinopathy. However, radiographic trochanteric cortical irregularities have high specificity (96–98%) for gluteal tendon abnormality on MRI correlation [8]. In cases of calcific gluteal tendinopathy, X-ray and ultrasound are the preferred diagnostic imaging modalities.

Ultrasound Sonographic evidence of GT may include tendon thickening, increased heterogeneity, loss of uniform fibrillar echotexture with or without focal hypoechoic regions indicative of tears, enthesopathy/cortical irregularity at the affected facet, intratendinous hyperechoic foci consistent with calcifications, neovascularization, and positive sonopalpation over the affected tendon(s). As previously discussed, trochanteric bursal distention is uncommon but frequently associated with GT when present. In cases of long-standing GT, muscle atrophy and fatty infiltration may be visualized. The absence or retraction of tendon fibers is indicative of a complete tear. Musculoskeletal ultrasound has a sensitivity of 79–100% and PPV of 95–100% for diagnosing GT and/or trochanteric bursopathy, comparable to MRI though operator dependent [9]. Patient body habitus is an important consideration with ultrasound evaluation.

MRI The earliest evidence of GT on MRI is often soft tissue edema surrounding the gluteus minimus and/or medius tendons, followed by tendon thickening and intratendinous signal intensity on T2-weighted imaging (Fig. 40.4) [10]. A focal absence of fibers suggests a partial tear, and complete discontinuity or bony avulsion at the greater trochanter indicates a complete tear. Additional evidence of GT includes fatty muscular atrophy, hypertrophy of the ipsilateral tensor fascia latae (TFL), and cortical irregularities. Because intratendinous calcifications have a hypointense appearance similar to that of the tendon, calcific tendinopathy is frequently underappreciated on MRI. Overall, MRI has a sensitivity of 73% and specificity of 95% for GT [11].

40.1.7 Treatments

40.1.7.1 Medical Management

Gluteal tendinopathy is often a self-limited condition with greater than 90% of patients responding to conservative care [12]. Conservative treatment includes patient education, relative rest, activity modification, icing, topical or oral NSAIDs (in patients with no contraindications), and physical therapy. NSAIDs are typically used for no more than 2–4 weeks at a time at the lowest effective dose.

40.1.7.2 Rehabilitation

A comprehensive physical therapy program should be initiated specifically focusing on strengthening of the hip abductors, isolating gluteus minimus and medius from TFL. Typically, this begins with isometric loading, progressing to eccentric strengthening and more dynamic movements including single-leg squats and lateral hops for advanced patients (Fig. 40.5) [13]. Finally, walk/jog progression and return-to-sport protocols should be gradually advanced as indicated. By correcting dynamic hip adduction, tension through the gluteal tendons and compression of the gluteal entheses by the overlying iliotibial band (ITB) are reduced. Given frequent compensatory move-

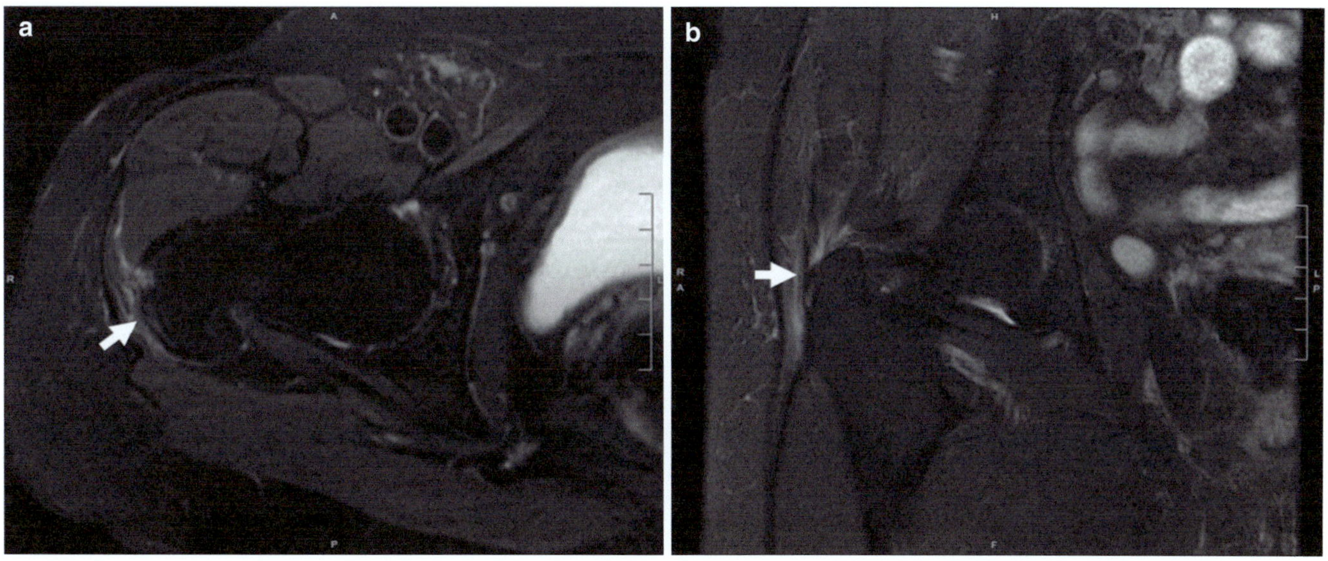

Fig. 40.4 Gluteus medius tendinopathy with partial-thickness insertional tear at the lateral facet of the greater trochanter (arrowhead) and mild surrounding edema on fat-suppressed T2-weighted axial (**a**) and coronal (**b**) MRI

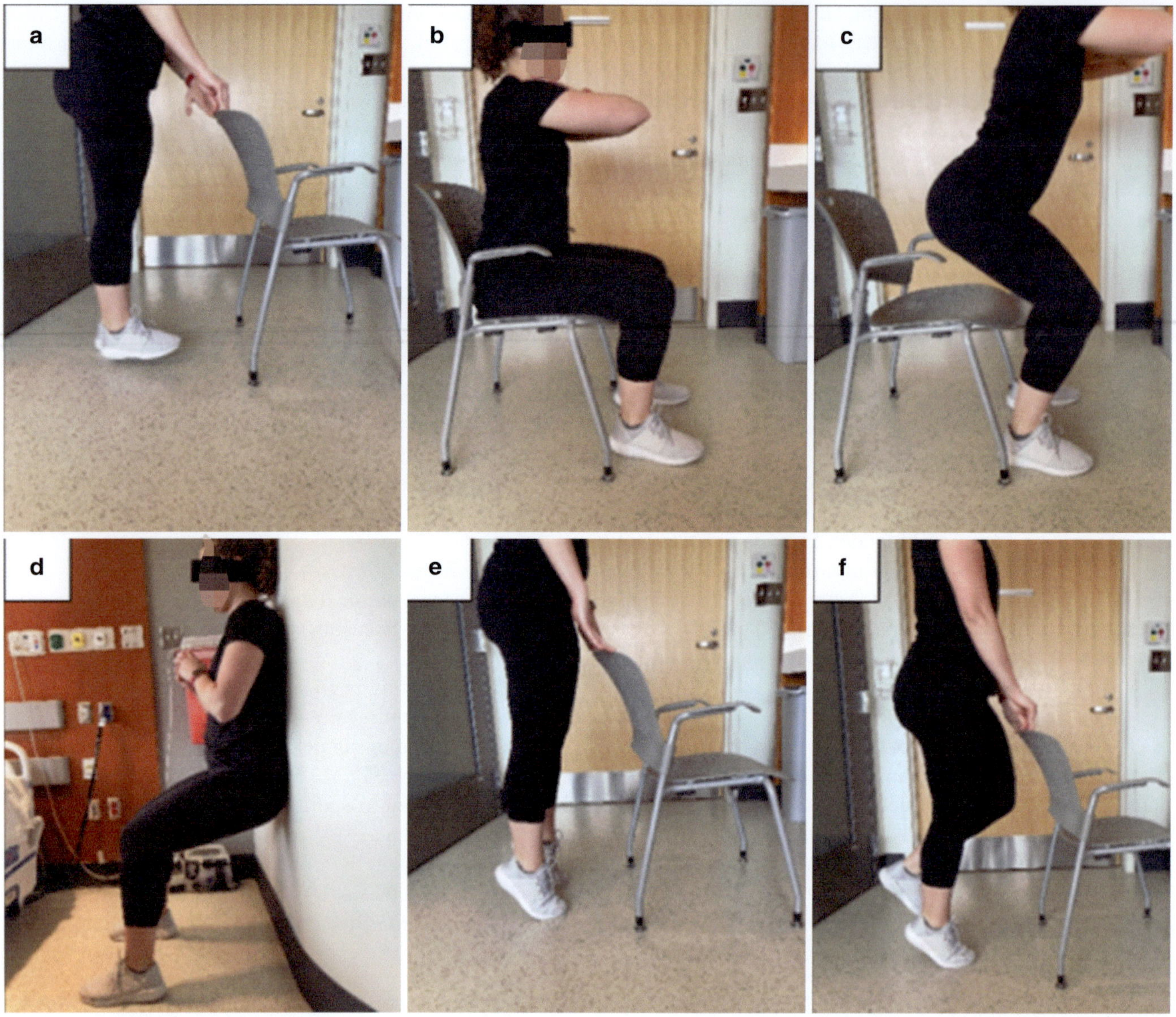

Fig. 40.5 Rehabilitation exercises for gluteal tendinopathy: hip hitch (**a**), standing unassisted (**b**, **c**), two-legged wall squats (**d**), two-legged calf raises (**e**), single-legged calf raises (**f**)

ment patterns, strengthening of the entire kinetic chain is also recommended, along with stretching and soft tissue work as needed.

40.1.7.3 Procedures

For patients with refractory symptoms, procedural interventions can be considered. Patient education, informed consent, and shared decision-making are important in all cases, particularly when treatment may confer out-of-pocket costs to the patients as is often the case with extracorporeal shockwave therapy (ESWT) and orthobiologic injections.

Corticosteroid injection (CSI) (CPT code 76942) Assuming no evidence of pre-existing gluteal tendon tear, a one-time ultrasound-guided CSI can be performed to ensure bursal rather than intra-tendinous infiltration. As for most tendinopathies, short-term pain reduction has been demonstrated with the use of steroid injection for GT. However, a randomized controlled trial (RCT) of 204 patients with GT found that 8 weeks of education plus exercise therapy had significant benefit over both steroid injection and wait-and-see approach for short-term pain and global improvement, as well as long-term global improvement at 1 year [14]. Long-term benefit has not been demonstrated for CSI, particularly when used in isolation. Further, potential risks of CSI must be considered, including progressive tendon tearing or rupture [15], particularly with repeat CSIs without image guidance.

Orthobiologic injection Ultrasound-guided injection of platelet-rich plasma (PRP) (CPT code 0232T) can be considered instead of steroid, sparing the tendon from steroid exposure with perhaps some regenerative properties. A recent RCT comparing PRP to steroid injection in patients with GT showed improved pain and function in the PRP group after 12 weeks of follow-up [16]. Evidence for other orthobiologic injectables including mesenchymal signaling cells is limited at this time.

Shockwave therapy (CPT 0101T) Another alternative treatment for GT is ESWT, which has been found to be more effective at mid- and long-term follow-up compared to steroid injection, producing comparable results to physical therapy, stretching and strengthening [17]. A recent randomized controlled trial demonstrated improved pain, function, and patient satisfaction with focused ESWT (3 weekly sessions, each including 2000 shocks with frequency of 5.0 Hz and total energy flux density of 0.20 mJ/mm^2) compared to placebo at 2 months with durability over the six-month study period [18]. Radial and combined ESWT protocols may also be considered.

Barbotage (CPT 20610) Barbotage, or ultrasound-guided percutaneous lavage, may be utilized for refractory calcific tendinopathy, though evidence specifically related to the gluteal tendons is limited. A variety of techniques are described, typically involving injection and aspiration of saline into the calcium deposit until it is disrupted or dissolved. The procedure is often followed by steroid injection to prevent post-procedure bursitis secondary to localized soft tissue calcium dispersion and resulting inflammation.

Percutaneous ultrasonic tenotomy (CPT 27006) Ultrasound-guided percutaneous tenotomy may be considered for refractory GT, including calcific gluteal tendinosis. This outpatient treatment utilizes ultrasonic energy with local irrigation to debride pathologic tissue. It has been shown to improve pain and functional outcomes up to 2 years post-treatment, though without a high level of evidence to date [2, 19].

40.1.7.4 Surgery

Surgery is generally not required for gluteal tendinopathy and is typically reserved for those with full- or high-grade partial-thickness tears that result in lumbopelvic instability or severe pain/functional impairment after greater than 6 months of non-surgical treatment [20]. Endoscopic approach is generally preferred to open approach in order to minimize tissue damage, shorten hospitalization, decrease postoperative pain, and improve rate of recovery. Surgery may involve debridement of the degenerative tissue, curettage of the bone surface, reattachment or direct repair of the tendon, and/or bursectomy with good pain and functional outcomes over a 2-year follow-up [20].

40.2 Iliotibial Band–Related Disorders

40.2.1 Synonyms

- Lateral/external snapping hip
- Lateral/external coxa saltans
- Iliotibial band syndrome (ITBS)
- Proximal iliotibial band friction syndrome

40.2.2 ICD-10 Codes

M76.30–M76.32

40.2.3 Description

Anatomy The ITB is a longitudinal fibrous band that originates at the iliac tubercle along the anterolateral iliac crest and TFL muscle proximally, serves as the insertion for much of the gluteus maximus, and travels the length of the lateral thigh before inserting at Gerdy's tubercle on the lateral tibial condyle. At the level of the greater trochanter, it passes just superior to the gluteal musculature and enthuses (Fig. 40.1). The function of the ITB is complex as it provides lower extremity joint stabilization dependent upon a variety of static and dynamic factors related to lumbopelvic, hip, and knee alignment.

40.2.3.1 External Snapping Hip or External Coxa Saltans

This condition has been reported in 5–10% of the general population with a much higher prevalence among athletes, particularly those engaging in activities involving extremes of hip motion such as dancers [21]. It is characterized by an audible and/or palpable snap occurring at the greater trochanteric region—most commonly arising from translation of the iliotibial band (ITB) over the greater trochanter—but more rarely caused by translation of the anterior fibers of the gluteus maximus over the greater trochanter. While the presence of an external snapping hip does not necessarily imply symptomatology, it is often attributed to repetitive overuse in the setting of suboptimal core and hip girdle biomechanics, similar to the risk factors for GT. As such, chronic translation over the greater trochanter can lead to thickening of the posterior fibers of the ITB or anterior gluteus maximus at its insertion on the ITB. This fascial thickening may further disrupt normal physiologic glide over the greater trochanter, potentially leading to more pronounced snapping, pain, partial tears, underlying frictional ITB bursal hypertrophy, and/or irritation of the vastus lateralis tendinous origin, all of which are encompassed by the broad term of *proximal ITB friction syndrome*. Additional risk factors may include coxa vara, increased intertrochanteric width, prominent greater trochanters, ITB/TFL tightness, generalized hypermobility, and connective tissue disorders. Finally, in rare cases, external snapping of the hip may be related to trauma.

40.2.4 Clinical Presentation

Patients often present with complaints of snapping and/or pain at the lateral hip, sometimes described as if their hip is dislocating. Provoking movements may be inconsistent for some patients, while others will be able to recreate the snapping on demand. When pain is present, it typically develops insidiously over months to years, is located at the greater trochanteric region, and is made worse during activities of end-range hip movement, walking, jogging, and cycling.

40.2.5 Physical Examination

A comprehensive musculoskeletal examination should be performed.

Gait evaluation Gait is typically normal; however, patients may complain of reproduction of lateral hip pain and/or snapping sensation at variable phases of the gait cycle.

Observation Inspection for swelling, erythema, asymmetry, or deformity is noted. Often, there will be no obvious outward abnormalities for disorders related to the ITB, but other observable risk factors can be assessed as previously described. If the patient is able to recreate snapping, an attempt should be made to directly visualize and/or palpate the snap for localization.

Palpation Palpation over the greater trochanteric region can be performed in any position that the patient is able to reproduce snapping symptoms. Further, tenderness may be present diffusely over the ITB including at its origin and/or anterior gluteus maximus border.

Range of motion (ROM) Full passive and active ROM should be present in ITB-related disorders, though reproduction of pain or even snapping may be present with a variety of movements. True passive ROM restriction generally indicates intra-articular hip pathology.

Sensory testing and reflexes Sensory examination and reflexes should be normal in the case of ITB-related disorders.

Motor testing Resisted hip abduction, both with concomitant hip flexion and hip extension, may reproduce lateral hip pain in ITB-related disorders given activation of the TFL and gluteus maximus muscles, respectively.

Joint testing Careful assessment of the hip, sacroiliac, and facet joints should be performed to differentiate ITB-related disorders from other differential diagnoses.

40.2.5.1 Special Maneuvers

FABER-external derotation test Snapping can be elicited by having the patient actively or passively move from the FABER position to extension, adduction, and internal rotation (Fig. 40.6a–c). Snapping may also be created by moving the patient from neutral to the FABER position.

Ober's test From a side-lying position with the affected side upward, the hip is passively extended and allowed to drop into adduction toward the exam table (Fig. 40.6d). Limited adduction implies ITB tightness, which can potentially contribute to external snapping hip.

Hula-hoop test From the standing position, the patient adducts and circumducts the affected hip while the examiner observes for snapping over the greater trochanter (Fig. 40.6e).

40.2.6 Diagnostic Evaluation

External snapping hip and proximal ITB friction syndrome are clinical diagnoses, but imaging can be a useful adjunct when the diagnosis is not readily apparent or in refractory cases.

X-ray As previously noted, radiographs of the hip are often useful to rule out osseous abnormalities. They are typically normal in isolated ITB-related disorders.

Ultrasound Dynamic ultrasound can definitively diagnose external snapping hip by allowing direct visualization of the ITB or anterior gluteus maximus fibers snapping over the greater trochanter, which may or may not be associated with ITB thickening or partial tearing.

MRI MRI can identify proximal thickening or tearing of the ITB, associated edema, or less frequently bursal hypertrophy (Fig. 40.7). Differentiating between ITB and gluteus maximus involvement can be helpful in determining prognosis, as patients with gluteus maximus involvement tend to have symptoms for a longer duration [22].

40.2.7 Treatments

40.2.7.1 Medical Management

Many people experience infrequent, asymptomatic snapping of the lateral hip. In these cases, no treatment is necessary. If

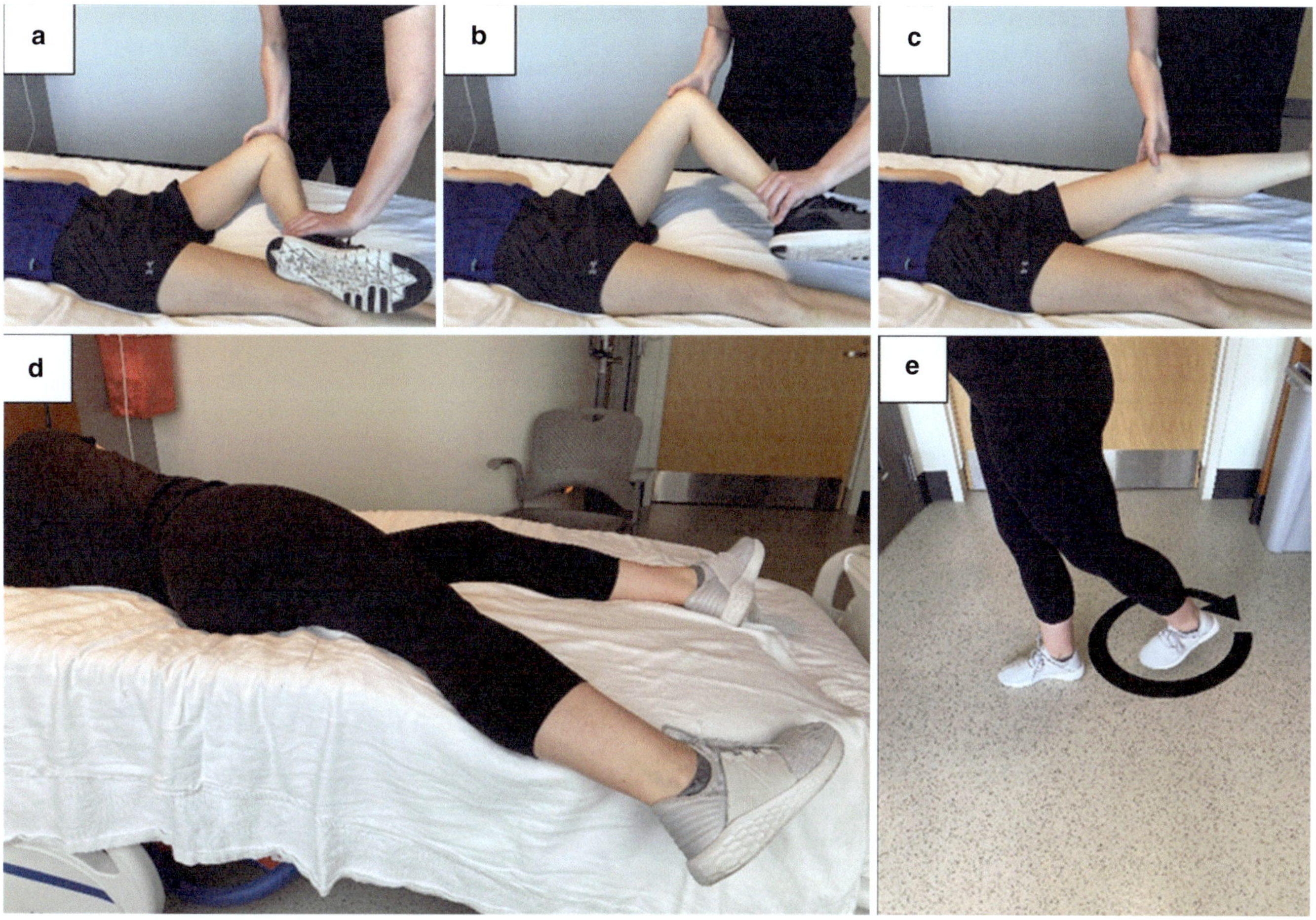

Fig. 40.6 Physical exam maneuvers for external snapping hip: FABER-external derotation test (**a–c**), normal Ober's test (**d**), hula-hoop test (**e**)

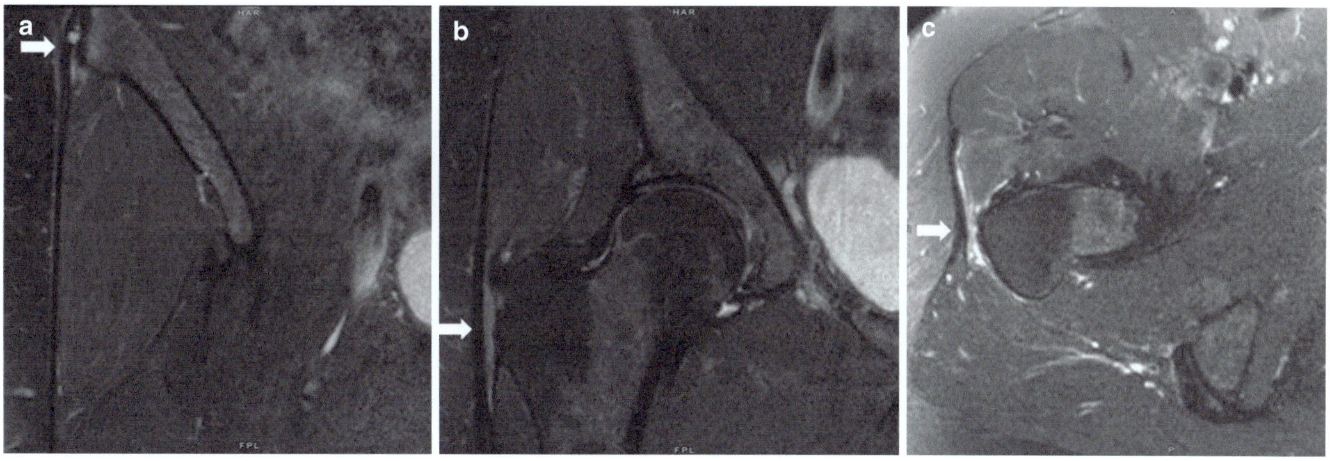

Fig. 40.7 Findings associated with proximal ITB syndrome including ITB thickening with partial tear and mild associated iliac tubercle bone marrow edema (arrow, **a**) and thickening at the level of the greater trochanter with the surrounding soft tissue edema (arrows, **b**, **c**) on coronal (**a**, **b**) and axial (**c**) fat-suppressed T2-weighted MRI

the snapping becomes symptomatic, a conservative care should be initiated, consisting of patient education, relative rest, activity modification, icing, topical or oral NSAIDS (if no contraindications exists), and physical therapy (PT). The vast majority of symptomatic patients respond well to conservative treatments alone.

40.2.7.2 Rehabilitation

PT should include a comprehensive evaluation of the kinetic chain as ITB-related disorders are impacted by postural, lumbopelvic, hip girdle, and knee mechanics. Often, there is overuse of the TFL as compared to the gluteal muscles, which can be addressed with exercises to specifically strengthen the gluteal muscles and stretch or lengthen the TFL. Gluteal strengthening will decrease dynamic hip adduction, preventing the greater trochanter from acting as a fulcrum compressing against the ITB and underlying soft tissues. Foam rolling and soft tissue work are often incorporated.

40.2.7.3 Procedures

For patients with refractory symptoms or limited ability to tolerate PT due to pain, steroid injection, orthobiologic injections, and ESWT may be appropriate, similar to GT. Currently, there is limited evidence related to the collective use of these interventions specifically for ITB-related disorders, and similar principles as discussed for GT should be considered.

40.2.7.4 Surgery

In the rare case that ITB-related disorders are refractory to non-operative treatment, surgery can be considered for ITB lengthening. In small studies, z-lengthening has shown good success in resolving snapping hip [23]. Endoscopic release, where a diamond-shaped defect is made through the ITB, has also demonstrated promising results over 2 years of follow-up [24]. Patients should be counseled regarding the potential for postoperative hip abductor weakness.

References

1. Chowdhury R, Naaseri S, Lee J, Rajeswaran G. Imaging and management of greater trochanteric pain syndrome. Postgrad Med J. 2014;90(1068):576–81.
2. Borgstrom H, McInnis KC. Female athlete hip injuries. Clin J Sport Med. 2022;32(1):62–71.
3. Birnbaum K, Siebert CH, Pandorf T, Schopphoff E, Prescher A, Niethard FU. Anatomical and biomechanical investigations of the iliotibial tract. Surg Radiol Anat. 2004;26(6):433–46.
4. Long SS, Surrey DE, Nazarian LN. Sonography of greater trochanteric pain syndrome and the rarity of primary bursitis. AJR Am J Roentgenol. 2013;201(5):1083–6.
5. Lequesne M, Mathieu P, Vuillemin-Bodaghi V, Bard H, Djian P. Gluteal tendinopathy in refractory greater trochanter pain syndrome: diagnostic value of two clinical tests. Arthritis Care Res. 2008;59(2):241–6.
6. Ortiz-Declet V, Chen AW, Maldonado DR, Yuen LC, Mu B, Domb BG. Diagnostic accuracy of a new clinical test (resisted internal rotation) for detection of gluteus medius tears. J Hip Preserv Surg. 2019;6(4):398–405.
7. Kaltenborn A, Bourg CM, Gutzeit A, Kalberer F. The hip lag sign – prospective blinded trial of a new clinical sign to predict hip abductor damage. PLoS One 2014;9(3). `.
8. Steinert L, Zanetti M, Hodler J, Pfirrmann CWA, Dora C, Saupe N. Are radiographic trochanteric surface irregularities associated with abductor tendon abnormalities? Radiology. 2010;257(3):754–63.
9. Westacott DJ, Minns JI, Foguet P. The diagnostic accuracy of magnetic resonance imaging and ultrasonography in gluteal tendon tears – a systematic review. Hip Int. 2011;21(6):637–45.
10. Kong A, Vliet A, Zadow S. MRI and US of gluteal tendinopathy in greater trochanteric pain syndrome. Eur Radiol. 2007;17(7):1772–83.
11. Cvitanic O, Henzie G, Skezas N, Lyons J, Minter J. MRI diagnosis of tears of the hip abductor tendons (gluteus medius and gluteus minimus). Am J Roentgenol. 2004;182(1):137–43.
12. Reid D. The management of greater trochanteric pain syndrome: a systematic literature review. J Orthop. 2016;13(1):15–28.
13. Ganderton C, Semciw A, Cook J, Moreira E, Pizzari T. Gluteal loading versus sham exercises to improve pain and dysfunction in postmenopausal women with greater trochanteric pain syndrome: a randomized controlled trial. J Women's Heal. 2018;27(6):815–29.
14. Mellor R, Bennell K, Grimaldi A, Nicolson P, Kasza J, Hodges P, et al. Education plus exercise versus corticosteroid injection use versus a wait and see approach on global outcome and pain from gluteal tendinopathy: prospective, single blinded, randomised clinical trial. BMJ. 2018;361:k1662.
15. Brinks A, Koes BW, Volkers AC, Verhaar JAN, Bierma-Zeinstra SMA. Adverse effects of extra-articular corticosteroid injections: a systematic review. BMC Musculoskelet Disord. 2010;11:206.
16. Fitzpatrick J, Bulsara MK, O'Donnell J, McCrory PR, Zheng MH. The effectiveness of platelet-rich plasma injections in gluteal tendinopathy: a randomized, double-blind controlled trial comparing a single platelet-rich plasma injection with a single corticosteroid injection. Am J Sports Med. 2018;46(4):933–9.
17. Korakakis V, Whiteley R, Tzavara A, Malliaropoulos N. The effectiveness of extracorporeal shockwave therapy in common lower limb conditions: a systematic review including quantification of patient-rated pain reduction. Br J Sports Med. 2018;52(6):387–407.
18. Ramon S, Russo S, Santoboni F, Lucenteforte G, Di Luise C, de Unzurrunzaga R, et al. Focused shockwave treatment for greater trochanteric pain syndrome: a multicenter, randomized, controlled clinical trial. J Bone Joint Surg Am. 2020;102(15):1305–11.
19. Baker CL Jr, Mahoney JR. Ultrasound-guided percutaneous tenotomy for gluteal tendinopathy. Orthop J Sports Med. 2020;8(3):2325967120907868.
20. Baker CL, Massie RV, Hurt WG, Savory CG. Arthroscopic bursectomy for recalcitrant trochanteric bursitis. Arthrosc – J Arthrosc Relat Surg. 2007;23(8):827–32.
21. Lewis CL. Extra-articular snapping hip: a literature review. Sports Health. 2010;2(3):186–90.
22. Kim CH, Lee SK, Kim JH, Yoon PW. External snapping hip: classification based on magnetic resonance imaging features and clinical correlation. Hip Int. 2022;32(1):118–123.
23. Provencher MT, Hofmeister EP, Muldoon MP. The surgical treatment of external coxa saltans (the snapping hip) by Z-plasty of the iliotibial band. Am J Sports Med. 2004;32(2):470–6.
24. White RA, Hughes MS, Burd T, Hamann J, Allen WC. A new operative approach in the correction of external coxa saltans: the snapping hip. Am J Sports Med. 2004;32(6):1504–8.

Hip Fractures and Dislocations

41

Kristian von Rickenbach, Adam Tenforde, and Haylee Borgstrom

41.1 Hip Stress Fracture/Bone Stress Injury

41.1.1 Synonyms

- Femoral neck stress fracture/bone stress injury
- Acetabular stress fracture/bone stress injury

41.1.2 ICD-10 Code

M84.35

41.1.3 Description

Anatomy The hip, or femoroacetabular articulation, is a ball-and-socket joint designed for weight-bearing. The femoral head and neck, along with the acetabulum, are rich in trabecular bone, which is likely more sensitive to relative energy deficiency in sport (RED-S) risk factors and resulting low bone mineral density compared to cortical-rich bone [7]. The superolateral border of the femoral neck is subject to high tensile forces, while the inferomedial border is subject to compressive forces (Fig. 41.1). Tension-side femoral neck stress injuries are classified as high-risk bone stress injuries (BSI) due to increased risk for displacement and resulting complications including delayed or non-union and avascular necrosis (AVN) [2]. Of note, hip abductor weakness alters force transmission through the femoral neck and acetabulum leading to increased tensile/compressive forces and joint contact pressures [8], potentially increasing risk for stress fractures and bone stress injuries.

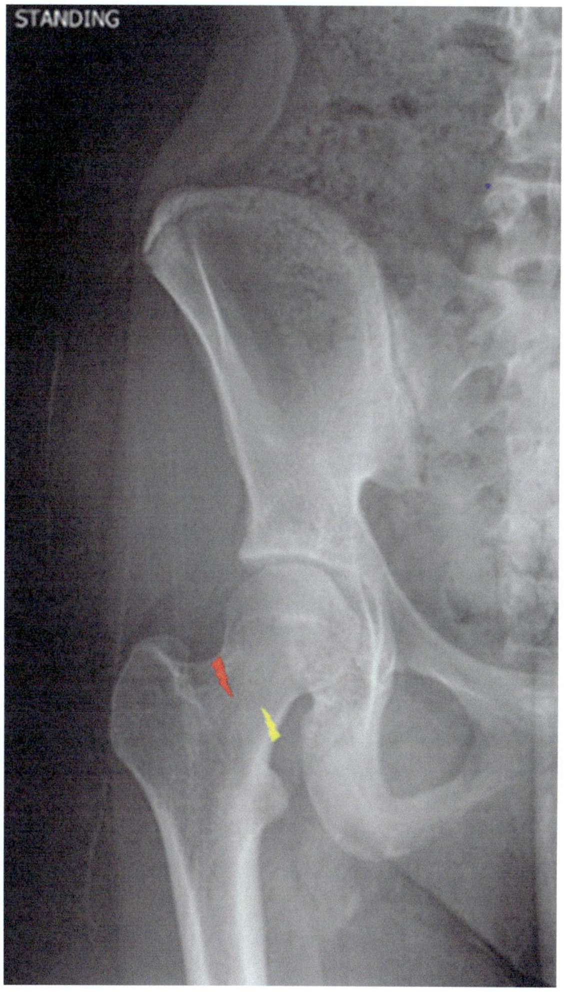

Fig. 41.1 Normal weight-bearing AP hip radiograph with typical locations for high-risk tension-sided (red) and compression-sided (yellow) femoral neck stress fractures

Stress fractures and *bone stress injuries* (BSI) of the femur and acetabulum are overuse injuries related to repetitive load, resulting in cumulative microtrauma and structural fatigue [1]. Thus, they typically occur in those participating in repetitive impact exercise, particularly long-distance run-

K. von Rickenbach · A. Tenforde
Department of Physical Medicine & Rehabilitation, Spaulding Rehabilitation Hospital, Harvard Medical School, Charlestown, MA, USA
e-mail: atenforde@mgh.harvard.edu

H. Borgstrom (✉)
Department of Physical Medicine & Rehabilitation, Spaulding Rehabilitation Hospital, Massachusetts General Hospital, Harvard Medical School, Boston, MA, USA
e-mail: hborgstrom@partners.org

© The Author(s), under exclusive license to Springer Nature Switzerland AG 2022

S. A. Mostoufi et al. (eds.), *Clinical Guide to Musculoskeletal Medicine*, https://doi.org/10.1007/978-3-030-92042-5_41

ners and military recruits, and are more common in females compared to males [1, 2]. Among athletes with bone stress injuries, femoral neck stress fractures are relatively uncommon, accounting for 3–5% of all stress fractures [2, 3]. However, recognition of femoral neck bone stress injury is important due to potential for serious sequelae including avascular necrosis (AVN) of the femoral head, so clinicians should maintain a high index of suspicion in the endurance athlete with hip pain. Acetabular stress fractures are far rarer still [4]. Bone metabolism is an intricate and highly dynamic process influenced by biomechanical, metabolic, anatomic, and other factors [5].

Etiology/risk factors The etiology for BSI is generally multifactorial. Biomechanical risk factors include volume and intensity of impact exercise, gait kinematics, and muscle strength and endurance [1]. Metabolic risk factors for BSI hinge on the concept of low energy availability encompassed by the concept of relative energy deficiency in sport (RED-S) [6], resulting in menstrual and neurohormonal dysregulation, low body mass index, micronutrient deficiency, and impaired bone health. Additional risk factors include coxa vara, acetabular retroversion, underlying bone or connective tissue disease, smoking, and high-risk medications including prolonged corticosteroid use [3].

41.1.4 Clinical Presentation

Patients with either femoral or acetabular BSI will typically present with an insidious onset of hip region pain. The location of pain is often poorly localized but is most commonly described in the anterior hip/groin region and proximal anterior thigh. Typically occurring in the setting of increased volume and/or intensity of impact exercise, pain is made worse with weight-bearing and/or impact activity and is alleviated by rest [2, 3]. As the severity of injury progresses, the patient may describe pain at rest and at nighttime. A thorough assessment of potential risk factors is vital and indicated as part of a complete history for suspected BSI in order to guide management and future prevention.

41.1.5 Physical Examination

Comprehensive musculoskeletal examination of the lumbar spine, sacroiliac joints, and bilateral hips is indicated given often overlapping referral patterns for these joints, along with lower extremity neurologic assessment to evaluate for possible neurologic etiology. Depending on findings, the examination may need to expand to assess for other potential sources of pain, including intra-abdominal or intra-pelvic etiologies.

Gait The patient may present with an antalgic gait, particularly in cases of high-grade injury [3].

Visual observation Inspection is generally normal in cases of bone stress injury, but asymmetries and alignment abnormalities should be noted as potential risk factors. Body habitus should be noted as a potential reflection of low energy availability and low body mass index and changes to the skin (callouses to suggest bulimia), hair (lanugo), or other findings that may suggest an underlying eating disorder.

Palpation Palpatory examination may be normal in the case of bone stress injury given deep location. However, it is not uncommon to have reactive regional myofascial pain or compensatory tendon overuse in the setting of antalgic gait with over 60% of patients with femoral neck stress fracture exhibiting non-specific anterior hip tenderness [3].

Range of motion (ROM) Pain with end range of motion, especially internal rotation, is present in nearly 80% of patients with femoral neck stress fractures [3]. Hip and lumbar spine ROM should be examined in all planes.

Sensory testing Sensory examination for bilateral L1-S1 dermatomes should be normal in the case of bone stress injury. Deficits should increase suspicion for neurologic etiology.

Deep tendon reflexes Bilateral lower extremity reflexes should be tested for patellar (primarily L4), medial hamstring (L5), and Achilles (S1) tendons. Reflexes shoulder be 2+ and symmetric in the case of bone stress injury.

Motor testing Manual motor testing for bilateral L2-S1 myotomes should be completed to assess for neurologic etiology. Pain may limit resisted hip flexion, extension, adduction, and abduction, but strength should be preserved distally in the case of bone stress injury. Resisted hip flexion may provoke pain in the associated lesser trochanteric bone stress injury, which may progress to femoral neck bone stress injury in advanced cases [9].

Joint testing As previously discussed, a thorough musculoskeletal evaluation of the lumbar spine and bilateral sacroiliac joints is indicated given frequently overlapping pain referral patterns.

41.1.5.1 Special Maneuvers

Intra-articular hip maneuvers Examination maneuvers correlated with intra-articular hip pathology are often positive in the case of femoral neck or acetabular stress injury including FADIR, FABER, log roll, and Stinchfield's (or resisted straight leg raise) tests [3]. These exam maneuvers are discussed in detail in the "Anterior Hip Disorders" chapter.

Weight-bearing or impact maneuvers While tests such as single-leg squat, hops, and stance are often positive in the case of femoral neck stress injuries, the potential risk for fracture propagation must be considered against their diagnostic utility [2]. Often, these tests can be deferred if the clinician suspects bone stress injury as imaging will be indicated.

Beighton score Testing for generalized hypermobility as a potential indicator of underlying connective tissue disease can be considered. Exam maneuvers included in this evaluation are described in detail in the "Anterior Hip Disorders" chapter.

41.1.6 Diagnostic Workup

X-ray Plain radiographs of the hips and pelvis are typically obtained as the initial screening tool for bone stress injury, though with low sensitivity on both initial evaluation (15%) and follow-up (50%) [2]. Radiographs can be useful for evaluating differential diagnoses including joint degenerative disease, calcific tendinopathy, and cam- or pincer-type morphology. Radiographic findings suggestive of femoroacetabular impingement may be associated with femoral neck bone stress injury [10].

Magnetic resonance imaging (MRI) MRI is the recommended imaging modality for assessment of bone stress injuries given a high sensitivity and specificity for even low-grade injuries. The earliest sign of bone stress injury is periosteal edema. As the grade of injury increases, bone marrow edema is appreciated on T2-weighted imaging, then as corresponding hypointense signal on T1-weighted imaging, finally followed by a discrete fracture line [11] (Fig. 41.2). Various grading systems are described for bone stress injuries, which have both diagnostic and prognostic value.

Musculoskeletal ultrasound Sonographic evaluation may reveal periosteal thickening or cortical irregularity in the presence of a femoral neck stress fracture, but MRI is the imaging modality of choice for diagnosis of bone stress injury.

Laboratory evaluation Basic blood work aimed at identifying metabolic contributors to impaired bone health should be completed particularly in the case of high-risk bone stress injury. This may include complete blood count, complete metabolic panel, inflammatory markers, iron studies, 25-hydroxyvitamin D level, reproductive hormone levels, and more. Specialist referral may be made for this testing depending on the expertise and comfort level of the clinician.

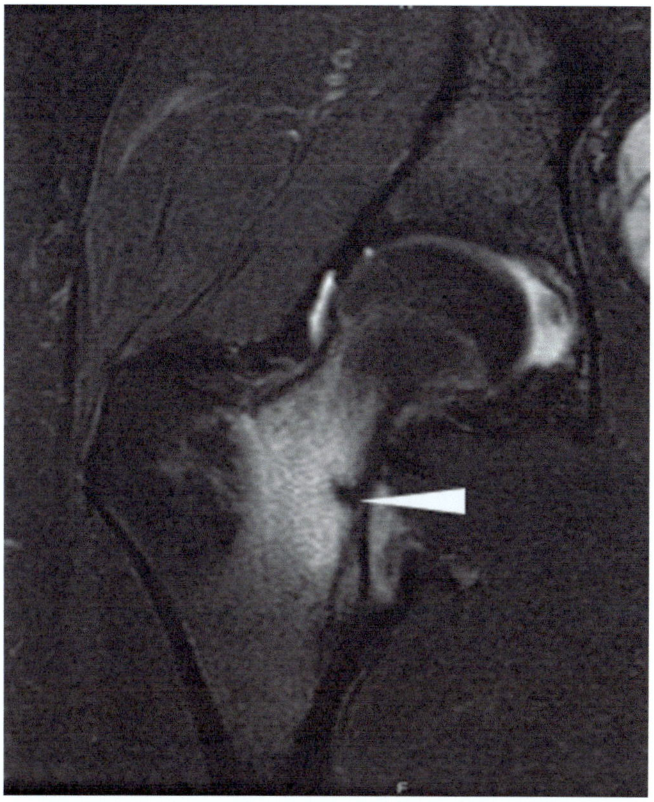

Fig. 41.2 Nondisplaced hypointense compression-side femoral neck stress fracture (arrowhead) with surrounding hyperintense bony edema on coronal T2-weighted MRI with fat suppression

Dual-energy X-ray absorptiometry (DXA) DXA may be considered to assess bone mineral density particularly in the setting of high-risk or recurrent bone stress injuries with associated RED-S risk factors. In pre-menopausal women and men younger than 50 years old, low bone mineral density is defined as age-matched Z-scores between −1.0 and −2.0 [12]. In post-menopausal women and men older than 50 years old, T-scores are used to diagnose osteopenia and osteoporosis.

41.1.7 Treatment

41.1.7.1 Medical Management

In the case of suspected femoral neck or acetabular bone stress injury, the patient should immediately be placed on crutches and adhere to non-weight-bearing status through the affected extremity until diagnostic imaging can be completed as discussed above. If necessary, pain control can be achieved with a multimodal approach including ice, topicals, acetaminophen, and short-course opioids if needed and after appropriate counseling. Non-steroidal anti-inflammatories may be avoided in the setting of fracture or BSI given theoretical risk for impaired bone healing. Identification and treatment of underlying metabolic contributors to impaired bone health are key as previously discussed. Vitamin D supplementation can be initiated in the case of hypovitaminosis D (less than 30 ng/mL). High-dose supplementation with 50,000 IU vitamin D3 weekly for 8 weeks may be considered, followed by 1000–2000 IU daily [13, 14]. Daily calcium intake of 1000–1200 mg daily is also recommended [14], primarily through dietary intake when possible. Because bone stress injuries are often multifactorial in etiology, a multidisciplinary team may be necessary to optimize fracture healing and prevention of recurrent injuries, including non-operative sport medicine, orthopedic surgery, physical therapy, endocrinology, eating disorder medicine, sport nutrition, sleep medicine, sport psychology, and more. Patient education is essential for successful treatment and prevention of bone stress injuries/stress fractures.

41.1.7.2 Rehabilitation

As with most bone stress injuries, rehabilitation begins with a period of weight-bearing and activity restriction based on the severity and location of bone stress injury. Compression-side femoral neck bone stress injuries can typically be managed non-operatively with 4–6 weeks of non-weight-bearing, physical therapy focused on core and gluteal strengthening, and gradual return to impact exercise. However, surgical consultation should be considered for fractures spanning greater than 50% of the femoral neck width [3]. As previously discussed, MRI grading can help to guide patient expectations related to return to sport with grade 1 through 4 injuries requiring an average of 7.4, 13.8, 14.7, and 17.5 weeks before return to run, respectively [15]. Nondisplaced acetabular stress fractures can be managed non-operatively with similar rehabilitation principles.

41.1.7.3 Procedures

Procedures are generally not required for the treatment of bone stress injuries.

Orthobiologic injections There is limited low-level evidence for the use of orthobiologics in the treatment of non-healing stress fractures, most commonly as augmentation during surgical management with none specifically focused on femoral neck or acetabular stress fractures [16].

Extracorporeal shockwave therapy (ESWT) There is limited low-level evidence supporting the use of ESWT for treatment of delayed or non-union stress fractures, generally in more superficial locations. More recently, focused ESWT has been demonstrated to reduce marrow edema in femoral head osteonecrosis [17]. This may be a consideration for refractory femoral neck and acetabular bone stress injuries, though higher-quality studies are needed.

41.1.7.4 Surgery

Tension-sided or displaced femoral neck and displaced acetabular stress fractures require urgent surgical evaluation given a high risk for complications. Surgical management of femoral neck and acetabular fractures is described in detail in a subsequent chapter. In the case of compression-side femoral neck or nondisplaced acetabular fractures, surgical intervention can often be avoided with a comprehensive non-operative treatment approach as described above.

41.2 Traumatic Hip Fracture

41.2.1 Synonyms

- Femoral neck fracture
- Intertrochanteric fracture
- Subtrochanteric fracture
- Acetabular fracture

41.2.2 ICD-10 Code

S72.00, S72.14, S72.23, S32.40

41.2.3 Description

Anatomy Proximal femur fractures can be categorized by their location, commonly as femoral neck, intertrochanteric (between the greater and lesser trochanters), or subtrochanteric (within 5 cm distal to the less trochanter) (Fig. 41.3). Femoral neck fractures are intra-capsular, whereas intertrochanteric and subtrochanteric fractures are extra-capsular. Acetabular fractures most commonly occur at the weight-bearing superior and posterior aspects of the acetabular dome.

Traumatic hip fractures of the proximal femur and acetabulum may occur in the setting of high-energy trauma, such as motor vehicle accident or less commonly collision sport, in young individuals, or as a result of low-energy trauma, primarily from falls, in older individuals [18, 19]. Increasing age, female sex, osteoporosis, disability, and more are risk factors for fracture in the aging population [18]. Among this same population, femoral neck and intertrochanteric fractures are most common, followed by subtrochanteric and

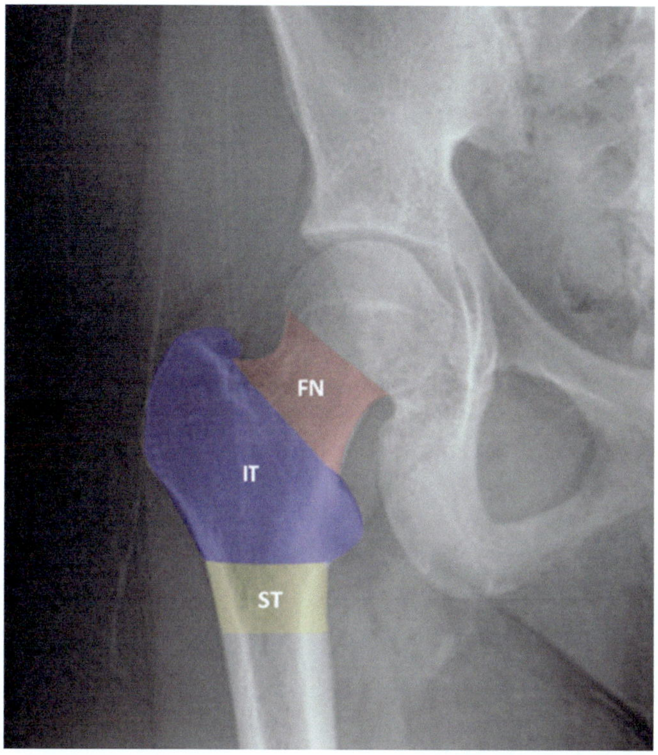

Fig. 41.3 Regions of intra-capsular femoral neck (FN, red) and extra-capsular intertrochanteric (IT, blue) and subtrochanteric (ST, yellow) hip fractures

acetabular fractures. In the National Football League (NFL), traumatic acetabular fractures are the most common hip fracture and may be associated with hip joint subluxation or dislocation. Though these injuries are rare, accounting for less than 2% of all hip injuries, they are second to only hip dislocations in terms of greatest time lost from sport at over 100 days [19]. Because of the high risk of complications including osteonecrosis of the femoral head, post-traumatic osteoarthritis, nerve injury, and heterotopic ossification, clinicians should have a high index of suspicion for proximal femur or acetabular fractures in the appropriate clinical scenario.

41.2.4 Clinical Presentation

Patients with traumatic proximal femur or acetabular fractures will typically present with an acute onset of groin pain and inability to bear weight on the affected limb after a high- or low-energy injury mechanism as previously described. These fractures may occur in the setting of polytrauma warranting emergency evaluation for other life-threatening associated injuries, or they may present as isolated injuries in otherwise medically stable patients amenable to workup in an urgent/expedited outpatient setting, which is the focus of this chapter. The differential diagnosis often includes hip dislocation, which is discussed in detail later in this chapter.

41.2.5 Physical Examination

Gait Most patients with proximal femur or acetabular fractures are not able to bear weight through the affected extremity and may present in an outpatient setting using an assistive device [20].

Visual observation In the case of displaced fractures, the affected limb is often shortened and externally rotated compared to the contralateral limb. There may be no obvious deformity in the case of nondisplaced fractures [20]. Additionally, ecchymosis is rarely present initially, but in cases of delayed presentation, it may appear in various distributions, including scrotal hematoma.

Palpation The deep structures of the proximal femur and acetabulum are not accessible by palpatory examination. However, the greater trochanter and other more superficial bony anatomy of the pelvic ring should be palpated for pain and/or crepitus. Additionally, palpation of the femoral, posterior tibial, and dorsalis pedis pulses, along with distal capillary refill, is mandatory to evaluate for possible associated vascular injury [20].

Range of motion (ROM) Hip ROM is typically limited by pain in all planes in the setting of proximal femoral or acetabular fractures.

Sensory testing Light touch should be tested in bilateral lower extremities throughout the L1-S1 dermatomes with special attention to the sciatic nerve distribution as this nerve can be injured in the case of displaced proximal femur and especially acetabular fractures.

Deep tendon reflexes The following lower extremity reflexes should be tested bilaterally as feasible based on patient positioning and pain: patellar tendon (L2-L4, L4 primary), hamstring tendon (L5), and Achilles tendon (S1).

Motor testing Manual muscle testing should be performed for L2-S1 myotomes, though often pain inhibition is present when testing more proximal muscle groups, especially those that cross the hip joint. As above, special attention should be paid to sciatic-innervated muscle groups, including knee flexors (tibial portion), ankle plantar flexors (tibial portion), and ankle dorsiflexors and evertors (fibular portion).

Joint testing Comprehensive musculoskeletal examination and screening of all joints including the spine are warranted to evaluate for possible associated traumatic injuries.

Special maneuvers Patients are often unable to tolerate exam maneuvers such as the log roll or straight leg raise due to pain in the setting of fracture [20].

41.2.6 Diagnostic Workup

X-ray Plain radiographs of the hips and pelvis should be obtained immediately in the case of suspected proximal femur or acetabular fracture with cross-table lateral and non-weight-bearing anteroposterior (AP) pelvis and Judet views [11]. These views can also assess hip dislocation as part of the differential diagnosis. If radiographs are negative, the patient should remain non-weight-bearing until further definitive diagnostic studies can be completed.

MRI In the case of negative radiographs, MRI is an appropriate test for further diagnostic evaluation and may reveal occult fracture or contusion with associated bone marrow edema, especially involving the trabecular bone, which may not be detected on computed tomography (CT) [11]. It may also reveal joint effusion, hemarthrosis, loose bodies, and labral, capsular, chondral, or ligamentum teres injuries. It is the diagnostic test of choice for associated soft tissue injuries as discussed in other chapters.

CT CT is also appropriate in the case of normal radiographs and can reveal more subtle cortical fractures and loose bodies and can assist with pre-operative planning [11].

41.2.7 Treatment

41.2.7.1 Medical Management

In the case of suspected proximal femur or acetabular fracture, the patient should remain non-weight-bearing until a definitive diagnosis is made. If the treating clinician is managing the patient in the field in the case of an injured athlete, the patient should be promptly transported to an emergency facility for expedited diagnosis and treatment of potential fracture. Multimodal pain management strategies can be utilized with consideration for avoidance of non-steroidal anti-inflammatories as described above.

41.2.7.2 Rehabilitation

Non-operative management and rehabilitation may be achieved in the case of nondisplaced or minimally displaced acetabular fractures that are stable for weight-bearing as determined by a surgeon. In general, 6–8 weeks of protected weight-bearing as tolerated with the use of crutches or a walker is recommended, along with physical therapy focused on core and gluteal strengthening and gait/mobility training, followed by a graduated increase in activity.

41.2.7.3 Procedures

Procedures are generally not required for the treatment of traumatic fractures.

41.2.7.4 Surgery

Surgical management is generally required for all traumatic femoral neck, intertrochanteric, and subtrochanteric fractures regardless of age, though approach may vary significantly based on patient-specific factors. Displaced acetabular fractures or those unstable for weight-bearing are also managed operatively. Specific surgical considerations, recommended approaches, and goals of post-operative rehabilitation are discussed in Chap. 42.

41.3 Hip Dislocations

41.3.1 Synonyms

Femoroacetabular dislocation/subluxation

41.3.2 ICD-10 Code

S73.0

41.3.3 Description

Anatomy The inherent stability of the hip as a true ball-and-socket joint makes dislocation rare. Additional supportive soft tissue structures include the labrum, capsule, reinforcing capsular ligaments including the iliofemoral (Y ligament of Bigelow), ischiofemoral, and pubofemoral ligaments, and the surrounding musculature. When dislocation does occur, there is a high risk for associated femoral and acetabular fractures, chondral, labral, and capsular injuries, and disruption of blood supply to the femoral head primarily from injury to the deep branch of the medial femoral circumflex artery leading to osteonecrosis.

Hip dislocations and subluxations occur infrequently and typically in the setting of high-velocity trauma. Thus, there is a high incidence of polytrauma in patients with hip dislocations, and concomitant acetabular fractures are described in 70% of cases [21]. The vast majority of hip dislocations occur posteriorly (Fig. 41.4), while only 10% or less occur anteriorly [21]. Motor vehicle accidents account for nearly

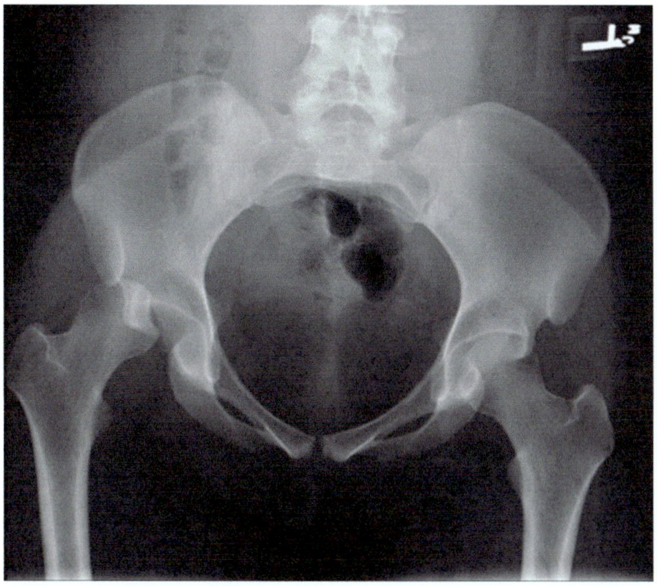

Fig. 41.4 AP radiograph reveals posterior dislocation of the right femoral head and likely intra-articular fracture fragment, possibly arising from the posterior acetabulum

all posterior hip dislocations, but a small percentage occur as a result of sport-related injuries or falls from height [21]. In the NFL, dislocations or subluxations account for just over 1% of hip injuries but result in the greatest time lost from sport at 126 days [19].

The mechanism of injury for posterior hip dislocations is most commonly a posteriorly directed axial load through a flexed, adducted, and internally rotated hip, often with a flexed knee, as is the case in a classic dashboard injury or fall during a tackle [19, 21]. Significant complications are associated with hip dislocations, including osteonecrosis of the femoral head, post-traumatic osteoarthritis, sciatic nerve injury, and heterotopic ossification [21].

41.3.4 Clinical Presentation

Patients with hip dislocations typically present with hip region pain, deformity, and inability to bear weight after trauma. Presentation can be similar to that of hip fractures, which may be concomitant, and polytrauma is common as previously discussed. Emergency assessment with initiation of advanced trauma life support (ATLS) is indicated in some scenarios, but the focus of this chapter is on medically stable patients with isolated hip injury.

41.3.5 Physical Examination

Gait Patients with hip dislocation are not generally able to bear weight through the affected limb and may present in an outpatient setting using an assistive device.

Visual observation For posterior hip dislocations, the affected limb is shortened compared to the contralateral side with the hip classically flexed, adducted, internally rotated. For anterior dislocations, the hip is classically in an extended, abducted, and externally rotated position [21].

Palpation There may be a palpable femoral head in the buttock region or the femoral triangle region based on direction of dislocation. Palpation of other bony anatomy and vascular examination must be completed as discussed in the hip fracture section.

Range of motion (ROM) Hip ROM is typically limited by pain in all planes with dislocation.

Sensory testing Light touch should be tested in bilateral L1-S1 dermatomes with special attention to the sciatic and femoral nerve distributions given risk for injury or impingement with posterior and anterior hip dislocations, respectively.

Deep tendon reflexes The following lower extremity reflexes should be tested bilaterally as feasible based on patient positioning and pain: patellar tendon (L2-L4, L4 primary), hamstring tendon (L5), and Achilles tendon (S1).

Motor testing Manual muscle testing should be performed for L2-S1 myotomes, though often pain inhibition is present, especially when testing proximal muscle groups that cross the hip joint. Special attention should be paid to sciatic-innervated muscle groups as described above for hip fractures, as well as femoral-innervated muscle groups including knee extensors.

Joint testing Comprehensive musculoskeletal examination and screening of all joints including the spine are warranted to evaluate for possible associated traumatic injuries.

Special maneuvers Patients are often unable to tolerate exam maneuvers such as the log roll or straight leg raise in the case of hip dislocation.

41.3.6 Diagnostic Workup

X-ray Plain radiographs of the hips and pelvis should be obtained immediately for suspected hip dislocation and are diagnostic (Fig. 41.5). Typical views are the same as described for hip fractures as above.

MRI, CT Post-reduction, advanced imaging with CT and/or MRI may reveal concomitant injuries or assist with preoperative planning as previously described for hip fractures. Hip fractures associated with dislocation are most commonly

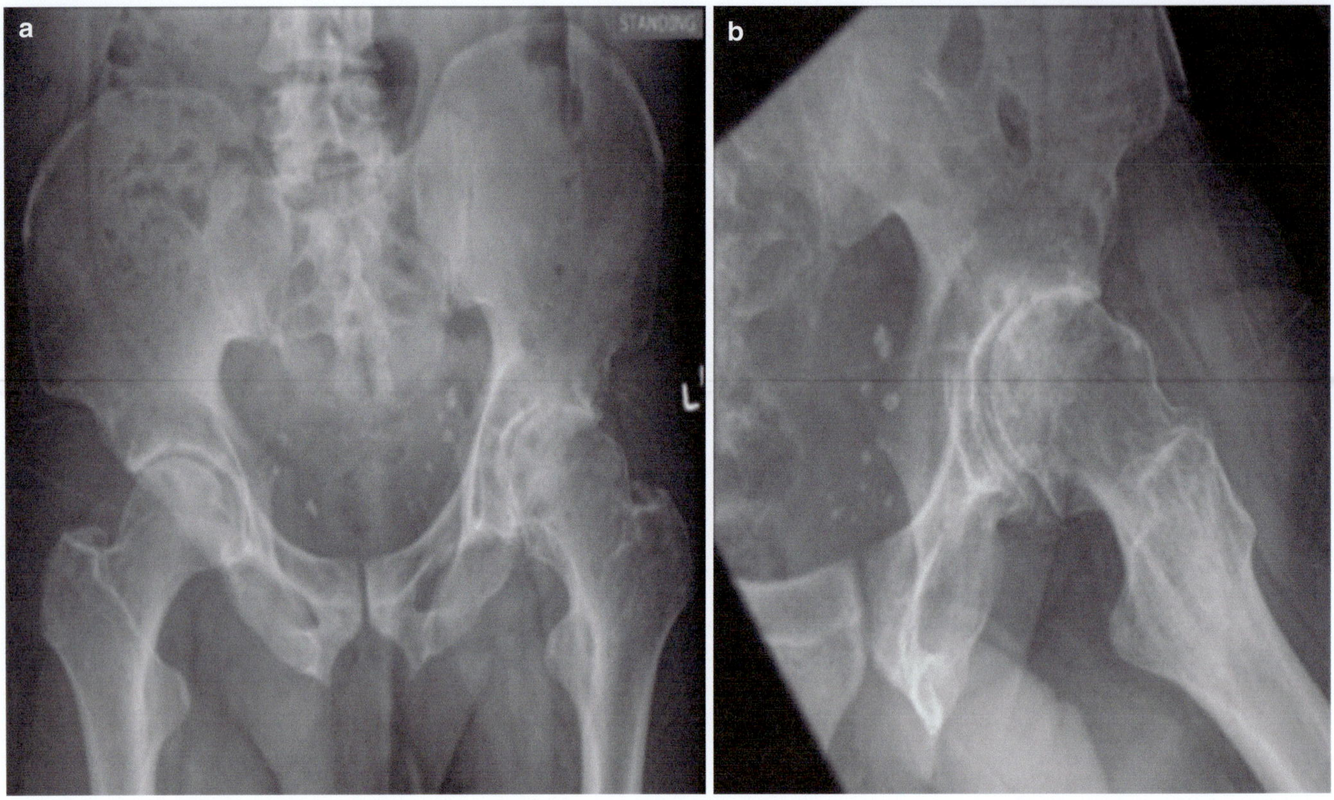

Fig. 41.5 Standing AP pelvis (**a**) and elongated femoral neck (**b**) radiographs demonstrating severe left hip osteoarthritis with associated severe joint space narrowing, osteophyte formation, subchondral sclerosis and cysts, and deformity of the femoral head

located at the superior femoral head or posterior acetabular lip. Associated capsular ligament injuries most commonly involve the femoral attachment of the iliofemoral ligament or the ischiofemoral ligament [11]. MRI should be considered 4–6 weeks post-dislocation to assess for early evidence of osteonecrosis with consideration of repeat MRI at 3 months for those with evidence of signal change in the marrow of the femoral head, earlier in the case of progressive pain [11, 22].

41.3.7 Treatment

41.3.7.1 Medical Management

In the case of suspected hip dislocation, the patient should remain non-weight-bearing until a definitive diagnosis is made. If the clinician is managing the patient in the field in the case of an injured athlete, the patient should be promptly transported to an emergency facility for expedited radiographic diagnosis, joint reduction with sedation, and post-reduction radiographs. Reduction within 6 hours decreases the risk for AVN [22]. If transport to an emergency facility could take longer than 6 hours or if the clinician is experienced, an attempt at immediate reduction can be made, keeping in mind the risk for further injury or pain especially in the setting of concomitant fracture. A variety of reduction techniques are described. Commonly for posterior dislocations, the clinician stands over the supine athlete, flexes the ipsilateral knee to 90°, and applies axial traction to the hip joint. An assistant is often needed to provide downward countertraction at the bilateral anterior iliac spines [22]. Multimodal pain management strategies should be utilized as previously described above. If closed reduction cannot be achieved, open surgical reduction may be necessary.

41.3.7.2 Rehabilitation

In the case of successful closed reduction, touch-down weight-bearing for a minimum of 4 weeks followed by progressive weight-bearing as tolerated is commonly recommended but may vary based on concomitant injuries. A physical therapy course focused on ROM, core and gluteal strengthening, and gait/mobility training should be initiated, followed by graduated return to activity/sport once full ROM and strength are achieved, along with no evidence of AVN on repeat imaging as discussed above [22].

41.3.7.3 Procedures

Procedures are generally not required for the treatment of hip dislocations, though ultrasound-guided femoral or fascia iliaca nerve blocks may be utilized to provide regional anesthesia to facilitate closed reduction techniques.

41.3.7.4 Surgery

Open reduction is indicated when closed reduction cannot be achieved. Additionally, operative management of associated injuries, including fractures or intra-articular loose bodies, may be required. Specific surgical considerations and postoperative management are discussed in detail in Chap. 42.

References

1. Warden SJ, Davis IS, Fredericson M. Management and prevention of bone stress injuries in long-distance runners. J Orthop Sports Phys Ther. 2014;44(10):749–65.
2. McInnis KC, Ramey LN. High-risk stress fractures: diagnosis and management. PM R. 2016;8(3 Suppl):S113–24.
3. Robertson GA, Wood AM. Femoral neck stress fractures in sport: a current concepts review. Sports Med Int Open. 2017;1(2):E58–68.
4. Williams TR, Puckett ML, Denison G, Shin AY, Gorman JD. Acetabular stress fractures in military endurance athletes and recruits: incidence and MRI and scintigraphic findings. Skeletal Radiol. 2002;31(5):277–81.
5. Datta HK, Ng WF, Walker JA, Tuck SP, Varanasi SS. The cell biology of bone metabolism. J Clin Pathol. 2008;61(5):577–87.
6. Mountjoy M, Sundgot-Borgen J, Burke L, Ackerman KE, Blauwet C, Constantini N, et al. International Olympic Committee (IOC) consensus statement on relative energy deficiency in sport (RED-S): 2018 update. Int J Sport Nutr Exerc Metab. 2018;28(4):316–31.
7. Tenforde AS, Parziale AL, Popp KL, Ackerman KE. Low bone mineral density in male athletes is associated with bone stress injuries at anatomic sites with greater trabecular composition. Am J Sports Med. 2018;46(1):30–6.
8. Inman VT. Functional aspects of the abductor muscles of the hip. J Bone Joint Surg Am. 1947;29(3):607–19.
9. Nguyen JT, Peterson JS, Biswal S, Beaulieu CF, Fredericson M. Stress-related injuries around the lesser trochanter in long-distance runners. AJR Am J Roentgenol. 2008;190(6):1616–20.
10. Goldin M, Anderson CN, Fredericson M, Safran MR, Stevens KJ. Femoral neck stress fractures and imaging features of femoroacetabular impingement. PM R. 2015;7(6):584–92.
11. Hegazi TM, Belair JA, McCarthy EJ, Roedl JB, Morrison WB. Sports injuries about the hip: what the radiologist should know. Radiographics. 2016;36(6):1717–45.
12. Nattiv A, Loucks AB, Manore MM, Sanborn CF, Sundgot-Borgen J, Warren MP, et al. American College of Sports Medicine position stand. The female athlete triad. Med Sci Sports Exerc. 2007;39(10):1867–82.
13. McCabe MP, Smyth MP, Richardson DR. Current concept review: vitamin D and stress fractures. Foot Ankle Int. 2012;33(6):526–33.
14. Williams K, Askew C, Mazoue C, Guy J, Torres-McGehee TM, Jackson JB III. Vitamin D3 supplementation and stress fractures in high-risk collegiate athletes - a pilot study. Orthop Res Rev. 2020;12:9–17.
15. Ramey LN, McInnis KC, Palmer WE. Femoral neck stress fracture: can MRI grade help predict return-to-running time? Am J Sports Med. 2016;44(8):2122–9.
16. Miller TL, Kaeding CC, Rodeo SA. Emerging options for biologic enhancement of stress fracture healing in athletes. J Am Acad Orthop Surg. 2020;28(1):1–9.
17. Zhao W, Gao Y, Zhang S, Liu Z, He L, Zhang D, et al. Extracorporeal shock wave therapy for bone marrow edema syndrome in patients with osteonecrosis of the femoral head: a retrospective cohort study. J Orthop Surg Res. 2021;16(1):21.
18. Rapp K, Buchele G, Dreinhofer K, Bucking B, Becker C, Benzinger P. Epidemiology of hip fractures : systematic literature review of German data and an overview of the international literature. Z Gerontol Geriatr. 2019;52(1):10–6.
19. Feeley BT, Powell JW, Muller MS, Barnes RP, Warren RF, Kelly BT. Hip injuries and labral tears in the national football league. Am J Sports Med. 2008;36(11):2187–95.
20. LeBlanc KE, Muncie HL Jr, LeBlanc LL. Hip fracture: diagnosis, treatment, and secondary prevention. Am Fam Physician. 2014;89(12):945–51.
21. Clegg TE, Roberts CS, Greene JW, Prather BA. Hip dislocations--epidemiology, treatment, and outcomes. Injury. 2010;41(4):329–34.
22. Skelley NW, McCormick JJ, Smith MV. In-game management of common joint dislocations. Sports Health. 2014;6(3):246–55.

Hip Surgeries

42

John Stelmach, Jomar Aryee, Chandler Berke, Steven Mennona, and Alfred J. Tria Jr

42.1 Femoroacetabular Impingement

Femoroacetabular impingement (FAI) is defined as an abnormal interface between the proximal femur and the acetabulum causing pain and articular degeneration [1]. FAI causing pain and activity limitation that is refractory to NSAIDs, injections, and physical therapy may be treated with surgery.

42.1.1 Operation

Options for treatment include arthroscopic debridement, osteoplasty, and in some cases labral repair. Arthroscopy allows the abnormal joint lesions, most commonly referred to as cam and pincer lesions, to be visualized. An osteoplasty is performed with a high-speed burr to remove the bone and recontour an optimal articular interface. In addition to bone resurfacing, labral tears are often present. Any damaged labral tissue may either be removed or be repaired depending on its viability. If the tissue is removed, the patient can generally bear weight as tolerated soon after the procedure. If it is repaired, the patient should be kept toe-touch weight-bearing for 4–6 weeks to allow for biological healing. Hip arthroscopy with osteoplasty has surpassed open hip dislocation and osteoplasty as the gold standard for the management of FAI [2].

42.1.2 Rehabilitation

At present, no universally agreed-upon protocol exists for post arthroscopic FAI rehabilitation, but there are some common principles across various protocols. Patients who undergo arthroscopic osteoplasty require a period of protected weight-bearing, up to six weeks, and are encouraged to perform early passive range of motion (PROM) exercises to limit stiffness [3]. As weight-bearing and range of motion advances, muscular strengthening is added to the rehabilitation protocol. Rehab progresses from submaximal isometric hip, thigh, and abdominal muscle exercises to resisted and eccentric exercises with a focus on the gluteal muscles (particularly gluteus medius) [4].

42.2 Hip Labral Tears

42.2.1 Operation

Surgery is indicated to repair labral tears when conservative measures do not control the patient's symptoms or when functional limitations are unsatisfactory. While the most common cause of labral tears is FAI, they may also be traumatic in etiology (i.e., hip dislocation, acetabulum fracture). If tears are not repairable, the labrum is removed with full weight-bearing as tolerated afterward. Labral tears are most commonly repaired through the use of arthroscopy with the use of bio-absorbable or permanent anchors. In some cases, articular cartilage damage is also present along with the labral tear. These are classified as chondral defects and are treated with microfracture. Multiple small holes are made in the defect to incite an inflammatory and healing response. Fibrocartilage ideally fills the defect and re-establishes the articular surface [5]. After microfracture, non-weight-bearing or toe-touch ambulation is necessary for at least 3–6 weeks to allow for the initial stages of fibrocartilage formation.

J. Stelmach · J. Aryee · C. Berke · S. Mennona
Department of Orthopaedics, Rutgers-Robert Wood Johnson Medical School, New Brunswick, NJ, USA
e-mail: cmi40@rwjms.rutgers.edu

A. J. Tria Jr (✉)
Department of Orthopaedics, Rutgers-Robert Wood Johnson Medical School, New Brunswick, NJ, USA

© The Author(s), under exclusive license to Springer Nature Switzerland AG 2022
S. A. Mostoufi et al. (eds.), *Clinical Guide to Musculoskeletal Medicine*, https://doi.org/10.1007/978-3-030-92042-5_42

42.2.2 Rehabilitation

Rehabilitation protocols following acetabular debridement or repair focus on progressive range of motion (ROM) and soft tissue flexibility with strengthening in the later phases. Most of the acetabular defects are located anterior or anterosuperiorly, thus limiting movements that stress this area. Initially, weight-bearing is limited to 50% for 7–10 days progressing to weight-bearing as tolerated for debridement. Labral repair patients are limited to toe-touch weight-bearing for 3–6 weeks. If the surgery involves additional procedures, such as microfracture, the weight-bearing restrictions can increase to 6 weeks. Early ROM is encouraged avoiding flexion and internal rotation of the hip to limit strain on the labral repair [6].

42.3 Hip Dysplasia

42.3.1 Operation

Adult dysplasia of the hip refers to an abnormal anatomical relationship of the acetabulum and the femoral head, most commonly resulting in a shallow acetabulum with decreased coverage. Treatment for this condition varies depending on severity of the deformity, patient age, and degree of joint damage or arthritis resulting from the deformity. Young patients may undergo pelvic osteotomy to rotate the acetabulum and increase femoral head coverage.

42.3.2 Rehabilitation

After surgery, protected weight-bearing is necessary for 6–8 weeks. Older patients with advanced arthritis typically undergo total hip arthroplasty (THA) with immediate postoperative weight-bearing.

42.4 Hip Osteoarthritis

The most common surgical treatment for persistent osteoarthritic pain is THA. Pelvic osteotomy and hip resurfacing may be performed in the early stages of disease for temporary relief. Younger patients and those who wish to preserve their native hip may look to these procedures for relief. Outcomes are enhanced when the procedure is performed soon after a failed course of conservative therapy [7].

42.4.1 Total Hip Arthroplasty

THA includes femoral head resection and acetabular reaming. The components can be a combination of metal, plastic, or ceramic and are fixated with or without cement. The common surgical approaches to THA include the posterior, direct anterior, direct lateral, and anterolateral [8]. The main goal of elective arthroplasty is early ambulation combined with adequate analgesia to allow the patient to be safely and rapidly discharged and minimize thromboembolic events. Weight-bearing after THA is supported for both cemented and cementless fixations [8]. All approaches have unique characteristics but should allow the patient to bear weight as tolerated immediately after surgery unless there is an adverse intra-operative event reported by the surgeon.

- *The posterior approach*: It has been the most approach and is associated with some increased risk of posterior dislocation and sciatic nerve palsy. Rehabilitation should avoid hip flexion and internal rotation for that reason. Stair climbing should be carefully monitored and sitting in a deep-seated chair should be avoided. The anterior approach has a higher risk of intraoperative femoral shaft fracture and anterior thigh numbness. Hip extension and external rotation may provoke an anterior dislocation; however, this is very rare.
- *Anterior approach*: The anterior approach to the hip is a safe, muscle-sparing, and fully extensible approach offering potentially great short- and medium-term advantages in total hip arthroplasty patient. Complications may include lateral femoral cutaneous nerve injury, and femoral fractures are more common in this approach as compared to posterior approach. The anterior approach operative time is longer but has a shorter time to discharge and a greater percentage of home discharge [9].
- *The lateral and anterolateral approaches*: It has a very low dislocation rate but carries a risk of abductor weakness. Physical therapy is started immediately after surgery for all approaches and continues for 4–6 weeks.

42.4.2 Pelvic Osteotomy

Pelvic osteotomy, or peri-acetabular osteotomy (PAO), includes multiple bone cuts around the acetabulum so that the articular surface can be rotated around the femoral head to change the contour and the coverage. Peri-acetabular osteotomy is indicated for the treatment of residual hip dysplasia to improve joint mechanics and can be classified as either reconstructive or salvage procedures. In some cases, the posterior column of the pelvis is preserved, and the patient may be weight-bearing as tolerated after surgery. If the posterior column is osteotomized during surgery, the patient will be toe-touch weight-bearing for a period of 6–8 weeks. The risk of dislocation after pelvic osteotomy is low and rarely requires precautions. Pelvic osteotomies are indicated for the pre-arthritic or mildly arthritic acetabulum or femoral head, whereas salvage procedures (including THA) are indicated for patients with established osteoarthritis and/or an incongruent hip joint that is less amenable to reorientation of the acetabulum [10].

42.4.3 Hip Resurfacing

Hip resurfacing is an alternative to THA and includes the young, active male with a sufficiently large femoral head size [11]. The femoral neck and some bone stock in the femoral head are preserved, while the outer cortex of the femoral head and the acetabulum are resurfaced. A metal-on-metal interface replaces the articular surface and weight-bearing as tolerated is allowed right after the procedure. Although rare, stress fractures of the femoral neck have been encountered within a year of surgery. Unexplained onset of pain with ambulation should bring this to mind.

42.5 Hip Dislocation

Ninety percent of all hip dislocations are posterior; however, they can occur in all four directions (anterior, posterior, superior, and inferior). The initial treatment is emergent closed reduction to decrease the rate of avascular necrosis of the femoral head [12]. Examination under anesthesia is sometimes performed after reduction to assess the stability of the hip joint. X-rays and CT scans should confirm concentric reduction without evidence of fracture or any intra-articular loose body.[19] In the stable simple dislocation, toe-touch weight-bearing is recommended for the first four weeks followed by progressive weight-bearing as tolerated [13].

Complex dislocations involving fracture of either the femoral head or the acetabulum are initially closed reduced pending the definitive surgical intervention. While waiting for the appropriate medical clearances, the reduction may require traction. The femoral head fractures require either open reduction and internal fixation (ORIF) or arthroplasty depending upon the configuration. After an ORIF, ROM can be started immediately with non-weight-bearing ambulation for 6–8 weeks until there is proper evidence of healing.[21] The acetabular fractures are reviewed in the next section.

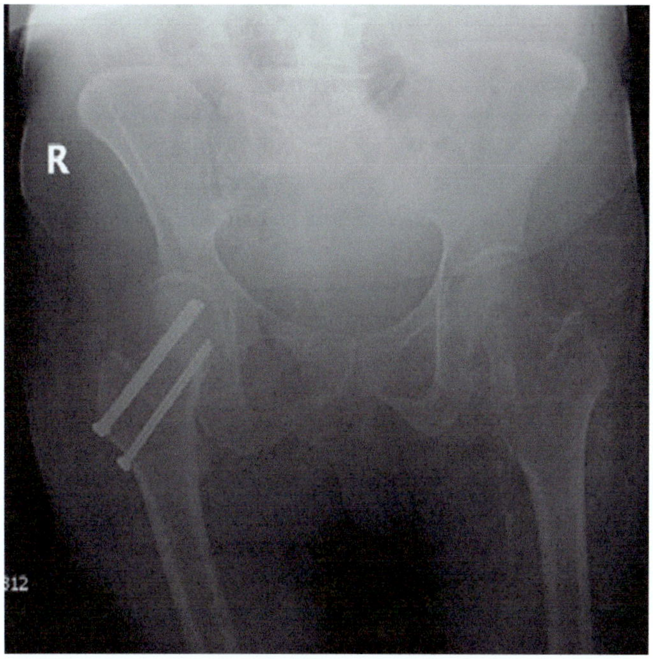

Fig. 42.1 Internal fixation of femoral neck fracture with cannulated screws. (Synthes 7.3 mm Cannulated Screws, Johnson and Johnson Medical Devices, West Chester, PA)

42.6 Hip Fractures

42.6.1 Femoral Neck Fracture

Operative management of proximal femoral fractures is based on patient activity level, anatomic location, and fracture displacement. The goal of fixation of all hip fractures is expedited weight-bearing as tolerated and ambulation. Anatomic reduction and internal fixation of femoral neck fractures are paramount in the younger patients to preserve the viability of the native hip. In the elderly, nondisplaced fractures of the neck of the femur may be treated with percutaneous internal fixation (Fig. 42.1), whereas displaced fractures require arthroplasty. The arthroplasty may replace the femoral head alone (hemiarthroplasty) or both the head and the acetabulum (THA) depending upon the degree of arthritic disease that is present. Severely displaced fractures of the femoral neck may require arthroplasty even in young patients if the viability of the femoral head is poor.

42.6.2 Intertrochanteric and Subtrochanteric Fracture

Injury at the intertrochanteric level or below in all age groups and activity levels is managed with percutaneous screw fixation, intramedullary nails (Fig. 42.2), or plate and screw fixa-

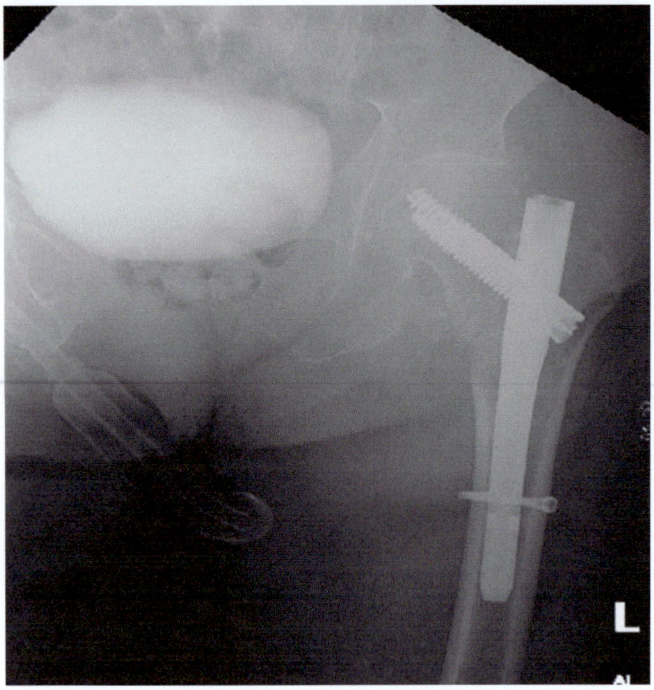

Fig. 42.2 Open reduction and internal fixation of intertrochanteric hip fracture with cephalomedullary nail. (Smith and Nephew Intertan™. Smith and Nephew, Memphis Tennessee.)

tion (Fig. 42.3) [14]. Immediate full weight-bearing is started if the construct is surgically stable. The rehabilitation of elderly hip fracture patients is highly challenging and extremely important to short- and long-term function of these individuals.

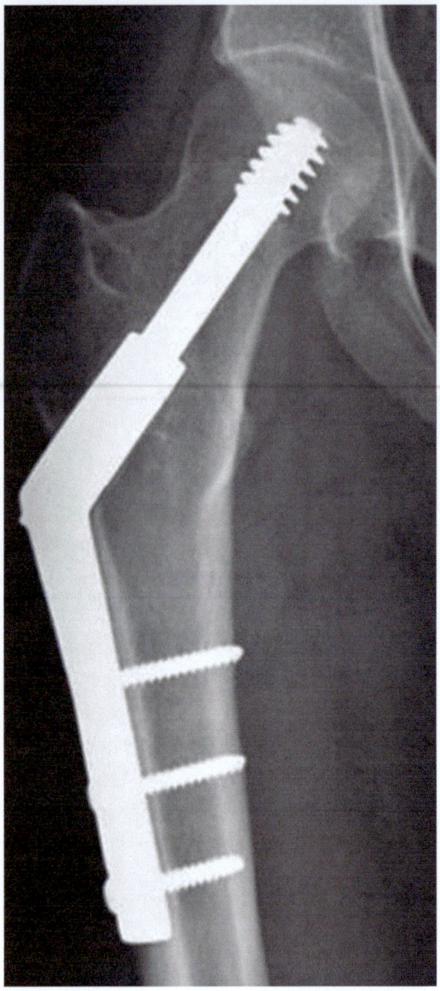

Fig. 42.3 Screw and side plate fixation for an intertrochanteric fracture. (Smith and Nephew, Compression Hip Screw™, Memphis, Tennessee.)

42.6.3 Acetabular Fracture

The majority of the weight-bearing surface of the acetabulum is located in the superolateral and posterior aspect of the dome. Fractures of the articular surface occur as a result of both high-energy mechanisms in young individuals and low-energy falls in osteoporotic patients. Goals of both operative and non-operative treatment include restoration of the articular surface, early ROM, and weight-bearing once bony healing has occurred. Acetabular fractures may be treated conservatively if the articular surface is well aligned and stable for weight-bearing ambulation. If an ORIF is required (Fig. 42.4), partial weight-bearing is necessary for the first 3 months [15]. Early ROM and core strengthening exercises can be started immediately after either approach.

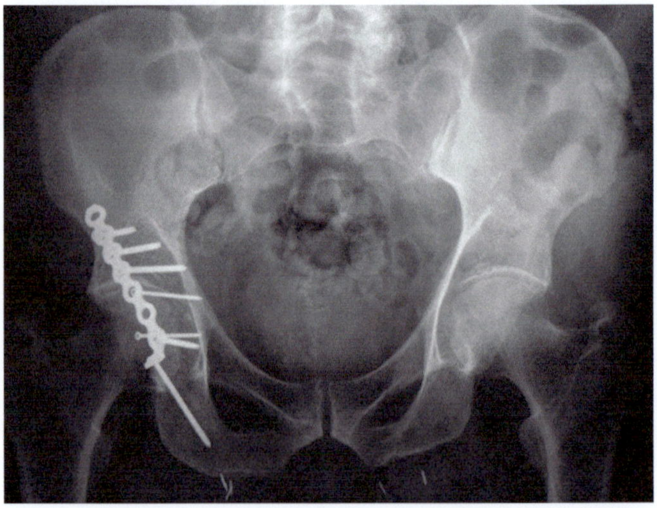

Fig. 42.4 Open reduction and internal fixation of a posterior wall acetabulum fracture via posterior approach. (Synthes 3.5 mm reconstruction pelvic plates, Johnson and Johnson Medical Devices, West Chester, PA.)

References

1. Jakobsen SS, Overgaard S, Søballe K, Ovesen O, Mygind-Klavsen B, Dippmann CA, Jensen MU, Stürup J, Retpen J. The interface between periacetabular osteotomy, hip arthroscopy and total hip arthroplasty in the young adult hip. EFORT Open Rev. 2018;3(7):408–17. https://doi.org/10.1302/2058-5241.3.170042. PMID: 30233816; PMCID: PMC6129960.
2. Bolarinwa SA, Aryee JN, Labaran LA, Werner BC, Browne JA. Does arthroscopic repair of femoroacetabular impingement pathology affect clinical outcomes after ipsilateral total hip arthroplasty? Hip Pelvis. 2020;32(1):35. https://doi.org/10.5371/hp.2020.32.1.35.
3. Grzybowski JS, Malloy P, Stegemann C, Bush-Joseph C, Harris JD, Nho SJ. Rehabilitation following hip arthroscopy – a systematic review. Front Surg. 2015;2. https://doi.org/10.3389/fsurg.2015.00021.
4. Enseki KR, Kohlrieser D. Rehabilitation following hip arthroscopy: an evolving process. Int J Sports Phys Ther. 2014;9(6):765–73. http://www.ncbi.nlm.nih.gov/pubmed/25383245. Accessed 6 Mar 2021.
5. McCarthy J, Noble P, Aluisio F V., Schuck M, Wright J, Lee J Ann. Anatomy, pathologic features, and treatment of acetabular labral tears. In: Clinical orthopaedics and related research. Lippincott Williams and Wilkins; 2003:38–47. https://doi.org/10.1097/00003086-200301000-00008.
6. Domb BG, Hartigan DE, Perets I. Decision making for labral treatment in the hip. J Am Acad Orthop Surg. 2017;25(3):e53–62. https://doi.org/10.5435/JAAOS-D-16-00144.
7. Murphy NJ, Eyles JP, Hunter DJ. Hip osteoarthritis: etiopathogenesis and implications for management. Adv Ther. 2016;33(11):1921–46. https://doi.org/10.1007/s12325-016-0409-3.
8. Kishida Y, Sugano N, Sakai T, et al. Full weight-bearing after cementless total hip arthroplasty. Int Orthop. 2001;25(1):25–8. https://doi.org/10.1007/s002640000221.
9. Galakatos GR. Direct anterior total hip arthroplasty. Mo Med. 2018;115(6):537–41.
10. Clohisy JC, Barrett SE, Gordon JE, Delgado ED, Schoenecker PL. Periacetabular osteotomy for the treatment of severe acetabular dysplasia. J Bone Jt Surg Ser A. 2005;87(2):254–9. https://doi.org/10.2106/JBJS.D.02093.
11. Lespasio MJ, Sultan AA, Piuzzi NS, et al. Hip osteoarthritis: a primer. Perm J. 2018;22. https://doi.org/10.7812/TPP/17-084.
12. Hougaard K, Thomsen PB. Traumatic posterior dislocation of the hip —prognostic factors influencing the incidence of avascular necrosis of the femoral head. Arch Orthop Trauma Surg. 1986;106:32–5. https://doi.org/10.1007/BF00435649.
13. Clegg TE, Roberts CS, Greene JW, Prather BA. Hip dislocations-epidemiology, treatment, and outcomes. Injury. 2010;41(4):329–34. https://doi.org/10.1016/j.injury.2009.08.007.
14. Peng SH, Wu CC, Yu YH, Lee PC, Chou YC, Yeh WL. Surgical treatment of femoral head fractures. Biom J. 2020;43(5):451–7. https://doi.org/10.1016/j.bj.2019.08.004.
15. Yu JK, Chiu FY, Feng CK, Chung TY, Chen TH. Surgical treatment of displaced fractures of posterior column and posterior wall of the acetabulum. Injury. 2004;35(8):766–70. https://doi.org/10.1016/j.injury.2003.09.036.

Part VIII

Knee

Section Editor
Timothy Tiu

43 Knee Disorder: Intra-Articular

Jennifer Soo Hoo, Gerard D'Onofrio, and Gisela Figueroa

43.1 ACL and PCL Injuries

43.1.1 Synonyms

- ACL tear
- ACL sprain
- PCL tear
- PCL sprain

43.1.2 ICD-10 Codes

S83.51–S83.52

43.1.3 Description

Injury to the anterior cruciate ligament (ACL) is one of the most common knee ligament injuries in sports. Injury to this ligament can span from sprain, partial tear, to complete rupture. In contrast, isolated injury to the posterior cruciate ligament (PCL) is uncommon and can be easily missed on physical examination.

Anatomy

- *ACL*: The ACL is a collagenous structure and spans from the medial wall of the lateral femoral condyle and crosses anteromedially to attach on the anterior aspect of the tibial articular surface. Its primary function is to act as a static stabilizer of the knee by resisting hyper extension, anterior tibial translation, and knee rotatory movements. It consists of two bundles: the anteromedial (AM) and posterolateral (PL), each identified by their relative insertion on the tibia. The anteromedial bundle tightens in flexion and the posterolateral bundle tightens in full extension. It has been shown that forces on the ACL are the greatest when knee is flexed about 30°. The main blood supply of the ACL is provided by a branch of the popliteal artery, middle genicular artery. Innervation comes from the branches of the tibial nerve including posterior articular nerve, which help aid in knee proprioception.
- *PCL*: The PCL is the other major intra-articular ligament of the knee. It spans from the anterolateral aspect of the medial femoral condyle and inserts on a depression on the posterior aspect of tibial plateau. The PCL is also composed of two bundles, the larger anterolateral bundle (ALB) and the smaller posteromedial bundle (PMB), which are best identified at their femoral locations. The PCL's primary function is to act as a stabilizer to posterior tibial translation in addition to secondary restraint to rotation, particularly between 90° and 120° of flexion. The PCL bears the most tension at 90° of flexion. The PCL shares neurovascular supply with ACL. Of note, the meniscofemoral ligaments (MFLs) are also associated with the bundles of the PCL in the majority of the population [1].

43.1.4 Clinical Presentation

ACL Injury

The classic presentation of an ACL injury is from a non-contact mechanism (70–80% cases) such as landing from a jump while cutting or a sudden deceleration in sports such as football, soccer, basketball, or alpine skiing. One such mechanism includes landing with an extended hip and knee, the knee in valgus, internal rotation of the tibia, and a pronated foot. In contact or traumatic injuries to the ACL, injuries are frequently associated with forceful valgus stress and usually

J. S. Hoo (✉)
Department of Rehabilitation Medicine, Weill Cornell Medicine, New York, NY, USA

New York Presbyterian, New York, NY, USA
e-mail: jes9343@med.cornell.edu

G. D'Onofrio · G. Figueroa
Department of Rehabilitation Medicine, New York Presbyterian, New York, NY, USA

© The Author(s), under exclusive license to Springer Nature Switzerland AG 2022

S. A. Mostoufi et al. (eds.), *Clinical Guide to Musculoskeletal Medicine*, https://doi.org/10.1007/978-3-030-92042-5_43

Table 43.1 Risk factors for ACL injury

Modifiable intrinsic	Modifiable extrinsic	Non-modifiable intrinsic
Body mass index	Equipment (footwear)	Gender (female)
Biomechanical & neuromuscular weakness	Playing surface (artificial turf)	Prior ACL injury
Pre-ovulatory phase of menstrual cycle in females not using oral contraceptives	Weather condition (dry condition)	Ligamentous laxity
Fatigue/conditioning	Type of sport	Tibial geometry
Decreased relative hamstring to quadriceps strength		Small and narrow intercondylar notch width
Decreased core strength and proprioception		Genetics

involve injury to other structures of the knee [2]. There has been a lot of research looking at the risk factors associated with ACL injury and the risk of injury is likely multifactorial in nature (see Table 43.1) [3, 4]. Patients often report immediate pain and instability after landing or cutting. It is often quite common for patients to report a “pop” and immediate swelling/hemarthrosis. It is also common to see a concomitant MCL and lateral meniscus injury as well. Athletes are typically not able to return to play after injury and have immediate difficulty weight-bearing.

PCL Injury

The classic presentation of PCL injury is either a posteriorly directed force to the anterior proximal tibia or knee hyperflexion with plantar flexion of the foot. Examples include the commonly seen “dashboard injury” in motor vehicle accidents where the proximal tibia hits the dashboard and is pushed posteriorly or sports injury where the athlete falls directly on their knee with their foot in plantar flexion. In other scenarios with hyperextension/hyperflexion or rotational injuries with varus/valgus stress, the PCL can be injured along with other structures of the knee. In contrast to ACL injuries, most patients do not report having felt or heard a “pop.” It’s also helpful to determine if the tear is acute or chronic as that will help management. As isolated PCL injuries are rare, it is important to determine if the PCL injury is part of a multi-ligament injury. Multi-ligament injuries usually have more swelling and instability [5].

43.1.5 Physical Examination

ACL Injury

A thorough history and physical exam are important when evaluating for a possible ACL injury. In acute presentation, a large effusion is commonly seen. Range of motion testing is often limited due to pain and guarding. Most common special tests used to evaluate include Lachman test, pivot shift test, and anterior drawer test.

*Lachman Test*This test has the highest sensitivity and specificity for diagnosing ACL injury. The patient lays supine with the quadriceps relaxed and the knee placed in 30° flexion. The examiner stabilizes the femur/thigh with one hand and grasps patient’s posterior aspect of proximal tibia and applies an anteriorly directed force. Increased anterior tibial translation with a soft endpoint compared to contralateral side indicates ACL injury [6, 7].

*Anterior Drawer Test*This test is not as sensitive or specific as the Lachman test but can help evaluate chronic ACL injury. The patient is supine with the hip flexed to about 45°, the knee flexed to about 90°, and the lower leg in neutral position with the foot resting on the table. The examiner stabilizes the patient’s foot with their thigh and places both hands behind the proximal tibia with the thumbs on the tibial plateau. The examiner then applies an anteriorly directed force to the proximal tibia and evaluates the amount of tibial translation. The amount of tibial translation on the injured side compared to the uninjured contralateral knee is compared, and increased anterior tibial displacement in side-to-side comparison is indicative of ACL injury [6, 7].

*Pivot Shift Test*This test can help identify rotational instability. This test is performed with the patient in supine position. The examiner grasps the heel of the involved extremity and internally rotates the knee and flexes the knee from full extension while using the other hand to apply valgus stress on the lateral side of proximal tibia. A positive test occurs when there is a sudden reduction in the anteriorly subluxed lateral tibial plateau beneath the lateral femoral condyle at about 30–40 degrees of flexion. This test has low sensitivity and is hard to perform in acute settings due to patient guarding [6, 7].

PCL Injury

A thorough history and physical exam are also important when evaluating for possible PCL injury. A complete neurovascular exam should also be completed. Physical exam may be difficult because of pain and swelling. On an acute exam, there may be swelling of the knee especially if it is part of multi-ligamentous injury. Bruising can point to a mechanism of injury (i.e., if there is bruising on tibial tuberosity from car accident). It is also important to evaluate for posterolateral corner (PLC) injury, which is commonly missed (see extraarticular knee disorders). Sometimes, a hematoma can be seen in the posterior knee from PCL tear. Range of motion testing can be restricted in acute settings due to pain and swelling. Most common special tests used to evaluate include posterior drawer test, posterior sag test, and quadriceps active test.

*Posterior Drawer test*This is the most accurate test to assess PCL integrity. This test is performed in the same position as the anterior drawer test with the patient laying supine and knee flexed to 90 degrees, with the examiner stabilizing the foot on table. The examiner is applying posteriorly directed force on the proximal tibia and evaluating the amount of tibial translation compared to the contralateral side and if a characteristic endpoint is seen. Of note, it is important to place the tibia in an anatomical neutral position before testing (normally the tibial plateau should be more than 1 cm anterior to the medial femoral condyle). The grading system is as follows: grade 1 (0–5 mm increased posterior tibial translation), grade 2 (6–10 mm increase translation), and grade 3 (more than 10 mm translation) [5, 8].

*Posterior Sag Test*The test is performed with the patient laying in supine with the examiner maintaining the hip and knee in 90° of flexion as the examiner holds the ankle/heel. This test is considered positive if the tibia sags down/posteriorly on the femur [5].

*Quadriceps Active Test*The test is performed with the examiner holding the knee in 90 degrees of flexion and stabilizing the foot. The patient is asked to contract their quadriceps muscle, and if it results in anterior translation of the tibia, this indicates PCL injury [5].

*Dial Test*This test can help diagnose combined PCL and PLC injuries. The test is performed with the patient positioned prone. The examiner then provides an external rotation force to both feet with the knees at 30° and then 90° of flexion. A side-to-side comparison difference of 10 ° or more is considered abnormal. Increased external rotation at 30° of knee flexion only indicates an isolated PLC injury, while increased external rotation at both 30° and 90° of knee flexion suggests a combined PCL and PLC injury [8].

43.1.6 Diagnostic Workup

ACL Injury

X-ray: In any acute injury, an anteroposterior (AP) and lateral X-ray is indicated to rule out any fracture or associated injuries. Two common X-ray findings that are commonly found in ACL injuries include tibial eminence fracture and Segond fracture, an avulsion fracture of the lateral capsule from the tibial plateau. In most cases, X-rays are normal aside from showing large effusion [2].

Magnetic resonance imaging (MRI): It is the gold standard for diagnosing ACL injury and any other concomitant ligamentous or meniscal injury that may be present. Adding oblique coronal and sagittal views that allow full-length views of ACL in one frame has helped increase accuracy of finding ACL injury on MRI. In most cases, there is characteristic bone bruise on the central lateral femoral condyle and posterior lateral tibial plateau [2].

PCL Injury

X-ray: Similar to ACL injuries, any acute knee injury should be evaluated with standard AP and lateral X-ray. They can be evaluated for posterior tibial subluxation and any fractures. A reverse-type second fracture, which is a cortical avulsion fracture off the medial tibial plateau, can also be seen with PCL tears. Stress views (anteroposterior and varus/valgus) can also be done to assess PCL and posterolateral corner laxity [5].

MRI: It is the gold standard for diagnosing PCL injuries. The PCL is best visualized in the sagittal plane but can also be seen on coronal and transverse views. In the case of isolated PCL tear, one study showed 69% occur in midsubstance and 27% occur proximally. A concomitant bone bruise is typically seen on anterior tibia [5].

43.1.7 Treatments

Medical Management

First-line treatment includes resting, icing, and elevating the leg to get the swelling to decrease. If tolerated, taking short-term anti-inflammatory medication (NSAIDs) can help decrease pain and swelling. Some patients may need crutches for the first 1–2 weeks or a brace to help stabilize the knee. For isolated PCL grade 1 or 2 injuries, protected weight-bearing in a knee extension brace is followed by rehabilitation.

Rehabilitation

- *ACL Injury Rehab*

  Whether conservative treatment is indicated depends on the extent of injury (partial or full tear) and what level of activity that patients would like to return to. Those with partial ACL tears can be managed conservatively. For those with complete ACL rupture, the current best available evidence does not indicate that an individual is at a greater risk of subsequent injury if they are managed with rehabilitation vs. ACL repair. Clinicians should suggest a period of rehabilitation before surgical decision-making for most patients with ACL rupture. There are many studies that found that pre-operative rehabilitation improves post-surgical outcomes in those who go on to have an ACL repair. Those who have functional instability after rehabilitation are likely to benefit from ACL repair [9].

  Physical therapy plays a key role in the rehabilitation of ACL injuries. In cases where surgery is being delayed or being managed nonoperatively, patients undergo exercise therapy programs or pre-habilitation, which has been found to improve knee function early post injury and 2 years after ACL reconstruction [10, 11]. The goals of nonoperative rehabilitation include decreased strain on ACL, decreased pain, edema management, improving range of motion and flexibility, increasing strength, improving balance and neuromuscular control, and plyometric training [10]. Compression, elevation, and cryotherapy are used to decrease edema. Range of motion, especially knee extension, should be assessed due to increased risk for limited extension post ACL reconstruction [12]. Hamstring and gastrocnemius stretching can also improve knee extension range of motion. It is important to make note that weight-bearing exercises produce smaller loads on the ACL compared to non-weight-bearing exercises and the ACL is loaded less at higher knee ranges of motion such as 50°–100° [13]. Quadriceps strength needs to be assessed and carefully progressed in open and closed chain environment. A deficiency in quadriceps strength of >20% has a significantly negative result on self-reported outcome 2 years post ACL reconstruction [10]. Neuromuscular electrical stimulation can be used to increase quadriceps strength along with exercise [14]. Neuromuscular control training including stability, perturbations, and proprioception must also be incorporated due to impairments in joint position sense post injury [10, 15]. Neuromuscular re-education can significantly decrease instability and improve knee function [16, 17]. Gait training is also incorporated due to compensatory patterns established due to pain and instability. Functional knee bracing may be useful in cases where there is ACL deficiency [18].

Clinical practice guidelines help guide the rehabilitation post ACL reconstruction. Guidelines such as those published by the American Physical Therapy Association (APTA), Royal Dutch Society for Physical Therapy (KNGF), and Multicenter Orthopaedic Outcomes Network (MOON) have been recommended [19]. Although these guidelines vary, there is agreement in immediate knee mobilization, early full weight-bearing, early open and closed chain exercises, strength and neuromuscular training, cryotherapy, and neuromuscular electrical stimulation. As range of motion and strengthening are progressed, the ACL must be protected during the healing process. The selection of exercises that limit strain on the ACL is important and should be based on the understanding that the ACL is under less physical load in the 50°–100° range of motion [13]. Continuous passive motion and functional bracing are not recommended [19].

- *PCL Injury Rehab*

  Non-surgical treatment is advised for patients with isolated grade 1 or 2 PCL injuries or those with grade 3 injuries but have mild symptoms and only participating in low-demand activities [8].
- PCL injuries treated either nonoperatively or operatively require physical therapy intervention. There are no set guidelines for treatment of nonoperative PCL injuries. However, the initial goal of treatment is protecting the healing ligament and reestablishing normal tibiofemoral positioning through initial immobilization subsequently by dynamic/functional bracing [20, 21]. Edema can be controlled by ice, compression, and elevation. Range of motion limitations are initially restricted to avoid sheering forces and additional strain on the PCL. Knee range of motion should be performed in prone position during the first few weeks to limit hamstring activation and posterior tibial sag [13, 21]. Loading of the PCL occurs less at lower knee ranges of motion. Open kinetic chain range of motion should initially be limited from 50° to 0° and closed kinetic chain range of motion should be limited from 0° to 50° [13]. Manual technique such as patellar mobilizations is incorporated to improve patellofemoral mobility [20]. Strengthening focuses on the quadriceps [13, 20, 21]. Neuromuscular electrical stimulation can be used to improve quadriceps strength. As quadriceps strengthening increases, neuromuscular training is integrated into the rehabilitation program to further improve knee stability and advance functional mobility over various surfaces at various speeds. Gait training is also required during the progression of weight-bearing as tolerated to full weight-bearing in order to normalize gait pattern without assistive device.

  There are no clinical practice guidelines for postoperative PCL rehabilitation. However, most protocols maintain the knee locked in extension in a long brace for 3–6 weeks along with weight-bearing precautions set by the surgeon to limit stress on the reconstructed PCL [21]. An assistive device such as axillary crutches may be initially required. Edema management is controlled by ice, compression, and elevation. There is disparity into how long isolated hamstring activation should be avoided to limit strain on the healing PCL from 6 weeks to 5 months [20]. Strength training focuses on the quadriceps [20, 21]. Neuromuscular electrical stimulation can be used to improve quadriceps strength. Neuromuscular reeducation is incorporated at approximately 6–8 weeks post-surgery [20].

Procedures

Arthrocentesis of hemarthrosis can be therapeutic and help immediate pain. There is also growing evidence that that the components of the hemarthrosis can be toxic to the joint and can lead to destruction of the intra-articular cartilage and degenerative arthritis, so immediate removal is recommended [22].

Surgery

- ACL Injury

  High-level athletes wanting to return to cutting sports and those who continue to have functional instability after rehabilitation are likely to benefit from ACL repair [9]. For more details, please see the chapter "Knee Surgeries."

- PCL Injury

  Those with grade 3 isolated PCL injuries who are involved in high-demand activities may benefit from surgery. In addition, those who still have functional instability despite conservative care or those with concomitant other ligamentous injuries or PLC injuries should have surgical evaluation. For more detail, please see chapter "Knee Surgeries."

43.2 Meniscal Injuries

43.2.1 Synonyms

- Meniscus tear
- Semilunar cartilage injury

43.2.2 ICD-10 Codes

S83.2, M23.3

43.2.3 Description

Meniscal injuries (semilunar cartilage injury) are very common and a cause of significant musculoskeletal morbidity. The menisci are important for normal function and health of the knee joint. The menisci can be damaged either during sport or through degenerative process.

Anatomy

Each of the medial and lateral compartments of the knee has a meniscus located in between the femur and tibia. The menisci are crescent-shaped wedges of fibrocartilage and allow effective articulation between the concave femoral condyles and relatively flat tibial plateau. They cover about 50–75% of the articular surface of the corresponding tibial plateau. The menisci function as load transmission from the soft tissue into the bone, decreasing the contact area, shock absorption, stability, nutrition, joint lubrication, and proprioception. Both medial and lateral menisci have anterior and posterior horns that anchor to the underlying bone. The peripheral part of the meniscus (red zone) is thick and convex and attaches to the knee joint capsule, while the central portion (white zone) is concave, thin, and unattached.

The medial meniscus is typically C-shaped and occupies approximately 60% of the articular contact area of the medial compartment. The posterior horn is significantly wider than the anterior horn. The anterior horn of meniscus attaches on the tibia anterior to the ACL, near the intercondylar fossa. The posterior horn is attached immediately anterior to the attachment of the PCL. The peripheral border of the medial meniscus merges with the knee joint capsule. The medial meniscus is subject to greater forces than lateral meniscus.

The lateral meniscus is almost circular in shape and is smaller and more mobile compared to the medial meniscus. It occupies about 80% of the articular surface. The anterior horn of the lateral meniscus attaches to the intercondylar fossa adjacent to the ACL, and the posterior horn inserts to the PCL and medial femoral condyle. There are meniscal variants that can occur. The most common is discoid meniscus most commonly located in the lateral compartment.

Overall, the menisci are relatively avascular structures with limited peripheral blood supply. The medial and lateral inferior and middle geniculate arteries (branches of popliteal artery) supply each meniscus. Radial branches from a perimeniscal plexus supply the anterior and posterior horns. Limited blood supply to the peripheral 10–25% lateral meniscus and 10–30% medial meniscus has important implications for healing. The bulk of meniscus nutrition comes from synovial diffusion or mechanical motion, especially in the avascular portion. The menisci receive innervation via the recurrent peroneal branch of the common peroneal nerve. These fibers are found primarily in the peripheral vascular zone covering the outer third of the meniscus [23].

43.2.4 Clinical Presentation

Meniscal tears are a very common source of pain and disability in the knee. For traumatic meniscal tears, they occur most commonly in males between ages 21 and 30 years of age. These can be seen in a sporting activity (i.e., soccer, rugby, football) or non-sporting activity (repetitive squatting). Medial meniscal tears are more common than lateral meniscal tears. Lateral meniscal tears occur most commonly in association with acute ACL tear. Its mechanism usually involves a twisting or shearing motion, with varus or valgus force directed on a flexed knee. Patients typically report taking a "wrong step." Other common mechanisms include cutting, deceleration, or landing from a jump. Acute traumatic meniscal tears can commonly occur with associated ligament or articular surface injury [23].

Degenerative tears are seen most commonly in the fourth through sixth decade. Some may not even be able to identify a specific inciting event or injury. They usually reflect cumulative stress and correlate with the presence of associated chondromalacia. There is an increase incidence of meniscal tears with increasing age. After the third decade of life, degenerative changes start to diminish the elasticity and make the meniscus more vulnerable to injury. Common symptoms produced by these tears include either medial or lateral knee pain and mild swelling. Immediate swelling is not frequently seen after isolated meniscal tear but could be present with a peripheral tear. A delayed effusion is more characteristic of this injury. Patients may experience "mechanical" symptoms such as locking, catching, grinding, or giving out. The frequency and severity of symptoms depend on the size and mobility of the meniscal tear [23].

43.2.5 Physical Examination

Full musculoskeletal examination is indicated in an acute knee injury. Commonly, the patient presents with an effusion and joint line tenderness. Patients often have an antalgic gait. Patients usually have full range of motion unless there is a displaced tear causing a mechanical block. They may have pain at end-range flexion or extension depending on where the tear is located. The most common special tests used to diagnose meniscal tears include McMurray test, Apley grind Test, and Thessaly test [24].

McMurray Test
This test helps detect occult tears of the posterior horns of the menisci. Patient is placed in a supine position with the knee fully flexed. The examiner then grabs the foot with one hand and steadies the knee with the other hand. To test for lateral meniscal tear, the tibia is rotated internally, and the knee is extended. To test for medial meniscal tear, the tibia is then externally rotated and extended. The test is considered positive if there is a palpable click or clunk but most commonly considered positive if it reproduces pain along the tested joint line. Of note, the test can only be performed when the patient has full knee flexion [24].

Apley Grind Test
The patient is positioned in the prone position for this test. The examiner flexes the patient's knee to 90° and then rotates the tibial externally in neutral loaded position, distraction position, and then compression. Increased pain in compression comparatively indicates meniscal tear. To test the lateral meniscus, the same test can be performed in internal rotation. In addition, a more acute knee flexion angle can help test the posterior horn [24].

Thessaly Test
The patient is asked to stand on the foot of the symptomatic side, which is fixed flat on the ground with the knee at a fixed angle (at first 5° and then at 20°). The patient then internally and externally rotates their body about three times. This should stress the meniscus. The test is considered positive with medial or lateral joint line discomfort or popping [24].

43.2.6 Diagnostic Workup

X-ray
All acute knee injury evaluation should include standing weight-bearing standard AP, posteroanterior at 45° (Rosenberg view), lateral, and merchant. These can be helpful to exclude bony pathologies and assess for the presence of degenerative changes [23].

MRI
MRI is the diagnostic modality of choice for evaluating the menisci with an accuracy range of 82–95%. The most commonly used sequences include spin-echo or fast spin-echo proton density with or without fat saturation, T1, and gradient echo. Radiologists will typically grade meniscal tears based on their appearance on MRI scan: grade 0 is normal, intact meniscus; grade I and grade II signals do not intersect superior or inferior articular surface of meniscus, but may represent meniscal degeneration; grade III signal intersects the superior and/or inferior articular surface of the meniscus and represents tear.

MRI can also be helpful to classify the type of meniscal tear by tear pattern. The main categories of meniscal tears include vertical longitudinal, radial (transverse), horizontal, complex (degenerative), and bucket-handle tears. Longitudinal, radial, and horizontal tears can progress to more complex tears. Degenerative tears occur gradually over time and are usually seen associated with osteoarthritis (OA). Extrusion of the meniscus can occur with certain tear types, particularly root tears and bucket-handle tears [25, 26].

43.2.7 Treatment

Medical Management
Initial nonoperative management is typically reserved for patients who do not have severely restricted range of motion, locking, or instability of the knee. After acute injury, management should include rest, ice, compression, and elevation. Patients can progress to full weight-bearing when tolerated [27].

Rehabilitation
Determination of conservative vs. surgical management depends on multiple factors including age, tear, type, activity intensity, instability, and response to treatment thus far. It is well established that peripheral meniscal tears can successfully heal without intervention, although poor intrinsic healing response is noted within the inner two-thirds of the meniscal tissue [27]. When meniscal function is compromised due to injury, the biomechanics of the knee is thrown off. There is increased stress on the cartilage in the joint, which can lead to cartilage loss, bony changes, and OA pro-

gression [26]. Multiple studies show that preservation of the meniscus is a first-line option given the multiple studies that show outcomes are worse after partial meniscectomy [28]. There have been multiple studies that show that outcomes after arthroscopic partial meniscectomy are no better than after conservative care.

Meniscal tears treated operatively or nonoperatively require physical therapy intervention. Clinical practice guidelines have been published through the American Physical Therapy Association (APTA), which help guide the rehabilitation process for both operative and nonoperative management of meniscal injury [29]. In patients with non-obstructive meniscal tears, physical therapy was found to be noninferior to arthroscopic partial meniscectomy for improving patient reported knee function over a 24-month follow-up period [30]. The goals of rehabilitation post meniscal injury are to decrease pain and edema, improve range of motion, increase strength, and improve balance. Rest, ice, compression, and elevation can control edema after acute injury. A 12-week exercise therapy program including neuromuscular and strength training should be considered for the rehabilitation of degenerative meniscal tears in middle-aged patients [31]. This 12-week program was found to increase quadriceps strength, improve lower extremity performance, and have the ability to maintain function 1 year post intervention. Supervised progressive range of motion and strength training of the hips and knees and neuromuscular training should be incorporated in treatment post meniscal tears [29]. Modalities such as neuromuscular electrical stimulation may be used to assist in progression of quadriceps strengthening. Aquatic therapy can be used as an adjunct to land-based therapy to improve strength and normalize gait. Progressive neuromuscular training over various surfaces along with unilateral concentric and eccentric strengthening exercises in both weight-bearing and non-weight-bearing environments should be included in the treatment plan [31].

There is no set protocol for postoperative rehabilitation of meniscal repairs [32]. However, there is agreement in early progressive weight-bearing and active and passive knee range of motion post meniscal surgery [29, 32]. Protecting the surgical site is suggested by limiting shearing and rotational forces at the knee. Post meniscectomy, it is recommended that a supervised in-clinic exercise program followed by progressive home program be a part of the treatment plan [29]. Guidelines published by the APTA suggest supervised progressive range of motion, strength training of the hips and knees, and neuromuscular training be incorporated to the treatment plan post meniscal surgery. Neuromuscular electrical stimulation can be included to improve quadriceps strength, functional performance, and knee function [29]. Gait training addresses any compensatory patterns of motion.

43.2.8 Procedures

Regenerative procedures for meniscal injuries have been more widely studied in the last few decades given there is still a treatment gap for helping those who do not respond to conventional treatment. Platelet-rich plasma (PRP) has fairly strong evidence in knee osteoarthritis, but current evidence for use in treatment of meniscal tears is still limited. PRP has the potential to use autologous source of healing and growth factors that could potentially help with healing of medial meniscal lesions and inhibit the negative inflammatory-mediated effects of osteoarthritis on chondrocytes. There is more limited evidence for use of mesenchymal stem cells and adipose-derived stem cells for treatment of these injuries [27].

Surgery

Surgical treatment of meniscal tears is recommended to patients with mechanical symptoms such as catching or locking or to help treat symptoms of pain if conservative treatment fails. Common surgical options include partial meniscectomy and direct meniscal repair. For more details, please see chapter "Knee Surgeries."

References

1. LaPrade CM, Civitarese DM, Rasmussen MT, LaPrade RF. Emerging updates on the posterior cruciate ligament: a review of the current literature. Am J Sports Med. 2015;43(12):3077–92.
2. Kaeding CC, Leger-St-Jean B, Magnussen RA. Epidemiology and diagnosis of anterior cruciate ligament injuries. Clin Sports Med. 2017;36(1):1–8.
3. Alentorn-Geli E, Myer GD, Silvers HJ, Samitier G, Romero D, Lazaro-Haro C, et al. Prevention of non-contact anterior cruciate ligament injuries in soccer players. Part 1: mechanisms of injury and underlying risk factors. Knee Surg Sports Traumatol Arthrosc. 2009;17(7):705–29.
4. Acevedo RJ, Rivera-Vega A, Miranda G, Micheo W. Anterior cruciate ligament injury: identification of risk factors and prevention strategies. Curr Sports Med Rep. 2014;13(3):186–91.
5. Verhulst FV, MacDonald P. Diagnosing PCL injuries: history, physical examination, imaging studies, arthroscopic evaluation. Sports Med Arthrosc Rev. 2020;28(1):2–7.
6. Decary S, Fallaha M, Belzile S, Martel-Pelletier J, Pelletier JP, Feldman D, et al. Clinical diagnosis of partial or complete anterior cruciate ligament tears using patients' history elements and physical examination tests. PLoS One. 2018;13(6):e0198797.
7. Benjaminse A, Gokeler A, van der Schans CP. Clinical diagnosis of an anterior cruciate ligament rupture: a meta-analysis. J Orthop Sports Phys Ther. 2006;36(5):267–88.
8. Wang D, Graziano J, Williams RJ 3rd, Jones KJ. Nonoperative treatment of PCL injuries: goals of rehabilitation and the natural history of conservative care. Curr Rev Musculoskelet Med. 2018;11(2):290–7.
9. Filbay SR, Grindem H. Evidence-based recommendations for the management of anterior cruciate ligament (ACL) rupture. Best Pract Res Clin Rheumatol. 2019;33(1):33–47.

10. Giesche F, Niederer D, Banzer W, Vogt L. Evidence for the effects of prehabilitation before ACL-reconstruction on return to sport-related and self-reported knee function: a systematic review. PLoS One. 2020;15(10):e0240192.
11. Eitzen I, Moksnes H, Snyder-Mackler L, Risberg MA. A progressive 5-week exercise therapy program leads to significant improvement in knee function early after anterior cruciate ligament injury. J Orthop Sports Phys Ther. 2010;40(11):705–21.
12. van Melick N, van Cingel RE, Brooijmans F, Neeter C, van Tienen T, Hullegie W, et al. Evidence-based clinical practice update: practice guidelines for anterior cruciate ligament rehabilitation based on a systematic review and multidisciplinary consensus. Br J Sports Med. 2016;50(24):1506–15.
13. Escamilla RF, Macleod TD, Wilk KE, Paulos L, Andrews JR. Cruciate ligament loading during common knee rehabilitation exercises. Proc Inst Mech Eng H. 2012;226(9):670–80.
14. Kim KM, Croy T, Hertel J, Saliba S. Effects of neuromuscular electrical stimulation after anterior cruciate ligament reconstruction on quadriceps strength, function, and patient-oriented outcomes: a systematic review. J Orthop Sports Phys Ther. 2010;40(7):383–91.
15. Relph N, Herrington L. The effect of conservatively treated acl injury on knee joint position sense. Int J Sports Phys Ther. 2016;11(4):536–43.
16. Anderson MJ, Browning WM 3rd, Urband CE, Kluczynski MA, Bisson LJ. A systematic summary of systematic reviews on the topic of the anterior cruciate ligament. Orthop J Sports Med. 2016;4(3):2325967116634074.
17. Zech A, Hubscher M, Vogt L, Banzer W, Hansel F, Pfeifer K. Neuromuscular training for rehabilitation of sports injuries: a systematic review. Med Sci Sports Exerc. 2009;41(10):1831–41.
18. Logerstedt DS, Scalzitti D, Risberg MA, Engebretsen L, Webster KE, Feller J, et al. Knee stability and movement coordination impairments: knee ligament sprain revision 2017. J Orthop Sports Phys Ther. 2017;47(11):A1–A47.
19. Andrade R, Pereira R, van Cingel R, Staal JB, Espregueira-Mendes J. How should clinicians rehabilitate patients after ACL reconstruction? A systematic review of clinical practice guidelines (CPGs) with a focus on quality appraisal (AGREE II). Br J Sports Med. 2020;54(9):512–9.
20. Winkler PW, Zsidai B, Wagala NN, Hughes JD, Horvath A, Senorski EH, et al. Evolving evidence in the treatment of primary and recurrent posterior cruciate ligament injuries, part 1: anatomy, biomechanics and diagnostics. Knee Surg Sports Traumatol Arthrosc. 2021;29(3):672–81.
21. Pierce CM, O'Brien L, Griffin LW, Laprade RF. Posterior cruciate ligament tears: functional and postoperative rehabilitation. Knee Surg Sports Traumatol Arthrosc. 2013;21(5):1071–84.
22. Lyons LP, Weinberg JB, Wittstein JR, McNulty AL. Blood in the joint: effects of hemarthrosis on meniscus health and repair techniques. Osteoarthr Cartil. 2021;29(4):471–9.
23. Fox AJ, Wanivenhaus F, Burge AJ, Warren RF, Rodeo SA. The human meniscus: a review of anatomy, function, injury, and advances in treatment. Clin Anat. 2015;28(2):269–87.
24. Chivers MD, Howitt SD. Anatomy and physical examination of the knee menisci: a narrative review of the orthopedic literature. J Can Chiropr Assoc. 2009;53(4):319–33.
25. Bronstein RD, Schaffer JC. Physical examination of the knee: meniscus, cartilage, and patellofemoral conditions. J Am Acad Orthop Surg. 2017;25(5):365–74.
26. Jacob G, Shimomura K, Krych AJ, Nakamura N. The meniscus tear: a review of stem cell therapies. Cells. 2019;9(1):92.
27. Chirichella PS, Jow S, Iacono S, Wey HE, Malanga GA. Treatment of knee meniscus pathology: rehabilitation, surgery, and orthobiologics. PM R. 2019;11(3):292–308.
28. Kopf S, Beaufils P, Hirschmann MT, Rotigliano N, Ollivier M, Pereira H, et al. Management of traumatic meniscus tears: the 2019 ESSKA meniscus consensus. Knee Surg Sports Traumatol Arthrosc. 2020;28(4):1177–94.
29. Logerstedt DS, Scalzitti DA, Bennell KL, Hinman RS, Silvers-Granelli H, Ebert J, et al. Knee pain and mobility impairments: meniscal and articular cartilage lesions revision 2018. J Orthop Sports Phys Ther. 2018;48(2):A1–A50.
30. van de Graaf VA, Noorduyn JCA, Willigenburg NW, Butter IK, de Gast A, Mol BW, et al. Effect of early surgery vs physical therapy on knee function among patients with nonobstructive meniscal tears: the ESCAPE randomized clinical trial. JAMA. 2018;320(13):1328–37.
31. Stensrud S, Roos EM, Risberg MA. A 12-week exercise therapy program in middle-aged patients with degenerative meniscus tears: a case series with 1-year follow-up. J Orthop Sports Phys Ther. 2012;42(11):919–31.
32. Spang Iii RC, Nasr MC, Mohamadi A, DeAngelis JP, Nazarian A, Ramappa AJ. Rehabilitation following meniscal repair: a systematic review. BMJ Open Sport Exerc Med. 2018;4(1):e000212.

Knee Disorders: Extra-Articular

44

S. Ali Mostoufi, Michael F. Saulle, Tony K. George, Charles Scott, Joseph Chin, and Yasmine Mostoufi

44.1 Anterior Knee Disorders

44.1.1 Quadriceps and Patellar Tendon Disorders

S. Ali Mostoufi

44.1.1.1 ICD 10 Code

- Quadriceps tendonitis M76.899
- Quadriceps tendon tear S76.119
- Patella tendonitis M76.50
- Patella tendon tear S86.819
- Osgood-Schlatter syndrome M92.529

S. A. Mostoufi (✉)
Department of Orthopedics and Rehabilitation, Tufts University School of Medicine, Boston, MA, USA

New England Spine Care Associates & Boston Regenerative Medicine, Cambridge, MA, USA
e-mail: Ali.Mostoufi@Tufts.edu

M. F. Saulle
Rehabilitation and Regenerative Medicine, New York Presbyterian Weill Cornell Medical Center, Columbia University Irving Medical Center, Tarrytown, NY, USA
e-mail: ms4798@cumc.columbia.edu

T. K. George
Restorative Orthopaedics Spine & Sports (ROSS) Institute, Somerset, NJ, USA

Department of Orthopaedics, Rutgers-Robert Wood Johnson Medical School, New Brunswick, NJ, USA

C. Scott
Rehabilitation and Regenerative Medicine, Columbia University Medical Center, New York, NY, USA
e-mail: cps2135@cumc.columbia.edu

J. Chin
Department of Physical Medicine and Rehabilitation, New York Presbyterian Weill Cornell Medical Center, Columbia University Irving Medical Center, New York, NY, USA

Y. Mostoufi
Landmark High, Beverly, MA, USA

44.1.1.2 Description

Anatomy

The extensor apparatus of the knee primarily consists of the proximal common tendon of the quadriceps femoris muscle (which itself is divided into rectus femoris, vastus lateralis, vastus intermedius, vastus medialis) and the distal portion named patellar tendon with its insertion into the tibial tuberosity. The rectus femoris originates at the ilium, thus crossing both the hip and knee joint along its course. This anatomy allows for the rectus femoris to assist with both hip flexion and knee extension. The remaining muscles originate on the femur and only help with knee extension [1]. The quadriceps femoris tendon is complex and has three layers from superficial to deep and, in combination with medial patellofemoral ligament and lateral patellofemoral ligament, helps stabilize the patella in both active and dynamic states. The tendon of the quadriceps muscle embeds the sesamoid bone "patella" and extends distally as patellar tendon to attach to the tibial tuberosity (Fig. 44.1). The term "jumper's knee" refers to disorders of patellar tendon. The disorders of the quadriceps tendon and the patellar tendon are unique and distinct [2].

Quadriceps Tendon and Patellar Tendon Disorders

Both quadriceps tendon and patellar tendon disorders are considered overuse injury, and although sports that require jumping are more prone to this injury, other sports with acceleration, deceleration, landing, and cutting could develop patellar tendinopathy and present for care [3]. Quadriceps tendon rupture tends to be more common than patellar tendon ruptures, particularly in individuals over the age 40 [4]. It is thought that the microtrauma to the patella is the backdrop to patellar tendinopathy. Sports such as volleyball, basketball, and track and field with hurdles all exert significant eccentric force on the quadriceps tendon and may result in repetitive stress and microtrauma leading to tendinopathy. It is a male-dominant condition; increased ligamentous laxity and hormonal changes in menstruating females may have some protective properties, hence lower rates of quadriceps

© The Author(s), under exclusive license to Springer Nature Switzerland AG 2022
S. A. Mostoufi et al. (eds.), *Clinical Guide to Musculoskeletal Medicine*, https://doi.org/10.1007/978-3-030-92042-5_44

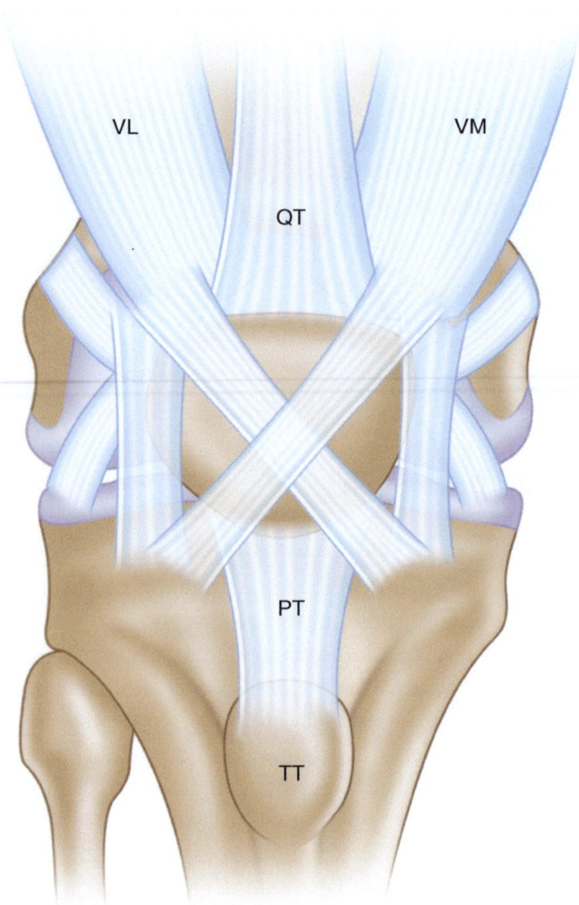

Fig. 44.1 Diagram of knee extensor apparatus with anterior vastus expansion. QT quadriceps tendon, PT patellar tendon, TT tibial tuberosity, VM vastus medialis, VL vastus lateralis. (Open access image. Adopted and modified from Ref. [1])

tendinopathy [5]. Risk factors include tightness of the hamstring and quadriceps muscle, restrictions in ankle dorsiflexion, coexistence of patella alta (high-riding patella) and abnormal patellar tracking, increased knee Q angle, ligamentous laxity, leg length discrepancy, abnormal foot arch (pes planus or varus), inappropriate frequency or intensity of training, and training on nonprofessional tracks [5–7]. Risk factors in nonathletes include high BMI and taller individuals. Specific risk factors for patellar tendinopathy leading to rupture may also include rheumatological disorders, chronic renal disease, diabetes, chronic corticosteroid intake, previous injuries, patellofemoral degeneration, and the use of certain antibiotic including fluoroquinolones [5–7].

The disorders of quadriceps tendon and patellar tendon can range from simple strain, tendinitis, to tendinosis with or without calcification and rupture. Blazina [5] developed the most accepted classification for quadricep tendinopathy, which is symptom presence with or without activity. Popkin-Golman developed the radiographic classification of quadriceps tendon injury which can be correlated to Blazina's classification. These can be used as an aid to treatment planning (Table 44.1) [8].

Table 44.1 The Blazina classification [5] and Popkin-Golman [8] classification of quadricep tendon injury

Blazina classification	Popkin-Golman radiographic classification	Treatment strategy
I pain only after sport	No tendon tear Tendon <8 mm	Brace, PT, NSAIDS, eccentric strengthening
II pain during and after sport Disappears with warmup Reappears when fatigue	<25% thickness tear	Brace, PT, NSAIDS, eccentric strengthening, +/− PRP
III pain during and after sport Unable to participate in sports at previous level	25–50% tendon tear	Brace, PT, NSAIDS, eccentric strengthening, +/− PRP Possible surgical repair if symptomatic >6 m
IV complete tendon rupture	>50% tendon tear	Brace, PT, NSAIDS, eccentric strengthening, +/-PRP Surgical intervention

Treatment strategy based on classification
PT physical therapy, *PRP* platelet-rich plasma

Osgood-Schlatter Syndrome

Also known as osteochondrosis, tibial tubercle apophysitis, or traction apophysitis, Osgood-Schlatter Syndrome (OSS) is a disorder with anterior knee pain in teenage athletes who have not reached skeletal maturity. Repetitive patellar tendon traction over the tibial tubercle leading to microvascular tears, fractures, and inflammation is thought to be the underlying cause [9]. Young athletes present in an atraumatic fashion, with gradual onset. Pain is focused on the tibial tuberosity (insertional site for the patellar tendon) due to repetitive stress on the knee extensor mechanism during jumping and sprinting. It is often self-limiting, treated with ice and nonsteroidal anti-inflammatory drugs (NSAIDs), as well as activity modification. Relative rest and lower extremity stretching regimen speed recovery and pain relief. If the pain persists, formal physical therapy may be warranted. In severe cases, brief immobilization is considered to reduce the stress on patellar tendon insertion. Surgery is rarely indicated but may be undertaken to excise the overlying bursa [10].

44.1.1.3 Presentation

Quadriceps Tendinopathy

Quadriceps tendon injuries are often acute. Chronic nontraumatic cases will present to an outpatient clinic or urgent care. In sports, classic presentation is the development of pain after injury at or above the superior pole of the patella. An athlete may report development of symptoms when kicking a ball, jumping, or initiating a sudden change in speed or direction while sprinting. Grading quadriceps strain may assist with further care. In grade 1 which is a milder presentation, the patient would have preserved strength with no palpable defect. In grade II, the patient would be in a moderate amount of pain with loss of strength and some palpable defect in the myotendinous junction, and in severe cases, a patient would be unable to extend the knee with a palpable defect in the distal quadriceps/myotendinous junction. An athlete may report lateral knee pain but also a loss of function at the time of injury and localized swelling in the rectus femoris myotendinous junction [11, 12].

Patellar Tendinopathy

Common presenting symptoms of patellar tendinopathy include anterior knee pain localized to the inferior pole of the patella with load-related pain that increases with the demand on the knee extensors. Other symptoms may include pain with prolonged sitting, squatting, and going up and down stairs. Pain may improve with warmups (repeated loading), but it can also increase as the degree and rate of tendon loading increases [13]. Disorders of the patellar tendon may range from tendinitis to tendinosis with calcification to incomplete or even complete tear. Pain presentation is localized distal to the patella and may extend to the tibial tuberosity. Injuries are often due to significant tensile forces on the tendon, and presentation could be acute (in the case of patellar tendon rupture and bony avulsion) versus chronic (due to repetitive microtrauma and tendinosis). Since attachment of the patellar tendon to the tibia is essential for normal gait, disruption to the tendon results in a significant functional loss and requires immediate surgical consultation [5].

44.1.1.4 Examination

Quadriceps Tendinopathy

Full musculoskeletal examination of the lower extremity and spine should be conducted with focus on the knee and extensor complex.

Inspection The entire knee should be inspected for the alignment, location of the patella, bruising, edema, and tolerance to weight bearing (most patients with quadriceps tendon tear would not be able to bear weight on the lower extremity).

Palpation The examiner should palpate the quadriceps muscle, myotendinous junction, and the portion of the tendon as it approaches the patella. In high-grade tears, a tendon gap may be palpable.

Knee extension function The patient's ability to extend the knee and raise his or her leg with the knee extended is impaired in full tendon tear, but in partial tear or acute tendon stress, function may also be impaired due to pain.

Ely test Evaluates rectus femoris flexibility. The patient lies prone as the affected knee is flexed (trying to touch the buttocks with the heel); a tight rectus muscle will cause the patient's hip joint to flex, resulting in the elevation of the affected buttock.

Patellar Tendinopathy

Pain is localized to the inferior pole of the patella and/or throughout the course of the entire patellar tendon. Athletes with patellar tendon pain tend to reduce the amount of knee flexion and appear stiff in their landing. In-office exam is similar to quadriceps tendon evaluation in which inspection and palpation should be done from the patella down to the insertional tibial tuberosity. Examiner should evaluate for local bruising, deformity, and any palpable gap in the tendon. In patients with Osgood-Schlatter Syndrome, the tibial tuberosity may be prominent at the baseline.

Special Test

Single-leg decline squat This is performed in standing position. Athletes are asked to stand on a 25° decline board with one leg. Then the athlete is asked to do a squat, and the maximal angle of knee flexion achieved is recorded. This is done both for the symptomatic and asymptomatic side. Pain reproduced with this test should be isolated to the patellar tendon from the lower pole to the tibial tuberosity. This test could be done as a diagnostic step or to monitor progress in rehab and tendon response to load.

44.1.1.5 Diagnostic Workup

The diagnostic imaging includes radiographs, MRIs, and various types of ultrasound techniques, such as grey scale, high resolution, color Doppler, and elastography [14]. Radiographs are readily available, inexpensive, and often the initial diagnostic tool for anterior knee pain. It could detect displacement of the patella superiorly (Fig. 44.2) in the case of tendon rupture or tibial avulsion, but other injuries including patella fracture can be detected rapidly which may lead to further advanced imaging/MRI for further delineation of the pathology.

Quadriceps Tendinopathy

X-rays may show abnormal position of the patella as well as fractures (Fig. 44.2). Both ultrasonography and MRI could be used in the workup of quadriceps tendinopathy, but in an acute trauma, when a patient is evaluated in the emergency room with suspicion of quadriceps tendon tear, an MRI is an appropriate diagnostic study. MRI has the ability to confirm diagnosis and specifies lesion type of complete or incomplete tear, avulsion, or intrasubstance tendon tear. Sports medicine physicians trained in ultrasound can quickly scan the quadriceps tendon at the time of injury which may lead to better sideline management and can dictate urgency of surgical referral/care.

Patellar Tendinopathy

Radiographs could be helpful in full tear of the patellar tendon with avulsion demonstrating superiorly displaced patella and avulsed fragments notable on plain radiographs. MRI of the patella should clearly demonstrate patellar tendon rupture and is considered the most sensitive imaging modality, with its ability to identify the exact location of the rupture. Ultrasound, although operator dependent, could be a useful tool at sideline or at outpatient clinic due to its portability and ability to visualize the quadriceps tendon complex and any tendon abnormality from chronic tendinosis to tear. In degenerated tendons, ultrasound findings include hypoechoic areas with neovascularization, but such findings could be also identified in symptom-free individuals with frequency as high as 10% (Fig. 44.3) [14]. Symptomatic athletes have an increased baseline ultrasound changes of hypoechoic segment as compared to non-symptomatic individuals based on the study by King et al. [14].

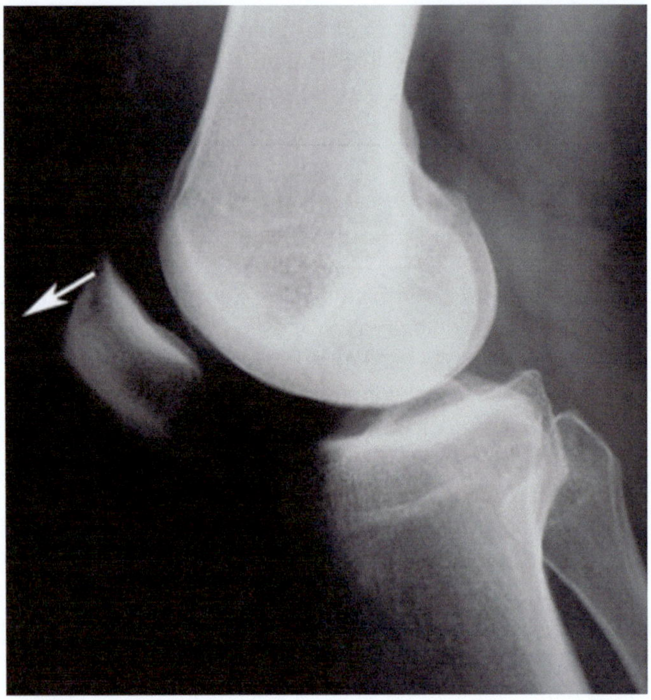

Fig. 44.2 Quadriceps tendon tear with forward shift of the proximal pole of the patella and patella baja. (Open access image from Ref. [1])

44.1.1.6 Treatment

Medical Management

Medical management of quadriceps and patellar tendinopathy could provide adequate symptom relief to patients with tendinitis or mild to moderate tendinosis without rupture. In the earlier stages of quadriceps tendinopathy, nonoperative care has shown superior outcomes compared to surgical treatment, which is typically reserved for later stages of disease or patients who have failed nonoperative measures [14]. Treatment options include pain relief with oral or topical NSAIDs, Tylenol, use of ice, and referral for PT. Manual treatments include myofascial manipulation of the knee extensor group, which has shown to have some positive pain reduction properties, both short-term and long-term [15]. It should be noted that in patients with severe quadricep tendinopathy, there is an increased risk of tendon rupture in individuals who have failed nonoperative treatment [16].

Rehabilitation

Pain relief is the initial goal of rehabilitation. This is followed by a progressive resistive strengthening exercise program, power exercises to improve the capacity in the stretch-shorten cycle, and finally functional return-to-sport training. Reducing an athlete's symptoms requires load management. Removing high-intensity drills, decreasing training volume, and reducing training frequency is advised to reduce the load on the tendon [13]. It is important to avoid complete cessation of tendon loading activities, as that will further

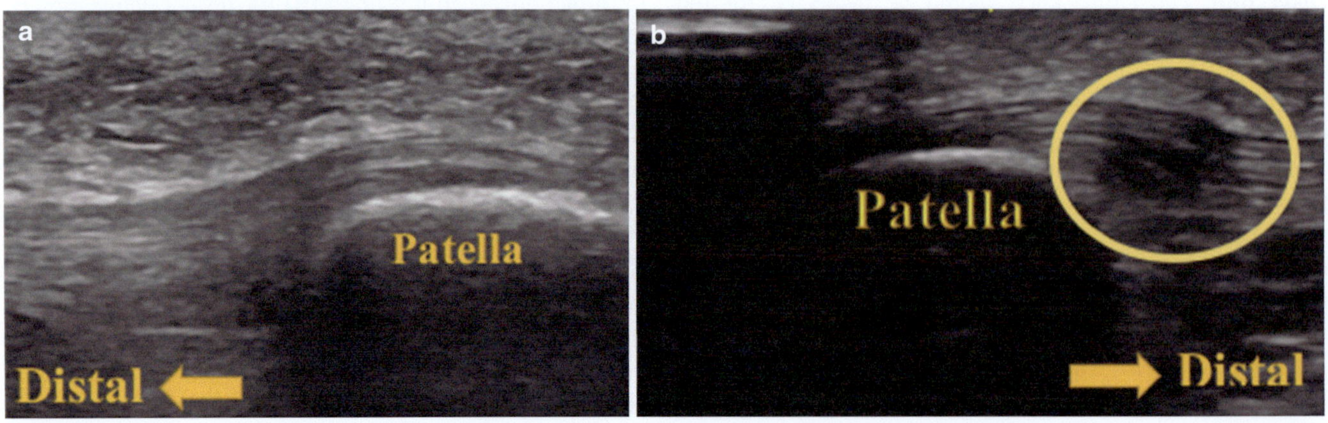

Fig. 44.3 US images of the patellar tendon. Image (**a**) shows normal echotexture of the left proximal patellar tendon. Image (**b**) is from the same patient with right proximal patellar tendinopathy, showing change in the echotexture with a hypoechoic thickened region

reduce the load capacity of the tendon. In terms of pain, sustained isometric contractions have been shown to be analgesic [17].

Manual Therapy Techniques
Myofascial manipulation of the knee extensor muscle group has had a positive effect on reducing pain in patellar tendinopathy patients in short-term and long-term follow-up [15].

Physical Therapy
There is no consensus on the rehabilitation approach. Progression from isometric exercise to an isotonic exercise, energy storage exercises (including jumping, acceleration, deceleration, and/or cutting), and finally, the progressive return to sport appears to be the most common approach for patella tendinopathy. Studies demonstrated that a training program of 6–12 weeks of duration, performing 2–3 sessions a week of eccentric exercises, can provoke enough stimulation to improve muscle function in different types of populations [18].

In general, *eccentric heavy low-resistance*, *isotonic*, and *isometric exercises* have been studied for patellar tendinopathy [19]. Heavy slow resistance isotonic exercises in people with patellar tendinopathy was investigated by Kongsgaard and colleagues, who compared the effects of a peritendinous corticosteroid injection to a decline squat eccentric exercise protocol and a heavy slow resistance protocol. All three groups showed improvements at 12 weeks; however, at 6 months, only the groups using the eccentric exercises and the heavy slow resistance exercises still showed sustained improvement. The heavy slow resistance group showed improved tissue normalization of the collagen and also demonstrated better clinical presentations than the eccentric group within the 12-week follow-up [20]. The *eccentric exercises* appear to have good short-term and long-term benefits. Eccentric exercises include bilateral weighted squats and unilateral declined squats [21].

Sport-Specific Rehab
Sport-specific functional strengthening should be incorporated in athletes' return to play treatment plan. Early drills should include low-impact activities such as hopping and jumping, progressing to agility movements. When introducing such exercises, athletic trainers and physical therapists should alternate between low-load, medium-load, and high-load exercise days to ensure safe return to play without reinjury [21].

Procedures
Steroid Injection
Some studies suggest that the chronic outcome of patients with peritendinous corticosteroid injection is worse as compared to those who received physical therapy treatment including eccentric decline squat training and heavy slow resistance training [20]. Bursitis may respond to steroid injection which should be performed with image guidance.

Platelet-Rich Plasma (PRP) Injection
In patients who have failed rehabilitation and oral agents, injection of PRP is considered for pain relief [22, 23]. Dallaudière et al. conducted a retrospective review of 408 patients with patellar tendinopathy treated by a single ultrasound (US)-guided PRP injection. They demonstrated an increased rapid tendon healing, satisfactory patient tolerance, and decreased size of the patellar tendon tear (9.2 mm at day 0 to 3.3 mm at week 6, $P < 0.001$) [24].

Shockwave Therapy
The benefit of the extracorporeal shockwave therapy was not seen as compared to placebo when applied to in-season jumping athletes with chronic patellar tendinopathy [25]. The effect of the shockwave therapy against PRP injection was studied, and both had positive pain relief properties in the first 2 months, but shockwave therapy did not have a beneficial outcome in 6- and 12-month follow-up as compared to the PRP group [26].

Surgery
Severe cases of quadricep tendinopathy, patellar tendinopathy, and ruptures require surgical repair. Arthroscopic and open surgical treatments have shown superior outcomes in advanced stage tendinopathy compared to nonoperative treatments [16]. The outcomes of surgical treatment of quadriceps tendinopathy have been studied extensively in athletes; however, there is a need for additional studies in the nonathlete population. For more details on surgical approach, please see Chap. 46.

44.1.2 Patellofemoral Pain Syndrome

S. Ali Mostoufi

44.1.2.1 ICD 10 Code
M22.2x9, M22.2x1, M22.2x2

44.1.2.2 Synonyms
- Chondromalacia patella
- Runner's knee
- Retropatellar pain syndrome
- Lateral facet compression syndrome

44.1.2.3 Description
Patellofemoral syndrome (PFPS) is one of the most common causes of anterior knee pain. Although known as the *runner's knee*, it is not exclusive to runners. It is also known as *retro-*

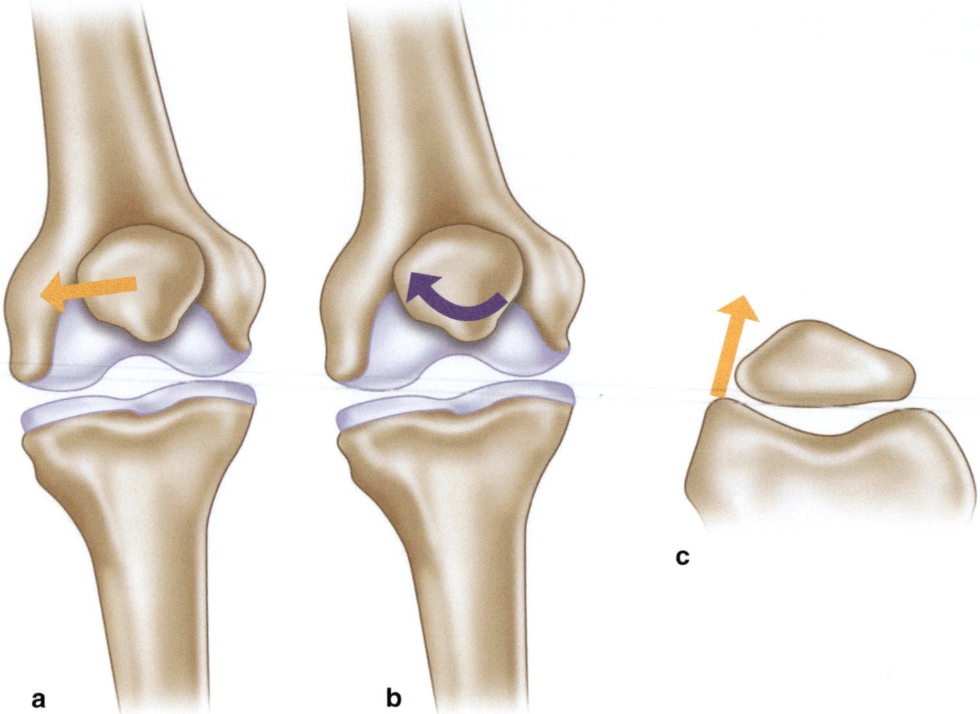

Fig. 44.4 Patient with patellofemoral syndrome has increased lateral shift (**a**), lateral splint (**b**), and increased lateral tilt (**c**) of the patella against the distal femur. (Adopted and modified from Ref. [27])

patellar pain syndrome or *lateral facet compression syndrome* since the pain is generated from the contact of osseous surfaces between the patella and distal femur. The exact etiology is unknown, but multifactorial etiology is commonly accepted.

PFPS is common in adults who jump, squat, or frequently climb stairs in the context of sports and/or daily activities [28]. It is more prevalent in females and is often associated with maltracking of the patella (valgus shift – Fig. 44.4) [27, 29]. Based on the study by Pal et al., maltracking of the patella may be due to delayed activation of the vastus medialis as compared to the vastus lateralis when the patient descends downstairs and climbs upstairs [30]. Studies also show that females with PFPS have decreased power in hip abduction, hip external rotation, and hip extension as compared with healthy controls; therefore, any weakness in such muscles may be a risk factor in developing PFPS (Table 44.2) [31]. Barton et al. showed that PFPS patients have a more pronated foot, more abduction forefoot, and increased rearfoot eversion in comparison with a healthy control group [32].

Table 44.2 Risk factor for patellofemoral syndrome [1, 8]

Malalignment of the lower patella	Malalignment of the lower extremity
Imbalance and muscle strength	Lower extremity overload
Trauma	Improper training practice
Foot deformities	Hip abductor weakness
Hindfoot eversion	Females
Improper sports techniques	Choice of equipment/footwear
Hamstring tightness	Lumbar pain/sacral inclination

44.1.2.4 Presentation

Anterior knee pain is the main complaint. Patients present with pain while running, jumping, squatting, and negotiating stairs. Symptoms are often aggravated by flexion of the knee. Pain may be exacerbated by sitting with the knee flexed for a longer time. The “movie theatre sign” describes patients with patellofemoral syndrome that prefer to sit at an aisle seat, where they can keep the knee extended and experience less pain. Some patients may report a giving way or a catching sensation in the knee which could be originating from ligamentous or femorotibial pathology. Associated symptoms could be swelling around the knee or a clicking sensation with knee flexion.

44.1.2.5 Examination

Inspection It should focus on observing any spine deformity, gait abnormality, pelvic obliquity, abnormal pelvic angle on sagittal view, Q angles of the lower extremity, position of the hindfoot, abnormal foot arch, muscle imbalance and atrophy, and redness and swelling around the knee joint.

Palpation It could be helpful to evaluate for tenderness of the quadriceps tendon and patellar tendon and any effusion, leading to a change of the knee and soft tissue around it. When testing knee range of motion, crepitus may be palpated.

MSK exam Full musculoskeletal examination of the spine pelvis and lower extremity should be performed. Examination testing includes bilateral lower extremity strength including hip abductors, quadriceps, and internal and external rotators of the hip, and a side-by-side comparison should be done. Evaluation includes the range of motion of the large joints including both hips, knees, and ankles. Focusing on the patella, the examiner may find an increased quadriceps angle, lateral and medial retinacular tenderness, crepitation of the patellofemoral joint, and reduced mobility of the patella [28].

Special Test

Single-Legged Squat

This test is commonly used for injury prevention screening or physical rehabilitation evaluation. It has also been applied to individuals with non-arthritic hip pain, patellofemoral pain syndrome, and knee osteoarthritis, among others. Excessive medial knee deviation during the eccentric phase of the squat is a common finding and, in patellofemoral syndrome, may be associated with increased anterior pain.

Clarke Test

It is also known as patellar grind test. The patient is positioned supine and the knee extended. The examiner will place the web space of his thumb and index finger against the superior pole of the patient's patella and will ask for an isometric quadriceps contraction. Pain sufficient to prevent the patient from maintaining a quadriceps contraction against resistance longer than 2 seconds is considered positive in suspected chondromalacia patella.

Ely Test

It evaluates rectus femoris flexibility. The patient lies prone as the affected knee is flexed (trying to touch the buttocks with the heel); a tight rectus muscle will cause the patient's hip joint to flex, resulting in the elevation of the affected buttock.

44.1.2.6 Workup

Radiographs

Radiographs are the first line for diagnostic testing. AP standing and lateral and sunrise views are often obtained. X-rays could identify abnormal patellar position (such as patellar alta or baja) as well as lateral/medial subluxations. The Insall-Salvati ratio and the Blackburne-Peel ratio (Fig. 44.5) are used by the radiologist measuring positioning of the patella against the trochlea as well as position of the distal pole of the patella compared to the horizontal line of tibial plateau [34]. There are a number of other patellofemoral joint measurements including patellar tilt, patellar subluxation, lateral trochlear inclination, trochlear depth, and sulcus angle that may be utilized when evaluating patients with patellofemoral syndrome [35].

CT and MRI

The cross-sectional imaging provides more detail on the morphology of the patella and the trochlea and provides a superior assessment of the soft tissue, cartilage, ligamentous structures, anterior patella enthesopathy, patellar tendon, quadriceps tendon, and the retinacular. It also provides information on the prepatellar fat pad and prepatellar and infrapatellar bursa. MRI of the knee in slight flexion can also image a medial plica, the extensor mechanism, the meniscus, and any synovial abnormality that could mimic the patellofemoral pain syndrome [35]. Dynamic testing would allow evaluation of the patellofemoral joint kinematics with focus on real-time interplay of the soft tissue and bony constraints. Thematic MRI and three-dimensional or four-dimensional CT are examples of dynamic testing, but they are not widely available and require expert radiologist and patient compliance [35].

44.1.2.7 Treatment

The majority of patients with PFPS respond to conservative care.

Conservative Care

Medication

Pharmacological therapy includes the use of NSAIDs to reduce nociceptive anterior knee pain. There may be some value in topical NSAIDs.

Bracing

Similar to taping, the brace will exert an external medially directed force counteracting the lateral patellar maltracking and as a result, may relieve pain.

Foot Orthotics

Both the pronated foot and hindfoot eversion have been linked to increased risk of patellofemoral syndrome. Orthotics that control the hindfoot and support the arch may be valuable in long-term management of patients with PFPS.

Physical Therapy

Exercises should address strengthening of hip girdle muscles, trunk stability, strength of the quadriceps versus the hamstrings and IT band. Active stretching exercises, squats, ergometer, static quadriceps exercises, active leg raises, leg press, and raising and lowering climbing exercises are part of this regimen [36].

Kinesio Taping

The main goal of this modality is to modify the tracking of the patella by applying strips of tape with a medially directed

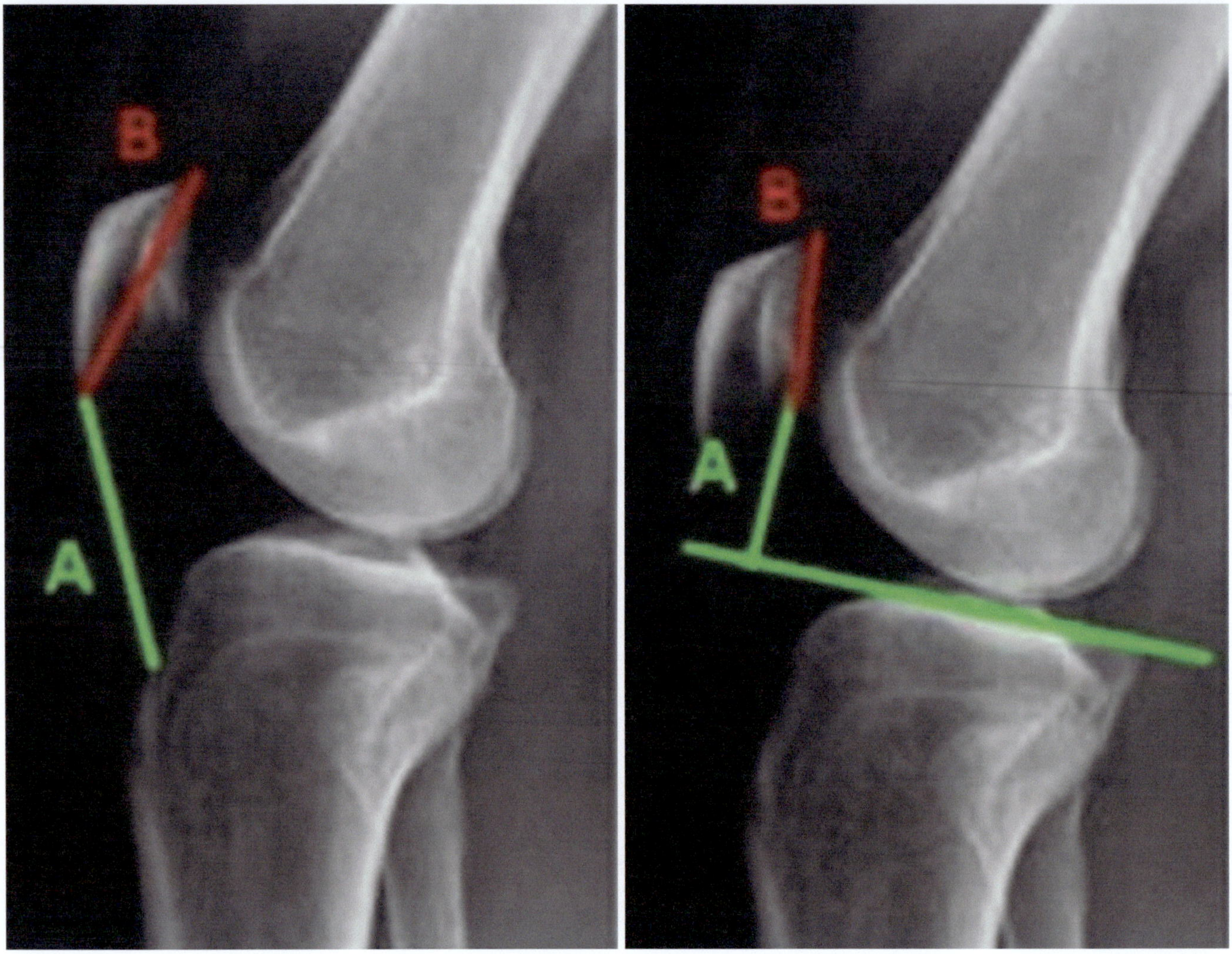

Fig. 44.5 The Insall-Salvati ratio on the left (measuring the positioning of the patella against the trochlea) and the Blackburne-Peel ratio on the right (relative position of the distal pole of the patella to the horizontal line of tibial plateau) are used by the radiologist in the workup of patellofemoral pain syndrome. (Image used with permission) [33]

force to counteract the lateral maltracking of the patella. Cowan demonstrated that this technique will promote earlier effect of the vastus medialis [37].

44.1.2.8 Surgery

Surgical intervention is rarely indicated. There are a multitude of procedures that can be considered for cases that fail to respond to all conservative measures. Most of these operations address the extensor mechanism alignment: the quadriceps mechanism, the tibial tubercle, or the medial patellofemoral ligament.

44.1.3 Patellar Instability

This topic is discussed in the Chap. 45.

44.1.4 Plica Syndrome

S. Ali Mostoufi

44.1.4.1 ICD 10 code

M67.50, M67.51, M67.52

44.1.4.2 Description

A plica is a band of thick, fibrotic tissue that extends from the synovial capsule of a joint. The knee is the joint most commonly affected by plica tissue. Knee plica are present in 50% of individuals [38]. With injury or repetitive use/overuse due to friction against the patella or the medial femoral condyle, the plica can thicken and can become inflamed and painful known as plica syndrome. The plica nomenclature is based on its location, such as suprapatellar, infrapatellar, lateral

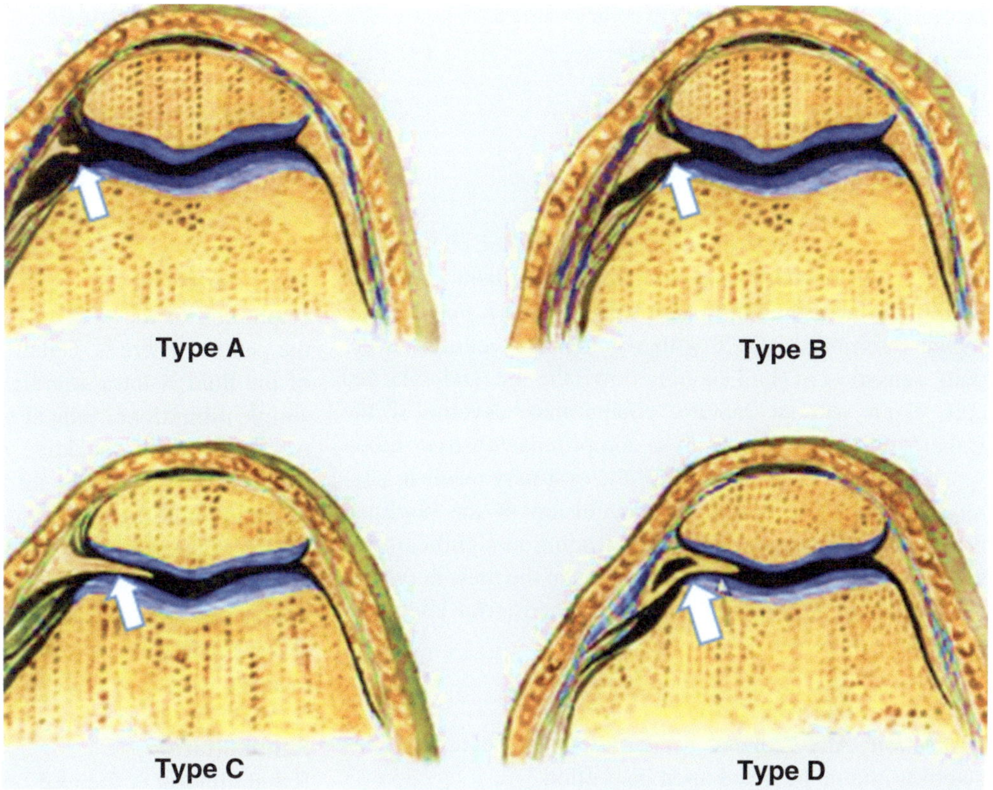

Fig. 44.6 Types of knee plica. (Original figure from Ref. [40], with permission from Springer Link)

plica, or the medial plica (which is the most commonly symptomatic location) [39]. There are four types of plica as seen in Fig. 44.6 based on the size and degree of impingement of the condyle.

44.1.4.3 Presentation and Examination

Patients with plica syndrome will experience pain on the anterior aspect of the knee associated with clicking or popping. Pain can be brought on by activities that load the patellofemoral joint (getting up from chair or sitting motion, going up and down the stairs, and squats). On a physical exam, taut bands may be found on palpation, but also special maneuvers such as the *Stutter test* can be helpful in diagnosis [39]. In the stutter test, the clinician would palpate the patella as the patient slowly extends the knee. The test is positive if a stuttering or ratcheting is noted between 45° and 60°.

44.1.4.4 Diagnostic Workup

The gold standard for diagnosis is arthroscopy, but studies show that physical exam has a 90% sensitivity and 89% specificity, ultrasound has 90% sensitivity and 83% specificity, and MRI has 77% sensitivity and 58% specificity for diagnosing plica syndrome [9].

44.1.4.5 Treatment

Types A and B are usually not symptomatic due to small size and if symptomatic, typically respond to conservative care. Types C and D are larger and likely symptomatic due to impingement on the medial femoral condyle. If NSAIDS and stretching exercises are not helpful, steroid injection of the plica can be tried prior to referral for arthroscopic resection.

44.2 Posterior Knee Disorders

44.2.1 Popliteal (Aka Baker's) Cyst

44.2.1.1 ICD 10 code

M71.20, M71.21, M71.22

44.2.1.2 Description

Anatomy Baker's cyst or popliteal cyst, also known as parameniscal cyst, is a cystic fluid collection within the popliteal fossa located in the posterior aspect of the knee which is associated with osteoarthritis of the knee or meniscal disease. Patients can be symptom-free or may present with tightness in the back of the knee, pain with motion, and acute pain if the cyst ruptures. Although more common in adults, it can develop in pediatrics as an isolated disease related to the hernia in the posterior knee joint synovium [41].

44.2.1.3 Presentation

Patients may report bulging or a palpable mass in the popliteal fossa when standing. The size of the mass may reduce as the patient flexes the knee to about 45° known as the Foucher's sign [41]. Often this condition is not associated

Table 44.3 Differential diagnosis of posterior knee pain

DVT	AV fistula
Baker's cyst	Abscess
Lymphadenopathy	Lymphadenopathy
Hematoma	Lipoma
Hemangioma	Distal hamstring tendinopathy

with any change in skin color although when ruptured, it could result in ecchymosis and redness. If there is a rapid accumulation of the fluid in the Baker's cyst, it may rupture which resembles a DVT with significant swelling, severe pain, sensation of fluid running down the leg, and enlarged calf. Even without rupture, edema may develop if the Baker's cyst is large enough to compromise/obstruct blood vessels. In rare cases, rupture of the cyst may result in posterior tibial nerve entrapment, occlusion of the popliteal artery, or compartment syndrome leading to significant leg swelling, possible foot drop, weakness in the toes, dysesthesias, and pain. Differential diagnosis of posterior knee pain is in Table 44.3.

44.2.1.4 Examination

Inspection Any redness, ecchymosis, and significant leg swelling should be noted upon inspection.

Gait The patient may have a normal gait, but in cases of ruptured cyst, the patient would be antalgic and may not be able to bear weight on the lower extremity.

Palpation The posterior knee should be examined to identify a palpable mass in the popliteal fossa. On standing, the Baker's cyst may protrude further, and it may be less notable when the knee is flexed at 45°.

44.2.1.5 Diagnostic Imaging

X-rays It will show corresponding osteoarthritis of the knee joint but cannot evaluate the Baker's cyst. Soft tissue edema may be noted on X-rays.

Ultrasound It can easily identify the Baker's cyst. The Baker's cyst develops between the medial head of the gastrocnemius and the semimembranosus tendon, and a slit-like communication stalk is noted between the base of the Baker's cyst and the knee joint (Fig. 44.7). Popliteal aneurysm may resemble Baker's cyst, and Doppler can easily identify vascular characterization of the lesion which is important if the clinician is planning on an aspiration procedure.

MRI MRI is the gold standard for the identification of Baker's cyst, and it is able to not only define the cyst but also differentiate from other mass lesions (Fig. 44.7).

44.2.1.6 Treatment

Medical Management

Non-compressive, asymptomatic cysts could be observed. If the inflammatory condition within the knee joint could improve with NSAIDs or intra-articular treatments, the Baker's cyst fluid accumulation may reduce over time.

Procedures

Aspiration of the cyst may provide adequate pain relief for the patient. There is a chance of recurrence since the source of the fluid is intra-articular and would not be treated with simple aspiration. Medical or procedural treatment related to osteoarthritis of the knee or the meniscal pathology can result in less inflamed intra-articular space and less fluid excretion into the cyst. Most aspirations are combined with delivery of steroids as an anti-inflammatory agent. Sclerosing agents including dextrose, ethanol, and doxycycline (sclerosing agents) have been used as an injection option for Baker's cyst after aspiration, but further studies are needed to evaluate the safety and effectiveness.

Rehabilitation

Rehabilitation is focused on the primary knee disorder that has led to the development of Baker's cyst. This is often either knee OA or knee meniscal disease; therefore, rehabilitation should focus on appropriate exercise and modalities related to those two conditions which is covered in Chaps. 43 and 53.

Surgery

Open and endoscopic surgical techniques are available for Baker's cyst resection. Surgeries in the knee are discussed in Chap. 46.

44.2.2 Plantaris Injury

S. Ali Mostoufi

44.2.2.1 ICD 10 code

S86.802, S86.801

44.2.2.2 Description

Plantaris is a small fusiform muscle of the superficial posterior leg, located between the popliteus and the lateral head of the gastrocnemius muscles, which can be absent in 10–20% of individuals [42]. It has traditionally been of most interest to surgeons as a donor site, with its tendon often being used as a graft for other tendon injuries including Achilles rupture. It is thin (<5 mm) and long (approximately 5 inches). It

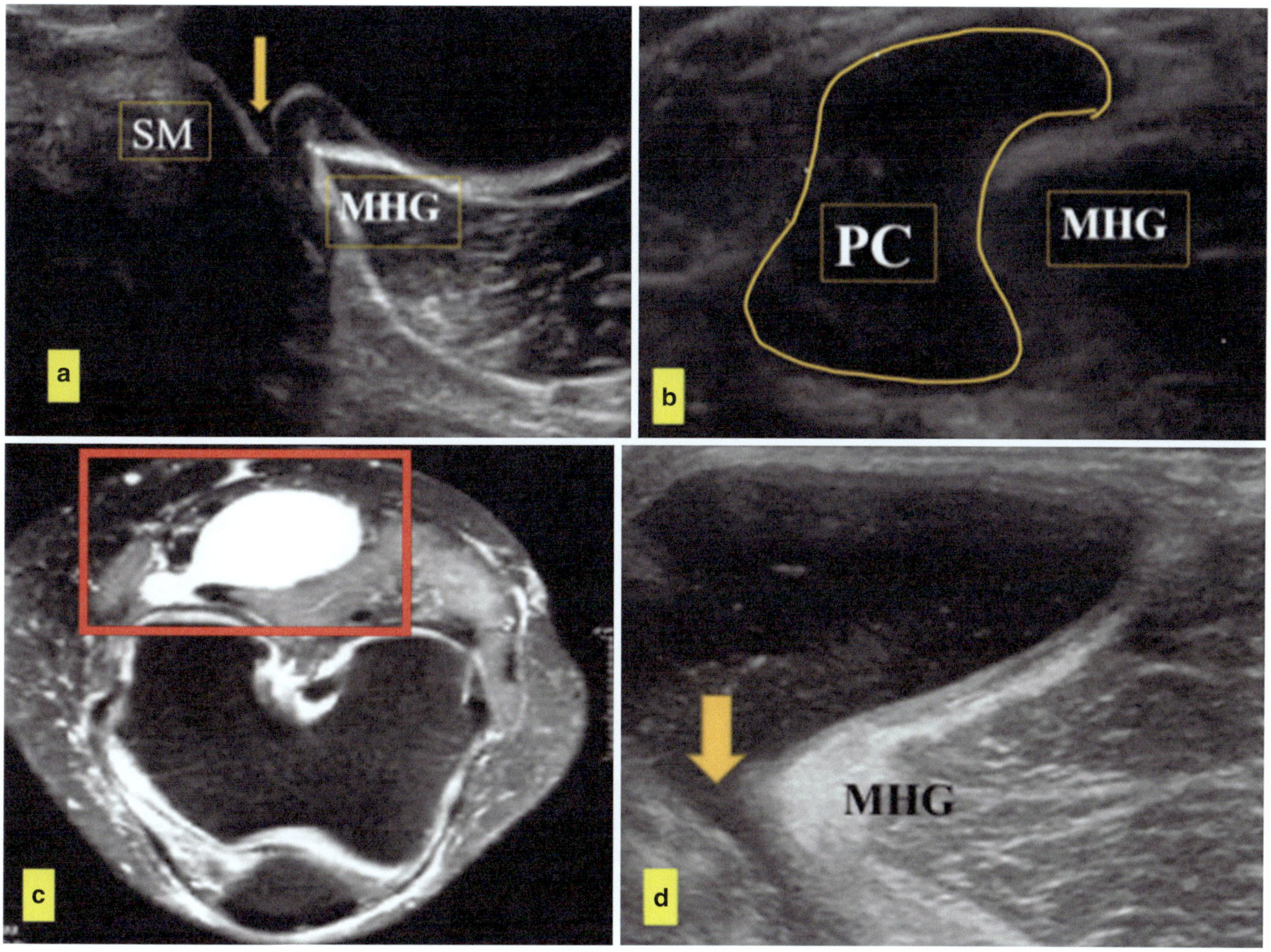

Fig. 44.7 The communication stock between the semimembranosus (SM) tendon and medial head of gastrocnemius (MHG) is highlighted by the arrows (**a** and **d**). Image (**b**) is a transverse US image showing a C-shaped popliteal cyst (PC) wrapped around the medial head of the gastrocnemius muscle. Image **c** shows T2 weighted image of a knee and a popliteal cyst is highlighted (**a** and **b** are from the author's library. Images (**c**) and (**d**) are courtesy of Keneth Mautner MD)

originates from the lateral supracondylar ridge of the femur and inserts into the posterior calcaneus (Fig. 44.8) through the calcaneal tendon (runs medial to the Achilles tendon) [42]. Plantaris assists with plantarflexion of the ankle and knee flexion. Injury to this structure occurs most frequently during running or jumping and usually results from an eccentric load placed across the ankle with the knee in an extended position [42]. It is not very common to have an isolated plantaris muscle injury as it is often associated with an injury to the medial head of the gastrocnemius and soleus [43]. There is potential relationship between the plantaris tendon injury and the development of Achilles tendinopathy [44].

44.2.2.3 Presentation

Posterior knee pain is the presenting symptom. Athletes report an incident in which they feel as if the posterior calf was struck by an object. Passive dorsiflexion and resisted plantarflexion elicit severe pain. Swelling in the region of the posterior knee and ankle and foot may be experienced by athletes. In most cases, pain becomes less severe after a few days of rest.

44.2.2.4 Examination

Inspection The posterior knee and posterior calf should be inspected for any bruising, swelling, and redness after injury. The Achilles tendon should be examined for any retraction or gapping. The distal hamstring muscle and its tendon should be examined for signs of injury.

Palpation The plantaris may be palpated in the popliteal fossa medial and superior to the lateral head of the gastrocnemius muscle. The tendon may be palpable at its distal calcaneal insertion with associated swelling as well as pain on passive dorsiflexion or resisted plantarflexion. In the popli-

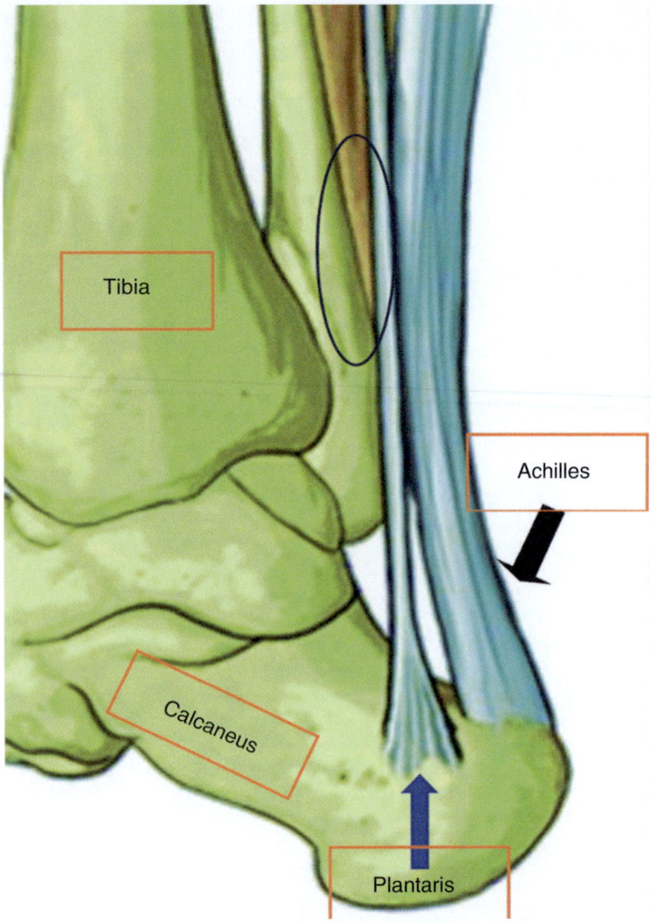

Fig. 44.8 Insertional relationship of plantaris and Achilles tendon. The circle highlights myotendinous junction which is the most common anatomic site for plantaris injury. (Adopted and modified from Dos Santos MA, Bertelli JA, Kechele PR, Duarte H. Anatomical study of the plantaris tendon: reliability as a tendo-osseous graft. Surg Radiol Anat. 2009 Jan;31)

teal fossa, any palpable masses should be noted, which may lead to other diagnoses such as Baker's cyst, soft tissue sarcoma, lipoma, and hematoma.

Musculoskeletal and Neurological Examination

A general musculoskeletal examination of the lower extremity including range of motion, strength, sensation, and reflexes should be conducted. Examination should also identify other pain generators that may be resembling injury to the plantaris muscle. Muscles and tendons of the posterior distal hamstring should be examined as well as the Achilles tendon. Plantaris pain may be elicited by passive dorsiflexion and resisted plantarflexion of the foot.

Special Test

The flexion compression test (Thomas test) clinically evaluates for Achilles' rupture which would present similarly to plantaris tear. Test is performed in prone, while both feet are just off the examination table. The examiner would compress the gastrocnemius muscle which should result in foot plantarflexion. If this test is negative, meaning that the Achilles tendon still flexes the foot, then the clinician would have a higher suspicion of the plantaris rupture.

44.2.2.5 Diagnostic Workup

Diagnosis is established by means of imaging with either an ultrasound or MRI. Although examination should focus on the plantaris, it should include evaluation of adjacent soft tissue and the knee joint as a differential diagnosis of plantaris.

Advanced imaging also can detect any abnormal mass, vascular abnormality, or potential infection in the region. The extent of the injury could be evaluated by MRI or ultrasound. MR finding includes abnormal T2 signal within the muscle at the myotendinous junction oriented toward the adjacent soft tissue [45]. Often complete plantaris rupture happens at the myotendinous junction with proximal retraction, and the muscle could be located in between popliteal tendons and the lateral head of the gastrocnemius muscle [42].

44.2.2.6 Treatment

Medial Management

The immediate treatment may include RICE (rest, ice, compression, elevation) and may include a brief period of immobilization. Medical management includes the use of NSAIDs for nociceptive pain, cryotherapy, and/or therapeutic ultrasound.

Rehabilitation

As with any other muscle injury, in the acute phase of injury, the objective is to prevent further damage, control inflammation, limit pain, and promote early mobilization. As the tissue heals and repairs, there is a degree of fibrosis and scarring that develops. It is important to proceed to an individualized strengthening, and proprioceptive rehabilitation. In terms of plantaris injury, there is no consensus on rehabilitation. Exercise programs should be gradual in progression. The initial phase includes stretching exercises, with progression to a strengthening program. The strengthening program first concentrates on antagonist muscles and then progresses to antagonist muscle (quadricep) [42].

Surgery

Isolated plantaris tendinopathy is almost always managed medically. In cases with thickened plantaris tendon adjacent to the medial aspect of the Achilles tendon with presentation of chronic painful mid-portion Achilles tendinopathy, removal of plantaris tendon and scraping of the ventral Achilles tendon have shown to be effective in symptom relief [46].

44.2.3 Posterolateral Corner Injuries

S. Ali Mostoufi

44.2.3.1 ICD 10 code

S89.90x, S89.91x, S89.92x

44.2.3.2 Description

Anatomy There are three layers of tissue in the lateral knee [47]. The iliotibial band and the biceps femoris are the most superficial. Beneath them, the patellar retinaculum and the patellofemoral ligament exist, and the deepest layer includes the lateral collateral ligament, fabellofibular ligament, the arcuate ligament, coronary ligament, popliteus tendon, the popliteofibular ligament, and finally the capsule of the knee joint (Fig. 44.9). The common fibular nerve lies between the first two superficial layers.

There are three major stabilizers of the lateral knee including the lateral collateral ligament (LCL), popliteus tendon, and popliteofibular ligament [47]. The LCL is the primary varus stabilizer of the knee and resists against the lateral stress on the knee joint [47, 48]. Other structures that contribute to lateral knee stability includes the capsule of the joint, arcuate ligament, fabellofibular ligament, the IT band, the lateral head of gastrocnemius, and the biceps femoris [48].

Injuries to the posterolateral corner (PLC) are traumatic injuries that are associated with lateral knee instability and usually present with a concomitant cruciate ligament injury, posterior cruciate being more common than anterior [49]. Among all the posterolateral injuries, 28% occurs in isolation, and if undiagnosed, it could lead to a failure in surgical outcome of ACL reconstruction surgery, which ultimately can lead to early degenerative changes of the joint [49, 50].

Etiology The most common mechanism of PLC injuries is a direct blow to the anteromedial knee [51], but hyperextension and noncontact varus stress can also injure the PLC [51]. Approximately 15–30% of injuries are associated with either vascular injuries or common peroneal nerve injury [48]. The Hughston and Fanelli grading for LCL instability has been used for diagnostic and therapeutic planning in PCL injuries (Table 44.4). A Hughston grade I is an FCL strain, grade II is a partial injury with moderate ligamentous

Table 44.4 Classification used for posterolateral corner instabilities [52]

Fanelli grading
Type A: 10° increase in external tibia rotation
Type B: 10° increase in external tibia rotation + slight varus relaxation 5–10 mm of the varus load test
Type C: 10° increase in external tibia rotation + severe valgus relaxation more than 10 mm on the valgus stress test
Hughston grading
Grade I: 0–5 mm gap in varus stress
Grade II: 6–10 mm gap in varus stress
Grade III: 10 mm or more gap in varus stress

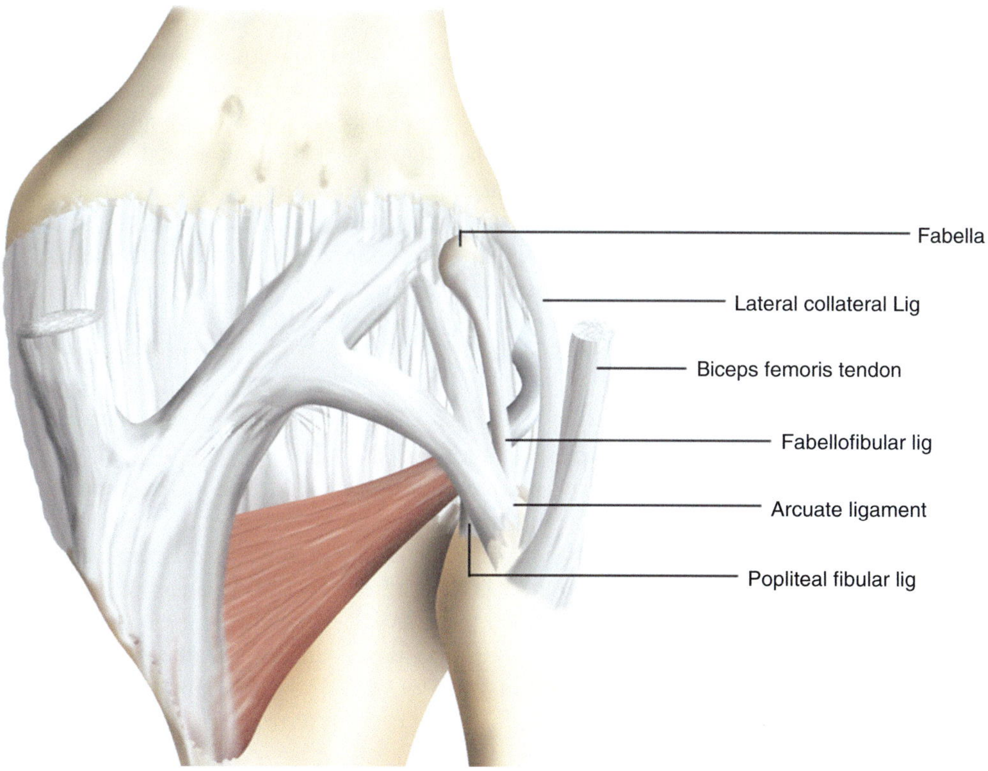

Fig. 44.9 The Posterolateral Ligamentous complex. (Creative Commons License. Case Courtesy of Assoc Prof Frank Gaillard, Radiopaedia.org, rID: 9330)

disruption, and grade III would be a full ligament disruption, resulting in measurable gap on varus stress of 10 mm or more [52].

44.2.3.3 Presentation

PLC injuries may present acutely or chronically with a history of sports injury, motor vehicle injury, or a fall [53]. Initially individuals may present with swelling and pain in the lateral and posterior aspect of the knee. If there is associated fibular nerve injury, sensory disturbance and ankle dorsiflexion weakness are also reported. Patients will note instability symptoms on weight bearing in extension during walking or on negotiating stairs [53]. In sports, athletes will report difficulty with pivoting and cutting [48, 53].

44.2.3.4 Examination

Focus examination of the knee includes examining all knee quadrants: the joint, tendon, and ligaments as discussed elsewhere in this chapter. On inspection, focal versus diffuse swelling, ecchymosis, tendon gaps, gait abnormality, ability to bear weight, and neurologic findings such as foot drop should be noted. Special tests can differentiate between injuries to the PLC as compared to other injuries to the knee.

Fibular Nerve Injury

As part of neuromuscular testing, the function of the peroneal nerve should be tested as this nerve traverses between the first and second layers. Injury to this nerve will result in altered sensation, pain, and ankle dorsiflexion weakness.

Special Tests

Varus Stress Test

Varus stress test (Fig. 44.18) is performed both in full extension and at 30° of flexion. The femur stabilized by the examiner with one hand which is also used to assess the amount of lateral compartment gapping. With his/her other hand, the examiner would hold the foot and ankle of the patient and apply a virus force. Lateral compartment gapping is tested in full extension and in 30° of flexion. Laxity of at 0° on varus stress indicates LCL and cruciate ligament injury. Lateral laxity of 30° indicates isolated LCL injury [48].

Dial Test

External rotation of the tibia relative to the femur is tested in the maneuver (Fig. 44.20). The dial test is performed on both knees at 30° and 90° of knee flexion with the subject in supine. The femur is fixed with one hand, while the ankle and foot are externally rotated. At 30°, if there is a 10° external rotation asymmetry, it is an isolated PLC injury. At 30° and 90° dial, if there is more than 10° external rotation asymmetry, likely both lateral collateral ligament and PLC are injured [48, 54].

Posterolateral Drawer Test

The posterolateral drawer test is performed when the hip is flexed at 45°, the knee is flexed at slightly less than 90°, and the foot is externally rotated at 10° to 15°. Combined posterior drawer and external rotation force when applied to the knee will result in posterior lateral translation and a positive test. This is due to lateral tibial externally rotating on the lateral femoral condyle [48, 54].

Reverse Pivot Shift Test

To perform this test, the patient should be supine with the knee flexed to near 90°. The knee joint line is palpated, a valgus load is applied through the knee, an external rotation force is applied to the tibia, and the knee is slowly extended. If the previously subluxated lateral tibial plateau reduces at approximately 35° to 40° of flexion, a clunk is noted, and this is a positive test. A positive reverse pivot shift has been reported to have a positive predictive value of 68% and a negative predictive value of 89%. A comparison to the contralateral knee is important as a positive test has been reported in 35% of uninjured knees [48, 54].

44.2.3.5 Diagnostic Imaging

Radiographs

Radiographs are used to rule out any fracture including fracture of the fibula or fracture of the femoral condyle. Both varus stress radiographs and standing long-leg AP radiographs are obtained.

Varus stress radiographs (bilateral varus stress XR in 20° flexion), in particular comparing side to side, can help to objectively determine the extent of the lateral and posterolateral knee injury [55]. Clinicians should suspect an isolated lateral collateral ligament injury if the opening on clinician-applied varus stress radiographs increases by approximately 2.7 mm (normal <1 mm) and a grade III posterolateral corner injury if values increase by approximately 4.0 mm.

Limb alignment and the weight-bearing axis should be evaluated using standing long-leg AP radiographs [48, 52].

MRI

It can identify the lateral collateral ligament, popliteus, and biceps tendon injuries, all of which contribute to the lateral stability of the knee.

44.2.3.6 Treatment

Nonoperative Care

Conservative care is indicated in mild grade I or isolated mid-substance grade II injury. Nonoperative management includes knee immobilization for 4 weeks and a rehabilitation program to follow [56]. Functional rehab includes quad strengthening [56]. In successful cases, athletes may return to training 2–3 months after injury.

Postoperative rehabilitation [57]: Patients will be non-weight-bearing for the first 6 weeks while in a knee immobilizer that can be removed for the range of motion exercises and hygiene. Physical therapy begins on postoperative day 1 which includes patient education, symptom management, knee motion, and quadriceps muscle activation. Knee flexion ROM is limited to 90° for the first 2 weeks and then is progressed gradually until full knee flexion is recovered. Hyperextension should be avoided, and patellofemoral joint mobilizations, peripatellar soft tissue mobilizations, and frequent quadriceps contractions should be incorporated to reduce postoperative stiffness.

Operative Care

Complete PLC lesions rarely heal with nonoperative treatment and are therefore treated surgically. Poor functional outcomes for nonoperatively treated grade III PLC injuries with persistent instability and degenerative changes have been reported [40, 58].

Generally, surgery would include direct PLC repair for isolated grade PLC tear with or without avulsion injuries. For higher grade tears, PLC hybrid reconstruction and repair may be suggested. If there are concomitant cruciate ligaments injuries, both PLC and cruciate ligament reconstruction are performed, and in select cases, valgus high tibial osteotomy is performed to correct bony alignment and to assure sustainable success of ACL and PCL reconstruction [40, 58]. For more details regarding surgery, please see Chap. 46.

44.2.4 Distal Hamstring Injuries

S. Ali Mostoufi

44.2.4.1 Description

Anatomy The semitendinosus, biceps femoris and the semimembranosus are the three muscles of the hamstring. The short head of the biceps originates from the lateral lip of the linea aspera and extends to the fibular head and the lateral condyle of the tibia. The long head of biceps femoris, semimembranosus, and semitendinosus all originate from ischial tuberosity. The long head of the biceps femoris has the same insertion with the short head of the biceps femoris. The semitendinosus inserts in the pes anserine location of the tibia, and the semimembranosus inserts into the medial tibial condyle. The long head of the biceps and the semitendinosus muscle have a common aponeurosis starting from the ischial tuberosity which extends a few inches below. The tibial nerve innervates the semimembranosus, semitendinosus, and long head of the biceps femoris, and the common peroneal branch of the sciatic nerve innervates the short head of the biceps femoris [59]. The hamstring muscles border the popliteal fossa, the distal biceps being lateral, and the semimembranosus and semitendinosus border is medial. The hamstring group functions as hip extenders as well as knee flexors [59].

Hamstring injuries peak at 16–25 years of age, and it is commonly related to sports where the hamstrings bear the most burden, with a rapid transition of its functional biomechanics at high speed like sprinting, soccer, football, track, and field sports [60, 61]. It can occur in elite and recreational athletes as well as weekend warriors. In addition to being highly prevalent, hamstring injuries are often slow healing and tend to recur, about 1/3 during the first year after the first injury [62]. From the statistical standpoint, the most common muscle in the hamstring group subjective to injury is the biceps femoris, followed by the semimembranosus and then the semitendinosus. Hamstring injury can be classified as a grade I (mild), grade II (moderate), and grade III (severe) (Table 44.5) [59].

Evidence suggests that right-left strength imbalances increase the likelihood of strains and sprains in the lower extremity. Furthermore, the contribution of factors such as flexibility, prior injury, joint laxity, and overall conditioning of the athlete may increase the risk of such injuries [63]. A ratio of at least 50–65% for hamstring strength compared with quadriceps strength is recommended to decrease the chance of sustaining a hamstring strain [64]. Identifying weakness in the hamstring muscles may allow the prediction of risk for muscle strain and allow a rehabilitation program to correct the problem before injury occurs [65].

44.2.4.2 Presentation

Pain in the posterior knee and distal hamstring is the main symptom, and the athlete may report a popping sound at the time of injury. A history of inadequate warmup or fatigue may be elicited from the patient. Another common scenario is for the athlete to feel tightness or an impending "pull" in the muscle during exercise and subsequently limit participation [60]. Difficulty with weight-bearing, antalgic gait, local swelling, and ecchymosis can be among presenting signs and symptoms.

44.2.4.3 Examination

In an acute event, examination is conducted at the athletic field. The athlete may grab the back of the thigh at the place

Table 44.5 Grading system for hamstring strain injuries

Grade I: Minimal disruption to the hamstring muscle fibers	Minimal pain, minimal functional impairment
Grade II: Partial-thickness tear, myotendinous junction	Moderate pain, loss of strength
Grade III: Full-thickness tear of the hamstring muscle or tendon	Severe pain, hematoma, significant loss of strength

of competition. There may be tenderness and palpable induration immediately after the injury particularly with complete tear. Ecchymosis and swelling are often present. The clinician should examine the hamstring tendon both in relaxed and mild tension. Given the anatomy of the region, it is possible that the significant defect is not palpated despite its presence. Examination for concurrent injuries in the lower extremity and spine and neurovascular structures should be conducted.

In an outpatient basis with milder hamstring injury, physical examination includes examination of the spine and neurovascular structures, as well as lower extremity muscles, tendons, hamstring muscles, and knee/hip joint examination. At the time of examination, strength and the range of motion of the affected hamstring should be tested and compared with those on the unaffected side. Ideally, the patient should be prone and the affected hip positioned at 0° of extension; then, knee flexion is assessed with resistance applied at the heel, the knee being in 15°, and 90° of flexion. Pain or weakness appreciated during the examination is considered a positive finding [61]. Hip flexion and knee extension should be examined, which may be limited by pain in patients with a hamstring injury [59].

Special Test

Straight leg raise testing should be performed, and the position of maximum tolerance should be noted which is a useful guide to the severity of the injury.

44.2.4.4 Workup

There is limited utility for X-rays, but radiographs can detect avulsion injuries or fractures. MRI would be a diagnostic test of choice which highlights high signal intensity abnormality on T2 weighted images pointing to edema or hemorrhage within the surrounding tissues or the hamstring muscles/tendon [59]. Ultrasonography could be performed at the sideline or in an outpatient clinic as a diagnostic tool for hamstring tendinopathy. Ultrasound allows dynamic assessment of the injured hamstring muscles, and any edema or hemorrhage is depicted by the echotexture on the ultrasound.

44.2.4.5 Treatment

Nonoperative Care

In the acute setting, crutches may be warranted for the more severe grade II and grade III hamstring strains. As with other injuries, rest, ice, compression, and elevation are still the preferred first aid in managing acute pain. Although the use of NSAIDs for the first 5–7 days is acceptable, a study by Almekinders et al. demonstrated that prolonged NSAIDS may interfere with repair and remodeling of regenerative muscle; therefore, it should be discontinued soon after [66]. Pivotal considerations in the regenerative process of the injured muscle are the quantity and quality of fibrous scar formation. The interaction between these two processes of muscle regeneration and fibrosis characterizes the effectiveness of the remodeling phase of muscle injury. Complete immobilization is not recommended as it will results in muscle atrophy and loss of flexibility and strength. Järvinen and Lehto studied and demonstrated that a short period of immobilization (5–7 days) is advantageous in limiting the extent of connective tissue proliferation at the site of injury [67].

Rehabilitation

A rehabilitation program that encompasses progressive agility and stabilization of the trunk exercises are more effective than a program emphasizing the isolated hamstring muscle [61]. A randomized controlled study in Swedish elite athletes with hamstring injuries found that a rehabilitation protocol emphasizing lengthening type of exercises is more effective than a protocol containing conventional exercises in promoting the time to return to sports [68]. Loss of flexibility is a characteristic feature of hamstring strains, and as part of rehabilitation, early stretching exercises should begin with gentle active stretching and progress to passive static stretching as the pain allows. Concurrent pain-free stretching exercises as well as strengthening exercises progressing from isometrics to isotonic and isokinetic are essential in regaining flexibility and strength in the hamstring muscle group [60]. The swimming pool and the stationary bike can also be useful in the early stage of rehabilitation because they allow pain-free motion and controlled resistance exercise. Once the muscle strength imbalance (hamstring-to-quadriceps ratio) has been corrected, the patient can return to play. It is acceptable to have a 10% difference between the injured and uninjured leg strength and nonoperative care [60].

Surgery

Indication for surgical procedure is complete rupture at origin or insertion of the hamstring muscle, bony avulsion with displacement of 2 cm or more. For more information on surgical treatments, please see Chap. 46.

44.3 Medial Knee Disorders

44.3.1 Pes Anserine Tendinopathy and Bursitis

S. Ali Mostoufi

44.3.1.1 ICD 10 code

M70.50

44.3.1.2 Description

The pes anserine bursa is located in between the proximal medial tibia and the insertion point of the semitendinosus, gracilis, and sartorius tendons (Fig. 44.10). Pes anserine bursitis is a clinical diagnosis associated with pain at the medial knee just below the joint line. Mechanical derangement, direct trauma, increased knee Q angle, obesity, and overuse have all been implicated in the development of pes anserine bursitis [69]. The association of pes anserine pain (but not necessarily bursitis) with concomitant osteoarthritis was noted in one study to be over 90% [70].

44.3.1.3 Clinical Presentation

Patients normally present with medial knee pain, just distal to the joint line, which is aggravated upon climbing stairs. In most cases they can put a finger on the exact location of the pain which should topographically correlate with pes anserine location.

44.3.1.4 Physical Examination

Full lower extremity exam and spine examination should be performed. Any abnormality in gait should be noted. Typical examination of the knee includes inspection, observation for edema, or skin changes. If there is associated osteoarthritis of the knee, swelling around the knee joint capsule and around the bursa may be visible to the naked eye. On palpation, the examiner will palpate the region of the pes anserine, medial joint capsule, and also posterior knee for fullness or masses. Concordant tenderness is noted at the pes anserine bursa with palpation. To rule out other associated knee disorders, typical knee examination should include range of motion, medial instability testing, lateral instability testing, testing for ACL and PCL injuries, and examination of the patella and patellar tendon.

44.3.1.5 Diagnostic Workup

Plain films Pes anserine bursitis (PAB) is a clinical diagnosis but could be confirmed with diagnostic ultrasound. Plain films are the initial imaging modality of PAB, identifying underlying bony abnormalities, including osteoarthritis.

MRI Advanced imaging including MRI is not necessary for PAB but could assist with identifying conditions that can be misdiagnosed as PAB including meniscal pathology, tendon pathology, medial collateral ligament pathology, and ACL and PCL tear. If pes anserine bursitis is noted on the MRI, it would be in a form of a fluid collection distal to the joint line and superficial to the medial collateral ligament, deep into the sartorius, gracilis, and semitendinosus.

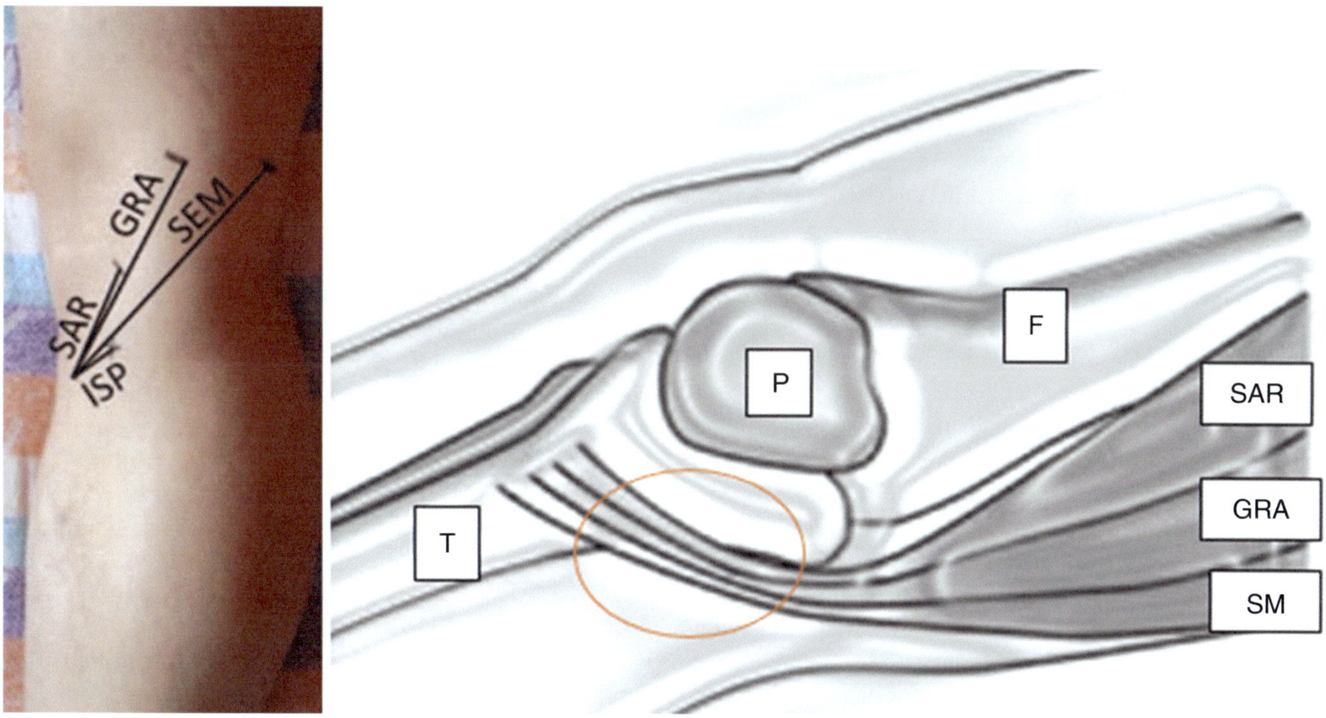

Fig. 44.10 Approximate path of the three muscles forming the pes anserine complex as it relates to the medial knee. The illustration demonstrates three muscles of sartorius, gracilis, and sartorius tendon joining to attach to the medial tibia. The circle is the location of the pes anserine bursa deep to the tendon. (Open source image from Zhong, Sheng et al. "The anatomical and imaging study of pes anserinus and its clinical application." Medicine vol. 97,152,018. Illustration by Yasmine Mostoufi)

Ultrasound In skilled hands, the bursa and insertional site for the muscles can be examined for signs of true bursitis including enlargement of a bursa, with an increased amount of anechoic fluid within it and an increased vascularity on Doppler. In chronic cases, thickening of the hyperechoic synovial wall may be seen.

44.3.1.6 Treatment

Medical Treatment
Most patients may be treated conservatively with oral NSAIDs, topical NSAIDs, and neoprene sleeve support and by avoiding activities that may aggravate the condition. Patients often benefit from local ice and leg elevation in the acute phase. For long-term improvement, recommendation on weight loss is appropriate.

Rehabilitation
Physical therapy is often prescribed by practitioners to work on muscle strengthening, range of motion restoration, gait training, soft tissue treatments, and transcutaneous electrical nerve stimulation (TENS) with goals of improvement of function. In terms of strengthening, quadriceps muscle groups and adductors of the thigh should be among the muscles targeted for strengthening.

Procedures

Injections
Injecting the pes anserine bursa could have diagnostic or therapeutic value. Diagnostic injection is performed as a way of identifying the exact source of medial knee pain. Therapeutic injections contain corticosteroid or platelet-rich plasma (PRP).

Lidocaine injection: Ultrasound-guided diagnostic pes anserine injection with small volume of anesthetics can help identify the source of medial knee pain. Pain relief for the half-life of anesthetic used can confirm pes anserine as a source of pain.

Steroid injection: In those cases that less aggressive treatment has not helped, ultrasound-guided bursa injection with corticosteroid could be considered. The procedure is done with ultrasonography to accurately place the needle in the plane of the bursa and not to inject any of the tendons. A study was performed to compare the effect of the physical therapy on pes anserine bursitis versus steroid injection without any PT. Both groups had significant improvement in all metrics tested, and there were no significant differences detected between the groups. In this study, pain relief was quicker in the steroid group due to known properties of the injectate [71].

PRP injection: Since the growth of regenerative medicine in musculoskeletal care, some practitioners provide patients with PRP injection instead of steroids. There is no structured study on the effectiveness of PRP specific to this condition.

Shockwave Therapy
SWT should also be considered in patients with pes anserine bursitis along with other rehabilitation efforts. A randomized clinical control trial comparing shockwave therapy to a sham treatment demonstrated positive effect for both pain relief and function in patients with pes anserine bursitis [72].

Surgery
Surgical procedures are often not necessary. In cases of calcific tendinitis, percutaneous ultrasound-guided debridement may be offered.

44.3.2 Medial Collateral Ligament Injury

S. Ali Mostoufi

44.3.2.1 ICD 10 code
S83.419, S83.412

44.3.2.2 Description
Anatomy: The anatomy of the medial knee could be thought of as three separate layers [73]. The superficial layer contains the skin, subcutaneous tissue and sartorius, and part of the patellar retinaculum. The middle layer consisted of semimembranosus and superficial fibers of the medial collateral ligament (MCL), the medial patellofemoral ligament, and part of the posterior oblique ligament. The deep layer includes most of the MCL fibers, posterior medial capsule, and the meniscotibial ligament (Fig. 44.10) [74].

Ligamentous injuries of the knees are approximately 40% of all the knee injuries of which medial collateral ligament is the most common [74]. MCL is a flat connective tissue, connecting the medial condyle of the tibia to the epicondyle of the femur, providing a valgus stability to the knee (Fig. 44.11). Injury often relates to sports in particular those with tackling. The medial collateral ligament (MCL) is commonly injured during an ACL rupture [75]. Approximately 78% of grade III MCL injuries consist of mixed ligamentous lesions, with an injury to the ACL occurring more than 95% of the time [75].

44.3.2.3 Clinical Presentation
Patients often point toward the area of pain and may also report a popping sensation at the time of injury. Although possible, this injury is not always associated with instability, and this may not be a presenting symptom. If the injury was related to a valgus force to the knee, ecchymosis of the skin may be noted both on the lateral knee (as a result of direct blow) and the medial knee (due to MCL injury). Particularly

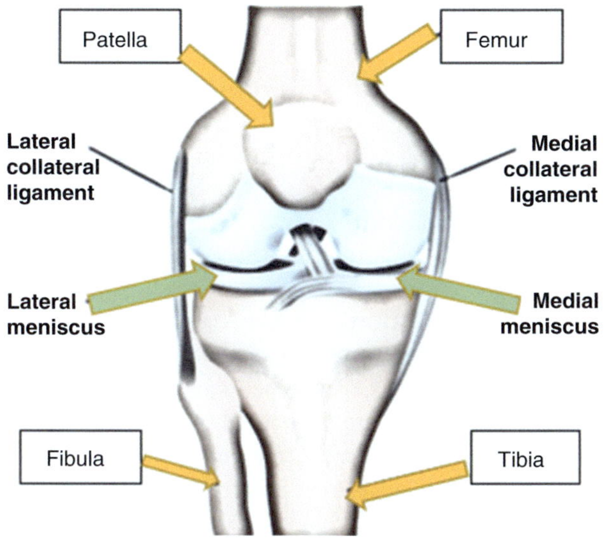

Fig. 44.11 The knee joint in an AP view identified the medial collateral ligament and lateral collateral ligament providing medial and lateral stability of the joint. (Original Illustration from Yorkshire knee clinic, modified by Yasmine Mostoufi)

Table 44.6 Differential diagnosis of medial knee pain

Pes anserine bursitis
Medial collateral ligament injury
Medial meniscus tear
Knee OA
Adductor tendinopathy
Lumbar radicular
ACL tear

when there is an ACL tear, or meniscal injury, there may be significant swelling and effusion. In an isolated MCL tear, weight-bearing may not be an issue, but when combined with ACL and meniscal tear, the patient is often antalgic. Palpation of medial joint space would be associated with reproduction of pain, anywhere from the joint line to the insertion to the tibia. Differential diagnosis of medial knee pain is in Table 44.6.

44.3.2.4 Examination

Inspection may demonstrate ecchymosis on the medial and lateral aspect of the knee (lateral due to direct helmet to knee contact). Swelling, soft tissue tenderness, and antalgic gait could be associated particularly when there is concomitant ACL and meniscal injury. Patients will complain about medial knee pain and may point to the location of the MCL. Complete knee evaluation should be performed to identify any associated injuries including testing for instability, testing for meniscal pathology, and a full neurological/musculoskeletal lower extremity exam. Spine is examined if referred pain is suspected.

Specialized Testing

MCL valgus stress test It will test the integrity of the MCL on valgus stress. It is performed with 30° knee flexion followed by a valgus force to the knee with the opposite hand, identifying any laxity. This would reproduce concordant pain and a sense of instability on testing. If medial laxity is found on examination when the knee is in full extension, it may point toward a more extensive injury potentially combined with cruciate ligament involvement [76].

44.3.2.5 Diagnostic Workup

Diagnosis of the MCL could be done clinically. Before MRI, the gold standard diagnostic tool was arthroscopy or surgical exploration [74]. Combining history, physical exam, ultrasonography, and MRI, most MCL could be diagnosed and effectively treated.

X-rays It is likely to be the first diagnostics modality in most knee pain including MCL. Occult fractures, avulsion fractures, and ossification emphysema are noted on X-ray. Stress radiographs can be performed to help with diagnosis.

MRI It is an excellent tool in detecting isolated MCL tears or MCL tear in association with ACL or meniscus tear. MRI is highly sensitive in detecting meniscal injury (91% lateral meniscus, 80.8% medial meniscus), and it is also specific (79% lateral meniscus, 85% medial meniscus) [77].

Ultrasound It is a fast, reliable, and relatively inexpensive modality that could be used both at sideline and in clinic which is able to identify MCL tears with high sensitivity up to 94% [78].

44.3.2.6 Treatment

Medical Management

Treatment of the MCL tear depends on the grade of injury (Table 44.7). For grade I or II, initial treatment includes use of NSAIDs to control pain and swelling, brace to avoid valgus stress to the knee (functional hinged knee brace), use of crutches immediately after the injury, and eventually partici-

Table 44.7 Grading of MCL injury [55, 56]

MCL injury grading
Grade I: Medial knee pain along the MCL with valgus stress
Mild injury, minor tear without loss of integrity of the MCL
Grade II: Medial knee pain along MCL + slight joint opening with firm endpoint
Moderate injury, incomplete tear, increased MCL laxity
Grade III: Medial knee pain along the MCL, significant joint space opening, no endpoint
Severe injury, complete tear, gross MCL laxity of MCL

pation in rehabilitation. Early return to sports is likely in grades I and II based on a study of high school football players who returned to sports on an average of 10.6 days for grade I and 19.5 days for grade II after MCL injury [79]. The most clinically significant complication of an MCL tear is the recurrence of injury [74].

Bracing It is not required for grade I injury, but grade II and grade III require functional hinged knee brace for up to 6 weeks [80].

Rehabilitation

Early initiation of range of motion exercises is encouraged particularly in grades I and II injuries. Prolonged immobilization without range of motion exercises may result in collagen degradation of the MCL and bone resorption at the insertion point of the ligament [80]. MCL grade I injuries can immediately proceed to early ROM rehab exercises. Grade II MCL injuries are placed in a protective brace but full ROM is allowed. Walking with the brace locked in full extension is allowed and is continued until the extension lag is improved. Physical therapy exercises include straight leg raise, quadriceps sets, and patellar mobilization. Closed kinetic chain exercises could be started after full weight-bearing is allowed [80].

Procedures

There is no indication for steroid injection in the setting of the tear. Clinicians may consider PRP or prolotherapy instead of steroids. There are limited studies on the efficacy of such regenerative treatments and MCL tears. In a study of effectiveness of PRP in MCL grade III tears, leukocyte-rich PRP injection in isolated MCL tear is found to be beneficial particularly when combined with rehabilitation [81].

Another study was done regarding the utility of intra-articular PRP injection in patients with refractory low-grade MCL injury. That particular study found an improvement in pain but also improvement/healing of the MCL tear in a 6-month posttreatment using MRI [82].

Surgery

Grade III injuries may lead to surgical correction particularly in athletes with return to play goal in which medial knee medial knee stability and rotational stability are crucial. Most of the grade III injuries are associated with ACL tears, requiring surgery. Surgical care requires reconstruction using allograft and autograft, and further detail could be reviewed in the "Knee Surgeries" chapter. Postoperative bracing locked a 30° flexion with touchdown weight-bearing for 3–4 weeks is recommended [78].

44.4 Lateral Knee Disorders

44.4.1 Iliotibial Band Syndrome

Michael F. Saulle, Charles Scott and Joseph Chin

44.4.1.1 ICD 10 code

M76.31, M76.32

44.4.1.2 Description

Iliotibial band (IT band) syndrome is a lateral knee condition frequently exacerbated with repetitive physical activities, such as running or cycling. Proximally, the tensor fascia lata (TFL) and gluteus maximus merge, providing fascial contributions to the IT band. At the mid-thigh, it associates with the linea aspera via the lateral intermuscular septum. Distally, it connects to the lateral femoral epicondyle with fibrous bands and inserts onto the patella and tibia at Gerdy's tubercle. The commonly held notion that repeated knee flexion and extension lead to IT band friction across the lateral femoral epicondyle at 30° of flexion (zone of impingement) has not been supported by anatomic studies [83, 84]. Rather, IT band movement around the lateral femoral epicondyle is restricted by fibrous bands. Altered tension of the TFL and hip musculature may compress the IT band around the lateral femoral epicondyle, resulting in compressive forces against the highly innervated deep fat pad as a source of pain [85]. Poor proximal hip control, genu valgus, and compromised rearfoot alignment all likely contribute to the altered biomechanics. Reduced hip control results in increased tibial internal rotation. As a result, the IT band distal attachment is moved more medially, augmenting compressive forces around the lateral femoral epicondyle. Gluteus medius weakness leads to increased thigh adduction, internal rotation, and increased valgus vector at the knee. This places the IT band under tension and may contribute to the compression of the lateral femoral epicondyle during foot contact when maximal deceleration occurs to absorb ground reaction force [86]. The differential diagnosis for IT band syndrome includes injury to the lateral collateral ligament, lateral compartment osteoarthritis, lateral meniscus injury, and posterolateral corner injuries and instability. Unlike a lateral collateral ligament injury which may present acutely after an injury, IT ban syndrome may present with increased volume in aerobic training. Differential diagnosis of lateral knee pain is in Table 44.8.

44.4.1.3 Clinical Presentation

IT band syndrome is associated with lateral knee pain and commonly occurs in cyclists, runners, and military recruits who run on cambered surfaces, down hills, or recently have increased their aerobic training volume [86, 87]. Patients may also complain of "crunching" at the lateral knee when using stairs or pedaling bicycles. While typically associated with physical activity, in later stages, pain may also occur even at rest.

44.4.1.4 Physical Examination

Observe for varus or valgus knee alignment when standing. Tenderness and/or crepitus may be palpable over the lateral epicondyle 2–3 cm proximal to the lateral joint line as the knee is passively ranged, in particular near 30° of flexion. Manual testing of hip abductor strength is helpful to assess neuromuscular control.

The Ober's test (Fig. 44.12) may be used to test for shortening of the TFL or gluteus maximus. The test is performed beginning with the patient lying on the unaffected side with hip and knee flexed 90°. The examiner then abducts and extends the affected leg while stabilizing the pelvis, and the thigh is then allowed to passively adduct. IT band tightness is minimal when adducted past horizontal, moderate when adducted to horizontal, and maximal if unable to adduct even to horizontal [84, 88].

Table 44.8 Differential diagnosis of lateral knee pain

Bicep femoris tear
Sprain or tear of the lateral collateral ligament
Sprain or tear of posterior cruciate ligament
Posterolateral corner injury
Lateral meniscus tear
Lateral compartment osteoarthritis

The Noble compression test may elicit pain at the LFC. When the patient is lying on his or her side, flex the knee to 90° on the affected side and apply pressure to the IT band over the LFC and extend the knee. The test is positive when the knee approaches 30° of flexion [87].

The modified Thomas test (Fig. 44.12) assesses the flexibility of the hip flexor group and may provide additional information about hip abductor and IT band tension. To perform this test, the patient lies supine with both knees maximally flexed to flatten the low back against the examination table. While holding the unaffected leg in hip and knee flexion, the affected leg is lowered, and the angle of hip flexion is observed. The test is positive when the patient is unable to maintain the lower back and sacrum against the table, maintain the hip in neutral, or if the hip remains in any degree of flexion [86]. Abduction of the hip in the terminal position is suggestive of TFL and IT band tension.

44.4.1.5 Diagnostic Workup

Knee radiographs (AP, lateral, and sunrise) may be used to rule out other causes of lateral knee pain but will not have specific findings for ITB syndrome. Diagnostic ultrasound may show thickening of the affected portion of the ITB (Fig. 44.13), while high-intensity signal can often be seen deep to the ITB on fluid-sensitive MRI sequences [84].

44.4.1.6 Treatments

Medical Management

Relative rest from contributory activities is recommended until pain resolution. Intermittent ice, NSAIDs, and targeted

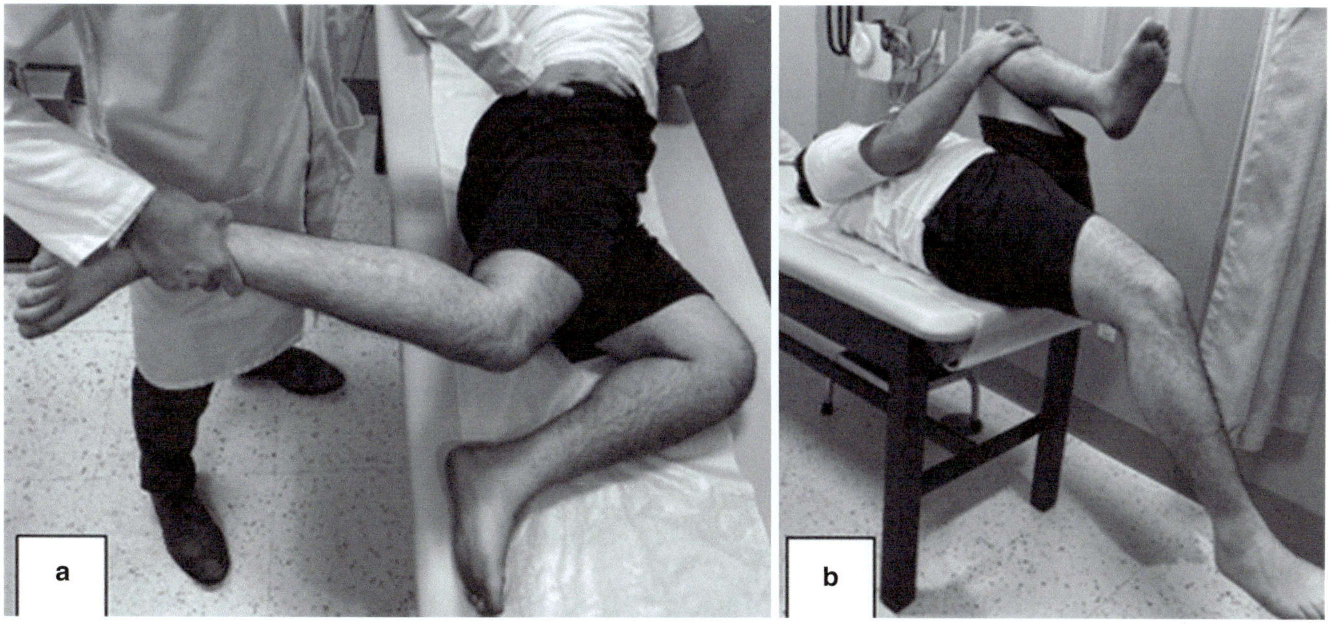

Fig. 44.12 Ober's test (**a**) and modified Thomas test (**b**). (Images from author's library)

corticosteroid injection may also provide relief from pain. Biomechanics should be addressed with shoe modifications, foot orthoses, and technical training. Graded return to activity is appropriate once pain has resolved, usually within 6–8 weeks of conservative treatment [85]. This may include a 6-week progressive running protocol, increasing frequency and intensity after 3–4 weeks and gradually adding hills/cambers if symptom-free while running on flat surfaces.

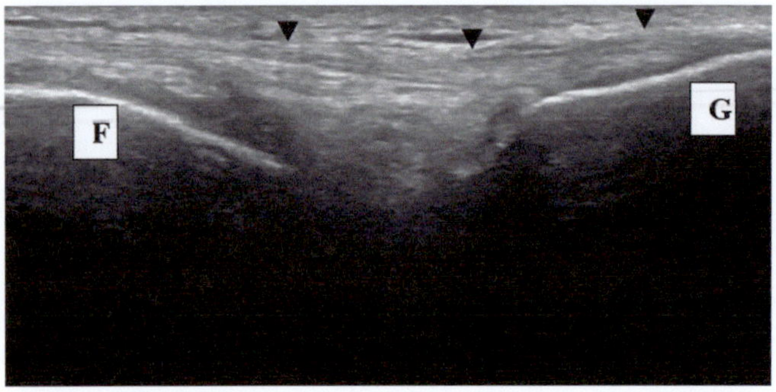

Fig. 44.13 This coronal image shows the iliotibial band (black arrowheads), distal femur (F), and Gerdy's tubercle (G). (Images from author's library)

Rehabilitation

A rehabilitation program will focus on posture, biomechanics, neuromuscular control, and focused stretching of the TFL and IT band. The standing IT band stretch (Fig. 44.14) can be performed by adducting and extending the symptomatic leg across the uninvolved leg. The trunk is then flexed to the opposite side until the stretch is felt. This can be performed with the arms overhead, at the side, or diagonally downward [87]. Foam rolling and deep tissue massage are used to address adhesions. Strengthening of hip abductors may involve concentric side-lying leg lifts (Fig. 44.15), single-leg balance, step-downs, and pelvic drop (Fig. 44.16) exercises. Additional, eccentric, multi-planar exercises include the modified matrix (Fig. 44.17), wallbangers, and frontal plane lunges [87]. Rehabilitation-based conservative treatment of IT band in runners has been demonstrated to be effective with return to pain-free running in approximately 6 weeks [86].

Procedures

Corticosteroids injected deep to the ITB at the lateral femoral condyle can reduce inflammation and pain to facilitate

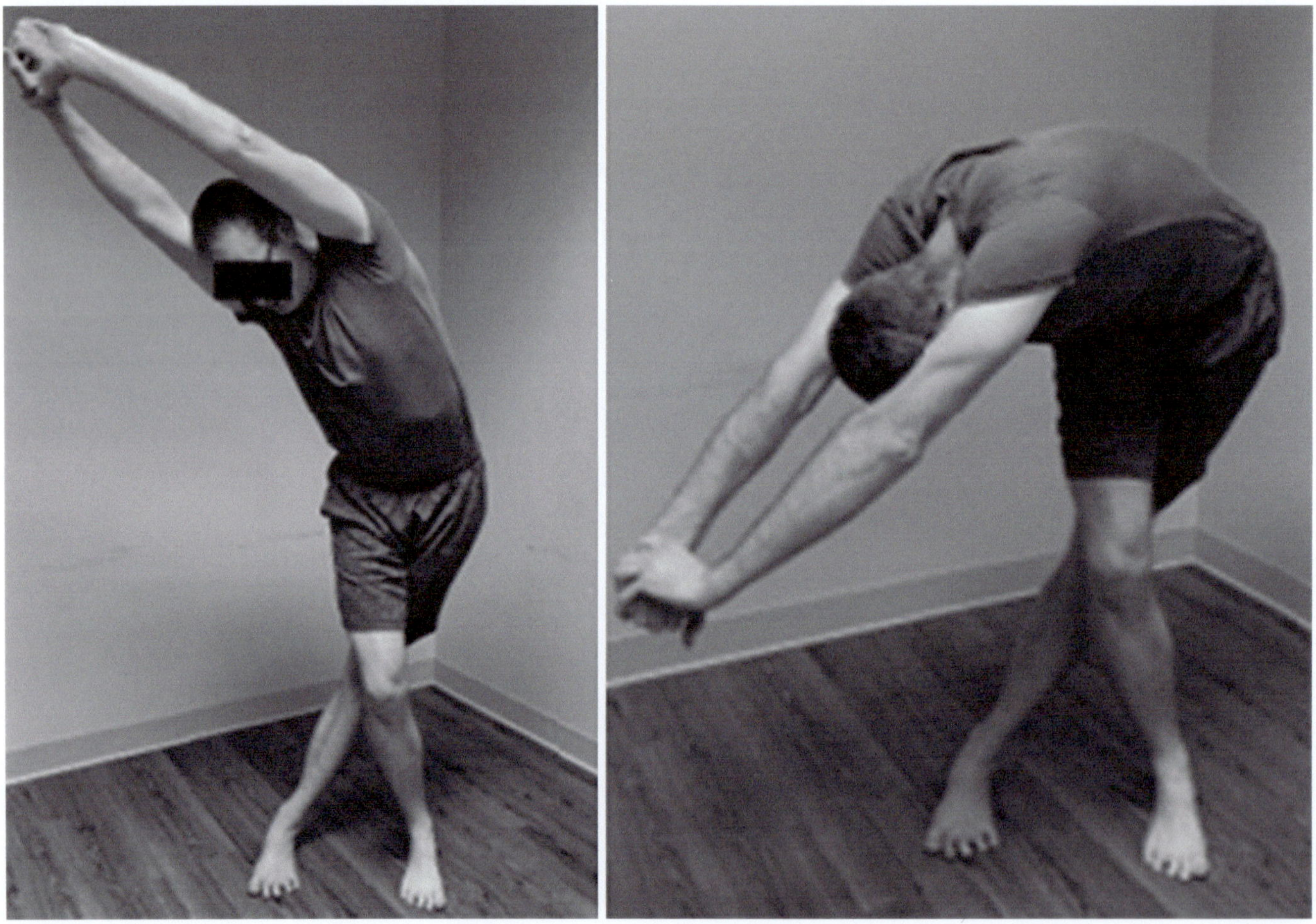

Fig. 44.14 ITB stretch. (Images from author's library)

participation in rehabilitation. Trigger point injection and dry needling of the gluteus maximus and gluteus medius have also been used [85].

Surgery

The surgical release of ITB may be considered if conservative management fails. Options include percutaneous ITB release, Z-plasty, ITB bursectomy, and arthroscopic ITB debridement [85].

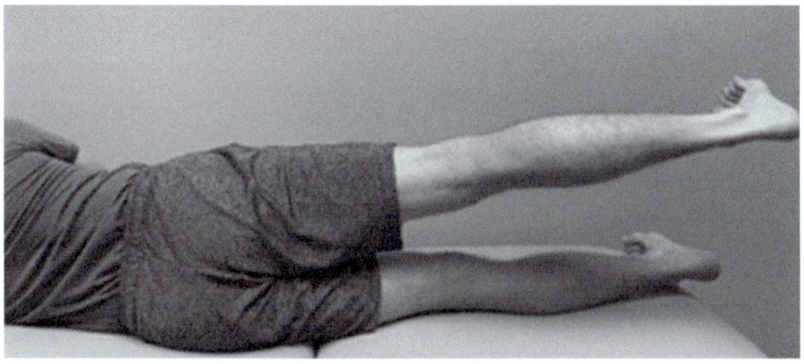

Fig. 44.15 Leg lifts. (Images from author's library)

44.4.2 Lateral Collateral Ligament Injury

Michael F. Saulle, Charles Scott and Joseph Chin

44.4.2.1 ICD 10 Code

- S83.429 Sprain of lateral collateral ligament of unspecified knee
- S83.421 Sprain of lateral collateral ligament of right knee
- S83.422A Sprain of lateral collateral ligament of left knee

44.4.2.2 Description

The lateral collateral ligament (LCL), also known as fibular collateral ligament (FCL), along with the popliteus and popliteofemoral ligament, functions to stabilize against varus gapping, external rotation, internal rotation, and posterolateral tibial translation. The LCL originates proximal and posterior to the lateral epicondyle and inserts at the lateral aspect of the fibular head, distal to the fibular styloid tip. The LCL acts as the primary restraint to varus instabil-

Fig. 44.16 Pelvic drops. (Images from author's library)

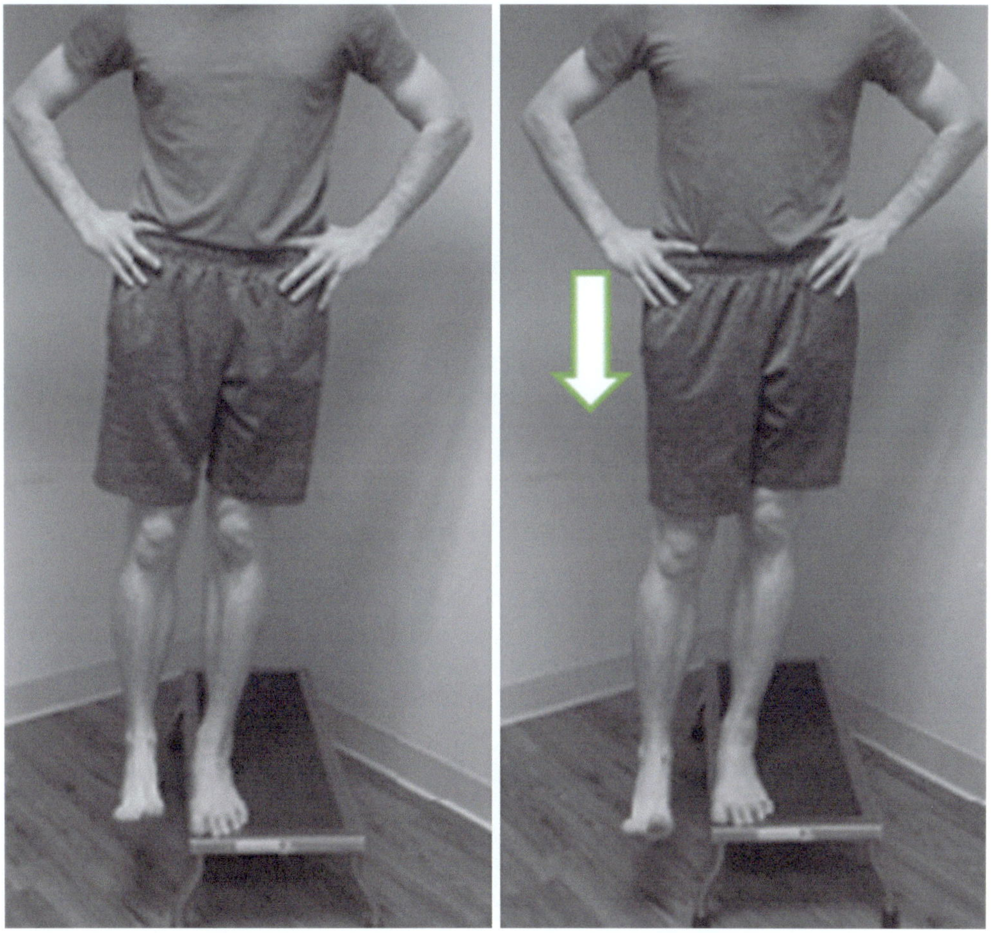

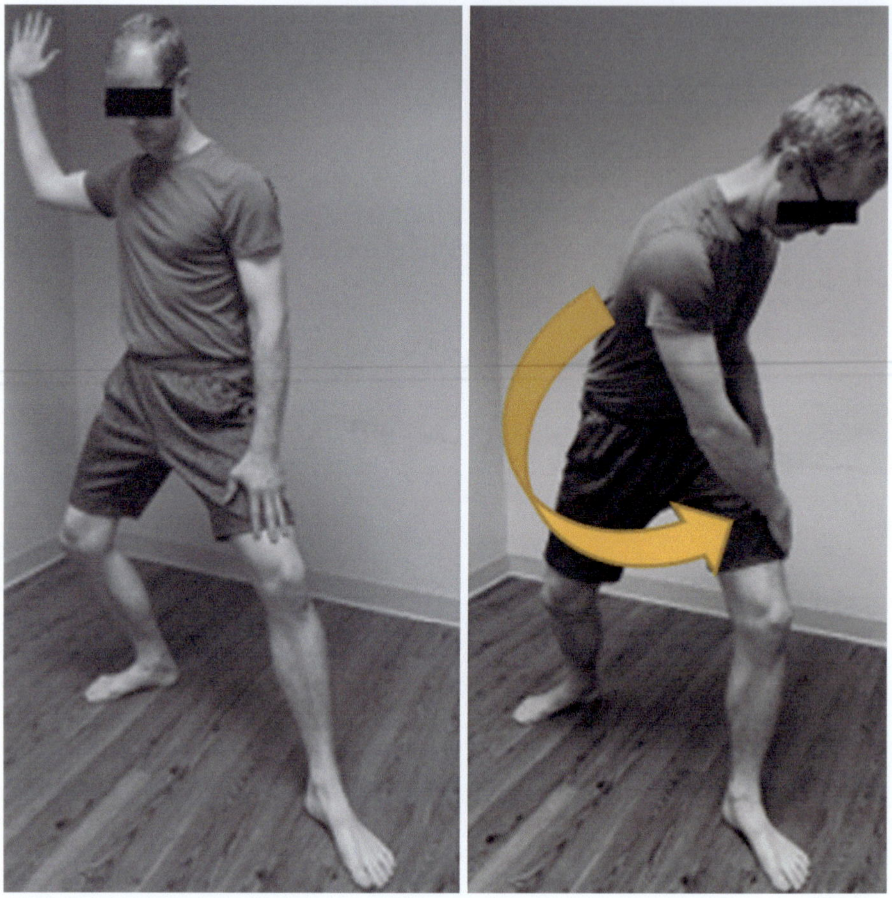

Fig. 44.17 Modified matrix. (Images from author's library)

ity. Peak forces are exerted on the LCL during full knee extension and external tibial rotation [7, 89]. Differential diagnosis for LCL injury includes LCL sprain, posterolateral corner injury, and lateral meniscus injury. LCL injury is unique given the sensation of lateral knee instability and is likely seen in the setting of acute trauma or repetitive cutting activities. Differential diagnosis of lateral knee pain is in Table 44.7.

44.4.2.3 Clinical Presentation

Patients with lateral collateral ligament (LCL) injuries may complain of pain or instability at the lateral knee. Symptoms typically onset shortly after a direct blow to the medial side of the knee, performing cutting activities, or hyperextension of the knee with or without contact. Injuries to the LCL are common in sports where quick changes of direction are required, such as football, hockey, soccer, and tennis [90].

44.4.2.4 Physical Examination

Figure-of-four position Lateral collateral ligament (LCL) tenderness may be present and can be facilitated with the figure-of-four position (Fig. 44.18), which allows direct palpation of the LCL. *Varus stress test*: Varus laxity is best observed at 30° of knee flexion for isolated injuries (Table 44.4, Fig. 44.18). This laxity may be present at full extension (0° of flexion) when there is injury to the lateral collateral ligament and anterior and posterior cruciate ligaments.

Varus laxity less than 5 mm is classified as a low-grade, 6–10 mm as a moderate-grade, and greater than 10 mm represents a high-grade injury. When high-grade LCL injury is present, injuries to other posterolateral corner structures and the cruciate ligaments should be excluded, as described earlier in this Chap. [90].

44.4.2.5 Diagnostic Workup

Diagnostic imaging may include weight-bearing and stress knee radiographs which may show lateral joint line widening. MR imaging can detect injury at the origin, midsubstance, and insertion of the ligament and can evaluate for injuries to other lateral knee structures [90]. MRI grading of lateral collateral ligament injury is as follows: (I) subcutaneous edema or fluid surrounding the ligament, (II) partial tearing with some fibers in continuity, and (III) complete tearing with no fibers in continuity [9, 91]. MRI may also demonstrate bone contusion within the medial compartment result-

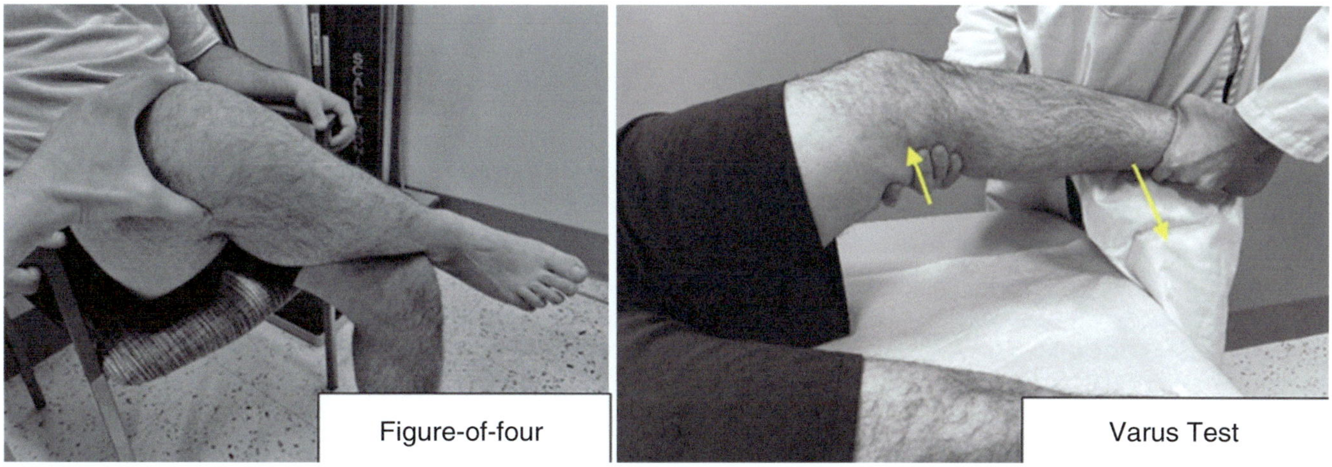

Fig. 44.18 Figure-of-four and varus stress test of the knee. (Images from author's library)

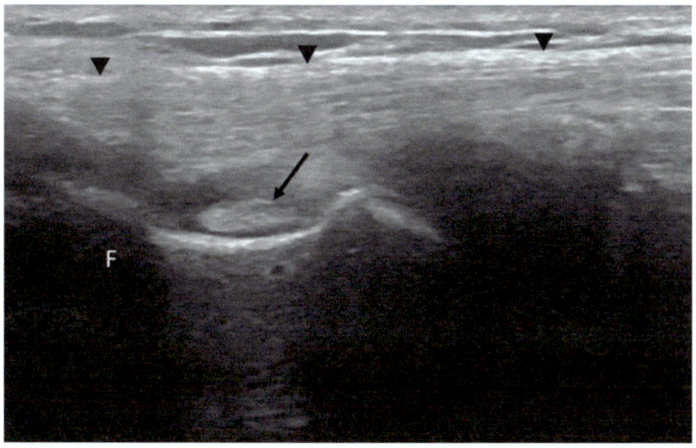

Fig. 44.19 This coronal oblique image shows the popliteus tendon (black arrows) with the lateral collateral ligament (black arrowheads) coursing superficially from its origin at the lateral femoral condyle (F). (Images from author's library)

ing from varus stress. The US is another valuable test for evaluating this tendon for abnormal echotexture (Fig. 44.19).

44.4.2.6 Treatments

Medical Management

Isolated grades I and II lateral collateral ligament (LCL) injuries can be managed conservatively with functional rehabilitation following a brief period of immobilization. For isolated grade III LCL tears, surgical management is associated with improved functional outcomes and earlier return to play [8, 90].

Rehabilitation

Nonoperative protocols include the use of a hinged knee brace until pain free with early passive and active prone knee flexion to prevent stiffness in the initial weeks post-injury. Lower extremity strengthening is initiated once pain has resolved. Patients may return to sport once there is full, pain-free range of motion and resolution of ligamentous laxity, typically at 4 weeks for grade I injuries and 10 weeks for grade II injuries. Following ligamentous reconstruction, a knee immobilizer is used for 6 weeks followed by aggressive quadricep strengthening. Hamstring strengthening is delayed until 4 months postoperatively, at which time a sport-specific therapy program may commence [91, 92].

Procedures

While there is limited literature discussing the use of PRP to treat LCL injury, leukocyte-rich PRP may have some utility in the treatment of ligamentous injury generally [93]. It is, therefore, reasonable to consider its use for treatment of isolated grade I and II injuries.

Surgery

Isolated ligamentous repair is indicated for acute grade III injuries when the ligament is avulsed from an attachment site; for example, a bioabsorbable suture may be used to anchor the LCL at its femoral attachment. For complete midsubstance tears with persistent instability, ligamentous reconstruction may be recommended. For example, a patellar tendon allograft may be used in an isometric reconstruction [90]. LCL injury and instability places other ligament reconstructions at risk of failure; lateral knee instability increases stress on the ACL and PCL reconstruction grafts. Therefore, in combined lateral soft tissue ligament knee and cruciate ligament injury, surgical repair or reconstruction of the LCL is essential [89]. Varus knee deformity with associated lateral instability may require osteotomy with ligament reconstruction [85].

44.4.3 Popliteus Injury

Michael F. Saulle, Charles Scott and Joseph Chin

44.4.3.1 ICD 10 Code

- M76.899 Popliteus tendonitis
- M66.109 Injury to popliteus muscle

44.4.3.2 Description

Despite its small size, the popliteus muscle is an important dynamic stabilizer of the posterolateral knee. This thin, triangular muscle originates at the popliteus sulcus of the lateral femoral condyle (LFC). After coursing through the popliteus hiatus, it passes beneath the lateral collateral ligament (LCL) and the tendon of the short head of the biceps femoris and then widens distally before inserting broadly over the proximal 10–12 cm of the posterior tibia superior to the soleal line. The proximal tendon originating at the LFC also contains aponeurotic fibers that blend with the joint capsule, the posterior horn of the lateral meniscus, and the fibular head [94, 95]. The popliteus muscle is innervated by the tibial nerve with contributions from the L4, L5, and S1 nerve roots.

The popliteus muscle acts as the primary medial rotator of the tibia during non-weight-bearing and helps to prevent excessive tibial external rotation during the swing phase of gait. During weight-bearing, its action results in lateral rotation of the femur, helping to unlock the fully extended knee in preparation for the swing phase [94, 96]. Together with other posterolateral stabilizers such as the posterior collateral ligament (PCL), the popliteus helps prevent posterior translation of the tibia relative to the femur. It may also play a role in the retraction of the lateral meniscus during knee extension, serving to prevent meniscal entrapment between the femur and tibia [94, 95, 97].

Isolated popliteus injury is less common than those that occur in the setting of complex posterolateral corner (PLC) injuries [96, 98]. Most isolated popliteal injuries are traumatic in origin, commonly involving strain or tear of the muscle-tendon unit. Tendon avulsion injuries at the LFC are commonly reported [96, 99]. Popliteus tenosynovitis and tendinopathy are the most frequently encountered overuse injuries. The intra-articular portion of the popliteus tendon is also susceptible to iatrogenic injury during knee arthroscopy. Differential diagnosis of popliteus injury is in Table 44.9.

Table 44.9 Differential diagnosis of popliteus injury

Iliotibial band syndrome
Distal biceps femoris tear/tendinopathy
Sprain or tear of the lateral collateral ligament (LCL)
Sprain or tear of the posterior cruciate ligament (PCL)
Posterolateral corner injury
Posterolateral rotatory instability
Lateral meniscus tear
Bone contusion
Proximal tibiofibular syndesmosis injury
Lateral knee compartment osteoarthritis
Lateral femoral condyle osteochondritis dissecans
Lateral tibial plateau fracture

44.4.3.3 Clinical Presentation

Traumatic popliteus injuries, including strain, rupture, or avulsion, commonly occur in field sports when varus force is applied to the knee with the tibia externally rotated, or with knee hyperextension or flexion with forced external rotation. These may present as an acutely swollen knee with posterolateral tenderness. Patients may describe subjective instability with the knee extended. Pain is reproduced with resisted tibial internal rotation [96]. Overuse injuries of the popliteus tendon, including tenosynovitis and tendinopathy, are more commonly described in runners. These injuries present as chronic posterolateral knee pain that may be clinically mistaken for a lateral meniscus injury. Runners may report reproduction of symptoms with fast downhill running. The popliteus may be subjected to increased stress during downhill gait as it serves to limit anterior displacement of the femur relative to the tibia and may also play a role in preventing forward rotation of the LFC on the tibia. Pain may also be noted with walking or running on uneven terrain or with descending stairs [94, 96].

44.4.3.4 Physical Examination

Although several physical examination maneuvers have been described to evaluate PCL injury, validated maneuvers to test the popliteus muscle-tendon unit in isolation are lacking. Reproduction of posterolateral pain with resisted tibial internal rotation is suggestive of popliteus injury. The shoe removal maneuver, performed by having the patient internally rotate the affected leg and attempt to push off the contralateral shoe, may also suggest injury to the popliteus [100]. When there is a clinical suspicion for popliteal injury, examination maneuvers to detect posterolateral rotatory instability should be performed. These include the dial test and the reverse pivot-shift test. The dial test is suggestive of PLC injury when passive external tibial rotation is increased by more than 10° compared to the opposite knee when the knee is tested in 30° of flexion. An increase in passive external tibial rotation by more than 10° in both 30° and 90° of knee flexion (Fig. 44.20) is suggestive of concurrent PLC and PCL injury [52]. The reverse pivot-shift test is performed by slowly extending the knee from a position of 90° of flexion while applying a valgus force and tibial external rotation. If a clunk is palpable as the lateral tibial plateau shifts from the position of posterior subluxation to its reduced position, the test is considered positive and indicates the presence of instability [52].

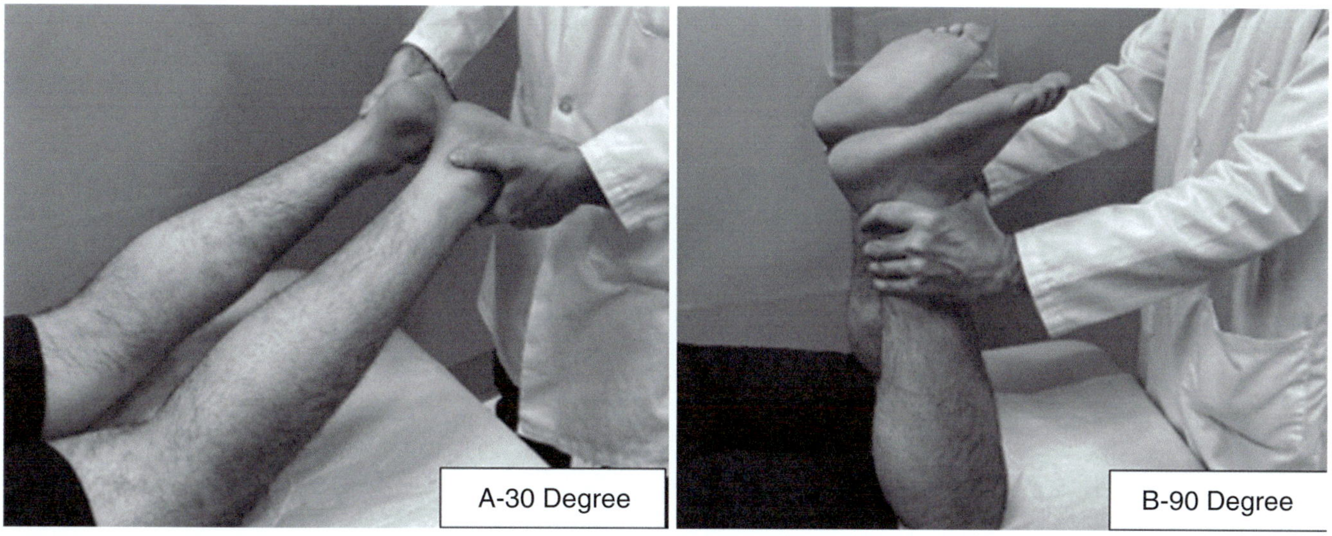

Fig. 44.20 Dial test at 30° (**a**) and Dial test at 90° (**b**). (Images from author's library)

44.4.3.5 Diagnostic Workup

When popliteus or posterolateral corner (PLC) injury is suspected, standard plain radiographs of the knee are initially obtained. In popliteus avulsion injuries, these may demonstrate a bony avulsion fragment at the level of the lateral femoral condyle [99]. Though technically challenging to obtain due to pain with acute injury, valgus stress films with the knee in 20° of flexion can suggest PLC injury when lateral tibiofemoral joint gapping occurs greater than 4 mm relative to the unaffected side [55].

Plain radiographs are generally not sufficient to diagnose and characterize complex knee injuries. Ultrasound can supplement soft tissue examination (Fig. 44.19). Magnetic resonance imaging (MRI) is indicated whenever posterolateral instability is noted on examination or posterolateral corner injury is suspected [52, 94]. Standard views are often sufficient, but coronal oblique views oriented in the plane of the popliteus tendon may allow for improved visualization of the PLC structures [52, 96]. Popliteus rupture may appear as irregularly contoured tendon and/or disorganized muscle fibers associated with surrounding high signal changes (edema) [18, 52]. Increased signal around or within the tendon on T2-weighted imaging is suggestive of tendonitis or tenosynovitis.

44.4.3.6 Treatments

Medical Management

Popliteus tenosynovitis and tendinopathy are initially treated conservatively with relative rest from precipitating activities, ice, compression, elevation, and nonsteroidal anti-inflammatory medications. Consensus is lacking around the treatment of isolated popliteal tendon rupture and avulsion, but a diversity of case reports and case series favors conservative treatment with bracing and rehabilitation in cases where instability is absent [96, 101, 102].

Rehabilitation

For isolated popliteus injury without instability, progressive functional rehabilitation focusing on eccentric quadriceps strengthening and lower extremity flexibility is recommended [103]. The rationale for strengthening the quadriceps is that a fatigued quadricep will strain the popliteus.

Procedures

As in other types of tendinopathy, the treatment of refractory popliteus tendinopathy has often involved peritendinous injection of corticosteroid. There is a growing interest in the utilization of PRP for the treatment of tendinopathy including popliteus tendinopathy and tenosynovitis.

Surgery

Popliteus injury occurring in the setting of high-grade PLC injury should be surgically addressed within 2–3 weeks of injury in order to prevent chronic posterolateral instability [11, 18, 52, 94]. Surgical management of injured primary PLC structures, including the popliteus, consists of repair when structures can be reduced to their point of origin. When reduction is not possible, reconstruction may be necessary.

44.4.4 Proximal Tibiofibular Joint Injury

Michael F. Saulle, Charles Scott and Joseph Chin

44.4.4.1 Synonyms

Reactive arthropathy of the tibiofibular joint, Rheumatoid arthritis of the tibiofibular joint.

44.4.4.2 ICD 10 Code

- S83.60XA Sprain of the superior tibiofibular joint and ligament
- S83.61XA Sprain of the superior tibiofibular joint and ligament, right
- S83.62XA Sprain of the superior tibiofibular joint and ligament, left
- M0209 Reactive arthropathy of the tibiofibular joint
- M06.9 Rheumatoid arthritis of the tibiofibular joint

44.4.4.3 Description

The proximal tibiofibular joint (PTFJ) is a synovial articulation composed of the posterolateral tibia and anteromedial portion of the fibula. Anatomic and radiographic studies show the PTFJ communicates directly with the tibiofemoral compartment of the knee joint in a varied percent of the population [104]. It is bound by a fibrous capsule along and stabilized by the anterior proximal tibiofibular ligament (APTFL), posterior proximal tibiofibular ligament (PPTFL), and more distally by the interosseous syndesmotic membrane (IOSM). The APTFL consists of three bands, providing greater thickness and tensile strength than the single broad band of the PPTFL [105, 106]. The APTFL stabilizes the joint when the ankle is plantarflexed and everted, while the PPTGL stabilizes the joint with ankle dorsiflexion, inversion, and knee flexion [105]. Both ligaments, along with the IOSM, provide rotational stability of the joint. The PTFJ has a variety of morphologic configurations accounting for variations in biomechanical stress, which led to the variable development of pathology [105]. The joint has three biomechanical functions: dissipation of torsional forces applied to the ankle, dissipation of lateral tibial forces, and providing tensile weight-bearing [105]. Mobility of the PTFJ is largely dependent on the adjacent knee and ankle joints. It is also important to note the proximity of the common fibular nerve to the PTFJ as it courses circumferentially and distal to the joint. Differential diagnosis of the proximal tibiofibular pain is in Table 44.10.

Table 44.10 Differential diagnosis of the proximal tibiofibular pain

Iliotibial band syndrome
Distal biceps femoris tear/tendinopathy
Sprain or tear of the lateral collateral ligament (LCL)
Sprain or tear of the posterior cruciate ligament (PCL)
Posterolateral corner injury
Posterolateral rotatory instability
Lateral meniscus tear
Bone contusion
Proximal tibiofibular syndesmosis injury
Osteosarcoma
Rheumatoid arthritis

44.4.4.4 Clinical Presentation

Isolated pathology at the proximal tibiofibular joint is rare, accounting for approximately 1% of all knee injuries [87]. It is often accompanied by ankle injuries or bony fractures of the lower leg. Instability, dislocation, osteoarthritis (OA), contusion, fracture, and cancer (osteosarcoma) are some of the reported issues affecting the PTFJ. Dislocation of the PTFJ is an uncommon and often missed diagnosis typically in the setting of lower extremity injury. Patients typically present with acute lateral knee pain following some form of high-energy trauma to the lateral leg. The patient may also report the injury occurred while landing on their leg with a rotated and flexed knee and a plantarflexed foot. These injuries occur mostly in the second to fourth decades and are associated with sports such as football, rugby, wrestling, gymnastics, long jumping, dancing, judo, and skiing. In contrast individuals with pain from PTFJ instability may have a history of lateral leg injury, but no acute trauma that precedes their presentation. They will complain of chronic intermittent lateral knee pain with some noting knee popping and transient nerve pain. The demographic for PTFJ instability will be similar as those with frank dislocations.

In some patients, instability may remain asymptomatic, leading to eventual progression to symptomatic PTFJ osteoarthritis (OA). PTFJ OA is uncommon and manifests in the fifth to sixth decades of life as either primary or post traumatic OA. Patients present with an insidious onset, typically with some relevant history of prior injury, dislocation, or surgery. Symptoms consist of well-localized lateral knee and leg pain that is worse with activities like standing and walking.

44.4.4.5 Physical Examination

Physical exam of the fibular head begins with side-to-side comparison of surface anatomy looking for any prominence, asymmetry, swelling, or masses. Palpation over the proximal tibiofibular joint is often confirmatory for pathology. Springing of the fibular head can help assess for instability, dislocation, and localized pain. In the case of the proximal tibiofibular joint dislocation (dependent on type), deformity and prominence of the fibular head will be present. On passive range of motion, there may be associated crepitations, popping, and limited knee extension. In those with lateral leg paresthesias, there may be a positive Tinel's sign at the fibular head or common fibular nerve palsy. Physical exam should also consist of careful evaluation of the foot and ankle as passive ankle movements may also precipitate lateral knee pain. The exam for PTFJ instability and OA will clinically appear similar with many of the aforementioned features with the exception of large bony deformity.

44.4.4.6 Diagnostic Workup

Initial imaging should consist of bilateral AP and lateral knee radiographs looking for increased interosseous gapping and associated fractures. When these images are inconclusive, MRI or CT imaging is indicated. Advanced imaging is needed when evaluating proximal tibiofibular joint dislocations to classify the dislocation type and help guide treatment. The Ogden classification describes four types of PTFJ dislocations (Table 44.11) [107, 108].

44.4.4.7 Treatments

Medical Management

Treatment of proximal tibiofibular joint dislocation is largely conservative, consisting of closed reduction and fixation with a *backslab splint* or brace followed by 2–6 weeks of immobilization and modified weight-bearing. Closed reduction for types III and IV dislocations, though challenging, may be attempted. Failure should prompt open reduction. Following reduction medical management consists of protection, rest, ice, compression, elevation, and NSAIDs. The medical management of PTFJ instability and OA consists of bracing, NSAIDs, topical anti-inflammatories, and activity modifications.

Rehabilitation

Physical therapy is recommended following the recommended 2–6 weeks of proximal tibiofibular joint immobilization following reduction. Focus should be directed at restoring proximal hip and core strength followed by closed-chain isometric quadricep strengthening with eventual progression to open-chain strengthening. Therapy should also be directed at restoring any alterations in foot and ankle mechanics following trauma to the PTFJ.

Procedures

For proximal tibiofibular joint OA, ultrasound or fluoroscopically guided corticosteroid injections can provide accurate delivery of medications for symptomatic relief. The role for regenerative treatments for proximal tibiofibular OA is unclear, though based on existing literature for knee OA, leukocyte-poor platelet-rich plasma (PRP) is a reasonable treatment option for OA and leukocyte-rich PRP for capsular ligaments [109]. Leukocyte-rich PRP may have some utility in the treatment and tightening of ligaments and may be considered for proximal tibiofibular capsular laxity [93]. There are no studies specifically looking at PRP and its application to this condition.

Table 44.11 Ogden classification of proximal Tib-Fib joint dislocation

Dislocation type	Description	Distinctions
Type 1	Subluxation	
Type 2	Anterior dislocation	Most common: accounts for 85% of dislocations
Type 3	Posteromedial dislocation	Associated peroneal nerve injury (neuropraxia)
Type 4	Superior dislocation	Associated tibia shaft fracture Associated peroneal nerve injury (neuropraxia)

Surgery

Surgery is indicated for proximal tibiofibular joint dislocation resulting in neurovascular compromise, recurrent dislocation, instability, or chronic pain. There are a variety of surgical approaches including open reduction, internal fixation, ligament reconstruction, and fibular head resection [107, 110]. In the setting of chronic instability and failed conservative care, proximal tibiofibular ligament reconstruction, specifically biceps rerouting and anatomic graft reconstruction, leads to improved outcomes with low complication rates [107]. If left uncorrected, chronic proximal tibiofibular instability can lead to OA, fibular nerve palsy, and chronic pain. In the setting of instability and osteoarthritis that have failed conservative care, arthrodesis may be indicated.

References

1. Saragaglia D, Pison A, Rubens-Duval B. Acute and old ruptures of the extensor apparatus of the knee in adults (excluding knee replacement). Orthop Traumatol Surg Res. 2013;99(1 Suppl):S67–76.
2. Nori S. Quadriceps tendon rupture. J Family Med Prim Care. 2018;7(1):257–60.
3. Fredberg U, Bolvig L, Jumper's knee. Review of the literature. Scand J Med Sci Sports. 1999;9(2):66–73.
4. Chhapan J, Sankineani SR, Chiranjeevi T, Reddy MV, Reddy D, Gurava Reddy AV. Early quadriceps tendon rupture after primary total knee arthroplasty. Knee. 2018;25(1):192–4.
5. Hsu H, Siwiec RM. Patellar tendon rupture. StatPearls. Treasure Island; 2021.
6. Lian OB, Engebretsen L, Bahr R. Prevalence of jumper's knee among elite athletes from different sports: a cross-sectional study. Am J Sports Med. 2005;33(4):561–7.
7. van der Worp H, van Ark M, Roerink S, Pepping GJ, van den Akker-Scheek I, Zwerver J. Risk factors for patellar tendinopathy: a systematic review of the literature. Br J Sports Med. 2011;45(5):446–52.
8. Golman M, Wright ML, Wong TT, Lynch TS, Ahmad CS, Thomopoulos S, et al. Rethinking patellar tendinopathy and partial patellar tendon tears: a novel classification system. Am J Sports Med. 2020;48(2):359–69.
9. Stubbings N, Smith T. Diagnostic test accuracy of clinical and radiological assessments for medial patella plica syndrome: a systematic review and meta-analysis. Knee. 2014;21(2):486–90.
10. Smith JM VM. Osgood Schlatter Disease. StatPearls [Internet] Treasure Island (FL). 2021(StatPearls Publishing).
11. Kary JM. Diagnosis and management of quadriceps strains and contusions. Curr Rev Musculoskelet Med. 2010;3(1–4):26–31.
12. Hughes CT, Hasselman CT, Best TM, Martinez S, Garrett WE Jr. Incomplete, intrasubstance strain injuries of the rectus femoris muscle. Am J Sports Med. 1995;23(4):500–6.

13. Kountouris A, Cook J. Rehabilitation of Achilles and patellar tendinopathies. Best Pract Res Clin Rheumatol. 2007;21(2):295–316.
14. King D, Yakubek G, Chughtai M, Khlopas A, Saluan P, Mont MA, et al. Quadriceps tendinopathy: a review-part 1: epidemiology and diagnosis. Ann Transl Med. 2019;7(4):71.
15. Pedrelli A, Stecco C, Day JA. Treating patellar tendinopathy with fascial manipulation. J Bodyw Mov Ther. 2009;13(1):73–80.
16. Kelly DW, Carter VS, Jobe FW, Kerlan RK. Patellar and quadriceps tendon ruptures–jumper's knee. Am J Sports Med. 1984;12(5):375–80.
17. Naugle KM, Fillingim RB, Riley JL 3rd. A meta-analytic review of the hypoalgesic effects of exercise. J Pain. 2012;13(12):1139–50.
18. Nunez FJ, Santalla A, Carrasquila I, Asian JA, Reina JI, Suarez-Arrones LJ. The effects of unilateral and bilateral eccentric overload training on hypertrophy, muscle power and COD performance, and its determinants, in team sport players. PLoS One. 2018;13(3):e0193841.
19. Purdam CR, Jonsson P, Alfredson H, Lorentzon R, Cook JL, Khan KM. A pilot study of the eccentric decline squat in the management of painful chronic patellar tendinopathy. Br J Sports Med. 2004;38(4):395–7.
20. Kongsgaard M, Kovanen V, Aagaard P, Doessing S, Hansen P, Laursen AH, et al. Corticosteroid injections, eccentric decline squat training and heavy slow resistance training in patellar tendinopathy. Scand J Med Sci Sports. 2009;19(6):790–802.
21. Frohm A, Saartok T, Halvorsen K, Renstrom P. Eccentric treatment for patellar tendinopathy: a prospective randomised short-term pilot study of two rehabilitation protocols. Br J Sports Med. 2007;41(7):e7.
22. Dragoo JL, Wasterlain AS, Braun HJ, Nead KT. Platelet-rich plasma as a treatment for patellar tendinopathy: a double-blind, randomized controlled trial. Am J Sports Med. 2014;42(3):610–8.
23. Filardo G, Kon E, Della Villa S, Vincentelli F, Fornasari PM, Marcacci M. Use of platelet-rich plasma for the treatment of refractory jumper's knee. Int Orthop. 2010;34(6):909–15.
24. Dallaudiere B, Pesquer L, Meyer P, Silvestre A, Perozziello A, Peuchant A, et al. Intratendinous injection of platelet-rich plasma under US guidance to treat tendinopathy: a long-term pilot study. J Vasc Interv Radiol. 2014;25(5):717–23.
25. Zwerver J, Hartgens F, Verhagen E, van der Worp H, van den Akker-Scheek I, Diercks RL. No effect of extracorporeal shockwave therapy on patellar tendinopathy in jumping athletes during the competitive season: a randomized clinical trial. Am J Sports Med. 2011;39(6):1191–9.
26. Vetrano M, Castorina A, Vulpiani MC, Baldini R, Pavan A, Ferretti A. Platelet-rich plasma versus focused shock waves in the treatment of jumper's knee in athletes. Am J Sports Med. 2013;41(4):795–803.
27. Petersen W, Ellermann A, Gosele-Koppenburg A, Best R, Rembitzki IV, Bruggemann GP, et al. Patellofemoral pain syndrome. Knee Surg Sports Traumatol Arthrosc. 2014;22(10):2264–74.
28. Bump JM, Lewis L. Patellofemoral syndrome. StatPearls. Treasure Island; 2021.
29. Wilson NA, Press JM, Koh JL, Hendrix RW, Zhang LQ. In vivo noninvasive evaluation of abnormal patellar tracking during squatting in patients with patellofemoral pain. J Bone Joint Surg Am. 2009;91(3):558–66.
30. Pal S, Draper CE, Fredericson M, Gold GE, Delp SL, Beaupre GS, et al. Patellar maltracking correlates with vastus medialis activation delay in patellofemoral pain patients. Am J Sports Med. 2011;39(3):590–8.
31. Prins MR, van der Wurff P. Females with patellofemoral pain syndrome have weak hip muscles: a systematic review. Aust J Physiother. 2009;55(1):9–15.
32. Barton CJ, Bonanno D, Levinger P, Menz HB. Foot and ankle characteristics in patellofemoral pain syndrome: a case control and reliability study. J Orthop Sports Phys Ther. 2010;40(5):286–96.
33. Narkbunnam R, Chareancholvanich K. Effect of patient position on measurement of patellar height ratio. Arch Orthop Trauma Surg. 2015;135(8):1151–6.
34. Verhulst FV, van Sambeeck JDP, Olthuis GS, van der Ree J, Koeter S. Patellar height measurements: Insall-Salvati ratio is most reliable method. Knee Surg Sports Traumatol Arthrosc. 2020;28(3):869–75.
35. Gulati A, McElrath C, Wadhwa V, Shah JP, Chhabra A. Current clinical, radiological and treatment perspectives of patellofemoral pain syndrome. Br J Radiol. 2018;91(1086):20170456.
36. Harvie D, O'Leary T, Kumar S. A systematic review of randomized controlled trials on exercise parameters in the treatment of patellofemoral pain: what works? J Multidiscip Healthc. 2011;4:383–92.
37. Cowan SM, Bennell KL, Hodges PW. Therapeutic patellar taping changes the timing of vasti muscle activation in people with patellofemoral pain syndrome. Clin J Sport Med. 2002;12(6):339–47.
38. Bellary SS, Lynch G, Housman B, Esmaeili E, Gielecki J, Tubbs RS, et al. Medial plica syndrome: a review of the literature. Clin Anat. 2012;25(4):423–8.
39. Kim SJ, Choe WS. Arthroscopic findings of the synovial plicae of the knee. Arthroscopy. 1997;13(1):33–41.
40. Griffith CJ, Wijdicks CA, Goerke U, Michaeli S, Ellermann J, LaPrade RF. Outcomes of untreated posterolateral knee injuries: an in vivo canine model. Knee Surg Sports Traumatol Arthrosc. 2011;19(7):1192–7.
41. Leib AD, Roshan A, Foris LA, Varacallo M. Baker's cyst. StatPearls. Treasure Island; 2021.
42. Spina AA. The plantaris muscle: anatomy, injury, imaging, and treatment. J Can Chiropr Assoc. 2007;51(3):158–65.
43. Froimson AI. Tennis leg. JAMA. 1969;209(3):415–6.
44. Pollock N, Dijkstra P, Calder J, Chakraverty R. Plantaris injuries in elite UK track and field athletes over a 4-year period: a retrospective cohort study. Knee Surg Sports Traumatol Arthrosc. 2016;24(7):2287–92.
45. Gopinath TN, Jagdish J, Krishnakiran K, Shaji PC. Rupture of plantaris muscle – a mimic: MRI findings. J Clin Imaging Sci. 2012;2:19.
46. Bedi HS, Jowett C, Ristanis S, Docking S, Cook J. Plantaris excision and ventral paratendinous scraping for Achilles tendinopathy in an athletic population. Foot Ankle Int. 2016;37(4):386–93. https://doi.org/10.1177/1071100715619989. Epub 2015 Dec 4. PMID: 26637273.
47. LaPrade RF, Ly TV, Wentorf FA, Engebretsen L. The posterolateral attachments of the knee: a qualitative and quantitative morphologic analysis of the Lateral Collateral Ligament, popliteus tendon, popliteofibular ligament, and lateral gastrocnemius tendon. Am J Sports Med. 2003;31(6):854–60.
48. Chahla J, Moatshe G, Dean CS, LaPrade RF. Posterolateral corner of the knee: current concepts. Arch Bone Jt Surg. 2016;4(2):97–103.
49. Geeslin AG, LaPrade RF. Location of bone bruises and other osseous injuries associated with acute grade III isolated and combined posterolateral knee injuries. Am J Sports Med. 2010;38(12):2502–8.
50. Harner CD, Vogrin TM, Hoher J, Ma CB, Woo SL. Biomechanical analysis of a posterior cruciate ligament reconstruction. Deficiency of the posterolateral structures as a cause of graft failure. Am J Sports Med. 2000;28(1):32–9.
51. LaPrade RF, Terry GC. Injuries to the posterolateral aspect of the knee. Association of anatomic injury patterns with clinical instability. Am J Sports Med. 1997;25(4):433–8.
52. Chahla J, Murray IR, Robinson J, Lagae K, Margheritini F, Fritsch B, et al. Posterolateral corner of the knee: an expert consensus

statement on diagnosis, classification, treatment, and rehabilitation. Knee Surg Sports Traumatol Arthrosc. 2019;27(8):2520–9.
53. Dean RS, LaPrade RF. ACL and posterolateral corner injuries. Curr Rev Musculoskelet Med. 2020;13(1):123–32. https://doi.org/10.1007/s12178-019-09581-3. PMID: 31884674; PMCID: PMC7083988
54. Cooper DE. Tests for posterolateral instability of the knee in normal subjects. Results of examination under anesthesia. J Bone Joint Surg Am. 1991;73(1):30–6.
55. LaPrade RF, Heikes C, Bakker AJ, Jakobsen RB. The reproducibility and repeatability of varus stress radiographs in the assessment of isolated Lateral Collateral Ligament and grade-III posterolateral knee injuries. An in vitro biomechanical study. J Bone Joint Surg Am. 2008;90(10):2069–76.
56. Kannus P. Nonoperative treatment of grade II and III sprains of the lateral ligament compartment of the knee. Am J Sports Med. 1989;17(1):83–8.
57. Kennedy MI, Bernhardson A, Moatshe G, Buckley PS, Engebretsen L, LaPrade RF. Fibular collateral ligament/posterolateral corner injury: when to repair, reconstruct, or both. Clin Sports Med. 2019;38(2):261–74. https://doi.org/10.1016/j.csm.2018.11.002. Epub 2019 Jan 19. PMID: 30878048.
58. Geeslin AG, LaPrade RF. Outcomes of treatment of acute grade-III isolated and combined posterolateral knee injuries: a prospective case series and surgical technique. J Bone Joint Surg Am. 2011;93(18):1672–83.
59. Rodgers CD, Raja A. Anatomy, bony pelvis and lower limb, hamstring muscle. StatPearls. Treasure Island; 2021.
60. Clanton TO, Coupe KJ. Hamstring strains in athletes: diagnosis and treatment. J Am Acad Orthop Surg. 1998;6(4):237–48.
61. Poudel B, Pandey S. Hamstring injury. [updated 2021 Aug 11]. In: StatPearls [internet]. Treasure Island (FL): StatPearls Publishing; 2021 January.
62. Heiderscheit BC, Sherry MA, Silder A, Chumanov ES, Thelen DG. Hamstring strain injuries: recommendations for diagnosis, rehabilitation, and injury prevention. J Orthop Sports Phys Ther. 2010;40(2):67–81.
63. Knapik JJ, Jones BH, Bauman CL, Harris JM. Strength, flexibility and athletic injuries. Sports Med. 1992;14(5):277–88.
64. Stafford MG, Grana WA. Hamstring/quadriceps ratios in college football players: a high velocity evaluation. Am J Sports Med. 1984;12(3):209–11.
65. Heiser TM, Weber J, Sullivan G, Clare P, Jacobs RR. Prophylaxis and management of hamstring muscle injuries in intercollegiate football players. Am J Sports Med. 1984;12(5):368–70.
66. Almekinders LC. Anti-inflammatory treatment of muscular injuries in sports. Sports Med. 1993;15(3):139–45.
67. Jarvinen MJ, Lehto MU. The effects of early mobilisation and immobilisation on the healing process following muscle injuries. Sports Med. 1993;15(2):78–89.
68. Askling CM, Tengvar M, Tarassova O, Thorstensson A. Acute hamstring injuries in Swedish elite sprinters and jumpers: a prospective randomised controlled clinical trial comparing two rehabilitation protocols. Br J Sports Med. 2014;48(7):532–9. https://doi.org/10.1136/bjsports-2013-093214. PMID: 24620041.
69. Sapp GH, Herman DC. Pay attention to the pes anserine in knee osteoarthritis. Curr Sports Med Rep. 2018;17(2):41.
70. Alvarez-Nemegyei J, Pelaez-Ballestas I, Goni M, Julian-Santiago F, Garcia-Garcia C, Quintana R, et al. Prevalence of rheumatic regional pain syndromes in Latin-American indigenous groups: a census study based on COPCORD methodology and syndrome-specific diagnostic criteria. Clin Rheumatol. 2016;35(Suppl 1):63–70.
71. Sarifakioglu B, Afsar SI, Yalbuzdag SA, Ustaomer K, Bayramoglu M. Comparison of the efficacy of physical therapy and corticosteroid injection in the treatment of pes anserine tendino-bursitis. J Phys Ther Sci. 2016;28(7):1993–7.
72. Khosrawi S, Taheri P, Ketabi M. Investigating the effect of extracorporeal shock wave therapy on reducing chronic pain in patients with pes anserine bursitis: a randomized, Clinical- Controlled Trial. Adv Biomed Res. 2017;6:70.
73. Warren LF, Marshall JL. The supporting structures and layers on the medial side of the knee: an anatomical analysis. J Bone Joint Surg Am. 1979;61(1):56–62.
74. Andrews K, Lu A, McKean L, Ebraheim N. Review: medial collateral ligament injuries. J Orthop. 2017;14(4):550–4.
75. Lee RJ, Margalit A, Nduaguba A, Gunderson MA, Ganley TJ. Risk factors for concomitant collateral ligament injuries in children and adolescents with anterior cruciate ligament tears. Orthop J Sports Med. 2018;6(11):2325967118810389. https://doi.org/10.1177/2325967118810389. PMID: 30480025; PMCID: PMC6249661
76. Memarzadeh AMJ. Medial collateral ligament of the knee: anatomy, management, and surgical techniques for reconstruction. Orthopaed Trauma. 2019;33(2):91–9.
77. Kim SH, Lee H-J, Jang Y-H, Chun K-J, Park Y-B. Diagnostic accuracy of magnetic resonance imaging in the detection of type and location of meniscus tears: comparison with arthroscopic findings. J Clin Med. 2021;10:606. https://doi.org/10.3390/jcm10040606.
78. Naqvi U, Sherman A. Medial collateral ligament knee injuries. StatPearls. Treasure Island; 2021.
79. Derscheid GL, Garrick JG. Medial collateral ligament injuries in football. Nonoperative management of grade I and grade II sprains. Am J Sports Med. 1981;9(6):365–8.
80. Vosoughi F, Rezaei Dogahe R, Nuri A, Ayati Firoozabadi M, Mortazavi J. Medial collateral ligament injury of the knee: a review on current concept and management. Arch Bone Jt Surg. 2021;9(3):255–62.
81. Bagwell MSWK, Colberg RE, Dugas JR. The use of serial platelet RICH plasma injections with early rehabilitation to expedite grade iii medial collateral ligament injury in a professional athlete: a CASE report. Int J Sports Phys Ther. 2018;13(3):520–5.
82. Zou G, Zheng M, Chen W, He X, Cang D. Autologous platelet-rich plasma therapy for refractory pain after low-grade medial collateral ligament injury. J Int Med Res. 2020;48(2):300060520903636.
83. Hadeed A, Tapscott DC. Iliotibial band friction syndrome. StatPearls. Treasure Island; 2021.
84. Strauss EJ, Kim S, Calcei JG, Park D. Iliotibial band syndrome: evaluation and management. J Am Acad Orthop Surg. 2011;19(12):728–36.
85. Brukner K. Clinical sports medicine. 4th edn. McGraw Hill. 2012.
86. Fredericson M, Cookingham CL, Chaudhari AM, Dowdell BC, Oestreicher N, Sahrmann SA. Hip abductor weakness in distance runners with iliotibial band syndrome. Clin J Sport Med. 2000;10(3):169–75.
87. Fredericson M, Wolf C. Iliotibial band syndrome in runners: innovations in treatment. Sports Med. 2005;35(5):451–9.
88. Baker RL, Souza RB, Fredericson M. Iliotibial band syndrome: soft tissue and biomechanical factors in evaluation and treatment. PM R. 2011;3(6):550–61.
89. James EW, LaPrade CM, LaPrade RF. Anatomy and biomechanics of the lateral side of the knee and surgical implications. Sports Med Arthrosc Rev. 2015;23(1):2–9.
90. Grawe B, Schroeder AJ, Kakazu R, Messer MS. Lateral collateral ligament injury about the knee: anatomy, evaluation, and management. J Am Acad Orthop Surg. 2018;26(6):e120–e7.
91. Bushnell BD, Bitting SS, Crain JM, Boublik M, Schlegel TF. Treatment of magnetic resonance imaging-documented isolated grade III lateral collateral ligament injuries in National Football League athletes. Am J Sports Med. 2010;38(1):86–91.

92. Yaras RJ, O'Neill N, Yaish AM. Lateral collateral ligament knee injuries. StatPearls. Treasure Island; 2021.
93. Le ADK, Enweze L, DeBaun MR, Dragoo JL. Current clinical recommendations for use of platelet-rich plasma. Curr Rev Musculoskelet Med. 2018;11(4):624–34.
94. Jadhav SP, More SR, Riascos RF, Lemos DF, Swischuk LE. Comprehensive review of the anatomy, function, and imaging of the popliteus and associated pathologic conditions. Radiographics. 2014;34(2):496–513.
95. Chuncharunee A, Chanthong P, Lucksanasombool P. The patterns of proximal attachments of the popliteus muscle: form and function. Med Hypotheses. 2012;78(2):221–4.
96. Guha AR, Gorgees KA, Walker DI. Popliteus tendon rupture: a case report and review of the literature. Br J Sports Med. 2003;37(4):358–60.
97. Hyland S, Varacallo M. Anatomy, bony pelvis and lower limb, Popliteus Muscle. StatPearls. Treasure Island; 2021.
98. Mirkopulos N, Myer TJ. Isolated avulsion of the popliteus tendon. A case report. Am J Sports Med. 1991;19(4):417–9.
99. Algazwi DAR, Tian QS, Elizabeth GL, Ellis ES, Teng VSY, Hallinan J. Isolated popliteus tendon avulsion fracture. Am J Phys Med Rehabil. 2019;98(11):e140–e1.
100. Radhakrishna M, Macdonald P, Davidson M, Hodgekinson R, Craton N. Isolated popliteus injury in a professional football player. Clin J Sport Med. 2004;14(6):365–7.
101. Koong DP, An VVG, Lorentzos P, Moussa P, Sivakumar BS. Non-operative rehabilitation of isolated popliteus tendon rupture in a Rugby player. Knee Surg Relat Res. 2018;30(3):269–72.
102. McKay SD, Holt A, Stout T, Hysa VQ. Successful nonoperative treatment of isolated popliteus tendon avulsion fractures in two adolescents. Case Rep Orthop. 2014;2014:759419.
103. Petsche TS, Selesnick FH. Popliteus tendinitis: tips for diagnosis and management. Phys Sportsmed. 2002;30(8):27–31.
104. Forster BB, Lee JS, Kelly S, O'Dowd M, Munk PL, Andrews G, et al. Proximal tibiofibular joint: an often-forgotten cause of lateral knee pain. AJR Am J Roentgenol. 2007;188(4):W359–66.
105. Alves-da-Silva T, Guerra-Pinto F, Matias R, Pessoa P. Kinematics of the proximal tibiofibular joint is influenced by ligament integrity, knee and ankle mobility: an exploratory cadaver study. Knee Surg Sports Traumatol Arthrosc. 2019;27(2):405–11.
106. Marchetti DC, Moatshe G, Phelps BM, Dahl KD, Ferrari MB, Chahla J, et al. The proximal tibiofibular joint: a biomechanical analysis of the anterior and posterior ligamentous complexes. Am J Sports Med. 2017;45(8):1888–92.
107. Ogden JA. The anatomy and function of the proximal tibiofibular joint. Clin Orthop Relat Res. 1974;101:186–91.
108. Iosifidis MI, Giannoulis I, Tsarouhas A, Traios S. Isolated acute dislocation of the proximal tibiofibular joint. Orthopedics. 2008;31(6):605.
109. Belk JW, Kraeutler MJ, Houck DA, Goodrich JA, Dragoo JL, McCarty EC. Platelet-rich plasma versus hyaluronic acid for knee osteoarthritis: a systematic review and meta-analysis of randomized controlled trials. Am J Sports Med. 2021;49(1):249–60.
110. Mamound A, Hoencamp R, Bosman WM, Leijnen M. Proximal tibiofibular joint dislocation: a rare entity. BMJ Case Rep. 2019;12(1)

45 Knee Dislocations and Fractures

Jennifer Soo Hoo, Gerard D'Onofrio, and Gisela Figueroa

45.1 Synonyms

Kneecap dislocations
- Dislocated kneecap
- Patellar subluxation
- Tibiofemoral dislocation
- Knee subluxation
- Knee dislocation
- Patellar fracture
- Tibial plateau fracture
- Proximal tibia fracture

45.2 Knee Dislocations (S83.0)

45.2.1 Description

45.2.1.1 Anatomy of Patellofemoral Joint

The patellofemoral joint is one of the three main compartments of the knee. See anterior knee section for more detail regarding anatomy. The role of this joint is to enhance the extensor mechanism of the knee by increasing the moment arm of the quadriceps tendon on the tibia, increasing mechanical efficiency. Stability of the patella in the trochlear groove is provided by static and dynamic stabilizers. The bony contour of the patellofemoral joint provides static stabilization. Further, the medial and lateral patellofemoral ligaments add stability. A hypoplastic patellar ridge, flat trochlea, or increased Q angle can all predispose the patella to dislocate.

The quadriceps tendon and patellar tendon (ligament) are the main dynamic stabilizers of the patellofemoral articulation. Rupture of the medial patellofemoral ligament results in unopposed pull from lateral structures, such as the tensor fascia lata, lateral patellofemoral ligament, and the quadriceps tendon superiorly [1]. Articular hyaline cartilage, mostly type II collagen, covers the trochlear groove and patellar facets. The lateral patellar nerve innervates the lateral-anterior border of the patella, with the medial plantar nerve innervating the patella at the medial-anterior portion. These are both distal branches of the femoral nerve [2]. The vascular supply of the patellofemoral joint is provided by the genicular arteries.

45.2.1.2 Anatomy of Tibiofemoral Joint

The tibiofemoral joint is formed by the articulation of the medial and lateral femoral condyles with the corresponding tibial plateaus. These articulations are covered by hyaline cartilage, comprised of type II collagen. The tibiofemoral articulation is inherently unstable as the bony morphology does not provide significant stability. Thus, the joint is stabilized by the medial and lateral collateral ligaments as well as the anterior and posterior cruciate ligaments. Muscles crossing the tibiofemoral joint, such as the hamstrings, gastrocnemii, quadriceps, popliteus, and tendons of the pes anserine complex, add dynamic stability [1].

Patellar dislocations are the most common type of the knee dislocated. They most often result due to an injured medial patellofemoral ligament. This results in a destabilized patella because the medial patellofemoral ligament is the dominant medial static stabilizer of the knee.

Tibiofemoral dislocations or knee joint dislocations are very rare but considered a surgical emergency. It is important to know how to identify and screen for these as they require rapid transport to the ER for further evaluation.

J. S. Hoo (✉)
Department of Rehabilitation Medicine, Weill Cornell Medicine, New York, NY, USA

Department of Rehabilitation Medicine, New York Presbyterian, New York, NY, USA
e-mail: jes9343@med.cornell.edu

G. D'Onofrio · G. Figueroa
Department of Rehabilitation Medicine, New York Presbyterian, New York, NY, USA

© The Author(s), under exclusive license to Springer Nature Switzerland AG 2022
S. A. Mostoufi et al. (eds.), *Clinical Guide to Musculoskeletal Medicine*, https://doi.org/10.1007/978-3-030-92042-5_45

45.2.2 Clinical Presentation

45.2.2.1 Patella Dislocation

Patellar dislocations often occur as a result of noncontact injury, during which twisting activities can result in dislocation of the patella. In contact circumstances, there may be a direct blow to the knee with valgus force that destabilizes the patella. Notably, there is a high rate of recurrence of these injuries, with approximately 50% of patients experiencing recurrent injuries. The main complaints after patellar dislocation are instability, locking of the knee, and pain. A lateralized patella can be appreciated with an altered contour of the knee joint. Rapid accumulation of swelling may occur due to the acute injury, and patients may note difficulty bearing weight through the knee. Predisposing factors are those such as patella alta (high-riding patella), as well as trochlear dysplasia or quadriceps dysplasia [3]. Patellar dislocations occur commonly in the second decade and are more common in females.

45.2.2.2 Tibiofemoral Dislocation

Patients with instability or pain should be evaluated for tibiofemoral dislocation, as it is a surgical emergency and concurrent vascular injuries and jeopardize the lower extremity. Specifically, the popliteal artery is at risk of injury during tibiofemoral dislocation as well as the common peroneal nerve. The incidence of neurologic injury with tibiofemoral dislocation ranges from 10% to 40%. Cruciate ligaments may be torn in tibiofemoral dislocations and indicate worse functional outcomes. Tibiofemoral dislocation usually occurs in high-impact trauma. A posteriorly directed force across the tibia can cause posterior dislocations, whereas hyperextension injuries tend to cause anterior dislocations (most common). Tibiofemoral dislocations cause injuries to multiple ligaments. Patients typically present with severe pain, instability, and may hear a "pop" during the injury. They are unable to return to sport. There may be gross deformity depending on if the knee stays dislocated. Depending on whether vascular or nerve supply is affected, there may be numbness/tingling, weakness, and skin color change. This is a true surgical emergency [4].

45.2.3 Physical Examination

45.2.3.1 Patella Dislocation

Inspection The examiner should appreciate abnormal contour of the knee joint and altered patellar alignment, which may be assessed with patellar tilt and inclination. A lateralized patella may be at the level of the patellar facets or superolaterally. Discoloration may be evident along the medial aspect of the patellar facets, where the medial patellofemoral ligament may have been injured.

Palpation Patients may have tenderness to palpation evident on the medial aspect of the patella, due to injury of the medial patellofemoral ligament.

Range of motion General range of motion may be limited due to traumatically associated hemarthrosis of the knee. Further, the range of motion of the patellae can be appreciated with increased patellar translation, and patients may demonstrate apprehension during passive movement of the patella by the examiner. Patients will have pain or exhibit apprehension, which indicates patellar instability or medial patellofemoral ligament or medial retinaculum injury [1].

45.2.3.2 Tibiofemoral Dislocation

Inspection If the knee doesn't spontaneously reduce, the knee joint can be obviously deformed with associated swelling and bruising.

Neurovascular assessment Neurovascular assessment should be the main focus of evaluation due to potential injury of the popliteal artery and common peroneal nerve. Thorough evaluation should be performed with focus on dermatomes, myotomes, capillary refill, skin color, skin temperature, and dorsalis pedis and posterior tibial pulses. Strength testing at the knee should be avoided due to likely substantial ligamentous and soft tissue damage during injury.

45.2.4 Diagnostic Workup

X-ray X-rays are the staple of diagnosis for patellar dislocation and aid to rule out associated osteochondral fractures. Radiographs of the knee should have anteroposterior, lateral (with appropriate condylar alignment), and skyline films. Patella alta or a high-riding patella can be appreciated on lateral films, and the skyline films help to determine patellar tilt and position relative to the trochlear groove. X-rays will indicate tibiofemoral malalignment in cases of tibiofemoral dislocation [1].

MRI MRI is of importance for tibiofemoral dislocations as well, as it helps to provide insight into ligament integrity. MRIs may be indicated if the patient has recurrent patellar dislocations and there is concern for associated ligamentous and meniscal injury that may have occurred during the injurious episode. There is usually a characteristic bruising pattern of the lateral femoral condyle and medial patella in patellar dislocations. Further, MRI may reveal disruption of the medial patellofemoral ligament at the medial femoral epicondyle insertion. MRI can also provide information about articular cartilage damage on the medial patellar facet and whether there are additional osteochondral lesions.

Vascular studies In cases of tibiofemoral dislocation, vascular studies such as an ankle-brachial index (ABI) and vascular angiography are of value because they can elucidate whether the dislocation caused injury to popliteal artery. ABI provides a measurement of blood pressure in the ankle versus in the arm, whereas the CT angiography would provide a gold standard picture of the vascular network at the knee and below [4].

45.2.5 Treatment

45.2.5.1 Medical Management

Acute management of an acute patella dislocation includes prompt reduction of the patella by flexing the hip to relax the tension on the patella exerted by the quadriceps and subsequently, extending the knee. After confirming there are no significant, concurrent injuries that require further investigation, management is largely conservative. The emphasis is on abating the acute injury with rest, ice, compression, and elevation. Short-term NSAIDs can be used, and bracing in a J-brace or patella-stabilizing sleeve may be beneficial for the first 2–4 weeks. Patients are permitted to be weight-bearing as tolerated and may use crutches to aid them ambulate [5].

Initial treatment for tibiofemoral dislocation includes immediate reduction and splinting of the knee in extension or in the most comfortable position. Subsequently, the patient should be immediately transported to the nearest emergency room.

45.2.5.2 Rehabilitation

Tibiofemoral Dislocation Rehab

As this is a surgical emergency, this should be taken to the ER, and rehabilitation should not be tried as first-line treatment.

Patella Dislocation Rehab

Rehabilitation is important for those who sustained acute or recurrent patellar dislocations and are treated nonoperatively. Variations in treatment interventions for nonoperative patellar dislocations exist. There are no standardized clinical practice guidelines for nonoperative physical therapy interventions. There is a lack of quality evidence to support the use of any specific nonoperative method for the treatment of patellar dislocations [6]. Variations in treatment interventions for nonoperative patellar dislocations exist. Treatment interventions initially consist of reducing pain and edema through ice, compression, and elevation.

- Immobilization: After an acute patellar dislocation, the most common form of treatment is knee immobilization into extension to allow for healing and decrease stress of the soft tissue structures at the knee. Various knee immobilization braces, splints, or cast are used with duration of immobilization ranging from 3 weeks or greater [6, 7].
- Exercises: Strengthening begins with improving quadriceps activation including vastus medialis oblique activation. Electrical stimulation can be used to improve quadriceps muscle activation. As edema decreases and early healing has occurred, range of motion is progressed along with strengthening [8]. Posterior and lateral hip strengthening can be incorporated to address any weakness associated with excessive femoral internal rotation. Flexibility training of the quadriceps and gastrocnemius muscles may help to optimize patellar alignment and tracking. As functional mobility progresses, a patellar stabilization brace can be used for increased stability [7, 8].
- Patellar taping can also be used to improve patellar alignment and tracking [6].
- Manual techniques including patellar mobilizations and soft tissue massage may be used to address any superior or lateral soft tissue restrictions at the knee to improve patellar alignment and tracking within the femoral groove.
- Orthotics may be considered to correct for excessive foot pronation and tibial internal rotation possibly contributing to patellar instability [8]. Physical therapy exercises should focus on quadriceps and vastus medialis oblique strengthening, core strengthening, and proprioceptive training after patellofemoral dislocation.

45.2.5.3 Surgery

Patients with recurrent patella dislocations may require evaluation from orthopedic surgery so that stabilization can be achieved without further injury to the knee joint from dislocations. There is a paucity of evidence regarding the threshold for surgical intervention after recurrent patellofemoral dislocations. Tibiofemoral dislocations are a surgical emergency and must be brought to the nearest emergency room immediately for evaluation by a surgeon. Please see Knee Surgery chapter for more details.

45.3 Knee Fractures (S82.1)

45.3.1 Description

Anatomy The tibial plateau is the most proximal tibial surface which articulates with the femur [9]. It is divided into two sections, lateral tibial plateau and medial tibial plateau. The tibial plateau is a weight-bearing surface for the lower extremity, and fractures may occur due to axial loading forces or a valgus/varus moment leading to mechanical axis malalignment [10]. The tibial plateau is supplied by the genicular nerves. The vascular supply of the knee is largely provided by the popliteal artery and the four anastomosing genicular arteries [16].

Two of the most common knee fractures include patella and tibial plateau fractures. Tibial plateau fractures may result from traumatic injury or bone insufficiency, whereas patellar fractures commonly occur from either a direct blow to the patella or a failed knee extensor mechanism.

45.3.2 Clinical Presentation

45.3.2.1 Tibial Plateau Fractures

Patients will present with pain on weight-bearing. They may also present with associated effusions and decreased range of motion. Discoloration of the skin may be evident due to local injury. If the mechanism of injury is a fall from height—a common mechanism of injury for tibial plateau fracture—patients may have pelvic or spinal injuries as well. The mechanism of injury can be both low energy in the form of insufficiency fractures in osteoporotic patients or high-energy association with a traumatic event. The fractures typically occur along the lateral condyle but may be bicondylar or along the medial condyle. Tibial plateau fractures may be associated with meniscal tears, anterior cruciate ligament tears, or vascular injuries. The injuries tend to occur in younger males or frail, elders with underlying osteoporosis [17]. In addition, tibial plateau fractures should be assessed for concomitant dislocation/relocation injury and neurovascular compromise.

45.3.2.2 Patellar Fractures

It may occur as a result of either a blow to the anterior knee or a failed extensor mechanism of the knee. Patients will be unable to extend the knee and will have pain and swelling localizable to the patella. The sesamoid patella can fail when an opposing force is acting to flex the knee. For patellar fractures, patients should be assessed for associated femoral neck injuries and knee dislocation [11]. Contact sport athletes such as football players are at risk for direct blows to the knee causing patellar fractures. Elderly patients with weakened bone may suffer patella fractures as a result of the forces exerted on the patella exceeding strength of the bone [16].

45.3.3 Physical Examination

Inspection Both tibial and patellar fractures may present with redness evident on inspection. Further, there may be a dome effusion around the patella, obscuring the margins of the patella [16].

Palpation Direct pressure to either the patella or tibial plateau will result in pain reproduction in cases when those structures are fractured. Compartment syndrome must be ruled out in the case of knee fractures and may be evident when compartments are not compressible as compared to the contralateral knee.

Range of motion Active range of motion for the quadriceps muscles may be impaired in patellar fractures due to failure of the extensor mechanism. The patella acts to increase leverage for the quadriceps, and thus, if it is fractured, the patient may be unable to complete knee extension range of motion testing. Tibial plateau fractures may also have compromised range of motion due to a knee effusion associated with the fracture.

Manual muscle testing Muscular strength is diminished in the setting of patellar fractures as the sesamoid patella acts to transmit forces generated by the quadriceps. This would be evident in knee extension manual muscle testing.

Provocative maneuvers A straight leg test may be used to test the extensor mechanism of the knee joint in cases of patellar fractures and ultimately provide insight into the integrity of the patellofemoral junction.

Gait analysis Patients with knee fractures will walk with an antalgic gait and attempt to offload the affected side. This may include reduced time in stance phase and exhibit failure to flex the knee throughout the stance phase of the gait cycle.

45.3.4 Diagnostic Workup

X-ray Plain films are essential for the diagnosis of tibial plateau and patellar fractures. A knee trauma series should be ordered for evaluation of patellar fractures and tibial plateau fractures [16]. X-rays are useful because they not only pick up fractures but may also demonstrate radiopaque blood in

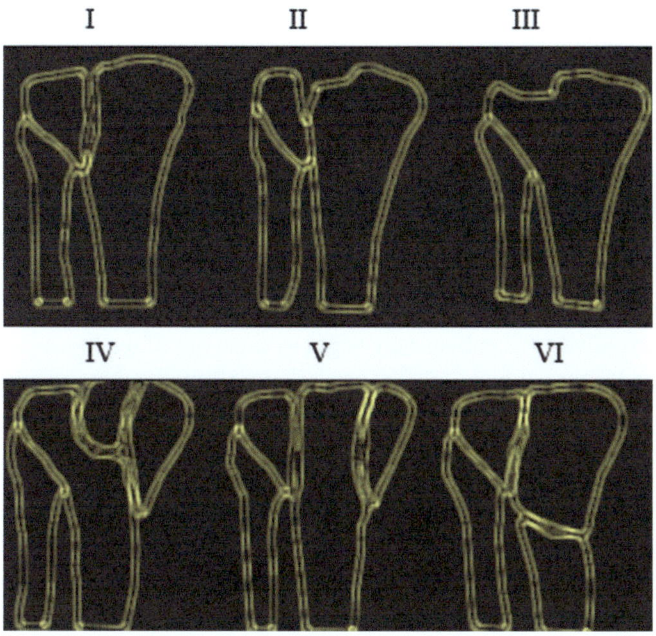

Fig. 45.1 The Schatzker classification system is used for tibial plateau fracture. (Modified Illustration by Yasmine Mostoufi)

hemorrhagic, traumatic effusions post-injury. Both anteroposterior and lateral knee X-rays are necessary to elucidate tibial plateau fractures and patellar fractures. The Schatzker classification system, used for tibial plateau fracture, is a six-grade classification (Fig. 45.1). Schatzker type I fractures and, occasionally, type II fractures are amenable to conservative treatment [17]. Patellar fractures can be classified as either displaced or nondisplaced. The displaced fractures generally have a step-off greater than 2 mm and a fracture gap greater than 1–4 mm [11].

CT Scan In the event clarity is needed after obtaining plain films, CT scans can provide a greater degree of insight into knee fractures. CT scans can be coupled with vascular imaging can evaluate vascular integrity. Figure 45.2 below shows an impaction fracture of the posteromedial tibial plateau in a patient with underlying bone demineralization.

45.3.5 Treatment

45.3.5.1 Medical Management

Tibial Plateau Fracture

Schatzker type I fractures and, occasionally, type II fractures are amenable to conservative treatment. Grade I fractures can be managed with knee immobilizers, hinged knee brace, or cast for 6–8 weeks as well as non-weight-bearing for 6–12 weeks [16]. More advanced grades require surgical intervention and may be permitted for greater range of motion postoperatively, but still require the patient to be non-weight-bearing for 12 weeks.

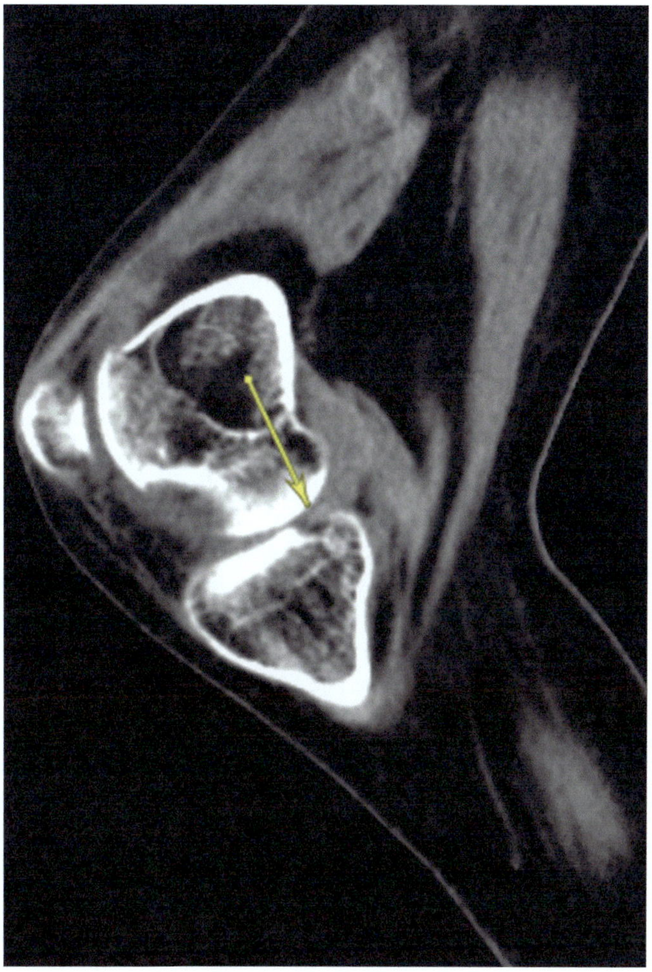

Fig. 45.2 CT scan showing impaction fracture of posteromedial tibial plateau

Patellar Fracture

Nondisplaced fractures with an intact extensor mechanism can be managed with a knee immobilizer for 6–8 weeks with active and active-assisted range of motion beginning at 1–2 weeks. Partial, early weight-bearing is recommended with the knee brace locked in extension [11, 16].

45.3.5.2 Rehabilitation

Tibial Plateau Fracture Rehab

Nonoperative tibial plateau fractures require physical therapy intervention. There is limited research published to guide the rehabilitation process. Goals of the acute phase are to protect the healing fracture. A long-hinged knee brace may be prescribed by the physician to decrease torsional forces at the knee and allow for safe mobilization [12]. While the brace may be unlocked to perform exercises, the patient may be instructed by the physician to lock the brace into extension during transfers and ambulation to provide stability at the knee. Weight-bearing precautions including duration and progression are provided by the physician ranging from non-weight-bearing to partial weight-bearing to offload the fracture sight. Pain and edema are treated with compression, elevation, and ice. Strengthening of quadriceps and gluteal isometrics are initially performed in open chain positions until the physician clears the patient for weight-bearing activities. Electrical stimulation may be used to increase quadriceps strength. Hip strengthening is initially performed with the knee brace locked in extension and may include straight leg raises in all planes of motion. Gastrocnemius strengthening using TheraBand can also be incorporated. The physician will guide the range of motion precautions. To decrease joint stiffness, active, active assist, and passive knee flexion/extension range of motion are performed during physical therapy sessions. Quadriceps, hamstrings, and gastrocnemius stretching can improve mobility of the affected lower extremity. Manual techniques such as patellar mobilizations and soft tissue massage help to improve knee range of motion and knee arthrokinematics. Once the patient has been cleared for weight-bearing at tolerated, closed chain strengthening such as step up/down exercises should be incorporated to progress lower extremity strength. Multi-surface and multiplane balance training is also included at this phase in order to improve lower extremity stability during functional mobility. Gait training is necessary to improve gait speed in various directions and progress the patient to ambulation without an assistive device or to a less restrictive device [12].

Patella Fracture Rehab

There are few published recommendations for physical therapy management. During the acute phase of injury, the goals of rehabilitation are to protect the healing fracture site and limit tensile loading through immobilization using bracing or casting into knee extension [13–16]. The duration of immobilization is physician-guided and ranges from 4 to 6 weeks [14–16]. Weight-bearing precautions and progression are provided by the physician and range from partial weight-bearing to weight-bearing as tolerated with knee brace locked in extension. Patients may use assistive devices such as bilateral axillary crutches or rolling worker to decrease pain with weight-bearing and improve standing balance during transfers and ambulation. Edema and pain are controlled through compression, elevation, and icing. Strengthening begins with quadriceps and gluteal isometrics with the knee brace locked in extension. As the fracture site demonstrates healing, the physician will clear the patient for gradual knee flexion passive, active assistive, and active range of motion. If there is minimal edema, moist heat can be used prior to range of motion to promote soft tissue extensibility [17]. Manual techniques such as patellar and tibiofemoral mobilizations may help to decrease joint stiffness and improve knee range of motion. Soft tissue massage to the surrounding structures of the knee can also increase the range of motion and decrease pain. Gait training initially begins by improving lower extremity weight acceptance. Once knee flexion range of motion is permitted, gait training is progressed to include swing phase training along with weight acceptance and loading in various directions. As quadriceps strength improves, the patient may begin to wean out of the brace per physician. Open- and closed-chain strengthening of hip extensors, hip abductors, quadriceps, hamstrings, and gastrocnemius will improve lower extremity stability. Aquatic therapy can also be used to improve range of motion and strength of the lower extremity. As range of motion and strength improve, patients progress to static and dynamic balance training on various surfaces and conditions to return the patient to their previous level of function including ambulation with the least restrictive assistive device or without an assistive device.

45.3.5.3 Surgery

Surgical intervention for knee fractures is necessary if there is a displaced patellar fracture and an advanced grade tibial plateau fracture. See Knee Surgery chapter for further details.

References

1. Thompson JC. Netter's concise orthopaedic anatomy. Elsevier. 2nd edn. 2016. p. 286–323
2. Waryasz GR, Mcdermott AY. Patellofemoral pain syndrome (PFPS): a systematic review of anatomy and potential risk factors. Dyn Med. 2008;14:1–14.
3. Moiz M, Smith N, Smith TO, Chawla A, Thompson P, Metcalfe A. Clinical outcomes after the nonoperative management of lateral patellar dislocations: a systematic review. Orthop J Sport Med. 2018;6(6):1–17.
4. Follow-up LLF, Jr RCS, Richter DL, Wascher DC. Knee dislocations. Orthop J. Sports Med. 2014;1–10.
5. Johnson DS, Turner PG. Management of the first-time lateral patellar dislocation. Knee [Internet]. 2019;26(6):1161–5. Available from: https://doi.org/10.1016/j.knee.2019.10.015.
6. Moiz M, Smith N, Smith TO, Chawla A, Thompson P, Metcalfe A. Clinical outcomes after the nonoperative management of lateral patellar dislocations: a systematic review. Orthop J Sports Med. 2018; https://doi.org/10.1177/2325967118766275.
7. Atkin DM, Fithian DC, Marangi KS, Stone ML, Dobson BE, Mendelsohn C. Characteristics of patients with primary acute lateral patellar dislocation and their recovery within the first 6 months of injury. Am J Sports Med. 2000;28(4):472–9. https://doi.org/10.1177/03635465000280040601.
8. Wilk KE, Davies GJ, Mangine RE, Malone TR. Patellofemoral disorders: a classification system and clinical guidelines for non-operative rehabilitation. J Orthop Sports Phys Ther. Elsevier. 1998;28(5):307–22.

9. Thompson JC. Netter's concise orthopaedic anatomy. Elsevier. 2nd edn. 2016. p. 286–323.
10. Mthethwa J, Chikate A. A review of the management of tibial plateau fractures. Musculoskelet Surg. 2018;102(2):119–27.
11. Melvin JS, Mehta S. Patellar fractures in adults. J Am Acad Orthop Surg. 2011;19(4):198–207.
12. Koval KJ, Helfet DL. Tibial plateau fractures: evaluation and treatment. J Am Acad Orthop Surg. 1995;3(2):86–94.
13. Bui CN, Learned JR, Scolaro JA. Treatment of patellar fractures and injuries to the extensor mechanism of the knee. JBJS Rev. 2018;6(10):e1. https://doi.org/10.2106/JBJS.RVW.17.00172.
14. Melvin JS, Mehta S. Patellar fractures in adults. Jam Acad Orthop Surg. 2011;19:198–207.
15. Cramer KE, Moed BR. Patellar fractures: contemporary approach to treatment. J Am Acad Orthop Surg. 1997;5:323–31.
16. Steinmetz S, Brügger A, Chauveau J, Chevalley F, Borens O, Thein E. Practical guidelines for the treatment of patellar fractures in adults. Swiss Medical Weekly 150 (2020): W20165. Web.
17. Exler Y. Patella fracture: review of the literature and five case presentations. J Orthop Sports Phys Ther. 1991;13(4):177–83.

Surgical Intervention in the Knee

46

Alfred J. Tria Jr, Casey Imbergamo, Daniel Haddad, and Andrzej Brzezinski

46.1 Knee Intra-articular Ligament Reconstruction (ACL, PCL)

46.1.1 ACL Surgery

46.1.1.1 Operation

Arthroscopy is a gold standard technique for addressing intra-articular knee pathologies. The treatment of anterior cruciate ligament (ACL) rupture is individualized, and surgical reconstruction of the ligament is typically implemented for those with a high activity level or with functional instability of the knee. Due to poor healing potential of the ACL, reconstructive techniques are utilized almost exclusively to address a complete tear of the ACL. The ligament can be reconstructed with autograft, allograft, or synthetic materials. Anatomic reconstruction of the ligament is achieved to restore anterior and rotational stability of the knee which prevents further meniscal and cartilaginous injuries

Autograft

Autograft selection includes most commonly the hamstrings (semitendinosus and gracilis), bone patellar tendon bone, and quadriceps tendon grafts. Clinical results do not differ based on autograft selection with weak evidence suggesting superior stability and graft incorporation with the use of a bone patellar tendon bone graft.

Allografts

An alternative option for ACL reconstruction, especially in less active patients over 40 years old, is the use of allografts. They are easily available and do not cause any donor site morbidity; however, an allograft can potentially provoke an immune response and is associated with a higher failure rate in young athletes. Good short- and mid-term results are also reported after using the new generation of synthetic grafts. Surgical technique includes passage of the graft into the joint through previously drilled tunnels and anchoring to the bone with interference screws, cross pins, or endobutton suspension techniques. Graft selection and fixation methods do not affect the rehabilitation protocol [1].

46.1.1.2 Rehabilitation: ACL

Postoperatively, patients undergo an accelerated rehabilitation program including immediate partial weight-bearing (PWB), early range of motion (ROM) with full passive extension, and progressive strengthening with an emphasis on closed chain movements. Open-chain movements such as seated leg extensions are avoided as they place excess stress on the graft as the extensor mechanism pulls the tibia anteriorly. Gait and proprioception training also seem to be beneficial for patients after ACL reconstruction. While historically some surgeons have recommended using a brace for return to sport postoperatively, it has been shown that bracing does not affect ROM, graft stability, or protection from subsequent injury [2].

46.1.2 PCL Surgery

46.1.2.1 Operation

Arthroscopic surgery is utilized in the treatment of posterior cruciate ligament (PCL) injuries. The PCL can be reconstructed with either an autograft, allograft, or synthetic material. Grafts can be harvested from the Achilles, patellar, hamstring, or anterior tibialis tendons. Postoperative rehabilitation for PCL reconstruction includes immediate PWB, early ROM in the prone position, and progressive resistance exercises (PRE) with a focus on quadriceps strengthening. Hamstring strengthening exercises such as hamstring curls are avoided in early rehabilitation as they pull the tibia posteriorly placing undue stress on the graft [3]. For PCL injuries, the knee should be protected with bracing, and sport activities should be limited for several months [4, 5].

A. J. Tria Jr (✉) · C. Imbergamo · D. Haddad · A. Brzezinski
Department of Orthopaedics, Rutgers-Robert Wood Johnson Medical School, New Brunswick, NJ, USA

© The Author(s), under exclusive license to Springer Nature Switzerland AG 2022
S. A. Mostoufi et al. (eds.), *Clinical Guide to Musculoskeletal Medicine*, https://doi.org/10.1007/978-3-030-92042-5_46

In the context of multi-ligamentous knee injuries, structures such as the lateral collateral ligament (LCL), medial collateral ligament (MCL), posterolateral corner (PLC), or posteromedial corner (PMC) may be damaged in addition to the cruciate ligaments. Nonsurgical treatment with a period of immobilization and restricted active and passive range of motion is a viable treatment option in selected group of patients (inactive, those with multiple comorbidities, or with contraindication to surgical intervention). Surgical intervention is preferred in younger, physically active patients and results in improved patient-reported outcomes [6, 7]. Surgical management must be tailored individually. Primary repair is utilized to address acute injury (<28 days) of non-cruciate ligaments, while reconstruction is preferred if surgery is delayed (>28 days).

46.1.2.2 Rehabilitation: PCL

Postoperative rehabilitation will vary based on the extent of injuries and methods of surgical repair or reconstruction utilized. The goal of rehabilitation is to maintain balance between stability and mobility of the knee. Protective braces and delayed weight-bearing until healing of collateral ligaments is recommended. Supervised early passive range of motion is utilized to prevent stiffness [6].

46.2 Knee Meniscal Injury

46.2.1 Operation

Meniscal injuries that fail initial conservative management can be addressed with surgical intervention. The primary goal with operative management is to restore the native structure, function, and biomechanics of the meniscus to prevent early development of osteoarthritis. With a few exceptions, an arthroscopic approach is utilized for meniscus surgery.

Meniscal injuries can often be repaired with suture devices; however, tears that are not amenable to repair (complex, degenerative, radial tear patterns) can be addressed with partial meniscectomy. Additionally, meniscal reconstruction can be considered in select patients with painful post-meniscectomy syndrome. Reconstruction techniques include meniscal allograft transplantation (MAT) or meniscus scaffold implantation with either a collagen or polyurethane-based scaffold. This is an ongoing area of novel research [8].

46.2.2 Rehabilitation

Rehab protocols vary depending on the treatment method. Following meniscectomy, accelerated rehabilitation protocols can be implemented which include immediate weight-bearing as tolerated (WBAT), early ROM, and progressive strengthening. A repaired or reconstructed meniscus needs to be protected for a period of 6 weeks with non-weight-bearing (NWB) ambulation and the knee locked in extension. Physical therapy should be focused on reducing pain and edema, restoring full extension with good quadriceps muscle control, and patella mobility. Supervised passive ROM exercise can start early after surgery with a goal of 90 degrees of knee flexion in the first 4 weeks, progressing to 120 degrees of flexion on postoperative week 8. Knee brace and crutches need to be utilized for about 6 weeks. After that time, gait and muscle strengthening exercises can be accelerated. Return to regular activity typically occurs at approximately 4–6 months [9].

46.3 Knee Cartilage Injuries

46.3.1 Operation

Various surgical techniques are utilized for the treatment of focal cartilage injury and depend on defect morphology (size, depth), location, patient-specific factors (age, activity level), and joint-related factors (stability, alignment, meniscus status). The goal of the surgery is to alleviate the symptoms, stop the progression of articular damage, restore the articular surface anatomy, and create an environment for healing [10]. Currently, the surgical options include palliative (debridement, marrow stimulation as abrasion arthroplasty, subchondral drilling, or microfractures) and reconstructive procedures (autologous chondrocyte implantation, osteochondral autografting, and fresh osteochondral allografting) [10]. The marrow stimulating techniques which can be performed arthroscopically are used to enhance the growth of fibrocartilage that fills the chondral defect. The goal of restorative techniques is to produce a hyaline-like articular surface and requires arthrotomy to be performed. Debridement and microfractures are recommended for high-demand patients with lesions <2.5 cm^2 or low-demand patients with lesions <4 cm^2. High-demand patients with lesions >2.5 cm^2 and others with cartilage defects >4 cm^2 may benefit from reconstructive options [10].

46.3.2 Rehabilitation

The objectives of physical therapy after cartilage restoration are to protect the repair, create an optimal environment for healing, and gradually restore the function of the knee. For the first 6 weeks after surgery, the knee needs to be immobilized in extension, and ROM needs to be limited to 60 degrees of flexion. The patient can ambulate with crutches and PWB, progressing to full weight-bearing (FWB) on postoperative week 6. Intermittent cyclic loading can be initiated early and progress through the rehabilitation program [11]. After 6 weeks, the knee ROM can be gradually increased until reaching full. The patient can work on gait and muscle strengthening exercises. Return to regular activity occurs at approximately 12 months. The rehab protocol can vary based on location and morphology of the defect with a more liberal protocol for small condylar lesions and a strict protocol for larger defects and those localized in the patellofemoral joint.

46.4 Knee Osteoarthritis

46.4.1 Operation

Knee osteoarthritis (OA) that has failed to respond to conservative management can be addressed with several surgical options. The type of surgical intervention depends on the severity and extent of the arthritic changes, as well as knee alignment and ligamentous status. Unicompartmental osteoarthritis in younger patients (<50 years) with stable knees can be treated with periarticular osteotomies or partial knee replacement. The best treatment option for advanced multicompartmental arthritis is total knee arthroplasty (TKA). The goal of the osteotomy is to unload an affected compartment alleviating the pressure on the cartilage and postpone the degenerative process. In patients with medial compartment OA, a valgus-producing high tibial osteotomy can be implemented. In case of lateral compartment disease, a distal femoral varus-producing osteotomy is recommended. Following an osteotomy, PWB is allowed immediately, with progression to unrestricted FWB within 6 weeks. Early ROM is also implemented for these patients [12]. Patients with unicompartmental disease may also be treated with unicompartmental knee arthroplasty (UKA). This procedure is an alternative to TKA and is thought to have fewer complications, faster recovery, and preservation of normal kinematics. UKA implants can have a fixed or a mobile-bearing design, both being viable options with successful patient outcomes [13]. TKA is utilized as a primary procedure for tricompartmental osteoarthritis of the knee or as a salvage procedure after failure of the other treatment options. For patients who undergo TKA, there are a variety of implants that can be utilized, including posterior stabilized (PS), posterior cruciate substituting (CS), posterior cruciate retaining (CR), and bi-cruciate retaining (BCR) implants. The standard knee arthroplasty implant typically consists of a cemented or non-cemented cobalt-chrome femoral component and a titanium tibial baseplate with a polyethylene liner. The patella can also be resurfaced with a polyethylene patellar button [14].

46.4.2 Rehabilitation

Following knee arthroplasty, patients require extensive rehabilitation starting on the same day as the surgery to regain ROM and function of the knee. Rehabilitation includes immediate WBAT with assistive devices, with progression to unrestricted FWB within 4 weeks. Early ROM is crucial, and 90 degrees of flexion should be obtained within 3–4 weeks following surgery. Exercises focusing on muscle strength (specifically of the quadriceps), gait, and balance should also be included in the rehabilitation process [15].

46.5 Knee Fractures

Fractures surrounding the knee joint can occur in the distal femur, proximal tibia, or patella. There is bimodal distribution of the fractures around the knee with high-energy trauma in younger individuals and lower-energy mechanisms in the elderly. The goal in treating these fractures is to restore the anatomy of the articular surface and provide stable fixation for early ROM [16].

46.5.1 Distal Femur Fractures

Distal femur fractures can be treated with open reduction internal fixation (ORIF) utilizing a weight-bearing construct, such as a locking plate or weight-sharing intramedullary (IM) devices. Following ORIF, depending on the fracture pattern, the patient may be made NWB or PWB with assistive devices. Progression to FWB typically occurs after 6 weeks. Additionally, arthroplasty with distal femoral replacement can be implemented for patients with fracture patterns that are not amenable to reconstruction or with preexisting osteoarthritis [16]. These patients undergo postoperative rehabilitation as described above for TKA.

46.5.1.1 *Rehabilitation:* Distal Femur Fractures

Early ROM and progressive resistance exercises should be incorporated into the rehabilitation protocol as well. Rehabilitation following IM nail placement depends on the stability of the fracture. Unstable fracture patterns (long oblique or spiral, comminuted) can be NWB for up to 6 weeks, while stable fracture patterns (minimally displaced, transverse, or short oblique) can be made PWB with assistance immediately after surgery, with progression to FWB when radiographic evidence of callus formation at the fracture site is present. Early ROM and progressive resistance exercises should also be incorporated into the rehabilitation process [17].

46.5.2 Proximal Tibia Fracture

Fractures of the proximal tibia can occur distal to the knee joint or extend into the articular surface in what is identified as a tibial plateau fracture. These fractures are treated with ORIF to restore the joint surface with absolute stability.

46.5.2.1 *Rehabilitation:* Proximal Tibia Fracture

Postoperatively, patients are placed in a hinged knee brace with early passive ROM and are made NWB or PWB for 3–4 months [18].

46.5.3 Patella Fracture

Fractures of the patella can be treated with ORIF techniques that include a tension band construct or screw fixation. For severe fractures that are not amenable to reconstruction, partial or complete patellectomy can be considered [19].

46.5.3.1 *Rehabilitation:* Fractures of the Patella

Following ORIF, PWB can be started with the knee locked in full extension. Range of motion exercises are slowly progressed with a goal of approximately 0–90 degrees of flexion by week 6 when FWB is typically instituted [20].

46.6 Knee Dislocation

Knee dislocations are traumatic injuries that require urgent reduction and assessment of neurovascular status, as they have a high rate of associated nerve (common fibular nerve) and vascular (popliteal artery) injury.

46.6.1 Operation

If closed reduction cannot be achieved, open reduction is indicated. Following reduction, most patients require surgical stabilization, followed by early ligamentous reconstruction within 3 weeks of initial injury. If the injury does not require an open arthrotomy, arthroscopic surgery is implemented for intra-articular pathology. See sections on ACL, PCL, and meniscal injuries. Open repair may be indicated for injuries to the PLC or PMC. There is a high complication rate after knee dislocation, and it is rare for the knee to return to a pre-injury state.

46.6.2 *Rehabilitation:* Knee Dislocation

Rehabilitation must be tailored to the pattern of injury, and the main goals are to protect the surgical repair, restore full passive extension, and maximize quadriceps function. Early restrictions are placed on weight-bearing and ROM, with incremental advancement after 6 weeks postoperatively [21]. The rehabilitation must be individually tailored to the extent of the injury and the surgical approach that was used.

References

1. Anderson MJ, Browning WM 3rd, Urband CE, Kluczynski MA, Bisson LJ. A systematic summary of systematic reviews on the topic of the anterior cruciate ligament. Orthop J Sports Med. 2016;4(3):2325967116634074. https://doi.org/10.1177/2325967116634074.
2. Wright RW, Fetzer GB. Bracing after ACL reconstruction: a systematic review. Clin Orthop Relat Res. 2007;455:162–8. https://doi.org/10.1097/BLO.0b013e31802c9360.
3. Kaufman KR, An KN, Litchy WJ, Morrey BF, Chao EY. Dynamic joint forces during knee isokinetic exercise. Am J Sports Med. 1991;19(3):305–16. https://doi.org/10.1177/036354659101900317.
4. Wright RW, Preston E, Fleming BC. A systematic review of anterior cruciate ligament reconstruction rehabilitation: part II: open versus closed kinetic chain exercises, neuromuscular electrical stimulation, accelerated rehabilitation, and miscellaneous topics. J Knee Surg. 2008;21(3):225–34. https://doi.org/10.1055/s-0030-1247823.
5. Pache S, Aman ZS, Kennedy M, Nakama GY, Moatshe G, Ziegler C, LaPrade RF. Posterior cruciate ligament: current concepts review. Arch Bone Jt Surg. 2018;6(1):8–18.
6. Cox CL, Spindler KP. Multiligamentous knee injuries - surgical treatment algorithm. N Am J Sports Phys Ther. 2008;3(4):198–203. PMID: 21509121; PMCID: PMC2953345.
7. Dedmond BT, Almekinders LC. Operative versus nonoperative treatment of knee dislocations: a meta-analysis. Am J Knee Surg. 2001 Winter;14(1):33–8. Erratum in: Am J Knee Surg 2001 Autumn;14(4):220. PMID: 11216717.
8. Doral MN, Bilge O, Huri G, Turhan E, Verdonk R. Modern treatment of meniscal tears. EFORT Open Rev. 2018;3(5):260–8. https://doi.org/10.1302/2058-5241.3.170067.
9. Spang RC III, Nasr MC, Mohamadi A, DeAngelis JP, Nazarian A, Ramappa AJ. Rehabilitation following meniscal repair: a systematic review. BMJ Open Sport Exerc Med. 2018;4(1):e000212. https://doi.org/10.1136/bmjsem-2016-000212.
10. Ozmeriç A, Alemdaroğlu KB, Aydoğan NH. Treatment for cartilage injuries of the knee with a new treatment algorithm. World J Orthop. 2014;5(5):677–84. https://doi.org/10.5312/wjo.v5.i5.677.
11. Hambly K, Silvers HJ, Steinwachs M. Rehabilitation after articular cartilage repair of the knee in the football (soccer) player. Cartilage. 2012;3(1 Suppl):50S–6S. https://doi.org/10.1177/1947603511413569.
12. Brinkman JM, Lobenhoffer P, Agneskirchner JD, Staubli AE, Wymenga AB, van Heerwaarden RJ. Osteotomies around the knee: patient selection, stability of fixation and bone healing in high tibial osteotomies. J Bone Joint Surg Br. 2008;90(12):1548–57. https://doi.org/10.1302/0301-620X.90B12.21198.
13. Lim JW, Cousins GR, Clift BA, Ridley D, Johnston LR. Oxford unicompartmental knee arthroplasty versus age and gender matched total knee arthroplasty - functional outcome and survivorship analysis. J Arthroplast. 2014;29(9):1779–83. https://doi.org/10.1016/j.arth.2014.03.043.
14. McGrory BJ, Weber KL, Jevsevar DS, Sevarino K. Surgical management of osteoarthritis of the knee: evidence-based guideline. J

Am Acad Orthop Surg. 2016;24(8):e87–93. https://doi.org/10.5435/JAAOS-D-16-00159.

15. Dávila Castrodad IM, Recai TM, Abraham MM, Etcheson JI, Mohamed NS, Edalatpour A, Delanois RE. Rehabilitation protocols following total knee arthroplasty: a review of study designs and outcome measures. Ann Transl Med. 2019;7(Suppl 7):S255. https://doi.org/10.21037/atm.2019.08.15.
16. Gangavalli AK, Nwachuku CO. Management of distal femur fractures in adults: an overview of options. Orthop Clin North Am. 2016;47(1):85–96. https://doi.org/10.1016/j.ocl.2015.08.011.
17. Kim J, Kang SB, Nam K, Rhee SH, Won JW, Han HS. Retrograde intramedullary nailing for distal femur fracture with osteoporosis. Clin Orthop Surg. 2012;4(4):307–12. https://doi.org/10.4055/cios.2012.4.4.307.
18. Prat-Fabregat S, Camacho-Carrasco P. Treatment strategy for tibial plateau fractures: an update. EFORT Open Rev. 2017;1(5):225–32. https://doi.org/10.1302/2058-5241.1.000031.
19. Gwinner C, Märdian S, Schwabe P, Schaser KD, Krapohl BD, Jung TM. Current concepts review: fractures of the patella. GMS Interdiscip Plast Reconstr Surg DGPW. 2016;5:Doc01. https://doi.org/10.3205/iprs000080.
20. Lazaro LE, Wellman DS, Sauro G, Pardee NC, Berkes MB, Little MT, Nguyen JT, Helfet DL, Lorich DG, et al. J Bone Joint Surg Am. 2013;95(14):e96 1–8. https://doi.org/10.2106/JBJS.L.00012.
21. Howells NR, Brunton LR, Robinson J, Porteus AJ, Eldridge JD, Murray JR. Acute knee dislocation: an evidence based approach to the management of the multiligament injured knee. Injury. 2011;42(11):1198–204. https://doi.org/10.1016/j.injury.2010.11.018.

Part IX

Ankle-Foot

Section Editor

Timothy Tiu

47 Anterior Ankle Disorders

Seyed Behrooz Mostofi, Abdolrahman Fazli, and Walter I. Sussman

47.1 Tibialis Anterior Tendinopathy

47.1.1 Synonyms

Anterior tibial tenosynovitis, *Anterior tibial tendonitis*, *Anterior tibial* tendinosis

47.1.2 ICD 10 Code

M76.819: Anterior tibial syndrome

47.1.3 Description

Tibialis anterior tendinopathy is acute or chronic changes of the tibialis anterior tendon, and it is frequently divided into mid-substance and distal type. Most tendon abnormalities are located within the first 3 cm proximal to the insertion [1].

Tibialis anterior tendinopathy can be spontaneous, traumatic, or associated with anterior ankle impingement/ankle OA. It has been reported in athletes, especially runners, where it is categorized as an overuse injury following an increase in training distance and with up- and downhill training [2]. Distal tibialis anterior tendinosis is predominantly reported in overweight women in the 50–70 years of age [3]. Grossly diseased tendon appears thickened and can lose its normal fibrillar architecture when scanned with ultrasound. Histologically, the tendon shows myxoid degeneration [4]. Longitudinal split tears and tenosynovitis can be detected by scanning the tendon, and in some cases distal bursitis is associated with tendinopathy. Differential diagnosis of tibialis anterior tendinopathy is in Table 47.1.

Table 47.1 Differential diagnosis of tibialis anterior tendinopathy

Differential diagnosis of tibialis anterior tendinopathy	
Anterior ankle impingement	Ankle joint or midfoot arthritis
Tibialis anterior bursitis	Tibialis anterior tendinosis
Tibialis anterior tendon rupture	Tibialis anterior tendinitis

47.1.3.1 Anatomy and Function

Tibialis anterior originates from the upper two-thirds of the lateral tibia, courses deep to the extensor retinaculum over the anterior ankle and inserts on the medial cuneiform and the first metatarsal bone, although variations in the distal insertions have been described [4]. The main synovial bursa associated with the insertion is located between the tendon and the medial cuneiform. The function of the tibialis anterior tendon is dorsiflexion of the ankle, supination and adduction of the foot, and support the suspension of the arch. It is innervated by a branch of the deep peroneal nerve, and blood supply arises from the anterior tibial artery and medial tarsal artery.

47.1.4 Clinical Presentation

Comprehensive musculoskeletal and neurologic examination should be conducted to evaluate the tendon but also to evaluate other causes of anterior ankle pain including radiculopathy. Patients typically present with a gradual onset of pain and swelling on the anterior aspect of the ankle joint and burning along the medial side of the midfoot. Active dorsiflexion of the foot against resistance is painful and limited. No sensory deficit is expected and, if detected, needs to be further investigated.

S. B. Mostofi (✉)
East Kent Hospitals University, NHS Foundation Trust, Canterbury, Kent, UK

Department of Orthopedics, Manipal Academy of Higher Education, Manipal, India

A. Fazli
Queen Elizabeth The Queen Mother Hospital, East Kent Hospitals University, NHS Foundation Trust, Margate, UK

W. I. Sussman
Department of Orthopedics and Rehabilitation, Tufts University School of Medicine, Boston, MA, USA

Boston Sports & Biologics PC, Wellesley, MA, USA

© The Author(s), under exclusive license to Springer Nature Switzerland AG 2022
S. A. Mostoufi et al. (eds.), *Clinical Guide to Musculoskeletal Medicine*, https://doi.org/10.1007/978-3-030-92042-5_47

47.1.5 Physical Examination

Swelling or palpable crepitus can sometimes be found along the course of the tendon. Active dorsiflexion of the foot against resistance is typically painful and limited. There is typically no loss of strength, but ankle dorsiflexion weakness should be of concern due to possible tendon tear or nerve impingement (spine or fibular nerve impingement).

47.1.5.1 Provocative Maneuvers

Tibialis anterior passive stretch test This is a provocative maneuver for tibialis anterior tendinosis [5]. During the test, ankle plantarflexion, hindfoot eversion, midfoot abduction, and pronation force is applied to the foot in an attempt to passively stretch the tibialis anterior tendon (Fig. 47.1). Pain at the tendon insertion site is considered to be a positive test.

47.1.6 Diagnostic Workup

X-rays Tibialis anterior tendinopathy is mostly clinical, but X-rays can rule out other pathology including ankle OA or osteophytosis resulting in anterior ankle impingement.

Ultrasound/MRI Ultrasound and MRI both can show the extent and severity of tendinopathy [1, 4]. US is widely available, portable, and can detect tenosynovitis, split tears, thickening of the tendon, and changes in tendon fibrillar pattern. In complex ankle injuries, MRI may be more appropriate and can be combined with contrast enhancement for further definition of pathology.

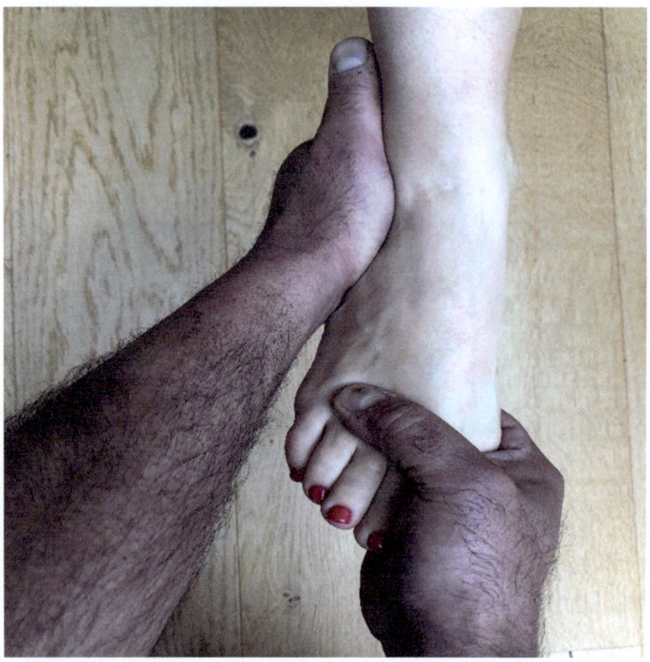

Fig. 47.1 Tibialis anterior passive stretch test

47.1.7 Treatment

47.1.7.1 Medical Management

Conservative management includes immobilization and modification of activities and modalities of physical therapy like therapeutic ultrasound and infrared treatment to reduce inflammation [6].

47.1.7.2 Procedures

For recurrent or nonresponsive cases of tenosynovitis and bursitis, peritendon corticosteroid injection has been reported to have good results [7]. US-guided platelet-rich plasma (PRP) injection can be considered for tenosynovitis, tendinosis, and tendinitis, but no studies specific to tibialis anterior tendinopathy have been conducted to date.

47.1.7.3 Rehabilitation

In nonoperative cases, many physical therapy strategies have been proposed to rehab tendinopathy. These include therapeutic ultrasound, extracorporeal shockwave therapy, low-level laser, iontophoresis, and non-electrotherapeutic modalities such as eccentric training and soft tissue techniques. There is no consensus of rehabilitation after procedural treatment such as PRP injection in particular intratendinous injections. Rehabilitation of the tendon after the operation can vary due to diverse surgical management and whether it is an open or endoscopic treatment.

47.1.7.4 Surgery

Surgical debridement of the tendon or repair with tendon augmentation, synovectomy, and/or bursectomy can be considered in cases not responding to conservative and procedural treatments. This can be done both as an open or endoscopic approach [8]. More information on foot and ankle surgery can be found in Chap. 52.

47.2 Anterior Ankle Impingement

47.2.1 Synonyms

- Ankle impingement
- Athlete's ankle
- Footballer's ankle (Soccer)
- Impingement exostoses

47.2.2 ICD 10 Code

M25.871, M25.872

47.2.3 Description

Morris and McMurray provided early descriptions of anterior impingement, coining the condition as "athlete's ankle" and "footballer's ankle," respectively [9, 10]. Anterior ankle impingement refers to a broad spectrum of pathology resulting in abnormal entrapment or impingement of traversing structures anterior to the tibiotalar joint during dorsiflexion resulting in pain or restricted motion. Differential diagnosis of anterior ankle impingement includes extensor tenosynovitis or rupture, synovial or ganglion cyst, and ankle osteoarthritis.

47.2.3.1 Anatomy and Etiology

Anatomically, anterior ankle impingement is defined as the ankle recess between the anterior tibial plafond and talar dome. There is an intra-articular triangular soft tissue (adipose tissue and synovium) at the anterior aspect of the ankle which is compressed above 15 degrees of dorsiflexion [11]. In the presence of anterior osteophytes, the space for this tissue is limited, and compression leads to chronic inflammation, synovitis, and capsuloligamentous hypertrophy. During dorsiflexion, the anterolateral border of the talus extends into the anterolateral recess, impinging bony or soft tissue structures. Anterolateral impingement occurs in a pyramidal space formed by the tibia, fibula, and ATFL. Anteromedial impingement occurs in the anteromedial recess formed by the talar dome/neck, medial malleolus, and deltoid ligament.

The etiology of anterior ankle impingement can be varied, often caused by bony and/or soft tissue structures of the anterior ankle including osteophytosis or exostosis. Anteromedial and anterolateral impingement have also been described [11]. The exact etiology of osteophyte/exostosis is not well described but is thought to be due to repetitive direct microtrauma leading to the formation of osseous spurs [12, 13]. These osteophytes then result in the irritation of the capsule and synovium. If osteophytes are present on both joint edges, then it is referred to as the "kissing lesion." Tibial osteophytes are more common and can have a corresponding through on the talar dome called "tram-line track" [14].

47.2.4 Clinical Presentation

Patients with anterior ankle impingement typically present with pain during dorsiflexion of the ankle accompanied by focal swelling. Exacerbating activities commonly include climbing stairs, running, uphill walking, ascending ladders, and deep squatting. With progression of the disorder, dorsiflexion pain may increase, range of motion may be restricted, and joint stiffness is noted.

47.2.5 Physical Examination

Examination should include both the foot and ankle. The ankle and foot are inspected for abnormal alignment, joint effusion, or soft tissue edema. The bone and soft tissue structures are systematically palpated to assess for localized tenderness. Anterior and anterolateral joint line pain is a hallmark of anterior ankle impingement syndrome. Forced dorsiflexion of the ankle generates pain by causing impingement between the bone spur of distal tibia and the neck of the talus.

47.2.6 Diagnostic Workup

X-rays Standard weight-bearing lateral X-rays, with the malleoli positioned perpendicular to the surface of the radiographic film, may be useful in the initial assessment of ankle impingement [15] (Fig. 47.2). Osteophytes/exostoses of the distal anterior tibia and dorsal talar neck may be present. Dynamic hyper dorsiflexion views can be considered to assess abnormal bony contact.

MRI Advanced imaging, such as MRI, can be useful to determine the presence of soft tissue pathology that may be causing ankle impingement. Furthermore, MRI allows the physician to rule out other potential diagnoses, including osteochondral lesions, loose bodies, and stress fractures. There is limited utility for CT if X-rays and MRI is available.

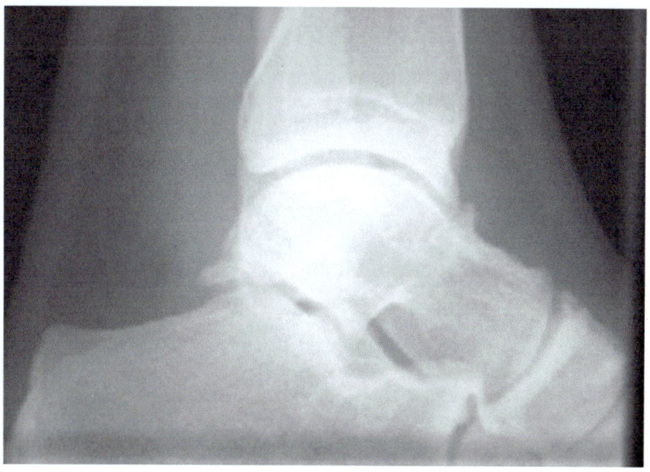

Fig. 47.2 Lateral view: anterior impingement showing the "kissing lesion" of the distal tibia and talar dome

47.2.7 Treatment

47.2.7.1 Medical Management

Nonsurgical treatment remains the initial approach to the management of both anterior and posterior impingement syndromes, despite limited evidence of its efficacy. For acute symptoms, a period of rest and an avoidance of provocative activities are recommended. Rest can be supplemented with ice, NSAIDs, or immobilization in a walking boot in severe cases. In chronic cases, shoe modifications, including heel lift orthoses to prevent dorsiflexion, have been utilized.

47.2.7.2 Rehabilitation

Physical therapy protocols focus on improving ankle stability and optimizing proprioception. In some cases, reduction of range of motion is noted and physical therapist will work with the patient to increase available range of motion in multiple planes including ankle dorsiflexion. Postoperative rehabilitation will follow surgeons' guidelines, and it depends on open versus arthroscopic approach.

47.2.7.3 Procedure

Some patients report improvements after intra-articular ankle steroid injection [16] which can be done with ultrasound or X-ray guidance. The primary objective is reduction in pain and perhaps improved participation in rehabilitation.

47.2.7.4 Surgery

Surgical intervention is generally indicated for cases which have not responded to nonoperative treatment. It involves debridement and removal of the osteophytes or impinged soft tissues or both. Open operative treatment of anterior ankle impingement has been demonstrated as effective but has also been associated with a number of complications like wound infection, damage to the nerves and vessels, and painful scars. Ankle arthroscopy has been growing in popularity with low complication rates [17]. More information on foot and ankle surgery can be found in Chap. 52.

47.3 Osteochondral Lesion of the Talus

47.3.1 Synonym

Osteochondral lesion of the talus, Osteochondritis dissecans of the talus, Transchondral fracture, Osteochondral fracture, Osteochondral defect

47.3.2 ICD 10 Code

- M93.271 – Osteochondritis dissecans, right ankle
- M93.272 – Osteochondritis dissecans, left ankle

47.3.3 Description

Osteochondral lesions of the talus are common injuries in recreational and professional athletes, with up to 50% of acute ankle sprains and fractures developing some form of chondral injury [18]. The talus is divided into three distinct regions: the body, neck, and head. Classically, osteochondral lesions are located in the dome of the body of the talus. There is limited vascular supply, limiting the healing potential for osteochondral injuries of the talus [19]. A variety of etiologies have been proposed, including local osteonecrosis, systemic vasculopathies, acute trauma, chronic microtrauma, endocrine or metabolic factors, degenerative joint disease, joint malalignment, and genetic predisposition. Many of these lesions are associated with traumatic events with a history of trauma documented in more than 75% of patients with osteochondral lesions of the talus [20].

Berndt and Harty classified transchondral lesion involving the subchondral bone into four different stages (Fig. 47.3):

- Stage I, a small area of compression of subchondral bone
- Stage II, a partially detached osteochondral fragment
- Stage III, a completely detached osteochondral fragment remaining in the crater
- Stage IV, a displaced osteochondral fragment

Medial lesions are more common and caused by inversion, plantarflexion, and lateral rotation injury of the tibia on the talus. They are also more posterior than lateral lesions, which are produced by inversion and strong dorsiflexion and are more anterior on the talar dome. Morphologically, medial lesions tend to be deeper and cup shaped, whereas lateral lesions are usually shallow and wafer shaped. Medial lesions usually are nondisplaced, and lateral lesions often are displaced. Although the incidence of osteochondral lesions of the talus has been reported as approximately 4% of all osteochondral lesions, the true incidence may be higher. Some studies have suggested that osteochondral lesions of the talus may occur in up to 50% of acute ankle sprains and fractures, particularly in association with sports injuries. Differential diagnosis of osteochondral lesion of the talus is in Table 47.2.

47.3.4 Clinical Presentation

Patients often have a delayed presentation, often 6–12 months after the initial trauma (ankle fracture or sprain). Patients typically describe a deep ankle pain provoked during or after load-bearing activities. Additional symptoms may include, but may not be limited to, stiffness, a locking or catching sensation (which can indicate a displaced fragment or

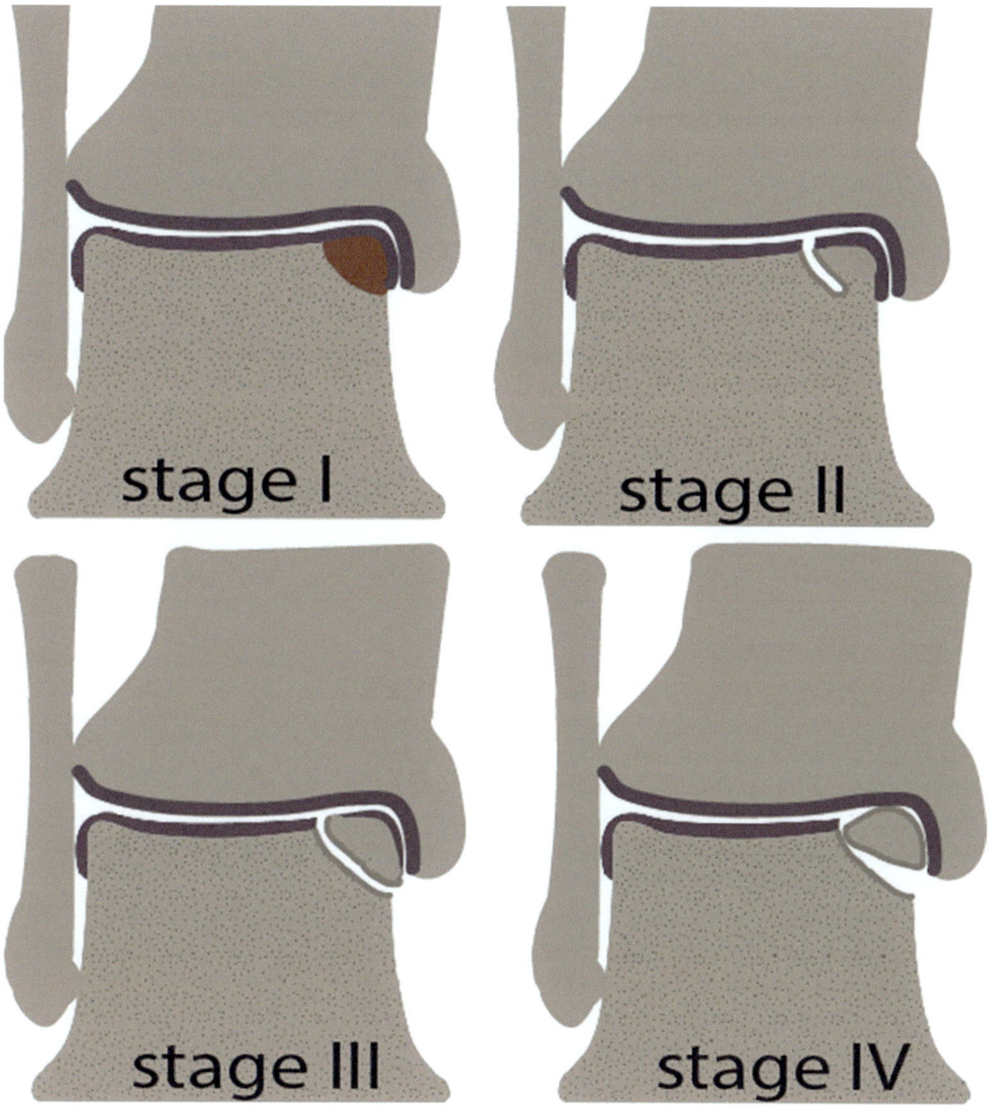

Fig. 47.3 Brandt and Harty classification of transchondral lesion involving the subchondral bone. (Illustration by Yasmine Mostoufi)

Table 47.2 Differential diagnosis of osteochondral lesion of the talus

Differential diagnosis of osteochondral lesion of the talus	
Occult fractures	Hindfoot coalitions or deformity
Syndesmotic injury	Lateral ankle instability
Peroneal tendinopathy	Ankle impingement
Ankle arthritis	Subtalar arthritis

pseudo-impingement due to the displaced cartilaginous flap), swelling (especially after activities), and reduced range of motion.

47.3.5 Physical Examination

Anterior ankle joint line tenderness may be present. The recognizable deep ankle pain can often be provoked by forcefully palpating the talar dome with the ankle in full plantar flexion. The lack of positive physical examination findings, however, does not exclude an osteochondral lesion since history and physical examination are often nonspecific and nondiagnostic. Persistent effusion, delayed synovitis, and locking or giving way of the joint 4–5 weeks after ankle injury are indications for radiographic examination.

47.3.6 Diagnostics Workup

X-rays Oblique and plantar flexion views that avoid tibial overlap generally show the osteochondral lesion more clearly than standard plain films [21]. Nearly half of osteochondral lesions of the talus were reported to be missed on radiographs by emergency department physicians, who usually make a diagnosis of "sprained ankle."

CT scan CT scan helps determine the exact size and location of the lesion and any related cystic lesions.

MRI Useful modality in patients with OCD with 96% sensitivity and 96% specificity [22].

47.3.7 Treatment

The treatment of an osteochondral lesion depends on a variety of factors, including the characteristics of the patient (activity level, general health, age) and the lesion (size, location) and associated degenerative changes.

47.3.7.1 Medical Management

Most nondisplaced osteochondral lesions initially should be treated conservatively with immobilization and physical therapy.

47.3.7.2 Rehabilitation

Type I and type II lesions and small grade 3 lesions may follow similar protocol during conservative treatment. This consists of immobilization (bracing) along with NSAIDs and non-weight-bearing status. If a patient is symptomatically improving, a gradual progressive weight-bearing- and exercise-based treatment may be added. Return to sports activity could be divided into multiple stages including walking, jogging, return to noncontact sport (running without swerving), and eventually return to contact sport (running with spurring and collision). Large grade 3 lesions and grade 4 lesions are generally considered operative candidates, and postoperative rehabilitation depends on the type of surgery performed. The age of the patient, body mass index, and the size of the osteochondral lesion may affect rehabilitation outcome. The postoperative rehabilitation protocols have not been uniformly determined. In arthroscopic-based surgeries, most published studies describe a period of early immobilization followed by up to 6 weeks of non-weight-bearing [23].

47.3.7.3 Procedures

PRP improves joint function and reduces pain in patients with osteochondral lesion [24]. In addition, inter-study comparison demonstrated that patients that received surgery along with PRP injections improved more than those that received PRP in isolation [24].

47.3.7.4 Surgery

Indications for operative treatment include failure of conservative management and completely avulsed and/or displaced fragments. Operative treatment may include debridement of the lesion with stimulation of the underlying subchondral bone (microfracture, drilling, abrasion, curettage), direct repair of the lesion (retrograde drilling and bone grafting, internal fixation), or repair of the lesion with osteochondral autografts or allografts or chondrocyte transplantation [19, 21]. Because of the difficulty of adequately filling the contours of the lesion, bone grafts have been used in conjunction with retrograde drilling to prevent articular collapse. More recently, surgical-grade calcium sulfate in a liquid form has been injected into the defect after drilling, and some authors have reported the use of a bone-marrow aspirate harvested from the iliac crest, centrifuged to isolate pluripotent cells, and mixed with the calcium graft to promote more rapid healing [19]. More information on foot and ankle surgery can be found in Chap. 52.

References

1. Mengiardi B, Pfirrmann CW, Vienne P, et al. Anterior tibial tendon abnormalities: MR imaging findings. Radiology. 2005;235:977–84.
2. Sammarco VJ, Sammarco GJ, Henning C, Chaim S. Surgical repair of acute and chronic tibialis anterior tendon ruptures. J Bone Joint Surg Am. 2009;91(2):325–32. https://doi.org/10.2106/JBJS.G.01386. PMID: 19181976.
3. Lemmens L, Van Beek N, Verfaillie S. Postoperative results of distal tibialis anterior tendinosis. Foot Ankle Surg. 2019:26. https://doi.org/10.1016/j.fas.2019.11.005.
4. Varghese A, Bianchi S. Ultrasound of tibialis anterior muscle and tendon: anatomy, technique of examination, normal and pathologic appearance. J Ultrasound. 2014;17(2):113–23.
5. Beischer AD, Beamond BM, Jowett AJ, O'Sullivan R. Distal tendinosis of the tibialis anterior tendon. Foot Ankle Int. 2009;30(11):1053–9.
6. Pedowitz D, Beck D. Presentation, diagnosis, and nonsurgical treatment options of the anterior tibial tendon, posterior tibial tendon, peroneals, and achilles. Foot Ankle Clin. 2017;22(4):677–87.
7. Laurell L, Court-Payen M, Nielsen S, Zak M, Fasth A. Ultrasonography and color Doppler in juvenile idiopathic arthritis: diagnosis and follow-up of ultrasound-guided steroid injection in the wrist region. A descriptive interventional study. Pediatr Rheumatol Online J. 2012;10:11. Published 2012 Apr 21. https://doi.org/10.1186/1546-0096-10-11.
8. Grundy JR, O'Sullivan RM, Beischer AD, et al. Operative management of distal tibialis anterior tendinopathy. Foot Ankle Int. 2010;31:212–9.
9. Morris LH. Report of cases of athlete's ankle. J Bone Joint Surg. 1943;25:22.
10. McMurray TP. Footballer's ankle. J Bone Joint Surg Br. 1950;32:68–9.
11. Berman Z, Tafur M, Ahmed SS, Huang BK, Chang EY. Ankle impingement syndromes: an imaging review. Br J Radiol. 2017;90:20160735.
12. Tol JL, van Dijk CN. Etiology of the anterior ankle impingement syndrome: a descriptive anatomical study. Foot Ankle Int. 2004;25:382–6.
13. Biedert R. Anterior ankle pain in sports medicine: aetiology and indications for arthroscopy. Arch Orthop Trauma Surg. 1991;110:293–7.
14. Robinson P, White LM, Salonen D, Ogilvie-Harris D. Anteromedial impingement of the ankle: using MR arthrography to assess the anteromedial recess. AJR. 2002;178:601–4.
15. van Dijk CN, Wessel RN, Tol JL, Maas M. Oblique radiograph for the detection of bone spurs in anterior ankle impingement. Skelet Radiol. 2002 Apr;31(4):214–21.

16. Nazarian LN, Gulvartian NV, Freeland EC, Chao W. Ultrasound-guided percutaneous needle fenestration and corticosteroid injection for anterior and anterolateral ankle impingement. Foot Ankle Spec. 2018;11(1):61–6.
17. Zekry M, Shahban SA, El Gamal T, et al. A literature review of the complications following anterior and posterior ankle arthroscopy. Foot Ankle Surg. 2018;S1268–7731(18):30079–1.
18. Murawski CD, Kennedy JG. Operative treatment of osteochondral lesions of the talus. J Bone Joint Surg Am. 2013;95(11):1045–54.
19. Looze CA, Capo J, Ryan MK, Begly JP, Chapman C, Swanson D, Singh BC, Strauss EJ. Evaluation and management of osteochondral lesions of the talus. Cartilage. 2017;8(1):19–30.
20. Rikken QGH, Kerkhoffs GMMJ. Osteochondral lesions of the talus: an individualized treatment paradigm from the Amsterdam perspective. Foot Ankle Clin. 2021;26(1):121–36.
21. McGahan PJ, Pinney SJ. Current concept review: osteochondral lesions of the talus. Foot Ankle Int. 2010;31(1):90–101.
22. Verhagen RA, Maas M, Dijkgraaf MG, Tol JL, Krips R, van Dijk CN. Prospective study on diagnostic strategies in osteochondral lesions of the talus. Is MRI superior to helical CT? J Bone Joint Surg Br. 2005;87(1):41–6.
23. Ferkel RD, Zanotti RM, Komenda GA, Sgaglione NA, Cheng MS, Applegate GR, Dopirak RM. Physical therapy and range-of-motion activities are usually started prior to weightbearing. Am J Sports Med. 2008;36(9):1750–62.
24. Yausep OE, Madhi I, Trigkilidas D. Platelet rich plasma for treatment of osteochondral lesions of the talus: a systematic review of clinical trials. J Orthop. 2020;18:218–25. https://doi.org/10.1016/j.jor.2020.01.046. PMID: 32071508; PMCID: PMC7013135.

48 Posterior Ankle Disorders

Seyed Behrooz Mostofi, Chu H. Chiang, Walter I. Sussman, and S. Ali Mostoufi

48.1 Achilles Tendon Disorders

48.1.1 ICD 10

- M76.61 Achilles tendonitis (bursitis), right
- M76.62 Achilles tendonitis (bursitis), left
- S86.011 Achilles rupture, right
- S86.012 Achilles rupture, left
- M65.28 Calcific Achilles tendinosis

48.1.2 Description

Achilles tendon pathology exists on a spectrum of disorders from tendinopathy to complete rupture and can involve the proximal myotendinous junction, midsubstance, or insertion of the tendon. Midsubstance Achilles tendinopathy is a painful overuse injury of the Achilles tendon and will be discussed in this section and insertional tendinopathy and Haglund deformity in the subsequent section.

Anatomy The Achilles tendon is a confluence of the gastrocnemius and soleus muscles. The gastrocnemius muscle crosses three joints, the knee, ankle, and the subtalar joint. This muscle provides the bulk of the definition and contour of the calf and is comprised of a higher proportion of fast-twitch muscle fibers in comparison to the soleus muscle [1, 2]. The second muscle, the soleus, crosses the ankle and subtalar joints. This muscle is predominantly involved in the maintenance of the posture of the leg. The gastrocsoleus complex is innervated by the tibial nerve. The Achilles tendon has no tendon sheath but has a highly vascularized paratenon. Healthy Achilles tendon inserts as a broad flat structure onto the posterior tubercle of the calcaneum. The fibers undergo a 90-degree internal rotation prior to insertion assisting its function by sporting potential energy via a recoil mechanism.

Etiology/pathophysiology Achilles tendinopathy is multifactorial which includes both intrinsic and extrinsic factors. Pathology is common in sports and daily life. While pathology is more likely to be seen with individuals who participate in physical activity such as running and jumping, it is not purely an athletic injury, as 65% of cases seen in a general practice setting are not sport related [3]. Extrinsic factors include training errors. Intrinsic risk factors include biomechanical abnormalities of the lower extremity (e.g., pes cavus, hyperpronation, varus deformity), increased age, corticosteroid use, diabetes, hypertension, obesity, gout, and fluoroquinolone antibiotic use. Enthesopathy due to rheumatologic spondyloarthropathy or autoimmune causes may also result in tendinopathy of the Achilles tendon. In 1976, Dr. Puddu and associates classified non-insertional Achilles tendinopathy into three stages as outlined in Table 48.1 [4].

Many terms have bene used to describe Achilles tendon pathology, including tendinitis, tendinosis, and paratenonitis. Recent histopathologic studies have shown a failed healing response, with reactive tendinopathy, tendon disrepair, and degenerative tendinopathy. The term tendinitis is now discouraged as it implies inflammatory activity, and histologically the tendon demonstrates a degenerative process instead of an inflammatory response. The term tendinopathy more accurately describes these intratendinous changes, including

S. B. Mostofi (✉)
East Kent Hospitals University, NHS Foundation Trust, Canterbury, Kent, UK

C. H. Chiang
Kent Surrey and Sussex Deanery, NHS Foundation Trust, Canterbury, Kent, UK

W. I. Sussman
Department of Orthopedics and Rehabilitation, Tufts University School of Medicine, Boston, MA, USA

Boston Sports & Biologics PC, Wellesley, MA, USA

S. A. Mostoufi
Department of Orthopedics and Rehabilitation, Tufts University School of Medicine, Boston, MA, USA

New England Spine Care Associates & Boston Regenerative Medicine, Cambridge, MA, USA

© The Author(s), under exclusive license to Springer Nature Switzerland AG 2022
S. A. Mostoufi et al. (eds.), *Clinical Guide to Musculoskeletal Medicine*, https://doi.org/10.1007/978-3-030-92042-5_48

Table 48.1 In 1976, Dr. Puddu and associates classified non-insertional Achilles tendinopathy into three stages

Puddu's classification of non-insertional Achilles tendon pathology
Paratenonitis: inflammation of the paratenon tissue
Paratenonitis with tendinosis: inflammation of the paratenon + degenerative tendon changes
Tendinosis: degenerative changes without inflammation. Rupture can occur

an increase in the number of tenocytes, disorganization and fragmentation of the collagen, and neovascularization.

Achilles tendon rupture accounts for 20% of all large tendon ruptures [5], and men are 2–12 times more prone to rupture than women [6]. There is a bimodal age distribution with the first peak between 25 and 40 years due to high sports injuries and the second peak in those >60 years old due to spontaneous rupture of degenerated Achilles tendons. Tears can be complete or partial.

48.1.3 Clinical Presentation

Heel pain is the primary symptom of Achilles pathology and can present with acute or a gradual onset of symptoms. Pain can be exacerbated with activity, but symptoms can progress, and patients may have pain at rest. Symptoms also can include stiffness and pain in the morning that improves throughout the day with mobilization.

Patients with an acute rupture often describe hearing a popping sound or have the feeling of being kicked in the back of the ankle. Patients typically will have difficulty weight-bearing and describe weakness.

48.1.4 Physical Examination

In cases of tendinopathy, pain with palpation of the Achilles tendon and fusiform thickening of the tendon may be present. In cases of Achilles tendon rupture, weakness, palpable defect, ecchymosis, and swelling may be present.

48.1.4.1 Special Tests

Thompson test squeezing the calf muscles while the patient is kneeling or lying face down with feet hanging unsupported. Squeezing the calf should cause contraction of the Achilles tendon, resulting in plantar flexion. If the Achilles tendon is completely ruptured, there will not be any apparent plantar flexion.

Matles test ask the patient to lie prone with her knees flexed to 90° with the feet relaxed. In a normal test, her feet will be in slight plantarflexion. Dorsiflexion of the foot is a positive test and indicates a ruptured Achilles tendon. False negative specialized testing may be present in cases with intact plantaris tendon or extrinsic foot flexors.

48.1.5 Diagnostic Workup

The diagnosis of Achilles tendinopathy or rupture is primarily clinical, but imaging can assist with diagnosis.

48.1.5.1 Plain Films

Routine orthogonal radiographs of the ankle can help reveal erosion of the cortical bone seen in inflammatory arthropathy, or calcification associated with inflammation that can be seen in the tendon or at the insertion.

48.1.5.2 Advanced Imaging

Advanced imaging in the form of ultrasound or magnetic resonance imaging (MRI) is useful for delineating the location of the tear when there is doubt (Fig. 48.1). Diagnostic ultrasound has an accuracy of 96% in diagnosing complete Achilles tendon ruptures (Fig. 48.2) and 75% accuracy in diagnosing partial ruptures compared to surgical correlation [7]. In Achilles tendinopathy, ultrasound is comparable to MRI [7]. MRI of Achilles tendon ruptures have reported the association of tendinosis in the tendon surround the rupture site [8] (Fig. 48.3a, b).

48.1.6 Treatment

48.1.6.1 Medical Management

Medical management of Achilles tendinopathy depends on the stage of the disease. In the early tendinitis/bursitis stage, treatment includes rest, ice packs, painkillers, and exercises to help to stretch and strengthen the Achilles tendon. Orthotics with heel elevation may reduce strain on the Achilles by shortening the pull of a tight gastrocnemius mus-

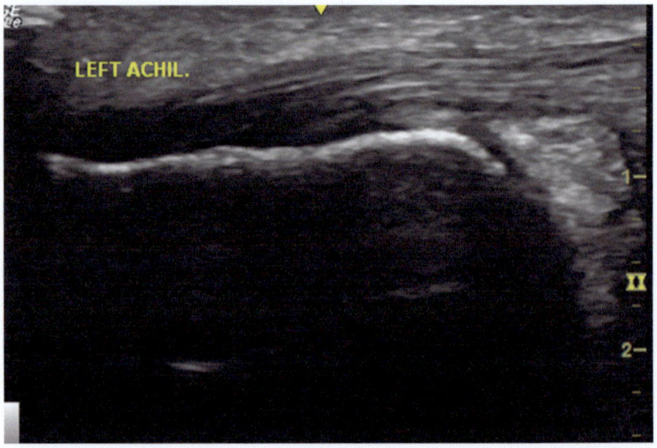

Fig. 48.1 A normal Achilles tendon and insertion onto calcaneus

cle on the tendon. For most people, the symptoms of Achilles tendinopathy usually clear within 3–6 months of starting treatment. In chronic tendinosis, NSAIDs may be less effective, but rehabilitation is recommended. In partial and full-thickness tear without retraction, initial plan of care should include pain management, short-term bracing, and involvement of orthopedic surgery for consultation, in particularly in full-thickness tear.

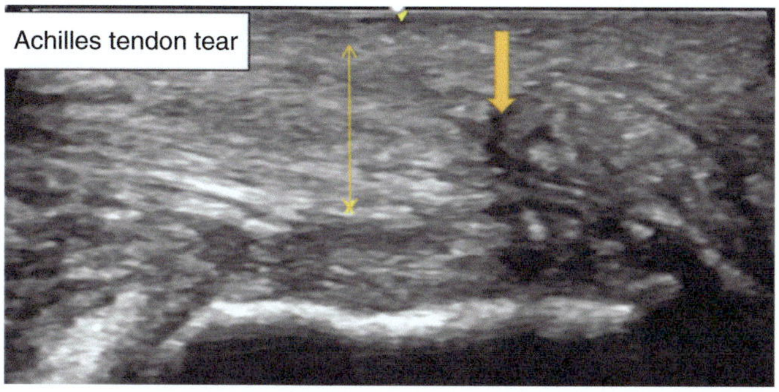

Fig. 48.2 US imaging demonstrating full tear of the Achilles tendon (thicker arrow) with retraction. Thickening of the Achilles tendon with tendinosis noted proximal to tear

48.1.6.2 Rehabilitation

Rehabilitation for Achilles tendon pathology is typically divided into four phases: (1) symptom management and load reduction, (2) recovery, (3) rebuilding, and (4) return to sport or activity. Loading of the tendon is generally introduced in the later phases. Eccentric resistance training exercises have been reported to be effective [9].

48.1.6.3 Procedure

Corticosteroid Injection

Corticosteroid injection in general is avoided due to concern of long-term effect such as atrophy and tendon rupture [10]. If a decision is made for a peritendon steroid injection in an acute inflammatory phase, with associated bursitis, practitioners should utilize image guidance to avoid tendon penetration.

Brisement

In athletes with midsubstance paratenonitis, brisement, or local anesthetic injection has been reported to be effective in 50% of patients after 2–3 serial injections. The hypothesis behind this technique is hydrodissection of the pseudosheath

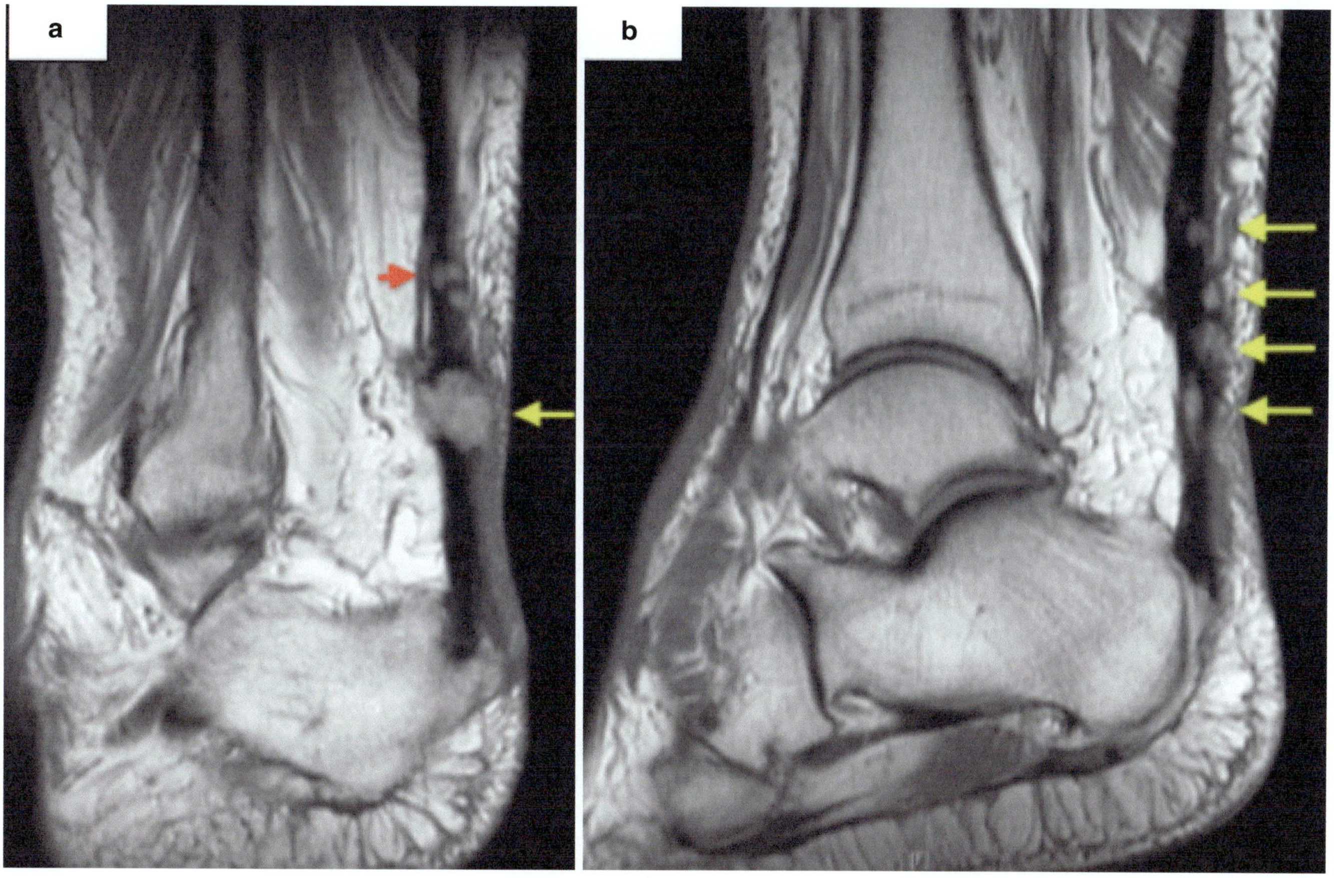

Fig. 48.3 (**a**) Achilles tendon rupture on MRI. Note the gap in the tendon marked by the yellow arrow. Please also note the associated tendinosis marked by the red arrow. (**b**) Surrounding Achilles tendinosis in the same patient marked by the yellow arrow

to break down the adhesions or disruption of the neovascularization [11]. Immobilization of the foot in a walking boot in neutral or slight plantarflexion with a mild lift can add value.

PRP Injection

The regenerative medicine literature is limited to platelet-rich plasma (PRP) and autologous whole blood injections, which can be considered in refractory cases. In a recent meta-analysis, there was no benefit of PRP over eccentric exercises or PRP vs placebo saline injection [12]. Fewer studies have examined PRP for insertional Achilles tendinopathy.

Extracorporeal Shockwave Therapy

Extracorporeal shockwave therapy (ESWT) utilizes acoustic shockwaves through the skin to target the affected tissue [13]. ESWT can be considered in midsubstance and insertional Achilles tendinopathy with collective studies suggesting overall efficacy [10]. There is no consensus on the best form and energy setting.

Percutaneous Ultrasonic Fasciotomy and Debridement

This procedure can be considered in refractory cases and has been shown to be beneficial for insertional Achilles tendinopathy and intratendinous calcification in small case series with a short-term satisfaction of 70% [14, 15], and the Tenex microtip (Tenex Health Lake Forest, CA) seems to have improved outcomes compared to manual percutaneous tenotomy with a needle [16]. High-volume injections (HVI) use a mixture of saline, anesthetic, and/or steroid injected along the interface of the Kager fat pad and midportion of the Achilles tendon and has a mechanical effect on adhesions between the tendon and peritendinous tissues. HVI were more effective when corticosteroid was included in the solution, indicating that corticosteroids may play a role in the efficacy of this treatment [10]. A recent RCT showed no benefit of HVI without cortisone [11].

48.1.6.4 Surgery

Surgical debridement for paratenonitis has been described but is a subject of much debate as resection part of the paratenon can potentially compromise the blood supply to the Achilles tendon placing it at further risk of rupture.

48.2 Insertional Achilles Tendonitis and Haglund Deformity

48.2.1 ICD 10

- M76.61 Achilles tendonitis (bursitis), right
- M76.62 Achilles tendonitis (bursitis), left
- M92.61 Haglund deformity, right
- M92.62 Haglund deformity, left

48.2.2 Description

Insertional Achilles tendinopathy pain occurs within 2 cm of the insertion and is often multifactorial and can involve the tendon, bone, and bursal tissue. When multiple sources of pain are involved, it can be challenging to identify the source of pain.

Anatomy The Achilles tendon inserts on the posterior-superior aspect of the calcaneus or the calcaneal tuberosity (Fig. 48.1). The retrocalcaneal and retro-Achilles bursa are located anterior and posterior to the tendon, respectively.

Etiology/pathophysiology The prominence of the postero-superior calcaneus is known as Haglund deformity. The etiology is often degenerative with repetitive microtrauma from overuse can lead to insertional Achilles tendinopathy. The etiology is often degenerative with repetitive microtrauma from overuse. Haglund deformity can cause degenerative changes of the Achilles tendon, retrocalcaneal bursitis, and intratendinous calcification known as Haglund syndrome. Associated enthesophytes or retro-Achilles bursitis can also cause heel pain and is associated with insertional Achilles tendinopathy. Differential diagnosis of insertional Achilles tendonitis is noted in Table 48.2.

48.2.3 Clinical Presentation

Patients with insertional tendinitis report pain focused on the bony prominence on the superior aspect of the calcaneum and difficulty in wearing shoes.

48.2.4 Physical Examination

On inspection of this area, a notable prominence to the posterior-superior aspect of the calcaneum can be present and is suggestive of a Haglund deformity. On palpation, patients with tendinitis will have pain on palpation of the insertion; this pain will be fixed in its location regardless of

Table 48.2 Differential diagnosis of insertional Achilles tendonitis

Achilles tendinopathy	Calcaneal stress fracture
Plantar fasciopathy	Simple bone cyst
Intraosseous lipoma	Retro-Achilles bursitis
Retrocalcaneal bursitis	Haglund syndrome
Baxter neuropathy	Tarsal tunnel syndrome
Heel pad syndrome	Achilles partial tear/complete tear

the position of the foot. This is in contrast to midsubstance Achilles tendinopathy where there is fusiform thickening, which moves proximally and distally with foot dorsiflexion and plantarflexion. It can be challenging to distinguish the source of pain on examination alone (i.e., isolated tendon pathology, Haglund syndrome, and retrocalcaneal or retro-Achilles bursitis). Associated retrocalcaneal bursitis can mimic posterior heel pain but can be differentiated by medial and lateral compression of the area just anterior and superior to the Achilles insertion.

48.2.5 Diagnostic Workup

Plane radiographs can reveal bone spurs, intratendinous calcifications, or a Haglund deformity. A Haglund deformity can be noted on a lateral image, and multiple radiographic criteria have been described. The parallel pitch lines is one method to radiographically diagnose Haglund deformity and is defined by measuring the pitch of the inferior calcaneum and drawing a parallel line along the tip of the posterior facet. Haglund deformity it noted when the superior surface of the calcaneus is found above the superior calcaneum [3] (Fig. 48.4).

MRI and CT scan can be helpful to assess soft tissue involvement and for surgical planning.

Labs: Rheumatology workup can be considered in cases of prominent enthesophytes to rule out seronegative arthropathy.

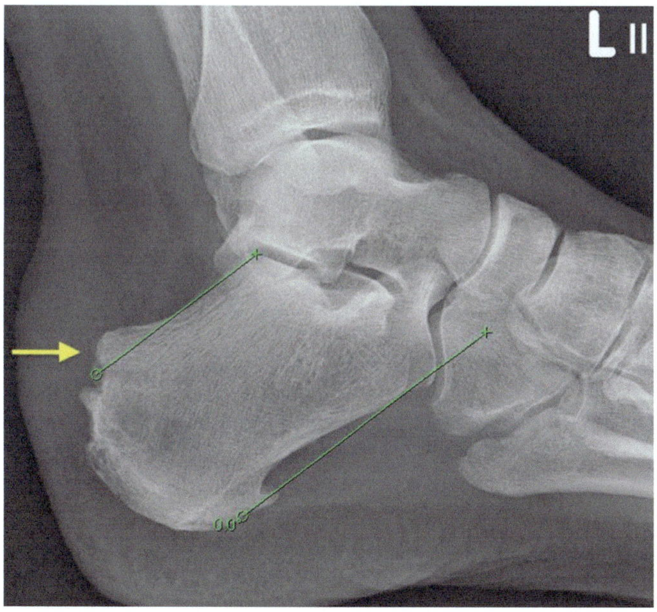

Fig. 48.4 Parallel pitch lines with posterior-superior exostosis of the calcaneum passing the superior pitch line. (Image courtesy of Amir Abbas Mostoufi, MD, Tehran IRAN)

48.2.6 Treatment

48.2.6.1 Medical Management

Initial conservative treatment includes nonsteroidal anti-inflammatory medications, rest and immobilization, and progressing to light activity and passive stretching. Patients with Haglund deformity or associated bursitis may benefit from a period of offloading of the affected area by wearing a backless shoe, and hindfoot malalignment associated with insertional pathology can be corrected by insoles if this is a provocative factor.

48.2.6.2 Rehabilitation

Physical therapy and extracorporeal shockwave therapy can be considered, but evidence is lacking.

48.2.6.3 Procedures

In cases with associated Haglund deformity, intra-tendinous calcification, and interstitial tendon partial tears orthobiologics or percutaneous treatments can be considered, but these lack randomized controlled trials on efficacy. Percutaneous resection of Haglund deformity has been reported in case reports using a 2–3 mm stab incision and ultrasonic surgical instrument that fragments and aspirates bone [14, 17]. Although promising and preserves the tendon, minimally invasive percutaneous tools is not well established and requires a physician highly skilled in interventional ultrasonography.

48.2.6.4 Surgery

Patients who fail conservative treatment due to degenerative tendinopathy and associated Haglund deformity, enthesophyte, or intra-tendinous calcification may need surgical management. Numerous methods and operative strategies have been described. Calcaneoplasty and resection of the retrocalcaneal bursa can be performed endoscopically. Open procedures involve violation of a part of the Achilles tendon, osteotomy to excise the deformity, and require a repair and a period of time immobilization to promote tendon healing. The literature has provided some debate on whether excision of the Haglund deformity is required [18].

48.3 Posterior Ankle Impingement (Os Trigonum Syndrome)

48.3.1 ICD 10

M26.82

48.3.1.1 Description

Posterior ankle impingement syndrome (Os trigonum syndrome) is when the os trigonum accessory ossicle becomes symptomatic from injury or repetitive overuse.

Table 48.3 Differential diagnosis of posterior ankle impingement

Shepherd fracture	Achilles tendinitis
FHL tendinitis or tenosynovitis	Retrocalcaneal bursitis
Osteochondritis dissecans	Subtalar coalition
Stress fracture	Sever's disease (calcaneal apophysitis)
Bone tumor (osteoid osteoma)	Peripheral nerve entrapment
Tarsal tunnel syndrome	Sural nerve entrapment

Os trigonum is the name for the most common accessory ossicle center of the posterolateral talar tubercle in the ankle. This accessory ossicle starts off as a secondary ossification center posterior to the posterolateral talus and becomes visible on radiographs at 8–10 years in females and 11–13 years in boys. This anatomic variant is typically asymptomatic; however, it can cause pain in patients with repetitive microtrauma and forced plantarflexion. A prominent or elongated posterolateral talar tubercle is known as a Stieda process and considered an anatomic variant. An os trigonum can also result from an acute fracture of the posterolateral tubercle or Steida process. The reported incidence is between 1% and 25% of the population [19]. This syndrome is more prevalent in dancers and is thought to be due to the time weight-bearing on their toes in end plantar flexion. Differential diagnosis of posterior ankle impingement is listed in Table 48.3.

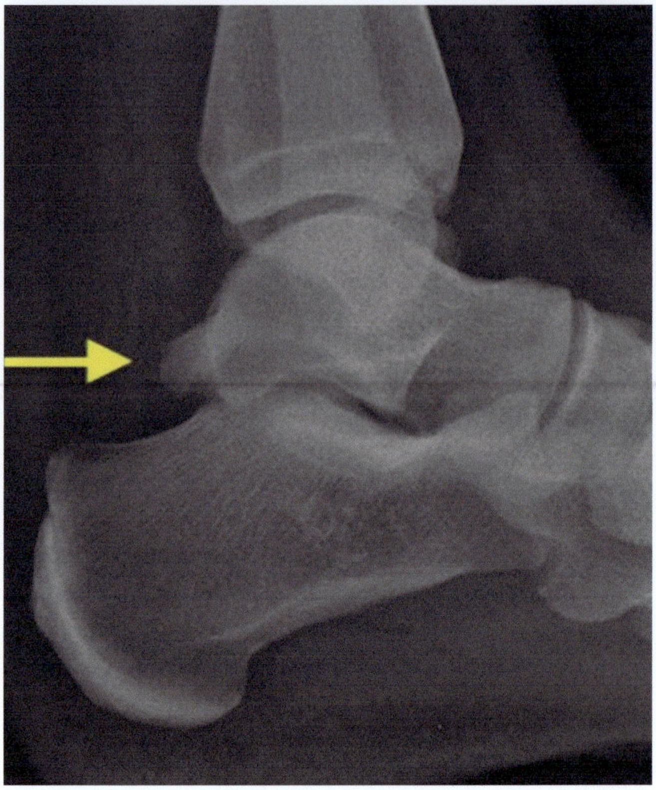

Fig. 48.5 Os trigonum marked by yellow arrow. Hard to tell if Steida process or os trigonum on this view

48.3.2 Clinical Presentation

The patient usually reports chronic or recurrent posterior ankle mechanical deep mechanical pain caused or exacerbated by forced plantar flexion or push-off activities, such as dancing, kicking, downhill running, sliding, and walking in shoes with high heels.

48.3.3 Physical Examination

There can be associated swelling and weakness in dorsiflexion. In some patients a bony prominence can be palpable. The symptoms can often be replicated with hyper plantarflexion of the ankle or dorsiflexion of the hallux.

Heel thrush test The physician pinches the talus between the posterior tibia and superior aspect of the calcaneus. Development of pain is considered a positive test.

48.3.4 Diagnostic Workup

48.3.4.1 Plain Films

Radiographs, particularly the lateral view, can demonstrate the prominence of the posterolateral talar process (Steida process) or accessory ossicle (Fig. 48.5).

48.3.4.2 MRI

Advanced imaging can help identify the presence of tissue and bony oedema, facture line, or associated tendinopathy.

48.3.5 Treatment

48.3.5.1 Medical Management

Initial treatment is with rest and nonsteroidal anti-inflammatory medications. Activity modifications and physical therapy can be undertaken to attempt to alleviate symptoms.

48.3.5.2 Rehabilitation

Physical therapy that included soft tissue therapy, stretching, and mobilizations of restricted joints of the lower kinetic chain should be done in conjunction with a progressive strengthening, balance, and proprioception program. In athletes, full ankle active ROM, strength, agility, and ability to perform acceleration/deceleration movements are needed to fully return to play [20].

48.3.5.3 Procedures

Corticosteroid injection can be attempted; however, the literature is limited, and a guided injection should be considered due to the proximity to the Achilles tendon.

48.3.5.4 Surgical Management

In cases where posterior impingement syndrome is a structure problem, conservative treatment can help control inflammation and improve symptoms, but surgery may be necessary in the active population, such as dancers or athletes, who wish to continue their sport. Surgical excision of the os trigonum or Steida process has been reported to be successful with patients returning to their presymptomatic level of activity and can be performed with an open, arthroscopic, or endoscopic approach [21].

References

1. Edgerton V, Smith J, Simpson D. Muscle fibre type populations of human leg muscles. Histochem J. 1975;7(3):259–66.
2. Noseworthy MD, Bulte DP, Alfonsi J. BOLD magnetic resonance imaging of skeletal muscle. Semin Musculoskelet Radiol. 2003;7(4):307–16.
3. de Jonge S, van den Berg C, de Vos RJ, et al. Incidence of midportion Achilles tendinopathy in the general population. Br J Sports Med. 2011;45(13):1026–8.
4. Puddu G, Ippolito E, Postacchini F. A classification of achilles tendon disease. Am J Sports Med. 1976;4(4):145–50.
5. Gillies H, Chalmers J. The management of fresh ruptures of the tendo achillis. J Bone Joint Surg Am. 1970;52(2):337–43.
6. Movin T, Ryberg A, McBride DJ, Maffulli N. Acute rupture of the Achilles tendon. Foot Ankle Clin. 2005;10(2):331–56.
7. Beard NM, Gousse RP. Current ultrasound application in the foot and ankle. Orthop Clin North Am. 2018;49(1):109–21.
8. Bäcker H, Wong T, Vosseller J. MRI assessment of degeneration of the tendon in Achilles tendon ruptures. Foot Ankle Int. 2019;40(8):895–9.
9. Beyer R, Kongsgaard M, Hougs Kjær B, Øhlenschlæger T, Kjær M, Magnusson SP. Heavy slow resistance versus eccentric training as treatment for Achilles tendinopathy: a randomized controlled trial. Am J Sports Med. 2015 Jul;43(7):1704–11.
10. Rhim HC, Kim MS, Choi S, Tenforde AS. Comparative efficacy and tolerability of nonsurgical therapies for the treatment of midportion Achilles tendinopathy: a systematic review with network meta-analysis. Orthop J Sports Med. 2020;8(7):2325967120930567.
11. van der Vlist AC, van Oosterom RF, van Veldhoven PLJ, Bierma-Zeinstra SMA, Waarsing JH, Verhaar JAN, de Vos RJ. Effectiveness of a high volume injection as treatment for chronic Achilles tendinopathy: randomised controlled trial. BMJ. 2020;370:m3027.
12. Liu CJ, Yu KL, Bai JB, Tian DH, Liu GL. Platelet-rich plasma injection for the treatment of chronic Achilles tendinopathy: a meta-analysis. Medicine (Baltimore). 2019;98(16):e15278.
13. Rompe J, Furia J, Maffulli N. Eccentric loading versus eccentric loading plus shock-wave treatment for midportion Achilles tendinopathy. Am J Sports Med. 2009;37(3):463–70.
14. Chimenti RL, et al. Percutaneous ultrasonic tenotomy reduces insertional Achilles tendinopathy pain with high patient satisfaction and a low complication rate. J Ultrasound Med. 2019;39(6):1629–35. Epub 2018 Oct.
15. Freed L, et al. Fasciotomy and surgical tenotomy for chronic achilles insertional tendinopathy: a retrospective study using ultrasound-guided percutaneous microresection. J Am Podiatr Med Assoc. 2019;109(1):1–8.
16. Testa V, Capasso G, Benazzo F, Maffulli N. Management of Achilles tendinopathy by ultrasound-guided percutaneous tenotomy. Med Sci Sports Exerc. 2002 Apr;34(4):573–80.
17. Sung K, Sussman WI. Minimally invasive resection of Haglund's deformity with percutaneous ultrasound guided treatment with TX bone device. Accepted *AIUM Meeting* 2021 for presentation.
18. Kang S, Thordarson DB, Charlton TP. Insertional Achilles tendinitis and Haglund's deformity. Foot Ankle Int. 2012;33(6):487–91.
19. Keles-Celik N, Kose O, Sekerci R, Aytac G, Turan A, Güler F. Accessory ossicles of the foot and ankle: disorders and a review of the literature. Cureus. 2017;9(11):e1881.
20. Soler T, Jezerskyte Banfi R, Katsmen L. The conservative treatment of posterior ankle impingement syndrome in professional ballet dancers: a literature review and experts consensus. European School of Physiotherapy. 2011.
21. Walsh K, Durante E, Moser B, Coetzee J, Stone MGR. Surgical outcomes of os trigonum syndrome in dancers: a case series. Orthop J Sports Med. 2020;8(7):232596712093876.

Lateral Ankle Disorders

49

Seyed Behrooz Mostofi, Chu H. Chiang, Walter I. Sussman, and S. Ali Mostoufi

49.1 Peroneal Tendinopathy

49.1.1 Synonyms

- Peroneal tendinosis
- Peroneal tendinopathy

49.1.2 ICD 10

- M76.71: Peroneal tendonitis, right leg
- M76.72: Peroneal tendonitis, left leg

49.1.3 Description

Peroneal tendon injuries are a potential cause of lateral ankle pain, and pathology may range from tendinopathy to ruptures, tears, and instability of the tendons.

S. B. Mostofi (✉)
East Kent Hospitals University, NHS Foundation Trust, Canterbury, Kent, UK

Department of Orthopaedics, Manipal Academy of Higher Education, Manipal, India

C. H. Chiang
Kent Surrey and Sussex Deanery, NHS Foundation Trust, Canterbury, Kent, UK

W. I. Sussman
Department of Orthopedics and Rehabilitation, Tufts University School of Medicine, Boston, MA, USA

Boston Sports & Biologics PC, Wellesley, MA, USA

S. A. Mostoufi
Department of Orthopedics and Rehabilitation, Tufts University School of Medicine, Boston, MA, USA

New England Spine Care Associates & Boston Regenerative Medicine, Cambridge, MA, USA

Anatomy The peroneus longus and peroneus brevis form the lateral compartment of the lower leg. The peroneus longus originates on the fibular head and upper ½ of the proximal fibula and is innervated by the superficial peroneal nerve. The peroneus brevis originates from the distal 2/3 of the fibula and intermuscular septum. The peroneal brevis tendon sits closer to the fibula as compared to the peroneal longus. At the level of the lateral malleolus, both tendons pass into the retro-malleolar groove and run deep the superior peroneal retinaculum (SPR). These forms an osteofibrous tunnel, and the tendons are surrounded by a common synovial sheath within the tunnel facilitating gliding within the sheath. The two tendons run lateral to the calcaneus with the peroneal longus above and the brevis below the peroneal tubercle where they are stabilized by a second retinaculum. The peroneus brevis then inserts onto the base of the fifth metatarsal, and the peroneus longus dives medially under the cuboid and inserts onto the base of the first metatarsal and medial cuneiform. The change of direction at this location places the tendon under stress.

Etiology/Pathophysiology Peroneal tendon pathology was previously considered uncommon, but cadaveric studies have reported tears in 11–38% of the cadevers [1]. It is now recognized that peroneal tendon pathology is a common cause of lateral ankle symptoms, although the true incidence of symptomatic tears is unclear. An MRI study of 294 patients with hindfoot pathology found a 35% incidence of radiological changes in the peroneal tendons, though these patients reported no symptoms or preceding injuries [2].

The predominant force for the peroneus brevis is eversion, and the peroneus longus induces plantarflexion and eversion. Several anatomic variations are associated with peroneal tendon pathology, including a low-lying peroneus brevis muscle belly, accessory peroneal muscles, shape of the retro-malleolar groove and os perineum. The incidence of os peroneum is estimated to be 4–30% and can be asymptomatic [3]. Fractures

© The Author(s), under exclusive license to Springer Nature Switzerland AG 2022

S. A. Mostoufi et al. (eds.), *Clinical Guide to Musculoskeletal Medicine*, https://doi.org/10.1007/978-3-030-92042-5_49

Table 49.1 Differential diagnosis of peroneal tendinopathy

Ankle sprain/ fracture	Stress fracture	Peroneal tendon dislocation
Os peroneum	Apophysitis of the fifth metatarsal	Peripheral neuropathy

Table 49.2 Classification of peroneal tendinopathy

Grade 1. Elevation of the SPR from the fibula along with periosteum
Grade 2. Progression of Grade 1 changes with the fibrocartilaginous area of tissue bordering the lateral aspect of the fibula
Grade 3. Avulsion of the cortical bone from the lateral fibula, allowing tendon displacement
Grade 4. Full tear of the SPR allowing peroneal tendons to dislocate

of the os peroneum can result in pain in the lateral aspect of the ankle as discussed later in this chapter.

Peroneal tendinopathy has been documented as an overuse injury with rupture of the superior peroneal retinaculum (SPR) noted in forceful contraction of the tendon during eccentric loading [4]. This can result in the more commonly reported dislocation of the peroneal tendons out of the sheath after a rupture of the overlying SPR. Peroneal tendinopathy has been classified by Eckert and Davis [4, 5], as noted in Table 49.2. Peroneal tendon tears can be difficult to distinguish from lateral ankle ligament injuries and tend to have a delayed diagnosis. In one study, only 60% of peroneal tendon disorders were accurately diagnosed at the initial evaluation [6]. Sammarco et al. reported an average duration of 7–48 months prior to diagnosis from the preceding injury [7]. Differential diagnosis of peroneal tendinopathy is in Table 49.1.

49.1.4 Clinical Presentation

Patients may present with a broad variety of symptoms. History should focus on recent or past injuries, and whether symptoms are mechanical versus inflammatory. Acute tears are likely to present with a sudden onset of pain and swelling. In subacute and chronic cases, patients typically present with complaints of worsening lateral ankle pain, which tend to be exacerbated with activity. This can result in the patient walking with an antalgic gait. Peroneus brevis pathology typically presents with pain around the distal fibula, whereas peroneus longus pathology presents with pain near the peroneal tubercle and cuboid tunnel.

49.1.5 Physical Examination

Inspection should focus on overall alignment as hindfoot varus may increase force on the peroneal tendons and predispose the patient to injury. Swelling and pain to palpation can occur anywhere along the course of the tendons, with retrofibular swelling commonly seen in peroneal brevis pathology and peroneal tubercle or cuboid tunnel pain seen in peroneal pathology [8].

The symptoms can be reproduced with resisted active dorsiflexion and/or eversion of the ankle. Pain on passive inversion and/or eversion may be indicative of severe tendinopathy. Circumduction may recreate tendon subluxation in cases of instability

49.1.6 Diagnostic Workup

Radiographs Standard weight-bearing radiographs of the foot and ankle with orthogonal view scan reveal other conditions, such as ankle fractures. A "fleck" sign lateral to the distal fibula is suggestive of avulsion of the SPR and may indicate tendon instability (Fig. 49.1).

Ultrasound Ultrasound has a reported accuracy of 90% in diagnosing peroneal tears; however, the reliability of ultrasonography is dependent on the user [9].

MRI MRI for distal peroneal tendons has been reported to be difficult due to the magic angle effect and may mask sub-

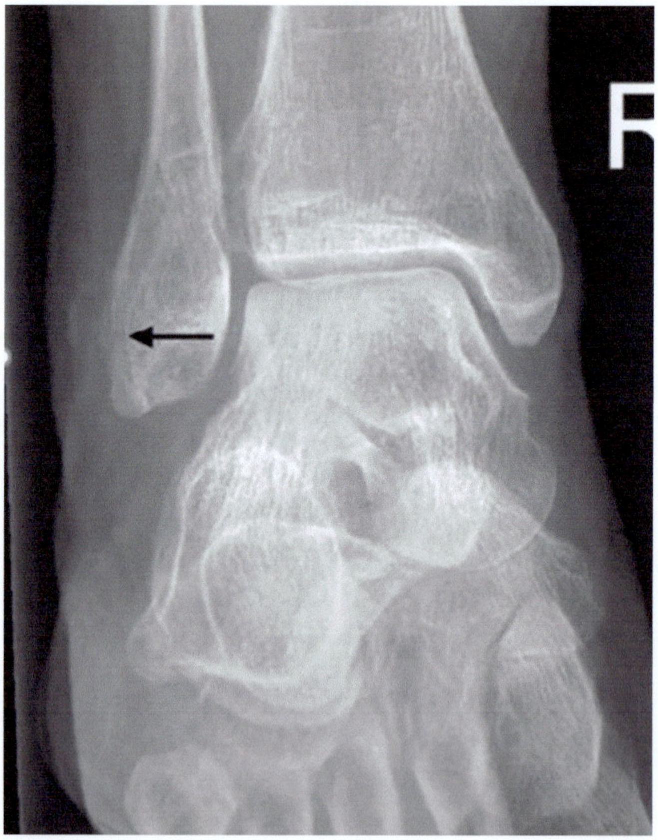

Fig. 49.1 Avulsion fracture lateral to the distal tip of the fibula (black arrow)

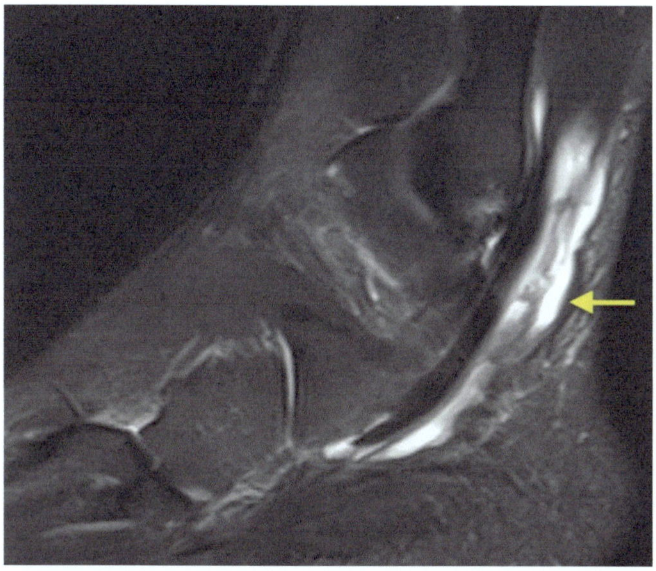

Fig. 49.2 Hyperintense signals along the course of the peroneal tendon sheath (yellow arrow)

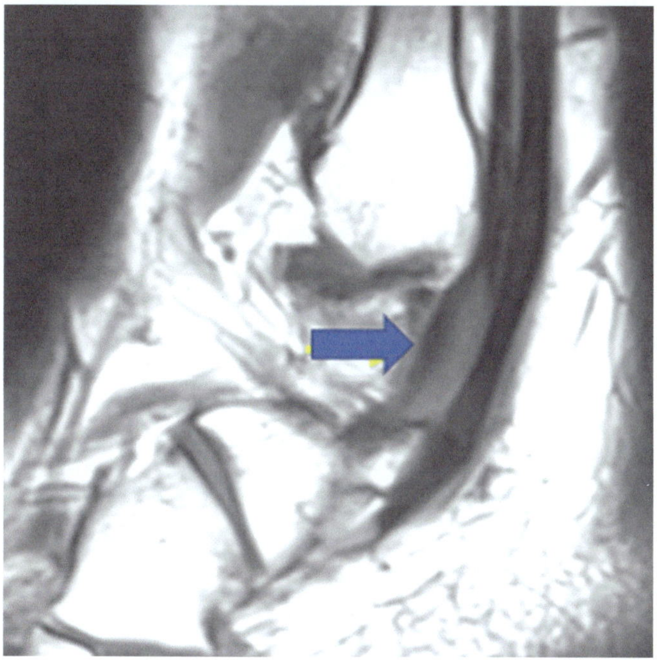

Fig. 49.3 MRI showing longitudinal tear in the peroneus brevis tendon (blue arrow)

tle changes of the tendon. This effect results in hyperintense signals when the tendon runs at a 55-degree angle to the scanner [10] (Figs. 49.2 and 49.3).

49.1.7 Treatment

49.1.7.1 Medical Management

Treatment should be tailored to the underlying pathology. Conservative management for peroneal tendinopathy includes offloading the affected limb, icing, bracing, or Kinesio taping and PT program.

49.1.7.2 Rehabilitation

Treatment for peroneal tendonitis includes a program of stretching, eccentric strengthening exercises, mobilization, proprioceptive, and balancing exercises. If symptoms are severe, a brief course of immobilization (cast or brace) may be necessary. After severe symptoms resolves, the patient begins a progressive rehabilitation program along with a gradual increase to full activity. Deep tissue friction massage, ultrasound, and electrical stimulation can also be included in the physical therapy [11]. In the case of tendon tear, postoperative rehabilitation follows a much slower progression and is directed based on type of surgery.

49.1.7.3 Procedures

In cases of peroneal tenosynovitis, corticosteroid injections have been suggested to manage inflammation followed by ankle immobilization to minimize the risk of tendon rupture [12]. There have been no studies comparing corticosteroid injection to medical management in peroneal tendinopathy.

49.1.7.4 Surgery

Surgical management of peroneal tendon tears can range from repair of short segment of the tear, tubularization of the tendon, or excision of the degenerative area [12]. The cases of chronic subluxation of the peroneal tendons can be addressed with either recreation of the retinaculum overlying the peroneal tendons or deepening the retromalleolar groove in which the tendons travel. Suh et al. in 2018 have reported good surgical outcomes from 34 patients studied retrospectively with no reports of recurrence of subluxation [13].

49.2 Os Peroneum Syndrome

49.2.1 Synonym

- POPS – painful os peroneum syndrome
- Painful os peroneum

49.2.2 ICD 10

M89.8X7

49.2.3 Description

The os peroneum is found within the peroneus longus tendon at the level of the calcaneocuboid joint. The small sesamoid bone can vary in size and be bipartite or multipartite. The os peroneum can be a source of pain and is associated with

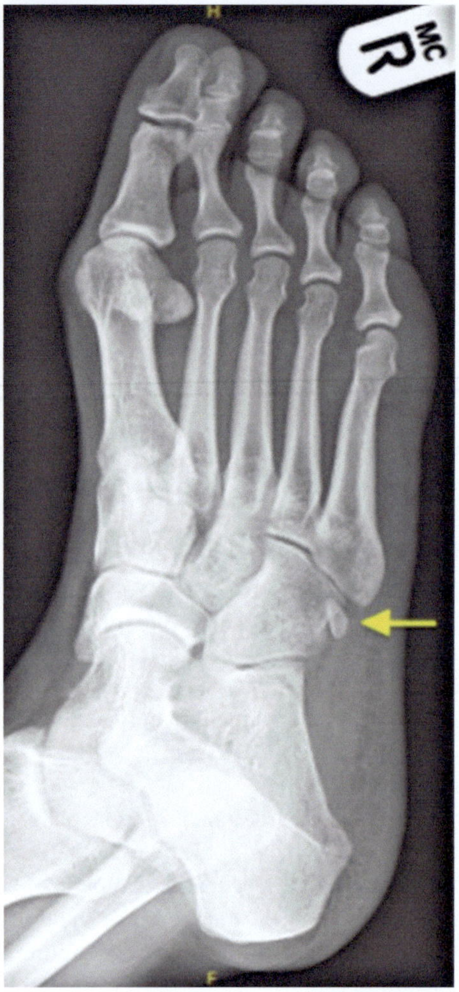

Fig. 49.4 Os peroneum is located distal to the calcaneocuboid joint (yellow arrow)

lesions of the peroneus longus tendon. Os peroneum are typically remnants of secondary ossification centers that have not fused. This ossicle is located near the calcaneocuboid joint as the tendon enters the tarsal tunnel (Fig. 49.4) and is one of the most common accessory ossicles in the body with an incidence of 9–20% and is bilateral in 60% of patients [14]. The os peroneum can appear similar to a cortical avulsion or soft tissue calcification. In peroneal longus tendon ruptures, the os peroneum can migrate with the tendon proximally or remain at site of the tear, depending on the site of tendon rupture. Differential diagnosis of this condition is outlined in Table 49.3.

49.2.4 Clinical Presentation

Patients often complain of pain near the lateral aspect of the midfoot at the level of cuboid. This can be acute, typically presenting after an ankle sprain or chronic overuse. On clinical examination, point tenderness can be noted over the lateral aspect of the midfoot. This pain is often exacerbated by physical activities.

Table 49.3 Differential diagnosis of os peroneum syndrome

Acute os peroneum fracture or a diastasis of a multipartite os peroneum	Arthritis of calcaneocuboid joint
Chronic (healing or healed) os peroneum fracture or diastasis of a multipartite os peroneum	Avulsion fracture/stress fracture base of the fifth metatarsal
Attrition or partial rupture of the peroneus longus tendon, proximal, or distal to the os peroneum	Iselin's disease (traction apophysitis of the base of the fifth metatarsal)
Cuboid fracture	Os vesalianum

49.2.5 Diagnostic Workup

Radiographs X-rays of the foot typically demonstrate the presence of an os peroneum; however, os peroneum can be asymptomatic, and correlation with clinical examination is mandatory as a bipartite os peroneum can be confused with an os peroneum fracture. Sharp cortical edges may indicate acute changes, and smooth cortical edges may indicate a chronic process [15].

MRI/US Magnetic resonance and ultrasound imaging can be utilized to visualize any pathology relating to the tendon.

49.2.6 Treatment

49.2.6.1 Medical/Procedural Care

Conservative management includes offloading the affected limb, icing, bracing or Kinesio taping, and PT program. Persistent symptoms can be managed with an injection under fluoroscopy, or ultrasound-guided injections can be used not only for therapeutic purposes but can be diagnostic to confirm the os peroneum is the source of the symptoms.

49.2.6.2 Surgery

Patients who are refractory to treatment can consider surgical management with excision of the os peroneum or surgical excision with tenodesis of the peroneal longus to the peroneus brevis tendon.

49.3 Os Subfibulare

49.3.1 Description

Os subfibulare is an accessory ossicle at the distal to the tip of the fibula. The os subfibulare is the result of an unfused

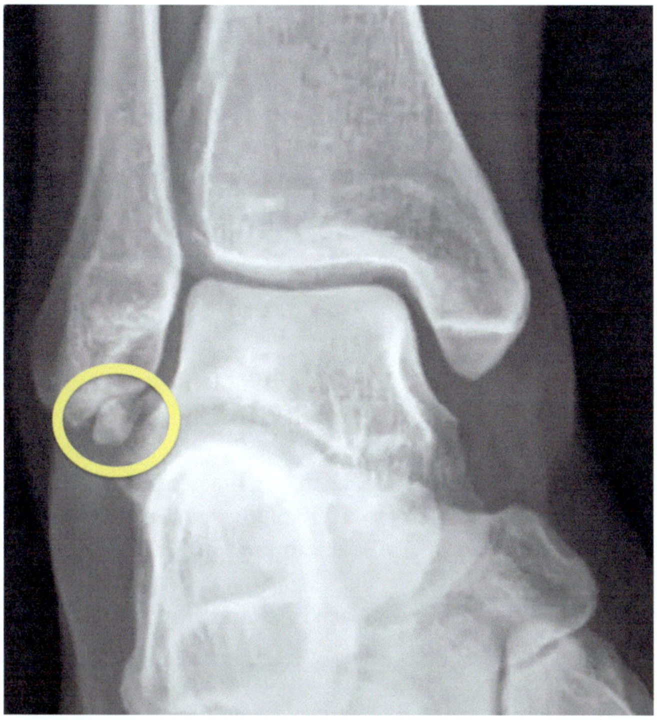

Fig. 49.5 Os subfibulare located distal to the tip of the fibula

accessory ossification center or avulsion fracture of the anterior talofibular ligament. These tend to be comma or round shaped on imaging. The os subfibulare is rare in comparison to the os peroneum with a prevalence of 1% [16]. The presence of this ossicle is often confused with a fracture of the lateral malleolus (Fig. 49.5).

49.3.2 Clinical Presentation

The os subfibulare can be symptomatic and present with local pain and lateral ankle instability. Acute traumatic or chronic inversion stress can result in an avulsion of the ossicle from the lateral malleolus and convert an asymptomatic ossicle to a symptomatic one. It can be difficult to differentiate between an os subfibulare and an avulsion fracture of the distal fibula. In acute injuries, these patients can have difficulty weight-bearing and would meet the Ottawa ankle criteria for ankle X-ray imaging in the emergency setting [17].

49.3.3 Physical Examination

Patients with chronic inversion injury can present with point tenderness over the ossicle. Chronic ankle instability often manifests as recurrent ankle sprains with and laxity on an anterior drawer test at the ankle joint.

49.3.4 Diagnostic Workup

Standard ankle X-rays (AP/lateral and mortise view) is sufficient for diagnosis. One should pay close attention to the cortical edge of the ossicle and determine whether it is sharp (an acute injury) versus smooth (chronic injury).

49.3.5 Treatment

Initial management would be conservative with nonsteroid anti-inflammatory medication and a period of immobilization. Patients who have persistent symptoms despite conservative treatment should be considered for possible surgical excision. This may be combined with a lateral ankle ligament reconstruction [18].

49.4 Sinus Tarsi Syndrome (STS)

49.4.1 Description

The sinus tarsi is an anatomical location that is anterior and inferior to the lateral malleolus. Sinus tarsi syndrome has been described as a result of lateral ankle stress resulting from excessive pronation at the subtalar joint due to instability [19]. Anatomically during this movement, the cuboid and lateral calcaneus compress the sinus tarsi. This results in swelling and inflammation.

49.4.2 Clinical Presentation

Classically, the patient presents with intermittent discomfort localized over the sinus tarsi (Fig. 49.6) without any sensory, motor, or vascular abnormality. Athletes with STS will typi-

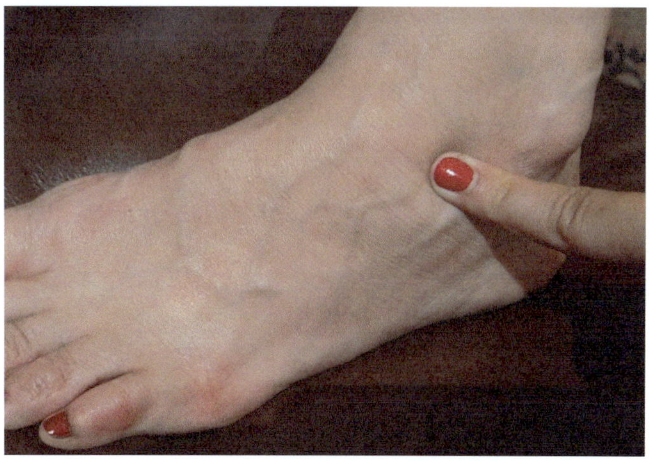

Fig. 49.6 Athletes localize discomfort over the sinus tarsi. (Image courtesy of Eva Mostoufi)

cally describe a feeling of instability of the foot and ankle that is provoked upon walking over uneven ground, stepping off a curb, or running or sprinting activities. Athletes involved with turning and jumping activities on firm surfaces will have the most difficulty [20].

49.4.3 Examination

Sinus tarsi area may become swollen and puffy on inspection. Assessment of standing posture in athletes with STS may demonstrate a pes planus posture. The walking gait of the patient may be altered as the patient will pronate the foot to avoid ground contact with the lateral aspect of the foot. Stability of the subtalar joint is assessed with medial and lateral subtalar joint glides [21].

49.4.4 Diagnostic Workup

Radiographs of the subtalar joint are usually performed with stress views (oblique-lateral views performed with the ankle and foot placed in inverted and supinated positions). Stress fluoroscopy is a method of visualizing the motions of the subtalar joint. Magnetic resonance imaging (MRI) is the best method to visualize the structure within the sinus tarsi. The most distinct finding for individuals with STS is a hyperintense T2 signal in the area for sinus tarsal adipose tissue as this represents an infiltration or replacement of this tissue with inflammatory cells and fibrotic tissue [22].

49.4.5 Treatment

Management of this syndrome is largely around symptomatic treatment with rest, compression, and elevation to reduce swelling. Local corticosteroid injections can be considered to manage the pain; however, surgery is not recommended for acute presentations. The literature has reported success in managing this condition with arthroscopic debridement of the sinus tarsi; however, it is to note that the arthroscopic procedure has altered the diagnosis in a significant number of cases potentially decreasing its actual effectiveness in management of sinus tarsi syndrome itself [19].

49.5 Fibula Nonunion

Fibula nonunion is one of the causes of lateral ankle pain. The details are covered under foot and ankle fracture/dislocation.

49.6 Ankle Sprain

49.6.1 Description

Lateral ankle sprains are the most common lower limb musculoskeletal injury incurred by individuals who participate in sports and recreational physical activities [23]. The prevalence of lateral ankle sprains among the general population is also substantial. Up to 70% of the general population report having incurred an ankle injury during their lifetime [24]. Individuals who incur an acute lateral ankle sprain injury have a twofold increased risk of reinjury in the year following their initial injury. Specifically, up to 75% of those who sprain their ankles will go on to develop chronic ankle instability. Later in life, patients with a history of a lateral ankle sprain and chronic ankle instability frequently develop posttraumatic ankle osteoarthritis [25]. There are different grading of ankle sprain, and the approach to care/return to play depends on the level of injury to the tendon (Table 49.4).

49.6.2 Clinical Presentation

A mechanism involving plantarflexion and inversion of the foot is suggestive of lateral ankle injury. More severe injuries with this mechanism also may involve the medial ankle. Syndesmosis and deltoid ligament injuries most commonly occur with an external rotation force applied to a fixed foot. The risk factors such as prior history of ankle sprains or ankle instability, specific sport or activity during which the injury occurred, playing surface, footwear, and the use of bracing or taping are important and should be investigated. The specific location of pain, presence of local or diffuse swelling, mechanical symptoms, and paresthesia should be elucidated.

Table 49.4 Grading of ankle sprain. Clinical judgments and examination dictates return to play which should be individualized

Grade	Ligament injury	Ecchymosis	Pain	Treatment	Return to play
I	None (stretched)	None or little	Minimal	PRICE/PT	2w
II	Incomplete tear	Moderate	Moderate	PRICE/PT/brace/taping	3–4weks
III	Complete tear	Severe	Severe	PRICE/PT/brace/taping Possible surgery	12 or more

49.6.3 Physical Examination

The clinical assessment of the integrity of the lateral ligaments of the ankle joint, as well as the ankle joint syndesmosis ligaments, is advocated. Lateral ligamentous stabilizers of the ankle joint are the anterior talofibular ligament, the calcaneofibular ligament, and the posterior talofibular ligament. The anterior talofibular ligament is the most commonly injured of these ligaments. Tenderness on palpation and/or stressing it by passive plantar flexion and inversion of the anterior talofibular ligament is indicative of injury to this ligament. The anterior drawer test is the most sensitive clinical stability test to assess for complete rupture of the anterior talofibular ligament.

Tenderness on palpation of the calcaneofibular ligament and/or stressing it by passive dorsiflexion of the ankle joint combined with passive inversion of the rearfoot is indicative of injury to this ligament.

The prevalence of ankle joint syndesmosis ligament injury (with or without concomitant lateral ligament involvement) has been reported to be 20%. Localized tenderness on palpation of the syndesmosis ligaments is the most sensitive clinical assessment test, while the squeeze test is the most specific clinical assessment test.

49.6.4 Diagnostic Workup

X-rays The primary purpose of plain films in the setting of acute ankle sprains is to rule out acute fracture.

Ultrasound The use of ultrasound for imaging the ankle is well described. Ultrasound allows clinicians to obtain dynamic views of the ankle to identify functional deficiencies or joint instability. But its accuracy in diagnosing acute ankle sprains is highly dependent on operator expertise.

MRI MRI remains the gold standard for imaging the ligamentous and intra-articular structures of the ankle. It is best for cases of persistent symptoms and chronic ankle instability to rule out osteochondral defects, missed syndesmotic injuries, or osseous injuries not identified on radiograph.

49.6.5 Treatment

49.6.5.1 Medical Management

Rest, ice, compression, and elevation, nonsteroidal anti-inflammatory drug, immobilization, and bracing are all part of conservative care. Lamb et al. [26] demonstrated that patients with severe ankle sprains who were immobilized in a below-knee cast or Aircast boot had a more rapid recovery.

49.6.5.2 Rehabilitation

Based on the findings of the systematic reviews ($n = 1417$) [27, 28] that compared structured exercise-based rehabilitation plus usual care versus usual care alone and supervised rehabilitation versus home exercise, there were no significant differences between treatment groups in terms of foot and ankle function, pain, subjective ankle instability, or subjective recovery. Theses systematic review showed significant reduction in ankle sprain recurrence in those who received exercise-based rehabilitation plus usual care compared with usual care alone at 7–12 months ($P = 0.0002$), but not at 3- to 6-month follow-up. In one systematic review, there was a significantly lower proportion of patients with recurrent ankle sprain in the supervised rehabilitation versus home exercise group, while in another study, no significant difference between groups was found [27, 28].

Randomized controlled trial found that compared with the traditional PRICE (protection, rest, ice, compression, and elevation) treatment, early mobilization using a stretch band ankle traction technique resulted in no significant differences in ankle strength, ankle function, pain, and number of days to returning to sport in children and adolescents ($P < 0.01$) [30]. Another randomized controlled trial compared Wii Fit™ exercise therapy with conventional physical therapy and with no therapy and found no significant differences between treatment groups for ankle function, pain, time to returning to sport, and self-reported satisfaction and effectiveness ($P \leq 0.01$) [31].

49.6.5.3 Procedures

There have been limited published data about the effect of the platelet-rich plasma (PRP) injections in acute ankle sprains. A single ultrasound-guided PRP injection to the AITFL and tibiofibular joint in addition to a standard rehabilitation protocol has proved to be effective [29].

49.6.5.4 Surgery

In chronic ankle instability, the modified Broström procedure is a commonly used surgical technique that involves the direct anatomic repair of injured lateral ligaments with reinforcement of the extensor retinaculum. Arthroscopy is commonly performed at the time of surgery to rule out concomitant intra-articular pathology.

References

1. Miura K, Ishibashi Y, Tsuda E, Kusumi T, Toh S. Split lesions of the peroneus brevis tendon in the Japanese population: an anatomic and histologic study of 112 cadaveric ankles. J Orthop Sci. 2004;9(3):291–5.
2. O'Neil J, Pedowitz D, Kerbel Y, Codding J, Zoga A, Raikin S. Peroneal tendon abnormalities on routine magnetic resonance imaging of the foot and ankle. Foot Ankle Int. 2016;37(7):743–7.

3. van Dijk PA, et al. The ESSKA-AFAS international consensus statement on peroneal tendon pathologies. Knee Surg Sports Traumatol Arthrosc. 2018;26:3096–107.
4. Eckert W, Davis E. Acute rupture of the peroneal retinaculum. J Bone Joint Surg. 1976;58(5):670–2.
5. Oden RR. Tendon injuries about the ankle resulting from skiing. Clin Orthop Relat Res. 1987;216:63–9. PMID: 3815972.
6. Dombek MF, Lamm BM, Saltrick K, Mendicino RW, Catanzariti AR. Peroneal tendon tears: a retrospective review. J Foot Ankle Surg. 2003;42:250–8.
7. Sammarco G. Peroneus longus tendon tears: acute and chronic. Foot Ankle Int. 1995;16(5):245–53.
8. Bahad S, Kane J. Peroneal tendon pathology. Orthop Clin N Am. 2020;51(1):121–30.
9. Grant TH, Kelikian AS, Jereb SE, McCarthy RJ. Ultrasound diagnosis of peroneal tendon tears. A surgical correlation. J Bone Joint Surg Am. 2005;87-A:1788–94.
10. Hayes C, Parellada J. The magic angle effect in musculoskeletal MR imaging. Top Magn Reson Imaging. 1996;8(1):51–6.
11. Coughlin M, Saltzman C, Anderson R, Mann R. Mann's surgery of the foot and ankle. Philadelphia: Saunders/Elsevier; 2014.
12. van Dijk P, Lubberts B, Verheul C, DiGiovanni C, Kerkhoffs G. Rehabilitation after surgical treatment of peroneal tendon tears and ruptures. Knee Surg Sports Traumatol Arthrosc. 2016;24(4):1165–74.
13. Suh J, Lee J, Park J, Choi W, Han S. Posterior fibular groove deepening procedure with low-profile screw fixation of fibrocartilaginous flap for chronic peroneal tendon dislocation. J Foot Ankle Surg. 2018;57(3):478–83.
14. Peacock KC, Resnick EJ, Thoder JJ. Fracture of the os peroneum with rupture of the peroneus longus tendon: a case report with review of the literature. Clin Orthop. 1986;202:223–6.
15. Nwawka OK, Hayashi D, Diaz LE, et al. Sesamoids and accessory ossicles of the foot: anatomical variability and related pathology. Insights Imaging. 2013;4(5):581–93. https://doi.org/10.1007/s13244-013-0277-1.
16. Monden S, Hasegawa A, Hio N, Taki M, Noguchi H. Arthroscopic excision of separated ossicles of the lateral malleolus. J Orthop Sci. 2013;18:733–9.
17. Stiell IG, Greenberg GH, McKnight RD, Nair RC, McDowell I, Reardon M, Stewart JP, Maloney J. Decision rules for the use of radiography in acute ankle injuries. Refinement and prospective validation. JAMA. 1993;269(9):1127–32. https://doi.org/10.1001/jama.269.9.1127.
18. Chun T, Park Y, Sung K. The effect of ossicle resection in the lateral ligament repair for treatment of chronic lateral ankle instability. Foot Ankle Int. 2013;34(8):1128–33.
19. Helgeson K. Examination and intervention for sinus tarsi syndrome. N Am J Sports Phys Ther. 2009;4(1):29–37.
20. Oloff LM, Schulhofer SD, Bocko AP. Subtalar joint arthroscopy for sinus tarsi syndrome: a review of 29 cases. J Foot Ankle Surg. 2001;40(3):152–7.
21. Heckman DS, Gluck SG, Parekh SG. Tendon disorders of the foot and ankle, part 1: peroneal tendon disorder. Am J Sports Med. 2009;37(3):614–25.
22. Lektrakul N, Chung CB, Yeong-man L, et al. Tarsal sinus: Arthographic, MR imaging, MR arthrographic, and pathological findings in cadavers and retrospective study data in patients with sinus tarsi syndrome. Radiology. 2001;219:802–10.
23. Gribble PA, Bleakley CM, Caulfield BM, Docherty CL, Fourchet F, Fong DT, Hertel J, Hiller CE, Kaminski TW, McKeon PO, Refshauge KM, Verhagen EA, Vicenzino BT, Wikstrom EA, Delahunt E. Evidence review for the 2016 International Ankle Consortium consensus statement on the prevalence, impact and long-term consequences of lateral ankle sprains. Br J Sports Med. 2016;50:1496–505.
24. Waterman BR, Owens BD, Davey S, Zacchilli MA, Belmont PJ Jr. The epidemiology of ankle sprains in the United States. J Bone Joint Surg Am. 2010;92:2279–84.
25. Hubbard-Turner T. Lack of medical treatment from a medical professional after an ankle sprain. J Athl Train. 2019;54(6):671–5. https://doi.org/10.4085/1062-6050-428-17.
26. Lamb SE, Marsh JL, Hutton JL, Nakash R, Cooke MW. Collaborative Ankle Support Trial (CAST Group) Mechanical supports for acute, severe ankle sprain: a pragmatic, multicentre, randomised controlled trial. Lancet. 2009;373(9663):575–81.
27. Feger MA, Herb CC, Fraser JJ, Glaviano N, Hertel J. Supervised rehabilitation versus home exercise in the treatment of acute ankle sprains: a systematic review. Clin Sports Med. 2015;34(2):329–46.
28. Iammarino K, Marrie J, Selhorst M, Lowes LP. Efficacy of the stretch band ankle traction technique in the treatment of pediatric patients with acute ankle sprains: a randomized control trial. Int J Sports Phys Ther. 2018;13(1):1–11.
29. Laver L, Carmont MR, McConkey MO, et al. Plasma rich in growth factors (PRGF) as a treatment for high ankle sprain in elite athletes: a randomized control trial. Knee Surg Sports Traumatol Arthrosc. 2015;23:3383–92.
30. Tran K, McCormack S. Exercise for the Treatment of Ankle Sprain: A Review of Clinical Effectiveness and Guidelines [Internet]. Ottawa (ON): Canadian Agency for Drugs and Technologies in Health; 2020 Apr 3. Available from: https://www.ncbi.nlm.nih.gov/books/NBK563007/.
31. Punt, Ilona & Ziltener, Jean-Luc & Monnin, Dominique & Allet, Lara. Wii Fit™ exercise therapy for the rehabilitation of ankle sprains: Its effect compared with physical therapy or no functional exercises at all. Scandinavian journal of medicine & science in sports; 2015. https://doi.org/10.1111/sms.12509.

Medial Ankle Disorders

50

Seyed Behrooz Mostofi, Abdolrahman Fazli,
and Walter I. Sussman

50.1 Posterior Tibialis Tendon Dysfunction (PTTD)

50.1.1 Synonym

- Tibialis posterior tendon tenosynovitis
- Tibialis posterior tendon rupture
- Tibialis posterior tendon dislocation
- Tibialis posterior tendonitis
- Posterior tibial tendon insufficiency
- Adult acquired flatfoot deformity

50.1.2 ICD 10 Code

- M76.821 – Posterior tibial tendinitis, right leg
- M76.822 – Posterior tibial tendinitis, left leg

50.1.3 Description

Posterior tibial tendon dysfunction (PTTD) is characterized by a collapse of the medial longitudinal arch and the prevailing cause of adult acquired flatfoot deformity. PTTD is progressive, and degeneration begins before clinical disease is apparent. It is more commonly seen in obese, middle-aged women and has been associated with diabetes, hypertension, obesity, previous surgery, seronegative spondyloarthropathies, and steroid use [1]. Estimates of prevalence range from 3.3% to 10% [2]. Multiple etiologies of PTTD have been described. A history of trauma may be present in up to 50% of cases and can include direct trauma to the tendon and is associated with ankle fractures [1]. Due to the short excursion of the tendon, even minor damage may render the tendon ineffective [1]. In degenerative cases, the hypovascular region of the medial malleolus may limit the healing potential. As the tendon loses function, there is a progressive collapse of the medial longitudinal arch and eventual valgus hindfoot alignment. Differential diagnosis of PTTD is given in Table 50.1.

Anatomy Tibialis posterior tendon originates from posterior aspect of proximal tibia, posteromedial fibula, and interosseous membrane. At the level of medial malleolus, it changes direction at almost 90° and has a broad attachment to the navicular tuberosity, but additional insertions in the hindfoot and midfoot have been described [3]. The tibialis posterior is the primary dynamic stabilizer of the medial longitudinal arch, and plantar flexes the ankle joint and inverts at the subtalar joint [4].

50.1.3.1 Classification

Different classification schemes have described the progressive stages of PTTD. Johnson and Strom introduced a classification system for PTTD which can guide in the treatment [4].

Table 50.1 Differential diagnosis of posterior tibialis tendon dysfunction

Deltoid ligament injuries	Spring ligament injury	Flexor retinaculum injury	Tarsal tunnel syndrome
Accessory flexor muscles	Subtalar coalition	Ligament tears	Tendon tears

S. B. Mostofi (✉)
East Kent Hospitals University, NHS Foundation Trust, Canterbury, Kent, UK

A. Fazli
Department of Orthopedics, Manipal Academy of Higher Education, Manipal, India

Queen Elizabeth The Queen Mother Hospital, East Kent Hospitals University, NHS Foundation Trust, Margate, UK

W. I. Sussman
Department of Orthopedics and Rehabilitation, Tufts University School of Medicine, Boston, MA, USA

Boston Sports & Biologics PC, Wellesley, MA, USA

© The Author(s), under exclusive license to Springer Nature Switzerland AG 2022
S. A. Mostoufi et al. (eds.), *Clinical Guide to Musculoskeletal Medicine*, https://doi.org/10.1007/978-3-030-92042-5_50

Stage I disease is characterized by swelling, pain, inflammation, and often effusion within the posterior tibial tendon sheath. Irritability is noted with passive eversion of the foot along the course of the posterior tibial tendon. Mild weakness to manual testing may be present; however, no deformity of the foot is demonstrated when compared with the opposite foot. The patient is able to invert the foot actively on a double leg-toe raise test and is able to perform a single leg-toe raise.

Stage II disease is characterized by the loss of function of the posterior tibial tendon and inability to perform a single leg-toe raise. The hindfoot remains flexible.

Stage III disease is characterized by the loss of function of the posterior tibial tendon, and a semirigid or rigid hindfoot deformity with valgus abduction occurs, and degenerative changes in ankle and subtalar joint may be apparent on radiographs.

Stage IV disease was described by Myerson et al. and involves valgus positioning and incongruence of the ankle joint in addition to stage III findings.

50.1.4 Clinical Presentation

Symptoms depend on the cause and severity of the condition. Patient presents with pain and swelling along the medial aspect of the foot and ankle and can radiate from the posteromedial aspect of the leg to the medial malleolus and navicular. Pain can be exacerbated with or worsen after activity. Range of motion of ankle may be restricted due to pain, and patients will often have pain when walking on toes or going up/down the stairs. As PTTD progresses, patients may have difficulty toe walking. In severe cases, with progressive collapse of the medial arch and valgus hindfoot deformity, pain maybe present over the lateral ankle due the distal fibula coming into contact with the lateral calcaneus.

50.1.5 Physical Examination

On examination, swelling along the route of the tendon may be present. Palpation of the tendon can be painful along its course. Patients may have pain with resisted inversion.

50.1.5.1 Provocative Testing

Single heel raise Patients can typically complete 8–10 repetitions of a single heel raise. In progressive stages, the patient cannot tip-toe on the affected side, and a positive test is when the patient had difficulty performing a single heel raise or weakness with multiple attempts.

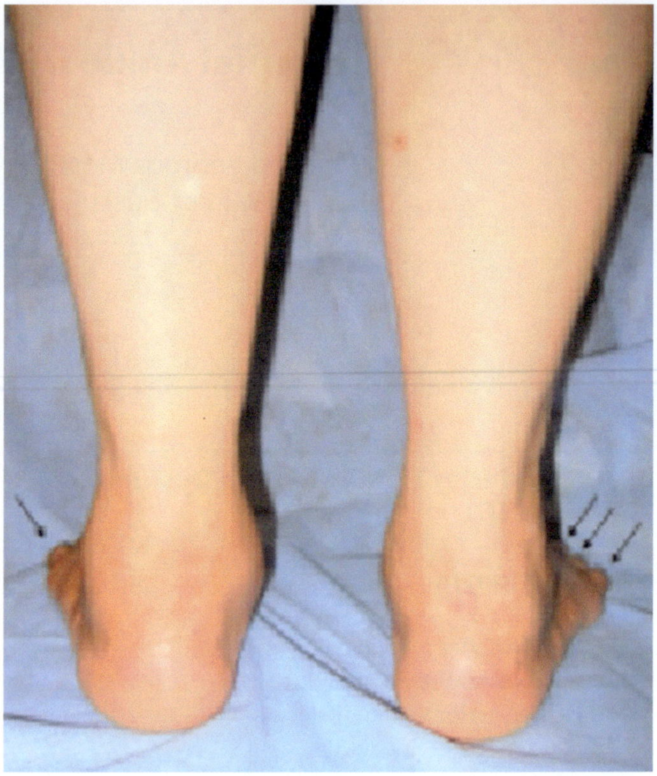

Fig. 50.1 Only one or two toes should be visible from behind. If more are seen, it is said that the too many toes sign is present (black arrows on the right). (From Rapid Orthopedic diagnosis, Springer; 2008 edition by Author S. Behrooz Mostofi, FRCS)

"Too many toes" sign In severe disease, there is collapse of the medial longitudinal arch and compensatory valgus heel deformity, midfoot abduction, and forefoot pronation. Inspection of the patient foot from behind will show a "too many toes" sign, and a positive test is when more than one or two toes are seen along the lateral aspect of the foot (Fig. 50.1).

50.1.6 Diagnostic Workup

50.1.6.1 Radiographs

Weight-bearing X-ray of the ankle and foot may demonstrate no significant changes in the first two stages of the disease. As the disease progresses, X-ray shows collapse of the medial longitudinal arch and degenerated changes of the midfoot. X-rays can show an increased talus-first metatarsal angle (normally 0°–10°). Loss of calcaneal pitch angle is another radiologic sign of progressive disease.

50.1.6.2 Ultrasound

Ultrasound can assess the posterior tibialis tendon, and an increase in tendon width greater than 6 mm is suggestive of tenosynovitis.

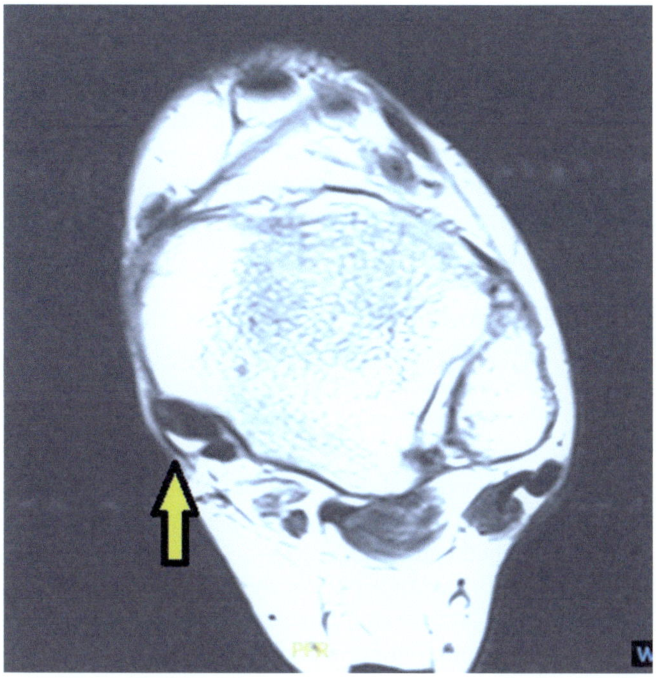

Fig. 50.2 Axial MRI showing inflammation and tear in the posterior tibial tendon. (Courtesy of Dr. Amir Abbas Mostoufi, MD, Tehran, Iran)

50.1.6.3 MRI/CT

MRI scan is very helpful as it can show inflammatory changes in the tendon sheath as well as longitudinal tears of the tendon (Fig. 50.2). Weight-bearing CT scan may be helpful in preoperative planning to correct the deformities.

50.1.7 Treatment

50.1.7.1 Medical Management

Treatment decisions vary according to the stage of the pathology. Conservative management is used in earlier stages (I and II) with a focus on strengthening and orthosis to maintain the shape of the foot and surgery in later stages to correct deformity seen in later stages.

Tenosynovitis (stage I) is treated with rest, nonsteroidal anti-inflammatory agents, and supportive modalities like walking boot, medial longitudinal arch support, ankle brace, or short leg walking cast. Preventing recurrence of stage I disease can be assisted with the use of an orthotic device that incorporates a medial heel wedge and medial forefoot post to place the hindfoot in neutral, decreasing force requirements for the posterior tibial muscle and tendon unit.

Conservative management of stage II disease is similar to stage I, but stage II is characterized by irreversible tendon changes with flattening of the medial arch. Treatment includes application of an orthotic device that has a medial post and an ankle-foot orthosis.

50.1.7.2 Procedures

Corticosteroid injections are controversial due to concerns that the injections may further jeopardize the tendon. If conservative treatment fails, platelet-rich plasma injection maybe beneficial, but the literature is lacking.

50.1.7.3 Rehabilitation

Stage I: After the acute inflammation of the tenosynovium subsides, rehabilitation of the calf and leg with physical therapy is often helpful. Success has been demonstrated with a comprehensive calf and leg rehabilitation program that emphasizes graduated isometric strengthening exercises and gastrocsoleus complex stretching [5]. Specialized rehabilitation may be required after tendon debridement and repair, tendon transfer, and reconstruction of the spring ligament and bony procedures/osteotomies according to surgeons' instructions.

50.1.7.4 Surgery

Surgery is reserved for recalcitrant cases, and open synovectomy remains the surgical treatment of choice for stage I disease, but tendoscopy has been reported to produce good results [6]. For stage II, surgical management typically requires tendon reconstruction. Stages III and IV: More advanced disease is characterized by progressive tendon degeneration and hindfoot arthropathy. Management is typically in the form of tendon debridement and repair, different tendon transfers, reconstruction of spring ligament, and bony procedures to correct deformity. The most common tendon transfer is that of flexor digitorum longus (FDL). Lateral column lengthening (LCL) and medial displacement of the tuberosity of the calcaneus (MDCO), a Z-shaped calcaneal osteotomy, or a combination of the two is the most commonly used osteotomies.

50.2 Flexor Hallucis Longus Tendinopathy (FHL)

50.2.1 Synonyms

- FHL tendinitis
- FHL tendinopathy
- FHL tendinosis
- FHL tenosynovitis
- Dancer's tendinitis

50.2.2 ICD 10 Code

- M65.871 Other synovitis and tenosynovitis, right ankle and foot
- M65.872 Other synovitis and tenosynovitis, left ankle and foot

50.2.3 Description

Flexor hallucis longus (FHL) tendinopathy is a painful condition due to inflammation of the FHL tendon. The FHL is the most common site of lower extremity tendon disorders in ballet dancers [7] and has become known as "dancer's tendinitis." The FHL generates power during gait, and individuals who perform repetitive push-off or plantar flexion can injure the FHL. Dancers tend to have symptoms for a longer period of time before seeking treatment than nondancers [7].

Anatomy The FHL originates from the lower 2/3 of the posterior fibula and interosseous membrane. As the tendon passes between the fibro-osseous tunnel at the back of the talus, it runs deep to the sustentaculum tali. The tendon crosses over the flexor digitorum longus at the level of the talonavicular joint, known as the knot of Henry, and then runs distally to insert on the first distal phalanx.

Etiology/Pathophysiology The FHL tendon is vulnerable at three areas along its course. The most common location is behind the medial malleolus. Pathology may also be found at the knot of Henry or at the base of the first metatarsal where the tendon passes beneath the sesamoid bones. Due to the anatomy, the FHL crosses several structures, and within this pulley system, the tendon can become inflamed and cause irritation and swelling. Reduced vascularity is also an important factor contributing to tendon degeneration and rupture under strain. When the tendon is thickened or a partial tear is present at the fibro-osseous tunnel below the sustentaculum talia, patients may described triggering. This condition is known as hallux saltans. When the tendon becomes completely fibrosed with stenosing tenosynovitis within the pulley system it can present with a pseudo hallux rigidus. Table 50.2 lists the differential diagnosis of flexor hallucis longus tendinopathy.

Table 50.2 Differential diagnosis of flexor hallucis longus tendinopathy

Medial plantar nerve pathology	Baxter's neuropathy	Tarsal tunnel syndrome	Achilles tendinopathy
Posterior ankle impingement	Myofascial pain	Medial malleoli stress fracture	Bursitis

50.2.4 Clinical Presentation

FHL tendinopathy presents as pain in the posteromedial aspect of the ankle both during ankle plantarflexion dorsiflexion motions, sometimes including "trigger toe," a snapping of the great toe when moving from ankle plantarflexion to neutral.

50.2.5 Examination

On clinical evaluation, assess for pain or crepitus along the FHL by placing the foot in plantarflexion and providing resistance to hallux flexion [8]. Triggering or crepitus of the tendon and tenderness along the sheath of the tendon when moving the great toe mimic the pain experienced while dancing and confirm the diagnosis.

Pain in the posterior aspect of the ankle when a patient assumes the plantarflexion position suggests a diagnosis of posterior impingement syndrome. Forceful passive plantar flexion of the relaxed foot (the plantarflexion test) reproduces the pain experienced while dancing, and this pain is the hallmark of posterior impingement syndrome.

50.2.6 Diagnostic Workup

Plain radiographs have no indication in this diagnosis except ruling out any bony or joint pathology. Ultrasound (Figs. 50.3 and 50.4) and MRI imaging can help with the diagnosis.

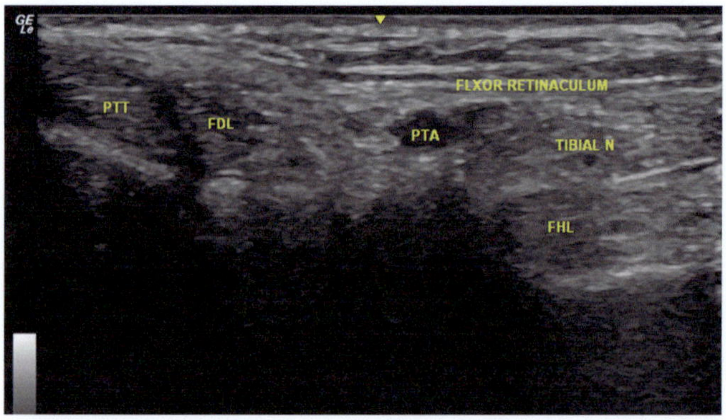

Fig. 50.3 Normal short access US image of FHL tendon, deep to the tibial nerve in the medial ankle. Posterior tibial artery (PTA), flexor digitorum longus (FDL), and posterior tibial tendon are all visualized in tis plane. (Image courtesy of S. Ali Mostoufi, MD, Boston Regenerative Medicine)

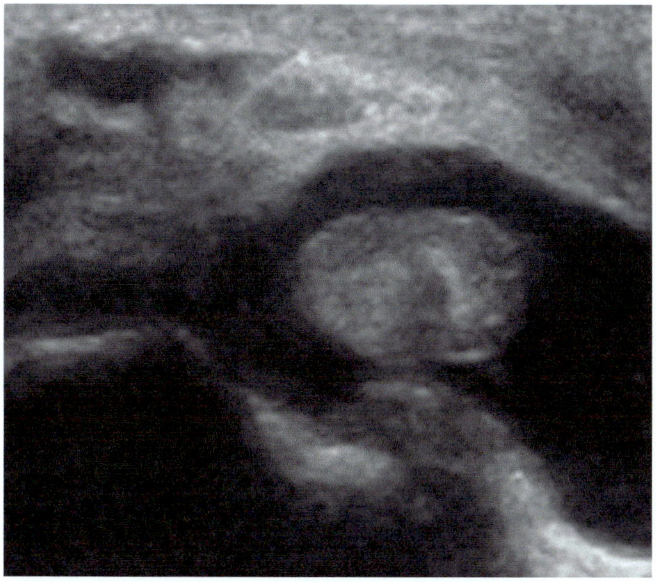

Fig. 50.4 Tenosynovitis of the flexor hallux longus at the knot of Henry, in a ballet dancer. Short axis focal fluid signal/distention of the tendon sheath. (Image courtesy of S. Ali Mostoufi, MD, Boston Regenerative Medicine)

50.2.7 Treatment

50.2.7.1 Medical Management

Management involves activity modification, cryotherapy, NSAIDs, and physiotherapy. For prolonged tendinopathy, short-term immobilization can be considered. Literature on treatment for FHL pathology is limited, and in one study of 81 patients, 64% demonstrated improvement with conservative management [9].

50.2.7.2 Procedures

As with other tenosynovitis cases, image-guided tendon sheath injection with steroid or PRP may provide pain relief and aid with rehabilitation. A period of immunization may be necessary to avoid tendon rupture after steroid injection. There is no indication for steroid injection in chronic tendinosis or tendon tear.

50.2.7.3 Rehabilitation

Rehabilitation of the FHL tendinopathy and tenosynovitis may include exercise-based treatment, often progressive in intensity. Strengthening exercises along the kinetic chain can help alleviate stress on the FHL ankle stability exercises with or without Kinesio taping may have value in the rehabilitation course. Initial rehab phase includes load management, modifying activities, and modifying training in athletes and dancers. In general, exercises and training should not aggravate the tendon and result in more pain. The combination of soft tissue massage, stretching, and foam rollers may assist with progression in rehabilitation. Physical therapists may utilize therapeutic ultrasound during rehabilitation courses.

50.2.7.4 Surgery

Open and endoscopic debridement has been discussed, but literature is limited. This condition is frequently persistent and disabling in dancers, and surgical tenolysis is frequently needed with good reported results [10].

50.3 Tarsal Tunnel Syndrome

50.3.1 Synonyms

Posterior tibial neuralgia

50.3.2 ICD 10 Code

- G57.51 – Tarsal tunnel syndrome, right lower limb
- G57.52 – Tarsal tunnel syndrome, left lower limb

50.3.3 Description

Tarsal tunnel syndrome (TTS) is an entrapment neuropathy of the tibial nerve in the tarsal tunnel. The tibial nerve branches that may be involved include the medial plantar nerve, lateral plantar nerve, Baxter's nerve (also known as the first branch of the lateral plantar nerve or inferior calcaneal nerve), and medial calcaneal nerve.

Anatomy The tarsal tunnel is a fibro-osseous tunnel within the posteromedial ankle and hindfoot in which the tibial nerve, posterior tibial artery, accompanying veins, posterior tibial tendon, flexor digitorum longus, and flexor hallucis longus tendons pass into the foot. The flexor retinaculum acts as the roof of this tunnel and extends from the medial malleolus to the medial side of the calcaneal tuberosity. Two regions of entrapment have been described: (1) in the proximal tarsal tunnel besides the flexor retinaculum and (2) in the distal tarsal tunnel at the medial intermuscular septum deep to the abductor hallucis muscle [11].

50.3.3.1 Etiology/Pathophysiology

In 50% of cases, TTS is idiopathic [11], but specific causes can include a space-occupying mass or systemic disorder. Sources of constriction beneath and adjacent to the tarsal tunnel can include bone fragments, tenosynovitis, ganglia, soft tissue encroachment in inflammatory arthritis, varicosities, neural tumors (neurilemmoma), perineural fibrosis, tarsal coalition, and after calcaneal osteotomies. Furthermore, a fixed valgus hindfoot can predispose to chronic traction neuropathy of the posterior tibial nerve or one of its branches.

The clinical diagnosis is made from the presence of dysesthesia in the distribution of the medial and lateral plantar nerves, the presence of Tinel's sign along the posteromedial ankle (paresthesias provoked by compression of the tarsal tunnel), tenderness of the nerve along its course (Valleix's phenomenon), and sensory or motor changes.

In this condition, the distribution of pain is not radicular; it is often described as being adjacent and distal to the tarsal tunnel. Symptoms may be similar to those of plantar fasciitis, but unlike plantar fasciitis, nerve entrapment symptoms do not resolve quickly. Making the diagnosis difficult as typical neurogenic symptoms are not always present and symptoms may be present at night, during exercise, or at rest. Symptoms can be confined to the lateral plantar nerve (Fig. 50.5), medial plantar nerve (Fig. 50.6), or medial calcaneal nerve.

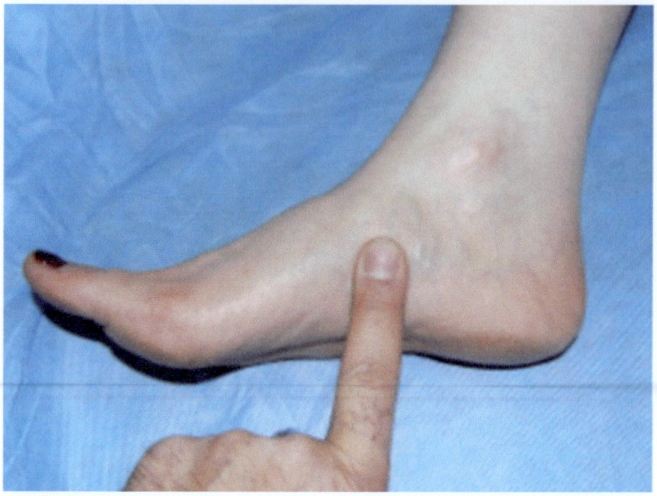

Fig. 50.6 Site of entrapment of medial plantar nerve by palpating the region of Henry's knot (plantar to the 1st TMT joint). (From Rapid Orthopedic diagnosis, Springer; 2008 edition, by Author S. Behrooz Mostofi, FRCS)

50.3.4 Physical Examination

A thorough, detailed examination, aided with a good patient history, improves diagnostic accuracy. Careful examination for subtle sensory abnormalities or differences in temperature, sweating pattern, and skin abnormalities may lead to the correct diagnosis. Although a common complaint of sensory abnormalities often are difficult to detect. Dryness and scaliness of the skin may be present over *only* the lateral or medial plantar nerve distribution. Atrophy of the abductor hallucis and/or abductor digiti minimi can be challenging to detect clinically but can be evident on advance imaging and

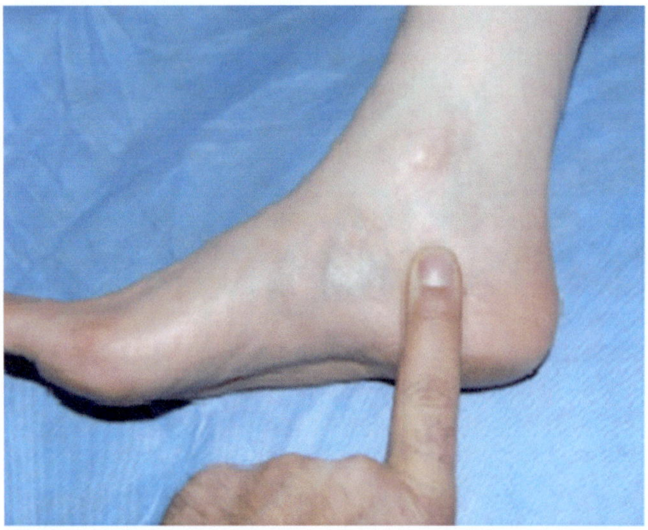

Fig. 50.5 Site of entrapment of lateral plantar nerve. (From Rapid Orthopedic diagnosis, Springer; 2008 edition, by Author S. Behrooz Mostofi, FRCS)

may be obvious when compared with the asymptomatic foot. Point tenderness of the medial heel in the soft spot at the lower edge of the abductor hallucis may indicate distal entrapment of the tibial branches.

50.3.4.1 Provocative Testing

Tinel's sign performed over the flexor retinaculum may indicate proximal entrapment.

Triple compression test Described by Abouelela and Zohiery, the triple compression test is performed with the ankle plantar flexed and the foot inverted (increasing the tarsal tunnel compartment pressures), and then a digital compression is applied over the tibial nerve.

50.3.5 Diagnostic Workup

Radiographs Plain radiographs demonstrate osseous abnormalities (e.g., fractures or talocalcaneal coalitions) that may contribute to tarsal tunnel symptoms.

Ultrasound High-resolution ultrasound is a reliable imaging modality to examine the tarsal tunnel and can identify compressive mass and swelling of the tibial nerve proximal to entrapment sites (Fig. 50.7). Axial cross-sectional area of the tibial nerve has shown an 81% sensitivity and 100% specificity for diagnosis of patients with clinical end electroneuromyography signs of TTS.

MRI scan is preferred because of the improved detail of the tarsal contents [12]. MRI has been shown to identify the cause of the tarsal tunnel syndrome in up to 88% of patients.

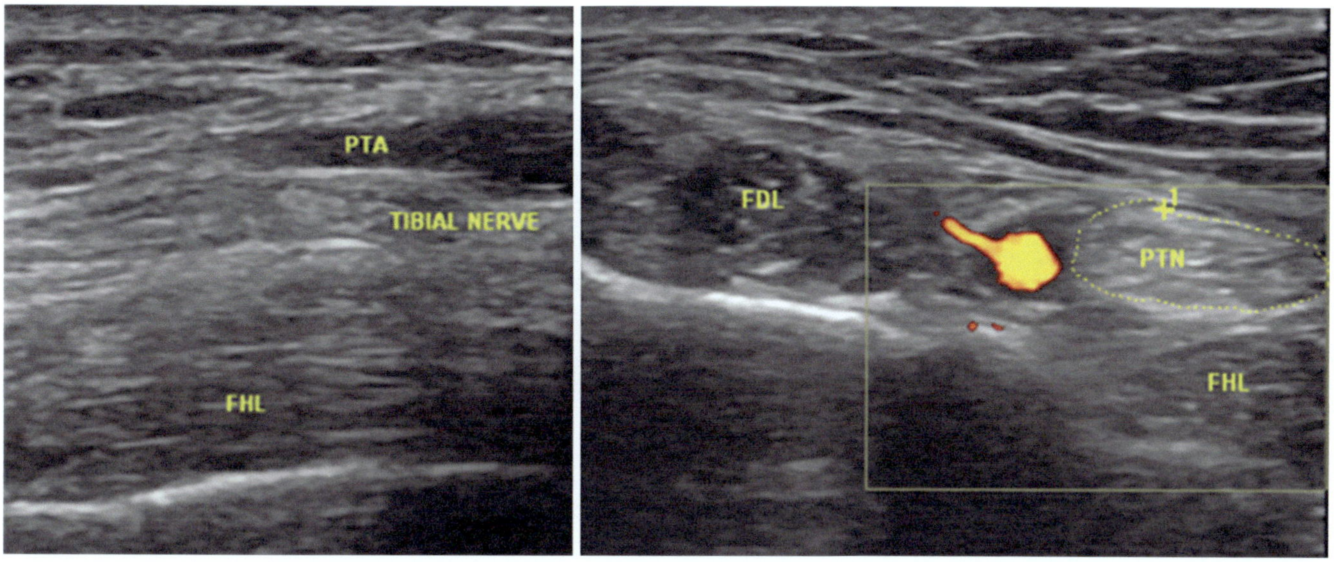

Fig. 50.7 Long axis sonogram (left) and short axis sonogram views of the tibial nerve in relation to the FHL and tibial artery at the tarsal tunnel. Tibial nerve measurements with signs of focal enlargement (circumferential in cross section) or linear measurement (in long axis) can be diagnostic for TT. (Image Courtesy of S. Ali Mostoufi, MD, Boston Regenerative Medicine)

More importantly, MRI aids with surgical planning by providing detailed characteristics and location of space-occupying lesions.

EMG Electrodiagnostic testing is indicated for any patient suspected of having compression of the tibial nerve beneath the flexor retinaculum and can assess for lumbar radiculopathy. In one study, 5% of patients with lower lumbar radiculopathy also suffered from tarsal tunnel syndrome, so these diagnoses are not exclusive [13].

50.3.6 Treatment

50.3.6.1 Medical Management

Treatment should be guided by the underlying cause of TTS. In idiopathic cases, conservative treatment should be the first line treatment. Initially, 6–12 weeks of ankle immobilization in a night splint, anti-inflammatory agents, and a wide, cushioned and comfortable shoe are recommended. If distal tarsal tunnel syndrome is suspected, an orthosis with a relief channel within the medial arch may be effective; a standard orthosis with a longitudinal arch may worsen symptoms.

50.3.6.2 Procedure

Symptoms caused by space-occupying lesions should be treated by addressing the underlying cause. Tenosynovitis and ganglion cysts can be treated initially with aspiration and/or corticosteroid injection.

50.3.6.3 Rehabilitation

Gentle exercises that move and "glide" the nerves may help reduce symptoms and improve function (nerve gliding). Strengthening activities for any muscles affected by TTS, such as the tibialis posterior muscle, may reduce symptoms and improve function. Physical therapist may utilize ankle taping, custom orthotic, or bracing to position the foot to decrease stress on the posterior tibial nerve.

50.3.6.4 Surgery

Patients with a space-occupying lesion or those that fail conservative measures may be a candidate for surgical release. Caution is recommended in advising surgical treatment of tarsal tunnel syndrome in patients who are older (60–80 years old), have post traumatic scarring within the tarsal canal, have no objective cause for symptoms (idiopathic), and those with protracted psychiatric illness [14]. More information on foot and ankle surgery can be found in Chap. 52.

References

1. Bubra PS, Keighley G, Rateesh S, Carmody D. Posterior tibial tendon dysfunction: an overlooked cause of foot deformity. J Family Med Prim Care. 2015;4(1):26–9.
2. Kohls-Gatzoulis J, Woods B, Angel JC, et al. The prevalence of symptomatic posterior tibialis tendon dysfunction in women over the age of 40 in England. Foot Ankle Surg. 2009;15:75–81.
3. Willegger M, Seyidova N, Schuh R, Windhager R, Hirtler L. The tibialis posterior tendon footprint: an anatomical dissection study. J Foot Ankle Res. 2020;13(1):25.

4. Johnson KA, Strom DE. Tibialis posterior tendon dysfunction. Clin Orthop Relat Res. 1989;239:196–206.
5. Kulig K, Reischl SF, Pomrantz AB, Burnfield JM, Mais-Requejo S, Thordarson DB, Smith RW. Nonsurgical management of posterior tibial tendon dysfunction with orthoses and resistive exercise: a randomized controlled trial. Phys Ther. 2009;89(1):26–37.
6. Grear BJ. Chapter 83. In: Campbell's operative orthopaedics. 2002. pp. 4154–4226.e10.
7. Hamilton WG. Dancer's tendinitis of the FHL tendon. Presented at the Second Annual Meeting of the American Orthopaedic Society for Sports Medicine, Durango, Colorado, July, 1976.
8. Lui TH, Chow FY. "Intersection syndrome" of the foot: treated by endoscopic release of master knot of Henry. Knee Surg Sports Traumatol Arthrosc. 2011;19:850–2.
9. Michelson J, Dunn L. Tenosynovitis of the flexor hallucis longus: a clinical study of the spectrum of presentation and treatment. Foot Ankle Int. 2005;26:291–303.
10. Corte-Real NM, Moreira RM, Guerra-Pinto F. Arthroscopic treatment of tenosynovitis of the flexor hallucis longus tendon. Foot Ankle Int. 2012;33(12):1108–12. https://doi.org/10.3113/FAI.2012.1108. PMID: 23199862.
11. Moroni S, Gibello AF, Zwierzina M, et al. Ultrasound-guided decompression surgery of the distal tarsal tunnel: a novel technique for the distal tarsal tunnel syndrome—part III. Surg Radiol Anat. 2019;41:313–21.
12. Frey C, Kerr R. Magnetic resonance imaging and the evaluation of tarsal tunnel syndrome. Foot Ankle. 1993;14:159–64.
13. Zheng C, Zhu Y, Jiang J, Ma X, Lu F, Jin X, Weber R. The prevalence of tarsal tunnel syndrome in patients with lumbosacral radiculopathy. Eur Spine J. 2016;25(3):895–905.
14. Grear BJ. Chapter 87. In: Campbell's operative orthopaedics. 2002. pp. 4345–4381.e3.

51 Foot and Ankle Dislocations and Fractures

Seyed Behrooz Mostofi, Abdolrahman Fazli, Woo A. Kim, and S. Ali Mostoufi

51.1 Ankle Fractures

51.1.1 Description

Ankle fractures are common in all age groups resulting from both high- and low-energy trauma [1]. The two most common age groups are physically active younger men and older women with frailty. Frail elderly patients are more likely to present following lower-energy trauma like a mechanical fall to the lower limb.

51.1.2 Classification

There are many different methods to classify acute ankle fractures. Assessing injuries accurately helps identify the extent of the injury and aids in formulating a management plan. Ankle injuries can be described by the number of malleoli fractured on imaging. For example, a trimalleolar ankle fracture involves medial, lateral, and posterior malleoli (Fig. 51.1). A common and practical classification, Danis-Weber, aims to classify an ankle fracture by describing its location in relation to the syndesmosis (Table 51.1). The interosseous membrane of the syndesmosis is formed by the tibia and fibula joining together, and this is further enforced by other ligaments.

51.1.3 Orthopedic Care

In more stable fractures (Weber A/isolated lateral malleolar fracture) or in younger patients, nonoperative management reportedly achieves similar functional outcomes to those treated with surgical fixation [1]. It has been broadly accepted that Weber B and C injuries are likely unstable, requiring internal fixation. Syndesmotic injury is linked with an unstable ankle joint injury. Unstable fractures with syndesmotic disruption will require surgical open reduction and internal fixation (ORIF). The lateral malleolus is fixed with a plate or nail, the medial malleolus with partial threaded screws, and the posterior malleolus is fixed with screws only or plate according to the size of the fragment (Fig. 51.2). The ankle is immobilized in a temporary plaster cast for the first 2 weeks for comfort, and then a range of motion exercises may start. Weight-bearing is determined according to the bone quality and fixation achieved during surgery. In younger patients with good bone stock and fixation, partial weight-bearing can begin after 2 weeks. Others may need a period of 6 weeks of non-weight-bearing.

S. B. Mostofi (✉)
Consultant Orthopaedic Foot and Ankle surgeon, East Kent Hospitals University, NHS Foundation Trust, Canterbury, Kent, UK

Visiting Professor, Department of Orthopedics, Manipal Academy of Higher Education, Manipal, India

A. Fazli
Department of Orthopedic, Queen Elizabeth The Queen Mother Hospital, East Kent Hospitals University, NHS Foundation Trust, Margate, UK

W. A. Kim
Department Of Orthopedics, Kent Surrey and Sussex Deanery, NHS Foundation Trust, Kent, UK

S. A. Mostoufi
Department of Orthopedics and Rehabilitation, Tufts University School of Medicine, Boston, MA, USA

New England Spine Care Associates & Boston Regenerative Medicine, Cambridge, MA, USA
e-mail: Ali.Mostoufi@Tufts.edu

© The Author(s), under exclusive license to Springer Nature Switzerland AG 2022

S. A. Mostoufi et al. (eds.), *Clinical Guide to Musculoskeletal Medicine*, https://doi.org/10.1007/978-3-030-92042-5_51

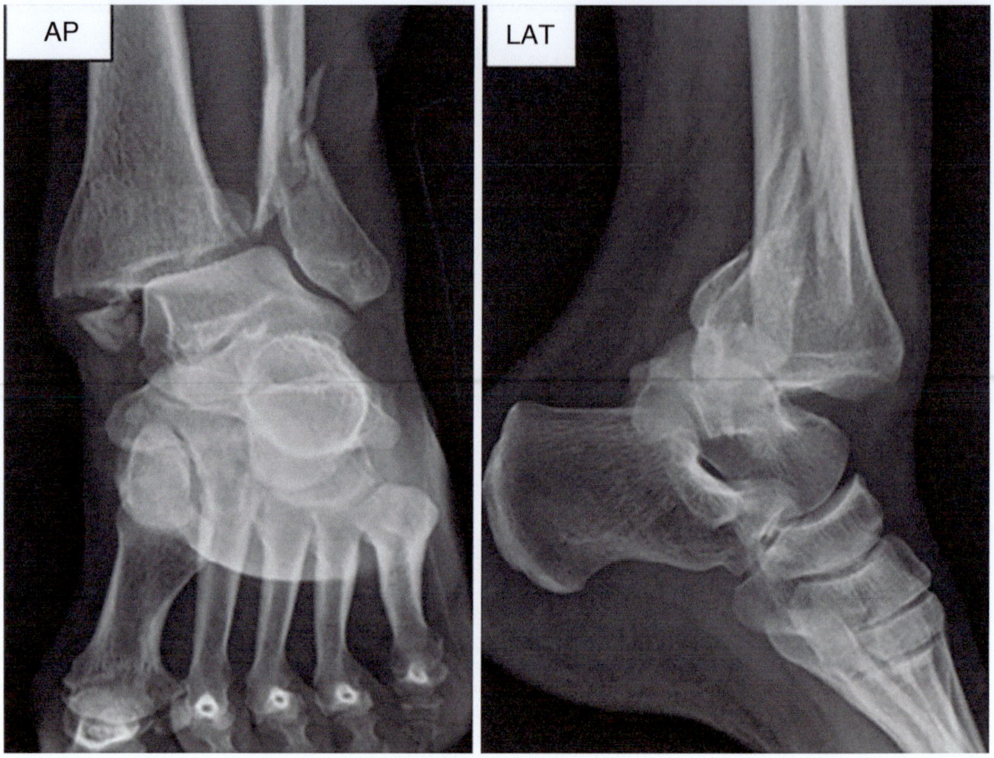

Fig. 51.1 Trimalleolar ankle fracture involves medial, lateral, and posterior malleoli. Lateral view of the same patient showing the ankle fractures with subluxation

Table 51.1 Danis-Weber classification of ankle fracture

Type of injury	Location of injury
Weber A	Below the syndesmosis
Weber B	At the level of syndesmosis
Weber C	Above the syndesmosis

51.1.4 Rehabilitation

Patients will require rehabilitation following a period of immobilization. The initial speed of recovery can be rapid, but often the healing process can take up to 2 years from initial injury [2]. Rehabilitation exercises are key to improving the patient's quality of life and restoring the dynamic function of the ankle joint.

51.2 Pilon Fractures

51.2.1 Description

Pilon fractures are high-energy injuries involving fractures of the articular surface of the distal tibial and occasional extension to the proximal diaphyseal bone. They are the result of axial loading with the talus being driven into the distal tibia [3]. Such high-energy fractures are typically associated with significant injury to the surrounding soft tissue envelope.

51.2.2 Classification

The fracture involves the tibial plafond and the distal tibial articular surface. Associated fractures of the fibula can be evident, with or without ankle dislocation. CT scan would further define the fracture pattern and assess for subluxation. Rüedi and Allgöwer [4] classified the fracture to three types outlined in Table 51.2.

51.2.3 Orthopedic Care

Pilon fractures are usually comminuted and unstable, requiring reconstruction of the joint surface anatomically to prevent arthritis in the future. Staged management of high-energy complex tibial pilon fractures is recommended since studies report acute ORIF through traumatized tissue was associated with high complication rate [5]. In staged treatment of open pillion fractures, the initial step is the application of external fixation and management of soft tissue swelling and wound care for the first 7–10 days, obtaining CT scan for ORIF planning followed by definitive ORIF using anatomic, locking plates. Perioperative complications include malreduction, inadequate fixation, and intra-articular penetration of hardware, all of which may be minimized by preoperative planning and meticulous operative techniques [3]. In some cases, with extensive soft tissue injury, soft tissue reconstruction utilizing free flap may be necessary.

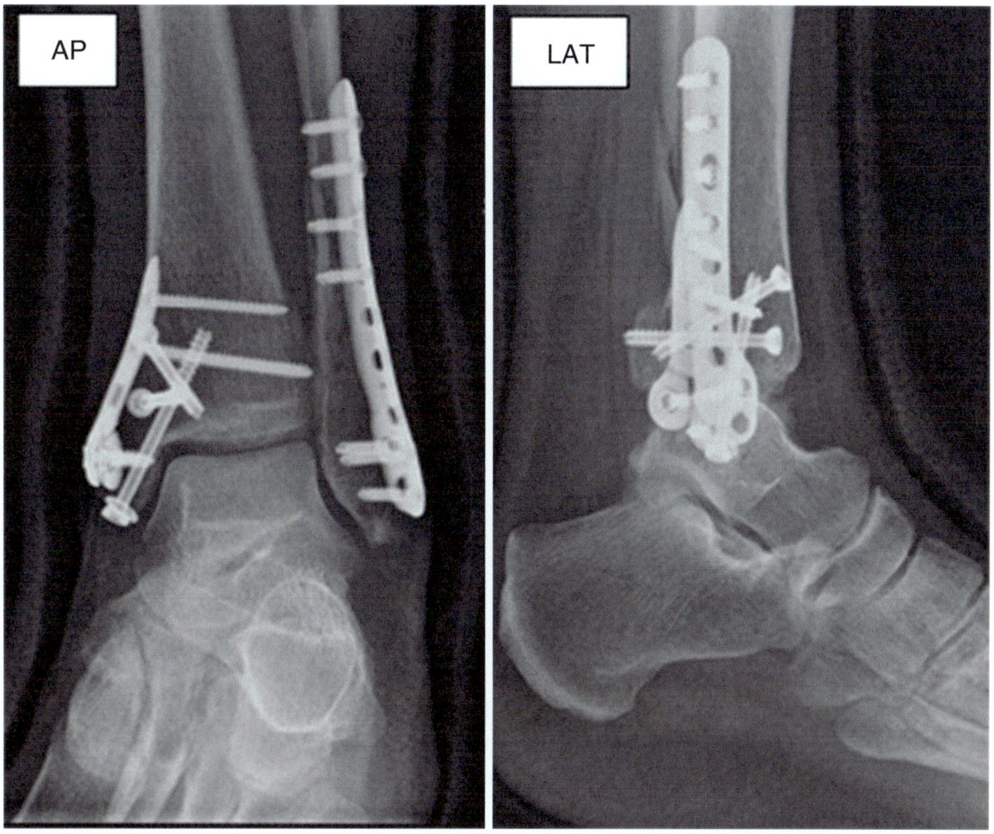

Fig. 51.2 AP and lateral view of the ankle after open reduction and internal fixation (ORIF)

Table 51.2 Rüedi and Allgöwer classification of Pilon fractures

Type 1	Nondisplaced intra-articular
Type 2	Displaced without comminution
Type 3	Displaced with comminution (most common)

51.2.4 Rehabilitation

Early postoperative mobilization is started in some cases, but weight-bearing is often delayed for 6 weeks to allow for bony healing.

51.3 Fracture of the Talus

51.3.1 Description

The talus is a crucial link between the leg and the foot, playing a vital role in normal ambulation. Motion of the foot and ankle is profoundly impacted by talar injuries. Talar fractures represent less than 1% of all fractures in the human body and between 3% and 6% of fractures in the foot.

Patients with talar fractures typically present after a high-energy injury such as a motor vehicle crash or fall from height and present with foot swelling, pain, or deformity. Fractures of the talus are challenging to manage, with historically poor outcomes and a high rate of complications. The talus has unique anatomic characteristics [6]; over one half of its surface is covered by articular cartilage, and it has no muscular attachments. The trochlea, or superior surface, articulates with the tibial plafond and is wider anteriorly such that maximal articular congruence of the ankle occurs in dorsiflexion. This superior articular surface extends both medially and laterally to articulate with the malleoli. The inferior aspect of the talus is predominantly covered with cartilage and has posterior, middle, and anterior facets, which correspond to the articular facets of the calcaneus. The lateral process of the talus is completely covered by cartilage and articulates with the distal end of the fibula. The posterior process of the talus contains the flexor hallucis longus tendon. The talus has a rich network of extra- and intraosseous anastomoses that is vulnerable to disruption from trauma. Its blood supply is from distal to proximal, so the risk of nonunion and avascular necrosis (AVN) is higher [6].

Fractures of the neck of the talus are the most common, accounting for 50% of all talus fractures due to forced dorsiflexion of the foot, which drives the weak trabecular bone of the neck of the talus against the stronger anterior tibial platform [6]. In approximately 25% of such fractures, supination of the hindfoot leads to medial neck comminution and medial malleolus fracture [6].

Table 51.3 Hawkins classification of talar neck fracture

Hawkins type 1	Nondisplaced talar neck fracture
Hawkins type 2	Talar neck fracture + either subluxation or dislocation of the subtalar joint
Hawkins type 3	Talar neck fracture + dislocation of tibiotalar and subtalar joint
Hawkins type 4	Talar neck fracture + subluxation or dislocation of the talonavicular joint

51.3.2 Classification

The most commonly used classification system for talar neck fractures was described by Hawkins (Table 51.3), and type 2 fracture is the most common.

51.3.3 Orthopedic Care

For high-energy injuries, the patient should undergo a detailed physical examination to identify associated injuries (extremity, spine). AP/lateral/mortise foot and ankle views are often the first diagnostic modality but due to the type of injury. CT scans are often indicated for comminution, detention of intra-articular fragments, and congruent reduction of the tibiotalar, subtalar, and talonavicular joints. When the talus is dislocated, an urgent reduction in the emergency room is indicated to reduce the risk of AVN. If reduction is unsuccessful, urgent surgical care is recommended. Displaced fractures of the talus are usually openly reduced and fixated with screws or plates. Ideal reduction is absolutely anatomical to minimize the risk of AVN and nonunion.

51.3.4 Rehabilitation

Postoperative rehabilitation is non-weight-bearing for at least 6 weeks, but range of motion can be started immediately after the operation.

51.4 Medial Malleolus Stress Fracture (M84.37, S82.5)

51.4.1 Description

This is a rare fracture seen in professional sportsmen mainly soccer players and runners. Stress fractures of the medial malleolus usually present as localized pain, swelling, and tenderness over the medial ankle. Initially, they may not be apparent on radiographs but usually can be demonstrated on bone scan CT or MRI. Often stress fractures become apparent on follow-up radiographs.

51.4.2 Orthopedic Care

Nonoperative and operative interventions have proven to be successful with regard to healing and return to play for medial malleolar stress fractures in the recreational and competitive athlete. However, early surgical care especially for elite athletes may result in early healing, decrease in symptoms, and quicker return to play [7].

Nonoperative treatment consists of non-weight-bearing immobilization, often with a prolonged period away from sport, and a more methodical and careful reintroduction to athletic activity [8]. Shelbourne et al. [9] recommended internal fixation for fractures that are immediately apparent on radiographs and cast immobilization for those only apparent on bone scans. Stress fractures of the medial malleolus have a high risk of progression to complete fracture, delayed union, or nonunion; therefore, aggressive treatment, including surgery, is often necessary.

51.4.3 Rehabilitation

Rehabilitation courses vary depending on nonoperative vs operative management.

51.5 Fibula Nonunion (S82.4)

51.5.1 Description

Ankle fractures are the most common fractures in the leg. These are often the result of a rotation force through the ankle with a foot in a fixed position. The incidence of fibula nonunion is not well described in the literature, but a systematic review performed in 2013 reported an incidence between 0.3% and 5.4% [10]. Nonunions can be divided into two types, hypertrophic or atrophic, depending on the appearance of callus formation on X-rays.

51.5.2 Presentation

The majority of patients present complaining of ongoing symptoms localized to the lateral aspect of the ankle despite treatment for their ankle injury. These patients can have prolonged swelling and point tenderness over the distal fibula. Complaints of recurrent ankle instability can also be noted. However, up to 20% of patients are asymptomatic, and the nonunion or delayed union is an incidental finding.

51.5.3 Diagnostic Workup

Initial imaging would be a standard set of ankle X-rays including an anterior-posterior, mortise, and lateral view weight-bearing views. This will often be able to show the ongoing presence of a fracture line through the distal fibula. Often a degree of callus can be noted; however, the patients will still be symptomatic. Further imaging would consist of computer tomography of the ankle to determine if there is any presence of bridging callus at the fracture site (Fig. 51.3).

51.5.4 Treatment

The management of fibula nonunion or delayed union is controversial in the literature. It has been reported that up to 50% of these patients will go on to union and has been thought of as a variant of delayed union [11]. The literature however does support the surgical fixation of patients with symptomatic nonunion of the distal fibula. This would take the form of open reduction and internal fixation of the fibula fracture with compression at the fracture site for hypertrophic nonunion with the addition of excision/refreshing of the atrophic edges of the fracture surface and bone grafting for atrophic nonunion (Fig. 51.4).

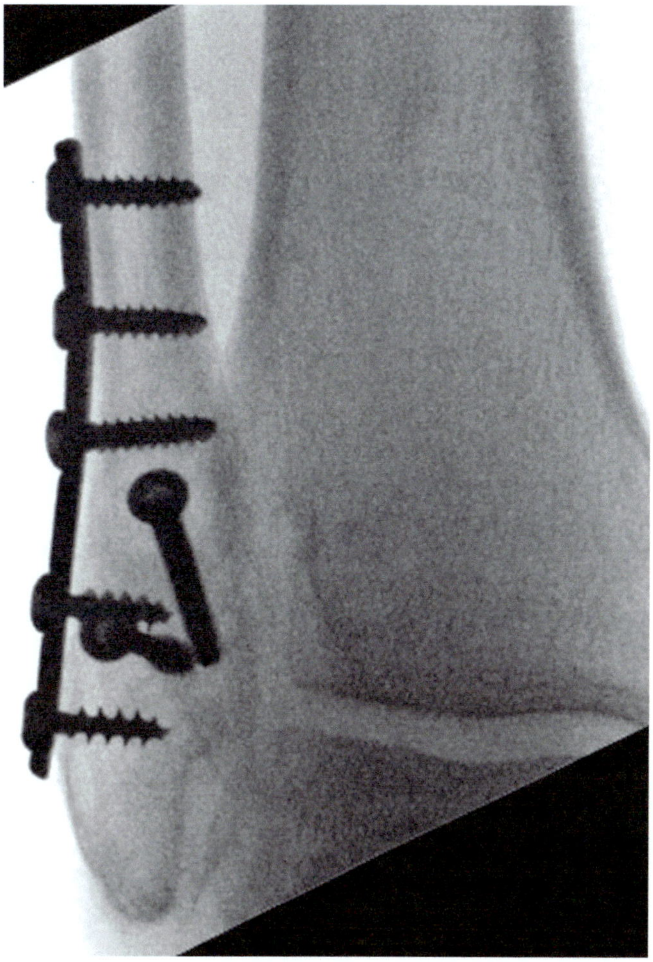

Fig. 51.4 Postoperative images of fibula nonunion treated with open reduction and internal fixation. (Courtesy of Mr. Louette, Kent and Canterbury Hospital, Canterbury, UK)

51.6 Foot Fractures

Foot fractures include the hindfoot bones (calcaneus, cuboid), midfoot (cuneiforms, navicular), and forefoot (metatarsals and phalanges). Metatarsal and toe fractures

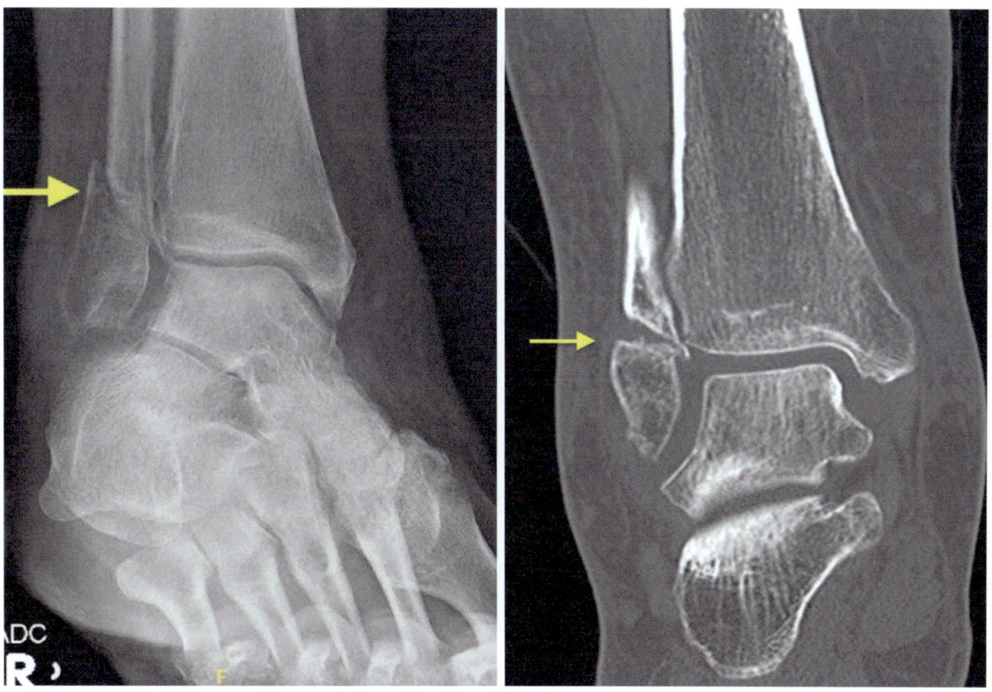

Fig. 51.3 Mortise view (left) of the right ankle showing distal fibula nonunion (yellow arrow), care to be taken to notice the well-corticated fracture margins CT scan (right) of the same patient revealing sclerotic fracture margins (yellow arrow)

are the most frequent injuries of the foot skeleton. Metatarsal fractures close to the base are nearly always associated with Lisfranc luxation and treatment must also take the instability of the tarsometatarsal joints into consideration [12].

51.6.1 Calcaneal Fracture (ICD 10 – S92.0)

Description The calcaneus is one of seven tarsal bones and is part of the hindfoot. The hindfoot articulates with the tibia and fibula creating the ankle joint. Calcaneal burst fractures most commonly occur during high-energy events leading to axial loading of the bone [13]. Falls from height and automobile accidents are the predominant mechanisms of injury. Stress fractures may occur with overuse or repetitive use, such as running. Most patients with calcaneus fractures are young, with the 20–39 age group the most common [13]. Calcaneal fracture is classified into *extraarticular fractures* (25%, avulsion injuries of either the calcaneal tuberosity from the Achilles tendon, the anterior process from the bifurcate ligament, or the sustentaculum tali) and *intraarticular fractures* (75% – the talus acts as a hammer or wedge compressing the calcaneus at the angle of Gissane [14]).

Orthopedic care Initial bony evaluation with AP, lateral, and axial plain films. Stress fractures such as those seen in runners would be best evaluated with a bone scan or MRI. Mondor's sign is a hematoma identified on CT that extends along the sole and is considered pathognomonic for calcaneal fracture [12]. In the initial phase of treatment, wound care and antibiotics are needed for contaminated wounds. Pain management, ice, elevation, and immobilization with splint are necessary with non-weight-bearing status in cases that outpatient management is recommended. For close fractures, particularly extra-articular fractures, 6–8 weeks of non-weight-bearing with gradual rehabilitation is advisable. Open surgical care is recommended for comminuted articular fracture, anterior process involvement, fracture dislocation, involvement of more than 25% of calcaneocuboid articulation, calcaneus body fracture with significant varus or valgus deformity, loss of calcaneal height, significant translation, and in cases of calcaneal tuberosity avulsion and displacement of the sustentaculum tali. Open reduction and stable internal fixation without joint transfixtion have been established as the standard treatment for displaced, intra-articular fractures [14]. There is a higher risk of wound complications after calcaneal fractures. The success rate also depends on several factors including bone quality, age, sex, smoking, and personality of the patient. Patients may develop subtalar joint arthritis and foot pain despite a good reduction and fixation.

Rehabilitation Postoperative rehabilitation is recommended with gradual increase in intensity after the patient has been cleared for weight-bearing, and bony healing has been confirmed.

51.6.2 Cuboid Fracture (ICD 10 – S92.2)

Description Cuboid fractures are usually associated with complex injuries of the foot, and isolated cuboid fractures are rare. It can occur as a result of a compression due to car accident or direct crush of the lateral and dorsum of the foot when a heavy object falls on the foot. It may also present as an avulsion fracture from an ankle sprain. It is often accompanied by Lisfranc fracture and dislocation [15].

Presentation Early detection of these fractures require a high degree of suspicion and often missed. Local swelling, antalgic gait, refusing to bear weight on the lateral aspect of the foot, may indicate cuboid fracture. Ecchymosis and deformity may point to calcaneocuboid joint involvement and instability. Direct palpation of the cuboid, the over lateral aspect of the midfoot reproduces pain.

Orthopedic care X-rays usually diagnose simple fractures, but advanced imaging including CT or MRI may be indicated particularly in stress fracture. Some practitioners with expertise in ultrasound may be able to detect these fractures on sonography. X-ray can differentiate between this entity and fractures of the fifth metatarsal, calcaneal avulsion fracture, Lisfranc injuries, tarsal coalition, and os peroneum injury which are all in the differential diagnosis. In most cases, supportive care is adequate for treatment of isolated cuboid fracture. This includes pain management, swelling control, elastic bandage or walking boot, and partial weight-bearing until symptom resolves. In severe cases, 4–6 weeks of immobilization with casting is necessary. Open cuboid fracture and articular displacement are among absolute indications for urgent ORIF management [16]. In cases with extensive skin lacerations, severe comminution and displacement of fragments, spanning external fixation, allows restoration of lateral column length [17].

51.6.3 Midfoot Fractures-Lisfranc (ICD S92.3)

Description The Lisfranc joint consists of the five tarsometatarsal joints that connect the forefoot to the midfoot. The Lisfranc ligament attaches the base of the second metatarsal to the first cuneiform. Lisfranc complex injuries vary in severity from simple strains to one or more tarsometatarsal joint dislocation with or without fracture. A Lisfranc fracture dislocation disrupts one or more tarsometatarsal joints and is associated with disruption of at least one ligament that stabilizes the midfoot. The mechanism of injury is either direct

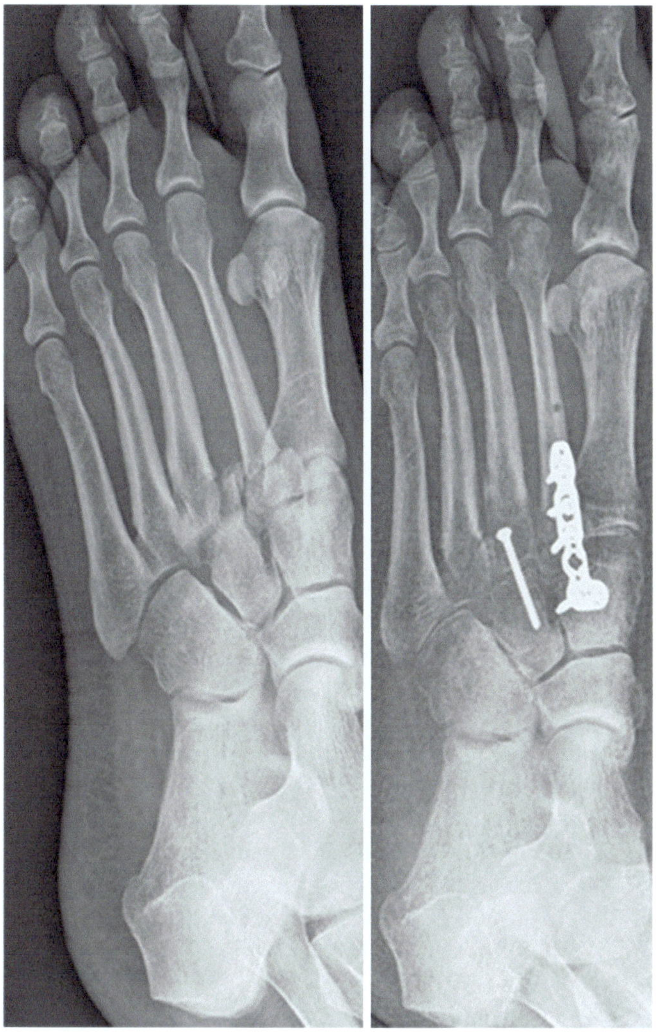

Fig. 51.5 Lisfranc's fracture/dislocation and oblique view after ORIF

blow or an indirect twisting force to the foot while in plantar flexion. AP, lateral, and oblique X-rays of the foot are indicated (Fig. 51.5), but these fractures could be missed requiring CT scan to identify disruption of the tarsometatarsal joint. If CT is not available, stress X-rays can be used.

Orthopedic care Dislocations often spontaneously reduce, but this injury usually requires open reduction with internal fixation (Fig. 51.5) or at times midfoot fusion. If surgery is not recommended, patients are immobilized with a cast and non-weight-bearing for ≥6 weeks.

51.6.4 Midfoot Fractures – Chopart (ICD S92.201)

Description Chopart fracture dislocation results from high-energy impact such as falling from heights, road collision producing a plantarflexion and inversion stress on the foot, and medial/superior dislocation along with fracture. The Chopart articulation was initially described in distal foot tumors, as a site for foot amputation. It corresponds to the center of the foot, allowing for articulation of the talocalcanealnavicular joint. The talonavicular or calcaneocuboid joints separate the hindfoot from the midfoot. Chopart fracture dislocation involves bony structures of navicular, cuboid, talus, and calcaneus [18].

Orthopedic care Given the complex nature of this injury, anatomical bone and joint reconstruction, addressing injured soft tissue, immediate joint reduction, and restoring bony alignment and avoiding complications including compartment syndrome, is the primary objective of surgical management [18, 19]. Fusion may become necessary if there is severe joint destruction but may result in impaired functional mobility of the foot [19].

51.6.5 Metatarsal Fracture (ICD 10 – S92.3)

A. *Proximal fifth metatarsal fracture* is a well-known fracture in high-performance athletes and dancers. There is an increased incidence of fifth metatarsal fracture observed in female dancers over 40, and a strong correlation was noted on this age group and low-energy trauma mechanism [20]. The so-called dancer's fracture [21] are long spiral fracture extending into the distal metaphyseal area.

   The blood supply characteristics and unique anatomy of proximal fifth metatarsal fracture makes a high risk of delayed union or nonunion of fractures occurring at the junction of the diaphyseal-metaphyseal. X-rays are diagnostic in detecting such fractures, but further imaging including CT scan may be indicated. Lawrence and Botte classified this fracture into three types/zones (Table 51.4,

Table 51.4 Lawrence and Botte classified proximal fifth metatarsal fracture

Lawrence and Botte classified proximal fifth metatarsal fracture (Fig. 51.6)
Avulsion fractures of tuberosity (Zone I)
Fractures at the metaphysis-diaphysis junction extending into the fourth-fifth intermetatarsal facet (Zone II)
Proximal diaphyseal fractures (Zone III)

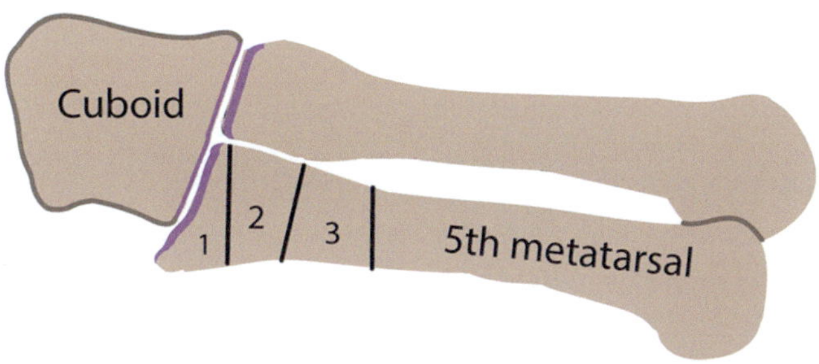

Fig. 51.6 Lawrence and Botte fracture zones. (Illustration by Yasmine Mostoufi)

Fig. 51.6), each corresponding to a prognosis and treatment strategy. For the fracture of Zone II and Zone III, percutaneous intramedullary screw or ORIF with a plate is the recommended management [20].

B. *Jones fracture:* This fracture is located at the metadiaphyseal junction, approximately 1.5–3 cm from the base of the fifth metatarsal and has a predominantly horizontal course. This fracture is prone to nonunion and almost always takes longer than 2 months to heal. X-rays/CT scan can detect Jones fracture. A non-weight-bearing cast for 6–8 weeks is needed to avoid displacement of the fracture. Intramedullary screw fixation is recommended for competitive athletes or in nonoperatively managed fractures when delayed union has occurred. ORIF may be needed in nonunion cases.

Most other metatarsal fractures can be treated conservatively with protective weight-bearing.

51.7 Toe Fracture

51.7.1 ICD 10

- Fracture of Lesser toes: S92.5
- Fracture Great toe: S392.4

51.7.2 Description

Toe fractures are common, comprising 3.6–8% of injuries to the lower extremity [22]. The big toe is the most commonly injured toe, representing the greatest proportion of all toe fractures [23] at 38–56%. Big toe fractures often involve distal phalanx resulting from direct crushing-type injury (dropping an object on the toe). Stabbing injury often involves interphalangeal joints and the resulting dislocations with or without intra-articular fracture [22]. If the toe is not fractured but only the ligaments around the toe are sprained due to hyperextension, this condition is called Turf toe, commonly seen in athletes playing on turf. Injuries to the hallux can result in long-term pain and disability if not properly diagnosed and treated.

51.7.3 Presentation

Fracture toe is associated with pain, swelling, and tenderness on examination and pain with gentle axial loading. X-rays are indicated if rotation deformity is noted or joint involvement is suspected. AP and oblique view of the hallux or individual toe can confirm fracture.

51.7.4 Management

Stable, nondisplaced toe fractures should be treated with buddy taping and a rigid-sole shoe to limit joint movement. In the case of displacement, reduction is necessary prior to buddy taping. Fracture dislocation, displaced intra-articular fracture, and unstable first toe fracture may result in circulatory compromise and significant soft tissue injury requiring surgical reduction and stabilization.

51.8 Ankle Dislocations

51.8.1 ICD: S93.0

51.8.1.1 Description

Ankle dislocations are a relatively common type of dislocation encountered in the emergency department. They exist in two forms: a true dislocation without fracture or a fracture-dislocation, occurring in the vast majority of cases [24].

A pure ligamentous dislocation has been reported to occur in multiple directions and by multiple mechanisms [25]. The most common injury pattern occurs when the ankle is maximally plantar-flexed with an axial load and forced inversion of the foot [26].

The more common ankle fracture-dislocation occurs via similar mechanics as non-dislocated ankle fractures. The most likely resulting fractures, bimalleolar and trimalleolar, often result from an abduction force and displacement of the talus which is how the ankle appears to be dislocated at the time of evaluation. Sometimes these dislocations will spontaneously reduce, leaving a malleolus fracture [27]. The ankle can be dislocated in five directions: anteriorly, posteriorly, laterally, medially, or superiorly. These descriptions describe the position of the talus when compared to the distal tibia.

51.8.1.2 Presentation

Ankle fracture dislocations most frequently occur in young males and are caused during road traffic accidents, sports trauma, or falls. These injuries typically result from high-energy trauma. On examination, it is important to note the direction of the foot relative to the ankle mortise, the presence/absence of the dorsalis pedis and posterior tibial pulses, capillary refill of the distal foot, other associated injuries of the foot, and localizing areas of tenderness and swelling. The sensory examination of the foot is mandatory. The examiner should also note the ability to flex and extend the toes. These important physical exam findings should be documented before and after the manipulation of the foot [26].

51.8.1.3 Orthopedic Care

The treatment goal is to obtain immediate anatomic alignment of the distal tibia and fibula, with a congruent tibiotalar joint. Ankle fracture dislocations are often treated operatively as they result in unstable bimalleolar and trimalleolar fractures. After a concentric reduction, these injuries can be approached in a similar way to unstable ankle fractures that did not result in a dislocation.

51.9 Toe Dislocation

51.9.1 ICD: S93.1

A toe dislocation occurs when the tissues, or ligaments, that hold the joint together are torn. Traumatic dislocations of lesser metatarsophalangeal joints and lesser interphalangeal joints are uncommon. Hyperextension with axial loading produces the injuries. Ipsilateral foot fractures or dislocations often occur and thus may compromise the outcome.

Thirty percent of dislocations of lesser metatarsophalangeal joints and virtually all lesser interphalangeal joints dislocations require open reduction; most often, the plantar plate prevents closed treatment of either group [27]. Postoperative course and rehabilitation should be in collaboration with surgeons. Splinting, taping, and an exercise program after recovery from surgery would likely be recommended which may include passive toe exercise, toe curl, towel scrunches, and marble pickups.

References

1. Beckenkamp PR, Lin C-WC, Chagpar S, Herbert RD, van der Ploeg HP, Moseley AM. Prognosis of physical function following ankle fracture: a systematic review with meta-analysis. J Orthop Sports Phys Ther. 2014;44(11):841–51.
2. Smeeing DPJ, Houwert RM, Briet JP, Kelder JC, Segers MJM, Verleisdonk EJMM, Leenen LPH, Hietbrink F. Weight-bearing and mobilization in the postoperative care of ankle fractures: a systematic review and meta-analysis of randomized controlled trials and cohort studies. PLoS One. 2015;10(2):e0118320.
3. Sirkin M, Sanders R, DiPasquale T, Herscovici D Jr. A staged protocol for soft tissue management in the treatment of complex pilon fractures. J Orthop Trauma. 2004;18(8 Suppl):S32–8. https://doi.org/10.1097/00005131-200409001-00005. PMID: 15472563.
4. Rüedi TP, Allgöwer M. The operative treatment of intra-articular fractures of the lower end of the tibia. Clin Orthop Relat Res. 1979;138:105–10.
5. Boraiah S, Kemp TJ, Erwteman A, Lucas PA, Asprinio DE. Outcome following open reduction and internal fixation of open pilon fractures. J Bone Joint Surg Am. 2010;92(2):346–52. https://doi.org/10.2106/JBJS.H.01678.
6. Buza JA, Leucht P. Fractures of the talus: current concepts and new developments. Foot Ankle Surg. 2018;24(4):282–90.
7. Irion V, Miller TL, Kaeding CC. The treatment and outcomes of medial malleolar stress fractures: a systematic review of the literature. Sports Health. 2014;6(6):527–30.
8. Orava S, Karpakka J, Taimela S, Hulkko A, Permi J, Kujala U. Stress fracture of the medial malleolus. J Bone Joint Surg Am. 1995;77(3):362–5.
9. Shelbourne KD, Fisher DA, Rettig AC, McCarroll JR. Stress fractures of the medial malleolus. Am J Sports Med. 1988;16(1):60–3.
10. Böstman O, Kyrö A. Delayed union of fibular fractures accompanying fractures of the tibial shaft. J Trauma. 1991;31(1):99–102.
11. McGonagle L, Ralte P, Kershaw S. Non-union of Weber B distal fibula fractures: a case series. Foot Ankle Surg. 2010;16(3):e63–7.
12. Petrisor BA, Ekrol I, Court-Brown C. The epidemiology of metatarsal fractures. Foot Ankle Int. 2006;27(3):172–4. https://doi.org/10.1177/107110070602700303.
13. Hordyk PJ, Fuerbringer BA, Roukis TS. Clinical management of acute, closed displaced intra-articular calcaneal fractures. Clin Podiatr Med Surg. 2019;36(2):163–71.
14. Davis D, Seaman TJ, Newton EJ. Calcaneus fractures. [Updated 2021 Aug 9]. In: StatPearls [Internet]. Treasure Island (FL): StatPearls Publishing; 2021.
15. Miller TT, Pavlov H, Gupta M, Schultz E, Greben C. Isolated injury of the cuboid bone. Emerg Radiol. 2002;9(5):272–7.
16. Borrelli J Jr, De S, Van Pelt M. Fracture of the cuboid. J Am Acad Orthop Surg. 2012;20(7):472–7.
17. Clements JR, Dijour F, Leong W. Surgical management navicular and cuboid fractures. Clin Podiatr Med Surg. 2018;35(2):145–59.
18. Klaue K. Treatment of chopart fracture-dislocations. Eur J Trauma Emerg Surg. 2010;36(3):191–5.
19. Swords MP, Schramski M, Switzer K, Nemec S. Chopart fractures and dislocations. Foot Ankle Clin. 2008;13(4):679–93, viii. https://doi.org/10.1016/j.fcl.2008.08.004. PMID: 19013402.
20. Schwagten K, Gill J, Thorisdottir V. Epidemiology of dancers fracture. Foot Ankle Surg. 2021;27(6):677–80. https://doi.org/10.1016/j.fas.2020.09.001. Epub 2020 Oct 21.
21. Cheung CN, Lui TH. Proximal fifth metatarsal fractures: anatomy, classification, treatment and complications. Arch Trauma Res. 2016;5(4):e33298. Published 2016 Jun 13. https://doi.org/10.5812/atr.33298.
22. Shibuya N, Davis ML, Jupiter DC. Epidemiology of foot and ankle fractures in the United States: an analysis of the National Trauma Data Bank (2007 to 2011). J Foot Ankle Surg. 2014;53(5):606–8.
23. York PJ, Wydra FB, Hunt KJ. Injuries to the great toe. Curr Rev Musculoskelet Med. 2017;10(1):104–12.
24. Wight L, Owen D, Goldbloom D, Knupp M. Pure ankle dislocation: a systematic review of the literature and estimation of incidence. Injury. 2017;48(10):2027–34.
25. Elsayed H, Thalava R, Afifi H, Khan M. Open ankle dislocation without associated malleolar fracture: review of the literature. Trauma Case Rep. 2017;8:20–3.
26. Agrawal AC, Raza HK, Haq RU. Closed posterior dislocation of the ankle without fracture. Indian J Orthop. 2008;42(3):360–2.
27. Brunet JA, Tubin S. Traumatic dislocations of the lesser toes. Foot Ankle Int. 1997;18:406–11.

52 Surgical Interventions in the Foot and Ankle

Seyed Behrooz Mostofi, Abdolrahman Fazli, Woo A. Kim, and S. Ali Mostoufi

52.1 Bony Trauma Surgery

Surgical procedures performed on the bone and joints are often related to injuries sustained in motor vehicle accidents, sports, or mechanical fall. Degenerative changes associated with pain and dysfunction may lead to surgical intervention as well. Surgical interventions in fracture require closed or open reduction of the broken bone and fixation of the fracture. Different methods are used to repair the fracture including Kirschner wires, screws, plates, and flexible or rigid intramedullary nails. Different plates including locking and anatomical plates are used. There are also different types of screws available with a variety of diameter, thread, and locking options.

52.1.1 Surgical Intervention: Ankle Fractures/Dislocations

Ankle fractures are common in all age groups, resulting from both high- and low-energy traumas [1]. The two most common age groups are physically active younger men and older women with frailty. Frail elderly patients are more likely to present following lower-energy trauma to the lower limb (i.e., mechanical fall). A common Danis-Weber classification (Table 52.1) describes ankle fracture by its location relative to the syndesmosis. Syndesmotic injury is linked with an unstable ankle joint injury.

Table 52.1 Danis-Weber classification of ankle fracture

Type of injury	Location of injury
Weber A	Below the syndesmosis
Weber B	At the level of syndesmosis
Weber C	Above the syndesmosis

52.1.1.1 Orthopedic Care

As opposed to Weber A stable fracture that could be managed nonoperatively, it is broadly accepted that Weber B and C injuries are likely to be unstable injuries and often require operative internal fixation (Fig. 52.1). Lateral malleolus is fixed with plate or nail and medial malleolus with partial threaded screws/plate; posterior malleolus is fixed with screws only or plate according to the size of the fragment. The ankle is immobilized in a temporary plaster cast for the first 2 weeks for comfort and then a range of motion exercises may start.

52.1.1.2 Rehabilitation

Weight-bearing is determined according to the bone quality and fixation achieved during surgery. In younger patients with good bone stock and fixation, partial weight-bearing can begin after 2 weeks. Others may need a period of 6 weeks of non-weight-bearing. Patients will require rehabilitation following a period of immobilization. The initial speed of recovery can be rapid, but often the healing process can take up to 2 years from initial injury [2]. Rehabilitation exercises are key to improving patients' quality of life and restoring the dynamic function of the ankle joint.

S. B. Mostofi (✉)
Consultant Orthopaedic Foot and Ankle surgeon, East Kent Hospitals University, NHS Foundation Trust, Canterbury, Kent, UK

Visiting Professor, Department of Orthopedics, Manipal Academy of Higher Education, Manipal, India

A. Fazli
Department of Orthopedic, Queen Elizabeth The Queen Mother Hospital, East Kent Hospitals University, NHS Foundation Trust, Margate, UK

W. A. Kim
Department Of Orthopedics, Kent Surrey and Sussex Deanery, NHS Foundation Trust, Kent, UK

S. A. Mostoufi
Department of Orthopedics and Rehabilitation, Tufts Orthopedics and Rehabilitation, Boston, MA, USA

New England Spine Care Associates & Boston Regenerative Medicine, Cambridge, MA, USA
e-mail: Ali.Mostoufi@Tufts.edu

© The Author(s), under exclusive license to Springer Nature Switzerland AG 2022

S. A. Mostoufi et al. (eds.), *Clinical Guide to Musculoskeletal Medicine*, https://doi.org/10.1007/978-3-030-92042-5_52

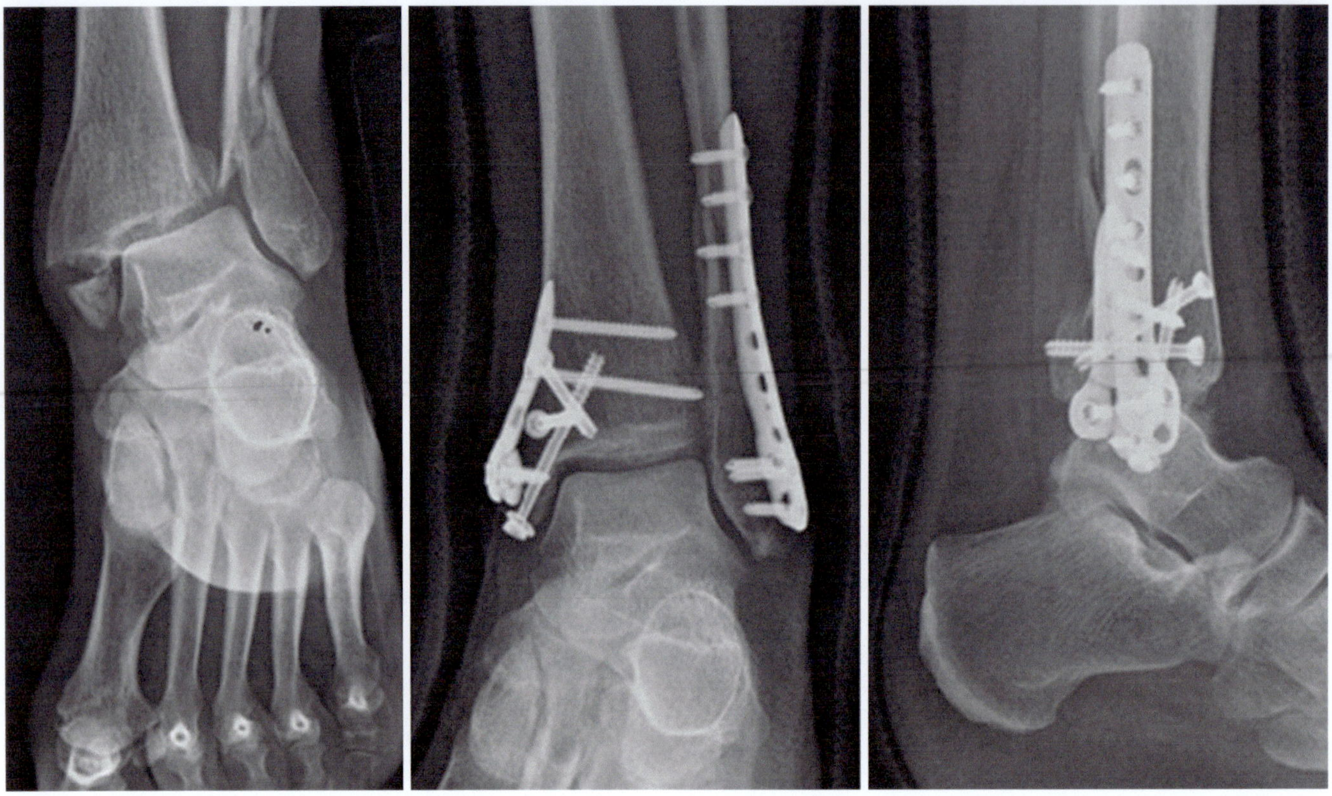

Fig. 52.1 AP/lateral view of the ankle, before and after open reduction and internal fixation (ORIF)

52.1.2 Surgical Intervention: Talar Fracture

The talus is a special bone, as its surface is more than 80% articular and its blood supply is from distal to proximal, so the risk of nonunion and avascular necrosis (AVN) is higher. Displaced fractures of the talus are usually openly reduced and fixed with screws or plates. Reduction must be absolutely anatomical to minimize the risk of already mentioned AVN and nonunion. Postoperative rehabilitation is not to bear weight for at least 6 weeks, but the range of motion can be started immediately after the operation.

52.1.3 Surgical Intervention: Pilon Fracture

Pilon fractures are high-energy injuries involving fractures of the articular surface of the distal tibial and occasional extension to the proximal diaphyseal bone. Rüedi and Allgöwer classified the fracture to three types [3] outlined in Table 52.2. Pilon fractures are usually comminuted and unstable, requiring reconstruction of the joint surface anatomically to prevent arthritis in the future. Staged management of high-energy complex tibial pilon fractures is recommended since studies report acute ORIF through traumatized tissue was associated with high complication rate [4]. Pilon fractures are fixed with anatomic, locking plates.

Table 52.2 Rüedi and Allgöwer classification of pilon fractures

Type 1	Nondisplaced intra-articular
Type 2	Displaced without comminution
Type 3	Displaced with comminution (most common)

Early rehabilitation is started in some cases, but weight-bearing is often delayed for at least 6 weeks. Soft tissue complications are more common in this type of injury because of poor soft tissue envelope in the distal third of the leg.

52.1.4 Surgical Intervention: Ankle Replacement

Total ankle replacement is a good treatment option for complete, end-stage ankle arthritis. It can restore joint function and make the patient mobile with little or no pain. There are, however, many contraindications to be considered. It is reserved for low-demand patients with severe arthritis. Longevity of the ankle replacements has improved significantly recently, achieving 75–90% at 10 years.

52.1.4.1 Operation

Anterior arthrotomy and capsulectomy are performed through an anterior, longitudinal incision between the extensor hallucis longus and anterior tibial tendons. After the tibial and the talar cut is performed, the trial components are inserted to check the alignment, stability, and joint motion, and the component position is confirmed by image intensification. The selected implants are then inserted, and the wound is closed and covered by a compressive dressing. In the case of malalignment, ligamentous instability, and concomitant osteoarthrosis of the distal joints, additional surgeries might be considered before prosthetic implantation. There are numerous implant designs [5], but the three-component mobile-bearing implants are most popular (Fig. 52.2). Relative contraindications include severe osteoporosis, poor bone quality, active infection, Charcot joint, and high BMI. Range of motion is allowed immediately after the operation; weight-bearing is dependent on the fixation method and the surgeon's preference but often restricted for 4–6 weeks.

52.1.4.2 Rehabilitation

After surgery, intensive outpatient physiotherapy begins which includes gait training, proprioception exercises, gradual increase to full weight-bearing, active and passive ankle ROM therapy, extension exercises, and therapy to strengthen the triceps surae muscle.

52.1.5 Surgical Intervention: Ankle Fusion

Ankle arthrodesis is a common treatment used for patients with end-stage ankle arthritis. Ankle arthrodesis has long been the traditional operative treatment for posttraumatic arthritis, rheumatoid arthritis, infection, neuromuscular conditions, and salvage of failed ankle arthroplasty. It remains the treatment of choice for patients in whom heavy and prolonged activity is anticipated. The surgical goal is to obtain bony union between the tibia and talus, adequate alignment, and improved ambulation function [6].

52.1.5.1 Operation

There are many variations in operative technique including different approaches (open or arthroscopic) and fixation methods (internal or external fixation) [7]. Fixation used ranges from screws to plate and nails (Fig. 52.3). Arthroscopic ankle arthrodesis is typically reserved for patients with little to no joint deformity. Open arthrodesis is best utilized for patients with moderate to severe deformity as this allows for better visualization for malalignment correction [6]. External fixation is typically indicated for complex patients with significant bone defects, limb length discrepancies, poor bone quality, and

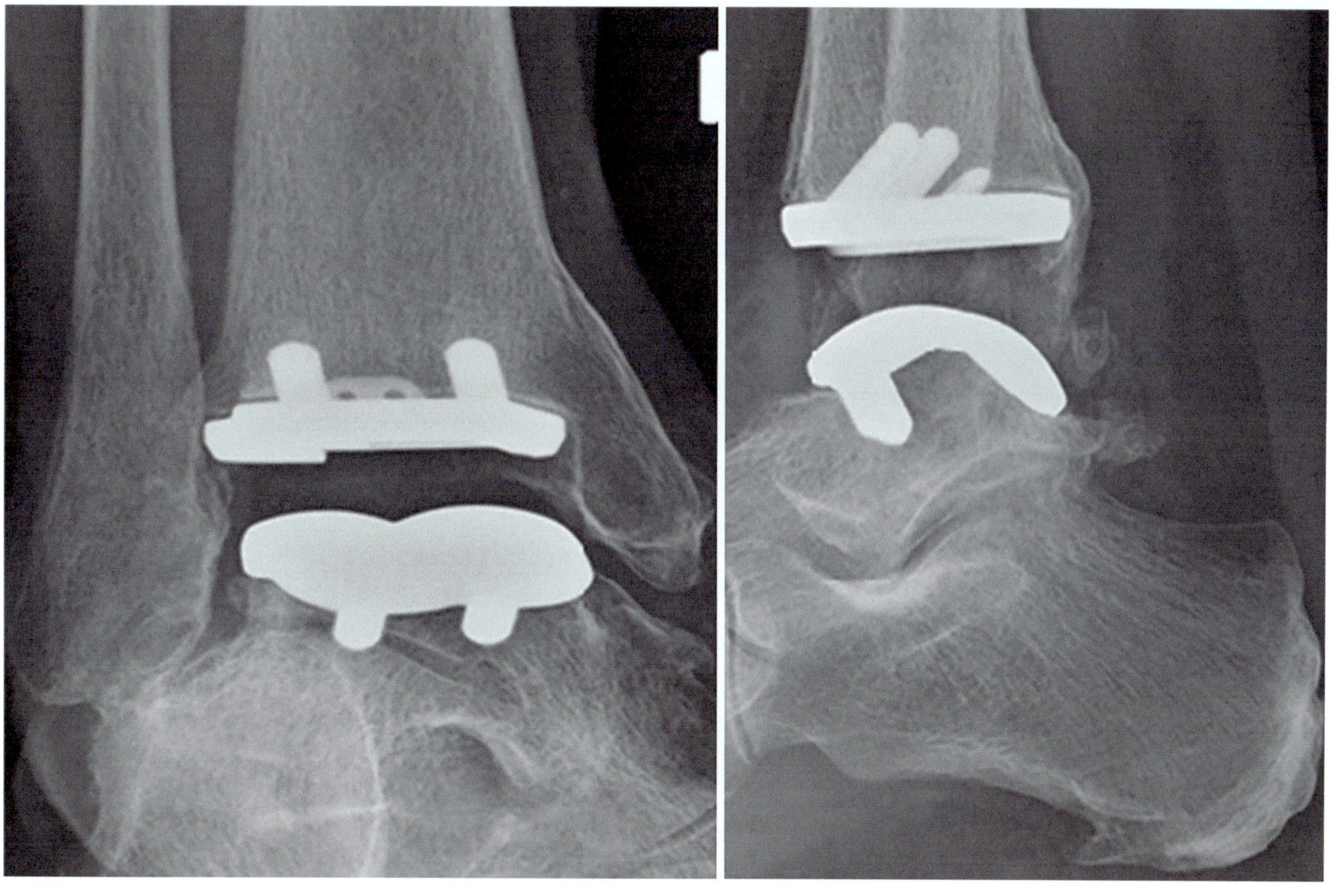

Fig. 52.2 Ankle joint replacement (AP and Lateral X-rays)

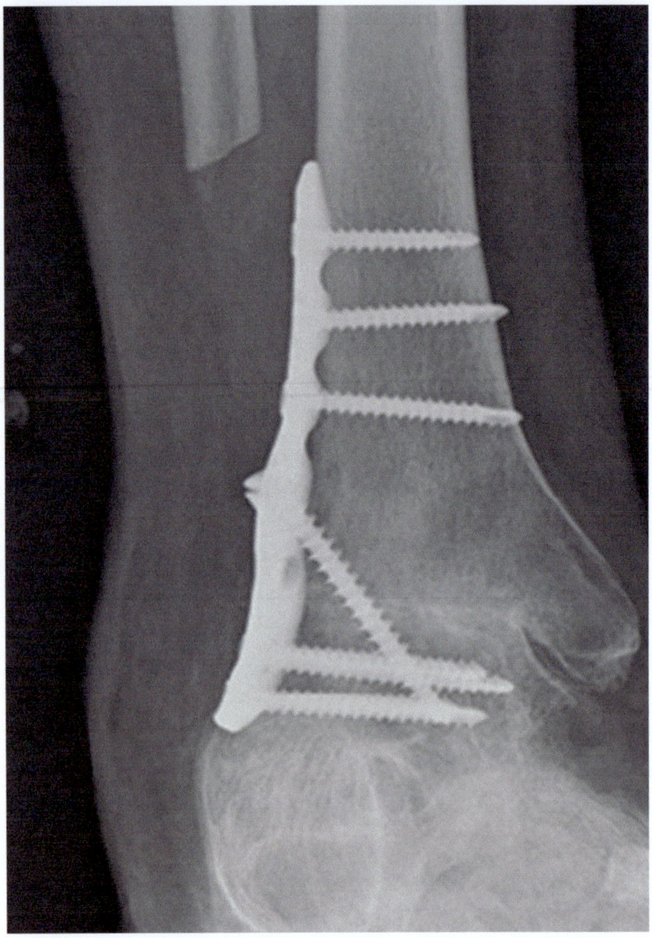

Fig. 52.3 AP view of ankle fusion with plate fixation

active or previous infection [6]. There is data to support a significantly higher rate of subsequent adjacent-joint arthrodesis in the open approach as compared to arthroscopic cohort [8].

52.1.5.2 Rehabilitation

The postoperative management depends on the method of fixation and preference of the surgeon.

52.1.6 Surgical Intervention: Foot Fractures/Dislocations

Fractures of the neck of the talus are the most common, accounting for 50% of all talus fractures due to forced dorsiflexion of the foot, which drives the weak trabecular bone of the neck of the talus against the stronger anterior tibial platform. In approximately 25% of such fractures, supination of the hindfoot leads to medial neck comminution and medial malleolus fracture. The most commonly used classification system for talar neck fractures was described by Hawkins (Table 52.3), and type 2 fracture is the most common.

Table 52.3 Hawkins classification of talar neck fracture

Hawkins type 1	Nondisplaced talar neck fracture
Hawkins type 2	Talar neck fracture + either subluxation or dislocation of the subtalar joint
Hawkins type 3	Talar neck fracture + dislocation of tibiotalar and subtalar joint
Hawkins type 4	Talar neck fracture + subluxation or dislocation of the *talonavicular joint*

When the talus is dislocated, an urgent reduction in the emergency room is indicated to reduce the risk of AVN. If reduction is unsuccessful, urgent surgical care is recommended. Displaced fractures of the talus are usually openly reduced and fixated with screws or plates. Ideal reduction is absolutely anatomical to reduce the risk of AVN and non-union. Postoperative rehabilitation is non-weight bearing for at least 6 weeks, but range of motion can be started immediately after the operation.

52.1.7 Surgical Intervention: Metatarsal Fractures

Most metatarsal fractures can be treated conservatively with protective weight-bearing. In a small number of cases, surgery is needed, and the fracture can be fixed with an intramedullary device or plate. Lisfranc's fracture dislocation must be mentioned as it represents dislocation of the tarsometatarsal joint and needs to be reduced anatomically and fixed accordingly (Fig. 52.4).

52.1.8 Surgical Intervention: Foot Fusion

Arthrodesis or fusion is the most common procedure done for arthritis or correction of deformities. It can involve one or more joints. Triple arthrodesis involves fusion of talonavicular, calcaneocuboid, and subtalar joints. A combination of screws and plates/staples are used to fix the joints. Below the knee, a cast is applied for at least 6 weeks. Non-weight-bearing is the standard for at least 6 weeks.

Fusion of the midfoot and forefoot follows the same principles as the hindfoot fusions. All of them are to relieve pain and correct deformity.

Fusion of the first metatarsal phalangeal joint (MTPJ) had been described as early as 1887 by Davies-Colley [9] and later by Clutton [10] in 1894 who concluded that stiffness of the first MTPJ, in an optimal position, would produce a long-standing and satisfactory result for patients with degenerative arthritis and hallux valgus (Fig. 52.5). The gold standard is still arthrodesis of the first MTPJ despite numerous options including partial or total replacement with metallic, ceramic, or silastic implants.

Resection arthroplasties of metatarsal head or proximal phalanges of metatarsophalangeal joints are sparingly used to correct deformities of the toes especially in a rheumatoid foot.

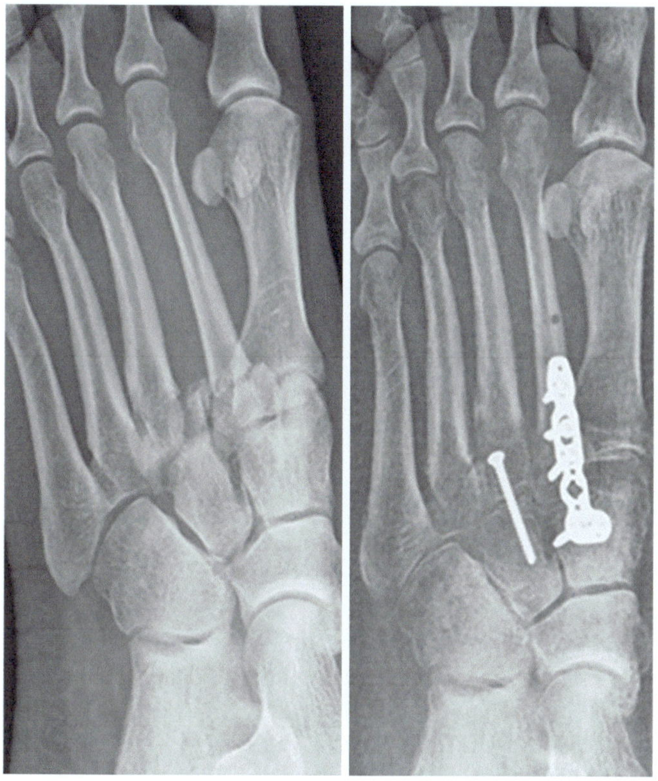

Fig. 52.4 Lisfranc's fracture/dislocation. Oblique view before and after ORIF

52.1.9 Surgical Intervention: Osteotomy

Corrective osteotomies are very common in the foot. Indications can be congenital as cerebral palsy deformities or acquired as pes planus. The most common osteotomies are calcaneal osteotomy to correct the hindfoot deformity. Lateral or medial column osteotomy to lengthen or shorten the column and correct the midfoot deformity.

Bunions or hallux valgus correction: Bunions are a common complaint, particularly among older female patients. They are characterized by progressive deformity at the metatarsophalangeal joint, resulting in a painful dorsomedial prominence. This may cause difficulties with shoe wear and contribute to falls in the elderly. Metatarsal osteotomies are needed to correct forefoot deformity (Fig. 52.6). More than 150 procedures have been described, and the most recommended is an open approach. More recently, a minimally invasive approach to bunion correction has gained popularity among some surgeons. Fixation of these osteotomies is done using screws and plates depending on the bone involved and the surgeon's preferences.

52.2 Soft Tissue Trauma Surgery

52.2.1 Acute Achilles Tendon Ruptures

Achilles tendon ruptures typically occur in two groups of patients. The first being high-performance athletes and is proposed to be secondary to a combination of underlying repetitive microtrauma and abnormally high loads placed through the tendon during eccentric loading. The second group of patients are middle-aged patients with a typical his-

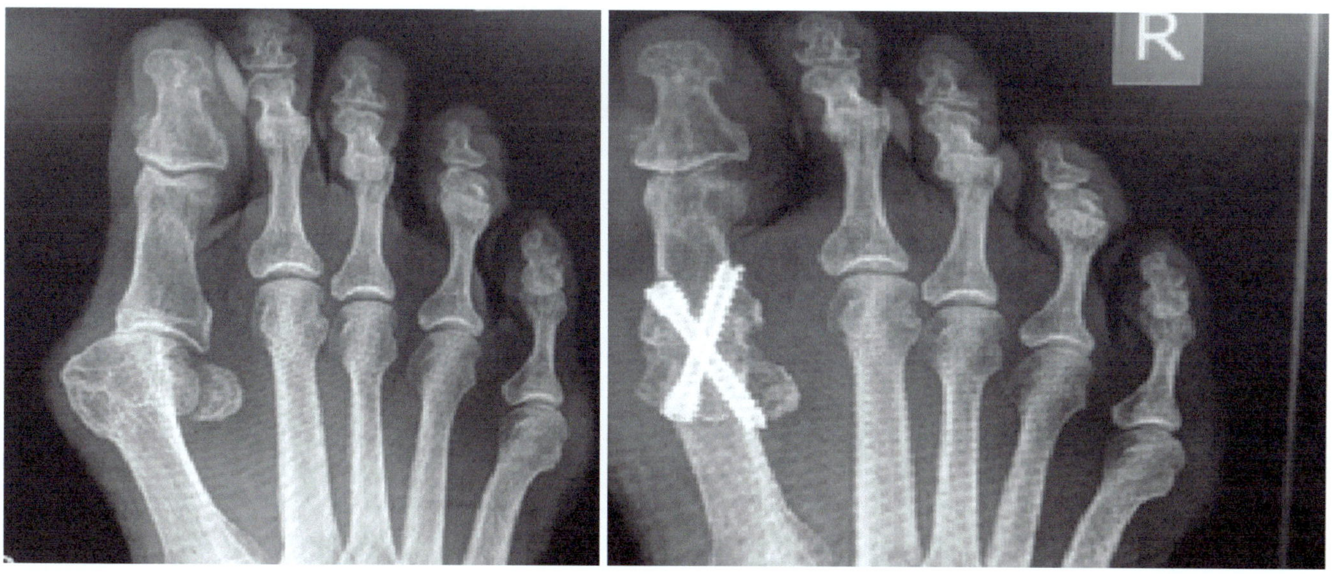

Fig. 52.5 Hallux valgus with arthritis of first MTPJ arthritis. Fusion of the first MTPJ with screws

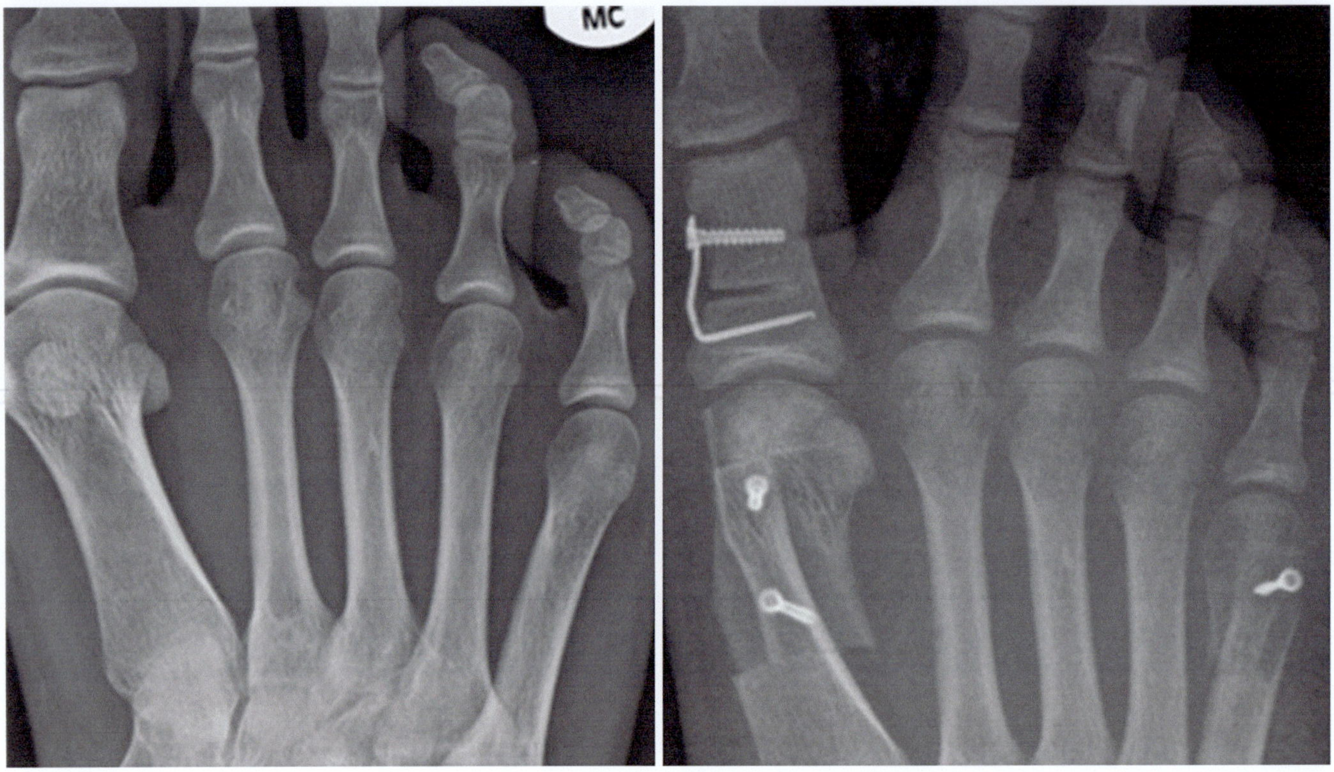

Fig. 52.6 AP view: hallux valgus deformity and bunionette deformity of the fifth ray before and after surgical correction

tory of occasional sports performance also known as the "weekend warrior." Unfortunately, the incidence of Achilles tendon ruptures has been rising. In 2005, Suchak et al. reported an incidence of 5.5–9.9 per 100,000 [11]. In 2017, Freedman et al. reported an incidence of 15 per 100,000 in women and 55 per 100,000 in men [12].

The exact mechanism of Achilles tendon ruptures is still an undergoing research as eccentric loading and microtrauma is only one aspect of the pathophysiology. Holmes et al. in 2007 proposed a metabolic component for Achilles tendon injury. They proposed a triad of hypertension, obesity, and diabetes to culminate in endothelial damage in the blood vessels, leading to tendon abnormalities. Additionally, they have reported an association with estrogen supplementation and Achilles tendon ruptures [13]. In support of the theory of an underlying metabolic component to Achilles tendon ruptures, it has been theorized that statins increase the risk of tendon rupture by impairing matrix metalloproteinase function [14]. Patient factors can also predispose the patient to tendon rupture. Inflammatory conditions such as rheumatoid arthritis, gout, and lupus also play a contributing role. Steroid medication and fluoroquinolone class of antibiotics have been associated with Achilles tendon rupture.

52.2.1.1 Orthopedic Care

A significant amount of literature has been published regarding the management of Achilles tendon ruptures. Initial management involves immobilizing the foot in a walking boot with wedges to place the foot in plantar flexion or placing the foot in an equine cast. A thorough discussion is then required to evaluate the patient for risk factors for tendon rupture and to establish the goals of treatment for that individual patient. Willets et al. reported equivalent functional outcomes with conservative and operative management [15]. The operative management provided better restoration of initial push-off strength; however, it subjects the patient to the risk of wound complications in the area.

52.2.1.2 Rehabilitation

Conservative treatment would entail early range of movement and controlled loading as this has been reported to have as good outcomes in comparison to operative management with protected weight-bearing in a walking boot with 20-degree heel inserts for 2 weeks which was subsequently advanced gradually to full weight-bearing at 4 weeks. The total duration of time in the boot was 8 weeks for patients [15]. Surgical repair of the Achilles tendon is a successful procedure but unfortunately risks the devastating complication of wound breakdown over the surgical incision site. Numerous methods for performing the repair have been described with new methods being introduced to promote minimally invasive repair techniques.

References

1. Beckenkamp PR, Lin C-WC, Chagpar S, Herbert RD, van der Ploeg HP, Moseley AM. Prognosis of physical function following ankle fracture: a systematic review with meta-analysis. J Orthop Sports Phys Ther. 2014;44(11):841–51.
2. Smeeing DPJ, Houwert RM, Briet JP, Kelder JC, Segers MJM, Verleisdonk EJMM, Leenen LPH, Hietbrink F. Weight-bearing and mobilization in the postoperative care of ankle fractures: a systematic review and meta-analysis of randomized controlled trials and cohort studies. PLoS One. 2015;10(2):e0118320.
3. Saad BN, Yingling JM, Liporace FA, Yoon RS. Pilon fractures: challenges and solutions. Orthop Res Rev. 2019;11:149–57. https://doi.org/10.2147/ORR.S170956.
4. Boraiah S, Kemp TJ, Erwteman A, Lucas PA, Asprinio DE. Outcome following open reduction and internal fixation of open pilon fractures. J Bone Joint Surg. 92(2):346–52. https://doi.org/10.2106/JBJS.H.01678.
5. Gougoulias NE, Khanna A, Maffulli N. History and evolution in total ankle arthroplasty. Br Med Bull. 2009;89(1):111–51. https://doi.org/10.1093/bmb/ldn039.
6. Yasui Y, Hannon CP, Seow D, Kennedy JG. Ankle arthrodesis: a systematic approach and review of the literature. World J Orthop. 2016;7(11):700–8. https://doi.org/10.5312/wjo.v7.i11.700.
7. Stone JW. Arthroscopic ankle arthrodesis. Foot Ankle Clin. 2006;11:361–8.
8. Morrey BF, Wiedeman GP. Complications and long-term results of ankle arthrodesis following trauma. J Bone Joint Surg Am. 1980;62:777–84.
9. Kelikian H. Arthrodesing operations in hallux valgus, allied deformities of the forefoot and metatarsalgia. Philadelphia: W.B. Saunders; 1965. p. 236–48.
10. Clutton in 1894 [2] H.H. Clutton treatment of hallux valgus. St Thomas Hosp Rep, 1894;22:1–12.
11. Suchak A, Bostick G, Reid D, Blitz S, Jomha N. The incidence of Achilles tendon ruptures in Edmonton, Canada. Foot Ankle Int. 2005;26(11):932–6.
12. Freedman B, Salka N, Morris T, Bhatt P, Pardes A, Gordon J, et al. Temporal healing of Achilles tendons after injury in rodents depends on surgical treatment and activity. J Am Acad Orthop Surg. 2017;25(9):635–47.
13. Holmes G, Lin J. Etiologic factors associated with symptomatic Achilles tendinopathy. Foot Ankle Int. 2006;27(11):952–9.
14. Pullar RC, Gadarla MR, Karas RH, Alsheikh-Ali AA, Thompson PD. Tendon rupture associated with simvastatin/exetimbie therapy. Am J Cardiol. 2007;100(1):152–3. https://doi.org/10.1016/j.amjcard.2007.02.068.
15. Willits K, Amendola A, Bryant D, Mohtadi N, Giffin J, Fowler P, et al. Operative versus nonoperative treatment of acute Achilles tendon ruptures. J Bone Joint Surg. 2010;92(17):2767–75.

Part X

MSK Topics

Section Editor

S. Ali Mostoufi

53 Osteoarthritis

William A. Berrigan, Oluseun Olufade, Kenneth Mautner, Jason L. Zaremski, Julio A. Martinez-Silvestrini, S. Ali Mostoufi, Ariana Mostoufi, Kristian von Rickenbach, Adam Tenforde, Haylee Borgstrom, Jennifer Soo Hoo, Gerard D'Onofrio, Figueroa Gisela, and Kyungje Sung

53.1 Shoulder OA

William A. Berrigan, Oluseun Olufade and Kenneth Mautner

53.1.1 ICD 10 Codes

Glenohumeral – M19.019

53.1.2 Synonyms

- Secondary osteoarthritis – shoulder (M19.219)
- Traumatic arthropathy – shoulder (M12.519)

53.1.3 Description

This section concentrates more on glenohumeral arthropathy, but the AC joint is part of the shoulder joint complex as well.

Glenohumeral osteoarthritis is defined as a progressive loss of articular cartilage resulting in bony erosion, increased pain, and decreased function. It is the third most commonly affected large joint behind the knee and the hip [1]. There are many primary risk factors for developing arthritis including age, genetics, sex, Caucasian race, and obesity. Secondary causes include avascular necrosis, infectious or crystalline arthropathy, prior trauma, and prior surgery [2]. The exact rate of progression of the disease in the shoulder is unknown but, in the knee, has been shown to have an annual progression rate of 2.8% [3].

AC joint The acromioclavicular joint although separate from the glenohumeral joint is considered part of the shoulder complex. It is prone to osteoarthritis and presents with anterior shoulder pain. AC arthropathy is often limiting factor with abducting the arm, using the arm overhead and moving the arm across the body to the opposite side. Clinically it is easy to diagnose given the location of the AC joint. NSAIDS, rehabilitation, localized injections, and rarely surgical intervention can treat pain associated with this disorder.

W. A. Berrigan
Clinical Sports Medicine Fellow, Department of Physical Medicine and Rehabilitation, Emory University School of Medicine, Atlanta, GA, USA

O. Olufade · K. Mautner
Department of Orthopaedics and Physical Medicine and Rehabilitation, Emory University School of Medicine, Atlanta, GA, USA

J. L. Zaremski
Divisions of PM&R, Sports Medicine, & Research, Department of Orthopaedics and Rehabilitation, UF Health, University of Florida, Gainesville, FL, USA

J. A. Martinez-Silvestrini
University of Massachusetts Medical School – Baystate, Longmeadow, MA, USA

S. A. Mostoufi (✉)
Department of Orthopedics and Rehabilitation, Tufts University School of Medicine, Boston, MA, USA

New England Spine Care Associates & Boston Regenerative Medicine, Cambridge, MA, USA
e-mail: ali.mostoufi@tufts.edu

A. Mostoufi
Concord Carlisle High school, Concord, MA, USA

K. von Rickenbach · A. Tenforde · H. Borgstrom
Department of Physical Medicine & Rehabilitation, Spaulding Rehabilitation Hospital, Harvard Medical School, Charlestown, MA, USA

J. S. Hoo · G. D'Onofrio · F. Gisela
Department of Rehabilitation Medicine, New York Presbyterian, New York, NY, USA

K. Sung
Department of Orthopedics and Rehabilitation Medicine, Tufts University School of Medicine, Boston, MA, USA

© The Author(s), under exclusive license to Springer Nature Switzerland AG 2022

S. A. Mostoufi et al. (eds.), *Clinical Guide to Musculoskeletal Medicine*, https://doi.org/10.1007/978-3-030-92042-5_53

53.1.4 Clinical Presentation

Symptomatic osteoarthritis is described as a progressive increase in pain that is localized posteriorly and deep within the joint. The pain is typically associated with pain at night, stiffness, reduced range of motion, and, as the disease progresses, causes functional limitations [4].

53.1.5 Physical Examination

Physical examination can reveal shoulder joint line tenderness +/− crepitus with a loss of range of motion, specifically in abduction and external rotation. It is important to exclude and consider other causes of shoulder pain that can cause a loss of active and passive range of motion such as calcific tendinopathy and idiopathic adhesive capsulitis.

53.1.6 Diagnostic Workup

Radiographs X-rays are the primary means of diagnosing osteoarthritis and can show joint space narrowing, osteophytes, subchondral sclerosis, and cystic changes (Fig. 53.1). The axillary and AP views with the arm at 45° of extension are best to identify narrowing. Advanced imaging beyond radiographs is often unnecessary but can provide information on concomitant labrum or rotator cuff pathology and be useful in preoperative planning [2].

53.1.7 Treatment

A trial of nonoperative management should be done as first-line treatment. Nonoperative strategies include activity modification, physical therapy to promote strength and flexibility, medications, corticosteroid injections, viscosupplementation, orthobiologics, and peripheral nerve stimulation.

53.1.7.1 Medical Management

Acetaminophen has been demonstrated to be both safe and effective at doses up to 3–4 g daily. NSAIDs can be used, but patients should be educated on side effects. Topical capsaicin has also been shown to be effective compared to placebo and offers an alternative and safe option for patients [5].

53.1.7.2 Rehabilitation

Rehabilitation programs are based on the individual's capabilities. Programs should include joint mobilization techniques, both passive and active, with gradual progression of mobility. Structure should include a physiotherapist-guided stretching program for the joint capsule, deltoids, rotators, trapezius, latissimus dorsi, biceps brachii, and neck musculature. Emphasis should then be placed on a gradual progression of strengthening exercises focused on shoulder and scapular stabilization. Exercises are progressed from isometric and isotonic movements to patient-tolerant weight exercises, eccentric contraction exercises, and open and closed kinetic chain techniques. A proper home exercise program with a combination of techniques should be taught for long-term maintenance [6].

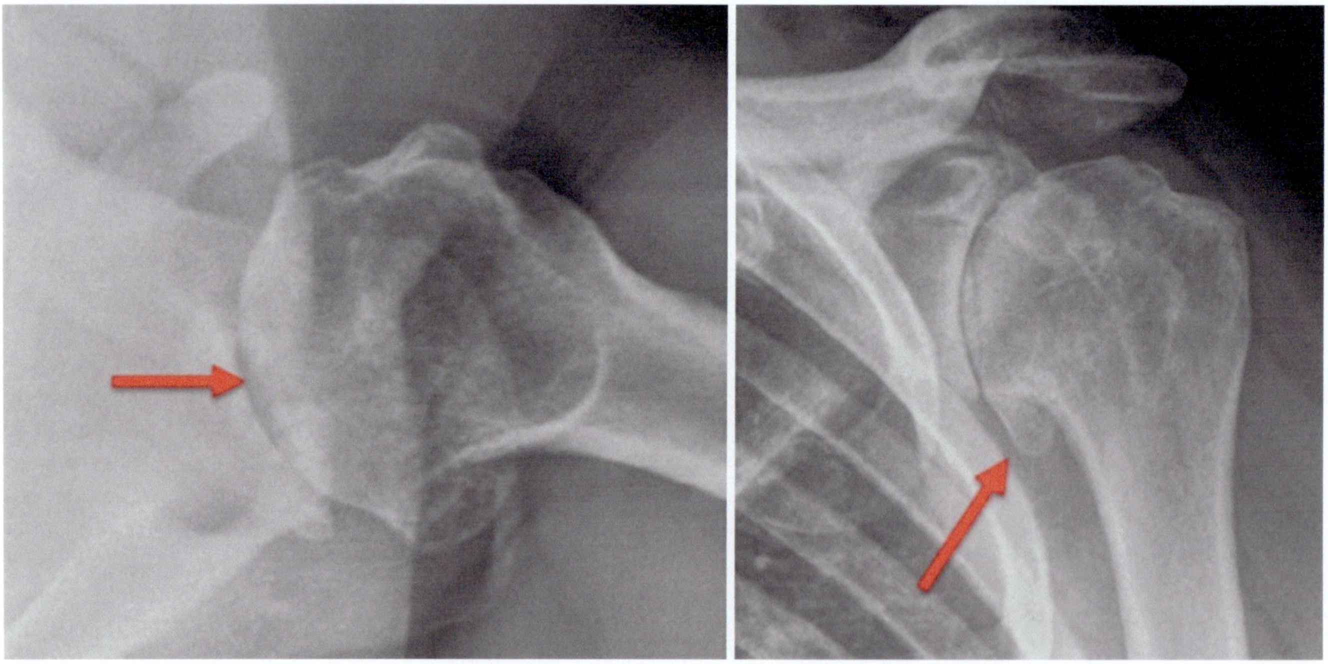

Fig. 53.1 Glenohumeral arthritis with loss of joint space (arrow) and inferior osteophyte (arrow)

53.1.7.3 Procedures

Corticosteroid Injections

The use of intra-articular corticosteroid injection is based on the effects of the corticosteroid on the synovium and surrounding tissue. Although a common practice, there is a lack of high-quality evidence for the indication of corticosteroid into the glenohumeral joint. One study showed an average pain relief of 4 months [7], while another demonstrated an improvement in outcomes at 3 months that was similar to that of hyaluronic acid [8]. Optimal dosage and volume have not been determined [9], and higher doses and duration are known to have detrimental effects on cartilage [10]. Due to its toxicity to joint cartilage, use of local anesthetics to dilute the steroid is discouraged, and saline should be used. US and X-ray can be used for needle placement (Fig. 53.2).

Viscosupplementation

Hyaluronic acid has proven efficacy in randomized clinical trials demonstrating both short-term and sustained pain relief for 6 months [8, 11].

Orthobiologics

Clinical trials on the use of platelet-rich plasma (PRP) and other cellular therapies for the glenohumeral joint are scarce and limited to case studies. Although there is high-level evidence for osteoarthritis of the knee, further studies are warranted to show efficacy for the glenohumeral joint [11, 12].

Peripheral Nerve Stimulation

Peripheral nerve stimulation of the axillary nerve/suprascapular nerve has shown promise for refractory shoulder pain in those that are not ideal candidates for surgery. Limited studies demonstrate high response rates with significant pain relief and decreased use of opiate medication. Higher-level studies are needed to further support its use in GH osteoarthritis [13–15].

53.1.7.4 Surgery

If nonoperative measures fail, many surgical options are available. For younger patients, joint preservation surgery is recommended and may include arthroscopic debridement, capsular release, and corrective osteotomy. Shoulder arthroplasty is recommended for severe osteoarthritis not responsive to conservative management, end-stage rotator cuff arthropathy, osteonecrosis, and previously failed joint preservation surgery. Postoperative recovery time usually includes resumption of normal activities of daily living by 6 weeks with return to athletic activities within 4 months [4]. For more detail on surgical interventions, please refer to Chap. 24.

53.2 Elbow OA

Jason L. Zaremski and Julio A. Martínez-Silvestrini

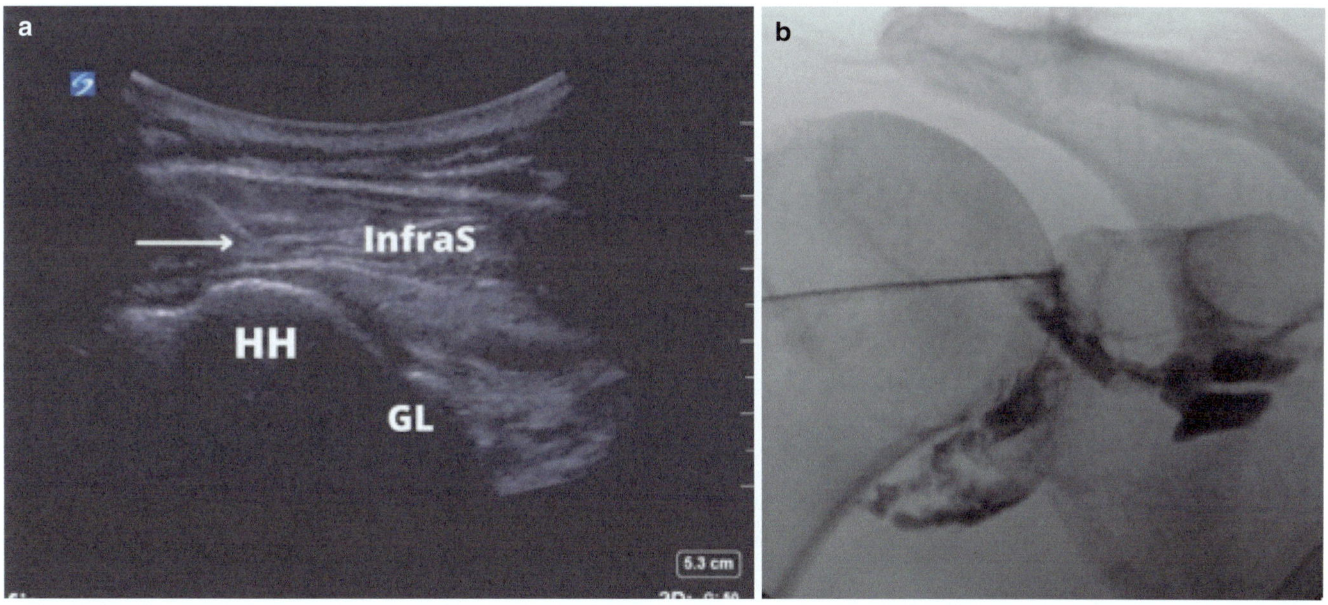

Fig. 53.2 Glenohumeral injection. (**a**) US-guided injection, a 5–2 MHz curvilinear probe is placed over the posterior aspect of the glenohumeral joint. Arrow indicates the needle in plane with the transducer. Humeral head (HH); posterior aspect of the glenoid (GL); Infraspinatus (InfraS). (**b**) Fluoroscope-guided needle placement and contrast enhancement are seen. (Fluoroscopic picture curtesy of S. Ali Mostoufi, MD Boston Regenerative Medicine)

53.2.1 ICD 10 Codes

M19.021, M19.022

53.2.2 Synonyms

Humeroulnar osteoarthritis

53.2.3 Definition

Osteoarthritis (OA) of the elbow may be primary (which is rare, as less than 2% of patients with elbow OA have primary elbow OA) or more commonly post-traumatic [16]. Risks for OA of the elbow are not only multifactorial (such as age, prior injury, overhead throwers, manual laborers) but also include genetic components [17]. Post-traumatic OA is more common in young males [18]. The average age of presentation is approximately 50 with a range of 20–70 years of age [19–21]. Due to the complexity of the elbow anatomy, one or multiple of the elbow joints may be involved.

53.2.3.1 Anatomy

The elbow joint is composed of three bones (humerus, radius, and ulna) and three joints (humeroulnar, proximal radioulna, and radiocapitellar joint). The humeral trochlea articulates with the ulnar olecranon, while the radius head articulates with both the proximal ulna (Fig. 53.3) and the humeral capitellum. Any or all these joints may be involved by degenerative joint changes.

53.2.4 Clinical Presentation

OA of the elbow typically presents with stiffness, decreased functionality (such as limited ROM), and pain. Occasionally, swelling and/or effusion may present as well. Patients will report that they have challenges performing everyday activities such as housekeeping [16]. There is also an association in the literature between the development of primary elbow OA and manual laborers that clinicians should be aware of when obtaining a vocational history [4]. Furthermore, clinicians should be aware of wheelchair ambulators, who have an increased risk of developing elbow OA due to the extensive loads on the elbow while maneuvering the wheelchair [19].

53.2.5 Physical Examination

A typical full physical examination of the elbow including inspection, palpation, active and passive range of motion, strength testing, neurovascular testing, and special tests should be performed. It is important to inquire prior to a physical examination if the patient has a history of elbow injury that may include bony injury (such as a fracture or osteochon-

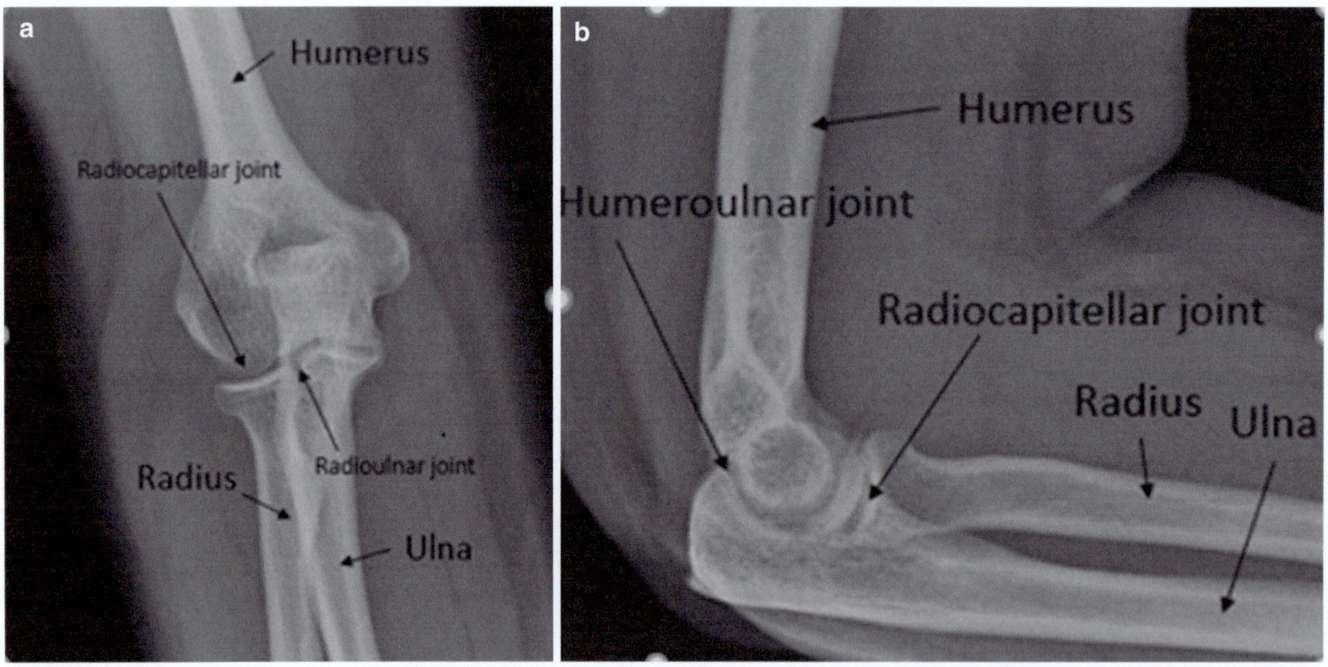

Fig. 53.3 (**a**) Anteroposterior X-ray view of the right elbow. The humerus, radius, ulna, radiocapitellar, and proximal radioulnar joints are also visible in this view. Osteoarthritis may affect one or more of the elbow joints. (**b**) Lateral X-ray view of the right elbow. The radiocapitellar and humeroulnar view are visible in this view

dral defects), prior instability (such as dislocation), and/or any surgical interventions. While inspecting the elbow, effusion may be observed. Fluid collections are usually identified at the lateral aspect, proximal or distal to the lateral epicondyle. Posterior elbow fluid collection may not be related to OA, but olecranon bursitis, which will be discussed in another chapter. Large joint effusions, redness, and increased temperature are uncommon in elbow OA. These findings may be a sign of elbow joint infection or gouty arthritis. Palpatory examination may confirm the presence of effusion, and patients may have tenderness at the radiocapitellar joint if that joint is the arthritic joint. The proximal radio-ulnar joint and humeroulnar joint are not easily palpated. In cases of severe humeroulnar joint, loose bodies at the posterior elbow may be palpated. In particular, it is important to pay attention to ROM since limited ROM will limit functionality. An early sign of elbow OA includes elbow contracture and loss of extension. Thus, clinicians should remember what normal elbow ROM is. For activities of daily living (ADLs), functional elbow active ROM is considered to be an angle of motion of 100° (30° of extension to 130° of flexion) and a 100° angle of forearm rotation (50° of pronation to 50° of supination) [16, 22]. Further, if there are limitations of ROM, it should be compared to contralateral side.

53.2.6 Diagnostic Workup

After a thorough history and physical examination has been completed, typically radiographs (Image 3) of the elbow are obtained to assess for potential extent of OA, if there are limitations of ROM on physical examination. Anterior-posterior and lateral images are typically sufficient for initial radiographic imaging [8]. If there is concern of loose bodies, in particular in the posterior compartments as well as the proximal radioulnar joints, advanced imaging (with computed tomography or magnetic resonance imaging arthrography) may be required [19, 23]. If there are any concerns of infection or gouty arthropathy, or if an effusion is present, one should consider a synovial fluid aspiration and analysis that includes cell count with differential, culture, and crystal analysis. While nonspecific, one may also consider obtaining C-reactive protein and erythrocyte sedimentation rate (CRP and ESR, respectively) as well as a chemical blood count with differential for further workup.

53.2.7 Treatments

53.2.7.1 Medical Treatment

Conservative treatment typically begins with relative rest, medications, and activity modifications. Nonsteroidal anti-inflammatory medication (NSAIDs) can be considered depending on preexisting medical conditions. Multiple NSAIDs are available, and the patient preference, previous experience, potential of adverse effects, and cost should be considered on the selection of these agents. If not contraindicated once a day, NSAIDs may be recommended to improve medication compliance. If the patient considers one of the NSAIDs ineffective, this not necessarily means all NSAIDs will be ineffective. It is known that individual response to equipotent NSAIDs doses is variable, for which changing an NSAID to a different agent should be considered. Adverse effects of NSAIDs include hypertension, gastrointestinal, renal, or hepatic toxicity. These agents are also usually contraindicated in patients with significant cardiovascular disease. Topical NSAIDs, for which in some patients in which oral NSAIDs are contraindicated, may be an alternative [24]. Topical NSAIDS have shown improvement in symptoms, pain, and ROM, yet their efficacy has short duration. Most adverse effects are local reactions, such as burning or redness. The systemic reactions observed with topical NSAIDs are typically minimal [24].

Acetaminophen (APAP) may be an alternative for patients in which NSAID use is contraindicated. The mechanism of action of APAP is poorly understood, most likely acting at the central nervous system.

Glucosamine and chondroitin have been studied predominantly in patients with OA in large weight-bearing joints and the knee and hip [25–27]. They are natural compounds found in the cartilage, and food supplements have been used in the management of OA with mixed results. They have a relatively safe profile, and no major interactions have been observed with these agents. Glucosamine could potentially alter glucose regulation, while chondroitin may have potential anticoagulant effects. These agents may need to be used with cautions in patients with poorly controlled diabetes mellitus, using anticoagulants or in patients with bleeding disorders [28].

53.2.7.2 Rehabilitation

The goals of rehabilitation are to decrease symptoms as pain and inflammation, maintain, and/or improve range of motion, strength, and function. To decrease pain and inflammation, modalities such as ice packs, ice massage, or cold compression pumps may be employed. Range of motion and stretching exercises, including pronation and supination of the elbow, are important to prevent elbow capsulitis or a "stiff elbow." Strengthening and functional exercises should also be considered according to symptoms tolerance. In patients with moderate to severe OA disease and resultant dysfunction, a supervised formal physical therapy (PT) may not be of great utility for patients and potentially exacerbate symptoms further as loose bodies, and osteophyte formation will result in loss of ROM, and PT will not improve ROM in this instance.

53.2.7.3 Procedures

Intra-articular corticosteroid injections may provide temporary pain relief and functional improvement. They are typically recommended in patients that have tried and failed conservative care as medications and PT or unable to participate in PT, due to uncontrolled pain. There is limited data that viscosupplementation has not been shown to be effective for elbow OA pain reduction [14]. Using local anesthetic as part of the intra-articular injectate adds diagnostic value and can differentiate the intra-articular source of pain from the referred pain [29]. There is growing interest in treating osteoarthritis with orthobiologics (including platelet-rich plasma (PRP), bone marrow aspirate concentrate (BMAC), dehydrated human amnion/chorion membrane allograft, and adipose-derived mesenchymal stem cells), but further research in safety and efficacy is still needed.

53.2.7.4 Surgery

If conservative measures such as relative rest, oral and topical medication, and injections fail, then referral to an elbow arthroplasty specialist would be indicated (see surgical intervention in the elbow).

53.3 Wrist and Hand OA

S. Ali Mostoufi and Ariana Mostoufi

53.3.1 ICD 10 Codes

- M19.039: Wrist OA – primary
- M19.139: Wrist OA – post trauma
- M19.239: Wrist OA – secondary

53.3.2 Synonyms

Carpometacarpal OA, Metacarpophalangeal OA, Interphalangeal OA, Osteoarthritis of the wrist, Wrist arthropathy

53.3.3 Description

53.3.3.1 Wrist OA

In humans, the wrist has a repetitive role in day-to-day activities, and as a result, it is predisposed to trauma and wear and tear, leading to osteoarthritis. The frequency of osteoarthritis at the wrist is approximately 13.6% and can result in dysfunction at home, at work, and during sports [30]. Most osteoarthritis of the wrist is age-related and develops in elderly population, although trauma particularly in younger adults can result in early OA development [31]. Trauma to the wrist injures the ligaments, fractures the bones, and increases the risk of OA over time [32]. Less common causes of wrist osteoarthritis include infection, steroid arthropathy, myelodysplastic disease, leukemic disorder, and crystal-induced arthritis [30].

53.3.3.2 Hand OA

Hand OA includes the first carpometacarpal joint (trapeziometacarpal), metacarpophalangeal joints, and distal and proximal interphalangeal joints. Hand osteoarthritis (OA) is a prevalent disease that can lead to substantial pain and physical disability. The Framingham study demonstrated that 27% of adults aged 26 and over have hand OA [33]. Distal interphalangeal joints demonstrate the highest osteoarthritis prevalence, while the proximal interphalangeal joint shows the lowest problems. In population diagnosed with hand OA, distal interphalangeal joints have 35% prevalence, third PIP has 18% prevalence, and first CMC has 21% prevalence [34]. Females have slightly higher problems than males [33]. Gender-specific hand dominance analysis demonstrates OA of second DIP and third PIP OA, presenting dominant hand [34].

53.3.4 Presentation

Wrist Pain is the primary complaint of a patient with wrist osteoarthritis, which could be exacerbated by the use of the wrist and improved with rest. Morning stiffness, swelling, and reduced range of motion can be associated with pain. Redness and warmth of the joints are often the presenting symptoms.

Hand Pain, swelling, morning stiffness, limited range of motion, difficulty with grip, and finger deformity are among the initial presenting symptoms. Osteoarthritis of the DIP joint is associated with joint enlargement, and nodular finding on examination is known as the "Heberden's node." Similar nodular finding of the DIPs is known as Bouchard's nodes [35]. Patients may have both Heberden's and Bouchard's nodes without any pain or swelling.

First CMC The trapeziometacarpal articulation has a saddle shape and is located at the base of the thumb. It is known as the basal joint and, among hand OA, requires a distinct recognition given the critical use of the thumb in almost all daily activities requiring the use of the hand. It is universally accepted that trauma age is a risk factor for hand OA, but other factors including obesity and manual occupation have been debated in the literature as risk factors (Fig. 53.6b) [33].

53.3.5 Physical Examination

53.3.5.1 Inspection

Wrist Swelling, deformity, redness, and any skin changes could be noted to help with differential diagnosis. In osteoarthritis, diffuse swelling in a circumferential pattern around the wrist and fingers is noted. Any deformity including dorsal subluxation of the ulnar head should be identified on inspection.

Fingers In examination of the fingers, ulnar or radial deviation of the digits and findings of nodules should be documented.

53.3.5.2 Palpation

Wrist For the examination of the wrist of the patient hold/support the wrist with both hands, place the wrist in slight flexion, and palpate the dorsal wrist with his/her thumbs. Instability of the joint could be tested in this position. During palpation, examine the radial styloid, ulnar styloid, distal radial ulnar joint, the hook of the hamate, and the anatomical location of the Guyon tunnel. Palpating just distal to the Lister tubercle is important to evaluate scaphoid.

Fingers Examination should be complete for Bouchard's nodes at the distal interphalangeal joints and Heberden's nodes in the proximal interphalangeal joints. These are nodular and hard and may feel like a bony bump (Fig. 53.4).

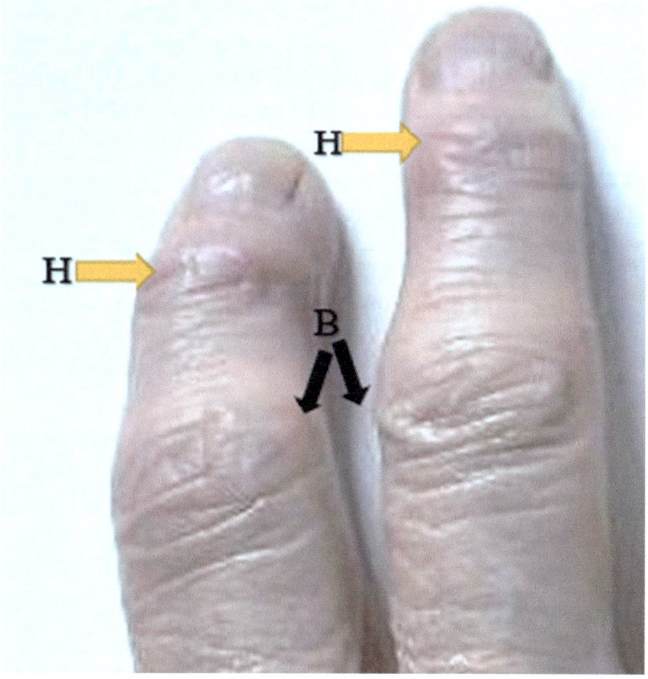

Fig. 53.4 Broussard's (B) and Heberden's (H) or hallmarks of osteoarthritis of the digits

53.3.5.3 Range of Motion

Wrist Deficits in range of motion should be noted. Normal range of flexion should be 60–80°, extension approximately 50–75°, ulnar deviation 30–45°, and radial deviation 15–25° [30].

Fingers Examination should evaluate the range of motion of the thumb and each digit individually. Metacarpophalangeal and interphalangeal joints should be tested. Functional range of motion of the metacarpophalangeal joint is 19–71°, proximal interphalangeal joint 23–87°, and interphalangeal joints 10–64° [36].

53.3.5.4 Neurological Examination

This includes upper extremity reflexes and sensory testing of the median, ulnar, and radial nerve distribution regions. Motor examination includes proximal arm, forearm muscles, intrinsic hand muscles, grip strength, pinch force, wrist flexion, wrist extension, wrist lateral deviation, wrist medial deviation, thumb flexion/extension, individual finger flexion /extension, flexion/extension of the metacarpophalangeal joints, abduction/adduction of the digits, and motor testing of longer/short finger flexors.

53.3.5.5 Special Testing

Tinel's sign A provocative test to assess diagnosis of median nerve compression at the wrist. This could be combined with ultrasonography, observation for thenar atrophy, sensory testing, and EMG for proper diagnosis.

Phalen test Also a provocative test which could be combined with Tinel's sign, EMG, and ultrasound for diagnosis of CTS, which is in the differential diagnosis for wrist OA.

Finkelstein test Performed in patients with medial wrist pain secondary to de Quervain's tenosynovitis (pain and swelling over the first compartment of the dorsal wrist). If the test is positive, it should be followed by diagnostic ultrasonography for signs of tenosynovitis.

Scaphoid shift test Also known as Watson test, it is a provocative maneuver to examine the dynamic stability of the scaphoid it is considered positive if it causes concordant pain. This test diagnoses injury to the scapholunate interosseous ligament.

Distal radial ulnar joint instability In order to evaluate volar instability of the wrist/radial ulnar joint, examiner will rest the distal radius and ulnar between the thumb and index of opposing hands and translates the radius relative to the ulna in the neutral, supination, and pronation positions.

Watson test/scaphoid shift test The patient will face the examiner, the elbow in 90° bend and the forearm in slight pronation. Watson test is performed by grasping the patient's hand from its ulnar aspect of the small metacarpal with the examiner's thumb on the palmar surface of the distal pole of the scaphoid. The examiner will then provoke dorsal subluxation of the proximal scaphoid over the dorsal rim of the radius, as the wrist is radially deviated. Examiner will passively move the wrist from ulnar deviation to radial deviation while observing the patient's response. Exerting pressure to the distal pole of the scaphoid is critical in order to prevent the scaphoid from flexing.

Carpometacarpal compression test In patients with lateral wrist/thumb pain, this test could elicit concordant pain originating from the first carpometacarpal joint. Test is performed by grabbing the patient's first metacarpal with one hand and the distal radius with the other, by applying longitudinal compression along the first metacarpal into the carpal bone and exerting axial compression of the carpometacarpal joint. A rotatory motion of the metacarpal could be performed as well, eliciting pain at the first CMC joint.

Ulnar collateral ligament testing The patient presenting with wrist/inner thumb pain (mostly traumatic) suspect Gamekeeper's thumb. The examiner would evaluate the UCL ligament by immobilizing the thumb metacarpal with one hand and the proximal phalanx with the other, while applying ulnar-directed force to the radial side of the joint to gap the thumb MCP joint on the ulnar side.

Thumb grind test Designed for evaluation of the osteoarthritis of the first carpometacarpal joint (trapeziometacarpal). The examiner grips the first metacarpal and exerts axial strain on the carpometacarpal joint while making rotational movements.

53.3.6 Diagnostic Workup

53.3.6.1 Plain Films

Plain radiograph of the wrist and hand/fingers is inexpensive, widely used, and highly diagnostic for osteoporosis of the wrist, hand, and finger. Osteoarthritis, most fractures, osteonecrosis, and erosions can be detected simply by X-rays. The hallmark of osteoarthritis of the fingers and hand includes marginal osteophyte formation, joint space narrowing (Fig. 53.5), sclerosis of the subchondral space, and cystic formations. If chondrocalcinosis is present, calcium pyrophosphate deposition compatible with pseudogout could be detected (Figs. 53.5 and 53.6).

53.3.6.2 Laboratory Testing

Standard laboratory testing including inflammatory markers (ESR, CRP) and rheumatoid factor should be ordered as standard workup for arthritic joints. Additional laboratory testing includes Lyme titer. If arthrocentesis is performed, synovial fluid could be analyzed including for inflammatory and crystal-induced arthritis.

53.3.6.3 MRI

Wrist and hand osteoarthritis could be simply detected with plain films, but if there is a suspicion of associated soft tissue injuries, tendon disorders, or instability, MRI may be indicated. MRI is sensitive for bone marrow abnormalities, synovitis and tenosynovitis, bursitis, ganglion cyst, infection, avascular necrosis, soft tissue mass, occult fracture, and ligamentum/tendon tear.

53.3.6.4 US

In the workup of the wrist/hand pain and wrist/hand OA, ultrasound is primarily used to identify any other abnormality that could resemble painful osteoarthritis including soft tissue disease. Ultrasound examination of the wrist and hand could be superior to other imaging methods in many aspects such as multidimensional character of this imaging modality, dynamic evaluation of both the joints and tendons, and precise assessment of the soft tissue. It is safe, there is no radiation, and it is portable and readily available in clinic or sideline. Ideally a transducer with >12 MHz frequency should be used for the wrist, hand, and finger examination.

Wrist US

The dorsal and palmar side of the wrist and hand should be evaluated. In the dorsal wrist, I–IV compartments of the wrist and its content should be carefully evaluated. Arteries, veins, and nerves of the wrist and hand and digits can be evaluated for abnormality. On the ventral side, median nerve, transcarpal ligament, and the carpal bones, metacarpals and phalangeal joints could all be evaluated in both static and dynamic forms. Evaluation of TFCC, midcarpal ligament, scapholunate ligament, and lunotriquetral ligament concludes ultrasonography of the wrist.

Fingers/Hand US

Ultrasonography is very sensitive in detecting tenosynovitis, trigger fingers, tendon tears, foreign body, and ganglion cyst and solid mass when evaluating fingers with ultrasound [37]. In osteoarthritis, degenerative findings could be detected with ultrasound, and dynamic testing can be performed.

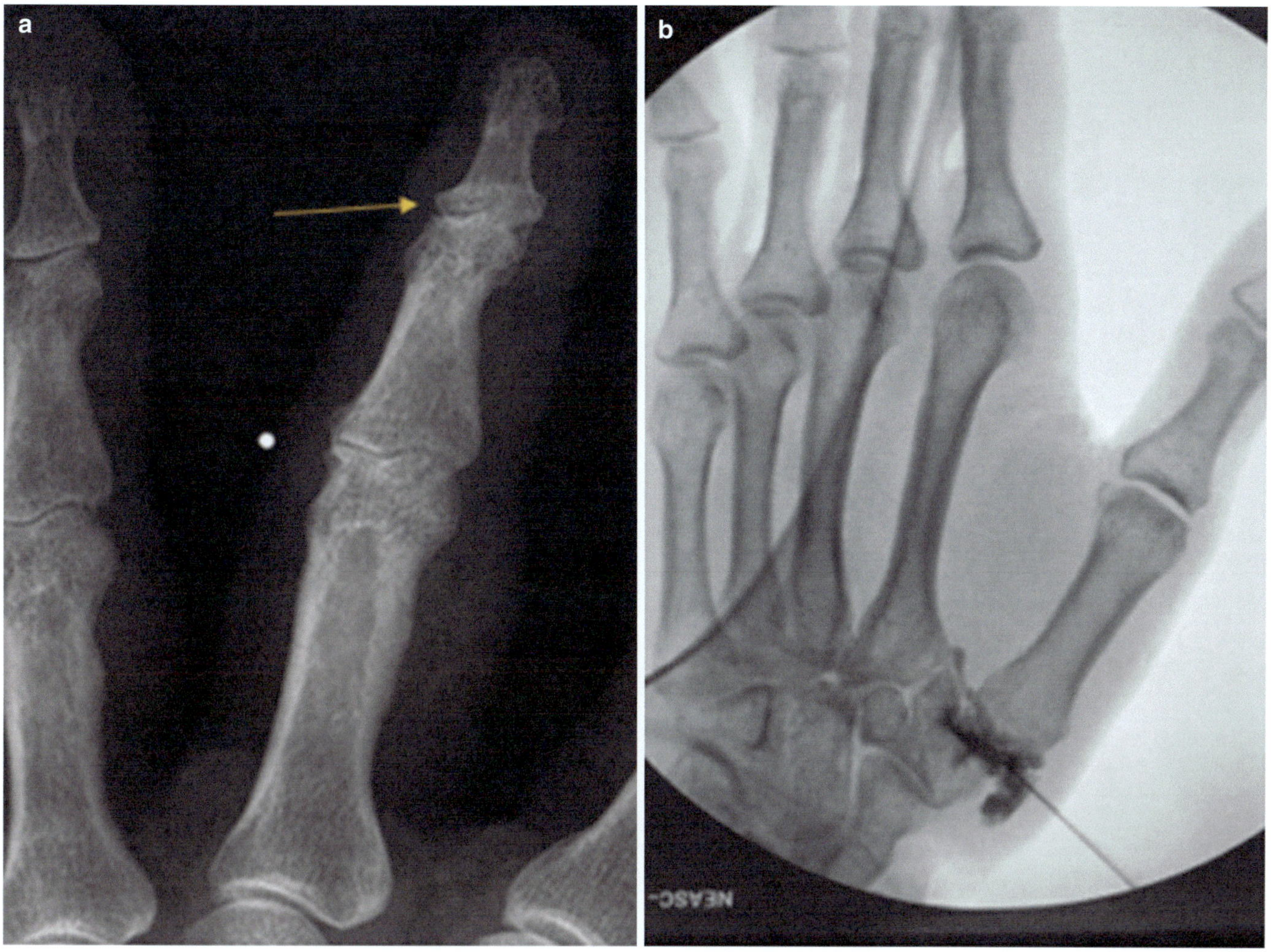

Fig. 53.5 (**a**) OA of the third distal interphalangeal joint (DIP with significant joint space narrowing). (**b**) Intraarticular injection of contrast into the first carpometacarpal joint (CMC) prior to injecting corticosteroid. (Images curtesy of S. Ali Mostoufi, MD Boston Regenerative Medicine)

53.3.7 Treatments

53.3.7.1 Medical Treatment

Conservative treatment typically begins with relative rest, medications, and activity modifications. Nonsteroidal anti-inflammatory medications (NSAIDs) can be considered depending on preexisting medical conditions. Acetaminophen (APAP) may be an alternative for patients in which NSAID use is contraindicated. Wrist splint and finger splints can assist with pain relief and improve function [37].

53.3.7.2 Rehabilitation

Guidelines from the European League Against Rheumatism (EULAR) recommend exercise therapy as a strategy for improving hand strength, but guidelines from the American College of Rheumatology (ACR) do not include exercise for hand OA. Hand exercise programs may comprise exercises designed to improve muscle strength, joint mobility, and/or joint stability [38]. Low-quality evidence shows small beneficial effects of exercise on wrist/hand pain and function and finger joint stiffness.

53.3.7.3 Procedures

Intra-articular injection of hyaluronic acid and cortisone relatively may provide short-term pain relief, but their long-term effect on pain and joint function is questionable [39]. They are typically recommended in patients that have tried and failed conservative care. Using local anesthetic as part of the intra-articular injectate adds diagnostic value and can differentiate the intra-articular source of pain from referred pain. There is growing interest in treating osteoarthritis with orthobiologics (including platelet-rich plasma (PRP), bone marrow aspirate concentrate (BMAC), dehydrated human amnion/chorion membrane allograft, and adipose-derived mesenchymal stem cells), but further research in safety and efficacy is still needed.

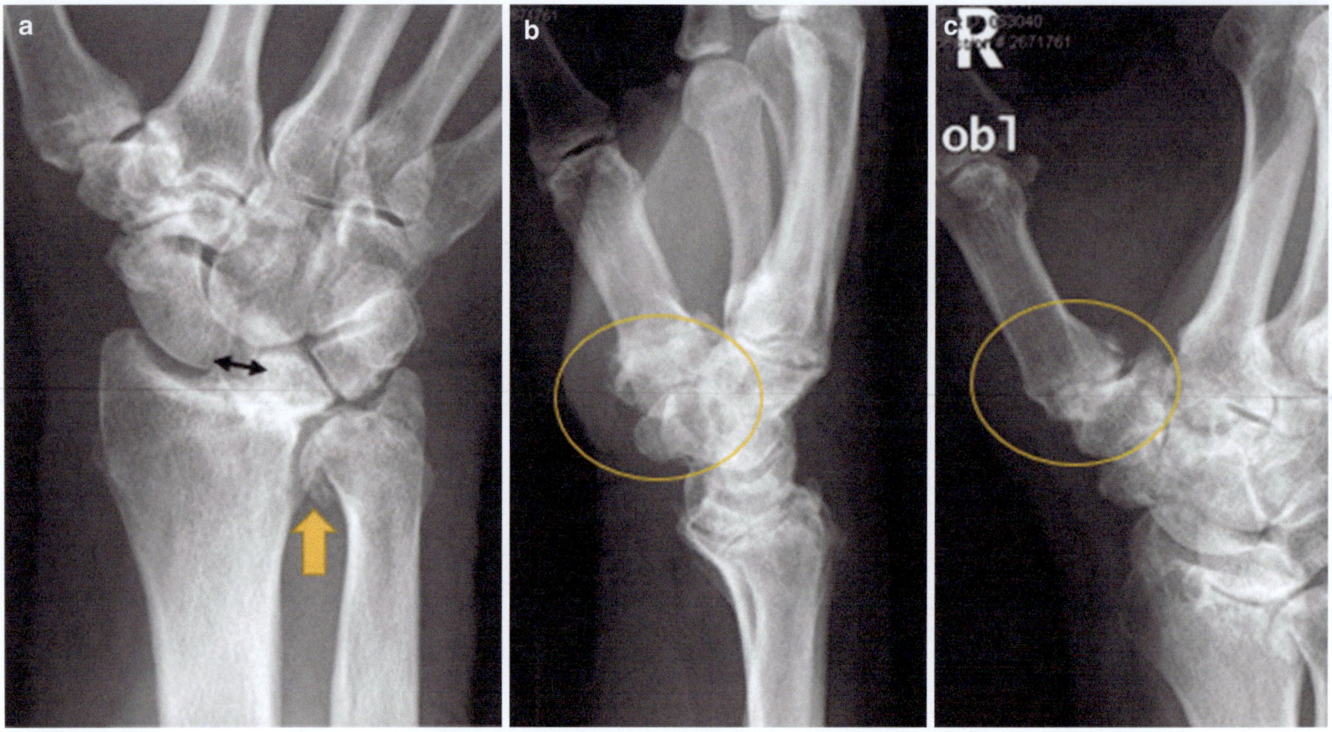

Fig. 53.6 (**a**) Osteoarthritis of the distal radial ulnar joint with opposing osteophyte formation. The double-sided arrow shows widening of the scapholunate distance. (**b** and **c**) Osteoarthritis of the first carpometacarpal joint with sclerosis of the trapezoid. (Fluoroscopic picture curtesy of S. Ali Mostoufi, MD Boston Regenerative Medicine)

53.3.7.4 Surgery

Wrist Surgery

Total wrist arthrodesis (fusion) has been the gold standard for managing advanced inflammatory and degenerative wrist arthritis. There is a recent trend toward motion-preserving surgery in the form of total wrist replacement. Wrist arthroplasty has been compared with wrist arthrodesis through retrospective-matched cohort studies in which the arthroplasty group showed better outcome in performing certain activities such as personal hygiene [40]. Pain scores, satisfaction, and complication rates were similar in both groups [40]. Studies are mix when it comes to functional outcomes when comparing arthroplasty to fusion.

Hand/Finger Surgery

For end-stage painful osteoarthritis of the hand and fingers, surgery may be recommended. Although joint replacement and arthrodesis are more common, denervation of the joints including trapeziometacarpal and finger joint denervation has shown to provide equally satisfactory pain relief. Given the high frequency of trapeziometacarpal osteoarthritis (first CMC), it is particularly of interest for arthroplasty. Studies on arthroplasty demonstrate 92% patient satisfaction, low complication rate, and a 5-year durability, making this treatment a reliable alternative to arthrodesis.

53.4 Hip OA

Kristian von Rickenbach, Adam Tenforde
and Haylee Borgstrom

53.4.1 Synonyms

Femoroacetabular osteoarthritis

53.4.2 ICD 10 Codes

- M16.10: Primary hip OA
- M16.11: Right hip OA
- M16.12: Left hip OA
- M16.7: Secondary hip OA

53.4.3 Description

Hip osteoarthritis (OA) is a multifactorial, degenerative process affecting not only the femoroacetabular articular cartilage but the entire joint and surrounding structures. Hip OA is common and is a leading cause of pain and disability worldwide [41]. The prevalence of symptomatic hip OA in

Table 53.1 Differential diagnosis of hip OA

Psoas tendinopathy	Femoral mononeuropathy
Lumbar radiculopathy	Sacroiliac pain (groin referral pain)
Pelvic pain	Fractures (pelvic/femoral/sacral)
Pelvic/sacral tumor	Hiatal hernia
Visceral pain	Spondylolisthesis (groin referral pain)

the United States is estimated at approximately 10% for those aged 55 years and older [42]. Hip OA may be primary (idiopathic), which is most common, or secondary (related to an underlying disorder or trauma). Risk factors for primary hip OA include advancing age, sex, obesity, ethnicity, and genetic predisposition [41, 43]. Men have increased prevalence of hip OA before the age of 50, while women have a higher prevalence thereafter [43]. Risk factors for secondary hip OA include trauma, metabolic or inflammatory disorders, and congenital or acquired hip deformities. While high-impact elite sport participation and certain occupations requiring heavy manual labor have been linked to hip OA [41], this association is likely due to increased risk for joint injury/trauma rather than joint loading itself. To date, there is no credible evidence to suggest that weight-bearing exercise leads to the development of OA. In fact, land-based exercise may be protective against OA and has been shown to improve pain and function in those with symptomatic hip OA [42, 44]. Differential diagnosis of hip OA is in Table 53.1.

53.4.4 Clinical Presentation

Hip OA typically presents with an insidious onset of anterior hip or groin pain. As discussed in the "Anterior Hip Disorders" chapter, patients may demonstrate the "C" sign and may describe complex referral patterns to the buttocks, thigh, and even beyond the knee. Joint stiffness is often worse in the morning and may impact activities of daily living, especially those that require excessive joint rotation such as donning socks or shoes. Weight-bearing activity, prolonged sitting, and transitional movements often exacerbate symptoms. Limping, mechanical symptoms, and sensation of weakness/instability may also be present as the severity of OA advances.

53.4.5 Physical Examination

Comprehensive musculoskeletal examination is needed to differentiate hip OA from other potential etiologies as discussed in preceding chapters.

- *Gait*: Patients with hip OA will often exhibit an antalgic gait with decreased stance phase on the affected side. Decreased cadence and short stride length related to restricted range of motion may also be appreciated. Trendelenburg gait may be present in the setting of concomitant gluteal muscular weakness [43].
- *Inspection*: Evaluate for posture, pelvic tilt, and leg length discrepancy noting any significant asymmetries which may be present as OA advances [43].
- *Palpation*: Palpatory examination may be normal for OA, though compensatory hip flexor tendon pain/dysfunction, gluteal and iliotibial band tendinopathy, and regional myofascial pain are common and described in preceding chapters.
- *Range of motion (ROM)*: Both passive and active ROM should be examined in all planes. In early hip OA, ROM may be preserved. Often, the first plane of motion to become restricted is hip internal rotation, but as OA advances ROM may become limited in all planes. Crepitus during ROM may be noted on exams.
- *Sensory testing*: Bilateral lower extremity sensory examination assessing L1-S1 dermatomes should be completed. Sensory exam should be normal in OA. If deficits are present, neurological diagnoses including lumbar radiculopathy should be considered.
- *Deep tendon reflexes*: Lower extremity reflexes should be tested, including the patella (L4 predominant), medial hamstring (L5), and Achilles (S1) tendons. Reflexes should be 2+ and symmetric in OA. Neurologic etiology should be considered in the case of deficits or asymmetries.
- *Motor testing*: Pain-limited weakness may be noted with manual muscle testing in the case of hip OA, especially with hip flexion and abduction. Strength assessment including L2-S1 myotomes should be completed to evaluate for possible neurologic etiology.
- *Joint testing*: A comprehensive assessment of the lumbar spine including facet joints and sacroiliac joints should be performed.

53.4.5.1 Special Maneuvers

Special maneuvers suggestive of intra-articular hip pathology, including OA, are described in detail in preceding chapters and include FABER, FADIR, log roll, Stinchfield's (or resisted straight leg raise) test, hop test, and scour test, among others (see chapter *Anterior Hip Disorders*). The most sensitive clinical tests for intra-articular hip pathology are flexion-abduction-external rotation (FABER: 82%) and flexion-adduction internal rotation (FADIR: 91%), while the most specific test is the Stinchfield's test (32%) [45]. In the Stinchfield's test, the patient lies supine and is asked to flex her hip to 20–30° with her knee fully extended and apply a resistive force. Pain in the anterior groin with this maneuver indicates a positive test.

53.4.6 Diagnostic Workup

X-ray Weight-bearing AP pelvis and lateral hip radiographs are the most frequently utilized imaging modality for diagnosis of hip OA. Severity of hip OA may be classified by various grading scales, most commonly with the Kellgren-Lawrence (KL) grading scale [43]. Radiographic findings indicative of hip OA includes joint space narrowing, osteophytes, subchondral sclerosis and cyst formation, and femoral head and acetabular deformity (Fig. 53.7). Importantly, radiographic presence of hip OA does not imply symptomatology. While the prevalence of radio-

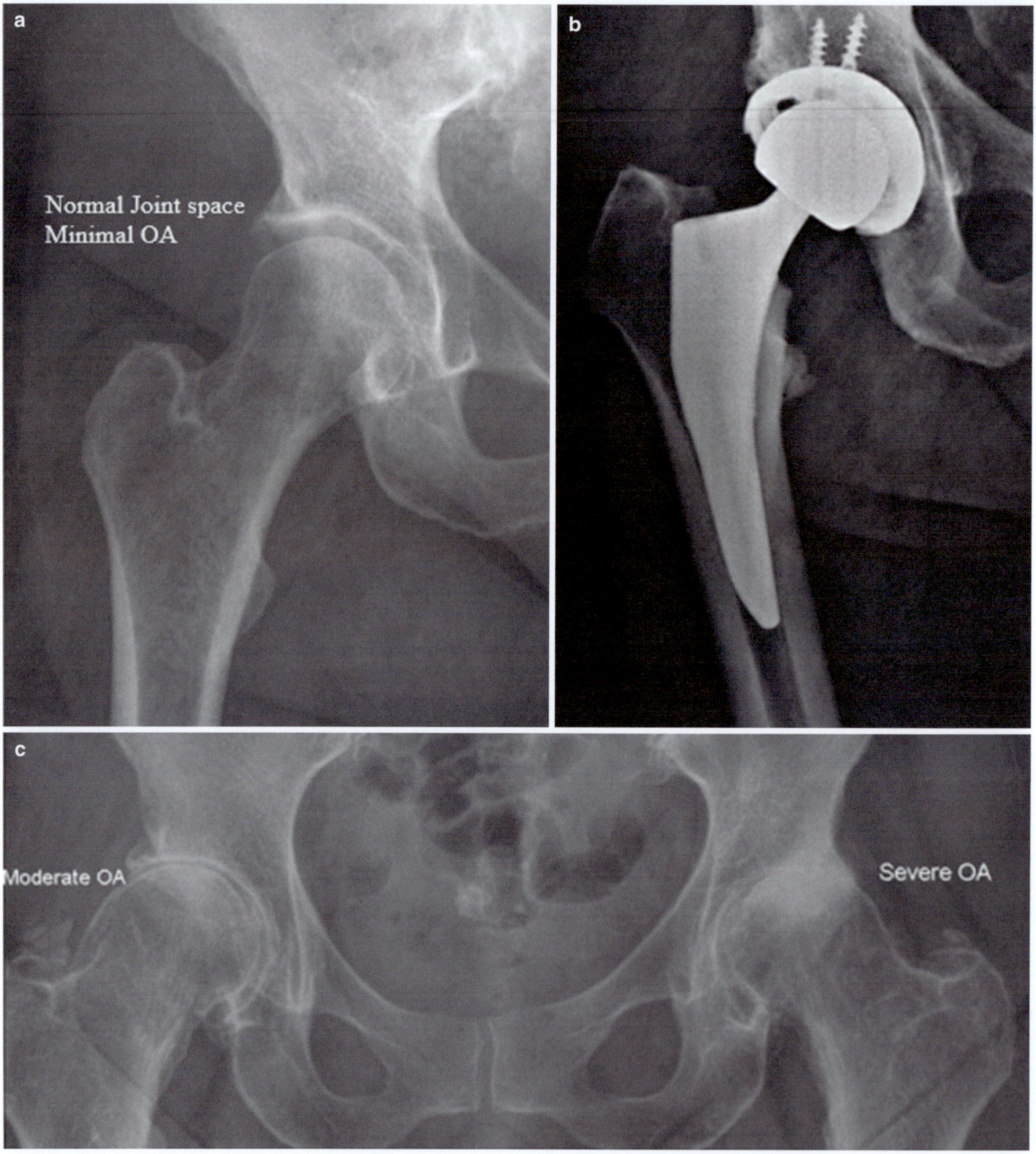

Fig. 53.7 OA of the hip joint. (**a**) Normal hip joint space. (**b**) Post arthroplasty. (**c**) On the left, moderate and on the right severe OA is noted with significant joint space narrowing and sclerosis. (Images curtesy of S. Ali Mostoufi, MD Boston Regenerative Medicine)

graphic hip OA has been described at nearly 30% [43], the presence of symptomatic hip OA is approximately 10% in those 55 years and older in the United States [42]. Similarly, symptom severity often does not correlate with radiographic grade.

MRI and CT Advanced imaging is typically not required for the diagnosis of hip OA. It can be presumed that all patients with clinically significant hip OA will have degenerative labral tears. Identification of these tears on MRI is not necessary and will not change management. However, MRI may be utilized for more detailed cartilage assessment in the setting of refractory pain or pain out of proportion to radiographic findings, evaluation of differential diagnoses and concomitant pathology, and guidance for further nonoperative treatment or operative planning.

53.4.7 Treatment

53.4.7.1 Medical Management

Conservative treatment for hip OA should include patient education, activity modification, ice/heat, physical therapy, dietary and weight loss recommendations (if appropriate), and consideration of pharmacologic therapy including acetaminophen, nonsteroidal anti-inflammatory drugs (NSAIDs), and topicals for concomitant myofascial pain. Supplementation with glucosamine and/or chondroitin have not been proven superior to placebo in the management of osteoarthritis [41].

53.4.7.2 Rehabilitation

Physical therapy is a mainstay of treatment for hip OA and should focus on developing an individualized program to improve core, gluteal, and circumferential hip strengthening, posture/pelvic alignment, balance, gait, and joint mobility [41, 43], keeping in mind that excessive stretching at end-range of motion is often irritating for the joint. Land-based exercise has been demonstrated to improve pain and function in symptomatic hip OA [42, 44]. As OA advances, impact exercise such as walking may exacerbate symptoms. Incorporation of non-impact aerobic exercise including cycling and swimming may be better tolerated as a means of promoting cardiovascular health and weight loss. An assistive device is often helpful [43]. A cane should be used in the contralateral hand and should fit the patient appropriately (height of greater trochanter, or 20–30° of elbow flexion).

53.4.7.3 Procedures

Corticosteroid injections (CSI) Ultrasound- or fluoroscopic-guided intra-articular hip CSIs are often utilized for the treatment of hip OA refractory to aforementioned conservative care (Figs. 53.8 and 53.9). A recent meta-analysis found that CSI for symptomatic hip OA resulted in greater pain reduction compared to placebo injection at 1 and 3 months [46]. Thus, CSI may provide temporary pain relief to allow improved tolerance of a combined physical therapy or home exercise program. The use of intra-articular steroid and local anesthetic injections should be weighed against concern for potential medication-related chondrotoxicity, particularly with repeat high-dose exposure.

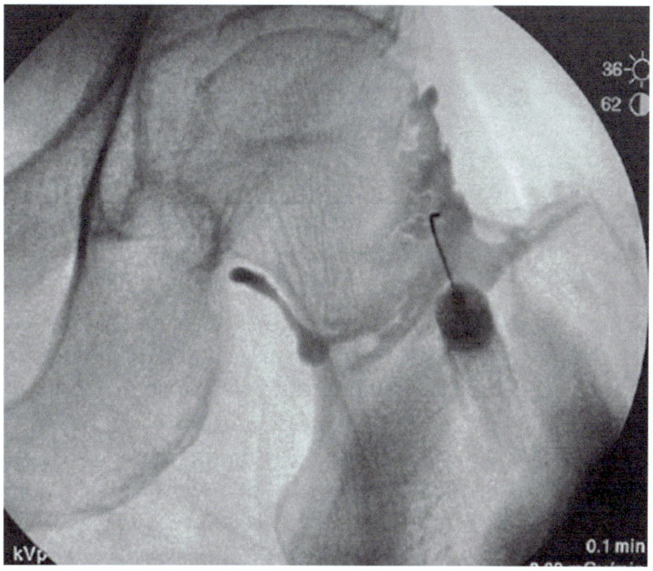

Fig. 53.8 Intra-articular injection of contrast media to confirm intra-articular needle placement in advance of steroid and normal saline delivery into the left hip joint to help with pain. (Image curtesy of S. Ali Mostoufi, MD)

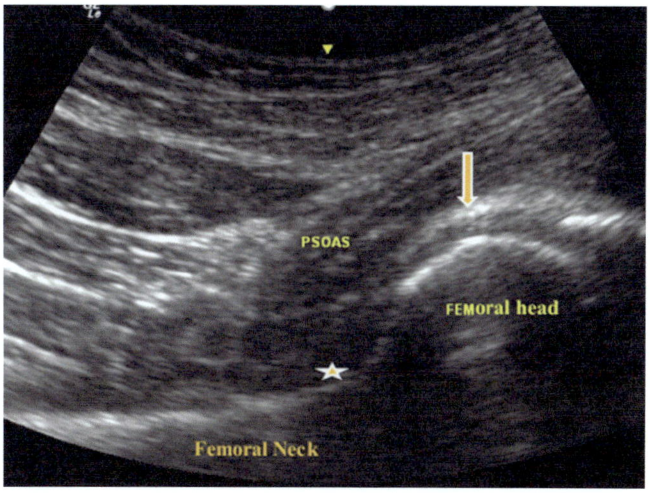

Fig. 53.9 Ultrasound can be utilized to perform intra-articular injection. Star demonstrates target for needle tip placement within joint capsule at the head and neck junction. Arrow shows the acetabulum and a portion of labrum. (Image curtesy of S. Ali Mostoufi, MD)

Hyaluronic acid (HA) injections HA injections, or visco-supplementation, may be considered for the treatment of refractory hip OA, though far less commonly compared to knee OA due to limited high-quality evidence and associated lack of insurance coverage. A recent meta-analysis of randomized controlled trials found HA provided superior pain relief compared to placebo injection at 1 and 3 months [46].

Orthobiologic injections There are limited high-level studies investigating the use of orthobiologic injections for the treatment of hip OA, including platelet-rich plasma (PRP) and adipose- or bone marrow-derived concentrates. PRP injection may have improved pain reduction at 6 months compared to control, CSI, or HA [46], though this has not been well-established. Micronized dehydrated human amnion/chorion membrane has demonstrated some success with OA-related knee pain (67% of individuals for 6 months), but the effectiveness and safety of this treatment for hip osteoarthritis are not studied systematically.

53.4.7.4 Surgery

Total hip arthroplasty (THA) is the most common surgical treatment for hip OA (Fig. 53.7). Surgical referral should be made in the case of refractory pain and/or functional limitation affecting quality of life, often in the setting of moderate to more advanced OA. Improved surgical outcomes have been demonstrated in patients with higher preoperative functional status [41], indicating the importance of preoperative rehabilitation and early referral after failure of nonoperative care. Specific surgical considerations for the treatment of hip OA along with postoperative management are discussed in detail in the following chapter. For detailed information on total hip replacement, please see Chap. 42.

53.5 Knee OA

Jennifer Soo Hoo, Gerard D'Onofrio and Gisela Figueroa

53.5.1 ICD 10 Codes

M17.1–M17.5

53.5.2 Description

Knee osteoarthritis (OA) is a degenerative condition of the knee joint resulting from periarticular tissue abnormalities, leading to failed tissue repair and cartilage loss. Knee osteoarthritis impacts all tissues within the joint, leading to detectable changes in tissue architecture and its metabolism and function. There are high rates of asymptomatic osteoarthritis, as symptoms do not necessarily correlate to disease extent on radiographs and the progression of disease varies greatly between patients.

Anatomy The knee joint is a hinged joint and is comprised of three different compartments: medial tibiofemoral, lateral tibiofemoral, and patellofemoral. The bones that contribute to these compartments are the femur, tibia, and patella. The medial and lateral femoral condyles articulate with corresponding tibial plateaus, and the knee capsule surrounds the entire joint and extends proximally into the suprapatellar pouch. Articular hyaline cartilage, mostly type II collagen, covers the femoral condyles, tibial plateaus, trochlear groove, and patellar facets. The knee is supplied by branches from the femoral, obturator, saphenous, tibial, and common fibular nerves. More specifically, the knee is innervated by the superior lateral, superior medial, and inferior medial genicular nerves. The vascular supply of the knee is largely provided by the popliteal artery and four anastomosing genicular arteries from the superior medial and superior lateral genicular arteries as well as the inferior medial and inferior lateral genicular arteries. There are additional anastomotic arteries contributing to the knee from the anterior tibial and posterior tibial arteries [41].

Knee OA is characterized by articular cartilage loss, but the disease extends to all aspects of the joint. Articular cartilage metabolism is influenced by mechanotransduction, leading to tissue remodeling. Improper excessive, or insufficient loading of articular cartilage, can lead to an imbalance of articular cartilage metabolic activity, leading to a depletion of extracellular matrix components and irreversible destruction of articular cartilage [42]. Differential diagnosis of Knee OA is in Table 53.2.

- Bone and Cartilage Changes in OA

  Subchondral bone adapts to mechanotransduction in a manner similar to, but more rapidly than, articular cartilage. For this reason, in osteoarthritis, the subchondral bone plate increases in volume and thickness known as *subchondral sclerosis*. Modification in osteoblastic and osteoclastic activity leads to bone lesions such as *subchondral cysts* and *osteophytes*. Osteophytes may also form at the joint margins via endochondral ossification. The synovial fluid and synovial membranes play a vital role in cartilage nutrition and may be adversely impacted by osteoarthritis, during which synovitis and inflamma-

Table 53.2 Differential diagnosis of knee osteoarthritis

Meniscal tear	Patellofemoral pain syndrome
Rheumatoid arthritis	Tibial plateau fracture
Septic arthritis	Osteochondritis dissecans
Ligament tear	Patellar bursopathies

tion may impact these tissues. Local inflammatory factors may cause *synovial hypertrophy* and painful synovitis.

- Soft Tissue Changes in OA

  Hoffa's fat pad, otherwise known as the *infrapatellar fat pad*, plays an important role in knee osteoarthritis as it is a local endocrine organ, serving to influence the joint microenvironment and playing a potential role in chronic knee pain. *Meniscus lesions* and injuries are commonly present in osteoarthritic knees, as alteration of meniscal function may lead to joint instability, abnormal loading, and development of arthritis. *Muscular tissues*, such as the quadriceps muscle, hamstrings, and hip muscles, play important roles in knee osteoarthritis, and patients with osteoarthritis may have increased intramuscular fat content in the quadriceps associated with knee cartilage loss. *Tendon and ligament* injuries can also hasten the onset of knee osteoarthritis [42].

53.5.3 Clinical Presentation

Common symptoms of knee osteoarthritis include knee pain, stiffness, swelling, reduced joint motion, crepitus, locking, pain rising from a chair or climbing stairs, and muscle weakness in the quadriceps. Risk factors for developing knee osteoarthritis include advanced age, previous knee injury or meniscus/ACL surgery, obesity, joint malalignment and instability, repetitive actions, and physical inactivity [42]. Women are more likely to develop knee osteoarthritis than men, which may be attributed to structural differences in females such as narrower femurs, greater Q angles, and differently sized tibial condyles.

A thorough history and physical examination of a patient with knee osteoarthritis may be sufficient for diagnosis. Patients can present with one or both knees affected, as well as other joints impacted by osteoarthritis. Pain is a common presenting symptom and is generally characterized as dull and worsened with activity and improved with rest. These symptoms can accompany feelings of morning stiffness, generally lasting less than 30 minutes. Generally, knee osteoarthritis does not present with warmth, swelling, and systemic inflammatory response symptoms, as it is a less-inflammatory process than septic or crystal arthropathies. Symptoms generally onset gradually in the fifth decade or beyond, but age is a variable contingent upon prior injuries. Patients may have coincident symptoms of locking and buckling as meniscal disease is commonly concurrent with knee osteoarthritis [43].

53.5.4 Physical Examination

53.5.4.1 Inspection

Patients with advanced knee osteoarthritis may have hypertrophy of the knee joint diffusely. Further, there may be altered joint alignment, due to a high prevalence of medial tibiofemoral osteoarthritis [44]. Preferential joint space narrowing, either at the medial or lateral tibiofemoral compartments may lead to resultant varus or valgus deformity of the knee evident in standing. An effusion may accompany osteoarthritis and may be discernible on inspection. Atrophy of the quadriceps can accompany advanced cases of knee osteoarthritis as well [42].

53.5.4.2 Palpation

Palpatory exam in patients with knee osteoarthritis may reveal joint line tenderness, indicating potentially superimposed meniscus pathology or localized pain due to osteophyte formation and loss of articular cartilage. Mobilization of the patella may indicate crepitus or pain if there is patellofemoral arthritis. Knee joint effusion may be present especially in acutely flared presentations. Generally, the affected knee is not warm or red.

53.5.4.3 Range of Motion

Range of motion may be limited in patients with advanced knee osteoarthritis and may be evidenced by contractures of muscles inserting around the knee joint. This mostly leads to a flexion contracture of the knee. Further, the entire arc of motion will reduce as osteoarthritis progresses and fibrosis of the joint capsule occurs. The normal range of motion is 0 for extension and 140° for flexion, both of which may be reduced in patients with advanced osteoarthritis [41].

53.5.4.4 Manual Muscle Testing

Dysfunction and atrophy of the quadriceps muscles associated with knee osteoarthritis may demonstrate knee extensor weakness on examination. The quadriceps may also be inhibited through arthrogenic inhibition if there is an associated effusion. Further, the hamstrings may be inhibited or altered if there is a knee flexion contracture. Hip musculature may also reveal weakness, potentially due to an altered kinetic chain.

53.5.4.5 Provocative Maneuvers

While there are no specific provocative maneuvers for knee osteoarthritis, maneuvers such as the McMurray and Thessaly tests may be used to examine meniscus pathology, which is commonly seen in knee osteoarthritis. Also, due to the pathogenesis of knee osteoarthritis and potential for other injuries inciting the process of cartilage degradation, testing for ligamentous laxity should be performed.

53.5.4.6 Gait Analysis

As pain is a common presenting symptom of knee osteoarthritis, the examiner should evaluate for an antalgic gait. In addition, there should be examination of the degree of knee flexion throughout stance phase, as this is an important determinant of gait stability, and reliance on genu recurvatum may indicate reluctance to load the quadriceps or quadriceps weakness, which may stem from nociceptive or arthrogenic inhibition.

53.5.5 Diagnostic Workup

53.5.5.1 X-Rays

Plain film radiographs play an important role in the diagnosis and treatment of osteoarthritis and are typically obtained while the patient is weight-bearing. Common findings include osteophytes, joint space narrowing, subchondral cysts, and subchondral sclerosis. In particular, the medial aspect of the joint may demonstrate joint space narrowing. X-rays commonly obtained are standing weight-bearing AP, Rosenberg view (PA radiograph with weight-bearing and 45° of flexion), and lateral and merchant views. These views provide insight into the different compartments of arthritis manifestation, which may be the patellofemoral compartment, medial tibiofemoral compartment, and lateral tibiofemoral compartments [41].

The Kellgren-Lawrence system is used to grade knee osteoarthritis on a 0–4 scale. Grade 0 is defined as absence of X-ray findings suggestive of osteoarthritis, whereas grade 4 indicates large osteophytes, marked narrowing of joint space, severe subchondral sclerosis, and definite deformity of bone ends (Fig. 53.10) [45].

53.5.5.2 MRI

Soft tissue imaging performed with MRI is a useful modality for evaluating knee pathology but has limited utility in the diagnosis and treatment of knee osteoarthritis. In particular, MRIs may be indicated if there are signs of concomitant meniscal pathology, where patients may have symptoms of locking, buckling, or an associated effusion.

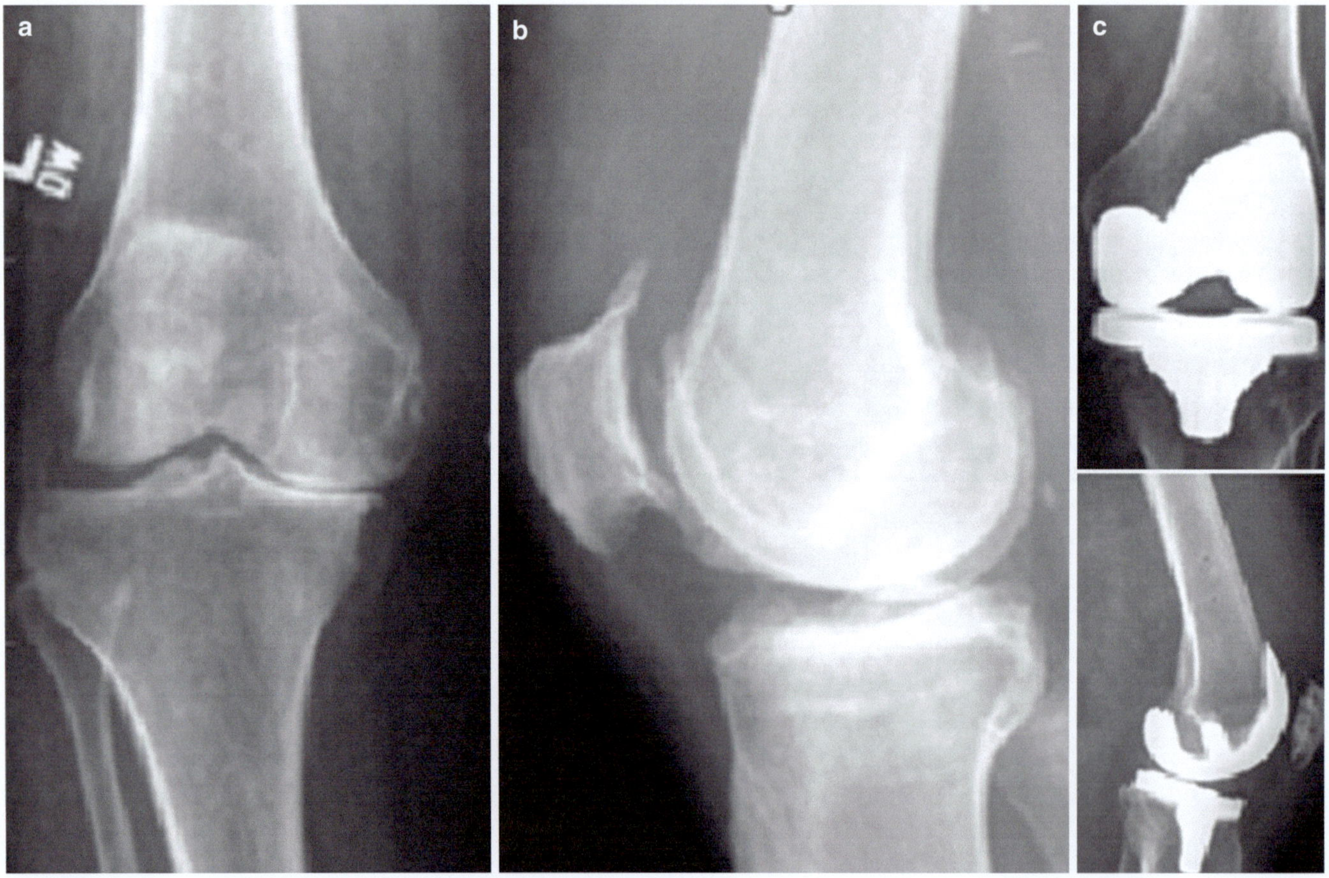

Fig. 53.10 Preoperative standing AP (**a**). Lateral (**b**) knee radiographs showing medial joint space narrowing, osteophyte formation, and subchondral sclerosis. (**c**) A right knee after arthroplasty. (Images curtesy of S. Ali Mostoufi, MD)

53.5.5.3 Ultrasound

Ultrasound evaluation of the knee can reveal effusions evident in the suprapatellar recess between the quadriceps fat pad and the quadriceps tendon. These may be appreciated with the patient supine and the knee slightly flexed, typically with a cylinder or towel roll supporting the posterior aspect of the knee. Osteoarthritis patients may present with isoechoic synovial hypertrophy and anechoic effusions [46].

Ultrasound of the posterior aspect of the knee joint in a patient with knee osteoarthritis can reveal a Baker's cyst between the semimembranosus and medial gastrocnemius tendons. Ultrasound of the lateral and medial knee joint lines can sometimes help to elucidate meniscal pathology that should be further evaluated with MRI if clinically indicated. Displacement of meniscal tissue can be appreciated dynamically. Possible other pathology that can be appreciated under ultrasound includes hypoechoic degeneration with anechoic clefts and osteophyte formation at the joint lines. In addition, ultrasound in transverse plane over the distal femur may demonstrate focal hyaline cartilage defects [46].

53.5.5.4 Arthrocentesis

Osteoarthritis with accompanying effusions can be aspirated, although this is not necessary for diagnosis. Synovial fluid can be analyzed for white blood cell count, with osteoarthritis patients typically having less than 2000/mL^3, while septic and inflammatory arthritis tend to have a higher concentration of white blood cells in synovial fluid [43].

53.5.6 Treatments

53.5.6.1 Medical Management

The medical management of knee osteoarthritis is conceptualized as a means to facilitate participation in physical therapy, reduce pain as a symptom of osteoarthritis, and increase physical activity.

- *Acetaminophen* is widely regarded as a first-line agent in symptomatic knee OA [47].
- *Topical NSAIDs* (e.g., diclofenac gel) can be used to mitigate pain.
- *Oral NSAIDs* (Cox-I or Cox-II inhibitors) in patients without contraindications (GI, renal, anticoagulated).
- *Glucosamine-chondroitin sulfate* supplements have mixed data but are generally considered not harmful.

53.5.6.2 Rehabilitation

Physical Therapy plays an important role in the rehabilitation of knee OA. The goal of rehabilitation is to optimize function including improving gait speed and decreasing the risk of falls. Treatment strategies address impairments such as edema, pain, muscle weakness, limited flexibility, decreased range of motion, and imbalance. There is high-quality evidence for improved knee extension and flexion strength with a low-intensity resistance program when compared to a control at short-term follow-up [48]. There is moderate-quality evidence for a large effect favoring high-intensity resistance programs [48]. A combination of hip and quadriceps strengthening exercises was found to be significantly more effective than quadriceps exercise alone for improving walking function (Fig. 53.11) [49]. Strengthening of the hip extensors, hip abductors, hip adductors, quadriceps, hamstrings, and gastrocnemius can help to reduce pain [50]. Gluteal strength training, Tai chi, and aerobics showed a significant reduction in the risk of falls [51]. Electrical stimulation can be used to enhance strength or decrease pain. Interferential current (IFC) was significantly effective in treatment of both pain intensity and change in pain score [52]. Moderate-quality evidence indicates that aquatic exercise might have small, short-term, and clinically relevant effects on pain, disability, and quality of life in individuals with knee and hip OA [53]. Bracing and foot orthoses can also be considered to decrease pain, joint stiffness, and improve balance; however, there is no strong evidence to support their long-term use [54]. Patients are provided with a home exercise program (HEP) for self-management and progression while on program. Large evidence of high-quality trials indicate home exercise programs with and without supervised clinic-based exercises to be effective in the rehabilitation of knee OA [55].

53.5.6.3 Procedures

The most commonly performed procedures are corticosteroid injections, viscosupplementation injections, neuromodulation and radiofrequency lesioning of genicular nerves. There has been emerging evidence and research looking into orthobiologics as a role in treating knee osteoarthritis.

Corticosteroid Injections

It provides an anti-inflammatory effect within the knee joint microenvironment, which may alter immune cell function and subsequently, pain. There are mixed data concerning the long-term effectiveness of intra-articular corticosteroid injections for knee osteoarthritis, and consideration must be made to use proper real-time imaging guidance in the form of ultrasound as opposed to blind palpatory technique [56]. Side effects of glucocorticoid administration include system absorption with resultant hyperglycemia, hypertension, insomnia, etc. Local effects include skin depigmentation, fat necrosis, and cutaneous atrophy. There is also evidence that shows corticosteroid and lidocaine use are chondrotoxic and may actually accelerate degeneration of the knee joint [57].

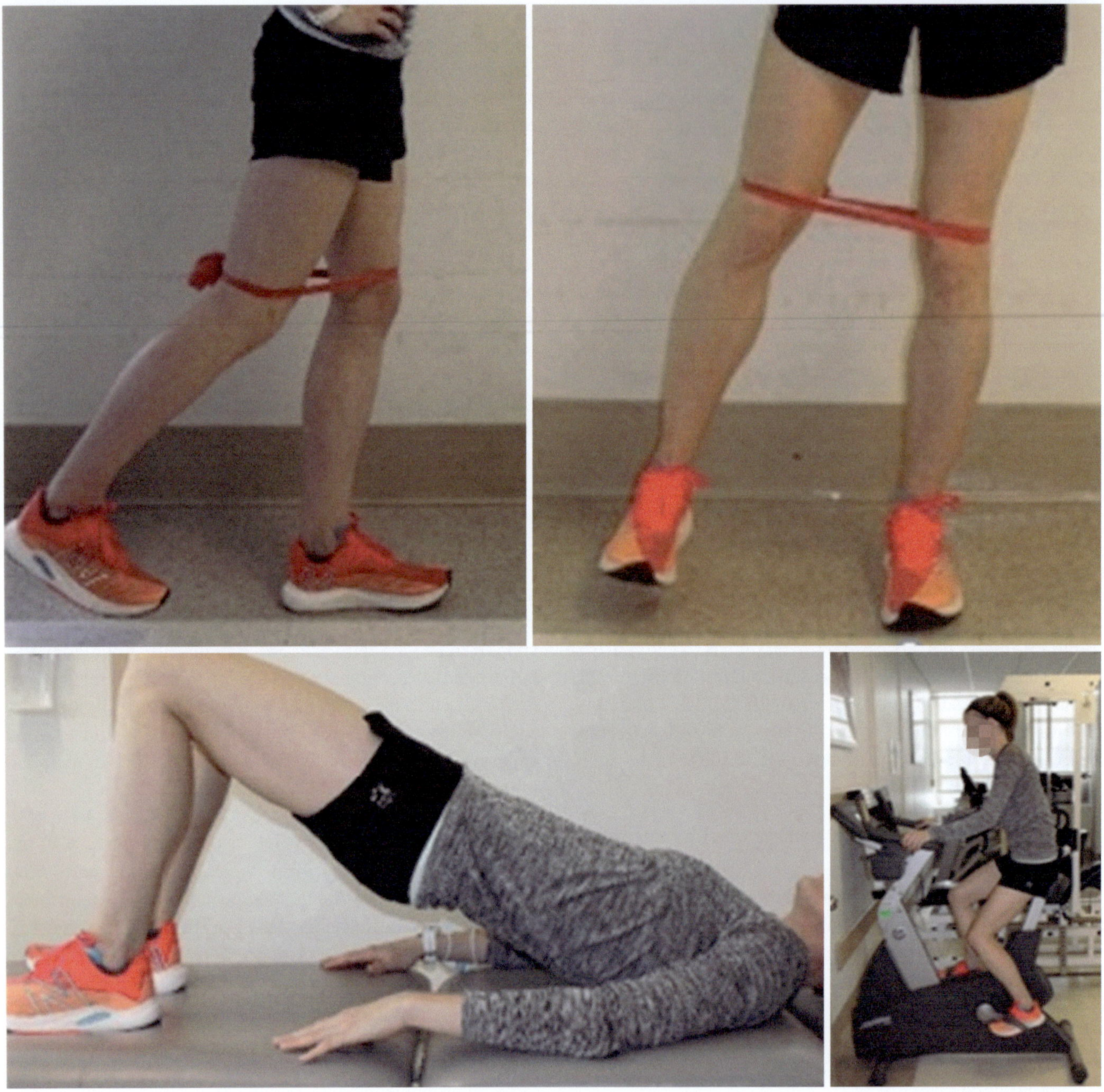

Fig. 53.11 A sample of PT exercises for knee OA. Exercises include stationary bike warm-up, hooklying bridge, resisted hip abduction, and resisted hip extension with TheraBand

Viscosupplementation

Hyaluronate or hyaluronan is a large viscoelastic glycosaminoglycan molecule that is found naturally in synovial fluid and cartilage. Hyaluronate injections help restore and spur generation of hyaluronate in synovial fluid. Hyaluronate acts as a lubricant and shock absorber. In osteoarthritic knees, the natural concentration of hyaluronate decreases. Injections can result in extended pain relief (several months). There are variable preparations of hyaluronate dependent on molecular weight, and their viability as a treatment may be related to their preparation – higher-molecular-weight hyaluronate preparations have shown clinical important reductions in pain [56].

Biologics

Various regenerative medicine therapies are growing in recognition for the treatment of knee OA.

- *Platelet-rich plasma (PRP)*: The proposed effect of PRP on the knee joint is that there is both a stimulation of local

chondrocytes as well as mitigation of inflammatory aspects of the condition. There is a growing literature base elucidating the benefit of leukocyte-rich or leukocyte-poor PRP. This is a safe procedure as it uses growth factors from patients' own blood [42, 56]. There is growing, high-quality evidence supporting the use of PRP in knee osteoarthritis.
- *Prolotherapy*: This is injection of a hypertonic solution that can be administered in both intra-articular and periarticular fashion. The premise of prolotherapy treatment for osteoarthritis is that it spurs a pro-inflammatory microenvironment that may in turn lead to a cascade of regenerative cytokines and restoration of cartilage thickness. There is mixed evidence regarding efficacy of this treatment option for OA.
- *Mesenchymal stem cells*: Both lipoaspirate concentrate and BMAC are proposed to provide minimal concentrations of mesenchymal stem cells and perhaps more importantly, deliver a litany of growth factors that can combat degenerative processes such as knee osteoarthritis. The literature for these treatments is growing and they are generally considered safe [42, 56].
- *Micronized dehydrated human amnion chorion membrane*: It is theorized that the human amniotic membrane contains growth factors and cytokines, which promote epithelial cell migration and proliferation, stimulate metabolic processes leading to collagen synthesis, and attract fibroblasts, while also reducing pain and inflammation [58]. Limited studies are available on effectiveness, but a recent study following patients for 6 weeks, 3 months, and 6 months postinjection showed 32%, 56%, and 65% improvement in mean Knee Injury and Osteoarthritis Outcome Score (KOOS) [58].

Genicular Knee Blocks and Radiofrequency Ablation (RFA)

Patients with knee OA and resultant pain and disability from the disease process may benefit from genicular knee blocks/RFA. This may also be an option for persistent knee region pain despite knee replacement surgery. Due to the neuronal innervation arising from multiple nerves such as the femoral, tibial, saphenous, obturator, and common peroneal nerves, practitioners can target these nerves as sites for diagnostic blocks and therapeutic ablations for refractory knee pain. Pain relief can be achieved by inhibiting the sensation of pain arising from the knee joint. The electromagnetic fields created at the distal end of an RFA needle can cause necrosis and denaturation of the fibers innervating the knee joint [56]. *In a* prospective, open-label, and controlled study, *comparing anesthetic-only injection* vs *RF ablation treatment of genicular nerve (patients followed for 6 months)*, the percentage of responders in the RF group was approximately 50% at 4 weeks, 30% at 12 weeks, and less than 10% at 6 months. Genicular RFA is a viable option for patients who are not responding to other conservative management although pain relief appears to be shorter as compared to RF ablation for medical branches performed for axial spine pain due to facet osteoarthritis [59].

Neuromodulation

Dorsal root ganglion stimulation, or genicular nerve stimulation, may be an option for nonoperable knee OA or for persistent post arthroplasty pain with neuropathic characteristics. The popularity of this modality is growing within pain management community, and despite its safety profile, effectiveness is yet to be proven on RCT studies.

53.5.6.4 Surgery

For those knee osteoarthritis patients not responding to conservative care and whose pain greatly impacts their function, total knee replacement can be considered. Please see "Surgical Knee" chapter for further detail.

53.6 Foot and Ankle OA

S. Ali Mostoufi and Kyungje Sung

53.6.1 ICD 10 Code

- M19.079: Ankle and foot OA – primary
- M19.179: Ankle and foot OA – traumatic
- M19.279: Ankle and foot OA – secondary
- M20.20: Hallux rigidus
- M20.10: Hallux valgus

53.6.2 Description

53.6.2.1 Ankle OA

Osteoarthritis is caused by joint degeneration (breakdown of articular cartilage in synovial joints) that eventually leads to pain and dysfunction [76]. Ankle and foot osteoarthritis may cause significant pain and impairments and may be more common than clinicians realize. Studies indicate that primary idiopathic osteoarthritis in the ankle is rare and that secondary osteoarthritis that follows rotational ankle fractures or recurrent ligamentous instability is much more common [60]. Obesity, by increasing mechanical stress, may also lead to a higher risk in developing lower limb osteoarthritis including OA of foot and ankle [76].

The most common cause of ankle osteoarthritis is trauma (malleolar, tibial, and talus fractures, ankle ligament lesions); the second common cause was secondary osteoarthritis (rheumatoid, hemochromatosis, hemophilia, clubfoot, avas-

Table 53.3 Differential diagnosis of ankle or foot osteoarthritis

L5/S1 radiculopathy	Tibialis anterior tendinitis
Stress fracture	Deltoid ligament tendinopathy
Peroneal tendinopathy	Anterior ankle impingement
Talus osteochondritis dissecans	Inferior tibiofibular joint disorder
Achilles tendinitis	Charcot foot
Gout/reactive arthritis	Plantar faucitis
Septic joint	Bursitis

cular talus, osteochondrosis dissecans, post infection), and lastly primary osteoarthritis [65]. Foot and ankle pain significantly increased the odds of developing other painful conditions including knee and spine duo to altered gait, so it is important to treat the ankle pain and help prevent chronic multifactorial pain [60]. Differential diagnosis of ankle osteoarthritis is given in Table 53.3.

53.6.2.2 Foot OA

Osteoarthritis of the midfoot and forefoot (metatarsophalangeal and toes) are common in older adults with slight preference toward females. OA of the foot joints results in pain, difficulty with weight-bearing, locomotor disability, poor balance, and risk of fall. Radiographic studies have demonstrated approximately 17% rate of osteoarthritis of the foot in ages 50 and up. Radiographic first MTP joint OA (hallux rigidus) most commonly occurred in isolation from the other joints in the affected foot, whereas OA in the midfoot joints tended to co-occur with OA in other joints in the same foot. Symptomatic osteoarthritis affect approximately 10% of the people at age 60 and above and apparently 15% of people age 45 and above [61].

In symptomatic foot OA, the most commonly affected individual joints in descending order are second cuneometatarsal, navicular first cuneiform, first MTP, first cuneometatarsal, and talonavicular joint. The Kellgren-Lawrence system is used to grade foot and toe osteoarthritis [62].

Most clinicians consider midfoot osteoarthritis as a separate medical entity as compared to first MTP OA due to differences in risk factors for development.

Midfoot OA

The most common area of midfoot injury is the Lisfranc joint complex. Risk factors for midfoot osteoarthritis includes female, lower socioeconomic class, older age, obesity, previous injury, and flat and pronated feet with increased plantar stress on the midfoot in particular on second CMT which has a high-frequency of OA [63].

First MTP OA

Hallux rigidus is a condition that refers to degenerative arthritis of the first metatarsophalangeal (MTP) joint. In this condition, the big toe will flex due to the plantar-flexed position of the proximal phalanx in relation to the metatarsal head, resulting in painful motion of the first MTP joint. Risk factors for this condition are flattened/pronated feet, ankle/subtalar joint eversion, ankle joint dorsiflexion, hindfoot valgus deformity more than 5°, excessive foot pronation, concomitant knee OA, finger interphalangeal joint OA, and first carpometacarpal OA [61, 65].

53.6.3 Clinical Presentation

53.6.3.1 Ankle OA

Ankle OA may present as morning pain or pain with prolonged sitting, antalgic gait, pain on weight-bearing, swelling, stiffness, reduced ROM, and sense of instability (posttraumatic cases). Pain may be located in distal shin, at the anterior crease of the ankle, back of the foot, medial or lateral malleoli area, or toward the foot. It may come and go, or there may be a chronic low level of pain with intermittent flare-ups.

53.6.3.2 Foot OA

Localized pain over the affected joint with weight-bearing, swelling, deformity of the joint, stiffness, and redness are all part of the presenting symptom of foot osteoarthritis. As part of the history, clinician should ask patient regarding pain duration, severity and quality, relationship to weight-bearing, location (plantar versus dorsal), radiation to a particular direction (e.g., toes or shin), alleviating factors, aggravating factors, time of the day in which pain is worse, walking ability in distance and time, ability to negotiate stairs, and previous treatment, whether they have been effective or not.

53.6.4 Examination

Gait Antalgic gait should be expected in significantly symptomatic foot and ankle pain. Patients would likely use a cane or other assistive devices when walking. Examination of the patient's shoe may demonstrate different patterns of wear, indicating abnormal contact of the foot with the ground.

Inspection Inspection should be done in barefoot, both in the standing position and examining the foot directly. Alignment of the ankle, foot, and hindfoot is best noted, barefoot, in standing position while the examiner is standing behind the patient. The examiner should observe any valgus/varus hindfoot deformity, hallux valgus, hallux valgus interphalangeus or hallux varus, claw toe, hammertoe, mallet toe foot pronation, supination, or pes planus and pes cavus abnormality, midfoot abduction, and forefoot pronation (Fig. 53.12), varus/valgus deformity of the knees, or scoliotic spine. Muscle atrophy is noted as well in the inspection phase.

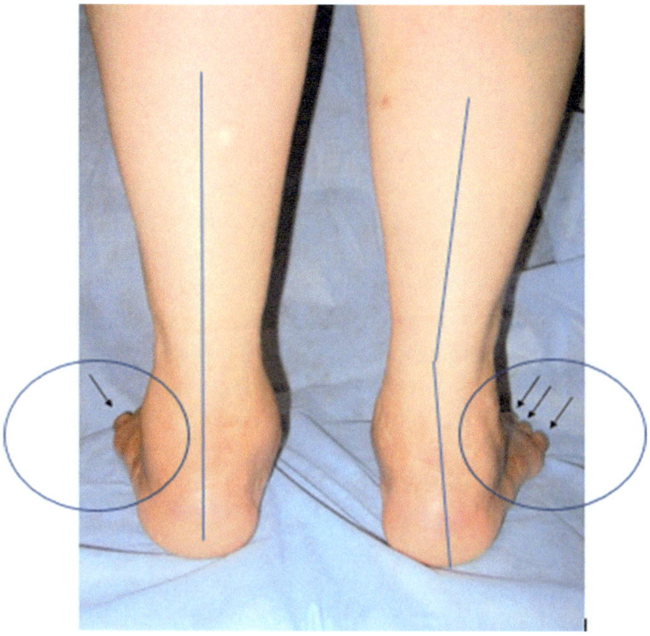

Fig. 53.12 Collapse of the medial longitudinal arch and forefoot pronation. Only one or two toes should be visible from behind. If more are seen, it is said that the "too many toes" sign is present (black arrows on the right). (Image curtesy of S. Behrooz Mostofi, FRCS)

Inspecting for skin abnormality, joint deformity, swelling and redness, pseudomotor abnormality, abnormalities in the nail, pronation and supination of the feet, and pes planus and pes cavus are all part of the inspection of the foot and ankle [66].

Palpation The examiner should palpate individual joints starting from the hindfoot to the forefoot and eventually to the toes while initially avoiding the most painful joint and further concentrating in isolating that particular painful joint. Passive and active range of motion should be noted. In examination of the first MTP, the examiner will evaluate for range of motion of the joint, and fixed versus reducible valgus of the big toe should be noted. Studies demonstrate high probability of osteoarthritis of the first MTP if examiner can detect dorsal exostosis, hard-end feel, crepitus less than 64° available dorsiflexion range of the first MTP along with 25 months of symptom history. The presence of three or more of these five features has a sensitivity of 88% and specificity of 71% [67].

Neurologic Lower extremity sensation should be tested to differentiate between painful ankle and foot OA from other medical conditions including peripheral neuropathy, stenosis, and radiculopathy. Motor strength should be tested including EHL (L5), ankle dorsiflexion, ankle eversion, extensor digitorum longus (digits 2–5), and flexor hallucis longus (curling toes). Reflexes should be tested as with any other neurological exam.

Table 53.4 Movements of the ankle joint [66]

Dorsiflexion	0–20°
Plantar flexion	0–50°
Inversion	0–35°
Eversion	0–15°

53.6.4.1 Ankle Exam

- Alignment: The normal ankle alignment is neutral. The examiner should evaluate for heel valgus angle.
- Passive and active ROM including supination and pronation of ankle and midfoot should be tested. In supination and pronation, ankle/foot moves in three planes. Supination is the combination of inversion, plantar flexion, and adduction. Pronation is the combination of eversion, dorsiflexion, and abduction. Deficits should be documented (Table 53.4).
- Too many toes. In a normal foot, you should not be able to see more than the fifth and fourth toes when the examiner looks at both ankles from behind. If there were more toes visible (third only or third and second), then it is called "too many toes" sign indicating an increased heel valgus angle (Fig. 53.12).
- Drawer test: It will test ankle stability and function of collateral ligaments.
- Talar tilt: It also tests the stability of the ankle, in particular the integrity of anterior talofibular and the calcaneofibular ligaments. The clinician would stabilize the distal part of the leg (just proximal to medial malleolus) with her nondominant hand while with the dominant hand, applies gradual inversion force to the hindfoot. The lateral talus should be palpated during maneuver to determine if the ankle joint is tilting.
- Silfverskiöld test: This test evaluates gastrocnemius contracture as a reason for posterior ankle pain/rigidity. The patient sits facing the examiner. The examiner will grasp the calcaneus with one hand, and with her other hand, the midfoot is locked into an anatomic position with the navicular aligned over the talus and the forefoot manipulated into plantar flexion or pronation.
- Squeeze test: It is designed to evaluate anterior inferior tibiofibular ligament sprain/injury in a patient with anterior ankle pain that resembles pain with OA. It is performed by squeezing then holding followed by quickly releasing the tibia and fibula just above the anterior tibiofibular ligament.

Midfoot exam The examiner should fully examine the midfoot by stabilizing the calcaneus and talus with one hand and move the foot with the other hand medially/abduction as well as laterally/abduction to observe any symptom reproduction. The motion of the first tarsometatarsal joint should be examined as well, in particular with patients who have hallux valgus.

Forefoot exam Metatarsophalangeal and interphalangeal joints are examined in forefoot examination. Each joint should be examined separately, and any deformity should be evaluated whether it is fixed or correctable.

53.6.5 Diagnostic Workup

53.6.5.1 Imaging: Ankle OA

Plain Films

X-rays are the gold standard for diagnosis of osteoarthritis. Weight-bearing AP and lateral views of the ankle and Mortise views are done for the assessment of osteoarthritis looking for joint space narrowing, osteophytes, and subchondral bone sclerosis. The Saltzmann view can be acquired for the evaluation of hindfoot alignment. The Kellgren–Lawrence score has been modified for the ankle joint (Table 53.5) [68]. A grade ≥1 is consistent with ankle osteoarthritis. Foot-specific atlas is another grading system developed by Menz et al. which assesses the weight-bearing foot in multiple views (dorsoplantar and lateral) and grade joint space narrowing and osteophytes [69].

Table 53.5 Modified Kellgren-Lawrence score of ankle OA

Grade 1	Osteophytes of questionable significance
Grade 2	Osteophytes on the medial malleolus
Grade 3	Osteophytes on the medial and/or lateral malleolus Moderate joint space narrowing <50%
Grade 4	Osteophytes on medial and lateral malleoli + tibiotalar joint margins Severe (>50%) joint space narrowing, tibiotalar sclerosis

Advanced Imaging

In the ankle OA, advanced imaging including MRI can detect joint effusion, synovitis, and bone marrow edema as a possible cause of pain. It can also detect underlying etiologies including ligament and tendon injuries, osteochondral lesions, and ankle impingement syndromes or postoperative changes. MR arthrography can be used in situations where there are no metallic components. CT arthrography is the imaging modality of choice in cartilage evaluation in the postoperative ankle joint to rule out early osteoarthritis.

53.6.5.2 Imaging: Foot OA

Plain films X-rays are the gold standard for diagnosis of foot OA. In the foot, weight-bearing AP, lateral, and internal rotation oblique radiographic views of the foot are helpful in the diagnosis (Fig. 53.13). Lateral weight-bearing radiographs may also demonstrate sagging of the medial column, either at the naviculocuneiform or at the talonavicular joint [70].

Advanced imaging Sophisticated testing including MRIs and CT scans may be necessary if soft tissue abnormalities are suspected or there are concerns regarding stress fracture, tumors, or lytic regions that may coexist along with the osteoarthritic changes seen on X-rays.

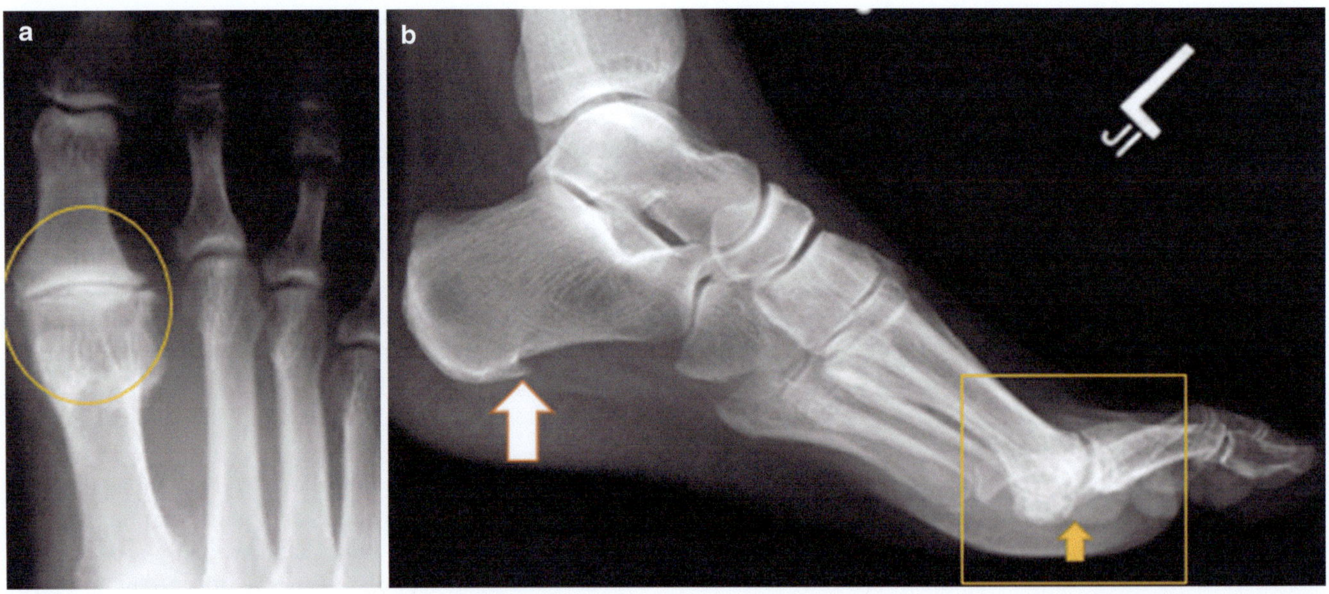

Fig. 53.13 (**a**) Severe OA of the first MTP joint. (**b**) The same OA on lateral view in addition to a small calcaneal spurring (thick arrow)

53.6.5.3 Ultrasound

US is portable, inexpensive, and could be valuable in evaluating foot and ankle pain in clinic or sideline. It could detect foot and ankle soft tissue abnormalities including tendons and ligaments and neurovascular structure. It could also evaluate the joints both in static and in dynamic fashion which provide valuable information that X-ray and MRI could not. Utilizing high-resolution probe, a great deal of information could be obtained particularly in midfoot and forefoot where most structures of interest are within 1-cm depth.

53.6.5.4 Diagnostic Injection

It may be difficult to identify the exact osteoarthritic joint that is causing patient's pain. In such cases, intra-articular diagnostic injection of anesthetic could provide valuable information and lead to more definitive treatment. Contrast-enhanced X-ray guidance or ultrasound guidance is necessary to confirm intra-articular placement in the target joint.

53.6.6 Treatment

53.6.6.1 Medial Management

The medical management of foot/ankle osteoarthritis is conceptualized as a means to facilitate participation in physical therapy, reduce pain as a symptom of osteoarthritis, and increase physical activity. In ankle and foot OA, based on clinical guidelines for knee and hip OA, research recommend education, exercise, and weight loss in the first line of recommended action. Regular exercise was found not to increase the risk for progression in foot and ankle osteoarthritis [69]. Low-impact aerobic exercise programs such as walking, biking, swimming, and other aquatic exercises may be best [77].

Mediations that can be incorporated in treatment plans are the following:

- *Acetaminophen* is widely regarded as a first-line agent.
- *Topical NSAIDs* (e.g., diclofenac gel) can be used to mitigate pain.
- *Oral NSAIDs* (Cox-I or Cox-II inhibitors) in patients without contraindications (GI, renal, anticoagulated).
- *Glucosamine-chondroitin sulfate* has limited data on effectiveness, but not harmful.

53.6.6.2 Rehabilitation

Rehab: Ankle OA

Strengthening, aerobic exercise, and weight loss may all help symptomatically manage pain related to ankle osteoarthritis [64]. Exercise is most effective when it consists of a combination of strength training (TheraBand exercises for gastrocnemius, soleus, tibialis anterior, and peronei), endurance training, active mobilizing exercises (ROM restoration, inversion, and eversion), balance and proprioceptive training (if there is instability), and functional exercises as they will combine several components simultaneously (one-legged stance, walk on uneven surfaces, climbing stairs) [72]. Some studies suggest hydrotherapy; swimming and water exercises are excellent for OA patients and provide pain relief and improve mobility [73]. Limited studies are available in the utility of electrotherapy, therapeutic ultrasound, laser, or electrotherapy in ankle OA. Education of the patient and self-management are both recommended.

Rehab: Midfoot and Forefoot OA

A number of rehabilitation strategies could be considered for painful osteoarthritis of the foot and toes. Rehab strategies in general includes therapeutical ultrasound, joint mobilization, stretching and strengthening exercises, application of cold packs, and electrical stimulation. In patients with first MTP OA, studies have shown that addition of sesamoid mobilization resulted in greater improvement in the first MTP range of motion, strength of toe flexor, and pain control [74]. Manipulation may also be performed in conjunction with other rehab modalities to maximize improvement although the therapeutic benefits of this technique appear to be limited to milder forms of the metatarsophalangeal OA [75].

53.6.6.3 Orthotics

Orthotics: Ankle OA

The objective of orthosis is to constrain the hindfoot motion in all planes while not impeding forefoot motion, for each ground condition. As a result, while walking on flat and uneven surface, the hindfoot remains stable and the patient experiences less pain. Custom-made ankle-foot orthosis (AFO), rigid hindfoot orthosis (HFO-R), and articulated hindfoot orthosis (HFO-A) are used in ankle OA. The AFO and HFO-R provide the best sagittal plane hindfoot motion restriction over all ground conditions [71].

Orthotics: Midfoot OA

The objective of orthotic is to facilitate the transfer of weight during gait, control excessive hindfoot eversion, and support the medial arch [61]. Both shoe-stiffening inserts and contoured foot orthoses have utility in individuals with midfoot OA. Examples include full-length flat carbon graphite inserts, rigid carbon fiber footplate insert, custom semi-rigid foot orthoses, and semi-custom root orthoses, and all were found to decrease pain [77]. Sneakers with rocker-bottom soles may help move pressure away from the midfoot and reduce symptoms [83].

Orthotics: First MTP OA

Contoured foot orthoses are commonly prescribed for people with first MTP joint OA; however, it is unknown whether these devices are effective in improving the symptoms associated with first MTP joint OA [81].

53.6.6.4 Procedures

Ankle and midfoot and forefoot intra-articular injections are done both for diagnostic and therapeutic purposes. Intra-articular placement of the needle should be done with X-ray visualization or with the use of ultrasound to be accurate and avoid complications (Fig. 53.14).

Recent cadaver studies have found that anesthetic drug leaks into adjacent joints in up to 20% of cases, thereby decreasing the selectivity of this diagnostic tool [82].

Similar to many other osteoarthritic conditions, for therapeutic purposes, the ankle and foot joints have been injected with a number of products including corticosteroid, hyaluronate, PRP, adipose or bone marrow mesenchymal cells, and prolotherapy. The goal of injectables are pain relief and improvement of function and increased tolerance to walking as well as increased participation in rehabilitation efforts. In general, the relative efficacy of all injectable therapies is far from definitive and warrants further high-quality comparative trials.

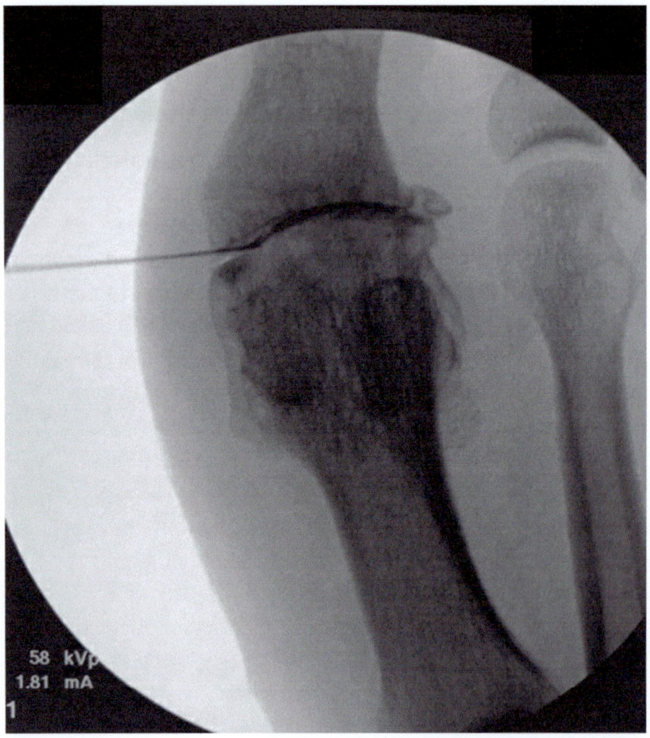

Fig. 53.14 X-ray-guided needle placement in the first metatarsophalangeal joint prior to injection or PRP. Contrast highlights correct needle placement

53.6.6.5 Steroid Injection

No placebo-controlled trials of intra-articular corticosteroid have been conducted for foot OA. Small studies regarding the effect of CSI on the midfoot shows ultrasound-guided corticosteroid injection resulted in pain relief in 78% of patients for 2 weeks, and only 15% of patient had sustained pain relief in 3 months [61].

53.6.6.6 Hyaluronan

- *Ankle*: A number of studies have been done including randomized control trial to compare steroid to platelet-rich plasma and mesenchymal stem cells for treatment of ankle pain. In such studies, corticosteroid injection had good but short-lived benefit or pain relief [78]. Evidence from small trials favors HA and PRP injections for the treatment of pain associated with ankle osteoarthritis. Injection of hyaluronic acid into the ankle joint improved ankle osteoarthritis scale for about 6 months as compared to saline injection ($n = 109$) [78].
- *MTP:* Small, randomized trial of patients with hallux rigidus reported that hyaluronan injection was more effective at reducing gait-related pain than corticosteroid injection [79]. Only randomized controlled trial so far undertaken found intra-articular injection of Hylan G-F 20 is no more effective than a placebo (saline) in reducing symptoms of first MTP OA ($N = 151$) [80].

53.6.6.7 Surgery

Surgical intervention may be indicated in patients with symptoms that have failed to respond to all nonsurgical therapy. More details regarding foot and ankle surgery is discussed elsewhere in the book.

Surgery: Medial Midfoot

Arthrodesis of the medial and middle columns is the mainstay of surgical treatment in persons with arthritis of the TMT and naviculocuneiform joint. Achievement of stability in the medial and middle columns requires that the first, second, and, potentially, third TMT joints be included in the arthrodesis along with the corresponding intercuneiform joints. A variety of plate and compression screws are used to achieve fusion [83].

Surgery: Lateral Midfoot

Data on surgical care for lateral midfoot is mixed. Few published studies suggest that arthrodesis of the more mobile lateral column should be performed, and several others suggest that bony fusion of these rays may lead to other complications including chronic lateral foot pain and an increased rate of nonunion or predisposition to fifth metatarsal fracture. A study by Raikin and Schon determined that arthrodesis of the fourth and fifth metatarsal joints can produce good outcomes in patients with lateral midfoot collapse, rocker-bottom deformity, and severe arthritic degeneration [84].

Surgery: First MTP OA

Both arthrodesis and hemiarthroplasty are performed for advanced osteoarthritis of the first metatarsophalangeal joint that is not responsive to nonoperative care. Controversy remains whether hemiarthroplasty or arthrodesis results in better postoperative outcomes. In a comparative study, the two groups had similar symptom intensity and degree of disability at greater than or equal to 1-year mark, although the patients were subjectively more pleased with the results after hemiarthroplasty [85].

References

1. Zhang Y, Jordan JM. Epidemiology of osteoarthritis. Clin Geriatr Med. 2010;26(3):355–69. https://doi.org/10.1016/j.cger.2010.03.001. Erratum in: Clin Geriatr Med. 2013 May;29(2):ix. PMID: 20699159; PMCID: PMC2920533.
2. Ansok CB, Muh SJ. Optimal management of glenohumeral osteoarthritis. Orthop Res Rev. 2018;10:9–18. Published 2018 Feb 23. https://doi.org/10.2147/ORR.S134732.
3. Leyland KM, Hart DJ, Javaid MK, Judge A, Kiran A, Soni A, Goulston LM, Cooper C, Spector TD, Arden NK. The natural history of radiographic knee osteoarthritis: a fourteen-year population-based cohort study. Arthritis Rheum. 2012;64(7):2243–51. https://doi.org/10.1002/art.34415. PMID: 22422507.
4. Millett PJ, Gobezie R, Boykin RE. Shoulder osteoarthritis: diagnosis and management. Am Fam Physician. 2008;78(5):605–11. PMID: 18788237.
5. Guedes V, Castro JP, Brito I. Topical capsaicin for pain in osteoarthritis: a literature review. Reumatol Clin. 2018;14(1):40–5. https://doi.org/10.1016/j.reuma.2016.07.008. English, Spanish. Epub 2016 Aug 27. PMID: 27575891.
6. Macías-Hernández SI, Morones-Alba JD, Miranda-Duarte A, Coronado-Zarco R, Soria-Bastida MLA, Nava-Bringas T, Cruz-Medina E, Olascoaga-Gómez A, Tallabs-Almazan LV, Palencia C. Glenohumeral osteoarthritis: overview, therapy, and rehabilitation. Disabil Rehabil. 2017;39(16):1674–82. https://doi.org/10.1080/09638288.2016.1207206. Epub 2016 Jul 14. PMID: 27416338.
7. Metzger CM, Farooq H, Merrell GA, Kaplan FTD, Greenberg JA, Crosby NE, Peck KM, Hoyer RW. Efficacy of a single, image-guided corticosteroid injection for glenohumeral arthritis. J Shoulder Elb Surg. 2021;30(5):1128–34. https://doi.org/10.1016/j.jse.2020.08.008. Epub 2020 Aug 25. PMID: 32858193.
8. Merolla G, Sperling JW, Paladini P, Porcellini G. Efficacy of Hylan G-F 20 versus 6-methylprednisolone acetate in painful shoulder osteoarthritis: a retrospective controlled trial. Musculoskelet Surg. 2011;95(3):215–24. https://doi.org/10.1007/s12306-011-0138-3. Epub 2011 May 13. PMID: 21567154.
9. Cushman DM, Bruno B, Christiansen J, Schultz A, McCormick ZL. Efficacy of injected corticosteroid type, dose, and volume for pain in large joints: a narrative review. PM R. 2018;10(7):748–57. https://doi.org/10.1016/j.pmrj.2018.01.002. Epub 2018 Jan 31. PMID: 29407227.
10. Wernecke C, Braun HJ, Dragoo JL. The effect of intra-articular corticosteroids on articular cartilage: a systematic review. Orthop J Sports Med. 2015;3(5):2325967115581163. https://doi.org/10.1177/2325967115581163. PMID: 26674652; PMCID: PMC4622344.
11. Blaine T, Moskowitz R, Udell J, Skyhar M, Levin R, Friedlander J, Daley M, Altman R. Treatment of persistent shoulder pain with sodium hyaluronate: a randomized, controlled trial. A multicenter study. J Bone Joint Surg Am. 2008;90(5):970–9. https://doi.org/10.2106/JBJS.F.01116. PMID: 18451387.
12. Rossi LA, Piuzzi NS, Shapiro SA. Glenohumeral osteoarthritis: the role for orthobiologic therapies: platelet-rich plasma and cell therapies. JBJS Rev. 2020;8(2):e0075. https://doi.org/10.2106/JBJS.RVW.19.00075.
13. Mansfield JT, Desai MJ. Axillary peripheral nerve stimulation for painful end-stage primary osteoarthritis of the shoulder: a case report. Neuromodulation. 2020;23(6):878–80. https://doi.org/10.1111/ner.13089. Epub 2019 Dec 16. PMID: 31845412.
14. Mansfield JT, Desai MJ. Axillary peripheral nerve stimulation for chronic shoulder pain: a retrospective case series. Neuromodulation. 2020;23(6):812–8. https://doi.org/10.1111/ner.13096. Epub 2020 Jan 13. PMID: 31930660.
15. Mazzola A, Spinner D. Ultrasound-guided peripheral nerve stimulation for shoulder pain: anatomic review and assessment of the current clinical evidence. Pain Physician. 2020;23(5):E461–74. PMID: 32967397.
16. Ravalli S, Pulici C, Binetti S, Aglieco A, Vecchio M, Musumeci G. An overview of the pathogenesis and treatment of elbow osteoarthritis. J Funct Morphol Kinesiol [Internet]. 2019. [cited 2021 Apr 11];;4(2):30.
17. Spector TD, MacGregor AJ. Risk factors for osteoarthritis: genetics. Osteoarthr Cartil. 2004;12(Suppl A):S39–44.
18. McAuliffe JA. Surgical alternatives for elbow arthritis in the young adult. Hand Clin. 2002;18(1):99–111.
19. Gramstad GD, Galatz LM. Management of elbow osteoarthritis. J Bone Joint Surg Am. 2006;88(2):421–30.
20. Stanley D. Prevalence and etiology of symptomatic elbow osteoarthritis. J Shoulder Elb Surg. 1994;3(6):386–9.
21. Morrey BF. Primary degenerative arthritis of the elbow. Treatment by ulnohumeral arthroplasty. J Bone Joint Surg Br. 1992;74(3):409–13.
22. Papatheodorou LK, Baratz ME, Sotereanos DG. Elbow arthritis: current concepts. J Hand Surg. 2013;38(3):605–13.
23. Savoie FH, O'Brien MJ, Field LD. Arthroscopy for arthritis of the elbow. Hand Clin. 2011;27(2):171–8, v–vi.
24. Wiffen PJ, Xia J. Systematic review of topical diclofenac for the treatment of acute and chronic musculoskeletal pain. Curr Med Res Opin. 2020;36(4):637–50.
25. Yang W, Sun C, He SQ, Chen JY, Wang Y, Zhuo Q. The efficacy and safety of disease-modifying osteoarthritis drugs for knee and hip osteoarthritis-a systematic review and network meta-analysis. J Gen Intern Med. 2021;36(7):2085–93.
26. Ogata T, Ideno Y, Akai M, Seichi A, Hagino H, Iwaya T, et al. Effects of glucosamine in patients with osteoarthritis of the knee: a systematic review and meta-analysis. Clin Rheumatol. 2018;37(9):2479–87.
27. Singh JA, Noorbaloochi S, MacDonald R, Maxwell LJ. Chondroitin for osteoarthritis. Cochrane Database Syst Rev. 2015;1:CD005614.
28. Martinez-Silvestrini J. Prescribing medications for pain and inflammation. In: Frontera WR, Herring SA, Micheli LJ, Silver JK, editors. Clinical sports medicine: medical management and rehabilitation, text with CD-ROM. Philadelphia: Elsevier; 2006. p. 512.
29. Sorani A, Campbell R. Image-guided elbow interventions: a literature review of interventional treatment options. Br J Radiol. 2016;89(1057):20150368.

30. Akhondi H, Panginikkod S. Wrist arthritis. [Updated 2021 Jul 8]. In: StatPearls [Internet]. Treasure Island: StatPearls Publishing; 2021. Available from: https://www.ncbi.nlm.nih.gov/books/NBK531497/.
31. Kurdi AJ, Voss BA, Tzeng TH, Scaife SL, El-Othmani MM, Saleh KJ. Rheumatoid arthritis vs osteoarthritis: comparison of demographics and trends of joint replacement data from the nationwide inpatient sample. Am J Orthop (Belle Mead NJ). 2018;47(7) [PubMed] [Reference list].
32. Lotz MK, Kraus VB. New developments in osteoarthritis. Posttraumatic osteoarthritis: pathogenesis and pharmacological treatment options. Arthritis Res Ther. 2010;12(3):211.
33. Lawrence RC, Felson DT, Helmick CG, Arnold LM, Choi H, Deyo RA, Gabriel S, Hirsch R, Hochberg MC, Hunder GG, Jordan JM, Katz JN, Kremers HM, Wolfe F, National Arthritis Data Workgroup. Estimates of the prevalence of arthritis and other rheumatic conditions in the United States. Part II. Arthritis Rheum. 2008;58(1):26–35. https://doi.org/10.1002/art.23176.
34. Wilder FV, Barrett JP, Farina EJ. Joint-specific prevalence of osteoarthritis of the hand. Osteoarthr Cartil. 2006;14(9):953–7. Epub 2006 Jun 8. PMID: 16759885.
35. Rees F, Doherty S, Hui M, Maciewicz R, Muir K, Zhang W, Doherty M. Distribution of finger nodes and their association with underlying radiographic features of osteoarthritis. Arthritis Care Res (Hoboken). 2012;64(4):533–8. https://doi.org/10.1002/acr.21586. PMID: 22213746.
36. Bain GI, Polites N, Higgs BG, Heptinstall RJ, McGrath AM. The functional range of motion of the finger joints. J Hand Surg Eur. 2015;40(4):406–11. https://doi.org/10.1177/1753193414533754. Epub 2014 May 23. PMID: 24859993.
37. El-Deek AMF, Hassan Dawood EMAEH. Role of ultrasonography in evaluation of tendons abnormalities in hand and fingers. Egypt J Radiol Nucl Med. 2019;50:108. https://doi.org/10.1186/s43055-019-0110-z.
38. Østerås N, Kjeken I, Smedslund G, et al. Exercise for hand osteoarthritis. Cochrane Database Syst Rev. 2017;1(1):CD010388. Published 2017 Jan 31.
39. Heyworth BE, Lee JH, Kim PD, Lipton CB, Strauch RJ, Rosenwasser MP. Hylan versus corticosteroid versus placebo for treatment of basal joint arthritis: a prospective, randomized, double-blinded clinical trial. J Hand Surg. 2008;33:40–8.
40. Berber O, Garagnani L, Gidwani S. Systematic review of total wrist arthroplasty and arthrodesis in wrist arthritis. J Wrist Surg. 2018;7(5):424–40. https://doi.org/10.1055/s-0038-1646956.
41. Thompson JC. Netter's concise orthopaedic anatomy. 2nd ed. Philadelphia: Saunders/Elsevier; 2016. p. 286–323.
42. Primorac D, Molnar V, Rod E, Jeleč Ž, Čukelj F, Matišić V, Vrdoljak T, Damir Hudetz HH, Borić I. Knee osteoarthritis: a review of pathogenesis and state-of-the-art non-operative therapeutic considerations. Genes (Basel). 2020;11(8):854–89.
43. Sharma L. Osteoarthritis of the knee. N Engl J Med. 2021;384:51–9.
44. Stoddart JC, Dandridge O, Garner A, Cobb J, van Arkel RJ. The compartmental distribution of knee osteoarthritis – a systematic review and meta-analysis. Osteoarthr Cartil [Internet]. 2021;29(4):445–55. Available from: https://doi.org/10.1016/j.joca.2020.10.011.
45. Kellgren JH, Lawrence JS. Radiological assessment of osteoarthosis. Ann Rheum Dis. 1957;(16):494.
46. Jacobson J. Fundamentals of musculoskeletal ultrasound, vol. 3. 3rd ed. Philadelphia: Elsevier; 2018. p. 308.
47. Bruyère O, Cooper C, Pelletier JP, Maheu E, Rannou F, Branco J, et al. A consensus statement on the European Society for Clinical and Economic Aspects of Osteoporosis and Osteoarthritis (ESCEO) algorithm for the management of knee osteoarthritis-from evidence-based medicine to the real-life setting. Semin Arthritis Rheum [Internet]. 2016;45(4):S3–11.
48. Zacharias A, Green RA, Semciw AI, Kingsley MIC, Pizzari. Efficacy of rehabilitation programs for improving muscle strength in people with hip or knee osteoarthritis: a systematic review with meta-analysis. Osteoarthr Cartil. 2014;22:1752–73.
49. Hislop AC, Collins NJ, Tucker K, Deasy M, Semciw AI. Does adding hip exercises to quadriceps exercises result in superior outcomes in pain, function and quality of life for people with knee osteoarthritis? A systematic review and meta-analysis. Br J Sports Med. 2020;54:263–71.
50. Melese H, Alamer A, Hailu Temesgen M, Nigussie F. Effectiveness of kinesio taping on the management of knee osteoarthritis: a systematic review of randomized controlled trials. J Pain Res. 2020;13:1267–76. Published 2020 May 28. https://doi.org/10.2147/JPR.S249567.
51. Xu Q, Chen B, Wang Y, Wang X, Han D, Ding D, Zheng Y, Cao Y, Zhan H, Zhou Y. The effectiveness of manual therapy for relieving pain, stiffness, and dysfunction in knee osteoarthritis: a systematic review and meta-analysis. Pain Physician. 2017;20:229–43.
52. Ekstrom RA, Donatelli RA, Carp KC. Electromyographic analysis of core trunk, hip, and thigh muscles during 9 rehabilitation exercises. J Orthop Sports Phys Ther. 2007;37(12):754–62. https://doi.org/10.2519/jospt.2007.2471.
53. Bartels EM, Juhl CB, Christensen R, Hagen KB, Danneskiold-Samsøe B, Dagfinrud H, Lund H. Aquatic exercise for the treatment of knee and hip osteoarthritis. Cochrane Database Syst Rev. 2016;3:CD005523. https://doi.org/10.1002/14651858.CD005523.pub3. Accessed 22 Mar 2021.
54. Raja K, Dewan N. Efficacy of knee braces and foot orthoses in conservative management of knee osteoarthritis. Am J Phys Med Rehabil. 2011;90(3):247–62. https://doi.org/10.1097/PHM.0b013e318206386b.
55. Anwer S, Alghadir A, Brismée JM. Effect of home exercise program in patients with knee osteoarthritis: a systematic review and meta-analysis. J Geriatr Phys Ther. 2016;39(1):38–48.
56. Billesberger LM, Fisher KM, Qadri YJ, Boortz-Marx RL. Procedural treatments for knee osteoarthritis: a review of current injectable therapies. Pain Res Manag. 2020;2020:1–11.
57. Jayaram P, Kennedy DJ, Yeh P, Dragoo J. Chondrotoxic effects of local anesthetics on human knee articular cartilage: a systematic review. PM R. 2019;11(4):379–400.
58. Alden KJ, Harris S, Hubbs B, Kot K, Istwan NB, Mason D. Micronized dehydrated human amnion chorion membrane injection in the treatment of knee osteoarthritis-a large retrospective case series. J Knee Surg. 2021;34(8):841–5. https://doi.org/10.1055/s--0039-3400951. Epub 2019 Nov 28. PMID: 31779034.
59. Ikeuchi M, Ushida T, Izumi M, Tani T. Percutaneous radiofrequency treatment for refractory anteromedial pain of osteoarthritic knees. Pain Med. 2011;12(4):546–51.
60. Paterson KL, Kasza J, Hunter DJ, et al. The relationship between foot and ankle symptoms and risk of developing knee osteoarthritis: data from the osteoarthritis initiative. Osteoarthr Cartil. 2017;25(5):639–46. https://doi.org/10.1016/j.joca.2016.12.003.
61. Roddy E, Menz HB. Foot osteoarthritis: latest evidence and developments. Ther Adv Musculoskelet Dis. 2018;10(4):91–103. https://doi.org/10.1177/1759720X17753337.
62. Roddy E, Thomas MJ, Marshall M, et al. The population prevalence of symptomatic radiographic foot osteoarthritis in community-dwelling older adults: cross-sectional findings from the Clinical Assessment Study of the Foot. Ann Rheum Dis. 2015;74:156–63.
63. Thomas MJ, Peat G, Rathod T, Marshall M, Moore A, Menz HB, Roddy E. The epidemiology of symptomatic midfoot osteoarthritis in community-dwelling older adults: cross-sectional findings from the Clinical Assessment Study of the Foot. Arthritis Res Ther. 2015;17(1):178. https://doi.org/10.1186/s13075-015-0693-3. PMID: 26166410; PMCID: PMC4499901.

64. National Clinical Guideline Centre. Osteoarthritis: care and management in adults. Clinic guideline CG177. Methods, evidence and recommendations. London: National Institute for Health and care Excellence; 2014.
65. Mahiquez MY, Wilder FV, Stephens HM. Positive hindfoot valgus and osteoarthritis of the first metatarsophalangeal joint. Foot Ankle Int. 2006;27(12):1055–9. https://doi.org/10.1177/107110070602701210. PMID: 17207432
66. Alazzawi S, Sukeik M, King D, Vemulapalli K. Foot and ankle history and clinical examination: a guide to everyday practice. World J Orthop. 2017;8(1):21–9. Published 2017 Jan 18. https://doi.org/10.5312/wjo.v8.i1.21.
67. Zammit GV, Munteanu SE, Menz HB. Development of a diagnostic rule for identifying radiographic osteoarthritis in people with first metatarsophalangeal joint pain. Osteoarthr Cartil. 2011;19(8):939–45. https://doi.org/10.1016/j.joca.2011.04.010. Epub 2011 May 12. PMID: 21619934.
68. Holzer N, Salvo D, Marijnissen A, et al. Radiographic evaluation of posttraumatic osteoarthritis of the ankle: the Kellgren-Lawrence scale is reliable and correlates with clinical symptoms. Osteoarthr Cartil. 2015;23(3):363–9.
69. Paterson KL, Gates L. Clinical assessment and management of foot and ankle osteoarthritis: a review of current evidence and focus on pharmacological treatment. Drugs Aging. 2019;36(3):203–11.
70. Patel A, Rao S, Nawoczenski D, Flemister AS, DiGiovanni B, Baumhauer JF. Midfoot arthritis. J Am Acad Orthop Surg. 2010;18(7):417–25. https://doi.org/10.5435/00124635-201007000-00004. PMID: 20595134.
71. Huang YC, Harbst K, Kotajarvi B, Hansen D, Koff MF, Kitaoka HB, Kaufman KR. Effects of ankle-foot orthoses on ankle and foot kinematics in patient with ankle osteoarthritis. Arch Phys Med Rehabil. 2006;87:710–6.
72. Peter WFH, Jansen MJ, Bloo H, et al. KNGF-richtlijn Artrose heup-knie. Supplement Nederlands Tijdschrift voor Fysiotherapie 120, 2010.
73. Reginster JY, Pelletier JP, Martel-Pelletier J, Henrotin Y. Osteoarthritis: clinical and experimental aspects. Berlin: Springer; 1999. p. 1–17.
74. Shamus J, Shamus E, Gugel RN, Brucker BS, Skaruppa C. The effect of sesamoid mobilization, flexor hallucis strengthening, and gait training on reducing pain and restoring function in individuals with hallux limitus: a clinical trial. J Orthop Sports Phys Ther. 2004;34(7):368–76. https://doi.org/10.2519/jospt.2004.34.7.368. PMID: 15296364.
75. Solan MC, Calder JD, Bendall SP. Manipulation and injection for hallux rigidus. Is it worthwhile? J Bone Joint Surg Br. 2001;83(5):706–8. https://doi.org/10.1302/0301-620x.83b5.11425. PMID: 11476310
76. Wilder FV, Barrett JP Jr, Farina EJ. Effect of regular exercise on the radiographic progression of foot osteoarthritis. J Am Podiatr Med Assoc. 2005;95(4):342–6.
77. Iagnocco A, Rizzo C, Gattamelata A, et al. Osteoarthritis of the foot: a review of the current state of knowledge. Med Ultrason. 2013;15(1):35–40.
78. Vannabouathong C, Del Fabbro G, Sales B, Smith C, Li CS, Yardley D, Bhandari M, Petrisor BA. Intra-articular injections in the treatment of symptoms from ankle arthritis: a systematic review. Foot Ankle Int. 2018;39(10):1141–50. https://doi.org/10.1177/1071100718779375. Epub 2018 Jun 18. PMID: 29909689.
79. Pons M, Alvarez F, Solana J, Viladot R, Varela L. Sodium hyaluronate in the treatment of hallux rigidus. A single-blind, randomized study. Foot Ankle Int. 2007;28(1):38–42.
80. Munteanu SE, Zammit GV, Menz HB, Landorf KB, Handley CJ, Elzarka A, Deluca J. Effectiveness of intra-articular hyaluronan (Synvisc, hylan G-F 20) for the treatment of first metatarsophalangeal joint osteoarthritis: a randomised placebo-controlled trial. Ann Rheum Dis. 2011;70(10):1838–41. https://doi.org/10.1136/ard.2011.153049. Epub 2011 Jul 25
81. Paterson KL, Hinman RS, Metcalf BR, Jones SE, Menz HB, Munteanu SE, Kasza J, Bennell KL. Foot orthoses for first metatarsophalangeal joint osteoarthritis: study protocol for the FORT randomised controlled trial. BMC Musculoskelet Disord. 2020;21(1):830.
82. Khosla S, Thiele R, Baumhauer JF. Ultrasound guidance for intra-articular injections of the foot and ankle. Foot Ankle Int. 2009;30(9):886–90.
83. Patel A, Rao S, Nawoczenski D, Flemister AS, DiGiovanni B, Baumhauer JF. Midfoot arthritis. J Am Acad Orthopaed Surg. 2010;18(7):417–25.
84. Raikin SM, Schon LC. Arthrodesis of the fourth and fifth tarsometatarsal joints of the midfoot. Foot Ankle Int. 2003;24(8):584–90. https://doi.org/10.1177/107110070302400803. PMID: 12956562.
85. Voskuijl T, Onstenk R. Operative treatment for osteoarthritis of the first metatarsophalangeal joint: arthrodesis versus hemiarthroplasty. J Foot Ankle Surg. 2015;54(6):1085–8. https://doi.org/10.1053/j.jfas.2015.06.019. Epub 2015 Aug 12. PMID.

Osteoporosis

54

Tony K. George and Jonathan M. Hagedorn

54.1 ICD-10

- Osteoporotic vertebral fracture M80.08xx
- Pathological vertebral fracture M84.48xx
- Pars fracture/spondylolysis M43.00
- Hip fracture M80.059
- Wrist fracture S62.109

54.2 Description

Osteoporosis is a diffuse demineralization of the bone. It is caused by an imbalance between bone production and resorption. Bone turnover increases later in life with decreasing sex hormones and can affect both sexes. Estrogen deficiency during menopause is a major risk factor for osteoporotic incidence. Although rare, children can be affected due to genetic or chronic diseases. Risk factors for osteoporosis are outlined in Table 54.1.

Insufficiency fracture is a result of bone demineralization, particularly in weight-bearing bones or spine.

Table 54.1 Common risk factors for osteoporosis

Common risk factors for osteoporosis [1]	
Estrogen deficiency	Chronic steroid use
Thyroid disorders	Malabsorption disorders
Anorexia	Cushing's syndrome
Chronic renal failure	Chronic antiepileptics use
Family history of fractures	Smoking
Alcohol intake	Females/White race
Age 50 or above	Early or on-time menopause

T. K. George (✉)
Restorative Orthopaedics Spine & Sports (ROSS) Institute, Somerset, NJ, USA

Department of Orthopaedics, Rutgers-Robert Wood Johnson Medical School, New Brunswick, NJ, USA

J. M. Hagedorn
Department of Anesthesiology and Perioperative Medicine, Division of Pain Medicine, Mayo Clinic, Rochester, MN, USA

Pathologic fractures are caused by the metastatic spread of cancer to the bone.

The femur, spine, and distal radius are common areas to fracture, and most of these occur from a fall. The femur has the highest incidence and also the highest predictability of fractures [2]. Fracture incidence is more common in females yet mortality is higher in males [3]. The thoracolumbar spine area at T10-L2 is the most common region of the spine affected by trauma due to the specific biomechanics of this segment.

Bone density testing combined with clinical risk scores, including Fracture Risk Assessment Tool (FRAX), can be used to predict which individuals are at high risk of fracture. The FRAX® algorithms give the 10-year probability of fracture. It incorporates several risk factors (which we described in Table 54.1) in calculating fracture risk.

54.3 Diagnostic Workup

54.3.1 Bone Density Testing

Dual-energy *X-ray* absorptiometry (DEXA) scans to measure bone mineral density (BMD) at the spine and hip have an important role in the evaluation of individuals at risk of osteoporosis. It is considered the gold standard for osteoporosis screening and recommended by the United States Preventive Services Task Force for women ages 65 and older [7]. Guidelines recommend earlier screening (age 50) in those with history of fracture and other clinical risk factors [8].

The result of this test allows clinicians to advise patients about the appropriate use of anti-fracture treatment. The z scores in the results enable BMD measurements to be compared between men and women of different ages and ethnic groups. The *T* scores compare the BMD measurements with those at an age when bone density is at its peak. The World Health Organization definition of osteoporosis and osteopenia used to interpret spine, hip, and forearm dual-energy X-ray absorptiometry scan results in postmenopausal White

© The Author(s), under exclusive license to Springer Nature Switzerland AG 2022
S. A. Mostoufi et al. (eds.), *Clinical Guide to Musculoskeletal Medicine*, https://doi.org/10.1007/978-3-030-92042-5_54

Table 54.2 The World Health Organization definitions of osteoporosis and osteopenia

The World Health Organization definitions of osteoporosis	
Normal	*T*-score ⩾ −1.0
Osteopenia	−2.5 < *T*-score < −1.0
Osteoporosis	*T*-score < −2.5
Established osteoporosis	*T*-score ⩾ −2.5 in the presence of one or more fracture

women (Table 54.2). Of regions susceptible to low scores, a low hip score has the highest predictivity for fractures [2].

54.3.2 X-Rays

X-rays are not used for the diagnosis of osteoporosis, but experienced radiologists can detect lower than normal bone density when visualizing X-rays. X-rays are used to detect fractures related to osteoporosis which commonly happens in the hip and the spine.

54.3.3 MRI

- Diagnostic MR: The postmenopausal women with osteoporosis exhibited a corresponding increase in vertebral marrow fat content as the bone density decreased. Bone marrow signal takes on a heterogeneous appearance with rounded focal fatty lesions replacing normal marrow with coalescence often occurring (*T1*: heterogeneously hyperintense, *T2*: variable signal). MR spectroscopy and diffusion-weighted magnetic resonance (indirect MRI methods) can assess vertebral marrow changes in postmenopausal women [12].
- MR and Fracture: It has high sensitivity and specificity (sensitivity 100% and specificity 85%) and is extremely useful for fracture diagnosis. MRI is superior and the preferred modality of choice in the diagnosis of stress fractures [9]. MR T_1, T_2, and STIR sequence imaging are utilized to visualize fracture lines from different exposures.

54.3.4 CT Scan

- Diagnostic CT: Quantitative CT can measure bone mineralization and BMD, which is usually done in the lumbar spine. In this modality, the tissue density of the analyzed volume is calibrated to units of equivalent concentration of a hydroxyapatite phantom in g/cm^3 yielding the BMD values.
- CT and Fractures: CT has sensitivity and specificity of 99% and 69% respectively. It is particularly useful for longitudinal fractures and stress fractures of the spine, of which a pars fracture is the most familiar. It is better than X-rays but not superior to MRI.

54.4 Presenting Symptoms

- Asymptomatic Osteoporosis

  Examination of a symptom-free/fracture-free individual with osteoporosis should be normal. Osteoporosis is only symptomatic when associated with fracture.
- Symptomatic Osteoporosis

  Patients with osteoporotic fractures would be in pain and will have mobility impairment. The setting of examination is often an emergency room in which an acute fracture has occurred either at the hip, wrist, spine, or any other long bone. Most hip and forearm fractures occur after a fall [4, 5], but the fractures of the spine/sacrum may be associated with less dramatic injury (sneeze, cough, misstep, etc.). In painful vertebral fractures, transition activities from lying to sitting or sitting to standing are often painful.

54.5 Physical Examination

Vertebral Fracture A classic presentation includes a female over the age of 50, thin-framed, and frail with a forward riding head and body tilt. A step-off may be present at the involved level of the compression fracture in the spine. Tenderness to palpation is present at the affected spinal level occurring at the thoracic or thoracolumbar junction, a common area of compression fractures around the spine. The range of motion could be compromised but can be insidious. In the spine, increased kyphotic angulation of the thoracic spine with step-off may be noted on visual inspection. In cases of prior compression fractures, advancing in anterior wedging presents as an exaggerated thoracic kyphosis and forward lean. Such postures, as expected, increase the risk of future falls, wedging, and new fractures.

Long Bone Fracture In hip/wrist/long bone fractures, deformed may be noted which would correspond to X-ray finding of the fracture. In hip fracture, shortened and externally rotated hip is often observed, and minor motion triggers pain. Antalgic gait may be present from stress injuries of the foot and ankle as would hip fractures [6]. Ecchymosis and soft tissue hematoma/swelling are often present with long bone fractures.

54.6 Treatments

54.6.1 Medical Management

- Calcium and vitamin D supplements are recommended for maintaining bone mineral density. Vitamin D recommendations for postmenopausal women are 800–1000 IU daily and 1200 mg for calcium [10]. Although important for BMD, their utility in preventing fractures is controversial. For those already at high risk, bisphosphonate therapy is initiated through oral or IV forms. Benefit is noted with discontinuation even after 5 years of bisphosphonate maintenance.
- Bracing: Indicated for stable fractures with no neurologic deficits. In most stable spine fractures, the purpose of the orthotic management effort is to relieve pain and discomfort and at the same time allow healing. Depending on the location of the fracture, brace is indicated to immobilize the segment, assist with pain relief, and improve function. For the lower thoracic spine through L1, thoraco-lumbosacral total-contact orthoses (TLSO) are utilized. For L2–5 compression fracture, lumbosacral orthosis may be adequate. Ideal brace should be light-weighted, easy wearing, and comfortable with compatible cushions. A graduated brace removal protocol is encouraged as fracture healing transitions from acute, to subacute, to chronic.
- Young patients with acute spondylolysis generally receive conservative management as their initial treatment. It consists of bracing, activity restriction, physical therapy, and pain control. Brace recommendation (TLSO) consists of 23 h a day usage for up to 6 months, with a subsequent six-month weaning period and physical therapy. Compliance is an issue with young brace wearers.
- Pain Management: Nociceptive pain often requires a short course of opioid management for optimal analgesia and basic mobility. In some cases, Tylenol and ice combined with bracing may be adequate. Nociceptive pain should resolve as the bone goes through its natural course of healing.

54.6.2 Rehabilitation

There is a diverse approach to rehabilitation after vertebral fracture. Most clinicians take the most conservative route, encouraging daily walks with thoracolumbar support, and introduction of pool therapy approximately 4 weeks after the incident of fracture. Most fractures solidify within 12 weeks after which a gentle progressive exercise program may add value in terms of mobility, paraspinal muscle strength, postural correction, and pain relief. Balance training should be introduced in patients with poor balance to prevent future fracture. In the studies available, there is uncertainty regarding the benefit of exercise to improve pain, self-reported physical function, and disease-specific quality-of-life metrics. Most studies demonstrated no clinically significant differences for these outcomes although pooled analysis showed a minor difference in favor of exercise [13]. After the expected course of healing for the vertebral fracture, regular exercises are encouraged including low-impact strengthening, weight-bearing exercises to maintain bone density, and patient education to avoid aggressive forward flexion, heavy lifting, axial load such as jumping, and overhead weight lifting and push-up/curl-ups [11].

54.6.3 Interventional Procedures

54.6.3.1 Vertebral Augmentation

Vertebral augmentation is a procedure in which fractured osteoporotic vertebrae are percutaneously injected with polymethylmethacrylate cement. The procedure is performed with or without the creation of a cavity using an expandable balloon. The procedure can also be performed after partial height restoration through percutaneously placed implantable devices, followed by injection of cement.

Indication and Contraindications

- Indications for vertebral augmentation include acute (<6 weeks) painful vertebral compression fractures (VCFs) resulting from osteoporotic, traumatic, and neoplastic etiologies. The most common cause of vertebral compression fractures is osteoporosis [26]. Options for bone augmentation are vertebroplasty, balloon kyphoplasty, and newer intraosseous implantable devices.
- Relative contraindications include VCF involving the posterior vertebral body cortex (posterior cortical breach) and patients experiencing only mild-to-moderate pain controlled with conservative measures.
- Absolute contraindications include lack of patient consent, unstable fractures, active infections both near and distant from the VCF, coagulation disorders, and complete vertebral collapse [27].

Literature Support

- Numerous studies have evaluated the effectiveness of vertebroplasty, balloon kyphoplasty, and intraosseous implantable devices. Early studies were nonrandomized and led to debate regarding the efficacy of vertebral augmentation procedures. In 2009, two studies were published questioning the benefits of vertebroplasty and kyphoplasty [14, 15]. However, more recently, substantial evidence has been published showing the beneficial clinical results of these treatments for patients with VCF, includ-

Table 54.3 The outcome comparison of different vertebral augmentation techniques

	Vertebroplasty	Kyphoplasty	OsseoFix®	SpineJack®	Kiva
Vertebral height change	No	Yes	Yes	Yes	Yes
Cement leakage	20–70%	4–13.7%	4%	5%	0.03%
VAS decrease	50%	45%	44%	55%	47%
ODI improvement	54%	55%	43%	30.9%	30.9%

Modified and simplified table from Long et al. [16]

ing improved pain relief, functional outcomes, and quality of life [16–21]. Table 54.3 provides a comparison of vertebral augmentation technique outcomes for height restoration, cement leakage, VAS, and ODI.

54.7 Types of Vertebral Augmentation

A. *Vertebroplasty*

Procedures are performed in an outpatient setting, with light conscious sedation, prophylactic antibiotics, and under local anesthesia. Procedures are performed in sterile fashion. There are two techniques for performing vertebroplasty, transpedicular and parapedicular approaches. The transpedicular approach is more common [22], but the parapedicular approach may be necessary when treating thoracic VCFs or when anatomically smaller pedicles are identified on preoperative imaging [23] (Fig. 54.1).

- *Transpedicular Vertebroplasty*

  The skin and vertebral periosteum are anesthetized, and a small vertical incision is made. For the transpedicular approach, the needle is inserted through the incision and placed at the 2 or 3 o'clock position on the right pedicle or the 9 or 10 o'clock position on the left pedicle. Using an orthopedic hammer, the needle is carefully tapped from the posterior surface of the pedicle, through the entire length of the pedicle, and into the vertebral body. The end position of the needle tip should be near the midline (coronal plane) and in the anterior one-third of the vertebral body (lateral views). The needle stylet is removed, and the injection system is attached. The medical cement is prepared and then injected through the needle into the vertebral body utilizing a slow injection method and fluoroscopy to ensure safety. Following placement of the cement, the needle is removed. The incision may be closed with a simple suture or steri-strips.

- *Parapedicular Vertebroplasty:*

  For the parapedicular approach, the needle entry position is lateral to the transpedicular positions, just outside of the pedicle. The needle will either enter the distal aspect of the pedicle or directly penetrate the vertebral body near the junction of the pedicle and vertebral body. The needle is advanced using an orthopedic hammer. Similar to the transpedicular approach, the end location of the needle tip should be the anterior one-third of the vertebral body, near the midline. The remainder of the procedure is identical to the description provided above.

- *Potential Complications of Vertebroplasty*

  Complications can be categorized into mild, moderate, and severe. Mild complications include temporary pain following the procedure and cement leakage into the adjoining disc space and paravertebral soft tissues. Moderate complications include post-procedural infection and cement leakage into the epidural space. Severe complications include cement leakage into the paravertebral vascular system, leading to pulmonary embolism, cerebral embolism, or cardiac perforation [25].

B. *Balloon Kyphoplasty and Radiofrequency Kyphoplasty*

- *Balloon Kyphoplasty*

  Procedures are performed in an outpatient setting, with light conscious sedation, prophylactic antibiotics, and under local anesthesia. Procedures are performed in sterile fashion with fluoroscopy/biplanar guidance. The patient is positioned prone on a radiolucent procedural table. The skin and vertebral periosteum are anesthetized with local anesthetic. A small vertical incision is made. The needle is inserted through the incision and placed at the 2 or 3 o'clock position on the right pedicle or the 9 or 10 o'clock position on the left pedicle. Using an orthopedic hammer, the needle is carefully tapped from the posterior surface of the pedicle, through the entire length of the pedicle, and into the vertebral body. The end position of the needle tip should be near the midline (coronal plane) and in the anterior one-third of the vertebral body (lateral views). The needle stylet is then removed, and a special balloon (bone tamp) is inserted and advanced into the vertebral body. The balloon is then inflated and compacts the bone to create a cavity and restore the height of the vertebral body. The balloon is deflated and removed. Following this, medical cement (polymethylmethacrylate) is prepared and injected through the needle into the previously prepared cavity within the vertebral body, utilizing a slow injection method and fluoroscopy to ensure safety and observation for cement leakage that may be visualized into the epidural veins, paravertebral soft tissues,

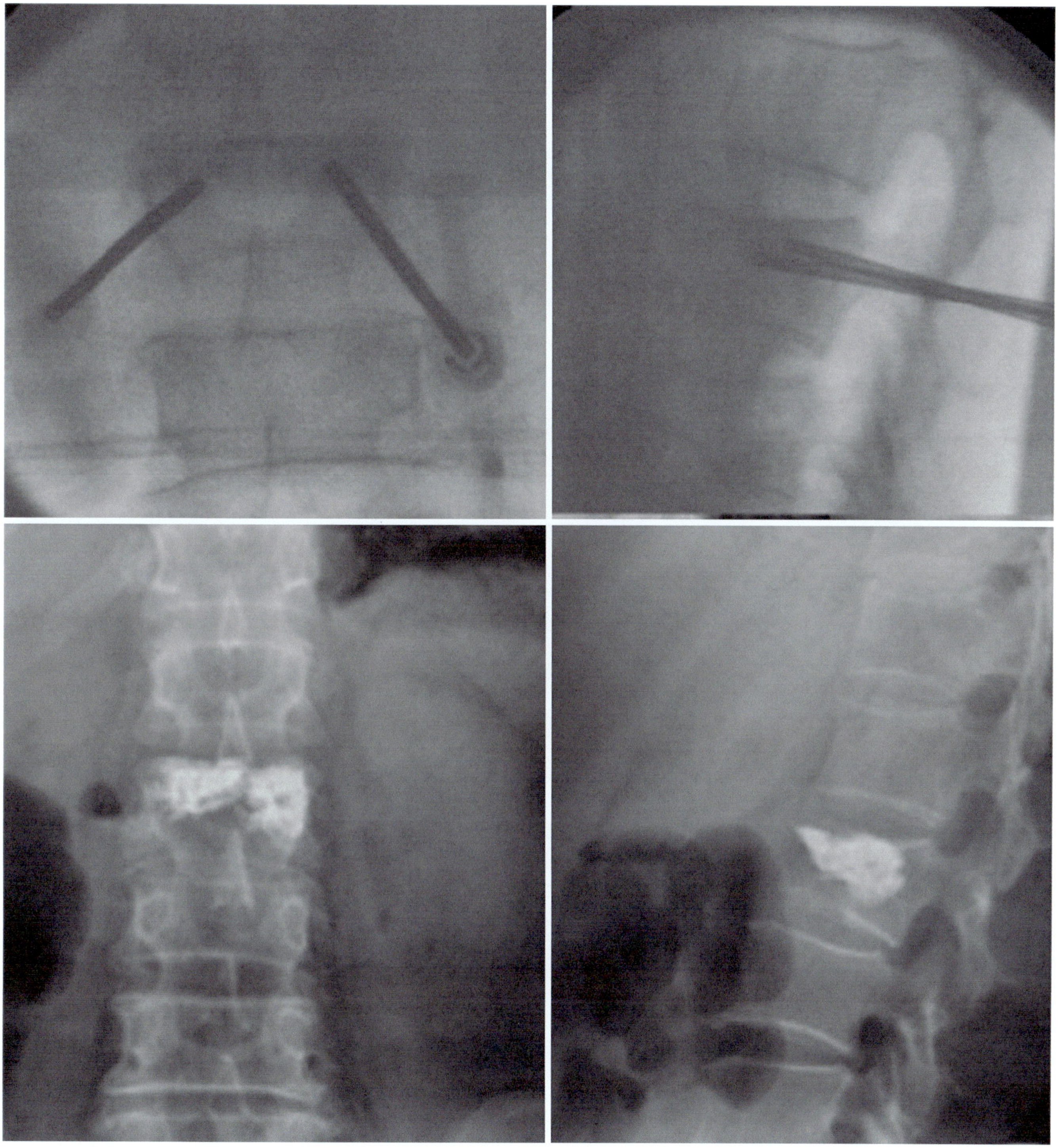

Fig. 54.1 The vertebroplasty procedure. Bilateral transpedicular needle placement confirmed on AP and lateral views, followed by injection of cement while monitoring for any cement leakage [24]. *(Image from authors library)*

disks, the intervertebral foramen, and spinal canal, in fractures with clefts. Following placement of the cement, the needle is removed. The incision may be closed with a simple suture or steri-strips (Fig. 54.2).

- *Radiofrequency Kyphoplasty*

  Radiofrequency kyphoplasty differs from balloon kyphoplasty in this regard – before cement injection, a steerable osteotome is placed into the vertebral body and creates channels in the cancellous bone. Then, the cement is heated using a radiofrequency source as it enters the delivery cannula, causing an abrupt increase in the cement viscosity to decrease cement leakage rates. The rest of the procedure is similar to balloon kyphoplasty.

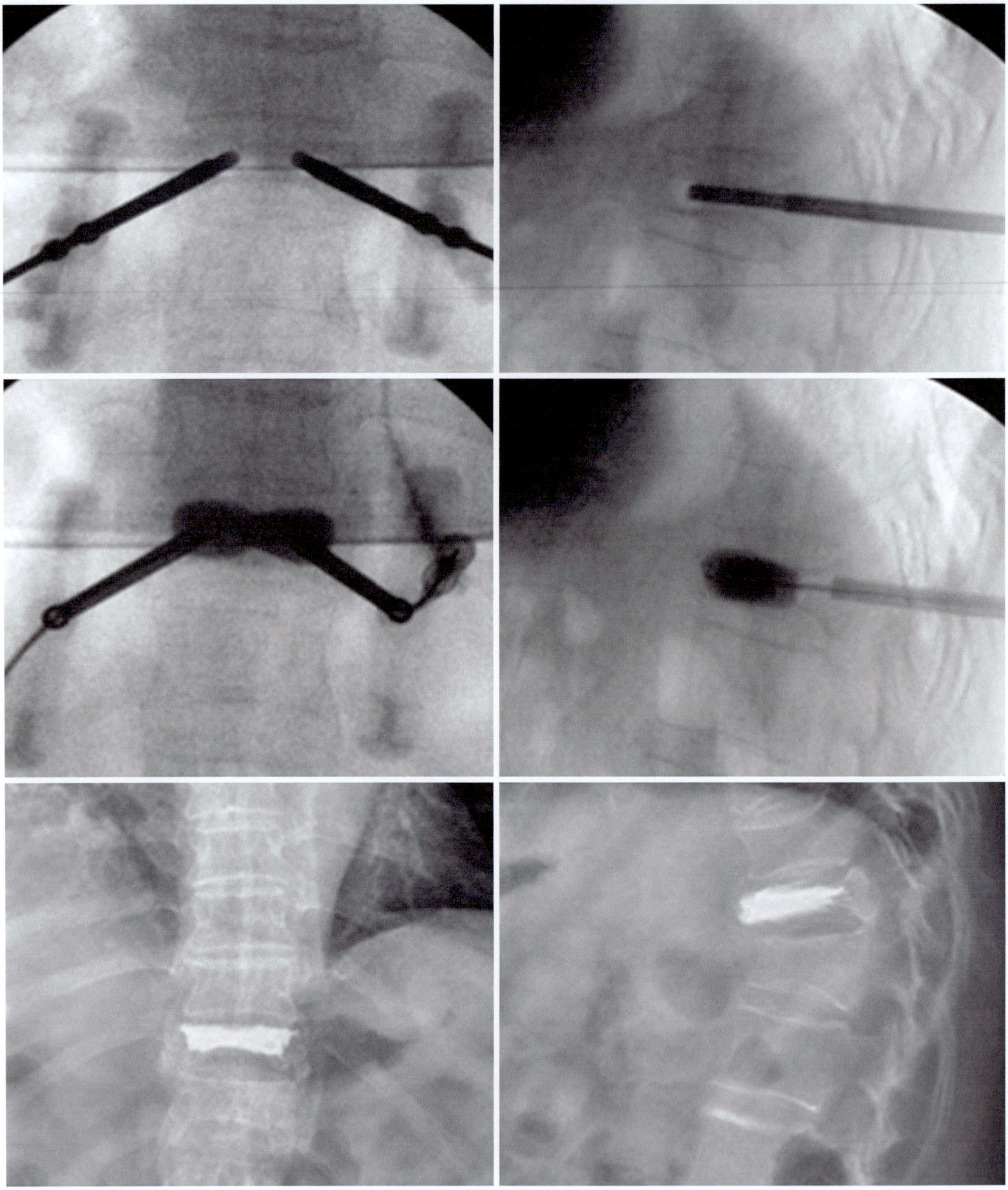

Fig. 54.2 Balloon kyphoplasty procedure. Bilateral, transpedicular needle/injection cannula placement is followed by balloon inflation. Once the final position of the balloon is confirmed, cement is injected, monitoring both AP and lateral views for any cement leakage

Comparison of Outcomes Between Balloon and Radiofrequency Kyphoplasty

A 2017 meta-analysis by Feng et al. reported the outcomes between balloon kyphoplasty and radiofrequency kyphoplasty [26]. They found the reduction of VAS score was 3.96 points greater in the radiofrequency kyphoplasty group compared to the balloon kyphoplasty group ($P = 0.007$). The procedural time was shorter in the radiofrequency kyphoplasty group compared to the balloon kyphoplasty group ($P = 0.01$). The radiofrequency kyphoplasty group had an additional 0.53 mm of anterior vertebral height restoration immediately after the procedure compared to the balloon kyphoplasty group ($P = 0.01$). There was a greater decrease of the kyphotic angle after radiofrequency kyphoplasty compared to balloon kyphoplasty, both immediately and 6 months after the procedure ($P = 0.002$ and $P < 0.00001$, respectively). There was no significant difference in the incidence of cement leakage between the two procedures ($P = 0.06$).

Potential Complications of Balloon and Radiofrequency Kyphoplasty

Similar to vertebroplasty, complications range from mild to severe and include temporary pain following the procedure, cement leakage into the adjoining disc space, paravertebral soft tissues, epidural space, and paravertebral vasculature, and post-procedural infection [27]. However, balloon kyphoplasty has been reported to have a higher rate of adjacent level fractures compared to vertebroplasty (0–7.8% versus 25–26%) [16]. It is theorized that height restoration and increased volumes of cement place additional stress on adjacent levels compared to vertebroplasty and radiofrequency kyphoplasty [28]. While radiofrequency kyphoplasty was introduced to reduce the risk of cement leakage, this has not been proven statistically significant in the published literature [26].

C. *Implantable Devices for Vertebral Fracture*

There are implantable devices for VCF treatment. They are generally utilized to restore anatomy, increase fixation strength, minimize cement requirements, and decrease cement leakage and protect patients from adjacent level fractures. These devices include OsseoFix Spinal System (Alphatec Holdings Inc., Carlsbad, CA), KIVA System (IZI Medical Products, Owings Mills, MD – Fig. 54.3), and SpineJack System (Stryker Corp., Kalamazoo, MI– Fig. 54.4), among others. In general,

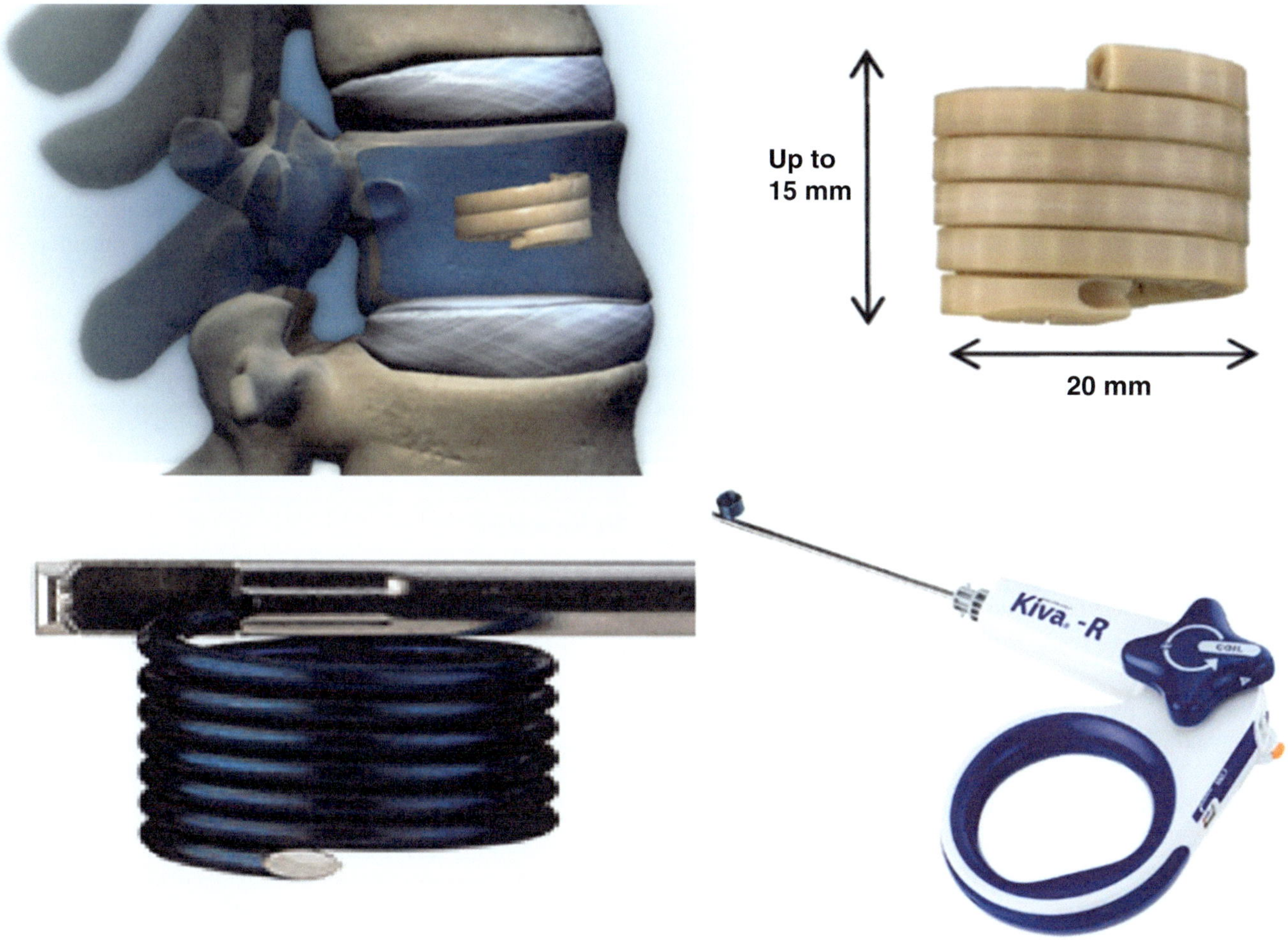

Fig. 54.3 The KIVA implant design and delivery hardware [29]. (Adapted from open source)

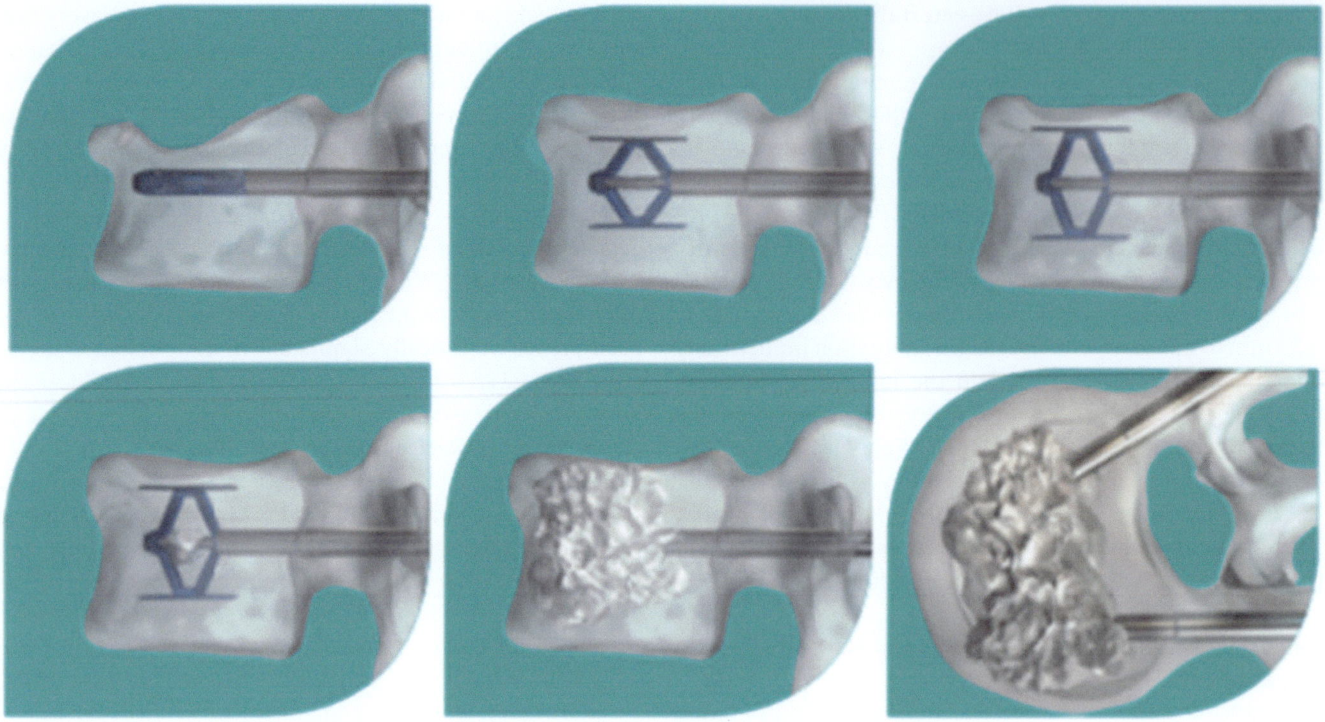

Fig. 54.4 The SpineJack implant design and implantation procedure [29]. (Adapted from open source)

these devices are placed in a transpedicular manner. Following deployment, the device and surrounding areas are filled with cement.

54.8 Post-augmentation Care and Rehabilitation

The recovery time period and progression will depend on a multitude of factors, including overall health, the number of treated vertebrae, and any complications during the procedure. In general, healthy people, fewer treated levels, and avoidance of complications allow a quicker recovery.

Post-augmentation Weeks 0–2

In the immediate postsurgical time period, the primary goal is to recover from the procedure and allow proper wound healing. Also, during this time, VCF inflammation and pain will generally improve. The patient should avoid stressing the spine by avoidance of bending, twisting, and lifting greater than 5 pounds. The patient should be encouraged to ambulate daily to increase exercise tolerance.

Post-augmentation Weeks 2–4

In Weeks 2–4, the introduction of lumbar strengthening and stability exercises should be performed, with a focus on lumbar extension exercises and postural retraining. The patient should increase ambulation distance and continue to avoid bending, twisting, and lifting greater than 5 pounds. Any bracing should be weaned and eventually discontinued.

Post-augmentation Weeks 4–8

It is considered recovery time period. The patient should resume full activities in a slow, controlled manner. The patient can begin lifting above 5 pounds but should limit carrying capacity if discomfort is felt. Return to work and full activities of daily living are expected. The patient should continue to perform home exercises focusing on lumbar and core strengthening. High-impact activities and anterior column loading should be avoided.

References

1. Cummings SR, Melton LJ. Epidemiology and outcomes of osteoporotic fractures. Lancet. 2002;359(9319):1761–7.
2. Nevitt MC, Cummings SR. Type of fall and risk of hip and wrist fractures: the study of osteoporotic fractures. The Study of Osteoporotic Fractures Research Group. J Am Geriatr Soc. 1993;41(11):1226–34.
3. Haentjens P, Magaziner J, Colon-Emeric CS, Vanderschueren D, Milisen K, Velkeniers B, Boonen S. Meta-analysis: excess mortality after hip fracture among older women and men. Ann Intern Med. 2010;152(6):380–90.
4. Shauver MJ, Yin H, Banerjee M, Chung KC. Current and future national costs to medicare for the treatment of distal radius fracture in the elderly. J Hand Surg Am. 2011;36(8):1282–7.

5. Hayes WC, Myers ER, Morris JN, Gerhart TN, Yett HS, Lipsitz LA. Impact near the hip dominates fracture risk in elderly nursing home residents who fall. Calcif Tissue Int. 1993;52(3):192–8.
6. MacKnight JM. Osteopenia and osteoporosis in female athletes. Clin Sports Med. 2017;36(4):687–702.
7. Miller PD, Zapalowski C, Kulak CA, Bilezikian JP. Bone densitometry: the best way to detect osteoporosis and to monitor therapy. J Clin Endocrinol Metab. 1999;84(6):1867–71.
8. Force USPST, Curry SJ, Krist AH, Owens DK, Barry MJ, Caughey AB, Davidson KW, Doubeni CA, Epling JW Jr, Kemper AR, et al. Screening for osteoporosis to prevent fractures: US preventive services task force recommendation statement. JAMA. 2018;319(24):2521–31.
9. Sofka CM. Imaging of stress fractures. Clin Sports Med. 2006;25(1):53–62, viii.
10. Cosman F, de Beur SJ, LeBoff MS, Lewiecki EM, Tanner B, Randall S, Lindsay R, National Osteoporosis F. Clinician's guide to prevention and treatment of osteoporosis. Osteoporos Int. 2014;25(10):2359–81.
11. Chilibeck PD, Vatanparast H, Cornish SM, Abeysekara S, Charlesworth S. Evidence-based risk assessment and recommendations for physical activity: arthritis, osteoporosis, and low back pain. Appl Physiol Nutr Metab. 2011;36 Suppl 1:S49–79.
12. Agrawal K, Agarwal Y, Chopra RK, Batra A, Chandra R, Thukral BB. Evaluation of MR spectroscopy and diffusion-weighted MRI in postmenopausal bone strength. Cureus. 2015;7(9):e327. Published 2015 Sep 21. https://doi.org/10.7759/cureus.327.
13. Gibbs JC, MacIntyre NJ, Ponzano M, Templeton JA, Thabane L, Papaioannou A, Giangregorio LM. Exercise for improving outcomes after osteoporotic vertebral fracture. Cochrane Database Syst Rev. 2019;7(7):CD008618. https://doi.org/10.1002/14651858.CD008618.pub3. PMID: 31273764; PMCID: PMC6609547.
14. Buchbinder R, Osborne RH, Ebeling PR, Wark JD, Mitchell P, Wriedt C, et al. A randomized trial of vertebroplasty for painful osteoporotic vertebral fractures. N Engl J Med. 2009;361(6):557–68.
15. Kallmes DF, Comstock BA, Heagerty PJ, Turner JA, Wilson DJ, Diamond TH, et al. A randomized trial of vertebroplasty for osteoporotic spinal fractures. N Engl J Med. 2009;361(6):569–79.
16. Long Y, Yi W, Yang D. Advances in vertebral augmentation systems for osteoporotic vertebral compression fractures. Pain Res Manag. 2020;2020:3947368.
17. Clark W, Bird P, Gonski P, Diamond TH, Smerdely P, McNeil HP, et al. Safety and efficacy of vertebroplasty for acute painful osteoporotic fractures (VAPOUR): a multicentre, randomised, double-blind, placebo-controlled trial. Lancet. 2016;388(10052):1408–16.
18. Hulme PA, Krebs J, Ferguson SJ, Berlemann U. Vertebroplasty and kyphoplasty: a systematic review of 69 clinical studies. Spine (Phila Pa 1976). 2006;31(17):1983–2001.
19. Klazen CA, Lohle PN, de Vries J, Jansen FH, Tielbeek AV, Blonk MC, et al. Vertebroplasty versus conservative treatment in acute osteoporotic vertebral compression fractures (Vertos II): an open-label randomised trial. Lancet. 2010;376(9746):1085–92.
20. Zhang Y, Shi L, Tang P, Zhang L. Comparison of the efficacy between two micro-operative therapies of old patients with osteoporotic vertebral compression fracture: a network meta-analysis. J Cell Biochem. 2017;118(10):3205–12.
21. Zhao S, Xu CY, Zhu AR, Ye L, Lv LL, Chen L, et al. Comparison of the efficacy and safety of 3 treatments for patients with osteoporotic vertebral compression fractures: a network meta-analysis. Medicine (Baltimore). 2017;96(26):e7328.
22. Robinson Y, Heyde CE, Försth P, Olerud C. Kyphoplasty in osteoporotic vertebral compression fractures--guidelines and technical considerations. J Orthop Surg Res. 2011;6:43.
23. Schupfner R, Koniarikova K, Pfeifer C, Grechenig P, Bakota B, Staresinic M, et al. An anatomical study of transpedicular vs. extrapedicular approach for kyphoplasty and vertebroplasty in the thoracic spine. Injury. 2020;52(Suppl 5):S63–9.
24. Lee JH, Jin Y. Surgical techniques and clinical evidence of vertebroplasty and kyphoplasty for osteoporotic vertebral fractures. Osteoporos Sarcopenia. 2017;3(2):82–9.
25. Al-Nakshabandi NA. Percutaneous vertebroplasty complications. Ann Saudi Med. 2011;31(3):294–7.
26. Feng L, Shen JM, Feng C, Chen J, Wu Y. Comparison of radiofrequency kyphoplasty (RFK) and balloon kyphoplasty (BKP) in the treatment of vertebral compression fractures: a meta-analysis. Medicine (Baltimore). 2017;96(25):e7150.
27. Taylor RS, Fritzell P, Taylor RJ. Balloon kyphoplasty in the management of vertebral compression fractures: an updated systematic review and meta-analysis. Eur Spine J. 2007;16(8):1085–100.
28. Ko BS, Cho KJ, Park JW. Early adjacent vertebral fractures after balloon kyphoplasty for osteoporotic vertebral compression fractures. Asian Spine J. 2019;13(2):210–5.
29. Long, et al. Advanced in vertebral augmentation systems for osteoporotic vertebral compression fractures. Pain Res Manag. 2020;19:3947368.

Rheumatic Disorders

55

Swetha Ann Alexander, Cathy Duddy, Abhijeet Danve, and Shiv T. Sehra

55.1 Fibromyalgia

55.1.1 Synonyms

Fibromyalgia Syndrome

55.1.2 ICD-10 Codes

M79.7

55.1.3 Description

Fibromyalgia is a common disorder with a prevalence of 2–8% and female-to-male ratio of 2:1 [1]. It is thought to be a disorder of increased pain perception to a normal stimulus in the central nervous system (CNS) through a process known as "pain centralization" [2]. Risk factors and triggers include a family history of fibromyalgia, environmental factors (viral illness, trauma, psychological stress), and the presence of other concomitant rheumatic disorders contributing to musculoskeletal pain (osteoarthritis, rheumatoid arthritis). Most patients with fibromyalgia also exhibit symptoms of fatigue, mood disorders, sleep disturbance, and memory impairment [3].

S. A. Alexander (✉)
Department of Internal Medicine, University of Connecticut, Farmington, CT, USA
e-mail: swetha.alexander@yale.edu

C. Duddy
Department of Physical Therapy, Mount Auburn Hospital, Harvard Medical School, Cambridge, MA, USA

A. Danve
Yale School of Medicine, New Haven, CT, USA

S. T. Sehra
Rheumatology Division, Mount Auburn Hospital, Harvard University, Cambridge, MA, USA

Harvard Medical School, Boston, MA, USA

55.1.4 Clinical Presentation

The 2016 revisions to the 2010/2011 American College of Rheumatology criteria for diagnosis of fibromyalgia combine a physician suspicion and patient-reported pain assessment (patient fills out the widespread pain index and symptom severity scale questionnaire) [4]. The hallmark of fibromyalgia is generalized pain in variable locations, with varying intensity of neuropathic quality (burning, numbness, tingling) at times. In addition, patients can have somatic symptoms like fatigue, sleep disturbances, brain fog ("fibro fog"), headache, depression, anxiety, irritable bowel syndrome, pelvic pain, and interstitial cystitis/painful bladder syndrome for more than 3 months.

55.1.5 Physical Examination

Physical exam can reveal increased pain on inflation of blood pressure cuff (sphygmomanometer-evoked allodynia) and increased tenderness on deep pressure over the joint as well as non-joint areas (tenderness only over the joints should raise suspicion for systemic autoimmune disease).

55.1.6 Diagnostic Workup

Fibromyalgia is a clinical diagnosis and lacks specific lab biomarkers. Initial workup including complete blood count, erythrocyte sedimentation rate, and C-reactive protein may be normal and helps eliminate an underlying inflammatory disorder. Other diagnostic workup includes checking thyroid-stimulating hormone (TSH), creatinine kinase (CK), and vitamin D. Antinuclear antibody and rheumatoid factor are not routinely recommended unless a concomitant inflammatory arthritis is suspected [5].

© The Author(s), under exclusive license to Springer Nature Switzerland AG 2022
S. A. Mostoufi et al. (eds.), *Clinical Guide to Musculoskeletal Medicine*, https://doi.org/10.1007/978-3-030-92042-5_55

55.1.7 Treatments

A diagnosis of fibromyalgia is often reassuring for the patient and helps them focus on treatment [6]. Management is usually multidisciplinary and centered around patient education and utilization of pharmacological and non-pharmacological treatment to optimize symptom control.

(a) *Medical Management:* The drugs are chosen based on patient's comorbidities and tolerance, and treating the underlying disease helps improve fibromyalgia symptoms. The general principle is to normalize the neurotransmitter activity responsible for the pain (decreasing activating neurotransmitters and increasing inhibitory neurotransmitters) [1]. The medications commonly used are tricyclic antidepressants (amitriptyline), serotonin-norepinephrine reuptake inhibitors (duloxetine, milnacipran, esreboxetine), gabapentin-like (gabapentin, pregabalin), gamma-hydroxybutyrate, low-dose selective serotonin reuptake inhibitors (fluoxetine, paroxetine, sertraline), low-dose naltrexone, and cannabinoids (nabilone). Opioids and nonsteroidal anti-inflammatory agents are not helpful for fibromyalgia pain and should not be prescribed [7].

(b) *Rehabilitation:* Proper exercise helps build strength, improve flexibility, and ultimately help with improving sleep. Education must be provided to avoid activities that worsen the pain. A good exercise routine may reduce the need for pain medication.

Recommended exercises

Aerobic: Low-impact exercises such as walking, biking, and elliptical machine

Strength training: Body weight exercise, dumbbell, weight machines, pool-based exercises

Flexibility: Static stretching, yoga, pilates (emphasizing pain-free range of motion)

(c) *Procedures*: No procedural treatment indicated

(d) *Surgery*: No surgical treatment indicated

55.2 Inflammatory Arthritis

55.2.1 Synonyms

Inflammatory Polyarthropathy, Inflammatory polyarthritis, Inflammatory arthritis of multiple joints

55.2.2 ICD-10 Codes

M05–M14

55.2.3 Description

Inflammatory arthritis is a broad term for patients with history and examination findings of joint pain and inflammation such as swelling, redness, warmth, and decreased function and mobility. These features are due to inflammation of the synovial membrane lining the joint cavity leading to fluid accumulation and hyperemia in the joints. Inflammatory arthritis can involve one (monoarthritis), few (oligoarthritis), or many (polyarthritis) joints.

In a patient with joint pain, the first step is to establish pathology within the joint (true articular) versus surrounding structures (periarticular) such as the bone, tendon, bursa, muscle, or remote structures (referred pain). Pain with active and passive movement usually indicates a true articular origin. Pain and point tenderness with active movement, but *no* pain with passive movement usually points to the nonarticular or periarticular origin of pain [8, 9].

Once articular or nonarticular diagnosis is established, it is important to distinguish inflammatory or noninflammatory joint pain next as this can focus the differentials and guide treatment decisions [10, 11]. The distinguishing features are displayed in Table 55.1.

Table 55.1 Distinguishing features between inflammatory and noninflammatory joint pain

Aspects to consider	Inflammatory pain	Noninflammatory pain
History	Systemic symptoms like fever, malaise, rash, eye involvement (uveitis), bowel disturbance (inflammatory bowel disease)	Not associated with systemic symptoms
Physical exam	Joint appear swollen, red, warm, and tender to touch with decreased mobility	Usually no swelling or tenderness but may show bony prominences and may have decreased mobility
Morning stiffness	Usually more than 1 h	Usually less than 1 h
Activity	Pain usually present at rest during acute flare-ups	Worse with weight-bearing and use
Pattern of joint involvement	Usually symmetric but can be asymmetrical	Asymmetric and usually involves weight-bearing joints
Lab work	ESR and CRP are usually elevated	ESR and CRP usually normal
Synovial fluid analysis	Greater than 2000 WBC/μL with the predominance of neutrophils in the acute phase and monocytes in the chronic phase	Usually less than 2000 WBC/μL with a predominance of monocytes

ESR erythrocyte sedimentation rate, *CRP* C-reactive protein, *WBC* white blood cell

Among inflammatory arthritides, those most commonly seen in clinical practice are rheumatoid arthritis (RA), spondyloarthritis, crystal arthropathies, and connective tissue disease-associated arthritis.

55.3 Rheumatoid Arthritis

55.3.1 Synonyms

Atrophic arthritis, Rheumatism, Rheumatic disease

55.3.2 ICD 10 Code

M06.9, M05.69

55.3.3 Description

Rheumatoid arthritis is a chronic systemic inflammatory disease affecting the joints as well as extra-articular structures such as eyes, lungs, skin, and nerves. RA has a worldwide prevalence of 5 per 1000 adults with a predominance among women [12]. The risk factors for developing RA include genetic predisposition (60%), smoking, infectious agents (microorganisms causing periodontal disease), and estrogen (RA is more prevalent in women than men) [13–15]. The pathogenesis of RA is due to synovial membrane inflammation which later on involves the underlying cartilage and bone leading to erosions [16].

55.3.4 Clinical Presentation

RA involves small and large joints predominantly of the peripheral skeletal system and may have extra-articular manifestations involving multiple organs (skin, eye, lung, heart, gastrointestinal system, nerves, and bone marrow). The most common presentation is gradual onset symmetric inflammatory polyarthritis of small joints of hands and feet. Occasionally RA can involve larger joints and mimic polymyalgia rheumatica especially in older adults. Some patients may have intermittent episodic arthritis (called palindromic rheumatism) before evolving into classical RA. The swelling is "soft" (due to synovitis) on palpation (in OA it is "hard"/bony) and fusiform (around the joint involved). No diagnostic criteria exist for RA [17]. Classic features suggestive of RA are joint pain and swelling over the metacarpophalangeal and/or metatarsophalangeal joints, with morning stiffness for greater than 30 min and positive autoantibodies.

Tables 55.2a and 55.2b *depicts the specific clinical features to look for while examining for suspected rheumatoid arthritis.*

Table 55.2a Articular manifestations of RA

Site of involvement	Specific feature
Cervical spine	Early disease shows neck stiffness with loss of range of motion (ROM). Severe erosive disease leads to C1–C2 instability and cervical myelopathy
Shoulders	Loss of range of motion in early and severe disease
Elbow	Flexion deformities in early RA, ulnar nerve compression
Hand	Wrists, mainly the metacarpophalangeal joint and proximal interphalangeal joint (PIP) with *sparing* of distal interphalangeal joint (DIP). Severe erosive diseases at these joints lead to swan-neck deformities and boutonniere deformity. Nerve entrapments lead to carpal tunnel syndrome (median nerve compressed) and Guyon's canal syndrome (ulnar nerve compressed) Tendon involvement leads to tenosynovitis, rheumatoid nodule formation, and tendon ruptures
Hip	Early RA is asymptomatic with gradual severity leading to groin pain on use of joint and restricted ROM
Knee	Popliteal (baker's) cyst formation
Foot and ankle	Involves the metatarsophalangeal joints (cock-up arthritis), talonavicular joint (leading to a pronated and everted foot) leading to gait dysfunction and significant pain. There is preservation of flexion and extension of the ankle in early RA. Nerve entrapment leads to tarsal tunnel syndrome (posterior tibial nerve involved)

Table 55.2b Extra-articular manifestations of RA

Organ	Specific feature
Skin	Rheumatoid nodules typically in active disease in bursae and along tendon sheaths; leukocytoclastic vasculitis with palpable purpura on exam
Eye	Keratoconjunctivitis sicca (dry eyes), episcleritis, scleritis
Lung	Cricoarytenoid joint involvement leading to laryngeal pain, interstitial lung disease with pleuritis unclear if due to RA versus treatment for RA
Heart	Pericardial effusion, valvular dysfunction, myocardiopathy, aortitis
GI	Xerostomia if associated with Sjogren's syndrome, ischemic bowel complications with rheumatoid vasculitis
Renal	Treatment of RA related to proteinuria (gold, penicillamine), interstitial renal disease (NSAID), papillary necrosis (chronic analgesic exposure)
CNS/PNS	Cervical spine instability, peripheral neuropathy due to nerve compression, vasculitis leading to mononeuritis multiplex
Hematologic	Hypochromic-microcytic anemia, Felty's syndrome (RA+ splenomegaly+ leukopenia+ leg ulcers), thrombocytopenia

NSAID nonsteroidal anti-inflammatory agent, *RA* rheumatoid arthritis

55.3.5 Diagnostic Workup

Rheumatoid arthritis is a clinical diagnosis with supportive lab work to confirm the suspicion.

Lab work Complete blood count to assess for anemia, leukopenia, or thrombocytopenia. Basic metabolic panel to assess for renal function due to medication induced renal dysfunction. Nonspecific inflammatory markers such as erythrocyte sedimentation rate (ESR) and C-reactive protein (CRP) can be used to trend response to treatment. Specific markers which aid in making a diagnosis are rheumatoid factor (RF) and anti-cyclic citrullinated peptide antibodies (anti-CCP) (which have greater than 90% specificity and are markers for erosive disease) [18].

55.3.5.1 Imaging

X-rays: Plain radiographs of the affected joints in early disease show soft tissue swelling and juxta-articular osteopenia. Later in disease progression, it can show marginal erosions (areas of bone loss) and cartilage destruction (joint space narrowing). Thus, radiographs especially of hands and feet are useful to diagnose and assess the progression of disease.

Ultrasound is more sensitive than plain radiographs to detect erosions, synovitis, and vascularity and can be used to monitor disease progression [19].

MRI is more sensitive than plain radiographs to detect erosions in the earlier stage of RA. In the later erosive stages, it also detects bone marrow edema and hypertrophic synovial tissue.

55.3.6 Treatment

The cornerstone of management is early identification of RA with prompt initiation of treatment to halt joint destruction. The 2015 ACR RA treatment guidelines recommend monitoring of the disease activity in response to treatment with Clinical Disease Activity Index (CDAI) and Disease Activity Score 28 (DAS28) which assess clinical symptoms, function, and overall well-being [20]. The goal of treatment is to achieve clinical remission (low disease activity) based on the above score.

(a) *Medical management*

The drugs used for RA treatment are disease-modifying antirheumatic drugs (DMARDs) which are synthetic type and biologics [21]. The synthetic types are (a) conventional drugs used initially and have proven to work (methotrexate, sulfasalazine, hydroxychloroquine, leflunomide) and (b) targeted therapy such as tofacitinib, upadacitinib, and baricitinib. Some of the commonly used biologic DMARDs used are etanercept, infliximab, certolizumab, golimumab, adalimumab, rituximab, tocilizumab, abatacept, sarilumab, and rituximab. Other drugs used are nonsteroidal anti-inflammatory drugs (NSAIDs) and glucocorticoids. Among the synthetic DMARD, methotrexate (MTX) is widely used and the first choice, while all other drugs are usually add-on therapies for nonresponders after maximizing the dose of MTX. Prompt referral to rheumatologists has shown better patient outcomes [22].

(b) *Procedures*: Arthrocentesis, if performed, will show inflammatory synovial fluid without crystals.

(c) *Rehabilitation:* Exercise goals are to improve joint mobility and muscle strength and maintain overall fitness. Exercise helps control flare-ups and can reduce pain and stiffness. Many RA patients suffer from accelerated muscle loss contributing to disability and poor quality of life. Exercise will build muscle strength and help maintain optimal function.

Recommended exercises

Aerobic: Low-impact exercises such as walking, biking, swimming, and dancing

Strength training: Body weight exercise, free weights, weight machines, TheraBands

Flexibility: Static stretching, yoga, pilates, Tai Chi

(d) *Surgery:* Surgery is usually reserved for complications of severe RA such as synovectomy, stabilization of unstable cervical vertebrae, carpal tunnel release, ruptured tendon repair, and total joint replacement in case of erosive disease

55.4 Spondyloarthritis

55.4.1 Synonyms

Axial spondyloarthritis, Ankylosing spondylitis, Spondyloarthritides, Spondyloarthropathy, and Spondyloarthropathies

55.4.2 ICD 10 Code

M14.89

55.4.3 Description

Spondyloarthritis encompasses a group of disorders involving inflammation of the axial skeleton (sacroiliac joint inflammation called sacroiliitis and spine inflammation called spondylitis), asymmetric peripheral joint inflammation, enthesitis/enthesopathy (inflammation at the point of tendon or a ligament attaching to the bone), dactylitis (uniformly swollen sausage-like digit), inflammatory eye disease, psoriasis, and genitourinary or gastrointestinal inflammation. Spondyloarthritides can be classified as axial (includes ankylosing spondylitis and non-radiographic axial spondyloarthritis) or peripheral (includes psoriatic arthritis, reactive arthritis, inflammatory bowel disease-associated arthritis). There can be overlapping features between axial and peripheral groups.

The pathogenesis of spondyloarthritis appears to be an abnormality in the innate immune system and T-cells causing increased cytokine production (tumor necrosis factor-alpha, interleukin-17, and interleukin-1) leading to joint damage in genetically predisposed individuals (positive HLA-B27).

55.4.4 Clinical Presentation and Physical Examination

The various subgroups of this disorder are listed below with their specific clinical features and treatment in Table 55.3.

Table 55.3 Features of various spondyloarthritides

Disease	Articular features	Extra-articular features	Clinical pearls	Treatment
Axial spondyloarthritis (AxSpa)	Inflammatory back pain (onset before age 45) with back pain that improves with activity, with involvement of the lower spine, sacroiliac (SI) joint, asymmetric oligoarthritis (hips and shoulders) enthesitis, dactylitis uncommon	Psoriasis; recurrent anterior uveitis, inflammatory bowel disease, restrictive pulmonary disease, osteopenia with risk of fragility fractures in setting of increased bone mineral density	Tenderness over the SI joints, reduction in spinal flexion, chest expansion and hip movement, hyperkyphosis of neck and thorax (hunching), loss of lumbar lordosis	First choice are NSAIDs. Tumor necrosis factor inhibitors (TNFI) in case of inadequate response to NSAIDs. Can also trial IL-17 inhibitors
Psoriatic Arthritis [23]	Five clinical subtypes have been seen: 1. Oligoarticular subtype (asymmetric ≤4 joints) 2. Polyarticular subtype (symmetric and similar to RA) 3. Distal subtype (involves DIP joints) 4. Arthritis mutilans (telescoping of digits) 5. Axial/spondyloarthritis subtype (involves spine and sacroiliac joints) Other features seen are enthesitis, dactylitis, tenosynovitis	Psoriasis (usual areas involved are hairline, ears, umbilicus, groin) usually before joint involvement, nail pitting and onychodystrophy	Morning stiffness present for more than 30 min better with activity, presence of joint line tenderness and effusion with less tenderness than other inflammatory arthritis and more deformity (arthritis mutilans)	1. csDMARD: methotrexate, leflunomide, sulfasalazine 2. bDMARD: TNFI agents (adalimumab, certolizumab, etanercept, golimumab, infliximab), IL-17 inhibitors (ixekizumab, secukinumab), anti-IL-12/IL-23 agents (ustekinumab), IL-23 inhibitors (guselkumab), JAK inhibitors (tofacitinib) 3. PDE4 inhibitor (apremilast)
Inflammatory bowel disorder (IBD)-associated arthritis	Spondylitis and sacroiliitis like AxSpa but not related to IBD activity, acute pauciarticular arthritis (mainly knee) associated with IBD flare, chronic polyarticular arthritis (mainly MCP) *not* associated with IBD flare, enthesitis, rarely dactylitis	Erythema nodosum, pyoderma gangrenosum, inflammatory bowel disease, bilateral chronic anterior uveitis, risk of vitamin D deficiency and fractures	Need to rule out septic arthritis due to increased risk	For IBD and arthritis relief, drug choices are sulfasalazine, azathioprine, 6-mercaptopurine, methotrexate, glucocorticoids, infliximab, and adalimumab.
Reactive arthritis	Acute onset asymmetric oligoarthritis which can lead to recurrent or persistent oligoarthritis; less occurrence of spondylitis, enthesitis, eactylitis	Keratoderma blennorrhagicum (hyperkeratotic skin changes on palms and soles), circinate balanitis (erythematous lesion with shallow ulcers on the penis), psoriatic nail changes, bilateral conjunctivitis, localized osteopenia	Usually presents 2–3 weeks after an inciting infection (can be of genitourinary or gastrointestinal source) and a majority are self-resolving and nonerosive arthritis	1. Treatment of inciting infection with appropriate antibiotics 2. Acute arthritis relief can be with NSAID and if no relief can use glucocorticoids (oral as well intra-articular) 3. Persistent symptoms can use sulfasalazine, methotrexate, or TNFI

AxSpa axial spondyloarthritis, *SI* sacroiliac, *IBD* inflammatory bowel disorder, *NSAID* nonsteroidal anti-inflammatory drug, *csDMARD* conventional synthetic disease-modifying antirheumatic drug, *bDMARD* biological disease-modifying antirheumatic drug, *IL-17 inhibitors* interleukin −17 inhibitors, *IL-12/IL-23* interleukin 12/interleukin 23, *MCP* metacarpophalangeal

55.4.5 Diagnostic Workup

Lab work: HLA-B27 seen in greater than 75% of the patients with spondyloarthritis is a helpful but not confirmatory test. About 6% of the US population has positive HLA B27, and only less than 10% develop spondyloarthritis [24]. ESR and CRP are usually elevated, but CRP is a better marker to assess radiographic progression and response to treatment [25, 26].

Imaging: Plain radiograph of the pelvis is useful to diagnose axSpA such as sacroiliitis. Sacroiliitis is characterized by false widening, erosions, sclerosis, and ankylosis of the sacroiliac joint. "Bamboo spine" appearance on spinal X-ray is typically seen in advanced ankylosing spondylitis due to bony bridges between the vertebrae. In psoriatic arthritis, the distal interphalangeal joints show destruction and overhanging growth by adjacent metacarpal/metatarsal giving a "pencil in a cup" appearance.

MRI of the pelvis is more sensitive than plain radiograph in the early stages of sacroiliitis with suggestive features such as bone marrow edema. We recommend using an MRI pelvis to evaluate for sacroiliitis in a young patient with inflammatory back pain and suspected axSpA. Routine use of X-ray lumbar spine is not recommended for initial evaluation for axSpA.

55.4.6 Treatments

The goal of treatment is to prevent progression of disease to preserve quality of life for extended periods. However, patient education on disease course and prognosis needs to be established early on.

(a) *Medical Management*: Please see Table 55.3.
(b) *Rehabilitation:* Physical therapy is key in improving the pain and stiffness in axSpa. Goals include improving posture and range of motion. Modalities such as hydrotherapy are utilized. Spinal manipulation should be avoided due to spinal fusion especially involving the cervical spine.
(c) *Procedures:* Arthrocentesis, if performed, will show inflammatory synovial fluid without crystals.
(d) *Surgery:* Joint replacement of affected joints may be necessary to prevent disability.

55.5 Crystal Arthropathies

Calcium or uric acid deposition in and around the joints evoking inflammation in the joints constitutes crystal-induced arthropathies. The most commonly seen is gout, and the others are calcium pyrophosphate disease (calcium deposition in cartilage) and basic calcium phosphate deposition (calcium deposition around the cartilage like "Milwaukee shoulder").

55.6 Gout

55.6.1 Synonyms

Crystal arthropathy, Gouty arthritis, Gout

55.6.2 ICD 10 Code

M11.9

55.6.3 Description

Hyperuricemia (serum uric acid ≥6.8 mg/dl) either from increased production or decreased excretion predisposes individuals to uric acid crystal deposition in the joints. About 16% of the US population has hyperuricemia, but gout occurs in a fraction of these patients. The risk factors for symptomatic gout are male sex, genetic predisposition, obesity, alcohol, and comorbid conditions (hypertension, hyperlipidemia, diabetes mellitus, chronic kidney disease).

55.6.4 Clinical Presentation

The natural history of gout manifestations is divided into three stages and patients can present in any stage.

1. Asymptomatic hyperuricemia: Elevated serum uric acid level on lab work but not overt symptoms like joint pain or kidney stones. A vast majority do not develop symptoms; however, a few risk factors like increasing age or increasing uric acid levels might lead to developing symptomatic features of gout.
2. Gout flares/acute intermittent gout: The first gout flare is typically monoarticular involving the lower extremity joints (especially the first metatarsophalangeal joint and this is known as "Podagra"). Usually it is triggered by a risk factor like trauma, surgery, dehydration, alcohol, drugs affecting the metabolism of uric acid, etc. Later in the course, the flares can be polyarticular involving multiple joints and can be associated with fever mimicking septic arthritis which needs to be ruled out. The gout flares occur in varying intervals with longer periods between attacks and as the disease progresses with shorter symptom-free intervals, where it is known as the intercritical gout phase.

3. Chronic recurrent tophaceous gout: Chronic frequent polyarticular attacks lead to persistent chronic arthritis. Long-standing disease leads to tophus formation (solid urate deposition with chronic inflammatory changes and joint destruction) especially over the extensors of the elbows, distal Achilles tendon, cartilage of ears, and distal interphalangeal joints of fingers.

55.6.5 Physical Examination

A joint with an initial gout flare is monoarticular, usually starts at night with a peak at 12–24 h, and is red, swollen, warm, and extremely tender with an inability to use the joint. A recurrent gout flare is similarly inflamed involving feet, ankles, knees, bursa, shoulder, sternoclavicular joint, and rarely even the spine.

Chronic long-standing gout shows tophus formation which appears chalky white and is not painful or tender.

55.6.6 Diagnostic Workup

Arthrocentesis and synovial fluid analysis are essential to confirm the diagnosis of gout. Synovial fluid analysis is inflammatory (WBC count between 10,000–100,000 μL) with neutrophil predominance. The gold standard for diagnosis is negatively birefringent needle-shaped uric acid crystals within neutrophils under polarized light microscopy.

Lab work can show nonspecific elevated ESR and CRP. Serum uric acid levels to demonstrate hyperuricemia are done 2 weeks after the gout flare subsides as levels can vary (can be normal) and cannot be interpreted accurately.

Imaging: Plain radiograph and MRI show changes in chronic gout like subcortical bone cysts and overhanging edges of cortical bone (due to bone erosions in the setting of tophi).

Ultrasound of joints can diagnose early gout and monitor response to treatment with a characteristic feature of "double contour sign" [27].

Dual-energy computed tomography can be used to differentiate uric acid deposition from calcium deposition.

55.6.7 Treatments

(a) *Medical Management:* Treatment of an acute gout flare aims to decrease the symptoms due to inflammation and can be achieved by colchicine, NSAIDs, and glucocorticoids (intra-articular injection, intramuscular depot form, oral short-course prednisone).

To prevent recurrent attacks of gout and joint destruction, lifestyle modification and reducing risk factors (stress, high BMI, alcohol intake) along with urate-lowering therapy are recommended. The urate-lowering therapy medications are allopurinol (first-line choice helps to reduce serum uric acid level), febuxostat (better choice in mild to moderate chronic kidney disease patients but avoid if patients have increased cardiovascular risk factors), probenecid (usually second line in combination with allopurinol to be avoided in patients with CKD and kidney stones), and pegloticase (used in recurrent severe tophaceous gout not responding to conventional therapy). Prophylaxis with colchicine, NSAIDs, or glucocorticoids is recommended for initial 3–6 months of urate-lowering therapy to prevent worsening of gout flares. Goal uric acid in a patient on urate-lowering therapy is less than 6 mg/dl.

(b) *Rehabilitation:* In the acute phase, resting the joint should be considered. In chronic cases, physical therapy can be considered to maintain ROM of the affected joint and improve function.

(c) *Procedures:* Arthrocentesis will reveal inflammatory synovial fluid. Visualization of appropriate crystals is the gold standard for diagnosis.

(d) *Surgery:* Occasionally tophi may be removed surgically, especially if they are at sites of repetitive trauma.

55.7 Osteoarthritis

55.7.1 Synonyms

Osteoarthritis

55.7.2 ICD-10 Codes

M15–M19

55.7.3 Description

This section covers osteoarthritis as a disorder. For details of osteoarthritis of upper and lower extremity joints, please refer to Chap. 53.

OA is a degenerative disease of the cartilaginous structures in the joint and the most common form of arthritis leading to significant pain and disability [28]. The risk factors implicated in the development of OA are increasing age, female sex, previous joint trauma, obesity, joint overuse due to occupation or vigorous exercise, smoking, quadriceps weakness, increased bone mass, and family history. These risk factors either acutely or cumulatively lead to abnormality in cartilage formation and joint injury. [29]

55.7.4 Clinical Presentation

The joints commonly involved in OA are knees, hips, first carpometacarpal (CMC) joint, distal (DIP) and proximal interphalangeal joints (PIP) of fingers, and facet joints of the cervical and lumbar spine. The pain from joint use is gradual and intermittent in onset but eventually becomes constant and debilitating. It is initially relieved with rest and analgesics. Patients experience morning stiffness usually less than 30 min and also gel phenomenon (stiffness with inactivity) which resolves within minutes. Joint involvement can have specific features; hand involvement leads to difficulty in dexterity; hip and knee involvement leads to gait and balance issues; spine involvement can lead to nerve compression symptoms.

55.7.5 Physical Examination

Affected joint demonstrates joint-line tenderness, loss of range of motion, crepitus, joint instability, and locking. Long-standing OA joints can have bony swelling (Bouchard in PIP and Heberden nodes in DIP) and squaring of CMC. Erosive OA can show signs of inflammation with warmth and joint effusion. Other causes such as septic arthritis and crystal-induced arthritis must be excluded by arthrocentesis.

55.7.6 Diagnostic Workup

55.7.6.1 Imaging

Plain radiographs do not correlate with symptoms and are not sensitive in early OA. Classic radiograph findings are asymmetric joint space narrowing, marginal osteophyte formation, and as the disease progresses, subchondral sclerosis, and cyst formation. In DIP and PIP, central erosions and cortical collapse may be seen. MRI and ultrasound are more sensitive to detect early changes in cartilage, but not routinely required. MRI is also useful to detect early changes in ligaments and meniscus.

55.7.6.2 Arthrocentesis

Arthrocentesis has a limited role in the diagnosis of OA. It can be done to exclude inflammatory arthritis, septic arthritis, or crystal-induced arthritis. Synovial fluid analysis is noninflammatory (white blood cell count is less than 2000 cells/mm^3) with predominant mononuclear cells.

55.7.7 Treatments

55.7.7.1 Medical Management

Medications can be used to provide symptom relief but not to reverse the disease process. Chronic conditions and co-existing medication regimes are to be factored to reduce drug toxicity. The choices are oral drugs such as acetaminophen, nonsteroidal anti-inflammatory agent (NSAID), duloxetine (efficacious in knee pain), and, in select situations, tramadol. Opioids are not preferred [30]. Local treatment can be in the form of intra-articular corticosteroid injection (useful if there are signs of inflammation or unable to take systemic therapy), viscosupplementation (injection of hyaluronan in the affected joint), closed tidal lavage (has shown similar efficacy to intra-articular corticosteroid injection and arthroscopic debridement), and topical therapies (NSAID, salicylates, capsaicin). Natural nutrition supplements available over the counter are glucosamine and chondroitin but lack sufficient data.

55.7.7.2 Rehabilitation

It begins with patient education to understand the disease process and set expectations. Individualized exercise regimen (nonimpact aerobic exercise, aquatic exercise regimen), weight loss, and assistive devices (braces, canes, walkers, splints) to carry out daily activities and provide symptomatic relief. Weight loss has proven to be beneficial only in knee osteoarthritis, while a combination of diet and exercise has proven to improve pain and function.

Physical Therapy

All patients benefit from participating in a home exercise program and physical therapy. Regardless of the underlying condition, the physical therapist instructs in the correct way to strengthen, stretch, and protect the involved joints. The exercise program should include aerobic (walking, biking, swimming), strengthening, and stretching exercises. If available, a water-based program is best as it can lighten the load on the joints while still providing resistance for the muscles to become stronger. A heated pool is very beneficial as warm water can soothe sore muscles.

Every exercise program is specific to the needs of the patient. The general recommendation is for patients to perform cardiovascular exercise 3–5×/week (30–60 min), strength train 2–3×/week (20–30 min), and stretch 3–7×/week (20–30 min). An increase in pain lasting more than 1 h after completing the routine is an indication of difficulty and should be reduced at the next session. An exercise program involving open and closed chain exercises will improve strength, flexibility, balance, and proprioception. Its result is less joint stiffness, better pain management, and better quality of life.

Recommended Exercises

Aerobic Walking, biking, swimming

Strength training Body weight exercise, free weights, weight machines, TheraBand

Flexibility Static and dynamic stretching, yoga, pilates

Participating in yoga, pilates, Tai Chi, and dance class are all great ways to reduce joint stiffness, build strength, and flexibility. Regular exercise can improve overall health, reduce the pain and stiffness associated with OA, and result in weight loss.

55.7.8 Procedures

- Intraarticular steroid injection. This is commonly performed in mild-moderate osteoarthritic joints and may reduce the inflammatory phase of the disease and reduce pain. From randomized controlled trials in OA patients, there is evidence that intra-articular corticosteroids are effective, but their benefit over placebo may be relatively short-lived, up to 4 weeks [31]. In a 2006 Cochrane review, the short-term efficacy of corticosteroids in knee OA has been confirmed [31]. Steroid should be diluted with saline and not with local anesthetics (LA), since all LA are cytotoxic to intraarticular cartilage.
- Viscosupplementation: Despite many clinical trials, the efficacy of HA is a matter of debate. The injectable hyaluronan products that are approved by FDA are sodium hyaluronate, Hylan G-F 20, and high-molecular-weight hyaluronan. Viscosupplementation is currently only indicated for knee OA.
- Intraarticular PRP: There is an increase in the utilization of PRP in managing pain in osteoarthritis. Systematic review and meta-analysis of RCT trials show that treatment of OA with leukocyte-poor PRP results in patient-reported positive outcomes and pain reduction for up to 1 year. However, there was no statistically significant difference between PRP and HA in pain reduction [32].
- Bone marrow-derived and adipose-derived stem cells: Stem cells are an important milestone in the field of tissue engineering and regenerative medicine. Stem cell therapy is considered to be a promising method to solve the regeneration of articular cartilage. Despite major interest and a growing body of evidence, there is limited research-backed support in the use of bone marrow- or adipose-derived mesenchymal stem cells for the treatment of OA. Ethical issues, regulatory obstacles to cell culture/expansion, high cost, poor cell localization, poor cell retention, and limited FDA-approved scaffolds are all major obstacles to research.

55.7.9 Surgery

Failure to respond to conventional therapy and exhibition of moderate to severe functional disability require surgical intervention such as total joint arthroplasty and cartilage repair and transplantation. Morbidly obese individuals with knee OA can trial bariatric surgery which has shown some evidence of knee OA improvement.

References

1. Clauw DJ. Fibromyalgia: a clinical review. JAMA. 2014;311(15):1547–55.
2. Williams DA, Clauw DJ. Understanding fibromyalgia: lessons from the broader pain research community. J Pain. 2009;10(8):777–91.
3. Phillips K, Clauw DJ. Central pain mechanisms in the rheumatic diseases: future directions. Arthritis Rheum. 2013;65(2):291–302.
4. Wolfe F, Clauw DJ, Fitzcharles MA, Goldenberg DL, Häuser W, Katz RL, Mease PJ, Russell AS, Russell IJ, Walitt B. 2016 revisions to the 2010/2011 fibromyalgia diagnostic criteria. Semin Arthritis Rheum. 2016;46(3):319–29.
5. Arora N, Gupta A, Reddy SB. Antinuclear antibody and subserology testing in the evaluation of fibromyalgia: a teachable moment. JAMA Intern Med. 2017;177(9):1369–70.
6. White KP, Nielson WR, Harth M, Ostbye T, Speechley M. Does the label "fibromyalgia" alter health status, function, and health service utilization? A prospective, within-group comparison in a community cohort of adults with chronic widespread pain. Arthritis Rheum. 2002;47(3):260–5.
7. Clauw DJ. Pain management: fibromyalgia drugs are 'as good as it gets' in chronic pain. Nat Rev Rheumatol. 2010;6(8):439–40.
8. Hoppenfeld S, Hutton R, Hugh T. Physical examination of the spine and extremities, vol. 798. New York: Appleton-Century-Crofts; 1976.
9. Sheon RP, Moskowitz RW, Goldberg VM. Soft tissue rheumatic pain: recognition, management, prevention. In: Soft tissue rheumatic pain: recognition, management, prevention. Philadelphia: Lea & Febiger; 1987. p. 332.
10. Shmerling RH, Fuchs HA, Lorish CD, Nichols LA, Partridge AJ, SanchezGuerrero J, Sands RA, Liang MH. Guidelines for the initial evaluation of the adult patient with acute musculoskeletal symptoms. American College of Rheumatology Ad Hoc Committee on Clinical Guidelines. Arthritis Rheum. 1996;39(1):1–8.
11. Pujalte GG, Albano-Aluquin SA. Differential diagnosis of polyarticular arthritis. Am Fam Physician. 2015;92(1):35–41.
12. Myasoedova E, Crowson CS, Kremers HM, Therneau TM, Gabriel SE. Is the incidence of rheumatoid arthritis rising?: results from Olmsted County, Minnesota, 1955-2007. Arthritis Rheum. 2010;62(6):1576–82.
13. Crowson CS, Matteson EL, Myasoedova E, Michet CJ, Ernste FC, Warrington KJ, Davis JM III, Hunder GG, Therneau TM, Gabriel SE. The lifetime risk of adult-onset rheumatoid arthritis and other inflammatory autoimmune rheumatic diseases. Arthritis Rheum. 2011;63(3):633–9.
14. Sugiyama D, Nishimura K, Tamaki K, Tsuji G, Nakazawa T, Morinobu A, Kumagai S. Impact of smoking as a risk factor for developing rheumatoid arthritis: a meta-analysis of observational studies. Ann Rheum Dis. 2010;69(01):70–81.
15. Okada Y, Wu D, Trynka G, Raj T, Terao C, Ikari K, Kochi Y, Ohmura K, Suzuki A, Yoshida S. Genetics of rheumatoid arthritis contributes to biology and drug discovery. Nature. 2014;506(7488):376–81.

16. Aletaha D, Smolen JS. Diagnosis and management of rheumatoid arthritis: a review. JAMA. 2018;320(13):1360–72.
17. Aletaha D, Neogi T, Silman AJ, Funovits J, Felson DT, Bingham CO III, Birnbaum NS, Burmester GR, Bykerk VP, Cohen MD. 2010 rheumatoid arthritis classification criteria: an American College of Rheumatology/European League Against Rheumatism collaborative initiative. Arthritis Rheum. 2010;62(9):2569–81.
18. Avouac J, Gossec L, Dougados M. Diagnostic and predictive value of anti-cyclic citrullinated protein antibodies in rheumatoid arthritis: a systematic literature review. Ann Rheum Dis. 2006;65(7):845–51.
19. Backhaus M, Burmester G, Sandrock D, Loreck D, Hess D, Scholz A, Blind S, Hamm B, Bollow M. Prospective two year follow up study comparing novel and conventional imaging procedures in patients with arthritic finger joints. Ann Rheum Dis. 2002;61(10):895–904.
20. Singh JA, Saag KG, Bridges SL Jr, Akl EA, Bannuru RR, Sullivan MC, Vaysbrot E, McNaughton C, Osani M, Shmerling RH. 2015 American College of Rheumatology guideline for the treatment of rheumatoid arthritis. Arthritis Rheumatol. 2016;68(1):1–26.
21. Smolen JS, van der Heijde D, Machold KP, Aletaha D, Landewé R. Proposal for a new nomenclature of disease-modifying antirheumatic drugs. Ann Rheum Dis. 2014;73(1):3–5.
22. Panush RS, Carias K, Kramer N, Rosenstein ED. Acute arthritis in the hospital: comparison of rheumatologic with nonrheumatologic care. J Clin Rheumatol. 1995;1(2):74–80.
23. Ritchlin CT, Colbert RA, Gladman DD. Psoriatic arthritis. N Engl J Med. 2017;376(10):957–70.
24. Hayward RJ, Machado PM. Classification criteria in axial spondyloarthritis: what have we learned; where are we going? Rheum Dis Clin. 2020;46(2):259–74.
25. Poddubnyy D, Haibel H, Listing J, Märker-Hermann E, Zeidler H, Braun J, Sieper J, Rudwaleit M. Baseline radiographic damage, elevated acute-phase reactant levels, and cigarette smoking status predict spinal radiographic progression in early axial spondylarthritis. Arthritis Rheum. 2012;64(5):1388–98.
26. Rudwaleit M, Listing J, Brandt J, Braun J, Sieper J. Prediction of a major clinical response (BASDAI 50) to tumour necrosis factor α blockers in ankylosing spondylitis. Ann Rheum Dis. 2004;63(6):665–70.
27. Rettenbacher T, Ennemoser S, Weirich H, Ulmer H, Hartig F, Klotz W, Herold M. Diagnostic imaging of gout: comparison of high-resolution US versus conventional X-ray. Eur Radiol. 2008;18(3):621–30.
28. Lawrence RC, Felson DT, Helmick CG, Arnold LM, Choi H, Deyo RA, Gabriel S, Hirsch R, Hochberg MC, Hunder GG. Estimates of the prevalence of arthritis and other rheumatic conditions in the United States: part II. Arthritis Rheum. 2008;58(1):26–35.
29. Goldring MB, Goldring SR. Articular cartilage and subchondral bone in the pathogenesis of osteoarthritis. Ann N Y Acad Sci. 2010;1192(1):230–7.
30. Krebs EE, Gravely A, Nugent S, Jensen AC, DeRonne B, Goldsmith ES, Kroenke K, Bair MJ, Noorbaloochi S. Effect of opioid vs nonopioid medications on pain-related function in patients with chronic back pain or hip or knee osteoarthritis pain: the SPACE randomized clinical trial. JAMA. 2018;319(9):872–82.
31. Prather H, Bonnette M, Hunt D. Nonoperative treatment options for patients with sacroiliac joint pain. Int J Spine Surg. 2020;14(Suppl 1):35–40. Published 2020 Feb 10. https://doi.org/10.14444/6082.
32. Garcia FL, Williams BT, Polce EM, Heller DB, Aman ZS, Nwachukwu BU, Nho SJ, Chahla J. Preparation methods and clinical outcomes of platelet-rich plasma for intra-articular hip disorders: a systematic review and meta-analysis of randomized clinical trials. Orthop J Sports Med. 2020;8(10):1–9.

Entrapment Syndromes

56

David P. Brown, Lei Lin, and Tomas Salazar

56.1 Carpal Tunnel Syndrome

56.1.1 Synonyms

Median neuropathy at the wrist

56.1.2 ICD-10 Codes

G56.00

56.1.3 Description

Carpal tunnel syndrome (CTS) is a median nerve compression neuropathy in the carpal tunnel. It is the most common entrapment neuropathy of the upper extremity.

Anatomy The median nerve arises from the C6–T1 nerve roots. Axons traverse all three trunks and then the medial and lateral cords. Sensation to the palmar lateral surface of the hand and the palmar thumb, index, middle, and lateral half of the ring finger is provided by the lateral cord. Axons from the medial cord provide innervation for median motor control of the hand with no sensory function; this includes the lumbricals 1 and 2, opponens pollicis, abductor pollicis brevis, and the flexor pollicis brevis (LOAF muscles). The carpal tunnel is bounded by the carpal bones and the transverse carpal ligament. The tunnel contains the four flexor digitorum superficialis tendons, the four flexor digitorum tendons, the flexor pollicis longus tendon, and the median nerve [2] (Fig. 56.1).

Carpal tunnel syndrome (CTS) can be an idiopathic process or a result of increased volume and pressure within the tunnel caused by specific disorders such as repetitive motion injuries, thyroid disease, congestive heart failure, renal failure, or masses including hematomas or tumors [1, 2]. In the last trimester of pregnancy, total body fluid volume may increase leading to increased carpal tunnel pressures. CTS associated with pregnancy may subside after delivery [3]. Other conditions which can cause tunnel compromise include fracture, arthritis, and rheumatoid tenosynovitis. Underlying conditions which can cause generalized peripheral neuropathies make individuals more prone to focal neuropathies like CTS. Differential diagnosis of CTS is outlined in Table 56.1.

Double crush syndrome occurs when radiculopathies, brachial plexopathies, or thoracic outlet syndrome occur with CTS. C6 and C7 radiculopathies must be considered in the differential diagnosis when considering CTS due to overlap of symptoms [1, 2].

56.1.4 Clinical Presentation

Classic CTS complaints include numbness and tingling of the thumb, index, and middle fingers. At times, due to referred pain, symptoms can extend into the ring and small fingers. Nocturnal pain and numbness are common. Symptoms can radiate proximally into the forearm as well. People may attest to weakness in grip and poor dexterity. Holding a phone, grasping a steering wheel, or repetitive motions can engender symptoms. In general, any activity leading to prolonged wrist flexion can generate numbness, tingling, and pain in patients with CTS [2].

56.1.5 Physical Examination

If the median nerve is only irritated (no axonal loss), the sensory examination may be normal. If sufficient axon loss has occurred, then sensation will be decreased in the median nerve distribution including the thumb, index finger, middle

D. P. Brown (✉)
Physical Medicine & Rehabilitation, Rutgers -Robert Wood Johnson Medical School, Electrodiagnostics & Sports Medicine, JFK, Johnson Rehabilitation Institute, Edison, NJ, USA
e-mail: DavidP.Brown@hmhn.org

L. Lin · T. Salazar
JFK, Johnson Rehabilitation Institute, Edison, NJ, USA
e-mail: Lei.Lin@hmhn.org

© The Author(s), under exclusive license to Springer Nature Switzerland AG 2022

S. A. Mostoufi et al. (eds.), *Clinical Guide to Musculoskeletal Medicine*, https://doi.org/10.1007/978-3-030-92042-5_56

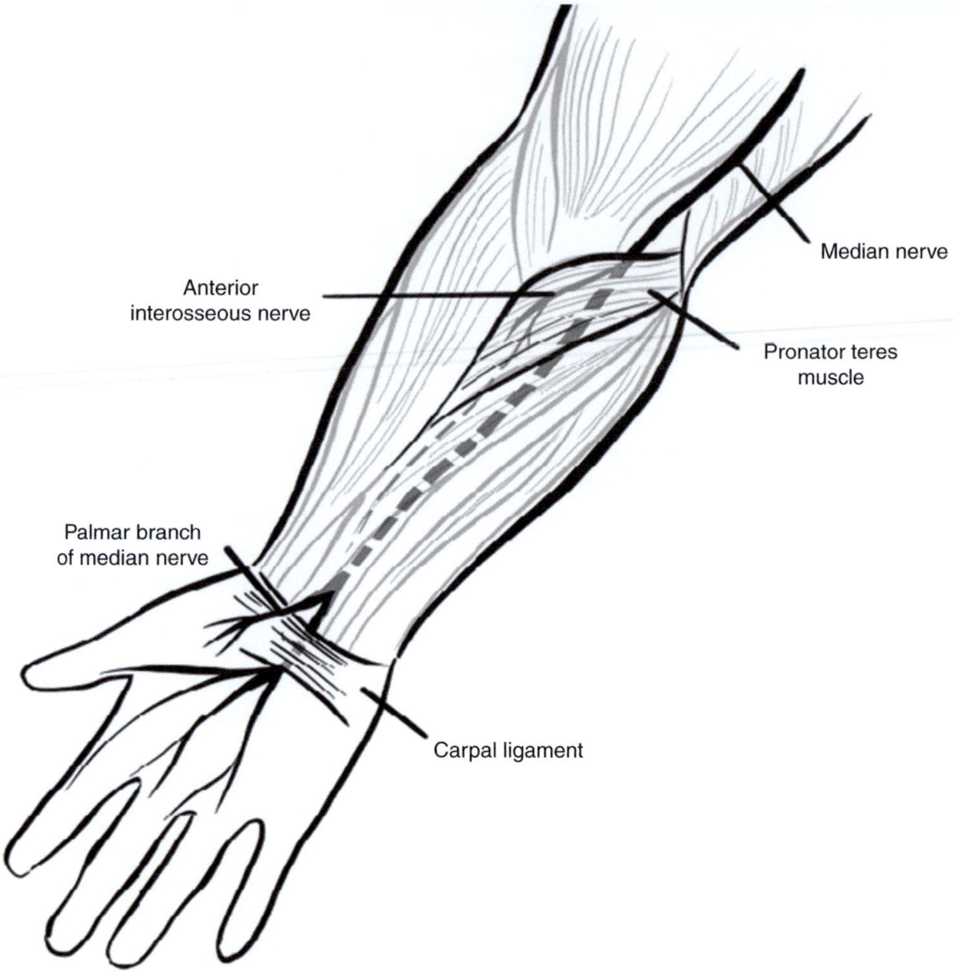

Fig. 56.1 Course of median nerve in the forearm and carpal tunnel

Table 56.1 Differential diagnosis of carpal tunnel syndrome

Brachial plexopathy	Anterior interosseous neuropathy
Cervical radiculopathy	Musculoskeletal disorders of hand and wrist
Generalized peripheral neuropathy	Pronator teres syndrome

finger, and the radially half of the ring finger. Motor function may be spared in mild to moderate cases. In more advanced CTS, thumb abduction weakness occurs, and atrophy of the abductor pollicis brevis may be seen.

As with all nerve entrapment cases, the examination including general inspection, palpation, range of motion, strength testing, deep tendon reflexes, and sensation of the upper limbs must take into account other possible causes for the presenting symptoms. *Tinel's sign* (mechanical tapping of the median nerve at the carpal tunnel) and *Phalen's test* (60-second maintained wrist flexion position eliciting median distribution paresthesias) are both provocative tests for CTS. Tinel's has about 65% sensitivity, and Phalen's test has about 85% sensitivity, and both have approximately 90% specificity for median nerve entrapment at the wrist [2, 24] (Fig. 56.2).

56.1.6 Diagnostic Workup

NCS and EMG are an extension of the physical examination. Sensory studies are more sensitive than motor studies. Median sensory distal latencies will be prolonged and should be compared to other nerves in the hand, either radial or ulnar. Antidromic studies will provide larger amplitudes. Axonal loss or conduction block will cause motor and sensory amplitude drop. Conduction studies of the median nerve through the forearm will help differentiate CTS from a more generalized peripheral neuropathy. EMG should sample C5–T1 selected muscles, the APB, and the cervical paraspinals [1].

Ultrasound is useful to assess the median nerve at the carpal tunnel proximal border (Fig. 56.3). At this site, the nerve will appear swollen (Fig. 56.4) and hypoechoic with a large cross-sectional area in comparison to the nerve more proximally [1]. Greater than $10mm^2$ at the carpal tunnel inlet is diagnostic for CTS [22].

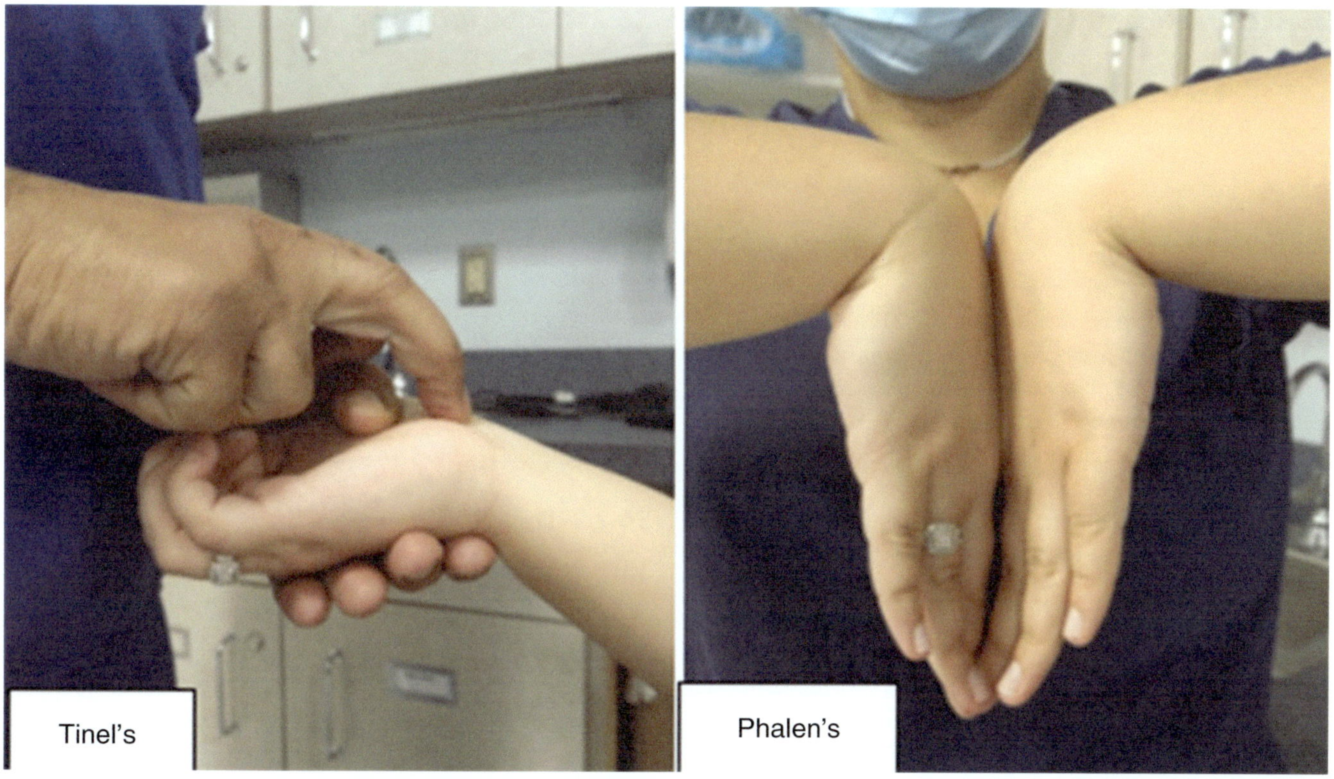

Fig. 56.2 Tinel's test (left) and Phalen's test (right) are part of CTS examination. (Courtesy of S. Ali Mostoufi, MD, Boston Regenerative Medicine)

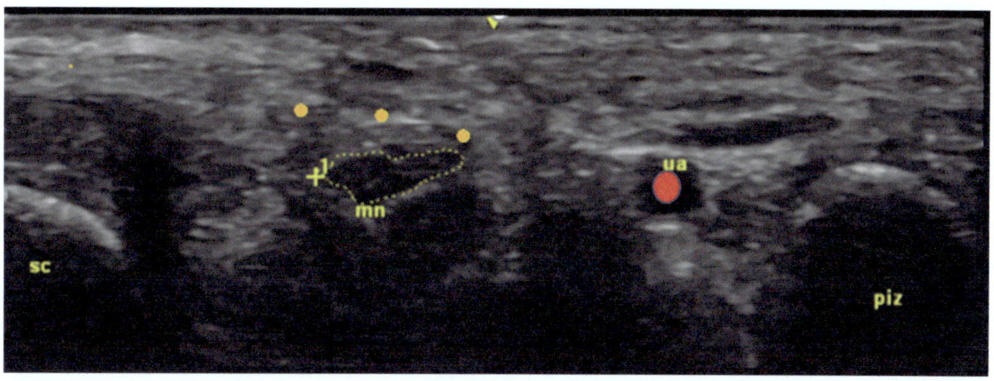

Fig. 56.3 Median nerve at carpal tunnel inlet with pisiform and scaphoid bony landmarks and the ulnar artery (UA). Transverse carpal ligament is marked as yellow dots superficial to MN. Measurement of the median nerve can be done at this site for diagnostic purposes. (Figure courtesy of S. Ali Mostoufi, MD)

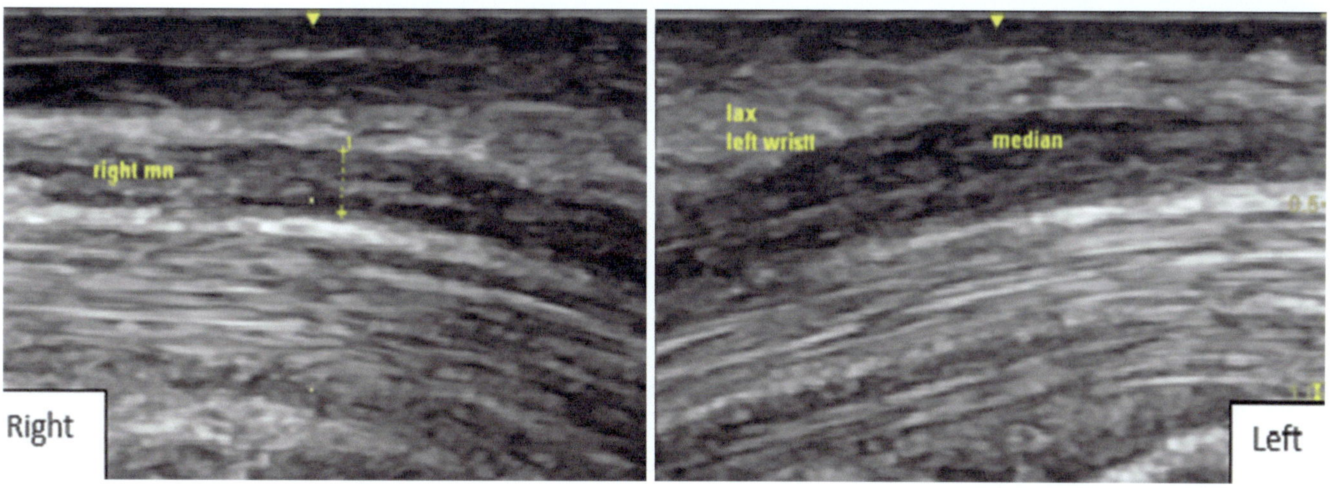

Fig. 56.4 Median nerve in long axis. Side-to-side comparison demonstrating enlargement of the left median nerve. (Courtesy of S. Ali Mostoufi, MD, Boston Regenerative Medicine)

56.1.7 Treatment

Conservative treatment is indicated in mild cases with no weakness, atrophy, or denervation on EMG. Orthotics: carpal tunnel splints usually worn at night

- Medications such as NSAIDs and diuretics
- Ergonomic modifications
- Image-guided steroid injections may provide some relief but may not be a permanent solution (Fig. 56.5).
- Hydrodissection has been used with some success in mild to moderate CTS. For more details, please see Chap. 32.
- Platelet-rich plasma injection into the carpal tunnel has been used with some success in mild to moderate CTS. For more details, please see Chap. 32.
- Ultrasound-guided percutaneous release of the carpal ligament has proved successful in mild to moderate CTS (Fig. 56.6). For more details, please see Chap. 32.

Surgical release is indicated for persistent numbness and pain despite conservative treatment. In CTS with severe muscle atrophy, surgical release does not have a high rate of success due to the extent of axon damage [2]. Surgical care is discussed in more detail in Chap. 37.

56.2 Anterior Interosseous Nerve Entrapment

56.2.1 Synonyms

- Anterior interosseous neuropathy
- Anterior interosseous syndrome
- Pure median motor neuropathy of the forearm

56.2.2 ICD-10 Codes

G56.10

56.2.3 Description

Anterior interosseous nerve (AIN) entrapment is a pure median motor neuropathy in the forearm. It is a less common median neuropathy and can be mistaken for brachial plexopathy or other proximal median neuropathies. AIN results in weakness in thumb and finger pinch strength. Trauma to the volar forearm is one possible cause. True entrapment of the AIN is rare [1, 2]. Differential diagnosis of AIN is outlined in Table 56.2.

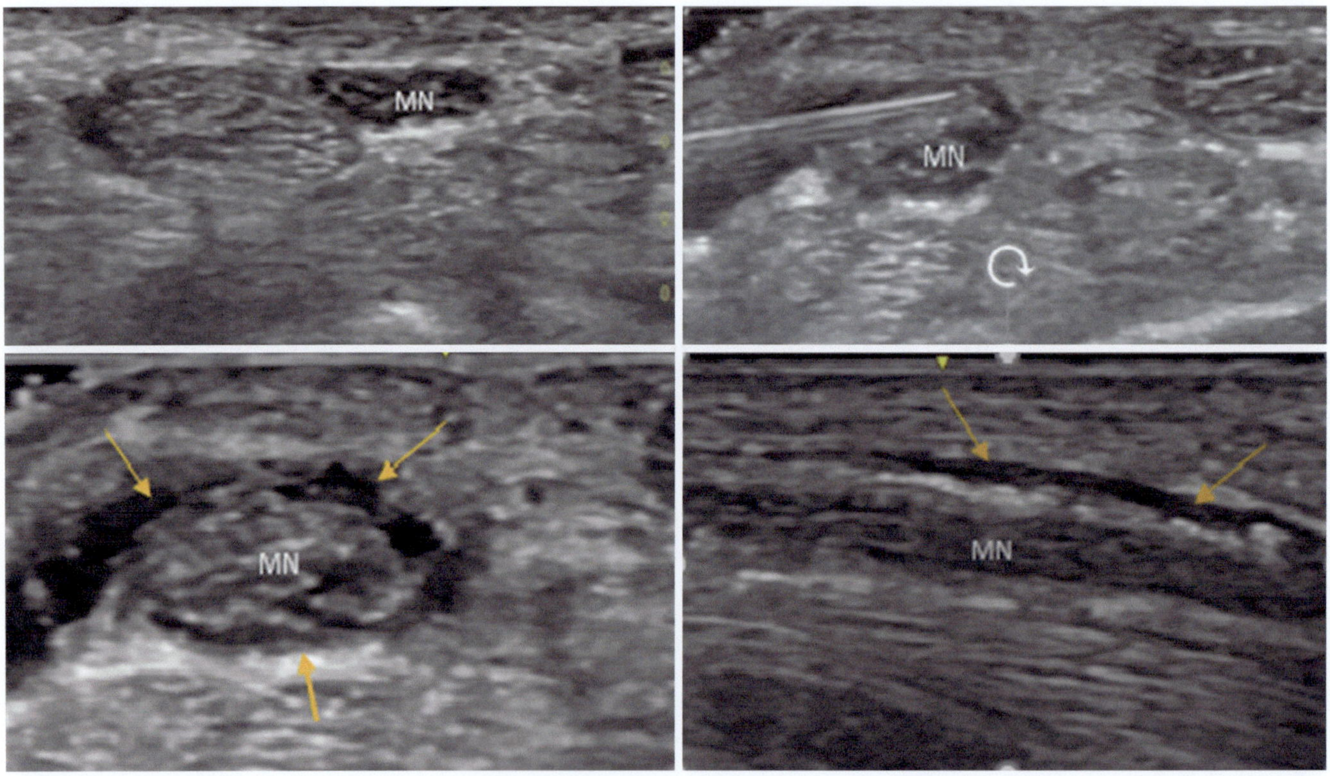

Fig. 56.5 CTS injection with US. Needle tip is placed between the transcarpal ligament and the median nerve. The correct injection flow should be confirmed in both short- and long-axis images. (Courtesy of S. Ali Mostoufi, MD, Boston Regenerative Medicine)

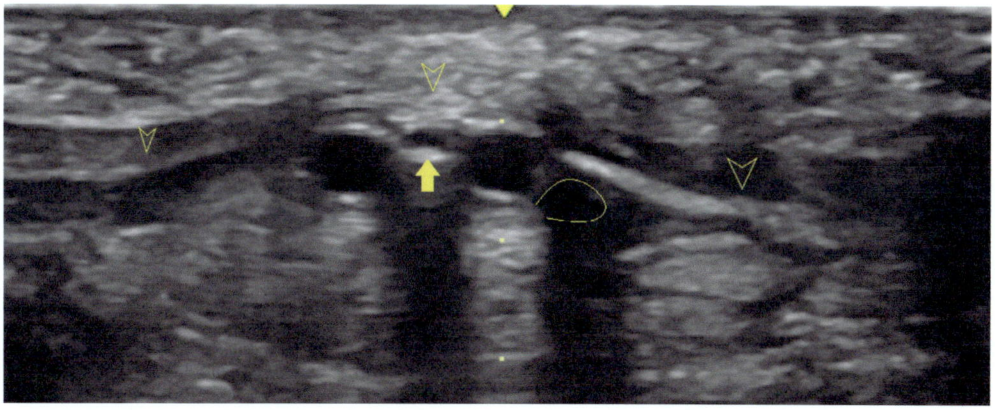

Fig. 56.6 Percutaneous US-guided CTS release. Triangles point to the transverse carpal ligament, and the arrows demonstrate the blade engaged in the ligament, The median nerve (circle) is displaced laterally and protected by an air chamber to avoid injury. (Courtesy of S. Ali Mostoufi, Boston Regenerative Medicine)

Table 56.2 Differential diagnosis of anterior interosseous syndrome

Brachial plexopathy	Multifocal motor neuropathy
Cervical radiculopathy	Muscle or tendon injury in the forearm
Carpal tunnel syndrome	Pronator syndrome

Anatomy Refer to the "Carpal Tunnel Syndrome" section for full median nerve anatomy. The AIN branches in the proximal forearm as a pure median motor nerve to innervate the flexor digitorum profundus I and II, the flexor pollicis longus, and pronator quadratus.

56.2.4 Clinical Presentation

AIN entrapment presents with severe pain in the forearm with no sensory loss. Weakness is evident in forming the letter "O" with the thumb, index, and middle fingers, due to denervation of the muscles of distal flexion of these digits [1].

56.2.5 Physical Examination

Inspection of the forearm may or may not reveal volar forearm atrophy. The patient may feel pain on the volar aspect of the proximal third of the forearm. Sensory should be intact for the upper limb. Weakness should be evident as noted above in thumb, index, and middle finger in flexion. Holding onto a single sheet of paper with just the fingertips can be challenging for these patients [4]. Upper limb reflexes should be normal. A thorough examination of the cervical neck and upper limbs is needed to rule out other causes.

56.2.6 Diagnostic Workup

Plain films Radiographs of the supracondylar humerus are indicated in AIN palsy, since 20% of fractures in this region will result in nerve palsy including AIN [23].

Electrodiagnostic studies are essential. Sensory and motor conduction studies of the median and ulnar nerves are needed to rule out other neuropathies and brachial plexopathy. EMG of the flexor digitorum I and II, flexor pollicis longus, and pronator quadratus are required and will show evidence of abnormalities. EMG of other muscles will rule in or out other nerve involvement.

Diagnostic ultrasound scans of the forearm may reveal nerve injury as swelling and increased heterogenicity. It can also show causes of entrapment including cysts, tumors, ischemia, hematomas, or fibrous bands [1].

56.2.7 Treatment

Conservative care involves stretching and strengthening of the forearm musculature. Surgical intervention may be needed for the release of fibrous bands or decompression of scar tissue or masses. Most patients improve without surgical intervention; recovery with conservative treatment may take up to 1 year after onset [4].

56.3 Pronator Teres Syndrome

56.3.1 Synonyms

- Median neuropathy at the pronator teres muscle
- Proximal median motor and sensory neuropathy of the forearm

56.3.2 ICD-10 Codes

G56.10

56.3.3 Description

Pronator teres syndrome is a median nerve entrapment at the pronator teres muscle affecting both motor and sensory function. The nerve is compressed at a fibrous arch connecting the two heads of the pronator teres muscle (Fig. 56.1). This

Table 56.3 Differential diagnosis of pronator syndrome

Anterior interosseous nerve syndrome	Generalized peripheral neuropathy
Brachial plexopathy	Forearm musculotendinous injury
Cervical radiculopathy	Multifocal motor neuropathy

results in weakness in all median innervated muscles of the forearm and hand distal to the pronator teres and numbness in the median nerve distribution. This is an uncommon neuropathy. The entrapment may be caused by activities requiring a high frequency of pronation. It may result from direct trauma or the development of a fibrous band [1, 2, 4]. Full median nerve anatomy is discussed in the CTS section. Differential diagnosis of pronator syndrome is outlined in Table 56.3.

56.3.4 Clinical Presentation

Pain may be felt in the volar proximal forearm. Weakness will be apparent in flexion of the thumb, flexion of the index and middle fingers, flexion of the wrist, and abduction and opposition of the thumb. Numbness will involve the lateral palmar hand, the palmar thumb, and the index and middle fingers.

56.3.5 Physical Examination

Examination may find atrophy of the volar forearm and pain upon palpation in the proximal volar forearm. Percussion over the pronator teres may cause radiating dysesthesias to the lateral palmar hand. Symptoms may be replicated with resisted pronation.

Weakness as noted above is apparent in wrist flexion; thumb, index, and middle fingers; and abduction and opposition of the thumb. Sensory will be diminished in the lateral palmar hand; the thumb; and the index, middle, and lateral half of the ring finger.

Deep tendon reflexes are normal. A thorough examination of the arm and cervical region is necessary to rule out other pathology.

56.3.6 Diagnostic Workup

EMG/NCS Electrodiagnostic studies are essential. Median nerve abnormalities will be present distal to the pronator teres. Axonal injury will result in low amplitudes for median motor and sensory function. EMG abnormalities will involve all median innervated muscles distal to the pronator teres. The median nerve function must be compared to other nerves to isolate abnormalities, in order to rule out other conditions.

Diagnostic Ultrasound of the forearm may help identify nerve swelling at the injury site or the presence of a fibrous band, mass, or hematoma [1].

56.3.7 Treatment

Conservative care includes stretching, soft tissue release techniques, and strengthening. Nonsurgical management with rest, nonsteroidal anti-inflammatory medications, and avoidance of troublesome activities are highly effective [4]. Corticosteroids can also be beneficial. Surgical release may be required to reduce scar tissue or fibrous bands, if conservative treatment fails, or if symptoms are caused by a mass [4].

56.4 Posterior Interosseous Nerve Syndrome

56.4.1 Synonyms

- Posterior interosseous neuropathy
- PIN syndrome

56.4.2 ICD-10 Codes

G56.80–G56.82

56.4.3 Descriptions

Posterior interosseous nerve (PIN) syndrome is a neuropathy at the forearm of the PIN. It occurs most frequently due to entrapment at the arcade of Frohse. Other potential etiologies, including the tendinous edge of the bordering tissues, adjacent muscles and vessels, ganglion cysts, tumor and other mass lesions, synovial pathologies, radial head fracture and Monteggia fracture-dislocation, and repetitive pronation/supination, may also cause compression of the PIN [1]. This is a rare diagnosis and can be difficult to distinguish from radial neuropathy occurring at the spiral groove [1, 5]. The differential diagnosis of PIN is listed in Table 56.4.

Anatomy The radial nerve is essentially derived from the C5 and T1 roots; radial fibers then travel through the posterior division of all three trunks and posterior cords of the brachial plexus. The radial nerve travels through the arm,

Table 56.4 Differential diagnosis of posterior interosseous neuropathy

Brachial plexopathy	Radial nerve palsy at spiral groove
Cervical radiculopathy	Radial tunnel syndrome
Lesions in the contralateral motor cortex	Wartenberg syndrome

wraps around the humerus in the spiral groove, descends into the lateral elbow, and divides into the superficial and deep branches proximal to the arcade of Frohse. The posterior interosseous nerve is the deep motor branch of the radial nerve. The radial nerve, after coursing anterior to the lateral epicondyle of the humerus, bifurcates into a superficial sensory and the PIN at the level of the radiocapitellar joint. After travelling through the radial tunnel, the PIN passes between the superficial and deep heads of the supinator muscle. After exiting the supinator canal, the PIN supplies the extensor compartment muscles of the forearm [1, 2, 5].

56.4.4 Clinical Presentation

Posterior interosseous neuropathy presents with paralysis, which can be partial or complete, involving some or all the posterior interosseous nerve-innervated muscle. In most instances, it is relatively acute over the course of several days to weeks. Pain in the elbow or proximal lateral extensor forearm is an inconsistent feature; when present, it is typically the initial symptom and short-lived, lasting for no more than 3 days.

56.4.5 Physical Examination

In posterior interosseous neuropathy, patients usually have weakness affecting the extensor carpi ulnaris, extensor digitorum communis, extensor digiti minimi, abductor pollicis longus, and extensor pollicis brevis. Typically, the extensor carpi radialis brevis and longus, supinator, brachioradialis, and triceps are not affected as they are innervated before the radial nerve divides.

Patients with PIN neuropathy have the characteristic presentation of finger drop with radial wrist deviation when attempting to extend the wrist and fingers, due to paralysis of the extensor carpi ulnaris and the unopposed contraction of the extensor carpi radialis longus and brevis. Patients should be able to weakly extend the wrist. Sensation should be intact, as the PIN has no sensory branches. Depending on the severity of injury, there may be a positive Tinel sign at the site of injury [1, 2, 5, 6]. As with all neuropathies, a full MSK/neuromuscular and cervical spine exam is required to rule out other etiologies.

56.4.6 Diagnostic Workup

Imaging studies can be useful if patients have bony structure abnormalities or mass lesions. *Electrodiagnostic studies* are key to this diagnosis. The study may show denervation signs in the muscles innervated by the posterior interosseous nerve, with sparing of muscles innervated by the radial nerve, including triceps, anconeus, brachioradialis, and extensor carpi radialis longus and brevis. Patients will have normal sensory nerve action potential of the superficial radial nerve [5].

Ultrasound may provide a convenient and complementary tool for diagnosis. Diagnostic neuromuscular ultrasound may demonstrate hypoechoic swelling of the PIN, while also providing direct visualization of the PIN throughout the entire supinator canal and adjacent anatomic structures. This enables the examiner to identify various potential causative lesions, as well as see possible secondary denervation atrophy of the affected muscles [6].

56.4.7 Treatment

Most patients without open trauma or mass lesions improve with conservative treatment, which can include splinting, NSAIDs, physical and occupational therapy, and activity modification [2]. Corticosteroid injections can also be beneficial [5]. For patients who fail 6 months of conservative treatment, surgical release of all five compression sites is recommended [5]. Rehabilitation should start soon after decompression with an early active range of motion. The patient may continue to see improvement for months after surgery [7].

56.5 Radial Tunnel Syndrome

56.5.1 Synonyms

- Radial neuropathy at the elbow
- Resistant tennis elbow

56.5.2 ICD-10 Codes

G56.30–G56.32

56.5.3 Descriptions

Radial tunnel syndrome is a radial nerve neuropathy at the elbow. It occurs as a result of chronic sporadic compression on the radial nerve by the radial head as it passes

Table 56.5 Differential diagnosis of radial tunnel syndrome

Biceps tendinopathy	Lesions in the contralateral motor cortex
Brachial plexopathy	Muscle tear of the extensor carpi radialis brevis
Cervical radiculopathy	Osteoarthritis of the radiocapitellar joint
Lateral epicondylitis	Posterior interosseous neuropathy

under the supinator. This is a debatable diagnosis, as patients do not have any signs or symptoms other than pain, and they have normal electrodiagnostic studies [1, 5, 8]. Table 56.5 details the differential diagnosis of radial tunnel syndrome.

Anatomy For complete anatomical overview of the radial nerve, please see the section "Posterior Interosseous Nerve Syndrome." The anatomical radial tunnel runs from the radial head to the inferior aspect of the supinator muscle. It is bordered by the supinator, extensor carpi radialis longus, extensor carpi radialis brevis, and brachioradialis muscle [8].

56.5.4 Clinical Presentation

Radial tunnel syndrome presents with pain over the radial proximal forearm, typically involving the dominant side. It is usually described as a dull ache, located deep in the extensor muscle mass, and may radiate proximally or distally into the arm and forearm respectively. Pain is usually worse at night or when the elbow is extended, forearm is pronated, or wrist is flexed [8].

56.5.5 Physical Examination

In radial tunnel syndrome, patients usually have tenderness over the radial nerve 3–5 cm distal to the lateral epicondyle and may be exacerbated with resisted forearm supination or wrist hyperextension [5, 8]. Pain while extending the middle finger against resistance has shown to be a strong clinical indicator of radial tunnel syndrome [8].

56.5.6 Diagnostic Workup

Electrodiagnostic studies are normal in radial tunnel syndrome but are still of value as clinically differentiating between radial tunnel syndrome and PIN syndrome is challenging. (PIN syndrome, as previously described, shows abnormalities on electrodiagnostic studies [5].)

MRI is usually also normal but could show muscle edema [8]. *Ultrasound* can be useful as it might demonstrate nerve edema; it can also help rule out other diagnoses such as lateral epicondylitis [8].

56.5.7 Treatment

Common conservative treatment methods include immobilization of the wrist with splinting, anti-inflammatory medication, ultrasound massage, and physical therapy. Activity modifications include avoiding prolonged elbow extension, forearm pronation, and wrist flexion. Nerve block has been beneficial in some patients. Surgical intervention is recommended if the symptoms do not improve with 3 months of conservative treatments [8]. Surgery usually also includes the release of the PIN [8].

56.6 Cubital Tunnel Syndrome

56.6.1 Synonyms

Ulnar neuropathy at the elbow

56.6.2 ICD-10 Codes

G56.21–G56.23

56.6.3 Description

Cubital tunnel syndrome is an ulnar neuropathy at the elbow. It is the second most common neuropathy affecting the upper extremity after carpal tunnel syndrome.

Anatomy The ulnar nerve comes from the C8 and T1 roots, with a minor part from C7. The nerve fibers go through the lower trunk and medial cord of the brachial plexus. The ulnar nerve descends through the medial arm toward the elbow. Here, it enters the ulnar groove between the medial epicondyle and the olecranon process. After traversing the ulnar groove, the nerve dives into the cubital tunnel by passing under the flexor carpi ulnaris. The tunnel is sometimes known as the humeral-ulnar aponeurosis [1, 2]. This path of the ulnar nerve is seen in Fig. 56.7.

Cubital tunnel syndrome is usually caused by chronic compression due to repeated elbow flexion traumatizing the nerve [1, 2]. Ulnar neuropathy at the elbow is also common in patients immobilized after surgery and during general anesthesia or coma. Congenitally tight cubital tunnels can also lead to compression [1]. In Table 56.6, the differential diagnosis of cubital tunnel syndrome is listed.

56.6.4 Clinical Presentation

Cubital tunnel syndrome typically presents with paresthesias, numbness, and/or pain in the ulnar cutaneous distribution, particularly the ring and pinky finger. This can be worsened at night due to elbow flexion while sleeping, but other actions that cause elbow flexion can also trigger the symptoms [2, 9]. As the condition worsens, motor strength diminishes, and patients can report clumsy hand function. Further advanced cases might also report hand deformities [9].

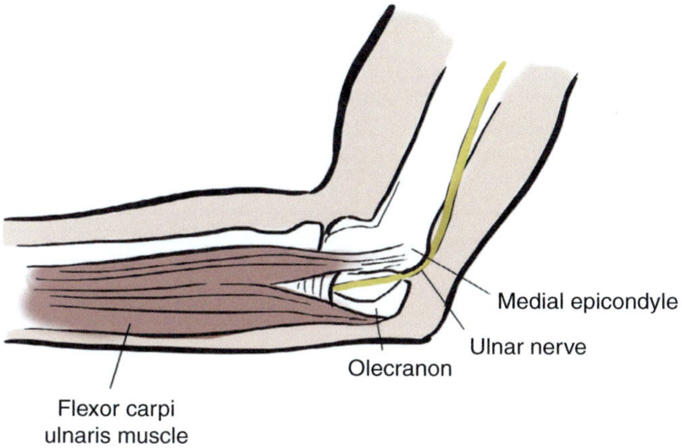

Fig. 56.7 Path of ulnar nerve traveling through the cubital tunnel. After traversing the ulnar groove, the nerve dives into the cubital tunnel by passing under the flexor carpi ulnaris

Table 56.6 Differential diagnosis of cubital tunnel syndrome

Amyotrophic lateral sclerosis	Superior sulcus tumor (Pancoast's tumor)
Lower cervical radiculopathy	Thoracic outlet syndrome
Spinal cord diseases	Ulnar neuropathy distal to the elbow

56.6.5 Physical Examination

Inspection of the hand can demonstrate atrophy of the intrinsic hand muscles. Strength testing can reveal weakness in the grip strength due to the involvement of the finger flexors. Flexion of the fifth digit at the distal interphalangeal joint is the best way to identify ulnar side involved muscle weakness [2]. Thumb adduction and flexion weakness can occur, but thumb abduction should not be involved [1]. Benediction posture, Wartenberg's sign, and Froment's sign are three examples of physical examination findings seen in more advanced cases (Fig. 56.8). Benediction hand, also known as claw hand deformity, is a hand positioned with metacarpophalangeal hyperextension and proximal and distal interphalangeal flexion of the fourth and fifth fingers [1, 9]. Wartenberg's sign is when the fifth finger on the involved hand is abducted at rest. Lastly, Froment's sign occurs when the patient is asked to pinch a piece of paper with their thumb and index finger. Due to intrinsic hand weakness, patients instead utilize the flexor pollicis longus and flexor digitorum profundus resulting in atypical flexion of the interphalangeal joints of those two fingers [1, 9]. Sensory exam can exhibit decrease in light touch over the ulnar half of the fourth finger and the complete fifth digit. No sensory changes in the forearm should be evident [1, 2, 9]. As with all suspected nerve entrapments, a complete neuromuscular examination of the involved extremity is vital to rule out other pathologies.

56.6.6 Diagnostic Workup

X-rays of the elbow to identify any bony abnormalities that might be causing a neuropathy can be helpful. If cervical radiculopathy or Pancoast tumor is of high concern, neck and chest radiographs, respectively, are recommended [9].

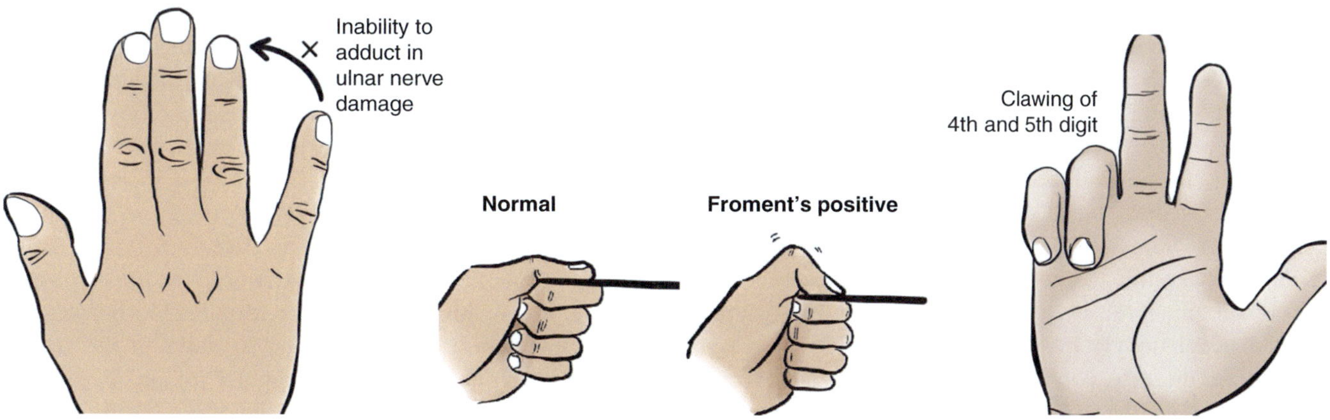

Fig. 56.8 Wartenberg's sign (left) is when the fifth finger on the involved hand is abducted at rest (unable to adduct due to ulnar nerve injury). Froment test (middle) examines ulnar neuropathy at the cubital tunnel. Benediction sign or claw hand deformity (right) is a hand positioned with metacarpophalangeal hyperextension and proximal and distal interphalangeal flexion of the fourth and fifth fingers

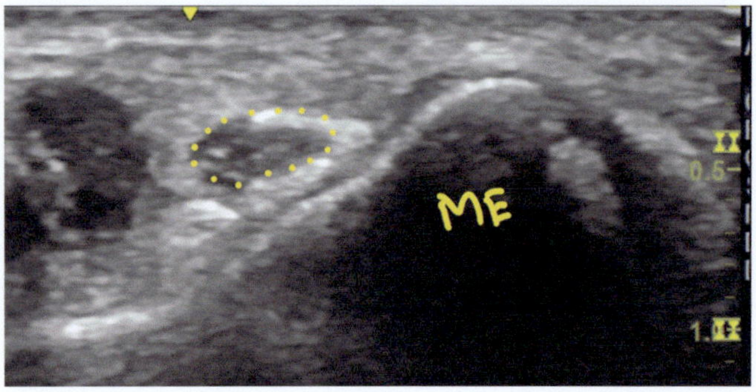

Fig. 56.9 Ulnar nerve highlighted in the cubital tunnel. Medial Epicondyle bony landmark is seen (ME). In dynamic US examination, subluxation of the ulnar nerve over the medial epicondyle can be easily seen. (Image courtesy of S. Ali Mostoufi, MD, Boston Regenerative Medicine)

Electrodiagnostic studies are key in identifying cubital tunnel syndrome. Nerve conduction studies need to include motor studies above and below the elbow to try and identify any demyelinating and/or axonal involvement across the elbow. Slowed conduction velocities, decreased amplitudes, and prolonged distal latency can be seen. Electromyography of both the ulnar-innervated muscles distal to the elbow and the muscles involved in C8 radiculopathy is necessary [2].

Ultrasound is a useful tool to easily follow the ulnar nerve through the arm. Flexing the elbow while observing the nerve at the elbow is a useful tool for identifying subluxation over the medial epicondyle (Fig. 56.9). Cross-sectional areas taken in the short axis can objectively determine if the nerve is edematous and enlarged [1].

56.6.7 Treatment

Conservative treatment should be initially attempted, with 50–90% of cases showing improvement [9, 10]. The program would include therapy, night splints, and patient education. Avoiding positions that provide direct pressure on the nerve at the elbow is of the utmost importance. Nightly elbow braces avoid hyperflexion and allow for inflammation to decrease. NSAID and steroid injections are sometimes attempted, but the evidence supporting their use is limited [9]. An ultrasound-guided steroid injection is demonstrated in Fig. 56.10. Surgery is necessary in advanced cases or after failing conservative treatment. Commonly used procedures are cubital tunnel release, ulnar nerve anterior transposition, or medial epicondylectomy, with medial epicondylectomy less utilized recently. Postsurgical physical therapy is recommended to help the patient regain strength and range of motion [9].

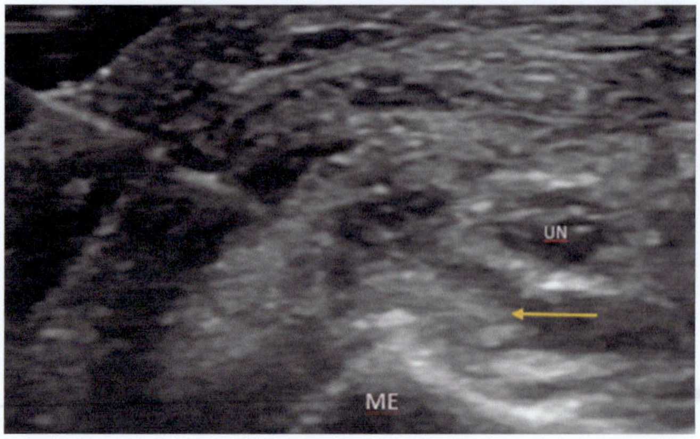

Fig. 56.10 US-guided perineural steroid injection of the ulnar nerve (UN) at the cubital tunnel. Needle tip (arrow) seen deep to the UN and slight hydrodissection is seen. Medial epicondyle's (ME) bony landmark is noted. (Courtesy of S. Ali Mostoufi, MD Boston Regen)

56.7 Suprascapular Nerve Entrapment

56.7.1 Synonyms

- Suprascapular neuropathy
- Suprascapular nerve palsy

56.7.2 ICD-10 Codes

G56.80

56.7.3 Description

Suprascapular nerve entrapment is a neuropathy due to compression of the suprascapular nerve. The nerve is most frequently injured at the suprascapular notch, but it can also be compressed at the spinoglenoid notch. Suprascapular nerve entrapment is also caused by rotator cuff tears with significant retraction, labral tears with cysts, and other mass lesions. Overhead activities are associated with suprascapular nerve entrapment [1, 11]. Table 56.7 describes the various diagnoses on the differential of suprascapular nerve entrapment.

Anatomy The suprascapular nerve arises from the upper trunk of the brachial plexus and receives innervation from the C5 and C6 roots. It travels posterior to the trapezius and clavicle on its path to the superior scapula. The nerve goes under the transverse suprascapular ligament at the suprascapular notch as it enters the scapular region. The transverse suprascapular ligament is the most likely site of entrapment. The suprascapular nerve then gives off motor fibers to the supraspinatus before heading towards the more laterally located spinoglenoid notch. After traversing under the spinoglenoid ligament, the nerve supplies motor innervation to the infraspinatus. Along its path, deep sensory innervation is given to the glenohumeral joint, acromioclavicular joint, and coracoacromial ligament. It rarely provides cutaneous sensation to the lateral arm [1, 2, 11]. See Fig. 56.11 for further the path of the suprascapular nerve in the posterior shoulder.

56.7.4 Clinical Presentation

Pain is typically the presenting complaint. Due to the deep sensory nerve branches of the nerve, patients complain of the pain feeling deep and dull as opposed to a more superficial pain. It can start in the upper scapula region with radiation to the shoulder. Shoulder movements can worsen the pain, particularly overhead activities. Patients also frequently report weakness with an aspect of shoulder fatigability. Usually, no inciting event is reported, but some might report frequent overhead activities [1, 11].

Table 56.7 Differential diagnosis of suprascapular nerve entrapment

AC joint injury	Neuralgic amyotrophy
Cervical radiculopathy and brachial plexopathy	Rotator cuff injury
Glenohumeral osteoarthritis	Shoulder labral tear

56.7.5 Physical Examination

With physical examination, inspection can discover atrophy of the supraspinatus and infraspinatus. Palpation over the suprascapular notch can yield tenderness. Patients can have weakness with shoulder abduction and external rotation due to the involvement of the supraspinatus and infraspinatus, respectively. Sensation should be intact as the suprascapular nerve does not have cutaneous involvement. Upper extremity reflexes should be normal. Site of entrapment changes the physical exam findings: entrapment after the supraspinatus is supplied (such as in entrapment at the spinoglenoid notch) would lead to normal shoulder abduction strength and no atrophy of the supraspinatus. A thorough exam of the cervical spine and shoulder is required to help narrow the diagnosis [11].

56.7.6 Diagnostic Workup

Electrodiagnostic studies are the gold standard for diagnosis. Despite there being no cutaneous distribution to test, the other sensory nerves in the arm should be tested to rule out brachial plexopathy. Motor conduction studies should be performed as well, with stimulation over Erb's point and recording the supraspinatus and infraspinatus. Motor studies may show decreased amplitudes and prolonged latencies. EMG of the supraspinatus and infraspinatus is key to diagnosing this disorder. Signs of denervation of those two muscles would point toward suprascapular neuropathy [1, 2].

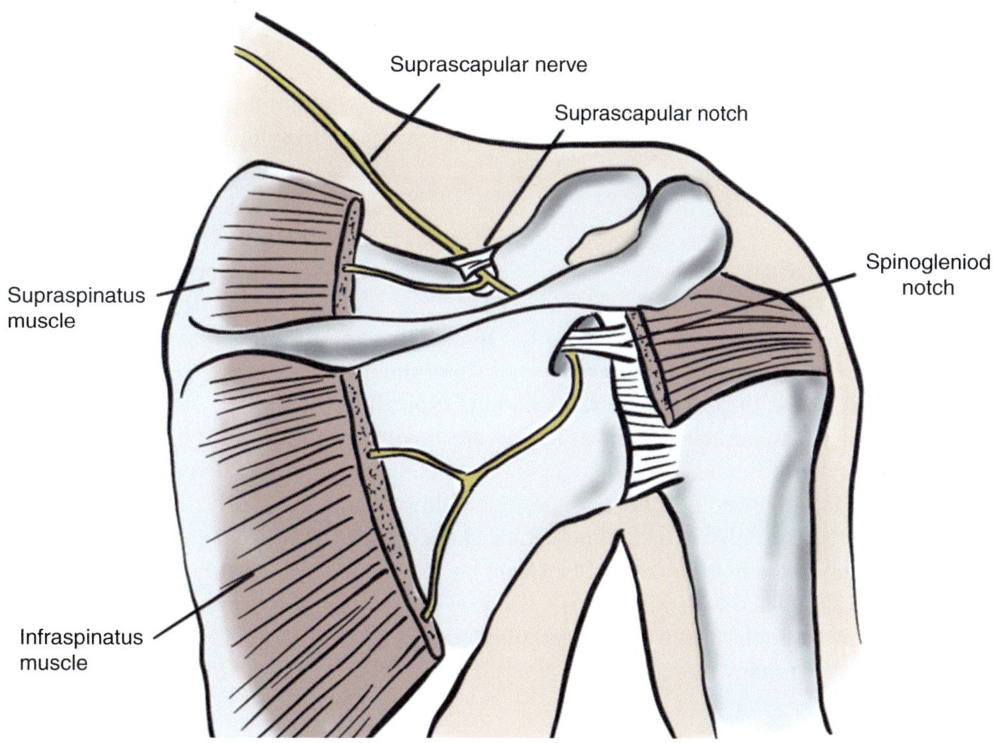

Fig. 56.11 Suprascapular nerve path in the posterior shoulder

Imaging Tests including radiographs, computed tomography, ultrasound, and magnetic resonance imaging can demonstrate the etiology of the entrapment, including fractures, ligament ossification, retracted rotator cuff tears, labral tears with cysts, and mass lesions [11].

56.7.7 Treatment

Conservative management involves avoiding overhead activities and utilizing physical therapy and nonsteroidal anti-inflammatory drugs. Physical therapy should focus on strengthening the shoulder and scapula musculature to improve motion and mechanics. If the patient fails conservative treatment or has a mass, then surgery is considered. These surgeries can decompress the entrapment and allow the nerve to heal. The surgical procedures can vary greatly based on the etiology of the problem and the location, but the release of the transverse scapular ligament is common [11]. If pain is a significant issue for the patient, then suprascapular nerve block or peripheral nerve stimulation are pain management treatment options [20] but they would not likely resolve any weakness.

56.8 Fibular Nerve Entrapment

56.8.1 Synonyms

- Peroneal neuropathy
- Foot drop
- Fibular neck entrapment

56.8.2 ICD-10 Codes

S84.10

56.8.3 Description

Fibular nerve entrapment is an injury to the fibular (peroneal) nerve at the fibular neck. The nerve travels superficially over the bone and is thus at risk at this location. Typically, both the deep and superficial peroneal nerves are involved [1]. Fibular nerve entrapment usually occurs after trauma or compression. Hospitalized patients with prolonged immobilization may develop it due to lack of positional changes and weight loss during the hospitalization. Frequent leg crossing has also been associated with peroneal nerve injury. While it is possible for the fibular nerve also to get impinged deep at the ankle, it is extremely rare and will therefore not be discussed in this section [1]. Table 56.8 details the differential diagnosis of fibular nerve entrapment.

Table 56.8 Differential diagnosis of fibular nerve entrapment

L5 radiculopathy	Peripheral neuropathy
Lumbosacral plexopathy	Sciatic neuropathy
Piriformis syndrome	Ischiofemoral impingement

Anatomy The common peroneal nerve runs within the sciatic nerve in the thigh after arising from the L4-S1 nerve roots and traversing the lumbosacral plexus. The sciatic nerves divide into the tibial nerve and common peroneal above the posterior knee. Sensory innervation is given off to the lateral knee via the lateral cutaneous nerve of the knee before the peroneal nerve passes over the fibular neck. At the neck, the future nerve fibers that become the deep peroneal nerve are closer to the bone, while the fibers for the superficial peroneal nerve are further away. The common fibular nerve splits into the superficial peroneal nerve and deep peroneal nerve after crossing the fibular neck. The superficial nerve gives sensation to the middle and lower lateral calf and also innervates the peroneus longus and brevis. It ends as cutaneous nerves giving sensation to the dorsal foot. The deep peroneal nerve innervates the tibialis anterior, extensor digitorum longus, extensor hallucis longus, and extensor digitorum brevis while also giving sensation to the area between the first and second toes [1]. Figure 56.12 demonstrates the path of the fibular nerve in the lower leg.

56.8.4 Clinical Presentation

Foot drop is a frequent presenting symptom. Patients report tripping while walking, ankle sprains, and foot slapping against the ground. About 80% of patients in one study reported sensory symptoms; pain was rare among the study group [12]. Loss of sensation occurs over the lateral distal leg and dorsal foot. Most present with acute onset of symptoms [12]. Recent significant weight loss causes the nerve to lose its protecting adipose tissue and could also be a part of the patient's history [1].

56.8.5 Physical Examination

Physical examination is a vital step in differentiating fibular nerve entrapment from L5 radiculopathy or other more global processes such as peripheral neuropathy. Peroneal neuropathy at the fibular neck leads to weakness in ankle dorsiflexion, foot eversion, and toe extension, but no weak-

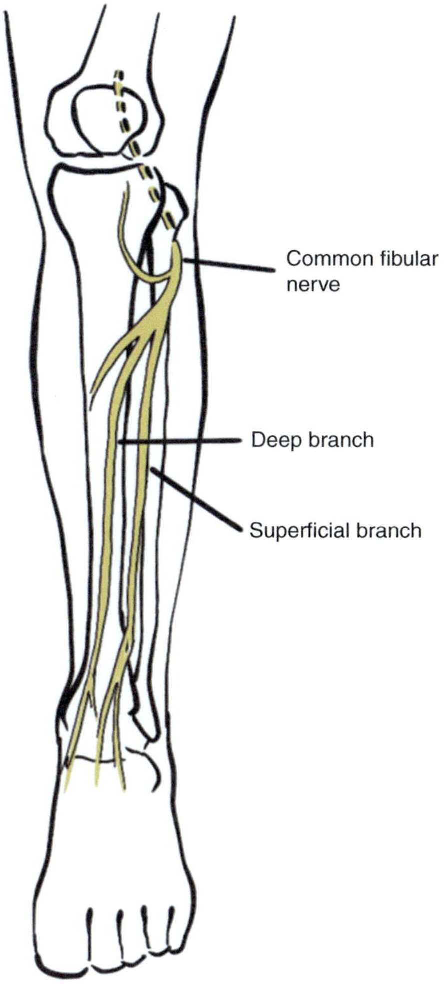

Fig. 56.12 Fibular nerve path and its branching in the lower extremity distal to the knee

ness in foot inversion. Patients should not have proximal muscle weakness either, so evaluating strength at the hip and knee is an important part of the physical exam. Sensation should be normal in the upper thigh and over the lateral knee but can be diminished over the lateral calf and dorsal foot. Reflexes should be intact. Gait analysis can reveal methods to clear the dropped foot: hip hike, foot circumduction, steppage gait [1].

56.8.6 Diagnostic Workup

Electrodiagnostic studies (EMG/NCS) are the most important test for diagnosing fibular nerve entrapment. Slowing or conduction block across the fibular neck on peroneal motor nerve conduction studies (NCS) would signal neuropathy at this location. Decreased amplitudes can also be seen in axonal loss. Recording at the tibialis anterior rather than extensor digitorum brevis can be more revealing in peroneal motor NCS [1, 12]. The sural and tibial nerves should be evaluated as well to rule out a more widespread process. EMG should target the peroneal innervated muscles but must also test sufficient muscles to rule out L5 radiculopathy, lumbosacral plexopathy, and sciatic neuropathy.

Ultrasound can be used if EMG/NCS does not pinpoint the location of the lesion or if a mass is suspected. MRI can also identify a mass lesion resulting in fibular nerve compression.

56.8.7 Treatment

Conservative management typically leads to improvement in patients. Physical therapy focusing on strengthening of the lower extremities is key as chronic foot drop positioning otherwise leads to plantarflexion contracture [13, 17, 18]. Ankle-foot orthosis (AFO) should be considered in patients with significant foot drop. Two examples are pictured in Fig. 56.13. Functional electrical stimulation is an alternative to an AFO and generally leads to improved patient satisfaction [19]. Padding can be added over the fibular head in patients with significant weight loss. Surgery for foot drop is typically only utilized in slowly progressing patients or those with masses identified [13]. One surgical option in cases of contractures is tendon transfer [17, 18]. For those with poor prognosis or more complete injuries, tibial nerve partial transfer to tibialis anterior has been successful [18].

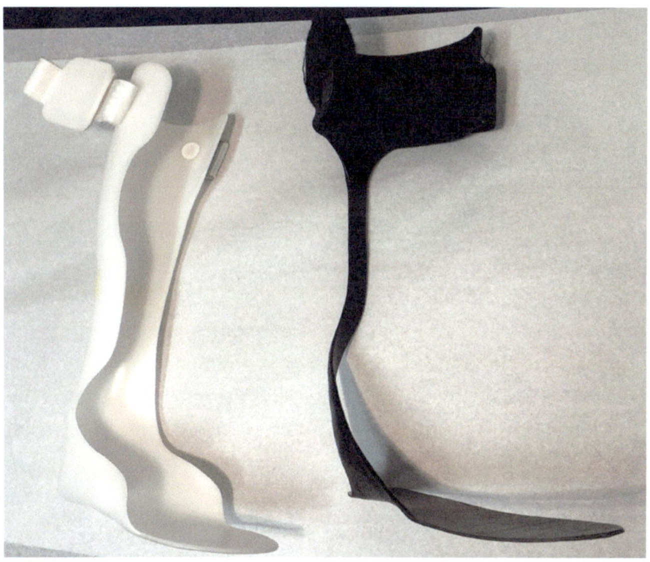

Fig. 56.13 Ankle-foot orthoses. A solid plastic AFO and a carbon fiber AFO are two options for patients with foot drop

56.9 Tarsal Tunnel Syndrome

56.9.1 Synonyms

- Tibial neuropathy
- Plantar neuropathy

56.9.2 ICD-10 Codes

G57.50

56.9.3 Description

Tarsal tunnel syndrome (TTS) is a neuropathy due to entrapment of the tibial nerve at the medial ankle. The nerve gets compressed as it travels under the flexor retinaculum posterior to the medial malleolus. TTS is rare, with most cases of an idiopathic etiology. Trauma has been associated with this entrapment. Masses can also cause impingement of the nerve [1, 13]. In Table 56.9, the differential diagnoses of tarsal tunnel syndrome are listed.

Anatomy The tibial nerve runs posterior to the medial malleolus and passes under the flexor retinaculum at the ankle, entering the tarsal tunnel. This tunnel is similar to the carpal tunnel in that it contains more than just the nerve; the tibial artery and vein pass through the tunnel along with the flexor hallucis longus tendon, flexor digitorum longus tendon, and tibialis posterior tendon. As the tibial nerve passes through the tunnel, it begins to separate into its three distal branches: the medial calcaneal sensory nerve, the lateral plantar nerve, and the medial plantar nerve. In some instances, the nerve does not divide until it exits the tunnel. The medial calcaneal sensory nerve is the sensory innervation of the heel. The lateral plantar nerve provides sensation to the lateral fourth toe and the fifth toe. It also has a motor component that innervates some of the intrinsic muscles of the foot such as the abductor digiti quinti pedis. The medial plantar nerve innervates the first three toes and the medial fourth toe while also innervating some of the intrinsic foot muscles including the abductor hallucis brevis and flexor hallucis brevis. The plantar nerves also provide sensory innervation to the sole of the foot [1, 13]. Figure 56.14 shows the relationship of the tibial nerve in the tarsal tunnel.

Table 56.9 Differential diagnosis of tarsal tunnel syndrome

Distal peripheral neuropathy	S1 radiculopathy
Lumbosacral plexopathy	Tendonitis of tibialis posterior
Plantar fasciitis	Calcaneal bone spur
Ankle osteoarthritis	Tendonitis of flexor hallucis longus, or flexor digitorum longus

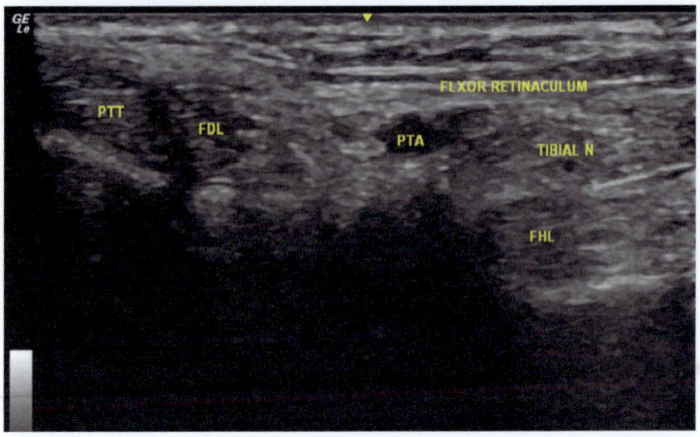

Fig. 56.14 Short access US image of the tarsal tunnel. Content of the tunnel noted deep to flexor retinaculum which includes posterior tibial artery (PTA) and vein, tibial nerve, and flexor hallux longus tendon (FHL). Posterior tibial tendon (PTT) and flexor digitorum longus (FDL) are also seen more anterior in this cross section against the bony medial malleoli

56.9.4 Clinical Presentation

Patients often present with pain around the medial ankle, with some radiation into the sole. It is typically characterized as a burning sensation [14]. Some complain of loss of sensation over the heel or sole and might have wounds as a result. Patients could also report a history of ankle sprains or fractures or could have a history of connective tissue disorders. Weakness is another presenting symptom but could be difficult for patients to notice; atrophy might be more easily noticeable to the patient [1].

56.9.5 Physical Examination

Inspection can yield atrophy of the intrinsic foot muscles. Strength is difficult to assess as the bulk of foot and toe strength comes from the larger muscles in the leg, which would not be affected by TTS. Decreased sensation over the sole of the foot could be the only significant abnormality on exam [1]. Tinel's sign over the tarsal tunnel can be checked, but it is unreliable [14]. Achilles' reflex should be normal, as it is innervated prior to the tarsal tunnel.

56.9.6 Diagnostic Workup

Electrodiagnostic studies are frequently utilized in diagnosing TTS. However, it is a technically difficult study to perform and lacks evidence on the proper techniques. Side-to-side comparison must be performed of the medial and lateral plantar nerves, recording over the abductor hallucis brevis and abductor digiti quinti pedis, respectively. Mixed studies can also be of diagnostic value. However, all three of these tests are frequently not obtainable in normal patients. Routine sural, tibial, and peroneal nerve studies should also be evaluated to rule out a more diffuse process. EMG of the foot muscles has many issues associated with it including patient tolerance, activation of the muscle, and infection risk [1, 13].

Ultrasound has been shown to be extremely useful in the TTS diagnosis process, as visualization of the tibial nerve in the tunnel is typically straightforward. Evaluating the nerve and its surroundings can demonstrate abnormalities with the nerve itself and nearby structures that might be impinging on the nerve. The plantar fascia can also be evaluated, as plantar fasciitis could be the actual cause of symptoms. MRI can also be used to observe mass lesions [1, 14].

56.9.7 Treatment

Conservative management with footwear modifications and nonsteroidal anti-inflammatory medications are the first steps. In some cases, tight-fitting shoes are the causative agent, and adjustment can relieve the symptoms.

US-guided tarsal tunnel corticosteroid injections with or without hydrodissection can provide symptomatic relief. Image guidance reduces the risk of tendon or neural injury during percutaneous injections [21]. Hydrodissection of the nerve can release it from scar tissue and relieve compression. Persistent symptoms or identified masses require surgical intervention [13]. Endoscopic release has been demonstrated as a successful technique that is simpler than more traditional open surgeries [15].

56.10 Femoral Nerve Entrapment

56.10.1 Synonyms

Femoral neuropathy

56.10.2 ICD-10 Codes

G57.20

56.10.3 Descriptions

Femoral nerve entrapment is a neuropathy that most typically causes knee extension weakness. When the nerve is injured more proximally, hip flexion will be weak as well. Femoral neuropathy can be caused by many conditions: retroperitoneal hematoma, compression at the inguinal ligament due to an iliopsoas bursal enlargement or hematoma, penetrating groin trauma, hip arthroplasty, poor lithotomy positioning, inadvertent clamping during femoral artery procedures, or pelvic surgery. Isolated femoral nerve entrapment is considered uncommon [1]. Table 56.10 lists other differential diagnoses that can present in a similar manner as femoral neuropathy.

Anatomy The femoral nerve arises from the L2, L3, and L4 nerve roots. Axons traverse the lumbar plexus. In the retroperitoneal space, the nerve travels between the psoas and iliacus muscles, then under the iliacus fascia in the pelvis. It enters the thigh below the inguinal ligament and lateral to the femoral artery. The femoral nerve innervates the psoas and iliacus in the pelvis. In the thigh, the nerve innervates the four quadriceps muscles: the vastus lateralis, vastus medialis, vastus intermedius, and rectus femoris. It also innervates the pectineus and sartorius muscles. Sensory branches supply medial sensation to the thigh from the medial cutaneous and intermediate cutaneous nerves. The distal medial thigh and medial lower leg sensation is supplied by the saphenous nerve which is a terminal branch of the femoral nerve [1, 16]. Figure 56.15 details the path of the femoral nerve through the thigh.

Table 56.10 Differential diagnosis of femoral neuropathy

Femoral amyotrophy	Multifocal motor neuropathy
L3/L4 radiculopathies	Hip/knee/pelvis disorders associated with pain or weakness
Lumbar plexopathies	Myopathies

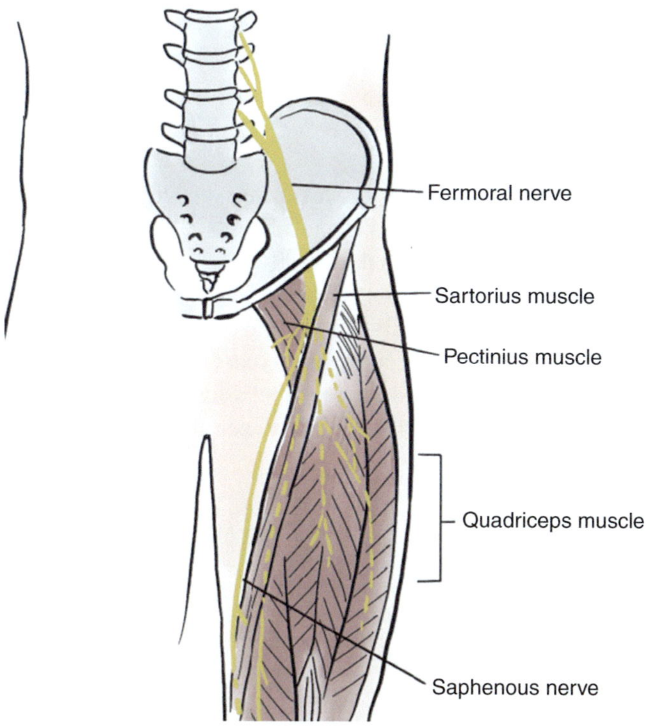

Fig. 56.15 Path of the femoral nerve through the proximal thigh

56.10.4 Clinical Presentation

Femoral nerve entrapment presents with weakness in knee extension. Buckling of the knee is common. Dragging the leg and weakness of the hip in flexion can occur with proximal nerve involvement. Some sensory involvement in the medial thigh and medial lower leg may be present.

56.10.5 Physical Examination

Examination will find weakness in knee extension and perhaps hip flexion with an absent or diminished patellar reflex. Sensory may be impaired in the medial thigh and medial lower leg [1]. A thorough examination of the lumbar region and lower limbs is needed to rule out other causes of weakness.

56.10.6 Diagnostic Workup

Electrodiagnostic studies are useful to diagnose and exclude other causes of weakness. A comparative side-to-side femoral motor study may show significant amplitude differences. EMG must sample at least two femoral innervated muscles and also muscles innervated by nerves outside of the femoral nerve in order to isolate a femoral neuropathy. Saphenous sensory studies may be helpful in the diagnosis but are often difficult to obtain [1, 16].

Ultrasound may reveal a swollen and heterogeneous appearing femoral nerve at the site of pathology or disruption of the nerve. It can also reveal masses and hematomas at the site of pathology [1].

56.10.7 Treatment

Treatment is dependent on the cause of the neuropathy. Conservative care includes therapeutic modalities, strengthening, and gait training with devices. Bracing includes the application of a knee-ankle-foot orthosis. Crutches or canes may also be needed for stability. Conservative management usually leads to some improvement within 2 years [16]. Surgical intervention may be required for decompression of hematomas or masses or to relieve scar tissue as in a neurolysis.

References

1. Preston DC, Shapiro BE. Electromyography and neuromuscular disorders E-book: clinical-electrophysiologic-ultrasound correlations. Amsterdam: Elsevier Health Sciences; 2020.
2. Amato AA, Russell JA. Neuromuscular disorders. 2nd ed. McGraw-Hill Education;2016:2–21. ISBN:9780071752503.
3. Padua L, Pasquale AD, Pazzaglia C, Liotta GA, Librante A, Mondelli M. Systematic review of pregnancy-related carpal tunnel syndrome. Muscle Nerve. 2010;42(5):697–702.
4. Dang AC, Rodner CM. Unusual compression neuropathies of the forearm, part II: median nerve. J Hand Surg Am. 2009;34(10):1915–20.
5. Bevelaqua AC, Hayter CL, Feinberg JH, Rodeo SA. Posterior interosseous neuropathy: electrodiagnostic evaluation. HSS J. 2012;8(2):184–9.
6. Djurdjevic T, Loizides A, Löscher W, Gruber H, Plaikner M, Peer S. High resolution ultrasound in posterior interosseous nerve syndrome. Muscle Nerve. 2014;49(1):35–9.
7. Kim DH, Murovic JA, Kim YY, Kline DG. Surgical treatment and outcomes in 45 cases of posterior interosseous nerve entrapments and injuries. J Neurosurg. 2006;104(5):766–77.
8. Moradi A, Ebrahimzadeh MH, Jupiter JB. Radial tunnel syndrome, diagnostic and treatment dilemma. Arch Bone Jt Surg. 2015;3(3):156.
9. Andrews K, Rowland A, Pranjal A, Ebraheim N. Cubital tunnel syndrome: anatomy, clinical presentation, and management. J Orthop. 2018;15(3):832–6.
10. Osei DA, Groves AP, Bommarito K, Ray WZ. Cubital tunnel syndrome: incidence and demographics in a national administrative database. Neurosurgery. 2017;80(3):417–20.
11. Boykin RE, Friedman DJ, Higgins LD, Warner JJ. Suprascapular neuropathy. JBJS. 2010;92(13):2348–64.
12. Katirji MB, Wilbourn AJ. Common peroneal mononeuropathy: a clinical and electrophysiologic study of 116 lesions. Neurology. 1988;38(11):1723–8.
13. Shapiro BE, Preston DC. Entrapment and compressive neuropathies. Med Clin N Am. 2009;93(2):285–315.
14. Samarawickrama D, Therimadasamy AK, Chan YC, Vijayan J, Wilder-Smith EP. Nerve ultrasound in electrophysiologically verified tarsal tunnel syndrome. Muscle Nerve. 2016;53(6):906–12.
15. Krishnan KG, Pinzer T, Schackert G. A novel endoscopic technique in treating single nerve entrapment syndromes with special attention to ulnar nerve transposition and tarsal tunnel release: clinical application. Oper Neurosurg. 2006;59(suppl_1):ONS-89.
16. Madani S, Doughty C. Lower extremity entrapment neuropathies. Best Pract Res Clin Rheumatol. 2020;34:101565.
17. Frontera WR, Silver JK, Rizzo TD. Essentials of physical medicine and rehabilitation e-book. Elsevier Health Sciences; 2018.
18. Giuffre JL, Bishop AT, Spinner RJ, Shin AY. Surgical technique of a partial tibial nerve transfer to the tibialis anterior motor branch for the treatment of peroneal nerve injury. Ann Plast Surg. 2012;69(1):48–53.
19. Bucklitsch J, Müller A, Weitner A, Filmann N, Patriciu A, Behmanesh B, Seifert V, Marquardt G, Quick-Weller J. Significant impact of implantable functional electrical stimulation on gait parameters: a kinetic analysis in foot drop patients. World Neurosurg. 2019;127:e236–41.
20. Gofeld M, Agur A. Peripheral nerve stimulation for chronic shoulder pain: a proof of concept anatomy study. Neuromodulation. 2018;21(3):284–9.
21. Lau JT, Daniels TR. Tarsal tunnel syndrome: a review of the literature. Foot Ankle Int. 1999;20(3):201–9.
22. Ziswiler HR, Reichenbach S, Vogelin E, Bachmann LM, Villiger PM, Juni P. Diagnostic value of sonography in patients with suspected carpal tunnel syndrome: a prospective study. Arthritis Rheum. 2005;52:304–11.
23. Vincelet Y, Journeau P, Popkov D, Haumont T, Lascombes P. The anatomical basis for anterior interosseous nerve palsy secondary to supracondylar humerus fractures in children. Orthop Traumatol Surg Res. 2013;99(5):543–7. https://doi.org/10.1016/j.otsr.2013.04.002. Epub 2013 Aug 2. PMID: 23916783.
24. Wiesman IM, Novak CB, Mackinnon SE, Winograd JM. Sensitivity and specificity of clinical testing for carpal tunnel syndrome. Can J Plast Surg. 2003;11(2):70–2. https://doi.org/10.1177/229255030301100205.

Plexopathies and Neuropathies

57

S. Ali Mostoufi, Tony K. George, Ogochukwu Azuh, Jeanie Cote, Emanuel Mostoufi, Kevin Zhang, Kyungje Sung, and Garett Lui

57.1 Intercostal Neuralgia

Kevin Zhang and S. Ali Mostoufi

57.1.1 Synonyms

- Intercostal neuropathy
- Intercostal neuritis

S. A. Mostoufi (✉)
Department of Orthopedics and Rehabilitation, Tufts University School of Medicine, Boston, MA, USA

New England Spine Care Associates & Boston Regenerative Medicine, Cambridge, MA, USA
e-mail: Ali.Mostoufi@Nespinecare.com

T. K. George
Restorative Orthopaedics Spine & Sports (ROSS) Institute, Somerset, NJ, USA

Department of Orthopaedics, Rutgers-Robert Wood Johnson Medical School, New Brunswick, NJ, USA

O. Azuh
Department of Physical Medicine and Rehabilitation, Memorial Healthcare, Owosso, MI, USA
e-mail: oazuh@memorialhealthcare.org

J. Cote
Department of Neurology/Neuroimmunology, Memorial Healthcare, Owosso, MI, USA
e-mail: jcote@memorialhealthcare.org

E. Mostoufi
Department of Neurology, University of Alberta School of Medicine, Calgary, CA, USA

K. Zhang
Departments or Orthopedics and Rehabilitation Medicine, Tufts University School of Medicine, Boston, MA, USA

K. Sung · G. Lui
Department of Orthopedics and Rehabilitation, Tufts Medical Center, Boston, MA, USA
e-mail: glui@tuftsmedicalcenter.org

57.1.2 ICD 10 Code

- G58.0

57.1.3 Description

Intercostal neuralgia is a painful condition originating from intercostal nerves. When the intercostal nerve is injured or inflamed, it will generate pain in that specific nerve distribution and along the edge of the adjacent rib, wrapping anteriorly. Intercostal neuralgia manifests as a neuropathic pain, which could be sharp, shooting, burning, or paresthesia, traveling along a single or multiple thoracic dermatome(s).

57.1.3.1 Anatomy

The term "intercostal" refers to the space between two ribs, starting from the costovertebral junction to the costosternal junction. Intercostal nerves arise from the anterior rami of thoracic spinal nerves at the respective level T1 through T11, while T12 is known as the subcostal nerve. Intercostal nerves are subdivided into typical and atypical nerves. *Typical intercostal nerve* stay within their intercostal space (T3–6), and *atypical intercostal nerves* (T1–2, T7–11) entirely or partially travel beyond the intercostal space and innervate locations such as the upper abdominal wall and axilla [6].

Typical intercostal nerves and the intercostal vessels travel under the inferior border of the rib with a fibrous sheath in the subcostal groove. The subcostal groove is between the innermost intercostal muscle and the internal intercostal muscle. The branches of typical intercostal nerves include gray rami communicantes (connect with the sympathetic chain), the muscular branches (innervates the intercostal muscles), the collateral branch, the lateral cutaneous branch, and the anterior cutaneous branch [7]. Atypical intercostal nerves T7–T11 and subcostal nerve have a similar path as the typical intercostal nerve but continue on to innervate the abdominal wall. These nerves take a 90-degree turn at the border of the rectus abdominis and are a common site

© The Author(s), under exclusive license to Springer Nature Switzerland AG 2022

S. A. Mostoufi et al. (eds.), *Clinical Guide to Musculoskeletal Medicine*, https://doi.org/10.1007/978-3-030-92042-5_57

of entrapment syndrome known as anterior cutaneous nerve entrapment syndrome [8].

57.1.3.2 Etiology

Although it can be idiopathic, common etiologies of intercostal neuralgia include direct nerve injury, stretching, entrapment, and inflammation [1]. Direct nerve injury can be due to physical trauma (penetrating injury, gun shot, displaced rib fracture) or iatrogenic (thoracotomy, median sternotomy, mastectomy, and chest tube placement). Stretching injuries can be from traction from pregnancy (gravid uterus). Intercostal nerve entrapment may be due to anatomical compression by neoplasm, sarcoidosis, and pleural mesothelioma. Inflammatory etiology of intercostal neuralgia is commonly from herpes zoster (HZ) infection (acute reactivation of dormant zoster virus) and/or chronic post-herpetic neuralgia [1]. Differential diagnosis of intercostal neuralgia is in Table 57.1.

The two most common and well-documented etiologies are thoracotomy and herpes zoster (HZ) infection.

1. Post-thoracotomy pain syndrome (PTPS) is defined as "pain that persists along a thoracotomy incision at least two months following the surgical procedure" [2]. Thoracotomy causes direct damage to the nerve or the surrounding structures, with subsequent scaring resulting in inflammation and entrapment. Systematic reviews have shown that approximately 50% of patient reports chronic pain after thoracotomy at 3 and 6 months [3]. Rogers et al. demonstrated that intercostal nerve injuries routinely occur due to rib retraction during thoracotomy by measuring intercostal nerve motor evoked potentials intraoperatively. Before and after entering the pleural space, intercostal nerves were functioning normally. After the rib retractor was removed, a total conduction block was seen in the nerve above and below the level of incision in most patients. Additionally, no intercostal nerve impairment was seen in a patient in which rib retractors were not used [4].
2. Herpes zoster (HZ) infection causes intercostal neuralgia acutely with reactivation and chronically with post-herpetic neuralgia. Reactivation and replication of dominant HZ virus in the dorsal root ganglia will cause inflammatory nerve damage along that dermatome. Inflammation or nerve damage leads to cytokine release and demyelination leaving the axons exposed, causing inappropriate upregulation and activation of ion channels and inappropriate action potentials generated, resulting in pain [5, 17]. Over time, this can lead to central sensitization resulting in continued pain despite resolution of the acute reactivation of the herpes zoster virus.

Table 57.1 Differential diagnosis of intercostal neuralgia

Thoracic radiculopathy
Cholecystitis
Costochondritis (Tietze syndrome)
Hepatic disease
Malignant neoplasm
Pleurisy
Pneumothorax
Referred pain (cardiac, pulmonary, vascular, GI)
Rib contusion or fractures

57.1.4 Clinical Presentation

When evaluating for intercostal neuralgia, history is of utmost importance. The condition manifests itself as a unilateral neuropathic pain, which could be described as sharp, shooting, tightness, burning, numbness, and paresthesia, traveling in a band-like pattern in a single or multiple thoracic dermatome. The pain can be worsened with physical activity and sharp body movements (i.e., rotation, lateral flexion, flexion, and extension). Also, patients can complain of pleuritic-type chest pain, referring under the scapula, upper back, and axilla. Timing of onset and specific events such as trauma, surgeries, and shingles can help with the differential. However, for some, the onset of pain may be more insidious with no identifiable preceding event.

57.1.5 Physical Examination

Visual inspection of the chest or abdominal may reveal skin discoloration, scar from prior surgeries, or healed shingles lesions (read or pale). Abdominal wall bulging can be a sign of intercostal nerve injury due to muscle weakness [1]. Sensory examination of the affected dermatomes may reveal sensory deficits as well as allodynia or hyperalgesia. Palpation over thoracic or upper abdomen may reproduce their usual neuropathic pain or accentuate it. Pain can be induced with trunk rotation, forward and lateral flexion, and/or extension.

57.1.6 Diagnostic Workup

Diagnostic workup should be conducted based on history and physical examination. In the cases of trauma, X-rays or CT or ultrasound scans can help with ruling out rib fractures, foreign bodies, as well as other cardiopulmonary or visceral pathologies. In patients with history of or suspicious of malignancies, MRIs may be considered. Ultrasound examination is useful in visualizing the intercostal nerve and potential site of compression. Clinicians use image-guided diagnostic intercostal nerve block as a specific diagnostic test for this condition, but addition of corticosteroid may provide therapeutic value as well.

57.1.7 Treatment

57.1.7.1 Medical Management

Initial management should be conservative and include pharmacological and non-pharmacological interventions. Topical medications have fewer systemic side effects and can be effective including topical analgesics, capsaicin cream, and transdermal lidocaine patch. Oral acetaminophen and nonsteroidal anti-inflammatory drugs can help with mild to moderate pain and especially with inflammatory cases. Typically, antiepileptics (such as gabapentin and pregabalin) are first-line in treating neuropathic pain in intercostal neuralgia and have low side effect profile. Alternative choices include tricyclic antidepressants such as amitriptyline and nortriptyline, although they have known anticholinergic side effects (dry mouth, constipation, sedation, and urinary retention). Other options include selective norepinephrine reputable inhibitors (such as duloxetine) and selective serotonin reputable inhibitors (such as fluoxetine). More severe or intractable intercostal neuralgia can be addressed with narcotics; however, this should be a temporizing measure while treating with other interventions. Non-pharmacological interventions include behavior therapy, acupuncture, and physical and occupational therapy.

57.1.7.2 Rehabilitation

Physical and occupational therapy can help with the management of intercostal neuralgia through desensitization techniques, relaxation therapy, exercises, and other modalities. Application of heat and cold therapy, kinesiology tape, and transcutaneous electrical nerve stimulation (TENS) can provide relief. In patients with lower thoracic nerve root involvement (traumatic), abdominal muscle weakness can be expected. Stretching and strengthening exercises should focus on the anterior and posterior chest muscles to improve posture and encourage deep breathing. Additionally, patients can become deconditioned due to the fear of avoidance behavior, thus it is important to maintain the patient's physical activity (Fig. 57.1).

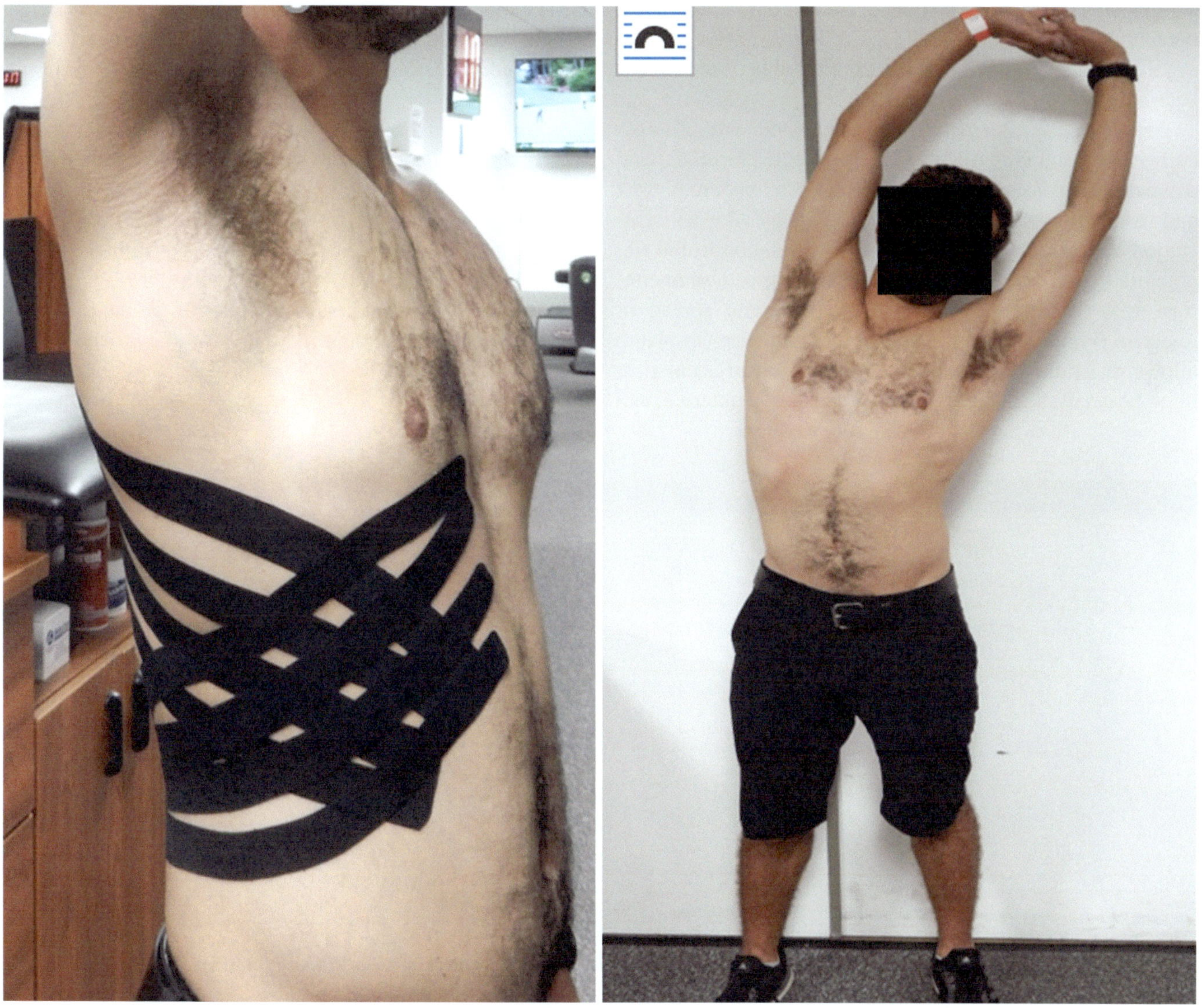

Fig. 57.1 Kinesiotaping and chest wall stretching. (Images courtesy of Dr. Tim Tiu, University of Miami)

57.1.7.3 Procedures

Intercostal Nerve Block

Landmark based or image-guided intercostal nerve block with anesthetics and steroid can provide immediate diagnostic value and therapeutic effect that may last several weeks. Fluoroscopy or ultrasound can be used as image guidance, both of which increase accuracy of needle placement and enhance safety.

For blind block (landmark-based), the most common site is at the angle of the rib about 7 cm lateral to the spinus process of target level in adults using a 1.5–2 inch (5 cm) 22–27 gauge (for single-shot injection) short-bevel needle. The needle is advanced until it contacts the rib typically at depth of less than 1 cm. The needle is then gently walked caudally off the rib. The needle is then advanced with a cephalad tilt angle until a subtle "give" or "pop" of the fascia of the internal intercostal muscle is felt. A peripheral nerve stimulator may aid in confirmation. After negative aspiration, local anesthetic and steroid are injected. Since this approach has a significant risk of pneumothorax, an alternative approach, placing the needle more parallel to the bottom of the rib, sliding the needle up underneath the inferior edge of the rib has been proposed [9].

Image-guided intercostal block can be done with fluoroscopy or ultrasound. It allows accurate needle placement and decreases the risk of complications such as pneumothorax and vascular uptake of injectate. Fluoroscopy allows visualization and localization of the needle in relation to the rib, potentially decreasing the risk of pneumothorax. Use of contrast will confirm the extravascular perineural spread of injectate (Fig. 57.2). Ultrasound needle guidance (in-plane) allows real-time visualization of pleura, two adjacent ribs, three layers of the intercostal muscles (external, internal, and innermost), and neurovascular bundle. Using ultrasound, while performing the block, dramatically decreases the risk of pneumothorax and vascular injury, as the needle tip is kept superficial to the pleura and away from vasculature. In addition, using ultrasound eliminates exposure to radiation, as compared to fluoroscopy guided blocks [10].

Pulsed Radiofrequency (RF) Lesioning

Pulsed RF is a nondestructive technique with utility in treating intercostal neuropathic pain with durable pain relief. Pulsed RF in intercostal neuralgia can provide significant improvement of postherpetic pain and patient's quality of life, however, duration of relief varies from study to study [10, 11]. The mechanism of pulsed RF is not well understood. A popular theory suggests rapidly changing electric fields produced by RF generators alter the transmission of pain signals via a pathway involving c-Fos, a so-called immediate-early gene. The c-Fos expression is not temperature-dependent but rather induced by pulsed electrical fields. Enhancement of noradrenergic and serotonergic descending pain inhibitory pathways is also postulated [10]. Pulsed radiofrequency can also be done with either fluoroscopy or ultrasound guidance.

Cryoablation

Cryoablation is another method of interrupting the peripheral nerve's ability to transmit pain by freezing it. One of the most common applications of cryoablation is in intercostal neuralgia. A 14-gauge angiocath is introduced underneath in the inferior edge of the rib with fluoroscopy [12]. A retrospective study showed the 60% of patients reported an immediate decrease in their pain after the procedure and approximately 50% had sustained relief 3 months afterward [13].

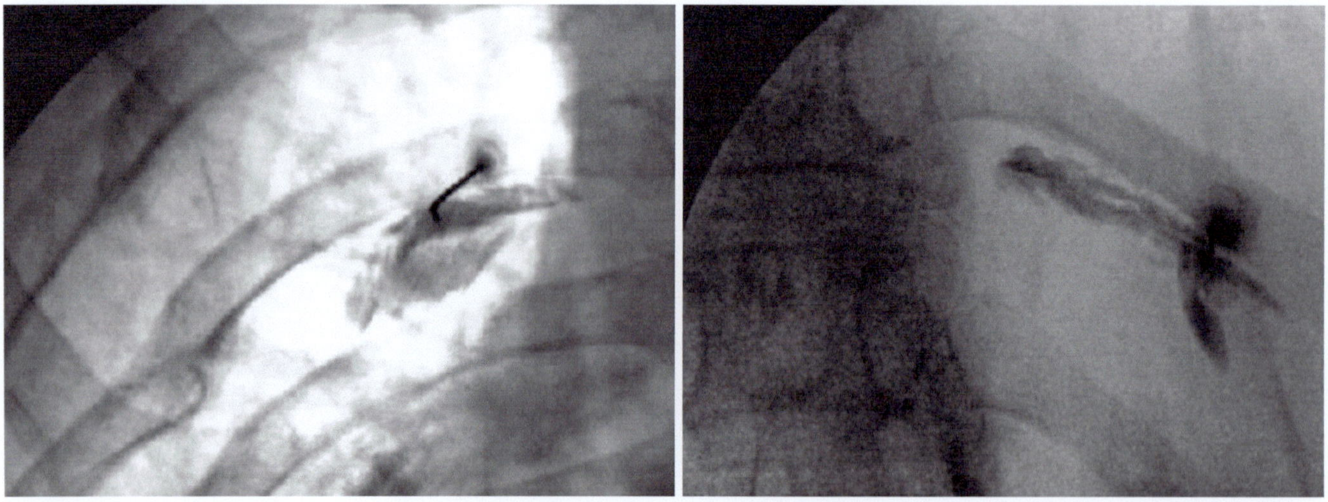

Fig. 57.2 Needle placement with contrast enhancement prior to RF ablation in patient with rib fracture. (Source: Authors film library)

Thermal Radiofrequency Ablation

Image-guided thermal RFA, a technique using heat generated from medium frequency alternating current (250–500 kHz), is used to induce cell death from coagulation necrosis. The technique and location of probe placement are similar to cryoablation. Case series have shown long-term pain relief for patients and serve as a possible intervention option [14]. Thermal RF may result in unpleasant dysesthesia, if partial burn is achieved.

Chemical Neurolysis

This is a rare method to treat intercostal neuralgia and may be considered in patients with malignancy involving the chest wall. Alcohol and phenol are the preferred agents, and both may be irritating to the surrounding tissue and cause initial increased pain [15].

Neuromodulation

Neuromodulation has been established as a non-pharmacological procedural option for neuropathic pain. It is separated into peripheral or central and noninvasive vs invasive neuromodulation. Peripheral noninvasive neurostimulation includes TENS, as discussed earlier. More invasive peripheral neuromodulation includes dorsal root ganglion (DRG) stimulation. Central neurostimulation includes spinal cord stimulator (SCS) [16]. The neuropathic component of intercostal neuralgia can be treated with neuromodulation after a successful trial lead placement resulting in significant pain relief and improved function. Both paresthesia based and high frequency neuromodulation techniques can be offered to patients.

57.1.7.4 Surgery

Surgery is rarely indicated. Surgical neurectomy, dorsal rhizotomy, or sensory ganglionectomy cause irreversible sensory and neurological deficits.

57.2 Phantom Limb Pain

Tony K. George

57.2.1 ICD-10

- G54.6

57.2.2 Synonyms

- Phantom limb syndrome

57.2.3 Definition

Phantom limb pain (PLP) is defined as unprovoked pain experienced in an amputated limb. It is a perception of neuropathic pain, paresthesia, or abnormal sensation in the dimension of a previously existing limb. Related but distinct is stump nociceptive pain localized to the residual limb provoked by pressure or traction. Previously known as phantom limb phenomenon, it was first described in 1551 by a French military surgeon on his treatise on gunshot wounds [18]. The phenomenon was understood to have distinct parts, i.e., phantom limb pain and phantom limb sensation.

Phantom limb pain (PLP) is commonly seen after limb amputations but also experienced after removal of organs including the breast, liver, testicle, or eye [19]. PLP is prevalent in up to 80% of post-amputee patients [3]. Limb amputations result from peripheral vascular disease, trauma, or malignancy, where amputations from diabetic-related vascular disease is a primary cause [20]. Diabetic patients often have preexisting pain in the limbs from peripheral neuropathy, and studies show pain prior to amputation is a risk factor for PLP [21]. Children with congenital limb deficiency or amputations experience phantom limb pain less frequently. Other risk factors for PLP include double amputations, shorter residual limbs, perioperative gangrene, and prolonged time interval between amputation and fitting of prosthesis.

Peripheral and central pathways influence PLP. Pain originates from developing neuromas around severed nerves during amputation. Disorganized axonal sprouting occurs at the distal end of the severed nerves, creating afferent impulses which ascend and reorganize the central pathways in the spinal cord and brain cortex. Through peripheral and central sensitization, neuronal reorganization occurs.

57.2.4 Clinical Presentation

Phantom limb is a subjective perception of neuropathic pain/sensation in the setting of an amputated limb. Phantom limb neuropathic symptoms include stabbing, burning, gnawing, and sharp tingling along with hyperesthesia and allodynia features located where the amputated limb preexisted. Patients may feel that the limb is still attached and working normally and may even perceive clothing and presence of rings/jewelry on the amputated limb.

57.2.5 Physical Examination

Inspection would reveal an amputated limb. Stump palpation or percussion may elicit painful responses from nearby neuroma. Skin texture may display hypertrophic changes with hyperesthesia or allodynia to light touch. Tenderness and warmth to touch with a palpable mass around the stump should raise concerns for heterotrophic ossification. Rarely a well circumscribed tender erythematous lesion may be an indication of choke syndrome from tight prosthesis.

57.2.6 Imaging

Radiographic testing is considered to rule out pain generators such as radiculopathy, tumor, or infection. Non-contrast MRI of lumbar spine is diagnostic for lumbar radiculopathy, and musculoskeletal ultrasound or MRI of extremity identifies soft tissue tumors and neuromas. For clinical suspicion of osteomyelitis, bone scan or MRI with contrast is the imaging modality of choice.

57.2.7 Treatment

57.2.7.1 Medical Management

Non-painful phantom limb sensation may not require treatment. Painful phantom limb requires a multidisciplinary approach starting with proper stump care in the acute and subacute settings after amputation. Crucial in early stages are edema control and skin care to prevent residual limb issues including pain. Graded motor imaging, mirror box therapy, and hypnosis have been effective in reducing phantom limb pain. Utilizing a mirror's reflective effects to visualize an absent limb helps brain reorganization and reduces aberrant sensory perception [22]. Pre-amputation counselling was associated with less likelihood of developing PLP, and desensitization with TENS unit can be effective for its management [23].

Medication appropriateness depends on the timeline from surgery to onset of PLP. The literature suggests PLP can arise a week after amputation [24]. During perioperative periods nociceptive pain predominates neuropathic pain. Evidence suggests opioid medications and IV ketamine are effective in optimizing pain control. Studies also suggest postoperative IV calcitonin may be effective in reducing onset of PLP [24]. Neuropathic medications are first-line medications for PLP where gabapentin has level II evidence for managing pain of intermediate chronicity [24]. With high incidence of depression in the amputee population, duloxetine is effective for its dual affective and neuropathic pain properties. Chronic opioid medication should be used with caution as preoperative opioid dependence is a risk for continuing dependence after amputation.

57.2.7.2 Procedures

Evidence is limited for interventional pain blocks including epidural injection or localized blocks to alleviate PLP; however, some evidence supports epidural anesthesia with bupivacaine or morphine perioperatively. Peripheral nerve stimulation, neuromodulation, and DRG stimulation may provide neuropathic pain relief in severe cases; however, data to support spinal cord stimulation is limited at this time [25].

57.2.7.3 Rehabilitation

Early rehabilitation improves function in the long run. Physical therapists work with the patient as early as the first few days after amputation and focus on transfers, stump management, proper prosthetics use, gait training, early ambulation, and continued strengthening of residual limb muscles and spine. Collaboration between prosthetist, physical therapist, occupational therapist, pain specialist, and PM&R specialist will result in the best overall outcome.

57.3 Genitofemoral Neuropathy

Emanuel Mostoufi

57.3.1 Synonyms

- Genitofemoral neuralgia
- Genitofemoral nerve entrapment
- Genitofemoral nerve compression

57.3.2 ICD 10 Codes

- G57.20–23

57.3.3 Description

Genitofemoral neuropathy (GFN) is characterized by cutaneous pain along the region of the inner thigh and groin typically caused by iatrogenic injury to the genitofemoral nerve. This condition often leads to chronic pain and significantly impacted quality of life in patients [26].

57.3.3.1 Anatomy

The genitofemoral nerve forms from the L1 and L2 ventral rami and gives rise to the genital and femoral branches after passing through the psoas muscle. The femoral branch pierces through the fascia lata, journeys through the femoral sheath, and provides cutaneous sensation to the anterior upper thigh. The genital branch travels through the inguinal canal and supplies sensation to the medial aspect of the thigh and the scrotum; the genital branch also provides motor innervation to the cremaster muscle in males and sensory innervation to the labia majora and mons pubis in females [27]. There is significant overlap in innervation between the genitofemoral, iliohypogastric, and ilioinguinal nerves; thus, it can be clinically difficult to distinguish which nerve is responsible for the patient's symptoms.

57.3.3.2 Etiology

The most common cause of GFN is iatrogenic often from direct injury or nerve entrapment from a surgical procedure.

Table 57.2 Differential diagnosis for genitofemoral neuropathy

Ilioinguinal neuropathy	Lumbar plexopathy
Iliohypogastric neuropathy	Inguinal hernia
Appendicitis	Salpingitis
Ovarian pathology	Epididymitis or orchitis

The most common surgical procedures associated with this condition are C-section, hysterectomy, trans-obturator surgery, and inguinal hernia repair. Other potential causes include postsurgical hematoma, or adhesions and psoas abscess/entrapment [28].

Differential diagnosis for genitofemoral neuropathy is given in Table 57.2.

57.3.4 Clinical Presentation

Patients with genitofemoral neuropathy present with inguinal pain or burning sensation with associated sensory changes in the region; the pain will often radiate to upper middle thigh and to the patient's genitalia (scrotum, vagina, labia majora) [27]. Standing, walking, and extension of the thigh may worsen symptoms, conversely lying down and flexion of the thigh provides relief.

57.3.5 Physical Examination

Visual Observation Observe the patient's preferred position of comfort which may include a bent over position (lumbar extension aggravates symptoms). Thorough inspection may reveal clues to rule in/out other diagnoses (e.g., visible defect from an inguinal hernia).

Palpation Given the proximity of the psoas muscle to the nerve, palpation of this muscle or its activation may worsen symptoms. In women, test for pain to palpation of the lateral vulva or the

Sensory Testing Test for sensory loss along the border of the abdomen and thigh, groin, anterior proximal thigh, and lateral scrotum or labia majora.

Range of Motion Assess for worsening of pain as the patient transitions from a seated to a standing position.

Reflexes Loss of cremasteric reflex (in males), assessed by stroking the inner part of the thigh in a downward direction, may be a finding in severe neuropathy [28].

57.3.6 Diagnostic Workup

EMG May be helpful in distinguishing lumbar plexopathy vs GFN (GFN should not have significant motor impairment) [27].

Ultrasound May reveal scarring along the nerve or local compression with nerve enlargement

MRI To assess for mass, abscess, or hematoma resulting in nerve entrapment

Response to Nerve Block No benefit is noted from selective ilioinguinal nerve or L1/L2 nerve block root block [29]. Patient may have symptomatic relief from US-guided genitofemoral nerve block. Hydrodissection may add some value and prolong the effect of the nerve block.

57.3.7 Treatment

57.3.7.1 Medica Management

Topical lidocaine patches, tricyclic antidepressants as first line. Other considerations include NSAIDs, anticonvulsants (gabapentin), SSRI/SNRIs, and N-methyl-D aspartate antagonists [27].

57.3.7.2 Procedures

Nerve block (corticosteroid + lidocaine), ultrasound-guided radiofrequency ablation or cryoablation of the nerve's myelin sheath and axon [30].

57.3.7.3 Surgery

Can be considered if limited response is noted from non-surgical management. Neurectomy of GFN can be performed via minimally invasive endoscopic retroperitoneal approach [27].

57.4 Ilioinguinal Neuropathy

Emanuel Mostoufi

57.4.1 Synonyms

- Ilioinguinal neuralgia
- Ilioinguinal nerve entrapment
- Ilioinguinal nerve compression

57.4.2 ICD 10 Codes

- G57.80–83

57.4.3 Description

57.4.3.1 Anatomy

The ilioinguinal nerve, a branch of the first lumbar nerve (L1), navigates through the transversus abdominis muscle and into the inguinal canal to supply sensory innervation to the superomedial region of the thigh, the pubis, the scrotum, and the labia majora [31].

57.4.3.2 Etiology/Pathophysiology

Ilioinguinal neuropathy is a common cause of lower abdominal pain which originates at the anterior superior iliac spine and radiates to the groin. Caused by entrapment of the ilioinguinal nerve, it is a rare but disabling cause of chronic neuropathic pain with the potential of significantly affecting quality of life [29]. The etiology of ilioinguinal neuropathy is usually iatrogenic, caused by injury to the nerve intraoperatively, i.e., during an inguinal hernia repair or other abdominal surgery. In the postoperative period, this condition may be caused by adhesions or formation of neuromas [29, 32]. Differential diagnosis for Ilioinguinal neuropathy is given in Table 57.3.

57.4.4 Clinical Presentation

Patients often present with tenderness to the iliac fossa which radiates to the groin, scrotum, labia majora, and the upper inner portion of the thigh [29]. They may also present with hyper/hypo- or dysesthesia distributed over the cutaneous regions innervated by the nerve (L1 dermatome). Finally, there may be a painful trigger point medial and below the anterior superior iliac spine. Aggravating factors include ambulation, hyperextension of the hip, and lying-in supine position; alleviating factors include hip flexion [29]. The symptoms of ilioinguinal neuropathy overlap with those of genitofemoral neuropathy making it difficult to distinguish these conditions from clinical examination alone.

57.4.5 Physical Examination

Visual Observation Observe the patient's preferred position of comfort which may include a bent over position (lumbar extension aggravates symptoms). Thorough inspection may reveal clues to rule in/out other diagnoses (e.g., visible defect from an inguinal hernia).

Palpation Palpate for tenderness inch medial and inferior to the anterior superior iliac spine (trigger point) [33].

Sensory Testing Test for sensory loss along the border of the abdomen and thigh, groin, anterior proximal thigh, and lateral scrotum or labia majora.

Range of Motion Assess for worsening of pain as the patient transitions from a seated to a standing position.

Table 57.3 Differential diagnosis for ilioinguinal neuropathy

Genitofemoral neuropathy	Lumbar plexopathy
Iliohypogastric neuropathy	Inguinal hernia
Appendicitis	Salpingitis
Ovarian pathology	Epididymitis or orchitis

57.4.6 Diagnostic Workup

1. *Response to nerve block:* Response to anesthetic injection into the area of maximum tenderness (the neurovascular foramina medial to the anterior superior iliac spine) indicates ilioinguinal nerve pathology [34].
2. *EMG*: Not specific for ilioinguinal pathology but may help in excluding other mimicking conditions, e.g., lumbar radiculopathy or plexopathy [35].
3. *MRI:* Mainly to exclude lumbar radiculopathy.

57.4.7 Management

Medical Management Topical lidocaine patches, tricyclic antidepressants. Other considerations include NSAIDs, anticonvulsants (gabapentin), SSRI/SNRIs, and N-methyl-D aspartate antagonists [27].

Procedures Ultrasound-guided nerve block; interrupts neuronal transmission leading to pain relief. It can serve both as a diagnostic tool and a therapeutic procedure [34].

Surgical Neurectomy of ilioinguinal nerve can be performed if other pain management techniques fail [32].

57.5 Lateral Femoral Cutaneous Neuropathy

Emanuel Mostoufi

57.5.1 Synonyms

- Meralgia paresthetica
- Anesthesia dolorosa of Lateral femoral cutaneous nerve
- Bernhardt-Roth syndrome
- Lateral femoral cutaneous nerve syndrome
- Lateral femoral cutaneous neuralgia

57.5.2 ICD 10 Codes

- G57.10–13

57.5.3 Description

Meralgia paresthetica is a condition that affects approximately 4.3 cases/10000 population and is characterized by burning pain, paresthesias, and sensory loss along the anterolateral thigh [36]. It is caused by compression of the lateral femoral cutaneous nerve, a primary sensory nerve, which travels from its origins at the lumbar plexus, emerges at the lateral border of the psoas major, passing under the inguinal ligament and eventually into the subcutaneous tissue of the anterior thigh [37]. The etiology of this condition can be divided into iatrogenic, idiopathic, and mechanical causes. Iatrogenic causes include damage to the nerve during surgery, most commonly hip joint replacement, and spine surgery and less commonly from laparoscopic appendectomies, C-sections, and gynecologic surgery. Idiopathic causes most commonly include diabetes mellitus, lead poisoning, alcohol use disorder, and hypothyroidism and obesity (pendulum abdomen), and finally mechanical compression of the nerve from tight seat belts, belts or restrictive clothing, sudden weight gain (pendulum abdomen), and pregnancy [38]. Differential diagnosis for lateral femoral cutaneous neuropathy is given in Table 57.4.

57.5.4 Clinical Presentation

The most common symptomatic description is unilateral burning pain, paresthesias, and sensory loss over the upper lateral thigh, with an acute to subacute onset over days to weeks [36]. As the lateral femoral cutaneous nerve provides only sensory innervation, there should be an absence of motor symptoms. Clinicians should pay attention to patients pointing to or rubbing their outer thigh to delineate the location of maximal discomfort or numbness. It is important to assess tight-fitting clothing (e.g., belts, tight stockings, tight pants, or leggings) and inquire about change in BMI, or pregnancy. Symptoms may be aggravated by prolonged standing or walking and alleviated by sitting.

57.5.5 Physical Examination

Visual Observation Observe the patient's preferred position of comfort which may include a bent over position. The patient may rub their lateral thigh indicating the location of discomfort (look for hair loss in this area from repeated rubbing) [36].

Table 57.4 Differential diagnosis for lateral femoral cutaneous neuropathy

Lumbar radiculopathy/plexopathy	Chronic appendicitis
Metastasis of iliac crest	Hip osteoarthritis
Pelvic tumors	Femoral neuropathy

Palpation The examiner may find allodynia or pain by palpating just medial to the anterior superior iliac spine.

Sensory Testing Test for unilateral sensory loss along the anterolateral thigh in an oblong pattern extending from the trochanteric region down to the lateral knee.

Special Tests

(a) Pelvic compression test: patient lying in lateral decubitus (symptomatic side facing up) with examiner applying downward pressure to the pelvis; an alleviation of symptoms is considered a positive test [39].
(b) Tinel sign: Repeated tapping just medial to the anterior superior iliac spine (where the lateral femoral cutaneous nerve passes deep to the inguinal ligament); a reproduction of symptoms is a positive test [40].

57.5.6 Diagnostic Workup

EMG While EMG studies of the LCNT can be helpful in diagnosis, there can be limitations in performing this procedure especially on patients with increased adipose tissue [41].

MRI Mainly to exclude lumbar radiculopathy.

Response to Nerve Block Response to anesthetic injection into the area where the LCNT exits the pelvis at the inguinal ligament is considered an affirmatory test for this condition.

57.5.7 Management

Medical NSAIDs, loosening of tight-fitting clothing/belts, and neuropathic medication are first-line treatments.

Rehabilitation No specific rehabilitation is indicated. Aerobic exercise with the goal of weight loss may be effective.

Procedures Ultrasound-guided nerve block or pulsed radiofrequency ablation may be offered. Hydrodissection of the nerve may have additional value, but this is not well studied.

Surgical Decompression of the lateral femoral cutaneous nerve can be performed if other pain management techniques fail [41].

57.6 Lumbosacral Plexopathy

Jeanie Cote, Ogochukwu Azuh and Kyungje Sung

57.6.1 Synonyms

- Lumbosacral plexus syndrome
- Lumbosacral plexus neuropathy
- Lumbosacral plexus neuritis
- Lumbosacral plexus disorder

57.6.2 ICD 10 Code

- G 54.1

57.6.3 Description

57.6.3.1 Anatomy

The lumbosacral plexus originates from the T12–S4 nerve roots and can be thought of comprising two plexi—the lumbar and the sacral (Figs. 57.3 and 57.4).

The lumbar plexus arises from the anterior rami of the L1–L4 root (a small contribution from T12). It gives rise to the iliohypogastric (T12–L1 roots), ilioinguinal (L1 root), genitofemoral (L1–2 roots), lateral femoral cutaneous (L2–3 roots), obturator (L2–L4 anterior division), and femoral nerves (L2–L4 posterior division). The obturator and femoral nerves are the major branches of the lumbar plexus and supply the muscles in the anterior and medial thigh, as well as sensation to these areas. The femoral nerve then branches into the saphenous nerve, which provides sensation to the anteromedial lower leg and foot.

The sacral plexus is made up of L5–S4 roots (an additional component from L4 root). Its major branches include the superior gluteal nerve (L4–S1), inferior gluteal nerve (L5–S2), sciatic nerve (L4–S2), posterior cutaneous nerve of the thigh (S1–3), and pudendal nerve (S1–S4) [42].

57.6.4 Types of Lumbosacral Plexopathy

When compared with brachial plexopathy, lumbosacral plexopathy is less common. This may be due to its position deep in the pelvis [45]. Clinically, lumbosacral plexopathies can be classified as affecting the lumbar or sacral plexus and whether the lesion is structural or nonstructural (i.e., causing mass effect) (Table 57.5).

Traumatic ethology such as penetrating (gunshot or puncture wounds) or high-velocity injuries are rare, likely due to the location of the plexus [42].

Nontraumatic etiologies make up most of the causes of lumbar plexopathy with the most common being diabetes mellitus (also referred to as diabetic amyotrophy, Bruns-Garland syndrome, proximal diabetic neuropathy, and diabetic lumbosacral radiculoplexus neuropathy) [45]. Pelvic or hip joint fractures may cause lumbosacral lesions; as can immune-mediated or inflammatory disorders. Neoplasms can lead to lumbar plexopathy as tumors may invade or extend into the plexus. Over 80% of the tumors are due to colorectal, urogenital, prostates, lymphoma, and retroperitoneal and pelvic sarcomas [42]. Metastatic disease from breast or lung cancer may result in lumbar plexopathy as well.

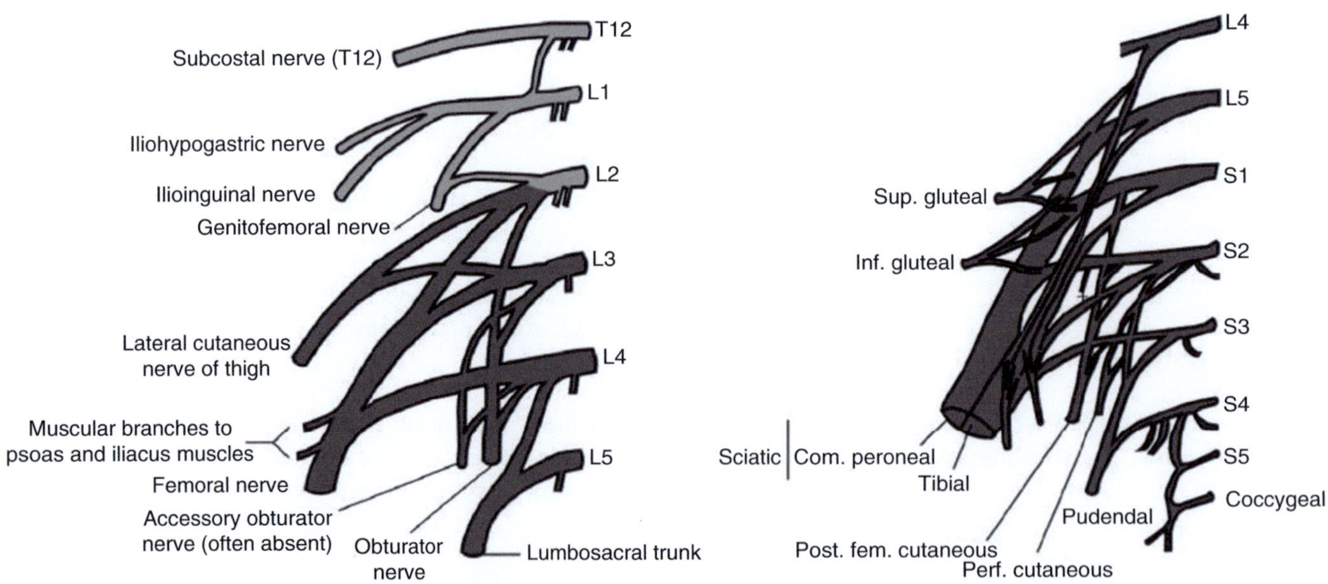

Fig. 57.3 Picture of the lumbosacral plexus. (From Neto et al. [57])

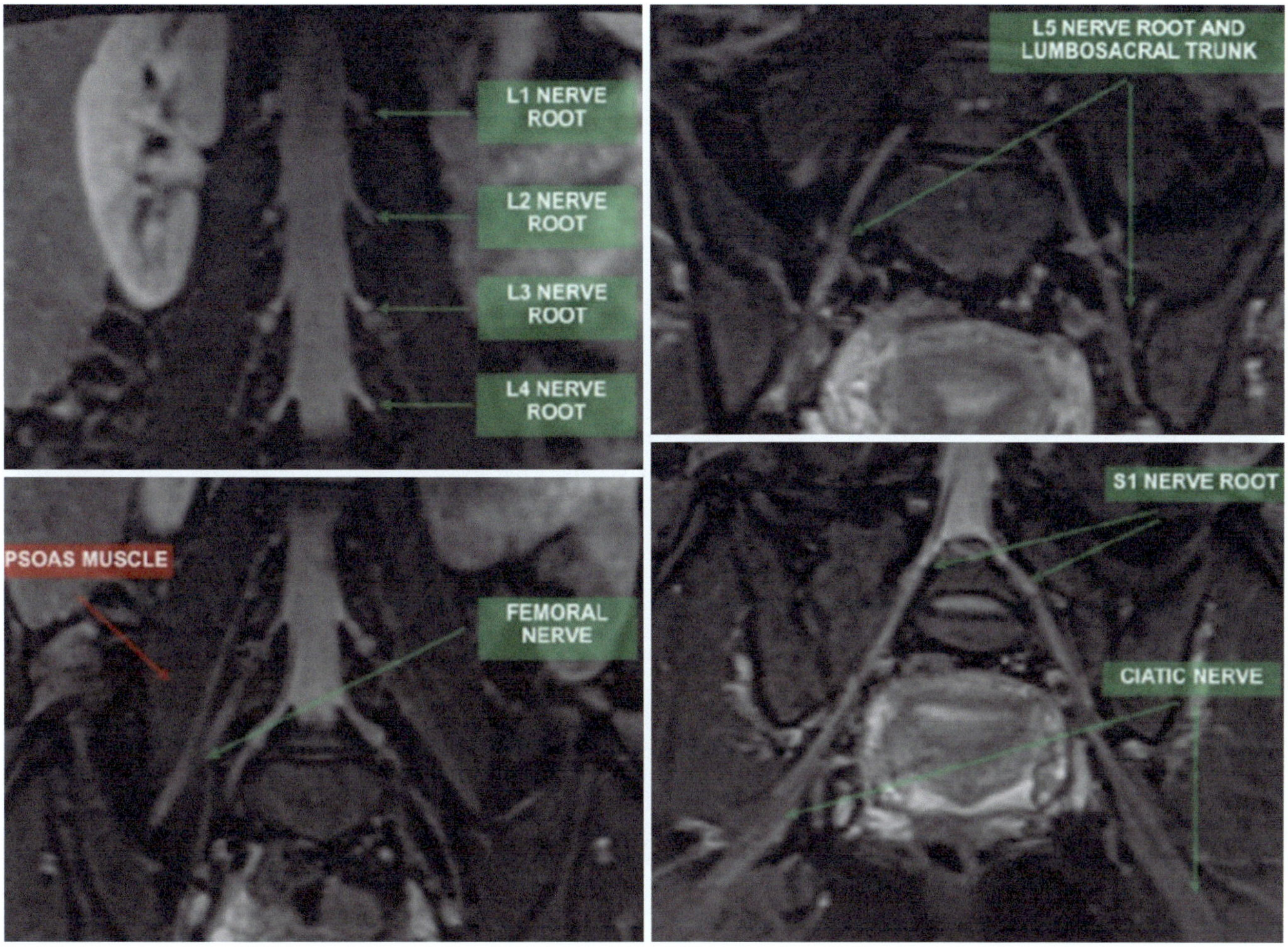

Fig. 57.4 MRI of lumbosacral plexus. Shows L1–L4 nerve roots, femoral nerve, L5, S1 nerve roots, and sciatic nerve. (From Neto et al. [57])

Table 57.5 Causes of lumbosacral plexopathy

Category	Examples
Trauma	Posterior hip dislocation, sacral fracture, penetrating (gunshot or puncture wounds), high-velocity injuries
Inflammatory/ idiopathic	Diabetic lumbosacral radiculoplexus neuropathy (LSPRN), nondiabetic LSRPN, diabetic amyotrophy, sarcoidosis, amyloidosis, postsurgical inflammatory neuropathy
Neoplastic	Metastatic disease (from breast or lung cancer), primary tumors (colorectal, cervix, uterus, ovary, prostate, lymphoma/leukemia, nerve sheath tumors, paraneoplastic, and retroperitoneal/pelvic sarcomas), endometriosis
Radiation	Radiation-induced lumbosacral plexopathy
Infection	Retroperitoneal abscess, psoas abscess, Lyme disease, VZV, *Borrelia burgdorferi*
Vascular	Retroperitoneal hematomas (in setting of bleeding disorder or anticoagulation use), internal iliac artery or common iliac (pseudo) aneurysm
Iatrogenic	Femoral artery catheterizations, abdominal or pelvic surgery, puncture for vascular access in groin
Pregnancy	Postpartum lumbosacral plexopathy

Radiation treatment for malignancy in the lower abdomen and pelvic region can also result in radiation plexopathy. Large retroperitoneal hematomas (in the setting of anticoagulation or bleeding disorders), large aneurysms, and abscesses may also cause lumbosacral plexopathy by compression of nerves. Iatrogenic causes such as groin puncture for vascular access, pelvic/abdominal surgery, or intraoperative patient positioning may also lead to injury of the lumbosacral plexus. Lumbosacral plexopathy can also occur during the later stages of pregnancy and sometimes during delivery when the lumbosacral trunk is compressed between the fetal head and the maternal pelvic rim [45]. Idiopathic plexitis (neuralgic amyotrophy) can occur, causing severe, asymmetrical leg pain, followed by asymmetrical multifocal

Table 57.6 Differential diagnosis of lumbosacral plexopathy

Amyotrophic lateral sclerosis (ALS)	Mononeuritis multiplex
Lumbar myelopathy	Multifocal motor neuropathy with conduction block
Lumbar radiculopathy	MSK disorder involving the hip, knee (i.e., avascular necrosis, hip fracture, osteoarthritis, bursitis, tendinitis)
Demyelinating disease	Lower extremity mononeuropathy
Intracranial pathology	Lower extremity complex regional pain syndrome
Spinal muscular atrophy	Peripheral vascular occlusive disease
Polyneuropathy	Infection: Guillain-Barré, chronic inflammatory demyelinating polyradiculoneuropathy, poliomyelitis

weakness and atrophy [47]. Differential diagnosis of lumbosacral plexopathy is given in Table 57.6.

57.6.5 Clinical Presentation

Common symptoms include pain, sensory loss, weakness, and muscle atrophy. For lumbar plexus lesions, pain can occur in the pelvis with radiation to the anterolateral and medial thigh region. The quadriceps, hip adductors, and hip flexors are primarily affected. With sacral lesions, pelvic pain can occur and will radiate posteriorly into the thigh and/or posterior-lateral calf. Weakness and sensory loss involve the posterior thigh, leg, and foot.

Timing of symptoms may differ depending on the etiology of the lumbosacral plexopathy. With trauma, weakness and sensory deficits often occur after an inciting event. Diabetic and nondiabetic lumbosacral radiculoplexus neuropathy share similar symptoms. Patients may experience "achy," "stabbing," or "burning" pain that may progress over days to weeks and spread to the thigh, leg, buttock, and back. It usually occurs unilaterally but can spread to the contralateral limb. This is followed by weakness and atrophy. Weight loss and autonomic symptoms such as orthostasis, constipation, and urinary and sexual dysfunction have been observed [54]. With neoplastic lumbosacral plexopathy, pain (dull and achy) usually occurs first; but for a small subset of patients, weakness or paresthesia may be the presenting symptoms [42]. In radiation-induced lumbosacral plexopathy, symptoms such as weakness, pain, and sensory loss can occur months to years after the radiation treatment. Symptoms in the setting of abscess or aneurysms formation may occur gradually (weeks to months), and pain and weakness usually happen in the proximal extremity. In iatrogenic cases (surgery, vascular procedures, femoral artery catheterizations), the onset and progression of symptoms will be rapid. In the case of maternal lumbosacral plexopathy, intermittent pain occurs first, and motor deficits such as a foot drop can appear; the symptoms dissipate after delivery and resolve within a few weeks [45]. Radiation-induced plexopathy generally presents as painless weakness.

57.6.6 Physical Examination

In addition to history, a complete neurological and musculoskeletal examination is key to diagnosing lumbosacral plexopathy. Inspection of lower limbs should be completed to observe for asymmetry and signs of muscle atrophy. A detailed sensory exam is paramount as many of the sensory nerves that arise from the lumbosacral plexus do not have standardized nerve conductions tests during electrodiagnosis [49]. Manual muscle strength, evaluation of reflexes, and dermatomes of the lower extremities can be tested bilaterally to see if any deficiencies exist. The patellar reflex may be decreased if the lumbar plexus is affected, and the hamstrings and Achilles' reflex may be diminished if the sacral plexus is involved (Table 57.7). In lumbosacral plexopathy, lower motor neuron signs such as decreased muscle tone, and lower extremity weakness can be seen [49]. Range of motion testing and provocative hip or knee can help exclude other MSK conditions that are in the differential diagnosis. Assessment of a gait pattern can highlight the affected muscles (i.e., foot drop), thereby helping to localize the lumbosacral plexus lesion.

57.6.7 Diagnostic Workup

57.6.7.1 Imaging

MRI is the imaging modality of choice when evaluating for plexus injuries or lesions. It can highlight intraneural anatomy and localize pathologic lesions in situations where physical exam and/or EMG findings are nonspecific [46] (Fig. 57.5). CT could be used to identify hematomas in the

Table 57.7 Clinical manifestations of lumbosacral plexus lesions

Location	Motor involvement	Sensory involvement	Reflex involved
Lumbar plexopathy (L2–L4 predominantly)	Quadriceps, iliopsoas, and hip adductor muscles (femoral and obturator nerves)	Lateral, anterior, and medial thigh Medial calf	Patella
Lower lumbosacral plexopathy (L4–S3)	Hip extensors (gluteus maximus), abductors and internal rotators (gluteus medius and tensor fascia lata) Hamstrings (peroneal and tibial nerves)	Posterior thigh Posterior-lateral calf Foot	Achilles

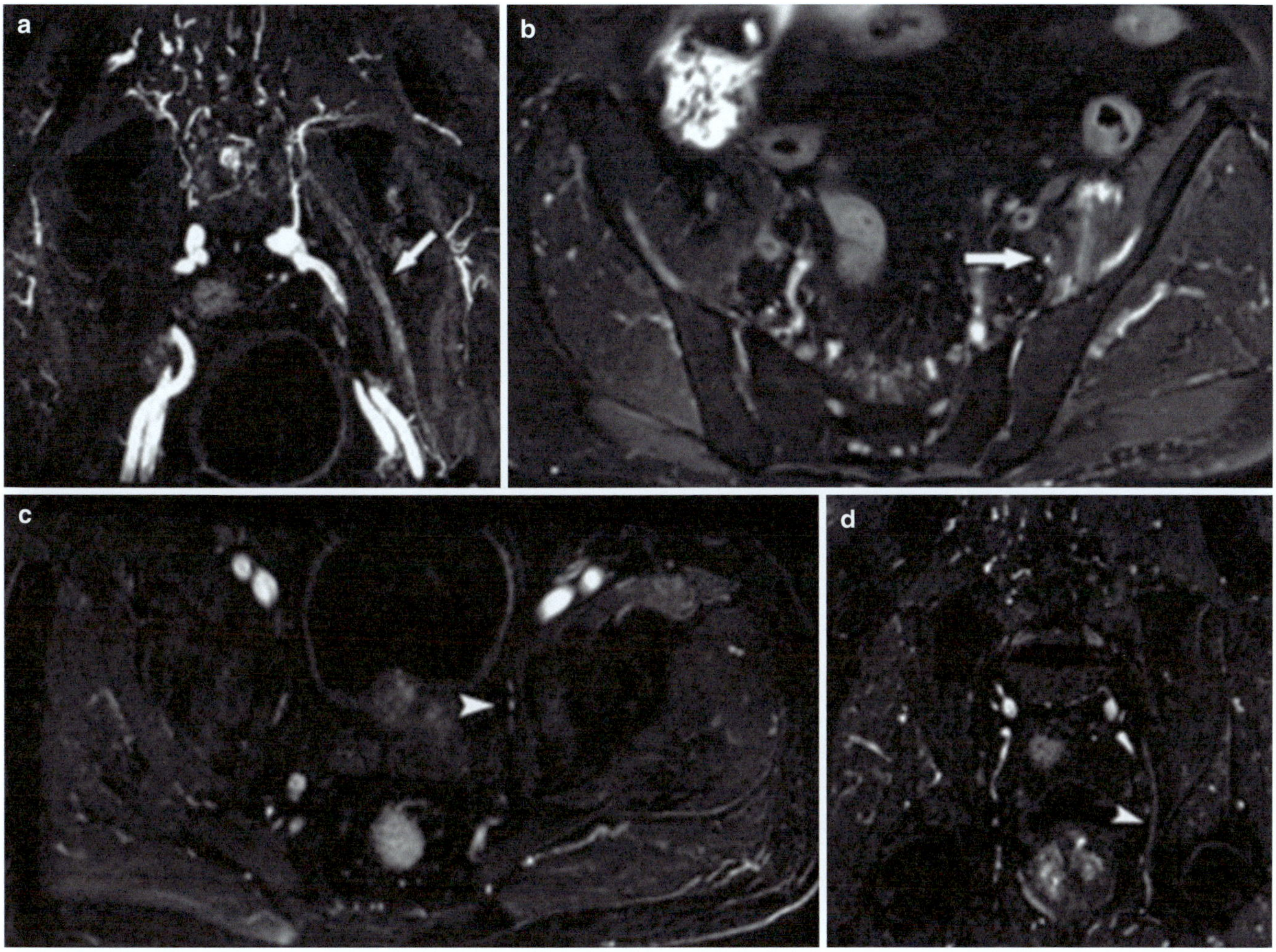

Fig. 57.5 MRN images in coronal STIR 3D SPACE MPR of patient with diabetic amyotrophy (**a**, **b**). L. femoral nerve (solid arrow) thickening with inflammatory signs and diffuse edema throughout its course. (**b**) Fluid is seen around the muscle and along the neural path (star). (**c**, **d**) Obturator nerve (arrowhead) is thickened with inflammation. (From Neto et al. [57])

pelvis or muscle; however, MRI is generally more sensitive. Imaging is especially important if there is concern for neoplastic involvement (primary or metastatic) [44] (Fig. 57.6). Due to the deep location of the lumbar and sacral plexus, structures may not be accessible by ultrasound [43].

57.6.7.2 Electrodiagnostic Testing

With the use of nerve conduction studies (NCS) and needle electromyography, electrodiagnostic testing is useful in localizing lesions to the lumbosacral plexus. It can also help exclude lumbosacral radiculopathy or peripheral mononeuropathies, characterize the pathophysiology of the nerve injury, and comment on the severity and prognosis of the injured nerve. Due to the technically challenging nature of acquiring NCS (i.e., body habitus or patients with normal low or absent SNAP amplitudes), it is always recommended to compare extremities for side-to-side differences.

Motor studies to be performed include the tibial and peroneal nerves. Femoral motor studies can also be performed for suspected lumbar plexopathies. Sensory nerve conduction studies to be performed are superficial peroneal and sural sensory studies. Saphenous studies can also be performed for suspected lumbar plexopathy. When suspecting meralgia paraesthetica, a lateral femoral cutaneous sensory study can be performed. Decreased or absent sensory nerve action potentials (SNAP) suggest the lesion is localized at or distal to the dorsal root ganglion. Furthermore, tibial and peroneal F responses and H reflexes could be performed to evaluate for a proximal lesion.

NCS alone cannot differentiate a mononeuropathy from a plexopathy; hence, needle EMG is required. Though one needs to sample a variety of distal and proximal muscles innervated by different roots and nerves, key muscles to take note of are gluteal, thigh adductors and paraspinal muscles. Gluteal muscles can differentiate sciatic neuropathy from

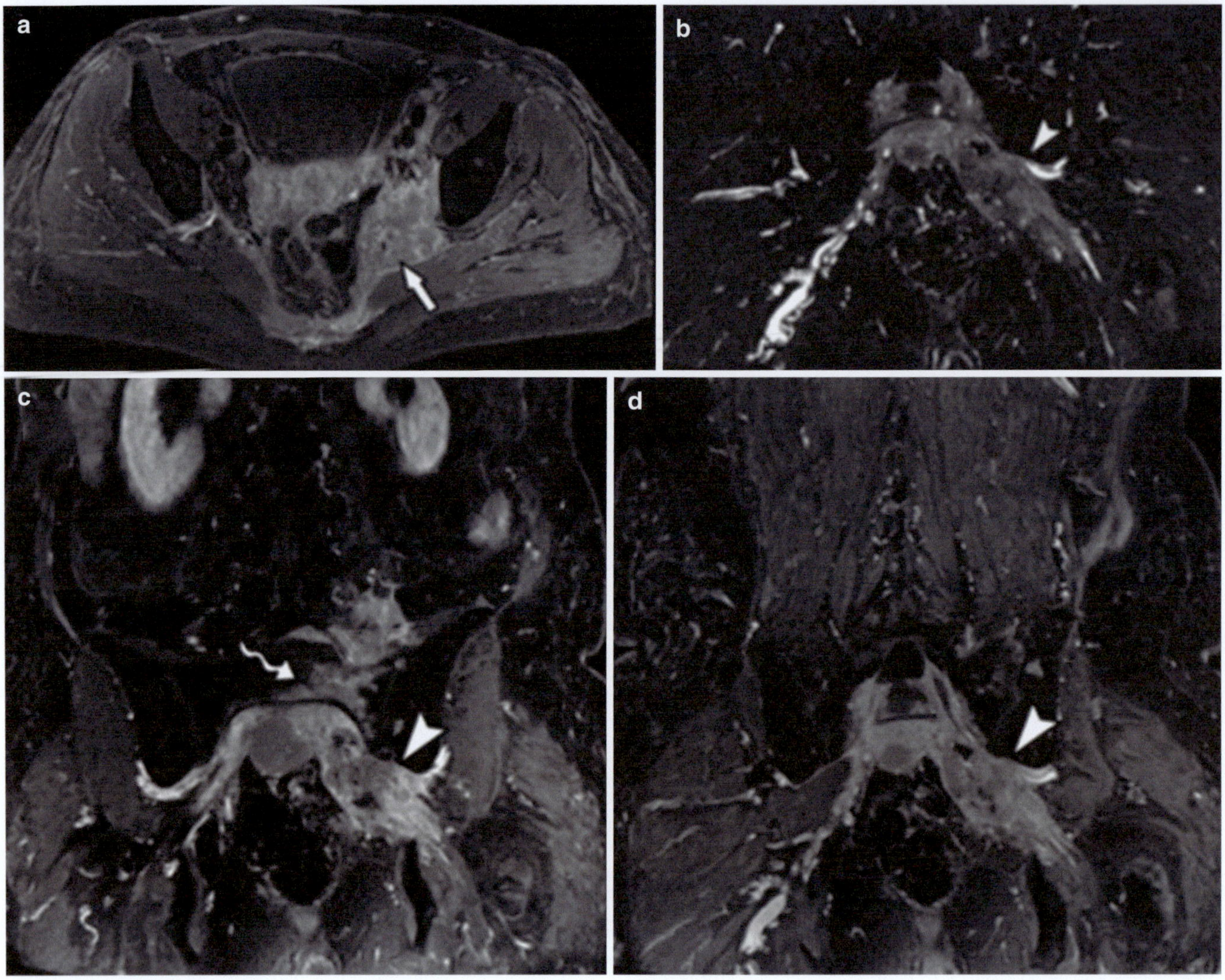

Fig. 57.6 MRN images in axial T1-weighted contrast-enhanced of patient with Hodgkin lymphoma (**a**) Large, lobular, contrasting, infiltrative mass (solid arrow) to L. neural foramina and emergent nerve roots of L4–L5 and L5–S1, and bilaterally, in S1–S2 to S4–S5. (**b–d**) Diffuse involvement of the L. sacral plexus, proximal segments of the obturator, pudendal, and sciatic nerves (arrowhead). There are also signs of bone infiltration (wavy arrow). (From Neto et al. [57])

lower lumbosacral plexopathy; thigh adductors can differentiate femoral neuropathy from lumbar plexopathy; and paraspinal muscles can differentiate nerve root from plexus lesions [53]. The findings of abnormalities on sensory NCS and the absence of lumbosacral paraspinal needle EMG findings lend itself to a diagnosis of lumbosacral plexopathy. Myokymic discharges are commonly found in radiation related lumbosacral plexopathy.

The optimal time for electrodiagnostic study is at least 3 weeks from symptom onset to allow enough time for Wallerian degeneration and denervation to occur. As nerves may take longer to heal and recover, serial electrodiagnostic studies may be necessary (over a period of 6 or more months) to make a definite prognosis in lumbosacral plexopathy [48].

57.6.7.3 Laboratory Studies

Depending on the suspected etiology, it may be prudent to acquire laboratory studies. In the case of hematoma or hemorrhage, trauma, or anticoagulation therapy, a complete blood count and coagulation panel will be helpful. In patients with diabetes, blood glucose and hemoglobin A1c may be helpful in assessing blood sugar control. Infectious etiologies may need to be ruled out with history of recent viral illness, skin involvement, or a history of inset bite. For suspected autoimmune or inflammatory diseases, inflammatory markers may be needed. Tests for neoplastic markers should be considered in suspected malignancy.

57.6.8 Treatments

57.6.8.1 Medical Management

Management of lumbosacral radiculopathy depends on the etiology. For diabetic and nondiabetic lumbosacral radiculoplexus neuropathy, the underlying cause is microscopic vasculitis leading to nerve ischemia. Though immunotherapy such as methylprednisolone, immunoglobulin, and plasma exchange has been trialed, there is no agreed upon consensus for or against its use as treatment [55]. With neoplastic lumbosacral plexopathy, radiation and chemotherapy are used to treat the malignancy. If the lumbosacral plexopathy is caused by an infectious cause, treating the infection will be indicated.

Symptomatic management for pain in the acute setting should focus on decreasing inflammation and neuropathic pain. This includes the use of medications such as NSAIDS and, if severe, usage of opioids [43]. Due to its addictive potential, one should be weary of long-term opioid use. For neuropathic pain, medications such as antiepileptics (gabapentin and carbamazepine), tricyclic antidepressants, or SNRIs can be tried.

57.6.8.2 Rehabilitation

The main goals of rehabilitation include preventing loss of function and maintaining range of motion. A dedicated home exercise program may be necessarily for patients with lumbosacral plexopathy to prevent loss of function, chronic pain and eventual debility. As weakness is commonly encountered, special focus on improving proximal lower extremity strength (including gluteus, adductor, hamstrings, and quadricep muscle groups) is key. Rehabilitation should focus on addressing muscular imbalances and maintaining range of motion. For those with difficulty ambulating, special attention should be placed on gait training in hopes of improving balance and gait. In some cases, assistive device (cane, walker) and braces may be required to offset weak muscles and provide ambulation support. Ankle-foot orthoses (AFOs) are especially important in cases of foot drop due to L4–L5 root injury affecting tibialis anterior, extensor digitorum longus and extensor hallucis longus. AFOs will allow patient to clear their foot during the swing phase of the gait cycle. Though cases of diabetic amyotrophy can be transient and prognosis is generally good, recovery can range from many months to 1–2 years [48, 53]. As there is no one definitive treatment option for radiation plexopathy, rehabilitation therapy may assist with symptom control, improve strength, and maintain function of the affected extremities [58, 59].

57.6.8.3 Procedures

For abscesses in the retroperitoneal region causing mass effect, this can usually be aspirated/drained through minimal invasive methods with interventional radiology (Fig. 57.7). In the case of lumbosacral plexopathy with intractable cancer pain, neuromodulation or permanent implantable intrathecal infusion pumps have been used for relief [50]. Nerve blocks with local anesthetics (i.e., bupivacaine, ropivacaine) to the lumbar and sacral plexus (e.g., psoas compartment block) are options as well for further pain control especially in the setting of trauma and/or planned surgery [51, 52]. For meralgia paresthetica, ultrasound-guided lateral femoral cutaneous nerve block can be diagnostic and provide pain relief. Pulsed radiofrequency ablation and more recently peripheral nerve stimulation have been used with some success for intractable pain [63, 64].

57.6.8.4 Surgery

In traumatic cases of lumbosacral plexopathy (Fig. 57.8), surgery may be indicated to repair intrapelvic structures and for distal nerve transfer to reinnervate femoral nerve function. Surgical repair is usually rare, as most traumatic plexopathies improve spontaneously and are treated conservatively. When surgery is attempted, repairing lumbar lesions seem to have better outcomes compared to sacral plexus injuries [45]. In the case of malignancy, surgical resection of the primary tumor is indicated. For terminal cancer pain, rhizotomy has been shown to be helpful [56]. Intrathecal drug infusion systems have also been successfully used in the setting of intractable cancer pain (using morphine) and a case of ischemic related lumbosacral plexopathy pain (using intrathecal baclofen) [50, 60, 61]. Spinal cord stimulators have also been used to control neuropathic pain secondary to traumatic lumbosacral plexopathy [62]. For retroperitoneal hematomas, this is usually managed conservatively with reversal of anticoagulation and administration of blood products. In cases of worsening hematoma or progressive neurologic loss, surgery may be warranted.

57.7 Brachial Plexopathy

Ogochukwu Azuh, Jeanie Cote and Kyungje Sung

57.7.1 Synonyms

- Brachial plexus syndrome
- Brachial plexus neuropathy
- Brachial plexus neuritis
- Brachial plexus disorder

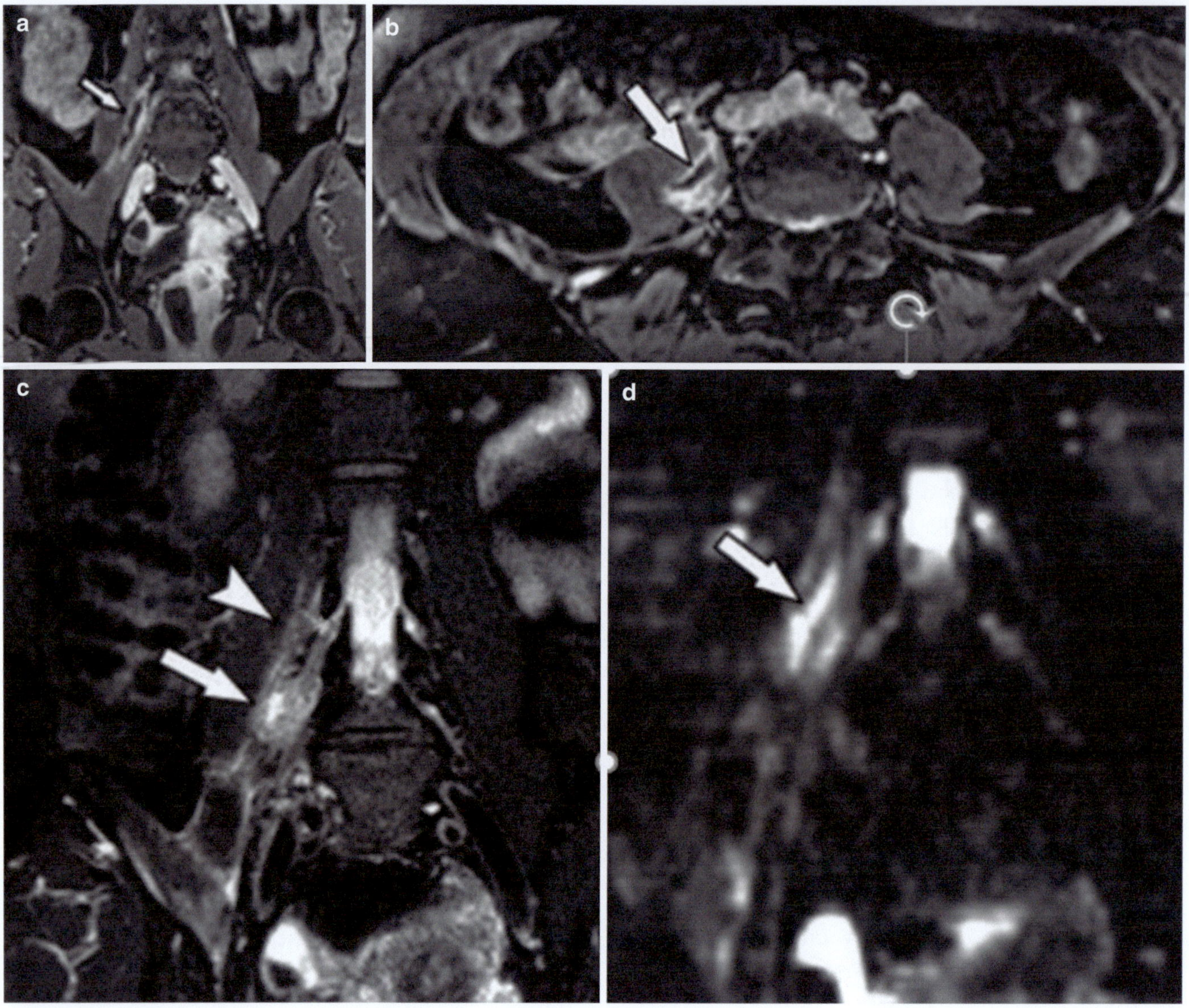

Fig. 57.7 MRN images in coronal T1VIBE post contrast of patient with fluid collection in R. iliopsoas muscle. (**a–d**) intense peripheral contrast enhancement imaging the fluid collection (solid arrow). (**d**) The L3 nerve root (arrowhead) presents signs of neuropathy. The R. L4 nerve root (star) is thickened and edematous w/ contrast enhancement throughout its course, up to the level of the inguinal region. (From Neto et al. [57])

57.7.2 ICD 10 Codes

- S143XXA, S143XXD, S143XXS

57.7.3 Description

Brachial plexopathy occurs when there is a lesion or injury to the brachial plexus. Common etiologies include trauma (most common with incidence between 44% and 77% of brachial plexus injuries [65, 66]), inflammatory causes, neoplasms, radiation, and idiopathic and anatomical variants. Differential diagnoses of brachial plexopathy are in Table 57.8, and common causes of brachial plexus are outlined in Table 57.9.

57.7.3.1 Anatomy

The brachial plexus (Fig. 57.9) arises from cervical nerve roots that emerge from the cervical spinal cord, travel down through the neck (the cervico-axillary canal), over the first rib, and into the axial area. The brachial plexus comprises of roots (C5–T1), trunks (upper, middle, and lower), divisions (three anterior, three posterior), cords (lateral, posterior, and medial), and terminal nerves. The roots and trunk are supra-

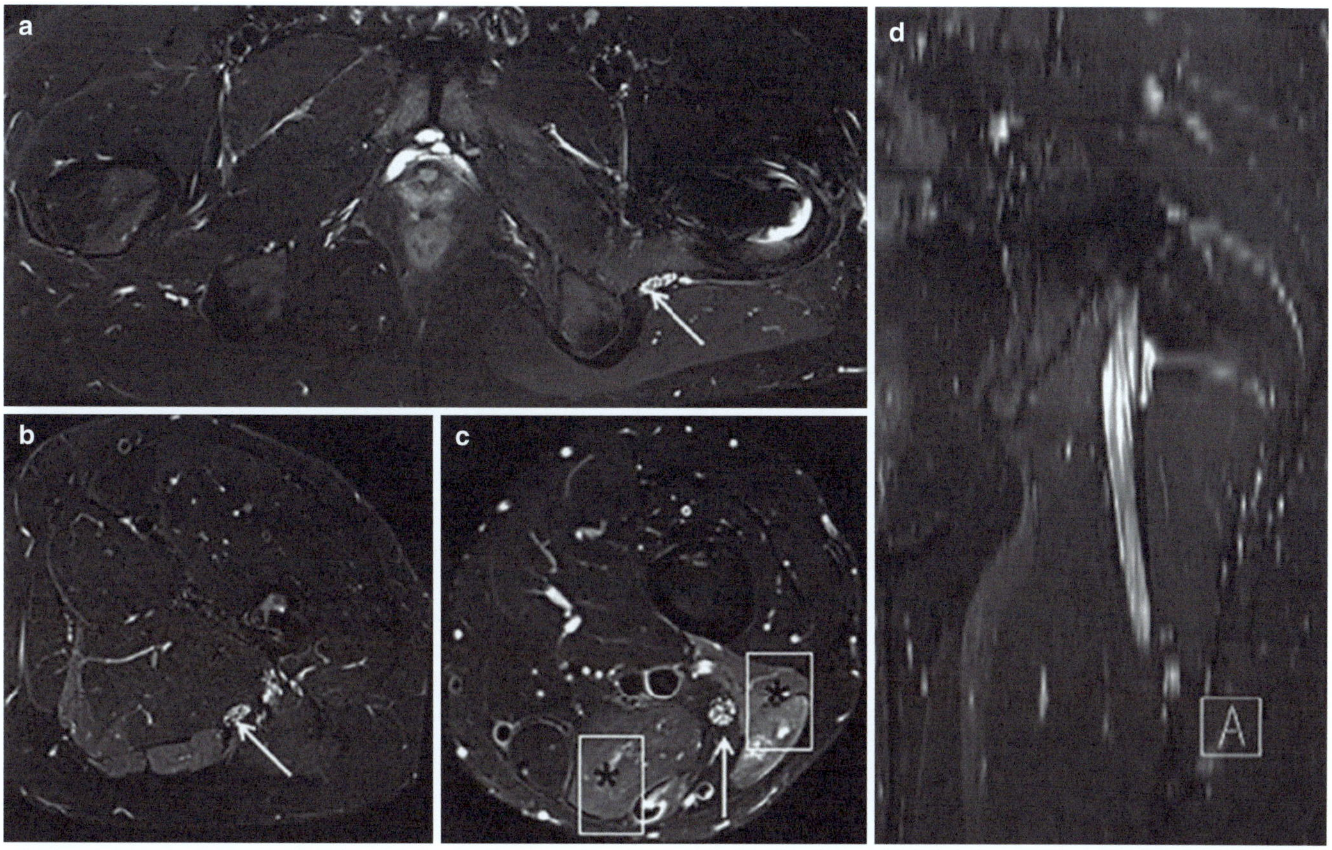

Fig. 57.8 L. femoral shaft fracture, sciatic nerve injury after road accident. (**a**) Axial T2-STIR at pelvic floor. (**b**, **c**) Sagittal oblique reformat. (**d**) Hyperintensity and enlargement of L. sciatic nerve. Arrows pointing to fascicular hypertrophy (**a–c**) with increased signal intensity of semimembranosus, semitendinosus, and long head of the biceps femuri due to acute denervation (**c**). (From Gasparotti et al. [47])

Table 57.8 Differential diagnoses of brachial plexopathy

Amyotrophic lateral sclerosis	Mononeuritis multiplex
Cervical myelopathy	Multifocal motor neuropathy with conduction block
Cervical radiculopathy	Musculoskeletal disorder involving the shoulder, elbow, or forearm (i.e., adhesive capsulitis, rotator cuff syndrome, bursitis, tendinitis)
Demyelinating disease	Upper extremity complex regional pain syndrome (CRPS)
Intracranial pathology	Upper extremity mononeuropathy

clavicular, and the cords and branches are infraclavicular. After exiting the cervical intervertebral foramina, the nerve roots will travel in between anterior and middle scalene muscle, and before reaching the clavicle, they will form the three trunks. The trunks will pass in between the clavicle and the first rib and form the three anterior and three posterior divisions. The divisions merge to produce three cords which are named according to their position in relation to the axillary artery. Each cord will further divide into the terminal nerves responsible for both the motor and sensory innervation of the arm.

Table 57.9 Causes of brachial plexopathy. (Revision of table from Shanina et al. [65])

Category	Examples
Trauma	High-velocity and penetrating injuries, birth (Erb's and Klumbke's), severe traction injury, root avulsion, compression (Rucksack palsy, Burner)
Inflammatory	Neuralgic amyotrophy (idiopathic and hereditary), diabetic cervical radiculoplexus neuropathy, postsurgical inflammatory plexopathy, hereditary neuralgic amyotrophy
Neoplastic	Metastatic disease, primary nerve tumors (Schwannoma), Pancoast tumor, paraneoplastic syndrome
Radiation	Radiation-induced plexopathy
Structural	Neurogenic thoracic outlet syndrome
Infection	Viruses: EBV, VZV, parvovirus B19, CMV, mumps, HIV, HSV, dengue, St. Louis encephalitis, Japanese B, WNV, HEV
	Bacteria and fungi: *Leptospira* sp., *Mycobacterium tuberculosis*, *Yersinia* sp., *Salmonella typhi*, *Coccidioides immitis*, *Borrelia burgdorferi*
Iatrogenic	Nerve blocks/ injections, post-thoracatomy traction, intra-operative surgical positioning, direct intraoperative nerve trauma
Ischemia	Polyarteritis nodosa, Behcet's, giant cell arteritis, hypersensitivity vasculitis, microscopic polyangiitis, Henoch-Schonlein purpura

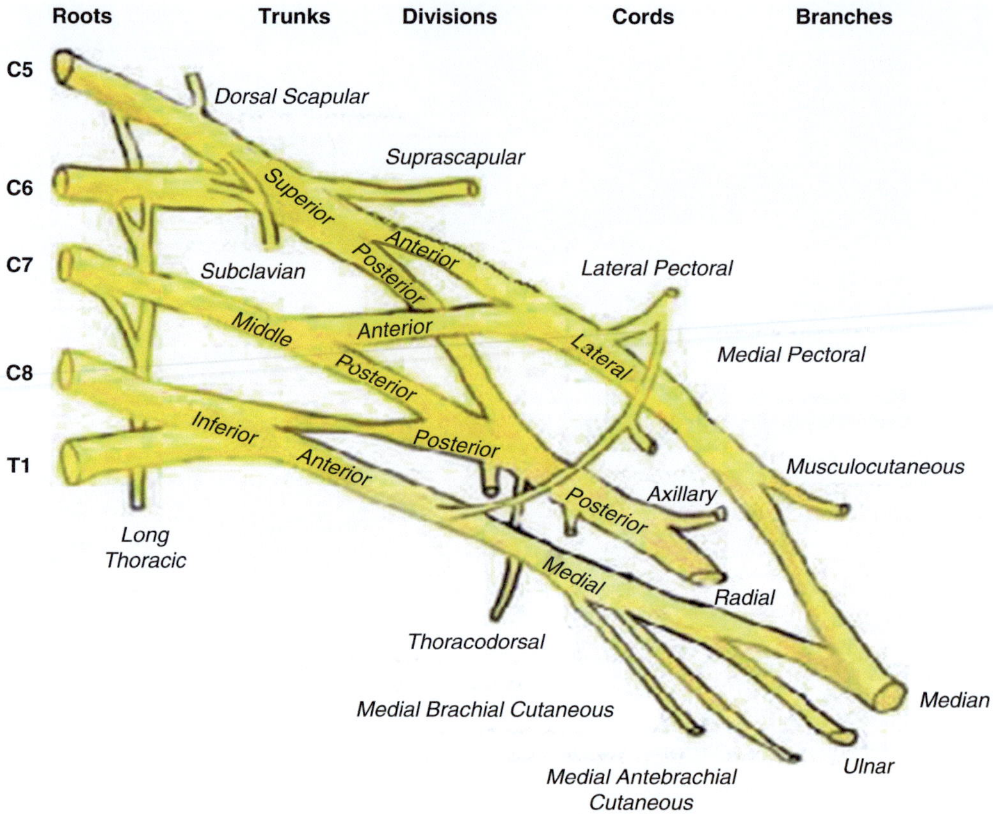

Fig. 57.9 Diagram of the brachial plexus. (From Hsu et al. [85])

57.7.3.2 Types of Brachial Plexopathy

Brachial plexopathies can be classified based on the region of the plexus affected. The supraclavicular area would involve the root and trunks, the retroclavicular region would affect the divisions, and the infraclavicular sites would compromise the cords and terminal nerves. An important detail to note that will affect treatment options is if the lesion is preganglionic, proximal to the dorsal root ganglion, or postganglionic, distal to the dorsal root ganglion. In a preganglionic injury, motor neurons can be separated from the spinal cord, but the sensory neurons may remain intact; this lesion will likely need nerve transfer for function to return. In a postganglionic injury, both sensory and motor neurons can be affected, and function may be restored spontaneously [67].

1. *Supraclavicular plexopathies* are more common, tend to be severe, and generally result in poorer outcomes. Supraclavicular plexopathy can also occur at birth, resulting in Erb's (affecting C5–7 roots) and Klumpke's palsies (C8–T1 roots). They can be subdivided into *upper* (C5 and C6 roots/upper trunk), *middle* (C7 root and middle trunk), and *lower* (C8 and T1 roots/lower trunk) injuries. This has clinical significance, i.e., upper supraclavicular plexopathies are usually in proximity to the muscles they innervate, usually related to demyelinating conduction block, and easily accessible to surgery. Hence, recovery tends to be more favorable [68]. Some examples include burner syndrome, rucksack paralysis, and classic postoperative paralysis. Middle supraclavicular plexopathies do not usually occur alone as it usually happens with either lower or upper supraclavicular plexus involvement. In both upper and middle supraclavicular plexopathies, closed traction is one of the main culprits [68]. In lower supraclavicular plexopathies, avulsion injuries are more common. Lower supraclavicular plexopathy disorders include true neurogenic thoracic outlet syndrome, postoperative disputed neurogenic thoracic outlet syndrome, post-median sternotomy plexopathy, and Pancoast syndrome.
2. *Retroclavicular plexopathies* usually do not occur alone as isolated injuries to this area is rare, and vascular damage is commonly present as well [66, 68].
3. *Infraclavicular plexopathies* can result after radiation to axillary lymph nodes, midshaft clavicular fractures, medial brachial fascial compartment syndrome, and glenohumeral dislocations and proximal humeral fractures. Examples of site-nonspecific brachial plexopathies includes neuralgic amyotrophy (Parsonage-Turner Syndrome or idiopathic plexopathy), primary and secondary neoplasms, radiation-induced, trauma, iatrogenic (after operations or nerve blocks), vasculitis, and infection.

57.7.4 Clinical Presentation

Depending on the etiology of the brachial plexopathy, most patients experience pain, weakness, and sensory disturbance in the affected upper extremity. Symptoms can develop rapidly (trauma), over days to weeks (i.e., brachial plexitis), or may develop slowly over month to years (i.e., neoplastic).

Pain is one of the cardinal symptoms, which can be excruciating. This neuropathic pain can be described as "achy," "stabbing," "burning" or "deep" in quality. Location of the pain depends on the specific area of the injured plexus. In an upper trunk injury, the pain may be present in the shoulder or upper arm, and in a lower trunk injury, the distal arm or hand may be involved.

Upper extremity weakness can be debilitating and result in functional loss. The myotomal weakness would reflect the specific site and severity of brachial plexus injury. Proximal arm weakness will likely develop in the setting of upper trunk involvement, and hand weakness will likely manifest with a lower trunk lesion. Muscle atrophy may be observed in subacute and chronic cases. With middle trunk injuries, deficits in elbow, wrist, and finger extensions will likely be present [69].

In supraclavicular lesions, a segmental (dermatome and myotome) pattern of motor and sensory loss may be observed. In infraclavicular injuries, non-segmental patterns are seen with involvement of terminal nerves [68].

Sensory disturbances include loss of sensation and symptoms such as tingling and pins and needle sensation. The distribution of sensory changes would depend on the location of the brachial plexus injury. In specific lower trunk plexopathies, Horner's syndrome may be present.

Table 57.10 Clinical manifestations of brachial plexus lesions

Location	Motor involvement	Sensory involvement	Reflex involvement
Upper trunk	All C5–C6 innervated muscles (e.g., Deltoid, biceps, brachioradialis, supraspinatus and infraspinatus)	Lateral arm Lateral forearm Lateral hand Thumb	Biceps Brachioradialis
Middle trunk	Triceps, flexor carpi radialis, pronator teres Mimics C7 radiculopathy	Middle finger Posterior forearm	Triceps
Lower trunk	All ulnar muscles C8–T1 innervated median nerve muscles (e.g., abductor pollicis brevis, flexor pollicis longus, flexor digitorum profundus) C8 innervated radial muscles (e.g., extensor indicis proprius, extensor pollicis brevis)	Medial arm Medial forearm Medial hand 4th–5th digits	None
Lateral cord	Biceps, flexor carpi radialis, pronator teres,	Lateral forearm Lateral hand, 1st–3rd fingers	Biceps
Posterior cord	All radial nerve muscles (include deltoid and latissimus dorsi)	Lateral arm Posterior arm Forearm Radial dorsal hand	Triceps Brachioradialis
Medial cord	All ulnar muscles C8–T1 innervated medial muscles	Medial arm Medial forearm Medial hand 4th–5th fingers	None

57.7.5 Physical Examination

For patients in whom a brachial plexus injury is suspected, a detailed neurological and musculoskeletal examination is of paramount importance. With the clinician looking for areas of motor, sensory and reflex changes as these usually can localize the location of the brachial plexus injury [53] (Table 57.10). Inspection of the affected limb can sometimes reveal atrophy of the affected muscles.

- *Supraclavicular injuries*: Shoulder may be adducted, internally rotated, and the elbow pronated. Percussion of the posterior triangle of the neck may elicit a tingling sensation (positive Tinel's sign) [66]. With suprascapular nerve injuries at the suprascapular notch, palpation can reveal localized pain and weakness of shoulder abduction and external rotation can be observed, or at the spinoglenoid notch with weakness of only shoulder external rotation. Dorsal scapular nerve injury will lead to scapular instability, and long thoracic nerve injury will demonstrate decreased scapular abduction [67].
- *Infraclavicular injuries*: This type of injuries will be associated with lesions of the axillary, suprascapular, and musculocutaneous nerves; hence, there may be defects with abduction of the shoulder, external rotation of the shoulder, and flexion of the elbow. Posterior cord injuries will likely affect the radial nerve, and there may be difficulty supinating the forearm and elbow/wrist/finger extensions.
- Sensory changes will also occur based on location of the brachial plexus injury and will likely result within the dermatome associated with the affected cervical roots.
- There may also be Horner syndrome (eyelid ptosis, meiosis, anhidrosis) with root avulsion injuries at the T1 root level [67].

57.7.6 Diagnostic Workup

57.7.6.1 Diagnostic Imaging

Imaging of the brachial plexus is an important tool, especially in the setting of trauma (i.e., root avulsion, hematomas), structural causes leading to compression, and neoplasms. Further, size or signal abnormalities may help indicate the existence of the brachial plexus disease. MRI is the image modality of choice to assess the brachial plexus (Fig. 57.10). Specifically, MR neurography has been found to have a high specificity (98–100%) and sensitivity of 41–71% in evaluation of brachial plexopathy [46, 70]. Other imaging studies that can be used include routine chest radiograph (helpful in assessing cervical rib for neurogenic thoracic outlet syndrome) (Fig. 57.11), CT scan (most useful in depicting a soft tissue mass or hematoma), ultrasound, and myelography (can identify a pseudomeningocele). In MRI imaging, increased T2 signal intensity, diffuse or focal enhancement, or enlargement or edema of nerve segments can all be seen within the brachial plexus [42].

57.7.6.2 EMG/NCS

Electrodiagnostic testing is a useful tool in evaluating the brachial plexus. A combination of motor and sensory nerve conduction studies (NCS) and needle electromyography (EMG) can help ensure the pathology is related to the brachial plexus, localize which section of the brachial plexus is involved, characterize the pathophysiology of the nerve injury and the amount of axon loss, and give insight into the state of nerve recovery or reinnervation. Some etiologies of brachial plexopathy result in focal electrodiagnostic findings (lower trunk in neurogenic thoracic outlet syndrome), or irregular findings within the nerve branches (Parsonage Turner syndrome).

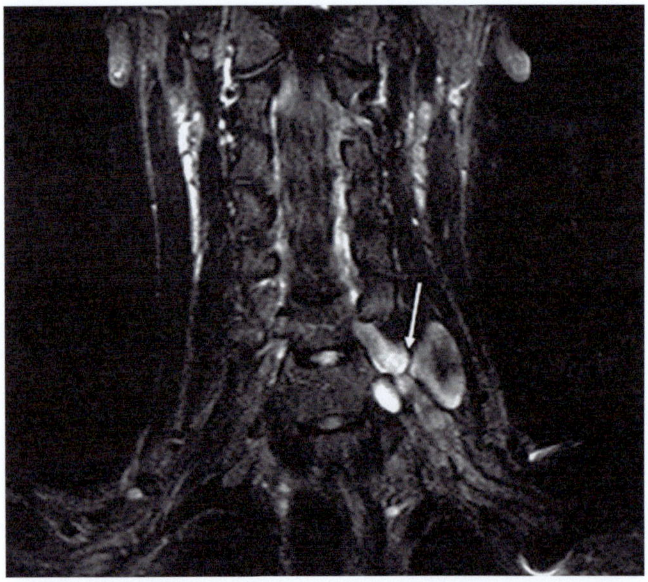

Fig. 57.10 MRN image of a traumatic injury of the left brachial plexus. White arrow showing neurotmesis of the L. C6 nerve root and stump neuroma. (From Gasparotti et al. [47])

Motor NCS can observe axonal loss (low compound muscle action potentials (CMAPs)). Anomalies may exist in the median and ulnar nerve with lower trunk or medial injuries. In upper trunk lesions, abnormalities may be present in musculocutaneous, suprascapular, or axillary nerves. Sensory NCS may show findings of low amplitude or absent response due to Wallerian degeneration to the sensory axons at or distal to the dorsal root ganglia. With needle EMG, irregularities will be seen in the muscles that are supplied by the specific injured portion of the brachial plexus. Fibrillation potentials and positive sharp waves will be seen in the setting of axonal loss and absence of complete reinnervation. There may be motor unit potential (MUP) changes depending on the progression of injury and timing of the EMG itself. Usually, in acute lesions, reduced recruitment of MUPs can be observed. In subacute to chronic injuries, there may be increased MUP amplitude, duration, and polyphasic waves. In severe cases, MUPs can be absent. Specific findings, such as myokymic discharges, can indicate radiation plexopathy [42, 53].

57.7.6.3 Laboratory Studies

Laboratory studies are not usually indicated in workup of brachial plexus injury as the most common cause is due to trauma. However, laboratory studies may be helpful in determining nontraumatic causes (i.e., autoimmune, metabolic, infectious, or oncological). Thus, tests for diabetes, inflammatory and neoplastic makers, connective tissue disease or systemic vasculitis may aid in diagnostic investigation.

57.7.7 Treatments

Management of brachial plexopathy depends on the etiology. Factors affecting prognosis are mechanism of injury, age, type of nerve (sensory, motor, or mixed), level of injury, duration of symptoms, time of surgical intervention, and other factors such as concomitant diseases (Table 57.11). In general, a multidisciplinary approach combining rehabilitation, medical, interventional, and surgical treatments is preferred.

57.7.7.1 Medical Management

Due to the painful nature of brachial plexopathy, pain management is crucial. Early-phase treatment should focus on decreasing inflammation and neuropathic pain. Common pain analgesics include NSAIDs, antiepileptics (e.g., gabapentin and carbamazepine), oral steroids, tricyclic antidepressants (e.g., nortriptyline and amitriptyline), and opioids.

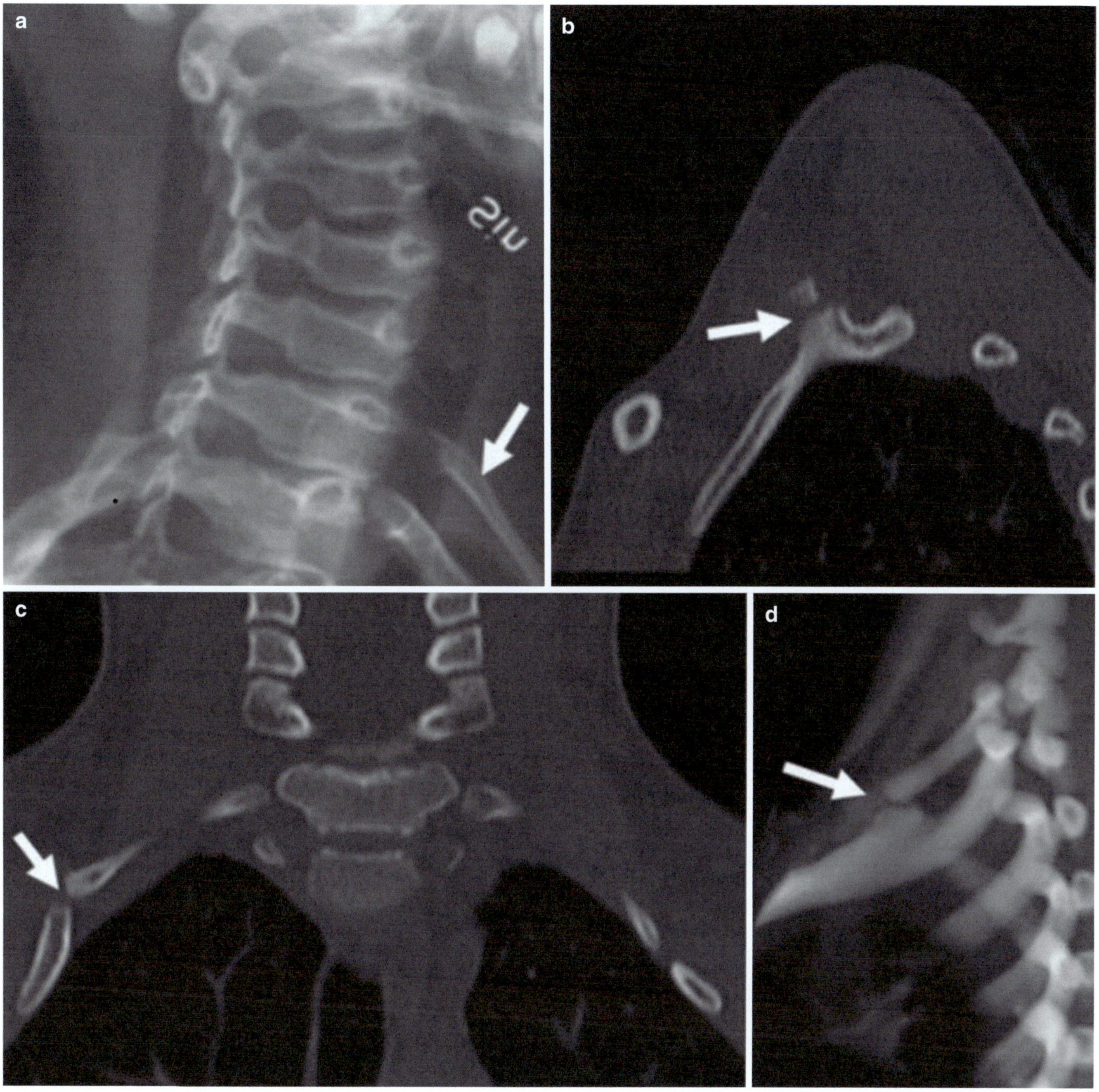

Fig. 57.11 (**a**) Plain radiograph oblique view showing R. cervical rib (arrow). (**b**) CT sagittal view. (**c**) CT coronal view. (**d**) 3D- reconstructed images. (**b–d**) showing pseudoarthrotic bony formation (arrows) between cervical rib and the first rib. (From Dahlin et al. [71])

Specific etiologies better lend themselves to initial management with medications prior to more invasive procedures such as surgery. In idiopathic brachial plexopathy, corticosteroid treatment given in the acute phase has been found to shorten the period of pain and hasten motor recovery [65]. Vascular brachial plexopathy (polyarteritis nodosa, Bechet's, giant cell arteritis, hypersensitivity vasculitis, microscopic polyangiitis, and Henoch-Schonlein purpura) can also be treated with steroids, IVIG, or plasmapheresis. Infectious brachial plexopathy involves treating the causative organism, whether it be a virus or bacteria. Brachial plexus birth palsy is initially managed by 1–2 weeks of elbow immobilization, followed by functional rehabilitation. In cases of neoplastic and paraneoplastic plexopathy, radiation, hormonal therapy, or chemotherapy is used for treatment of the offending mass or metastases. With radiation-induced plexopathy, surgical procedure may be more beneficial [65, 72]. The use of microsurgery for nerve transfer to the musculocutaneous nerve to improve elbow flexion has been reported [73].

57.7.7.2 Rehabilitation

Rehabilitation plays an important role in decreasing both short- and long-term effects of brachial plexopathy. The main goals of rehabilitation include preventing loss of function and maintaining range of motion. This can be achieved by prevention of muscle atrophy and secondary deformities, recovery of sensation deficits, limiting developmental disregard, and postoperative care [66].

To combat muscle atrophy, one starts with passive muscle stretching. Electrical stimulation, applied to injured nerve or denervated muscles, can also be used to recover muscle size and function. This is then followed by isokinetic and resistance exercises. These physiotherapy/occupational therapy options can be used in combination with orthoses (i.e., whole arm flail splint, elbow and hand splints, serial casting) to limit contractures and decreased range of motion. Therapeutic ultrasound, transcutaneous electrical nerve stimulation (TENS), and scar massage have been found to be helpful with muscular contractures. The use of TENS to painful extremities can also aid in neuropathic pain control.

Table 57.11 Prognostic factors of recovery after brachial plexopathy

Factor	Result
Mechanism of injury	High-energy injuries have worse prognosis Avulsion injuries have worse prognosis than acute ruptures Worse prognosis with concomitant vascular injury
Age	Better prognosis in young patients
Type of nerve	Exclusively sensory or motor nerves have better functional recovery than mixed nerves
Level of injury	Supraclavicular lesions have worse prognosis than infraclavicular Upper trunk lesions have the best prognosis
Pain	Patients with persistent pain for more than 6 months after traumatic injury have less possibility for recovery
Time of surgical intervention	Fibrosis and degeneration of target organs at the time of surgical intervention are related to poor prognosis
Other factors	Concomitant diseases (infections, etc.) are related to worse prognosis

From Sakellariou et al. [67]

For sensory derangements after peripheral nerve injury, tactile exercises like touching different shapes and textures with eyes closed or opened, localizing stimuli, or enhanced treatments (e.g., sensor glove system) can be used to retrain the sensory system. For those exhibiting developmental disregard (desire to not actively use the impaired limb), the use of constrained-induced movement therapy (CIMT) can be effective. This is achieved by limiting the non-affected limb, with a glove or sling, for most of the day, and intensively exercising the affected limb for up to 6 h a day for 2–3 weeks [66].

The goal of rehabilitation should be to return patients as fast and safe as possible to daily life activities. In addition, physical therapy plays an important role in preventing and relieving pain. Failure of rehabilitation can lead to upper extremity weakness, chronic pain, and eventual functional impairment.

57.7.7.3 Procedures

For associated musculoskeletal ailments (i.e., shoulder pain from subluxation due to muscle weakness), localized corticosteroid injections can be considered. For those who develop refractory neuropathic pain, acupuncture, peripheral and sympathetic nerve blocks, or neuromodulation can be effective (Fig. 57.12). Neuromodulation relies on the gate control theory [74–76]. Choi et al. discussed the use of combined spinal cord stimulator (SCS) and peripheral nerve stimulation (PNS) to control pain from brachial plexopathy [74].

For pain related to thoracic outlet syndrome, Botox injections to the anterior scalene, pectoralis minor, and subclavius muscle have been found to be helpful in controlling pain [77,

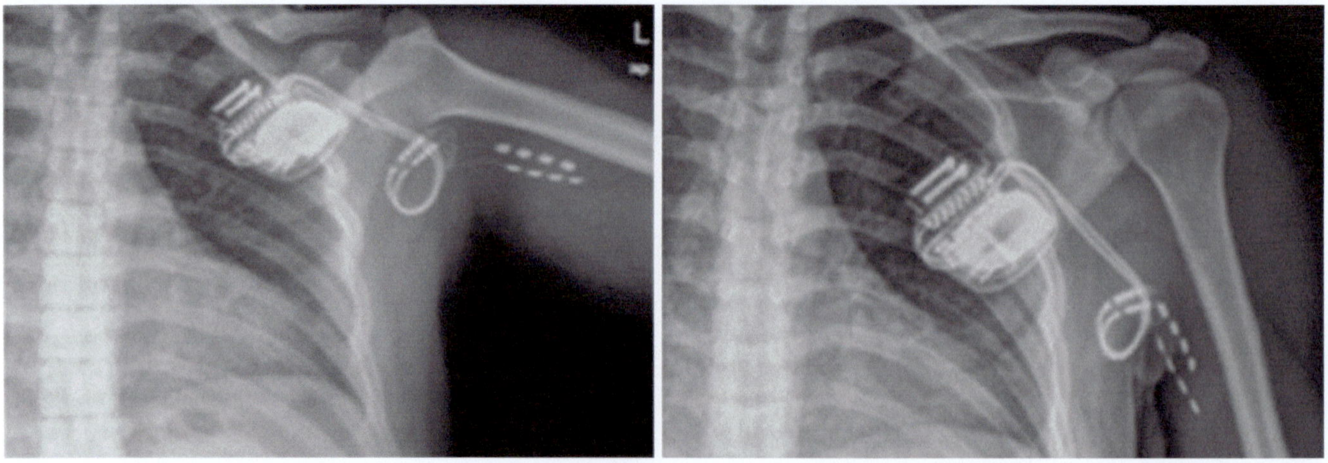

Fig. 57.12 Radiograph of position of leads to the brachial plexus (radial and median nerve). (From Stevanato et al. [84])

78]. In addition, a good response to Botox injections to the above muscles may indicate favorable outcomes in surgical repair of thoracic outlet syndrome [79]. Though rarely used, chemical neurolysis with alcohol or phenol to the trunks (upper, middle, lower) has also been described in literature for treatment of cancer-related pain [80, 81]. With the expected permanent loss of motor and sensory function, patient selection is paramount [81]. Ultrasound and electrostimulation guided pulsed radiofrequency treatment to the root of C6 has been trailed for neoplastic brachio-plexopathy with at least 67% decrease in NRS scores at the 2-month follow-up period [82].

57.7.7.4 Surgery

In the treatment of traumatic brachial plexopathy, surgery is the treatment of choice. For avulsion, penetrating and vascular injuries, immediate surgical intervention is required to achieve maximal improvement. This includes neurolysis, nerve repair, nerve transfer or grafting, tendon transfer, free functioning muscle transfer, brachial plexus reimplantation, and arthrodesis. After prognostication of nerve injury is achieved with EMG, a common window for nerve transfer to occur is approximately 3–6 months after the traumatic event.

For brachial plexus birth palsy, surgical procedures such as nerve grafting or transfer and extra-plexus neurotization (severe cases) may be indicated 3–6 months after the initial insult depending on motor and functional recovery [69]. In idiopathic neuralgic amyotrophy, nerve grafts or nerve transfers become an option for severe cases if refractory symptoms do not improve 6 months after onset [83].

In cases of true neurogenic thoracic outlet syndrome, one can attempt surgical removal of the offending agent (i.e., first cervical rib and taut band or scalene muscle) to achieve decompression. Complete surgical resection is indicated in primary tumors causing brachial plexopathy with sparing use of nerve grafts to assist with recovery (Fig. 57.13). In radiation-induced plexopathy, surgery is preferred to mechanically release radiation fibrosis, improve vascularization with flap coverage, and improve function with nerve grafting and muscle/tendon transfers [72].

57.8 Thoracic Outlet Syndrome

Garett Lui and S. Ali Mostoufi

Keywords
Thoracic outlet syndrome; Cervical rib; Costoclavicular syndrome; Scalene anticus syndrome

57.8.1 Synonyms and ICD

- Vascular thoracic outlet syndrome (G54.0)
- Neurogenic thoracic outlet syndrome (G54.0)
- Venous thoracic outlet syndrome of subclavian vein (I87.1)
- Arterial thoracic outlet syndrome due to cervical rib (G54.0)
- Brachial plexus disorders (G54.0)
- Cervical rib syndrome (Q76.5)
- Costoclavicular syndrome (G54.0)
- Scalenus anticus syndrome (G54.0)

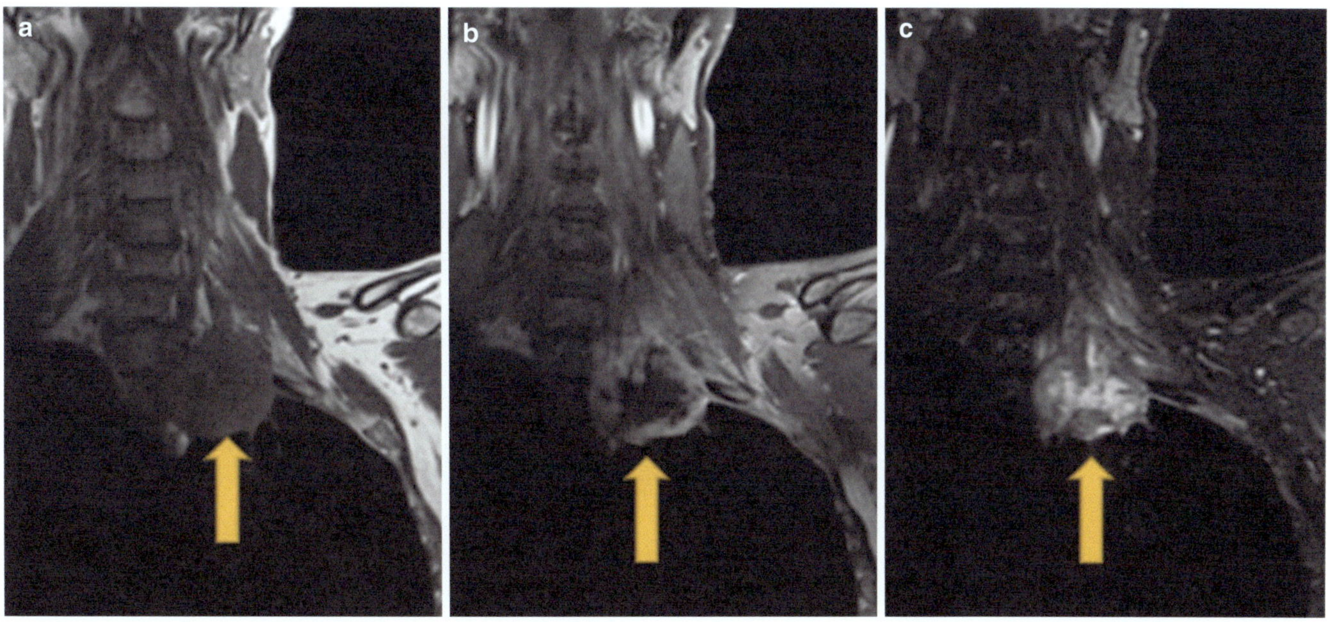

Fig. 57.13 (**a**) Coronal T1 (**b**) Contrast-enhanced T1 (**c**) and STIR images showing superintense, heterogenous enhancing lesion in left lung apex (Pancoast tumor) involving the L C7, C8, and T1. (From Gasparotti et al. [47])

57.8.2 Description

Thoracic outlet is a space created by the borders of the supraclavicular fossa to the axilla passing between the clavicle and first rib. Thoracic outlet syndrome (TOS) describes a collection of syndromes that occur due to compression of neurovasculature as they pass from the supraclavicular fossa to the axilla at one or multiple distinct sites. Differential diagnosis of thoracic outlet syndrome is given in Table 57.12.

To diagnose TOS, a clinician must use a combination of history, physical, and potentially several diagnostic modalities, as each case presentation may vary depending on which neurovascular structures are involved. Typically, the involved structures include the brachial plexus, subclavian vein, and subclavian artery that are each implicated in development of neurogenic TOS (nTOS), venous TOS (vTOS), and arterial TOS (aTOS), respectively. Venous TOS is also known as Paget-Schroetter syndrome or McCleery syndrome.

True neurogenic TOS is neurological abnormalities confirmed by electrodiagnostic studies. Disputed neurogenic TOS is neurological abnormalities not confirmed by electrodiagnostic studies. If left untreated, nTOS can lead to muscle atrophy in addition to pain and paresthesias, while vTOS and aTOS can lead to ischemia, thromboembolic events, gangrene, and limb loss.

Within the thoracic outlet, these neurovascular structures can be compressed within the *interscalene triangle*, the *costoclavicular space*, and the *retropectoralis minor space*. These three sites can become narrowed by cervical ribs, anomalous ligaments, or accessory muscles, post-traumatic scarring, altered posture or biomechanics, congenital extensions of the C7 transverse process or cervical ribs, anomalous ribs, vascular abnormalities, and postoperative complications such as hematomas and abscesses [86, 87].

- The interscale triangle, also known as the costoscalene hiatus, comprises the anterior and middle scalene muscles and the first rib, between which the trunks of the brachial plexus and subclavian artery can be compressed. Historically this had been known as *scalene anticus syndrome*.
- The costoclavicular space contains the divisions of the brachial plexus and subclavian vessels, which can be compressed by the subclavius muscle, costocoracoid ligament, and clavicle anterolaterally, and the first rib medially, with the scalene muscles and scapula posteriorly.
- The retropectoralis minor space that contains the cords of the brachial plexus and axillary vessels, made of the pectoralis minor anteriorly, the second to fourth ribs posteriorly, and the coranoid process superiorly.

Table 57.12 Differential diagnosis of thoracic outlet syndrome

Cervical radiculopathy
Cervical dystonia
Myofascial pain syndrome/fibromyalgia
Peripheral nerve compression neuropathy
Complex regional pain syndrome
Brachial plexopathy (idiopathic) or secondary

57.8.3 Clinical Presentation

Clinically, neurogenic TOS presents with upper extremity paresthesias, numbness or weakness, non-radicular pain, or heaviness. Venous TOS presents with spontaneous upper extremity swelling, activity-related sense of heaviness with or without cyanosis, and pain that may be felt in the upper extremity or deeper into the patient's shoulder or chest. Arterial TOS is the rarest of the three entities and presents with signs of ischemia such as non-radicular pain, paresthesias, weakness, and temperature-related pallor [88, 89].

nTOS is the most common of the three forms of TOS. In one single-center American study, the incidence of NTOS was 2–3 per 100,000 individuals, while vTOS occurred in 0.5–1 per 100,000 cases, and aTOS was even less common [90]. Risk factors for TOS include congenital abnormalities, trauma, or functionally acquired causes of compression such as repetitive overhead movements.

There is no standardized diagnostic criteria or treatment of TOS [91]. A recent committee of the Society for Vascular Surgery has attempted to establish a preferred set of terminology. For example, to classify the anatomical sites of compression, nTOS may be differentiated from neurogenic pectoralis minor syndrome, while terminology to describe the disease course include persistent TOS, recurrent TOS, and secondary TOS [92]. The Consortium for Outcomes Research and Education of TOS developed a consensus-based criteria to diagnose nTOS, including requiring at least 3 months duration of symptoms, anatomical distribution of symptoms, and meeting at least one feature in four of five categories: principal symptoms, symptom characteristics, clinical history, physical exam, and provocative maneuvers [93].

57.8.4 Physical Examination

Inspection One should first note the appearance of skin and nails and signs of muscle atrophy or edema. Ischemic ulcers or discoloration may be present in aTOS. Pulses should be examined.

Palpation It must include evaluation for tenderness at the interscalene triangle and pectoralis minor.

Spine Exam Examination for TOS should also include a thorough cervical spine examination to exclude pathology caused by cervical spondylosis, radiculopathy, or facet arthropathy. This includes sensory, manual motor testing, and deep tendon reflex testing.

Special Test (Fig. 57.14a–d) When assessing a patient with provocative maneuvers, multiple maneuvers should be performed to decrease the rate of false positives that occur when using a single maneuver. Specificity increased further with additional maneuvers. Positive test will be the symptomatic arm of the affected side.

- *The Adson test* (sensitivity 94%, specificity 18–87% [96], false positive 51% rate [97]) tests subclavian artery compression between anterior and middle scalene. It is performed by palpating for a diminishing pulse of the affected extremity while it is resting on the patient's thigh, while the patient hyperextends the neck, turns to the affected side, and inspires.
- *The Wright hyperabduction test* (high false positive rate in the general population [98]) tests subclavian artery compression by pectoralis minor. It performed by abduction of bilateral shoulder and flexion of elbows to 90°, while the clinician feels for obliteration of the radial pulse.
- The Roos test is performed by asking the patient to abduct bilateral shoulders and flex bilateral elbows to 90°, followed by clenching fists intermittently for 3 min [99].
- *Costoclavicular test* tests compression of subclavian artery between clavicle and first rib. It includes retraction of the shoulder of the affected limb, with elbow extension and protrusion of the chest. A positive costoclavicular test is reduction in the radial pulse after 1 min.
- *The Upper Limb Tension* Test (ULTT) aims to stretch the brachial plexus and reproduce cervicobrachial pain by first having a seated patient in similar position as the EAST; then if the patient remains asymptomatic, the patient's elbows are extended and hands pronated, with optional addition of wrist extension and head tilt away from the affected side.

In a study by Rayan and Jensen, 91% of the 100 healthy subjects without any known upper extremity musculoskeletal disorders were found to have at least 1 positive physical exam maneuver, between the Adson, costoclavicular, and hyperabduction maneuvers [94]. Conversely, the utility of combining just two provocative maneuvers was highlighted by a series by Gillard et al. that showed that the combined specificity of Adson test and Roos test was 82%, while individually they were 76% and 30%, respectively [95].

57.8.5 Diagnostic Workup

57.8.5.1 Plain Films

In terms of imaging, all patients should undergo chest and cervical spine plain radiography to evaluate for osseous abnormalities including cervical rib and, in some cases, lung apex tumors. CT being best at evaluating bony causes of compression such as abnormalities of cervical spine transverse processes or abnormalities of clavicles or ribs or lung tumors.

57.8.5.2 CT/MR/Angiography

Both CT and MRI are often used together, with CT being best at evaluating bony causes of compression such as abnormalities of cervical spine transverse processes or abnormalities of clavicles or ribs, while evaluation with MRI is better suited for evaluation of soft tissue abnormalities, vascular abnormalities, or postoperative complications such as hematomas, abscesses, chylomas, or granulomas [87]. MRI with contrast is recommended when tumor or infection is suspected [87]. While imaging of the brachial plexus has not yet been proven to correlate with outcomes, magnetic resonance neurography (MRN) has been increasingly studied, which allows for improved visualization of nerve morphology [90, 100]. To directly visualize compression or inflammation of the brachial plexus and soft tissues, as well as vascular obstruction, patients are then likely to undergo CT angiograms and MRIs [100]. To evaluate vascular abnormalities from aTOS, catheter-based angiography has largely been replaced by computed tomography angiography (CTA) and magnetic resonance angiography (MRA) [89]. In vTOS, catheter-based venogram may be preferred over CTA or MRA if a patient presents within 6 weeks of onset of symptoms [88].

57.8.5.3 Ultrasound

Ultrasound is a reliable means of diagnosing this etiology when combined with provocative testing and patient history. Dynamic capabilities of ultrasound by visualizing thoracic outlet while placing the patient in provocative maneuvers can identify blood flow deficits /nerve compression at the site of compression [103]. Presence of a "wedge-sickle sign" that is highly sensitive for fibromuscular compression of the lower trunk [101]. Thrombosis in the axillary and subclavian veins from vTOS can be detected with duplex ultrasound; however, a negative study cannot rule out vTOS (21% false negative rate); therefore, when vTOS is suspected, anticoagulation should be started promptly [88].

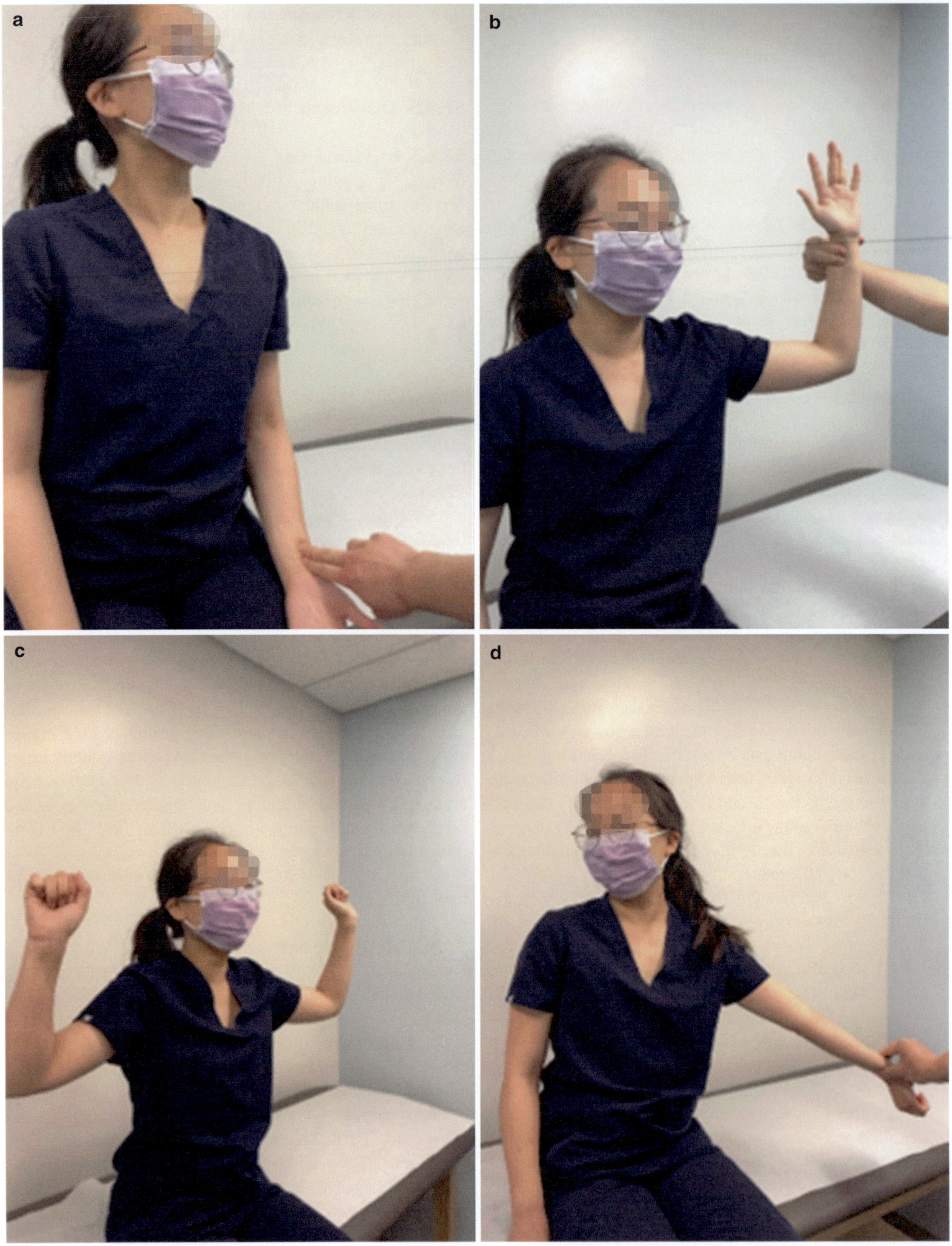

Fig. 57.14 (**a**) Adsons, (**b**)Wright, (**c**) Roos, and (**d**) ostoclavicular test for TOS

57.8.5.4 EMG

Most nTOS is caused by a fibrous band that extends from a cervical rib to the first thoracic rib that entraps the lower trunk [102]. EMG/NCS can help differentiate nTOS from plexopathy, neuropathy, and cervical radiculopathy although this can also be normal in nTOS [104].

57.8.5.5 Diagnostic Injections

1. Anterior scalene TPI: Earlier study by Lum et al. reported that positive response to lidocaine injections to the anterior scalene muscle can be predictive of successful transaxillary decompression in nTOS patients older than 40 years of age [10].
2. Botox injection (Fig. 57.15): While botulinum toxin injections have been used for treatment of nTOS, they are of diagnostic value as well. Recent study by Donahue et al. [91] showed that ultrasound-guided botulinum toxin injections to the anterior scalene and pectoralis minor muscles may be indicated in patients under consideration for surgery for nTOS in so far that short-term symptomatic improvement from the injections correlates with favorable long-term outcomes after surgeries, the majority of which were anterior scalenectomy with first-rib resections.

57.8.6 Treatment

57.8.6.1 Medical Management

Nonoperative management is considered initially for neurogenic TOS and asymptomatic arterial TOS with demonstrated compression of subclavian artery but no evidence of arterial degeneration. Conservative management includes patient education, relaxation techniques, postural correction, work/school ergonomics, activity modifications including limiting repetitive overhead activities. NSAIDS, muscle relaxants, and adjunct medications may be of some value.

57.8.6.2 Rehabilitation

A course of 4–6 weeks of PT should almost always be an appropriate first step. In one prospective observational cohort study that first treated nTOS patients with 4–6 weeks of PT alone, 31% of the 130 patients achieved satisfactory improvement in symptoms [105].

57.8.6.3 Procedures

For cases refractory to a course of PT, there is limited evidence for therapeutic injections. In the most recent Cochrane systematic review of treatments for TOS, there was only one nonsurgical intervention studied with a randomized control trial that met the minimum requirement for a follow-up period of at least 6 months [106]. In contrast to the favorable diagnostic use of botulinum toxin injections, a study by Finlayson et al. did not show significant change in pain, strength, or disability from treatment of scalene muscles with botulinum toxin injections versus saline in patients of no particular type of TOS (112). This intervention only provided a statistical significant improvement in patients' paresthesias after 6 months [106].

57.8.6.4 Surgery

nTOS

Surgical decompression should be pursued promptly in cases of acute progression of weakness or acute signs of vascular occlusion or embolism.

There are three main surgical approaches used to decompress the brachial plexus: transaxillary, supraclavicular, or posterior approaches. In a randomized control trial, a significant reduction of pain with transaxillary first rib resection was reported [106]. A separate systematic review showed

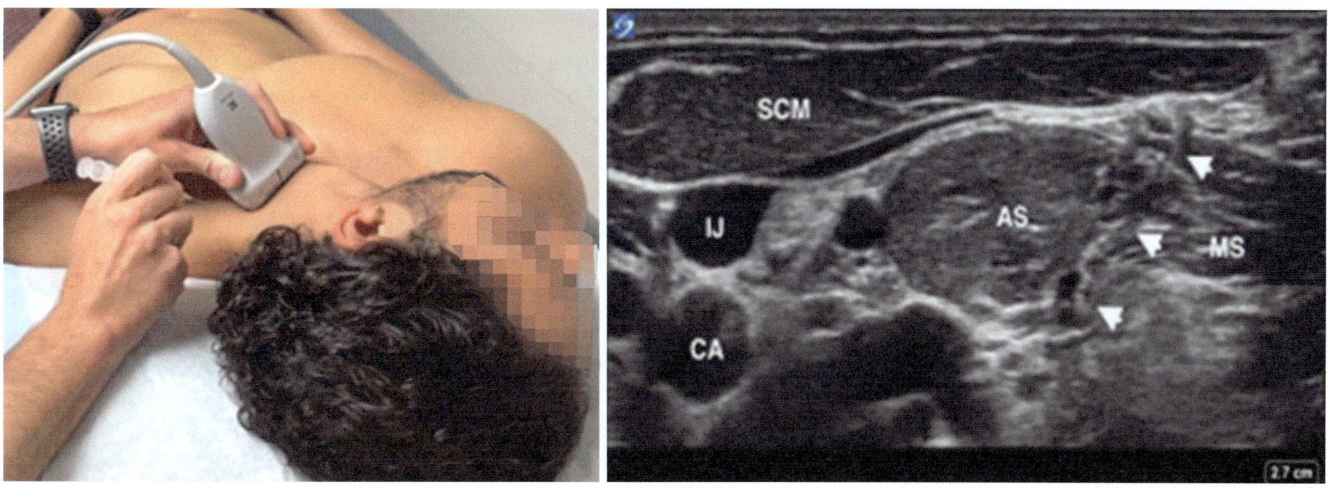

Fig. 57.15 Anterior/middle scalene ultrasound-guided injection. (Image courtesy of Robert L Bowers, DO, PhD, Mayo Clinic)

that for nTOS, between transaxillary first rib excision (TAFRE), supraclavicular first rib resection with scalenotomy (SCFRE), and supraclavicular release with leaving the first rib intact (SCR), the SCR had the greatest probability of success, although the difference was not statistically significant [107].

vTOS and aTOS

Surgical decompression of vTOS is considered in most cases. Balloon angioplasty can be pursued earlier, but it is not a definitive treatment, and ultimately patients with vTOS will require surgery. Otherwise, if they are poor surgical candidates, long-term anticoagulation is the only alternative [88]. Either thrombectomy or catheter-directed thrombolysis is performed for varying degrees of acute limb ischemia resulting from aTOS. Then depending on the severity of any potential aneurysm that can form distal to the point of stenosis, initial removal of thrombi is then followed by rib resection with or without aneurysm resection [89].

57.9 Complex Regional Pain Syndrome (CRPS)

Tony K. George

57.9.1 Synonyms

- Reflex sympathetic dystrophy
- Causalgia
- CRPS-I
- CRPS-II

57.9.2 ICD 10 Code

- G90.50

57.9.3 Description

CRPS is a painful expression of an identifiable or non-identifiable nerve injury triggered by trauma [108]. Fracture is the most common cause, and others include iatrogenic insults from surgery or casting and individually inflicted sprains or burns among others [109]. CRPS may not be well circumscribed and typically has poorly defined margins. Over time, through unresolved sensitization, its painful margins could enlarge. Its features have led to two classifications: CRPS types I and II. CRPS type II is easier to identify, where a specific sensory nerve injury is involved. Motor weakness may be present in a minority of cases and with coinciding dermatomal involvement identifies the nerve involved. CRPS type I is poorly localized and identified through patient history, clinical signs, and symptoms. The overwhelming majority comprise CRPS type I cases [110]. CRPS unique feature is autonomic dysfunction that distinguishes this pain from others. C-fiber nerves are particularly involved and influence edema and autonomic responses. Although peripherally mediated initially, it progresses to involve complex central and sympathetic pain pathways.

Anyone could be predisposed to CRPS, yet it has a preponderance to develop in women and those with upper extremity and high-trauma injuries [110]. Once afflicted, children and teenagers recover better. Comorbidities retarding recovery include diabetes, smoking, and chemotherapy, where its effects already have deleterious effects on nerve function and prolonging recovery.

57.9.4 Clinical Presentation

CRPS typically occurs in an extremity. It presents with a painful presentation out of proportion to provoking stimuli. Its features include pain with hyperalgesia, allodynia, dysesthesia, and skin textures changes. Depending on acuity of injury, skin presentations may be warm or cold [111]. Warm signs include erythema, hyperemia, and edema, and cold signs include pale, blue, and blotchy skin presentation. Others include shiny or scaly appearance of skin, abnormal nail or hair growth, signs of edema, and skin temperature change. Stiffness and muscle impairments may be due to disuse atrophy or directly from nerve injuries.

57.9.5 Physical Examination

Skin manifestations are the most common signs presenting in CRPS pain. Depending on acuity, they would include edematous and erythematous extremities, whereas in later stages sweaty and dusky extremities are more common. Pain is the most common symptom, and its unique manifestations including hyperalgesia, allodynia, and dysesthesias elicited through palpation provoking feedback response from patient. Excessive hair or nail growth or the lack of such may be visible and should be compared with the contralateral limb. Subtle temperature changes may be felt (either warm or cold) through palpation of the involved limb and comparison with the contralateral limb. Motor strength and comparison may reveal subtle strength deficits of the involved extremity.

57.9.6 Diagnostic Workup

CRPS is a clinical diagnosis. The Budapest criteria aids the diagnosis of CRPS (Table 57.13) [112]. Embedded in its cri-

Table 57.13 Budapest criteria for CRPS diagnosis. A sign is counted only if it is observed at the time of diagnosis

Budapest criteria: Clinical diagnostic criteria for CRPS
1. Continuing pain, which is disproportionate to any inciting event.
2. Must report at least one symptom in three of the four following categories: Sensory: reports of hyperalgesia and/or allodynia Vasomotor: reports of temperature asymmetry and/or skin color changes and/or skin color asymmetry Sudomotor/edema: reports of edema and/or sweating changes and/or sweating asymmetry Motor/trophic: reports of decreased range of motion and/or motor dysfunction (weakness, tremor, dystonia) and/or trophic changes (hair, nails, skin)
3. Must display at least one sign at time of evaluation in two or more of the following categories: Sensory: evidence of hyperalgesia (to pinprick) and/or allodynia (to light touch and/or deep somatic pressure and/or joint movement) Vasomotor: evidence of temperature asymmetry and/or skin color changes and/or asymmetry Sudomotor/edema: evidence of edema and/or sweating changes and/or sweating asymmetry Motor/trophic: evidence of decreased range of motion and/or motor dysfunction (weakness, tremor, dystonia) and/or trophic changes (hair, nails, skin)
4. There is no other diagnosis that better explains the signs and symptoms.

teria are sensory, motor, sudomotor, and vasomotor findings typically seen in CRPS presentations. Developed by the International Study of the Association of Pain, it is 99% sensitive and 68% specific [11].

Certain tests indirectly aid in its diagnosis. Ultrasound guidance can visualize injured nerve, triple phase bones scans reveal bone resorption, and nerve conductions studies could aid in identifying affected nerves.

Equally important is clinical judgement ruling out alternate diagnoses having overlapping features such as occult fractures, DVT, diabetic neuropathy, and autoimmune etiologies masquerading as CRPS.

57.9.7 Treatments

57.9.7.1 Medical Management

There is no specific FDA-approved drug; however, neuropathic medications are given assuming nerve mediation from C-fiber involvement. Medications such as gabapentin, Lyrica, Cymbalta, amitriptyline, and nortriptyline and transdermal patches such as lidocaine, NSAID, and capsaicin are often tried however with limited literature to support efficacy. In the acute inflammatory phase, corticosteroids and bisphosphonates may reduce inflammation and bone turnover [113, 114]. In cases of intractable CRPS, ketamine infusions have been promising in the right setting, but further studies are needed [115].

57.9.7.2 Rehabilitation

The focus of rehabilitation is restoring micro or macro functional deficits from CRPS. Physical therapy goals include maintaining flexibility, strength, desensitization, and improving circulation. Graded motor imagery and mirror therapy utilize visualization of moving nonpainful parts to help brain reorganization and desensitization of the affected body part with good effect [116].

57.9.7.3 Procedures

Stellate ganglion and lumbar sympathetic blocks help diagnostic purposes; however, its therapeutic relief is short-lived. Urgency for long-term solutions has led to exploration of spinal cord stimulation (SCS) with effective outcomes. In recent years, better understanding of dorsal root ganglions (DRG) role in pain modulation has led to DRG stimulation with studies, such as the ACCURATE study, demonstrating superiority over traditional SCS in effectively managing CRPS mediated pain [117].

57.9.7.4 Surgery

Surgical management is generally not recommended, and the roles of sympathectomy and limb amputations are controversial.

References

1. Olamikan S, Gulati A, Trescot AM. Intercostal nerve entrapment: Chest Wall. In: Peripheral nerve entrapments: clinical diagnosis and management. Switzerland: Springer; 2016. p. 279–90.
2. Gerner P. Postthoracotomy pain management problems. Anesthesiol Clin. 2008;26(2):355–67, vii. https://doi.org/10.1016/j.anclin.2008.01.007.
3. Bayman EO, Brennan TJ. Incidence and severity of chronic pain at 3 and 6 months after thoracotomy: meta-analysis. J Pain. 2014;15(9):887–97.
4. Rogers ML, Henderson L, Mahajan RP, Duffy JP. Preliminary findings in the neurophysiological assessment of intercostal nerve injury during thoracotomy. Eur J Cardiothorac Surg. 2002;21(2):298–301.
5. Jeon YH. Herpes zoster and postherpetic neuralgia: practical consideration for prevention and treatment. Korean J Pain. 2015;28(3):177–84. https://doi.org/10.3344/kjp.2015.28.3.177. Epub 2015 Jul 1
6. Nguyen KD, Choudhri HF, Macomson SD. The intercostal nerve as a target for diagnostic biopsy. J Neurosurg. 2018;128(4):1222–5. Retrieved Apr 20, 2021, from https://thejns.org/view/journals/j--neurosurg/128/4/article-p1222.xml
7. Glenesk NL, Rahman S, Lopez PP. Anatomy, thorax, intercostal nerves. [Updated 2020 Jul 27]. In: StatPearls [Internet]. Treasure Island: StatPearls Publishing; 2021.
8. Fazekas D, Doroshenko M, Horn DB. Intercostal neuralgia. 2021 Feb 8. In: StatPearls [Internet]. Treasure Island: StatPearls Publishing; 2021.
9. Dureja GP. Intercostal neuralgia: a review. J Neurol Transl Neurosci. 2017;5(1):1076.
10. Makharita MY, El Bendary HM, Sonbul ZM, Ahmed SES, Latif MA. Ultrasound-guided pulsed radiofrequency in the manage-

ment of thoracic postherpetic neuralgia: a randomized, double-blinded, controlled trial. Clin J Pain. 2018;34(11):1017–24.
11. Ke M, Yinghui F, Yi J, Xeuhua H, Xiaoming L, Zhijun C, Chao H, Yingwei W. Efficacy of pulsed radiofrequency in the treatment of thoracic postherpetic neuralgia from the angulus costae: a randomized, double-blinded, controlled trial. Pain Physician. 2013;16(1):15–25. PMID: 23340530
12. Byas-Smith MG, Gulati A. Ultrasound-guided intercostal Panda N, Donahue DM. Evaluation of patients cryoablation. Anesth Analg. 2006;103(4):1033–5.
13. Green CR, de Rosayro AM, Tait AR. The role of cryoanalgesia for chronic thoracic pain: results of a long-term follow up. J Natl Med Assoc. 2002;94(8):716–20.
14. Engel AJ. Utility of intercostal nerve conventional thermal radiofrequency ablations in the injured worker after blunt trauma. Pain Physician. 2012;15(5):E711–8.
15. Kang J, Liu Y, Niu L, Wang M, Meng C, Zhou H. Anesthesia upstream of the alcoholic lesion point alleviates the pain of alcohol neurolysis for intercostal neuralgia: a prospective randomized clinical trial. Clinics (Sao Paulo). 2020;75:e1296.
16. Szok D, Tajti J, Nyári A, Vécsei L. Therapeutic approaches for peripheral and central neuropathic pain. Behav Neurol. 2019;2019:8685954.
17. Devor M. Sodium channels and mechanisms of neuropathic pain. J Pain. 2006;7(1 Suppl 1):S3–S12.
18. Price DB, Twombly NJ. The phantom limb phenomenon: a medical, folkloric, and historical study: texts and translations of 10th to 20th century miracle accounts of the miraculous restoration of lost body parts. Washington, DC: Georgetown University Press; 1978.
19. Hansen DM, Kehlet H, Gärtner R. Phantom breast sensations are frequent after mastectomy. Dan Med Bull. 2011;58(4):A4259.
20. Ziegler-Graham K, MacKenzie EJ, Ephraim PL, Travison TG, Brookmeyer R. Estimating the prevalence of limb loss in the United States: 2005 to 2050. Arch Phys Med Rehabil. 2008;89(3):422–9.
21. Kehlet H, Jensen TS, Woolf CJ. Persistent postsurgical pain: risk factors and prevention. Lancet. 2006;367:1618–25.
22. Batsford S, Ryan CG, Martin DJ. Non-pharmacological conservative therapy for phantom limb pain: a systematic review of randomized controlled trials. Physiother Theory Pract. 2017;33(3):173–83. https://doi.org/10.1080/09593985.2017.1288283.
23. Cruccu G, et al. EFNS guidelines on neurostimulation therapy for neuropathic pain. Eur J Neurol. 2007;14(9):952–70.
24. McCormick Z, Chang-Chien G, Marshall B, Huang M, Harden RN. Phantom limb pain: a systematic neuroanatomical-based review of pharmacologic treatment: neuroanatomical-based review of pharmacologic treatment of phantom limb pain. Pain Med. 2014;15(2):292–305.
25. Gilmore CA, Ilfeld BM, Rosenow JM, Li S, Desai MJ, Hunter CW, Rauck RL, Nader A, Mak J, Cohen SP, Crosby ND, Boggs JW. Percutaneous 60-day peripheral nerve stimulation implant provides sustained relief of chronic pain following amputation: 12-month follow-up of a randomized, double-blind, placebo-controlled trial. Reg Anesth Pain Med. 2020;45:44–51.
26. Parris D, Fischbein N, Mackey S, Carroll I. A novel CT-guided transpsoas approach to diagnostic GFN block and ablation. Pain Med. 2010;11:785–9.
27. Cesmebasi A, Yadav A, Gielecki J, Tubbs RS, Loukas M. Genitofemoral neuralgia: a review. Clin Anat. 2014;28(1):128–35. https://doi.org/10.1002/ca.22481.
28. Acar F, Ozdemir M, Bayrakli F, Cirak B, Coskun E, Burchiel K. Management of medically intractable genitofemoral and ilioinguinal neuralgia. Turk Neurosurg. 2013;23:753–77.
29. Starling JR, Harms BA. Diagnosis and treatment of genitofemoral and ilioinguinal neuralgia. World J Surg. 1989;13:586–91.
30. Campos NA, Chiles JH, Plunkett AR. Ultrasound-guided cryoablation of genitofemoral nerve for chronic inguinal pain. Pain Phys. 2009;12:997–1000.
31. Ndiaye A, Diop M, Ndoye JM, Konaté I, Ndiaye AI, Mané L, Nazarian S, Dia A. Anatomical basis of neuropathies and damage to the ilioinguinal nerve during repairs of groin hernias. (about 100 dissections). Surg Radiol Anat. 2007;29(8):675–81.
32. Kim DH, Murovic JA, Tiel RL, Kline DG. Surgical management of 33 ilioinguinal and iliohypogastric neuralgias at Louisiana State University Health Sciences Center. Neurosurgery. 2005;56(5):1013–20.
33. Meulen BC, Peters EW, Wijsmuller A, Kropman RF, Mosch A, Tavy DL. Acute scrotal pain from idiopathic ilioinguinal neuropathy: diagnosis and treatment with EMG-guided nerve block. Clin Neurol Neurosurg. 2007;109:535–7.
34. Gofeld M, Christakis M. Sonographically guided ilioinguinal nerve block. J Ultrasound Med. 2006;25(12):1571–5.
35. Cho HM, Park DS, Kim DH, Nam HS. Diagnosis of ilioinguinal nerve injury based on electromyography and ultrasonography: a case report. Ann Rehabil Med. 2017;41(4):705–8.
36. Ivins GK. Meralgia paresthetica, the elusive diagnosis: clinical experience with 14 adult patients. Ann Surg. 2000;232(2):281–6.
37. Uzel M, Akkin SM, Tanyeli E, et al. Relationships of the lateral femoral cutaneous nerve to bony landmarks. Clin Orthop Relat Res. 2011;469(9):2605–11.
38. Parisi TJ, Mandrekar J, Dyck PJ, et al. Meralgia paresthetica: relation to obesity, advanced age, and diabetes mellitus. Neurology. 2011;77(16):1538–42.
39. Nouraei SA, Anand B, Spink G, et al. A novel approach to the diagnosis and management of meralgia paresthetica. Neurosurgery. 2007;60(4):696–700.
40. Parmar MS. Hiphuggers' tingly thighs. CMAJ. 2003;168(1):16.
41. Grossman MG, Ducey SA, Nadler SS, et al. Meralgia paresthetica: diagnosis and treatment. J Am Acad Orthop Surg. 2001;9(5):336–44.
42. Rubin DI. Brachial and lumbosacral plexopathies: a review. Clin Neurophysiol Pract. 2020;5:173–93.
43. van Alfen N, Malessy MJ. Diagnosis of brachial and lumbosacral plexus lesions. Handb Clin Neurol. 2013;115:293–310.
44. Planner AC, Donaghy M, Moore NR. Causes of lumbosacral plexopathy. Clin Radiol. 2006;61(12):987–95.
45. Wilbourn AJ. Plexopathies. Neurol Clin. 2007;25(1):139–71.
46. Bykowski J, Aulino JM, Berger KL, Cassidy RC, Choudhri AF, Kendi AT, Kirsch C, Luttrull MD, Sharma A, Shetty VS, Than K, Winfree CJ, Cornelius RS. ACR appropriateness criteria®Plexopathy. J Am Coll Radiol. 2017;14(5S):S225–33.
47. Gasparotti R, Shah L. Diseases of the brain, head and neck, spine 2020–2023: diagnostic imaging. Switzerland: Springer International Publishing; 2020.
48. Williams FH, Johns JS, Weiss JM, Weiss LD, Kim CT, Strommen JA, Rashbaum IG. Neuromuscular rehabilitation and electrodiagnosis. 1. Mononeuropathy. Arch Phys Med Rehabil. 2005;86(3 Suppl 1):S3–S10.
49. Stankowski JA. Electrodiagnosis of plexopathy. PM R. 2013;5(5 Suppl):S50–5.
50. Greenberg HS, Taren J, Ensminger WD, Doan K. Benefit from and tolerance to continuous intrathecal infusion of morphine for intractable cancer pain. J Neurosurg. 1982;57(3):360–4.
51. Capdevila X, Coimbra C, Choquet O. Approaches to the lumbar plexus: success, risks, and outcome. Reg Anesth Pain Med. 2005;30(2):150–62.
52. Fusco P, Di Carlo S, Paladini G, Scimia P, Petrucci E, Marinangeli F. The perpendicular sacral plexus block: an alternative approach to the sacral plexus. Minerva Anestesiol. 2019;85(5):562–3.
53. Preston D, Shapiro B. Electromyography and neuromuscular disorders. 4th ed. Philadelphia: Elsevier; 2020.

54. Dyck PJB, Windebank AJ. Diabetic and nondiabetic lumbosacral radiculoplexus neuropathies: new insights into pathophysiology and treatment. Muscle Nerve. 2002;25:477–91.
55. Chan YC, Lo YL, Chan ES. Immunotherapy for diabetic amyotrophy. Cochrane Database Syst Rev. 2017;7:CD006521.
56. Son BC, Yoon JH, Kim DR, Lee SW. Dorsal rhizotomy for pain from neoplastic lumbosacral plexopathy in advanced pelvic cancer. Stereotact Funct Neurosurg. 2014;92(2):109–16.
57. Neto FJM, Filho ENK, Miranda FC, Rosemberg LA, Santos DCB, Taneja AK. Demystifying MR neurography of the lumbosacral plexus: from protocols to pathologies. Biomed Res Int. 2018;2018:9608947.
58. Jaeckle KA. Neurological manifestations of neoplastic and radiation-induced plexopathies. Semin Neurol. 2004;24(4):385–93.
59. Ozçakar L, Kara M, Erol O, Kaymak B, Akinci A, Taşkiran C, Ayhan A. A reappraisal on the management of lumbosacral plexopaties in gynaecological malignancies: where do the physiatrists stand? Int J Gynecol Cancer. 2005;15:915–7.
60. Zuniga RE, Schlicht CR, Abram SE. Intrathecal baclofen is analgesic in patients with chronic pain. Anesthesiology. 2000;92(3):876–80.
61. Enneking FK, Chan V, Greger J, Hadzić A, Lang SA, Horlocker TT. Lower-extremity peripheral nerve blockade: essentials of our current understanding. Reg Anesth Pain Med. 2005;30(1):4–35.
62. Choi KC, Son BC, Hong JT, Lee SW. Spinal cord stimulation for the neuropathic pain caused by traumatic lumbosacral plexopathy after extensive pelvic fracture. J Korean Neurosurg Soc. 2005;38(3):234–7.
63. Philip CN, Candido KD, Joseph NJ, Crystal GJ. Successful treatment of meralgia paresthetica with pulsed radiofrequency of the lateral femoral cutaneous nerve. Pain Physician. 2009;12(5):881–5.
64. Langford B, Mauck WD. Peripheral nerve stimulation: a new treatment for Meralgia Paresthetica. Pain Med. 2021;22(1):213–6.
65. Shanina E, Liao B, Smith RG. Brachial Plexopathies: update on treatment. Curr Treat Options Neurol. 2019;21(5):24.
66. Smania N, Berto G, La ME, Melotti C, Midiri A, Roncari L, Zenorini A, Ianes P, Picelli A, Waldner A, Faccioli S, Gandolfi M. Rehabilitation of brachial plexus injuries in adults and children. Eur J Phys Rehabil Med. 2012;48(3):483–506.
67. Sakellariou VI, Badilas NK, Mazis GA, Stavropoulos NA, Kotoulas HK, Kyriakopoulos S, Tagkalegkas I, Sofianos IP. Brachial plexus injuries in adults: evaluation and diagnostic approach. ISRN Orthop. 2014;2014:726103.
68. Ferrante MA. Brachial plexopathies: classification, causes, and consequences. Muscle Nerve. 2004;30(5):547–68.
69. Abid A. Brachial plexus birth palsy: management during the first year of life. Orthop Traumatol Surg Res. 2016;102(1):S125–32.
70. Crim J, Ingalls K. Accuracy of MR neurography in the diagnosis of brachial plexopathy. Eur J Radiol. 2017;95:24–7.
71. Dahlin LB, Backman C, Düppe H, Saito H, Chemnitz A, Abul-Kasim K, Maly P. Compression of the lower trunk of the brachial plexus by a cervical rib in two adolescent girls: case reports and surgical treatment. J Brach Plex Periph Nerve Inj. 2009;4:14.
72. Chang EI, Rose MI, Rossi K, Elkwood AI. Microneurosurgical treatment options in peripheral nerve compression syndromes after chemotherapy and radiation treatment. J Surg Oncol. 2018;118(5):793–9.
73. Tung TH, Liu DZ, Mackinnon SE. Nerve transfer for elbow flexion in radiation-induced brachial plexopathy: a case report. Hand (N Y). 2009;4(2):123–8.
74. Choi JH, Choi SC, Kim DK, Sung CH, Chon JY, Hong SJ, Lee JY, Moon HS. Combined spinal cord stimulation and peripheral nerve stimulation for brachial plexopathy: a case report. Pain Physician. 2016;19(3):E459–63.
75. Frederico TN, da Silva FT. Peripheral nerve stimulation of the brachial plexus for chronic refractory CRPS pain of the upper limb: description of a new technique and case series. Pain Med. 2020;21(Suppl 1):S18–26.
76. Goroszeniuk T, Kothari SC, Hamann WC. Percutaneous implantation of a brachial plexus electrode for management of pain syndrome caused by a traction injury. Neuromodulation. 2007;10(2):148–55.
77. Lee GW, Kwon YH, Jeong JH, Kim JW. The efficacy of scalene injection in thoracic outlet syndrome. J Korean Neurosurg Soc. 2011;50(1):36–9.
78. Torriani M, Gupta R, Donahue DM. Botulinum toxin injection in neurogenic thoracic outlet syndrome: results and experience using a ultrasound-guided approach. Skelet Radiol. 2010;39(10):973–80.
79. Donahue DM, Godoy IRB, Gupta R, Donahue JA, Torriani M. Sonographically guided botulinum toxin injections in patients with neurogenic thoracic outlet syndrome: correlation with surgical. Skelet Radiol. 2020;49(5):715–22.
80. Liu CW, Flamer D. Supraclavicular brachial plexus Neurolysis for a malignant peripheral nerve sheath tumor: a case report. A A Pract. 2018;11(11):309–11.
81. Loh T-H, et al. Brachial plexus chemical Neurolysis with ethanol for cancer pain. Case Rep Med. 2018;2018:1–3.
82. Arai YC, Nishihara M, Aono S, Ikemoto T, Suzuki C, Kinoshita A, Ushida T. Pulsed radiofrequency treatment within brachial plexus for the management of intractable neoplastic plexopathic pain. J Anesth. 2013;27(2):298–301.
83. Akane M, Iwatsuki K, Tatebe M, et al. Anterior interosseous nerve and posterior interosseous nerve involvement in neuralgic amyotrophy. Clin Neurol Neurosurg. 2016;151:108–12.
84. Stevanato G, Devigili G, Eleopra R, Fontana P, Lettieri C, Baracco C, Guida F, Rinaldo S, Bevilacqua M. Chronic post-traumatic neuropathic pain of brachial plexus and upper limb: a new technique of peripheral nerve stimulation. Neurosurg Rev. 2014;37:473–80.
85. Hsu PC, Chang KV, Mezian K, et al. Sonographic pearls for imaging the brachial plexus and its pathologies. Diagnostics (Basel). 2020;10(5):324.
86. Kuynh L, Kennedy DJ. Physical examination of the cervical spine. In: Malanga GA, Mautner K, editors. Musculoskeletal physical examination: an evidence-based approach; 2016. Accessed 29 Apr 2021. http://public.ebookcentral.proquest.com/choice/publicfullrecord.aspx?p=4622956.
87. Khalilzadeh O, Glover M, Torriani M, Gupta R. Imaging assessment of thoracic outlet syndrome. Thorac Surg Clin. 2021;31(1):19–25. https://doi.org/10.1016/j.thorsurg.2020.09.002.
88. Cook JR, Thompson RW. Evaluation and management of venous thoracic outlet syndrome. Thorac Surg Clin. 2021;31(1):27–44. https://doi.org/10.1016/j.thorsurg.2020.08.012.
89. Nguyen LL, Soo Hoo AJ. Evaluation and management of arterial thoracic outlet syndrome. Thorac Surg Clin. 2021;31(1):45–54. https://doi.org/10.1016/j.thorsurg.2020.09.006.
90. Illig KA, Rodriguez-Zoppi E, Bland T, Muftah M, Jospitre E. The incidence of thoracic outlet syndrome. Ann Vasc Surg. 2021;70:263–72. https://doi.org/10.1016/j.avsg.2020.07.029.
91. Donahue DM, Godoy IRB, Gupta R, Donahue JA, Torriani M. Sonographically guided botulinum toxin injections in patients with neurogenic thoracic outlet syndrome: correlation with surgical outcomes. Skelet Radiol. 2020;49(5):715–22. https://doi.org/10.1007/s00256-019-03331-9.
92. Illig KA, Donahue D, Duncan A, et al. Reporting standards of the Society for Vascular Surgery for thoracic outlet syndrome. J Vasc Surg. 2016;64(3):e23–35. https://doi.org/10.1016/j.jvs.2016.04.039.
93. Thompson RW. Development of consensus-based diagnostic criteria for NTOS. In: Illig KA, Thompson RW, Freischlag JA, Donahue DM, Jordan SE, Edgelow PI, editors. Thoracic out-

let syndrome. London: Springer; 2013. p. 143–55. https://doi.org/10.1007/978-1-4471-4366-6_21.
94. Rayan G, Jensen C. Thoracic outlet syndrome: provocative examination maneuvers in a typical population. J Shoulder Elb Surg. 1995;4(2):113–7. https://doi.org/10.1016/S1058-2746(05)80064-3.
95. Gillard J, Pérez-Cousin M, Hachulla É, et al. Diagnosing thoracic outlet syndrome: contribution of provocative tests, ultrasonography, electrophysiology, and helical computed tomography in 48 patients. Joint Bone Spine. 2001;68(5):416–24. https://doi.org/10.1016/S1297-319X(01)00298-6.
96. Marx RG, Bombardier C, Wright JG. What do we know about the reliability and validity of physical examination tests used to examine the upper extremity? J Hand Surg Am. 1999;24(1):185–93. https://doi.org/10.1053/jhsu.1999.jhsu24a0185.
97. Gergoudis R, Barnes RW. Thoracic outlet arterial compression: prevalence in normal persons. Angiology. 1980;31(8):538–41. https://doi.org/10.1177/000331978003100805.
98. Raaf J. Surgery for cervical rib and scalene anticus syndrome. J Am Med Assoc. 1965;157:219.
99. Plewa MC, Delinger M. The false-positive rate of thoracic outlet syndrome shoulder maneuvers in healthy subjects. Acad Emerg Med. 1998;5(4):337–42. https://doi.org/10.1111/j.1553-2712.1998.tb02716.x.
100. Jones MR, Prabhakar A, Viswanath O, et al. Thoracic outlet syndrome: a comprehensive review of pathophysiology, diagnosis, and treatment. Pain Ther. 2019;8(1):5–18. https://doi.org/10.1007/s40122-019-0124-2.
101. Farina R, Foti PV, Conti A, et al. The role of ultrasound imaging in vascular compression syndromes. Ultrasound J. 2021;13(1):4. https://doi.org/10.1186/s13089-020-00202-6.
102. Preston DC, Shapiro BE. Electromyography and neuromuscular disorders: clinical-electrophysiologic-ultrasound correlations. 4th ed. Cham: Elsevier, Inc; 2020.
103. Leonhard V, Caldwell G, Goh M, Reeder S, Smith HF. Ultrasonographic diagnosis of thoracic outlet syndrome secondary to brachial plexus piercing variation. Diagnostics (Basel). 2017;7(3):40. Published 2017 Jul 4. https://doi.org/10.3390/diagnostics7030040.
104. Panda N, Donahue DM. Evaluation of patients with neurogenic thoracic outlet syndrome. Thorac Surg Clin. 2021;31(1):55–9. https://doi.org/10.1016/j.thorsurg.2020.09.005.
105. Balderman J, Abuirqeba AA, Eichaker L, et al. Physical therapy management, surgical treatment, and patient-reported outcomes measures in a prospective observational cohort of patients with neurogenic thoracic outlet syndrome. J Vasc Surg. 2019;70(3):832–41. https://doi.org/10.1016/j.jvs.2018.12.027.
106. Povlsen B, Hansson T, Povlsen SD. Treatment for thoracic outlet syndrome. In Cochrane Neuromuscular Group, editor. *Cochrane database of systematic reviews*. Published online 26 Nov 2014. https://doi.org/10.1002/14651858.CD007218.pub3
107. Yin ZG, Gong KT, Zhang JB. Outcomes of surgical management of neurogenic thoracic outlet syndrome: a systematic review and Bayesian perspective. J Hand Surg Am. 2019;44(5):416.e1–416.e17. https://doi.org/10.1016/j.jhsa.2018.06.120.
108. Petersen PB, Mikkelsen KL, Lauritzen JB, Krogsgaard MR. Risk factors for post-treatment complex regional pain syndrome (CRPS): an analysis of 647 cases of CRPS from the Danish patient compensation association. Pain Pract. 2018;18(3):341–9.
109. Beerthuizen A, Stronks DL, Van't Spijker A, Yaksh A, Hanraets BM, Klein J, Huygen F. Demographic and medical parameters in the development of complex regional pain syndrome type 1 (CRPS1): prospective study on 596 patients with a fracture. Pain. 2012;153(6):1187–92.
110. de Mos M, de Bruijn AG, Huygen FJ, Dieleman JP, Stricker BH, Sturkenboom MC. The incidence of complex regional pain syndrome: a population-based study. Pain. 2007;129(1–2):12–20.
111. Marinus J, Moseley GL, Birklein F, Baron R, Maihofner C, Kingery WS, van Hilten JJ. Clinical features and pathophysiology of complex regional pain syndrome. Lancet Neurol. 2011;10(7):637–48.
112. Harden RN, Bruehl S, Stanton-Hicks M, Wilson PR. Proposed new diagnostic criteria for complex regional pain syndrome. Pain Med. 2007;8(4):326–31.
113. Chevreau M, Romand X, Gaudin P, Juvin R, Baillet A. Bisphosphonates for treatment of complex regional pain syndrome type 1: a systematic literature review and meta-analysis of randomized controlled trials versus placebo. Joint Bone Spine. 2017;84(4):393–9.
114. Kalita J, Misra U, Kumar A, Bhoi SK. Long-term prednisolone in post-stroke complex regional pain syndrome. Pain Physician. 2016;19(8):565–74.
115. Connolly SB, Prager JP, Harden RN. A systematic review of ketamine for complex regional pain syndrome. Pain Med. 2015;16(5):943–69.
116. Smart KM, Wand BM, O'Connell NE. Physiotherapy for pain and disability in adults with complex regional pain syndrome (CRPS) types I and II. Cochrane Database Syst Rev. 2016;2:CD010853.
117. Deer TR, Levy RM, Kramer J, Poree L, Amirdelfan K, Grigsby E, Staats P, Burton AW, Burgher AH, Obray J, et al. Dorsal root ganglion stimulation yielded higher treatment success rate for complex regional pain syndrome and causalgia at 3 and 12 months: a randomized comparative trial. Pain. 2017;158(4):669–81.

Alternative Medicine: Musculoskeletal Applications

58

Arthur Jason De Luigi

58.1 Description of Complementary and Alternative Medicine (CAM)

Facing rising health care costs, patients and providers have begun to seek nontraditional treatments to manage their pain and improve function. These nontraditional treatment options are typically classified as "complementary and alternative medicine." Alternative treatments are typically interpreted as "nontraditional" or "nonconventional" medicine outside of the scope of Western medicine. Additionally, when these alternative treatment methods are used in conjunction with traditional treatments, they are termed "complementary medicine." There is not a "true" definition of CAM because the spectrum of what the medical community deems as alternative is broad and the field is constantly evolving as new options are developed and introduced into the health care system. Over time, these "alternative" options have begun to gain acceptance by both patients and providers, which further blurs the lines between what is considered "alternative" versus "conventional."

CAM usage is prevalent in the United States and crosses cultural, ethnic, and racial boundaries. Many of these treatments have been brought to the United States and Western medicine by other cultures as they have been used in these other cultures for generations. Despite the widespread use elsewhere and the growing popularity in Western medicine, there remains a relative paucity of quality evidence-based medicine on the various CAM treatment options demonstrating effectiveness.

Population-based studies have confirmed the increasing popularity of CAM treatments for MSK conditions. Callahan and colleagues reviewed over 2000 patients from primary care (n = 1077) and specialty clinics (n = 1063) in North Carolina and found that 90.5% of patients treated by specialists and 82.8% by primary care physicians had tried complementary therapy for arthritis symptoms [1]. Another study evaluating racial and ethnic differences in CAM utilization rates for osteoarthritis revealed that African Americans (89%) were most likely to report CAM use, followed by Asians (83%), Hispanics (81%), and Caucasians (78%) [2]. A study by Herman and colleagues identified that 90% of Hispanic or non-Hispanics White adults with osteoarthritis had attempted usage, and 69% were still currently using CAM [3]. However, there was no significant difference in current CAM usage between Hispanics (66%) and non-Hispanics (68%) [4].

CAM has proposed utility for a wide variety of ailments and diseases, but this chapter will focus on the utilization of CAM for symptoms associated with musculoskeletal (MSK) injuries and conditions. Table 58.1 outlines a sample of CAM treatments which will be discussed below.

Table 58.1 Examples of complementary and alternative medicine

Acupuncture	Pharmacopuncture
Laser acupuncture	Electroacupuncture
Moxibustion	Laser therapy
Transcutaneous electrical nerve	Massage

58.2 Acupuncture

Acupuncture is probably the most recognized and widely used alternative treatment. It is an integral part of the practice and theory of traditional Chinese medicine. In traditional Chinese medicine, the body has 365 divisions and 12 meridians [5]. Acupuncture involves the insertion and manipulation of needles in specific points of the body along the 12 meridians, depending on the condition being treated [5].

One of the major challenges in acupuncture research is in the design of an appropriate placebo control group. Compared to trials of new medications where double blinding is the accepted standard, acupuncture has more difficulty with study design and blinding. This is particularly a challenge to

A. J. De Luigi (✉)
Department of Physical Medicine & Rehabilitation, Mayo Clinic Arizona, Phoenix, AZ, USA

Sports Medicine, Mayo Clinic Arizona, Mayo Clinic School of Medicine, Phoenix, AZ, USA

© The Author(s), under exclusive license to Springer Nature Switzerland AG 2022
S. A. Mostoufi et al. (eds.), *Clinical Guide to Musculoskeletal Medicine*, https://doi.org/10.1007/978-3-030-92042-5_58

have both the acupuncturist and patient being blinded to the treatment being given [5]. Despite these limitations, acupuncture is still the most widely studied CAM treatment for MSK conditions (Table 58.2). Another challenge is the variance and lack of standardization between numerous approaches and nomenclatures (standard, conventional, constitutional acupuncture). Without a standard definition or protocol that has been implemented between studies, it is challenging to accurately compare efficacy across multiple studies. This heterogeneity of treatment makes systematic reviews a challenge to determine the comparative efficacy of acupuncture [6–13]. Recent Cochrane reviews evaluated the use of acupuncture for numerous conditions including peripheral joint osteoarthritis [6, 7], concluding that acupuncture demonstrated statistically significant benefits for the treatment of peripheral joint osteoarthritis of the knee, hip, or hand in sham-controlled trials [6, 7]. Kwon and colleagues completed a systematic review and meta-analysis of acupuncture for peripheral joint osteoarthritis with significant effect of acupuncture compared with sham acupuncture [8]. However, there are different cultural and regional approaches to acupuncture which can provide additional challenges. For example, a subset of acupuncture, known as *Sasang* constitutional acupuncture, is utilized in Korea based on the yin and yang theory and on Confucianism. This philosophy classifies humans into four constitutions: [1] sensitivity to certain groups of herbs and medicines, [2] equilibrium among internal organic functions, [3] physical features, and [4] psychological characteristics. Systematic reviews have been performed as well to compare constitutional versus standard acupuncture. The results of these reviews demonstrated that constitutional acupuncture is effective compared to standard acupuncture [9].

Another subset and variance with acupuncture is the use of concomitant electrostimulation, commonly known as electroacupuncture. Electroacupuncture was compared to traditional acupuncture in another review including 10 trials of acupuncture for knee osteoarthritis. The review concluded that both methods are effective in the treatment of pain and physical dysfunction [10]. Another review by Lev-Ari and colleagues identified two large randomized controlled trials (RCTs) showing that acupuncture serves as an effective complement to standard care by improving function and providing pain relief in patients with knee osteoarthritis [11]. Ezzo and colleagues completed a systematic review that included seven trials and 393 patients with knee OA. The results of this review indicated that there is strong evidence for pain reduction with acupuncture compared to acupuncture [12].

One of the biggest challenges is a lack of consensus regarding the optimal treatment frequency and dose of acupuncture. However, a review of 13 randomized controlled trials determined that optimal results occur with high body temperature, high expectations, minimum of four needles, electroacupuncture, electrical stimulation to needles placed in muscle, and a course of at least 10 treatments [13].

There are several RCTs evaluating acupuncture for the treatment of osteoarthritis compared to a variety of treatments and sham acupuncture. Traditional Chinese acupuncture was compared to sham acupuncture in 455 patients with knee osteoarthritis who were randomized into three groups (waiting list, high expectations of success by acupuncturist, or neutral expectations). The study found that there is a statistically significant difference in pain reduction and satisfaction in the acupuncture group with high expectations [14]. These findings suggest that the acupuncturist's style and behavior may affect the patient's response [14]. Manual acupuncture and electroacupuncture were compared to sham acupuncture in 34 patients with knee osteoarthritis resulting in a statistically significant improvement in pain compared to sham in both treatment groups [15]. Another study of 32 patients with knee osteoarthritis was randomized into four treatment groups: acupuncture, transcutaneous electrical nerve stimulation (TENS), both, and topical poultice (control) with significant reductions in pain intensity and improvement of knee function in the acupuncture, TENS, and combined treatment groups [16]. In an open study in which 30 patients were randomized into either acupuncture, acupuncture with medication, or medication alone followed by acupuncture 5 weeks later, all three groups showed significant improvement after the course of acupuncture [17]. Wang and colleagues randomized 63 patients with knee osteoarthritis into a treatment group combining acupuncture with blood-letting versus routine acupuncture and found no significant difference between the groups [18].

Beyond the above research on osteoarthritis, there are other studies assessing the efficacy of acupuncture on a variety of musculoskeletal conditions. Some of these studies are on vague or widespread pain, whereas others have a focal condition or injury being treated.

Acupuncture has been studied for its use in tendon, muscle, and joint pathologies. A single-blinded randomized controlled trial by Lathia et al. evaluated the efficacy of acupuncture for chronic shoulder pain. The study included 31 patients with osteoarthritis or rotator cuff tendonitis who were randomized into three treatment groups: individualized acupuncture points, fixed/standard acupuncture points, or sham non-penetrating acupuncture. Each subject received 12 treatments and was followed for 6 weeks. All three groups had improvement after 6 weeks, but it was only clinically significant in groups 1 and 2 [19]. Another RCT of 68 participants looked at true versus sham acupuncture for shoulder impingement with significant differences in pain and function at 3 months in the patients with true acupuncture compared to sham [20].

Table 58.2 Acupuncture in MSK medicine

	Method	Diagnosis	Study size	Intervention	Control	Outcome measures	Result
Lee MS, Ernst E (2011) [6]	Review	Peripheral joint osteoarthritis	NA	Acupuncture	Various	Various	Effective for peripheral joint osteoarthritis
Wang SH et al. (2010) [18]	RCT	Knee osteoarthritis	63	Routine acupuncture on affected side 3 times/ week for 4 weeks in combination with blood-letting once a week for 4 weeks	Routine acupuncture only	WOMAC, clinical therapeutic effects (pain index, physiological integral scores, joint stiffness index)	Total effective rates were 87.5% (treatment) vs. 90.32% (control). No significant difference found between two groups in therapeutic effects
Manheimer E et al. (2010) [7]	Cochrane review	Peripheral joint osteoarthritis	16 trials (3498 patients): 12 RCTs knee OA, 3 RCTs hip OA, 1 mix hip/knee OA	Acupuncture	Sham; supervised education; home exercises/advice leaflet; supervised exercise	Pain and function	Acupuncture statistically significant improvement in short-term pain and function vs. sham control; borderline statistical significance at 6 months; clinically relevant short- and long-term improvements in pain and function compared to education/home exercise/ advice leaflets, and supervised exercise
Suarez-Almazor et al. (2010) [14]	RCT	Knee osteoarthritis	455	Traditional Chinese acupuncture (TCA)	Sham acupuncture	Joint-Specific Multidimensional Assessment of Pain (J-MAP), WOMAC, satisfaction scores	No statistically significant differences between TCA and Sham; however, both groups had significant reductions in J-MAP and WOMAC
Lee et al. (2009) [9]	Review	Knee osteoarthritis (1 RCT)		Constitutional acupuncture (CA)	Standard acupuncture	Various	Favorable effects on pain reduction with CA vs. standard
Taechaarpornkul et al. (2009) [25]	RCT	Knee osteoarthritis	70	Six-point group: six acupuncture pts	Two-point group: two acupuncture points	WOMAC at baseline, week 5, 9, and 13	Mean total WOMAC score at weeks 5 and 13 of patients in both groups showed no statistical significance. Electro-acupuncture to 2 local pts. may be sufficient to treat knee OA
Jubb et al. (2008) [15]	RCT	Knee osteoarthritis	68	Manual acupuncture, electro-acupuncture	Sham acupuncture	WOMAC, self-reported pain scale, EuroQol score, plasma beta-endorphin	Significantly greater improvement on WOMAC and pain with acupuncture group compared to sham; no difference on EuroQol or plasma beta-endorphin levels
Selfe TK, Taylor AG (2008) [10]	Review	Knee osteoarthritis	10 trials (1456 participants)	Acupuncture	Various	Various	Acupuncture is an effective treatment for pain and physical dysfunction associated with knee osteoarthritis
Itoh et al. (2008) [16]	Pilot study	Knee osteoarthritis	32	Acupuncture, acupuncture and TENS, TENS	Topical poultice	VAS, WOMAC	Acupuncture, TENS, and acupuncture with TENS reported lower VAS and WOMAC compared to control. Significant reduction in pain intensity and knee function shown with combining acupuncture with TENS

(continued)

Table 58.2 (continued)

	Method	Diagnosis	Study size	Intervention	Control	Outcome measures	Result
Lev-Ari et al. (2007) [11]	Review	Knee osteoarthritis	Two phase 3 RCT	Acupuncture	Various	Various	Acupuncture improves function and provides pain relief of knee osteoarthritis. Effective complementary treatment to standard care
Vas J, white A (2007) [13]	Review	Knee osteoarthritis	13 RCT	Acupuncture, electro-acupuncture, manual acupuncture, percutaneous electrical stimulation	Various	Various	Optimal results: High patient expectation, minimum of four needles, electro-acupuncture, strong electrical stimulation to needles in muscle, and at least ten treatments
Kwon et al. (2006) [8]	Review	Peripheral joint osteoarthritis	18 RCT (10 trials manual, 8 electro-acupuncture)	Acupuncture, electro-acupuncture	Sham acupuncture	Various	Significant effect of manual acupuncture compared to sham. However, heterogeneity of electro-acupuncture trials prevented meaningful meta-analysis
Tukmachi et al. (2004) [17]	Open RCT	Knee osteoarthritis	30	Manual and electro-acupuncture alone (A), acupuncture with medication (B), medication for 5 weeks then acupuncture (C)	NA	VAS, WOMAC	Highly significant improvement in pain (VAS) with groups A and B, but no change in group C. Similar significance on WOMCA
Ezzo et al. (2001) [12]	Review	Knee osteoarthritis	7 trials (393 patients)	Acupuncture	Sham acupuncture	Pain, function, global improvement, imaging	Strong evidence that acupuncture is more effective than sham in relieving pain. Inconclusive evidence for function
Lathia et al. [19]	RCT	Chronic shoulder pain due to rotator cuff tendinitis or osteoarthritis	31	Individualized acupuncture points, fixed/standard acupuncture points	Sham acupuncture	Pain, function	All three groups had improvement after 6 weeks, but only the two treatment groups had clinically significant improvement
Rueda Garrido et al. [20]	RCT	Shoulder impingement	68	Acupuncture	Sham acupuncture	Pain, function	Significant differences in pain and function at 3 months in treatment group compared to the control group
Zhou et al. [21]	Systematic review/ meta-analysis	Lateral epicondylitis	10 RCTs (796 patients)	Acupuncture, medications, blocking therapy	Sham acupuncture	Pain, function	Increased clinical efficacy of acupuncture compared to the other treatment modalities and sham acupuncture
Zhang et al.	RCT	Achilles tendinopathy	64 patients	Acupuncture	Eccentric exercises	Pain, function	Significant differences in pain and function at in 8, 16, and 24 weeks in treatment group compared to the control group
Clark et al. [23]	Systematic review	Plantar fasciitis	Eight studies (five RCT and three nonrandomized)	Acupuncture, NSAIDs, dexamethasone injections, night splints, stretching	Variety	Pain, function	Clinical improvement especially when combined with standard treatments

A systematic review and meta-analysis were performed to evaluate acupuncture for lateral epicondylitis. A total of 10 RCTs were included with a collective total of 796 patients resulting in increased clinical efficacy with acupuncture compared to sham acupuncture, medicine therapy, and blocking therapy [21].

Acupuncture has also been evaluated to treat chronic Achilles tendinopathy. An RCT was performed with 64 patients being randomized in an acupuncture group vs a control group that completed eccentric exercises. There was a significant improvement in both pain and function at 8, 16, and 24 weeks for the acupuncture group compared to the control [22]. The efficacy of acupuncture for plantar fasciitis has also been assessed through a systematic review concluding that acupuncture is an effective treatment for the condition and that the evidence is comparable to other commonly used interventions, such as stretching, night splints, and dexamethasone [23].

Overall, there is significant heterogeneity of acupuncture treatment regimens and inclusion criteria throughout the literature which makes a definitive conclusion difficult. However, there was consistency in the literature that acupuncture shows statistically significant benefits for pain and function compared to sham acupuncture for the treatment of osteoarthritis.

58.3 Electroacupuncture (Percutaneous Electrical Nerve Stimulation)

Electroacupuncture (EA), also known as percutaneous electrical nerve stimulation (PENS), is a form of acupuncture utilizing a small electric current passed between pairs of acupuncture needles. Similar to traditional acupuncture, there are a variety of acupuncture regimens differing in the number of treatment points. It has been postulated that there are endocrinological changes influenced by electroacupuncture. This was demonstrated in a randomized controlled study with significant improvement of pain, function, increase in plasma beta-endorphin, and a fall in plasma cortisol compared to sham acupuncture [24]. Comparatively in another RCT, there was a non-statistically significant improvement in pain in subjects receiving both two and six acupuncture points [25].

Electroacupuncture has been compared to oral diclofenac in an RCT of 60 patients with hip osteoarthritis. There was marked improvement of pain and joint function in both groups but greater changes in the electroacupuncture group [26]. Another comparison of electroacupuncture with diclofenac in 186 patients with knee osteoarthritis demonstrated a significant improvement in pain and function with electroacupuncture compared to placebo and diclofenac [27]. Electroacupuncture has also been compared with hyaluronic acid injections in 245 patients with knee osteoarthritis with results slightly favoring electroacupuncture without any significant difference of the therapeutic effects between the two groups [28].

Electroacupuncture has also been compared with TENS and patient education in 24 patients with knee osteoarthritis. There were reductions in knee pain in both the electroacupuncture and TENS groups when compared to the education-only group [29]. Another study of 100 patients with knee OA compared EA, TENS, and ice massage demonstrated that all three methods decreased pain and stiffness [30].

Electroacupuncture was compared to hydrotherapy in the treatment of hip osteoarthritis with 45 patients revealing improvements in pain, functional activity, and quality of life with EA and hydrotherapy both individually and in combination [31]. Lastly, a broad systematic review was completed looking at any MSK disorder of the extremities. This review found that EA was superior to exercise for Achilles tendinopathy, superior to placebo for shoulder pain and plantar fasciitis [32]. The results of these studies (Table 58.3) provide a significant foundation of evidence which is promising for the use of electroacupuncture for the treatment of osteoarthritis.

58.4 Pharmacopuncture and Laser Acupuncture

Pharmacopuncture and herbal acupuncture are needle therapies that integrate acupuncture and herbal therapies. A minute amount of herbal extraction is injected in affected areas to maximize the efficacies of both acupuncture and herbal medicine. In a study of 60 patients with knee OA treated with pharmacopuncture using root bark of *Ulmus Davidiana Planch* (UDP) or *normal saline acupuncture*, the pharmacopuncture was more effective in pain improvement although without significant differences in the other outcome measures (Table 58.4) [33]. A systematic review and meta-analysis including 16 studies were conducted on the use of pharmacopuncture for patients suffering pain related to lumbar disc herniations. The results of the review were equivocal; however, the meta-analysis revealed that pharmacopuncture has a significant improvement in pain and function [34].

Bee venom acupuncture (BVA) is a type of herbal acupuncture exerting both pharmacological actions from the bee venom as well as a mechanical effect from acupuncture stimulation (Table 58.5). Lee and colleagues performed a review of the literature to evaluate evidence regarding the effectiveness of BVA for arthritis showing that BVA was promising in the treatment of arthritis; however, there is limited evidence demonstrating the efficacy of BVA in arthritis [35]. Kwon and colleagues investigated direct administration of bee venom into acupoints of patients with knee OA and demon-

Table 58.3 Electroacupuncture in MSJK medicine

	Method	Diagnosis	Study size	Intervention	Control	Outcome measures	Result
Sheng XP, Fan TY (2010) [26]	RCT	Hip osteoarthritis	60	Electroacupuncture	Diclofenac	VAS	Both groups had marked reduction of VAS pain scores; however, VAS reduction was markedly greater in the electroacupuncture
Wu et al. (2010) [28]	RCT	Knee osteoarthritis	245	Electroacupuncture	Intra-articular hyaluronic acid injection	Knee symptom score, contents of cytokines	Knee symptoms scores and contents of cytokines were significantly lowered in both groups, but to a greater extent in the electroacupuncture group
Ashin et al. (2009) [24]	RCT	Knee osteoarthritis	40	Electroacupuncture	Sham acupuncture	VAS, WOMAC, plasma beta-endorphin and cortisol levels, self-assessment of pain intensity	Significant improvement in WOMAC and VAS, significant rise in plasma beta-endorphin, and a significant fall in plasma cortisol in the acupuncture group
Ng et al. (2003) [29]	RCT	Knee osteoarthritis	24	Electroacupuncture (EA), TENS	Control	NRS, Timed Up-and-Go Test (TUGT)	Significant reduction of NRS in both EA and TENS groups, TUGT score in EA group significantly lower than control; however, no significant change between TENS and control
Sangdee et al. (2002) [27]	RCT	Knee osteoarthritis	193	Electroacupuncture, diclofenac, combined	Placebo	VAS, WOMAC, Lequesne's functional index, 50 feet walk time	Improvement in VAS significantly greater in EA compared to diclofenac or placebo, significant improvement in Lequesne's with EA compared to placebo, significant improvement in WOMAC between combined and placebo
Stener-Victorin et al. (2004) [31]	RCT	Hip osteoarthritis	45	Electroacupuncture, hydrotherapy, combination with patient education	Patient education alone	VAS, Disability Rating Index (DRI), Global self-rating Index (GSI)	6 month ache and pain reduction in EA group, 3 month with hydrotherapy, disability improved 6 months in both EA and hydrotherapy, quality of life improved 3 months for EA and hydrotherapy; No changes with education alone
Yurtkuran M, Kocagil T (1999) [30]	RCT	Knee osteoarthritis	100	TENS, EA, Ice	Placebo	Pain at rest, stiffness, 50 feet walk time, quadriceps muscle strength, knee flexion degree	TENS, EA, and Ice are effective in improving all objective parameters compared to placebo
Cox et al. (2016) [32]	Systematic review	General MSK (Achilles tendinopathy, plantar fasciitis, shoulder pain)	15 studies	Electroacupuncture	Placebo (shoulder pain, plantar fasciitis), exercises (Achilles)	Pain and function	EA is superior to exercises for Achilles tendinopathy and superior to placebo for shoulder pain and plantar fasciitis

Table 58.4 Pharmacopuncture in MSK medicine

	Method	Diagnosis	Study size	Intervention	Control	Outcome measures	Result
Kim et al. (2010) [33]	RCT	Knee osteoarthritis	60	Pharmacopuncture using Ulmus davidiana Planch (UDP)	Normal saline injections	VAS, WOMAC, SF 36	Pharmacopuncture was more effective in pain improvement than normal saline injections although there were not significant differences in functional outcome measures
Byun et al. (2021) [34]	Systematic review/ meta-analysis	Lumbar disc herniations	16 studies	Pharmacopuncture	Placebo, exercises	Pain and function	Significant improvement of pain and function

Table 58.5 Bee venom acupuncture

	Method	Diagnosis	Study size	Intervention	Control	Outcome measures	Result
Lee et al. (2005) [35]	Review	Osteoarthritis	15 trials	BVA	Various	Various	2 RCT and 3 uncontrolled trials showed BVA effective. There is limited evidence regarding efficacy of BVA in arthritis
Kwon et al. (2001) [36]	Comparative	Osteoarthritis		BVA	Traditional acupuncture	Pain relief, computerized infrared thermography (IRT)	Significant pain relief and IRT score with BVA compared to traditional acupuncture
Shen et al. (2020) [37]	Systematic review/ meta-analysis	Chronic shoulder pain		BVA	Placebo	Pain and function	May be beneficial

Table 58.6 Laser acupuncture

	Method	Diagnosis	Study size	Intervention	Control	Outcome measures	Result
Zhao et al. [39]	RCT	Knee osteoarthritis	40	Laser acupuncture-moxibustion	Sham	WOMAC at wk. 2 and 4	Significant improvement in WOMAC at 2 weeks but not at 4 in weeks in treatment compared to sham
Yurtkuran et al. (2007) [41]	RCT	Knee osteoarthritis	52	Laser acupuncture	Placebo laser therapy	VAS, 50 foot walk test, knee circumference (KC), medial tenderness score (MTS), WOMAC, Nottingham Health Profile (NHP)	There was statistically significant improvement with both groups in all outcome measures; however, when groups compared to each other, the only improvement that the treatment group was superior was KC

strated a majority (82.5%) of subjects receiving BVA reported substantial pain relief compared with traditional acupuncture therapy (55%). The therapeutic efficacy was favorable irrespective of disease duration (acute, subacute, or chronic stage), arthritic type (unilateral or bilateral knee OA), and radiological severity [36]. A systematic review and meta-analysis regarding BVA for chronic shoulder pain (variety of diagnosis) suggested that this modality may be beneficial [37]. Lastly, another RCT regarding BVA for chronic low back pain is being investigated [38].

Low-level laser acupuncture involves the application of low-level laser photic energy, photobiomodulation, to acupuncture points [40]. There has only been one study on laser acupuncture (Table 58.6). Yurtkuran and colleagues conducted a double-blind, RCT comparing laser acupuncture to sham laser for the treatment of knee osteoarthritis. Both groups revealed statistically significant improvements in all outcome measures; however, there was a clear superiority in the treatment group in the reduction of periarticular swelling [41]. Currently, there is an insufficient volume of quality evidence to support the use of pharmacopuncture or laser acupuncture for osteoarthritis, and additional high-quality studies are necessary.

58.5 Moxibustion

Moxibustion is a form of heat treatment in traditional Chinese medicine that stimulates specific acupuncture points. The term moxibustion is a combination of the word moxa (Japanese mogusa-mugwort) and combustion ("burning") and thus the "the burning of mugwort."

Current literature review on moxibustion for the treatment of osteoarthritis revealed multiple studies and reviews (Table 58.7). In the review of the literature by Choi and colleagues, a subgroup analysis showed significant effects of moxibustion compared with medication therapy in patients with knee osteoarthritis [42]. A review by Lee and colleagues suggested significant pain reductions for indirect moxibustion in osteoarthritis compared with medication therapy [43]. The largest sample size in this review was the case series of 563 patients being treated with moxibustion and acupuncture for knee osteoarthritis. The results of this case series revealed that 75% of the patients achieved a pain reduction of 45% or greater with both treatments [44]. An observational study by Fu and colleagues on the therapeutic effect of moxibustion on knee osteoarthritis with a total effectiveness of 97.5% of the 34 patients, although there was no control [45]. A study

Table 58.7 Moxibustion in MSK medicine

	Method	Diagnosis	Study Size	Intervention	Control	Outcome measures	Result
Choi et al. (2011) [42]	Review	Rheumatic conditions	14 RCTs	Moxibustion	Varied	Varied	All RCTs of low methodological quality Meta-analysis of eight RCTs suggest favorable effects compared to medications. Subgroup analysis show significant effects compared to medications in knee osteoarthritis subgroup
Lee et al. (2010) [43]	Review	Pain	14 RCTs	Moxibustion	Varied	Varied	Two RCTs suggested significant pain reduction for indirect moxibustion in OA compared to medications
Zhang QR, Fu WB (2010) [46]	RCT	Knee osteoarthritis	62	Moxibustion with acupuncture	Acupuncture	VAS, WHOQOL-BREF, Lysholm knee joint motor functions scale	Improvement of VAS and Lysholm in both groups; however, degree of improvement was superior with combination of moxibustion and acupuncture. No statistical significance in WHOQOL-BREF in either group
Su et al. (2009)	RCT	Knee osteoarthritis	65	Moxibustion	Infrared therapy	Lysholm, pain score, joint ROM, joint stability, up, and down stairs score	Improvement in all measures in moxibustion group compared to infrared
Cao et al. (2009)	RCT	Knee osteoarthritis	90	Moxibustion	Control	WHOQOL-BREF, Lysholm	Significantly higher WHOQOL-BREF and Lysholm with moxibustion
Ding el al (2009) [48]	RCT	Knee osteoarthritis	90	Moxibustion	Western medicine (ibuprofen), waiting group (no treatment)	WOMAC, SF-16	No significant difference in moxibustion vs. western medicine, no significant difference in pre- and post-treatment WOMAC or SF-16 scores between moxibustion or western medicine, both groups superior to waiting
Li et al. (2008) [47]	RCT	Knee osteoarthritis	90	Monkshood cake moxibustion	Medication (Xianling Gubao capsules)	VAS, index of severity of OA (ISOA) scale	Significant improvement in both groups, but significant difference with moxibustion compared to medication
Fu et al. (2007) [45]	Observation	Knee osteoarthritis	34	Moxibustion	None	Pain, joint mobility, stair activity	10 cases cured, 14 cased markedly effective, 9 effective, 1 ineffective
Vas et al. (2004) [44]	Case series	Knee osteoarthritis	563	Moxibustion	Acupuncture	Pain intensity and frequency, daily dose of analgesic and anti-inflammatory medications	75% achieved a pain reduction of 45% or more in both groups
	Systematic review/ meta-analysis	Low back pain due to herniation		Moxibustion	Multiple controls	Pain and function	Favorable results, but studies demonstrated potential high risk of bias

of 62 patients was randomized into treatment with moxibustion and acupuncture versus acupuncture alone. While both groups demonstrated improvement in VAS and Lysholm knee joint motor function scores, the group receiving both treatments had a superior degree of improvement [46]. Li and colleagues completed an RCT evaluating the clinical effect of moxibustion for the treatment of knee osteoarthritis and found that 80% of patients treated with moxibustion had improvement compared to 53% with medication [47]. Another RCT of 90 patients divided into three groups: warming needle moxibustion, Western medicine (oral NSAID medication), and a waiting group; the total effective rate of moxibustion was 83% compared to 60% in the western medicine group; however, both were significantly better than the waiting group [48]. A systematic review and meta-analysis of moxibustion for low back pain due to lumbar disc herniation concluded that these studies had a high risk of bias and further studies were necessary to determine efficacy [49]. Significant heterogeneity exists in the study designs, particularly with the preparation and administration of moxibustion. Therefore, although evidence exists supporting the use of moxibustion for the treatment of osteoarthritis, it is favorable, but far from conclusive.

58.6 Transcutaneous Electrical Nerve Stimulation (TENS)

Transcutaneous electrical nerve stimulation (TENS) is the use of electrical current via attached electrodes to treat pain. There are a wide variety of frequencies that can be applied ranging from high frequency (>50 Hz) with an intensity below motor conduction to low frequency (<10 Hz) which produces muscle contraction. This wide variety of treatment intensities leads to significant heterogeneity in the treatment protocols utilized in the literature (Table 58.8). Law and colleagues attempted to determine the optimal stimulation frequency to reduce pain due to knee osteoarthritis and did not reveal any difference after 2 weeks of treatment at 2 Hz, 100 Hz, or 2/100 Hz [50]. A study by Cheing and colleagues attempted to determine the optimal stimulation duration to provide analgesia for osteoarthritic knee pain and found that 40 min of TENS provided the greatest magnitude and duration of pain reduction [51].

Recent reviews on TENS for knee osteoarthritis identified a total of 18 studies of 813 patients with knee osteoarthritis and initially revealed a large effect on pain relief, but after reanalyzing the data and correcting for design flaws, they concluded that TENS was no more effective than fake stimulation [52, 53]. A Cochrane review on TENS for Knee OA was conducted by Osiri and colleagues including seven trials with a total of 194 patients that received either TENS or placebo and demonstrated TENS yielded significant pain relief [54].

An RCT of 100 women with bilateral knee osteoarthritis was performed comparing individual and combined treatments with hot pack, short-wave diathermy, ultrasound, and TENS with a significant improvement in pain and function with TENS plus hot pack [55]. Another study comparing TENS, therapeutic ultrasound, and superficial heat did not find any statistical significance between the groups on pain, function, strength, or quality of life [56]. One study has shown that TENS may improve range of motion (ROM) and function for a short period, but the results were not sustained at 10 days [57].

In an RCT of 60 patients comparing intra-articular hyaluronic acid to TENS, there was statistically significant improvement in both groups; however, the improvement in functional scores was greater in the hylan group [58]. TENS has also been compared to nonsteroidal anti-inflammatory medication and placebo, with no significant differences between any of the treatments [59]. Another RCT compared TENS with paracetamol and showed a slight nonsignificant difference favoring TENS [60].

The most significant limitation in the review of the TENS literature is the wide range of treatment duration and intensities resulting in varying results. Despite the significant heterogeneity in the studies, TENS appears to be effective in pain relief of osteoarthritis; however, more studies are necessary to determine the most effective treatment regimen and appropriate patient selection.

58.7 Laser Therapy

Low-level laser therapy (LLLT), also known as *photobiomodulation*, refers to the use of red-beam or near-infrared lasers with a wavelength between 600 and 1000 nm and wattage from 5 to 500 milliwatts (compared to surgical lasers at 300 Watts). When LLLT is applied to the skin, the low-level lasers do not produce any sensation, nor do they burn the skin. The low-level laser is absorbed by human skin, and it is hypothesized that the laser light can penetrate deeply into the tissues where it has a photobiostimulative effect. The exact mechanism of its effect is unknown, but hypotheses have included improved cellular repair and stimulation of the immune, lymphatic, and vascular systems.

A review of the literature (Table 58.9) was conducted to evaluate the evidence supporting LLLT to treat the symptoms of osteoarthritis. The meta-analysis by Brosseau and colleagues in 2000 identified 13 trials in patients with either rheumatoid arthritis or osteoarthritis. In the OA studies, there were a total of 197 patients that were randomized. The pooled estimate did not show significant differences in pain,

Table 58.8 TENS in MSK medicine

	Method	Diagnosis	Study size	Intervention	Control	Outcome measures	Result
Rutjes A (2010) [52]	Review	Knee osteoarthritis	18 trials (813 persons)	TENS	Various	Various	Large effect on pain relief, moderate improvement of function; however, only small trials and larger trial is needed
Rutjes et al. (2009) [53]	Cochrane review	Knee osteoarthritis	18 trials (813 persons)	TENS	Various	Various	Inconclusive due to small trials of questionable quality
Cetin et al. (2008) [55]	RCT	Knee osteoarthritis	100	TENS, short wave diathermy, ultrasound	Hot packs +/−isokinetic exercise	VAS, Lequesne index	Pain and disability index scores were significantly reduced in each group compared to the control group; particularly TENS and diathermy
Eyigor et al. (2008) [56]	RCT	Knee osteoarthritis	45	TENS, ultrasound	Superficial heat and exercise	VAS, Lequesne index, WOMAC, 20 meter walk test, SF36	Both treatment groups had significant improvement on activity VAS, 20 m walking test, Lequesne index, WOMAC, and most of the sub-scores of SF36 comparted to control group
Cheing GL, Tsui AY (2004)	RCT	Knee osteoarthritis	Two groups	TENS	Placebo TENS	VAS, Timed Up and Go Test (TUGT), knee ROM	TENS produced a significantly greater increase in maximum knee ROM comparted to placebo, moderate correlation in reduction of pain scores, no significant difference on TUGT
Paker et al. (2006) [58]	RCT	Knee osteoarthritis	60	TENS	Hyaluronic acid injection	VAS, WOMAC, Lequesne index, SF36	Statistically significant improvement on WOMAC with both TENS and injection from baseline, pain relief sustained for 6 months in both groups, no change in physical function and SF36
Law PP, Cheing GL (2004) [50]	RCT	Knee osteoarthritis	34	TENS	Placebo TENS	VAS, TUGT, knee ROM	Significant pain reduction, TUGT time, and knee ROM between treatment and control
Cheing GL et (2003) [51]	RCT	Knee osteoarthritis	38	TENS	Placebo TENS	VAS	40 minutes of TENS is optimal treatment duration providing statistically significant pain reduction compared to placebo
Osiri et al. (2000) [54]	Cochrane review	Knee osteoarthritis	7 trials (294 patients)	TENS	Various	Various	TENS and acupuncture like TENS provide significantly better pain reduction compared to placebo
Lewis et al. (1994) [59]	RCT	Knee osteoarthritis	36	TENS, NSAID	Placebo TENS, placebo drug, double placebo	Pain diary	No significant difference across all groups, but NSAID plus placebo TENS more effective than double placebo
Lewis et al. (1984) [60]	Double blind cross over	Knee osteoarthritis	30	TENS	Placebo TENS	VAS	Length of pain relief significantly longer compared to placebo
Taylor et al. (1981)	Double blind cross over	Knee osteoarthritis	10	TENS	Placebo	Pain relief	Statistically significant pain relief with TENS compared to placebo

joint tenderness, joint mobility, or strength, but there was statistically significant heterogeneity in the treatment regimens (wavelength, site of application, duration) [61]. Another Cochrane review by Brosseau and colleagues in 2007 expanded the initial review and focused only on OA. A total of seven trials were included, with 184 patients randomized to laser and 161 to placebo laser. The results of the Cochrane review were the same as the initial review and did not find any significant improvement in any of the outcome measures, except one study demonstrated significant improvement of

Table 58.9 Laser in MSK medicine

	Method	Diagnosis	Study size	Intervention	Control	Outcome measures	Result
Zhao et al. (2010) [39]	RCT	Knee osteoarthritis	40	Laser acupuncture-moxibustion	Sham	WOMAC at wk. 2 and 4	Significant improvement in WOMAC at 2 weeks but not at 4 weeks in treatment compared to sham
Brosseau et al. (2007) [64]	Cochrane	Osteoarthritis	Seven RCTs (345 patients)	Low-level Laser Therapy (LLLT)	Placebo laser	Pain, joint tenderness, ROM	No significant difference in any outcome measures, except one study found significant improvement of knee ROM
Brosseau et al. (2005) [65]	RCT	Hand osteoarthritis	88	Low-level Laser Therapy (LLLT)	Placebo laser	Pain relief, morning stiffness, functional status, finger ROM, grip strength	No significant difference in any measures (except CMC opposition ROM) in LLLT vs. sham
Brosseau et al. (2000) [61]	Meta-analysis	Osteoarthritis	13 RCTs (RA and OA-386 total patients of which 197 OA)	Laser	Placebo laser	Pain, morning stiffness, function, ROM	In OA patients, no significant effects on any outcome measure
Hegedus et al. (2009) [63]	RCT	Knee osteoarthritis		LLLT	Placebo laser	VAS, thermography, joint flexion, circumference, pressure sensitivity	Significant improvement in pain relief and pressure sensitivity in treatment group

Table 58.10 Massage in MSK medicine

	Method	Diagnosis	Study size	Intervention	Control	Outcome measures	Result
Yib YB, Tam AC (2008) [67]	RCT	Knee pain	59	Aromatic (1% *Zingiber officinale* and 0.5% *Citrus sinensis*) massage, olive oil massage	No massage	WOMAC, pain, stiffness	Superior improvement with aromatic massage compared to both control and placebo groups at 1 week, but not sustained at 4 weeks
Perlman et al. (2006) [66]	RCT	Knee osteoarthritis	68	Swedish massage	Delayed intervention	WOMAC, VAS	Significant improvement in WOMAC and VAS

knee range of motion [62]. An RCT by Hegedus and colleagues was completed after these reviews showing that there was a significant improvement of pain, knee circumference, and pressure sensitivity as well as improvement in thermographic measurements suggesting an effect on the microcirculation for the treatment group [63]. Additionally, an RCT of LLLT for the treatment of hand osteoarthritis did not demonstrate significant improvement versus placebo for pain relief, stiffness, nor function [65].

Despite some positive findings, there are four important factors that significantly increase the heterogeneity of the literature and thus dilute the applicability of the results: wavelength, treatment duration, dosage, and site of application. This practical data and appropriate patient selection need to be further clarified to elucidate the efficacy of LLLT for OA.

58.8 Massage Therapy

Massage therapy is utilized for several musculoskeletal conditions. One of the limiting factors in evaluating the efficacy of massage therapy is the vast heterogeneity in treatment techniques. Overall, there is a paucity of evidence-based literature on massage therapy for the treatment of osteoarthritis (Table 58.10). Perlman and colleagues randomized 68 adults to Swedish massage versus no treatment and demonstrated significant improvements in pain and function in those receiving massage [66]. Another study evaluated aroma-massage therapy with ginger and orange oil to massage with olive oil and revealed that there was significant improvement of physical function and pain in the aroma massage therapy group at 1 week that was not sustained at 4 weeks [67]. At the current time, there is insufficient evidence to support massage therapy for the treatment of the symptoms of osteoarthritis.

58.9 CAM for OA

As discussed above, there are several limitations in the evidence-based review of CAM for osteoarthritis. One of the more interesting aspects is that there is a paucity of literature in English peer-reviewed journals, particularly modalities that originated in Chinese medicine. Other major issues include the heterogeneity of treatment regimens and patient selection and the lack of consensus regarding an exact treatment making a true comparison extremely difficult. Despite these limitations, the evidence is promising with several CAM for the treatment of osteoarthritis and other musculoskeletal conditions. Although more studies with a homogenous treatment regimen are necessary, the current evidence is favorable for acupuncture, electroacupuncture, moxibustion, and TENS for musculoskeletal conditions and osteoarthritis in particular. Given how frequently massage is used for musculoskeletal conditions and in particular soft tissue pain, the lack of published literature on this treatment was unanticipated. The current evidence is clear that LLLT is ineffective for osteoarthritis, and there is insufficient evidence for pharmacopuncture, BVA, and massage for osteoarthritis and other musculoskeletal conditions.

References

1. Callahan LF, Wiley-Exley EK, Mielenz TJ, et al. Use of complementary and alternative medicine among patients with arthritis. Prev Chronic Dis. 2009;6(2):A44.
2. Katz P, Lee F. Racial/ethnic differences in the use of complementary and alternative medicine in patients with arthritis. J Clin Rheumatol. 2007;13(1):3–11.
3. Herman CJ, Allen P, Hunt WC, et al. Use of complementary therapies among primary care clinic patients with arthritis. Prev Chronic Dis. 2004;1(4):A12.
4. Herman CJ, Dente JM, Allen P, Hunt WC. Ethnic differences in the use of complementary and alternative therapies among adults with osteoarthritis. Prev Chronic Dis. 2006;3(3):A80.
5. White AR, Filshie J, Cummings TM. Clinical trials of acupuncture: consensus recommendations for optimal treatment, sham controls and blinding. Complement Ther Med. 2001;9(4):237–45.
6. Lee MS, Ernst E. Acupuncture for pain: an overview of Cochrane reviews. Chin J Integr Med. 2011;17(3):187–9.
7. Manheimer E, Cheng K, Linde K, et al. Acupuncture for peripheral joint osteoarthritis. Cochrane Database Syst Rev. 2010;(1):CD001977.
8. Kwon YD, Pittler MH, Ernst E, et al. Acupuncture for peripheral joint osteoarthritis: a systematic review and meta-analysis. Rheumatology (Oxford). 2006;45(11):1331–7.
9. Lee MS, Shin BC, Choi SM, Kim JY. Randomized clinical trials of constitutional acupuncture: a systematic review. Evid Based Complement Alternat Med. 2009;6 Suppl 1:59–64.
10. Selfe TK, Taylor AG. Acupuncture and osteoarthritis of the knee: a review of randomized, controlled trials. Fam Community Health. 2008;31(3):247–54.
11. Lev-Ari S, Hasner A, Amir H, et al. Acupuncture as complementary medicine in patients with osteoarthritis of the knee. [Original in Hebrew]. Harefuah. 2007;146(5):354–7, 406
12. Ezzo J, Hadhazy V, Birch S, et al. Acupuncture for osteoarthritis of the knee: a systematic review. Arthritis Rheum. 2001;44(4):819–25.
13. Vas J, White A. Evidence from RCTs on optimal acupuncture treatment for knee osteoarthritis--an exploratory review. Acupunct Med. 2007;25(1–2):29–35.
14. Suarez-Almazor ME, Looney C, Liu Y, et al. A randomized controlled trial of acupuncture for osteoarthritis of the knee: effects of patient-provider communication. Arthritis Care Res (Hoboken). 2010;62(9):1229–36.
15. Jubb RW, Tukmachi ES, Jones PW, et al. A blinded randomised trial of acupuncture (manual and electroacupuncture) compared with a non-penetrating sham for the symptoms of osteoarthritis of the knee. Acupunct Med. 2008;26(2):69–78.
16. Itoh K, Hirota S, Katsumi Y, et al. A pilot study on using acupuncture and transcutaneous electrical nerve stimulation (TENS) to treat knee osteoarthritis (OA). Chin Med. 2008;3:2.
17. Tukmachi E, Jubb R, Dempsey E, Jones P. The effect of acupuncture on the symptoms of knee osteoarthritis--an open randomised controlled study. Acupunct Med. 2004;22(1):14–22.
18. Wang SH, Xu MZ, Cui SY, Guo YQ. Randomized controlled clinical trials on treatment of knee osteoarthritis with acupuncture combined with blood-letting therapy. [Original Article in Chinese]. Zhen Ci Yan Jiu. 2010;35(2):129–33.
19. Lathia AT, Jung SM, Chen LX. Efficacy of acupuncture as a treatment for chronic shoulder pain. J Altern Complement Med. 2009;15(6):613–8.
20. Rueda Garrido JC, Vas J, Lopez DR. Acupuncture treatment of shoulder impingement syndrome: a randomized controlled trial. Complement Ther Med. 2016;25:9207.
21. Zhou Y, Guo Y, Zhou R, et al. Effectiveness of acupuncture for lateral epicondylitis: a systematic review and meta-analysis of randomized controlled trials. Pain Res Manag. 2020;2020:8506591.
22. Zhang B, Zhong L, Xu S, Jiang H, Shen J. Acupuncture for chronic Achilles tendinopathy: a randomized controlled study. Chin J Integr Med. 2013;19(12):900–4.
23. Clark RJ, Tighe M. The effectiveness of acupuncture for plantar heel pain: a systematic review. Acupunct Med. 2012;30(4):298–306.
24. Ahsin S, Saleem S, Bhatti AM, et al. Clinical and endocrinological changes after electro-acupuncture treatment in patients with osteoarthritis of the knee. Pain. 2009;147(1–3):60–6.
25. Taechaarpornkul W, Suvapan D, Theppanom C, et al. Comparison of the effectiveness of six and two acupuncture point regimens in osteoarthritis of the knee: a randomised trial. Acupunct Med. 2009;27(1):3–8.
26. Sheng XP, Fan TY. Comparative observation on hip osteoarthritis treated with electroacupuncture and medication. [Original in Chinese]. Zhongguo Zhen Jiu. 2010;30(12):982–4.
27. Sangdee C, Teekachunhatean S, Sananpanich K, et al. Electroacupuncture versus diclofenac in symptomatic treatment of osteoarthritis of the knee: a randomized controlled trial. BMC Complement Altern Med. 2002;2:3.
28. Wu MX, Li XH, Lin MN, et al. Clinical study on the treatment of knee osteoarthritis of Shen-Sui insufficiency syndrome type by electroacupuncture. Chin J Integr Med. 2010;16(4):291–7.
29. Ng MM, Leung MC, Poon DM. The effects of electro-acupuncture and transcutaneous electrical nerve stimulation on patients with painful osteoarthritic knees: a randomized controlled trial with follow-up evaluation. J Altern Complement Med. 2003;9(5):641–9.
30. Yurtkuran M, Kocagil T. TENS, electroacupuncture and ice massage: comparison of treatment for osteoarthritis of the knee. Am J Acupunct. 1999;27(3–4):133–40.
31. Stener-Victorin E, Kruse-Smidje C, Jung K. Comparison between electro-acupuncture and hydrotherapy, both in combination with patient education and patient education alone, on the symptomatic treatment of osteoarthritis of the hip. Clin J Pain. 2004;20(3):179–85.
32. Cox J, Varatharajan S, Cote P. Effectiveness of acupuncture therapies to manage musculoskeletal disorders of the extremities: a systematic review. J Orthop Sports Phys Ther. 2016;45(6):409–29.
33. Kim EJ, Jang MK, Yoon EH, et al. Efficacy of pharmacopuncture using root bark of Ulmus davidiana planch in patients with knee osteoarthritis: a double-blind randomized controlled trial. J Acupunct Meridian Stud. 2010;3(1):16–23.
34. Byun DY, Kim H, Han SH, Kim KW, et al. Pharmacopuncture for lumbar herniated intervertebral disc: a systematic review and meta-analysis. Complement Ther Clin Pract. 2021;43:101369.

35. Lee JD, Park HJ, Chae Y, Lim S. An overview of bee venom acupuncture in the treatment of arthritis. Evid Based Complement Alternat Med. 2005;2(1):79–84.
36. Kwon YB, Kim JH, Yoon JH, et al. The analgesic efficacy of bee venom acupuncture for knee osteoarthritis: a comparative study with needle acupuncture. Am J Chin Med. 2001;29(2):187–99.
37. Shen L, Lee JH, Joo JC, et al. Bee venom acupuncture for shoulder pain: a systematic review and meta—analysis of randomized controlled trials. J Pharmacopuncture. 2020;23(2):44–53.
38. Seo BK, Lee JH, Sung WS, et al. Bee venom acupuncture for the treatment of chronic low Back pain: study protocol for a randomized double-blinded, sham-controlled trial. Trials. 2013;14:16.
39. Zhao L, Shen X, Cheng K, et al. Validating a nonacupoint sham control for laser treatment of knee osteoarthritis. Photomedicine and laser surgery. 2010;28(3):351–356. https://doi.org/10.1089/pho.2009.2511.
40. Vargas JT. Low level laser acupuncture. Med Acup. 2005;16(2):38–41.
41. Yurtkuran M, Alp A, Konur S, et al. Laser acupuncture in knee osteoarthritis: a double-blind, randomized controlled study. Photomed Laser Surg. 2007;25(1):14–20.
42. Choi TY, Kim TH, Kang JW, et al. Moxibustion for rheumatic conditions: a systematic review and meta-analysis. Clin Rheumatol. 2011;30(7):937–45.
43. Lee MS, Choi TY, Kang JW, et al. Moxibustion for treating pain: a systematic review. Am J Chin Med. 2010;38(5):829–38.
44. Vas J, Perea-Milla E, Méndez C. Acupuncture and moxibustion as an adjunctive treatment for osteoarthritis of the knee--a large case series. Acupunct Med. 2004;22(1):23–8.
45. Fu Y, Kang MF, Chen RX, Zhang B, Zhang HF. Observation on the therapeutic effect of painless festering moxibustion on knee osteoarthritis. [original in Chinese]. Zhongguo Zhen Jiu. 2007;27(7):513–5.
46. Zhang QR, Fu WB. Osteoarthritis of knee joint treated with acupuncture and moxibustion. [Original in Chinese]. Zhongguo Zhen Jiu. 2010;30(5):375–8.
47. Li JW, Xiang SY, Ma ZY, Feng YB, Tong HY, Geng HP, Jin J, Su X. Clinical observation on cake-separated mild-warm moxibustion for treatment of knee osteoarthritis. [Original in Chinese]. Zhongguo Zhen Jiu. 2008;28(1):17–9.
48. Ding MH, Zhang H, Li Y. A randomized controlled study on warming needle moxibustion for treatment of knee osteoarthritis. [Original in Chinese]. Zhong Zhen Jiu. 2009;29(8):603–7.
49. Wang Y, Zhang H, Xiz L, et al. Effectiveness and safety of moxibustion in treatment of lumbar disc herniation: a systematic review and meta-analysis. J Tradit Chin Med. 2019;39(5):599–608.
50. Law PP, Cheing GL. Optimal stimulation frequency of transcutaneous electrical nerve stimulation on people with knee osteoarthritis. J Rehabil Med. 2004;36(5):220–5.
51. Cheing GL, Tsui AY, Lo SK, Hui-Chan CW. Optimal stimulation duration of TENS in the management of osteoarthritic knee pain. J Rehabil Med. 2003;35(2):62–8.
52. Rutjes A. TENS for knee osteoarthritis. J Evid Based Med. 2010;3(1):54.
53. Rutjes AWS, Nüesch E, Sterchi R, et al. Transcutaneous electrostimulation for osteoarthritis of the knee. Cochrane Database Syst Rev. 2009;(4):CD002823.
54. Osiri M, Welch V, Brosseau L, et al. Transcutaneous electrical nerve stimulation for knee osteoarthritis. Cochrane Database Syst Rev. 2000;4:CD002823. Update in Cochrane Database Syst Rev. 2009;(4):CD002823.
55. Cetin N, Aytar A, Atalay A, Akman MN. Comparing hot pack, short-wave diathermy, ultrasound, and TENS on isokinetic strength, pain, and functional status of women with osteoarthritic knees: a single-blind, randomized, controlled trial. Am J Phys Med Rehabil. 2008;87(6):443–51.
56. Eyigör S, Karapolat H, Ibisoğlu U, Durmaz B. Does transcutaneous electrical nerve stimulation or therapeutic ultrasound increase the effectiveness of exercise for knee osteoarthritis: a randomized controlled study [Original in Turkish]. Agri. 2008;20(1):32–40.
57. Law PP, Cheing GL, Tsui AY. Does transcutaneous electrical nerve stimulation improve the physical performance of people with knee osteoarthritis? J Clin Rheumatol. 2004;10(6):295–9.
58. Paker N, Tekdös D, Kesiktas N, Soy D. Comparison of the therapeutic efficacy of TENS versus intra-articular hyaluronic acid injection in patients with knee osteoarthritis: a prospective randomized study. Adv Ther. 2006;23(2):342–53.
59. Lewis B, Lewis D, Cumming G. The comparative analgesic efficacy of transcutaneous electrical nerve stimulation and a non-steroidal anti-inflammatory drug for painful osteoarthritis. Br J Rheumatol. 1994;33(5):455–60.
60. Lewis D, Lewis B, Sturrock RD. Transcutaneous electrical nerve stimulation in osteoarthrosis: a therapeutic alternative? Ann Rheum Dis. 1984;43(1):47–9.
61. Brosseau L, Welch V, Wells G, et al. Low level laser therapy for osteoarthritis and rheumatoid arthritis: a meta-analysis. J Rheumatol. 2000;27(8):1961–9.
62. Brosseau L, Welch V, Wells G, et al. Low level laser therapy (classes I, II and III) for treating osteoarthritis. Cochrane Database Syst Rev. 2004;(3):CD002046. Update in Cochrane Database Syst Rev. 2007;(1):CD002046.
63. Hegedus B, Viharos L, Gervain M, Gálfi M. The effect of low-level laser in knee osteoarthritis: a double-blind, randomized, placebo-controlled trial. Photomed Laser Surg. 2009;27(4):577–84.
64. Brosseau L, Robinson V, Wells G, Debie R, Gam A, Harman K, Morin M, Shea B, Tugwell P. WITHDRAWN: Low level laser therapy (Classes III) for treating osteoarthritis. Cochrane Database Syst Rev. 2007;18;(1):CD002046. https://doi.org/10.1002/14651858.
65. Brosseau L, Wells G, Marchand S, et al. Randomized controlled trial on low level laser therapy (LLLT) in the treatment of osteoarthritis (OA) of the hand. Lasers Surg Med. 2005;36(3):210–9.
66. Perlman AI, Sabina A, Williams AL, et al. Massage therapy for osteoarthritis of the knee: a randomized controlled trial. Arch Intern Med. 2006;166(22):2533–8.
67. Yip YB, Tam AC. An experimental study on the effectiveness of massage with aromatic ginger and orange essential oil for moderate-to-severe knee pain among the elderly in Hong Kong. Complement Ther Med. 2008;16(3):131–8.

59 Osteopathic Medicine: Musculoskeletal Applications

Laura Griffin and Darren C. Rosenberg

59.1 ICD 10 Codes

- M99.00 Segmental & somatic dysfunction of head region
- M99.01 Segmental & somatic dysfunction of cervical region
- M99.02 Segmental & somatic dysfunction of thoracic region
- M99.03 Segmental & somatic dysfunction of lumbar region
- M99.04 Segmental & somatic dysfunction of sacral region
- M99.05 Segmental & somatic dysfunction of pelvic region
- M99.06 Segmental & somatic dysfunction of lower extremity
- M99.07 Segmental & somatic dysfunction of upper extremity
- M99.08 Segmental & somatic dysfunction of rib cage
- M99.09 Segmental & somatic dysfunction of abdomen & other regions CPT Codes
- 98925-29 Osteopathic manipulative treatment (OMT based on number of regions treated)

59.2 Description

Osteopathic manipulation is a component of osteopathic medicine comprising palpatory diagnosis and manipulative treatment based on three tenets: the structure and function of the body are reciprocally interrelated; the body has self-healing and self-regulating mechanisms; and the patient should be treated as an integrated entity incorporating physical, mental, and emotional elements.

Andrew Taylor Still, MD, who developed osteopathy and introduced it in 1874, did not view osteopathic treatment in isolation. Rather, osteopathic principles and techniques were to be integrated into the practice of all physicians as a complementary system of diagnosis and treatment. The 2012 National Health Interview Survey showed that chiropractic or osteopathic manipulation is the fourth most commonly used form of all complementary health approaches [1].

Osteopathic manipulative medicine (OMM) is the application of osteopathic philosophy, structural diagnosis, and use of osteopathic manipulative treatment in the diagnosis and management of the patient. Osteopathic manipulative treatment (OMT) is the therapeutic application of manually guided forces by an osteopathic physician to improve physiologic function and/or support homeostasis that has been altered by somatic dysfunction [2]. An osteopathic structural examination focuses on the patient's musculoskeletal system, with attention to posture and the motion of the spine and other joints. Palpatory examination is performed to evaluate asymmetry, changes in tissue texture, restriction of motion, and tenderness in the joints, muscles, ligaments, tendons, and fascia. An abnormal finding is called somatic dysfunction.

The ability to use palpation to detect somatic dysfunction is both a psychomotor and sensorimotor skill essential for osteopathic diagnosis and treatment. OMT is used to treat somatic dysfunction, with the goal of reducing pain, removing motion restrictions, improving mechanical function, or supporting the healing of an injury. Palpation is also used to evaluate a patient's response to OMT as well as other interventions such as physical therapy, medications, and injections.

Somatic dysfunction can be diagnosed by testing the patient's range of motion both passively and actively both at regional levels as well as in individual joints and spinal seg-

L. Griffin (✉)
Osteopathic Principles and Practices Department, Kentucky College of Osteopathic Medicine, University of Pikeville, Pikeville, KY, USA
e-mail: lauragriffin@upike.edu

D. C. Rosenberg
Physical Medicine and Rehabilitation, Harvard Medical School, Boston, MA, USA

Osteopathic Manipulative Medicine, Spaulding Rehabilitation Network, Boston, MA, USA
e-mail: Drosenberg@mgh.harvard.edu

© The Author(s), under exclusive license to Springer Nature Switzerland AG 2022

S. A. Mostoufi et al. (eds.), *Clinical Guide to Musculoskeletal Medicine*, https://doi.org/10.1007/978-3-030-92042-5_59

ments. A normal physiologic barrier is reached at the end of the active range of motion, while a passive range of motion carries the joint further to the anatomic barrier. However, somatic dysfunction creates a restrictive barrier that is reached before the normal physiologic barrier, and OMT is directed at restoring normal motion by improving or eliminating these restrictive barriers. Restoring normal motion may improve the body's self-healing capacity by enhancing arterial flow to and venous and lymphatic drainage from the tissues in the area. On a global level, maintaining optimal function of the thoraco-abdomino-pelvic cylinder and free motion of the diaphragm allows for better blood flow, tissue oxygenation, and lymphatic drainage for the whole body. A somatic dysfunction of the thoraco-abdomino-pelvic cylinder is believed to interfere with the body's self-healing and self-regulating mechanisms.

59.3 Methods of Osteopathic Manipulative Treatment (OMT)

There are multiple OMT methods used in patient care. A direct technique engages the restrictive barrier and carries the dysfunctional joint or tissue through that barrier such that normal, symmetrical motion is approached or completely restored. Indirect techniques move away from the restrictive barrier, thereby decreasing the tension in the tissues causing the dysfunction and presumably inhibiting the spinal reflex causing increased muscle hypertonicity. Some techniques are considered combined treatment methods in which the initial positioning of the tissues is away from the restrictive barrier then changing to a direct force to restore normal motion. Techniques can also be classified as active or passive. An active technique requires the patient to voluntarily perform a physician-directed motion, whereas in passive techniques, the patient needs only to stay relaxed.

59.3.1 High-Velocity/Low-Amplitude (HVLA) Technique

HVLA (Fig. 59.1), also known as thrust technique, is what is typically thought of when considering "manipulation." It is a passive, direct treatment in which a thrust is delivered quickly, over a very short distance to restore specific joint motion. This is always performed within the joint's normal range of motion, never moving past the anatomic barrier. With precise positioning of the involved joint, this can be done with minimal force. The thrust may or may not produce an audible "popping" sound, known as joint cavitation [3], but its presence does not indicate resolution of the somatic dysfunction, and its absence does not mean the thrust did not achieve the desired result. Like most osteopathic techniques, the principle of HVLA can be applied in most joints of the spine, ribs, pelvis, and extremities and is useful when a firm barrier or "hard end feel" is perceived on palpation.

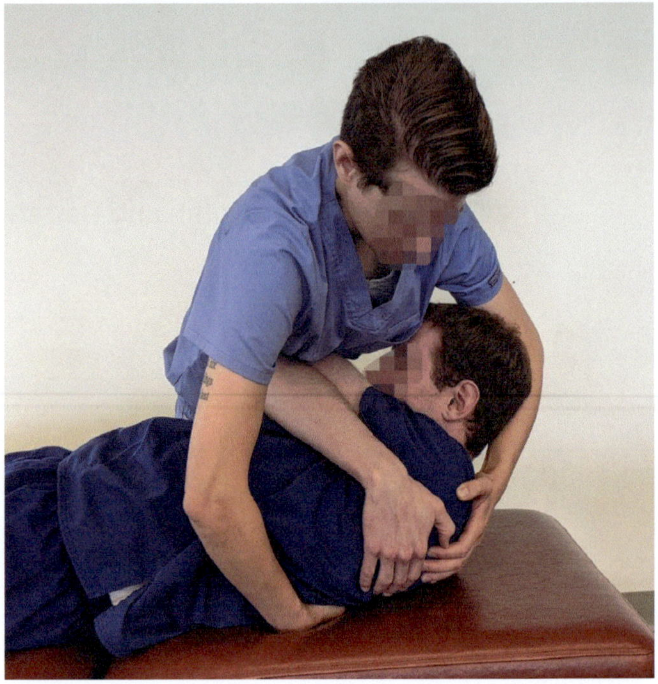

Fig. 59.1 High-velocity/low-amplitude (HVLA) technique (thrust technique)

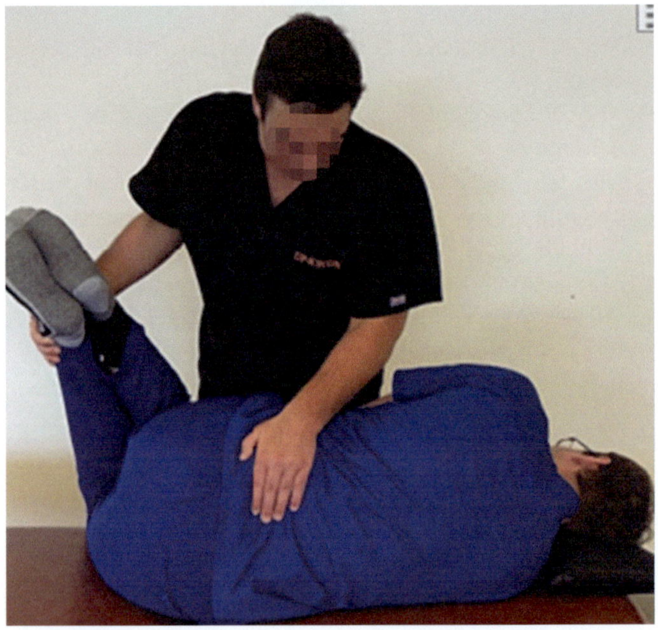

Fig. 59.2 Muscle energy technique

59.3.2 Muscle Energy Technique (MET)

MET (Fig. 59.2) is a direct, active technique in which the physician engages the restrictive barrier, holding the involved joint in a controlled position while the patient resists the physician's force isometrically for a few seconds at the physician's direction. After the tissues are allowed to relax for a short period, the new barrier is then engaged, and the technique is repeated until normal motion is restored. Muscle energy is well tolerated and is useful when a direct technique is needed, but there are contraindications to HVLA. It does require that the patient have enough strength to provide the necessary resistance and the ability to understand and respond to the physician's instructions.

Articulatory technique (Fig. 59.3) is a direct, passive technique in which the involved joint is moved through a moderate to a wide range of motion at a slow pace. The barrier can be engaged in a single movement, or the practitioner can use a repetitive springing motion to engage the barrier multiple times until normal motion is restored.

59.3.3 Myofascial Release (MFR)

MER (Fig. 59.4) technique is a passive technique that can be done in either a direct or indirect fashion, based on physician preference and patient tolerance. Indirect MFR and other indirect techniques are often used in cases in which directly engaging the barrier may be too painful or cause reflex spasm, such as when the patient has suffered an acute injury. MFR utilizes a constant force and ongoing palpatory feedback to reduce tension in the dysfunctional muscles and related fasciae.

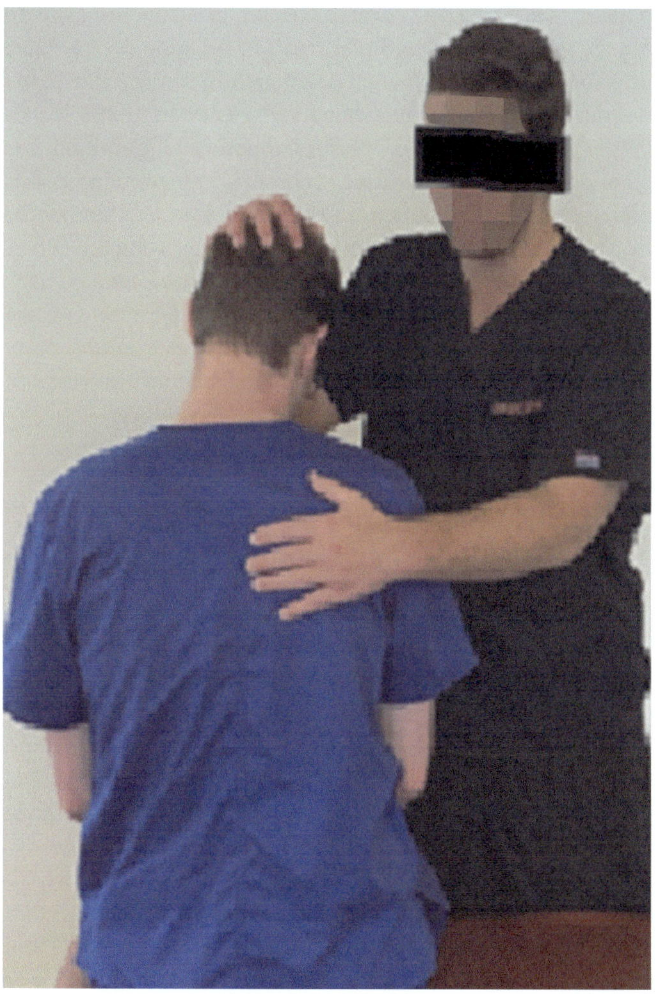

Fig. 59.3 Articulatory technique

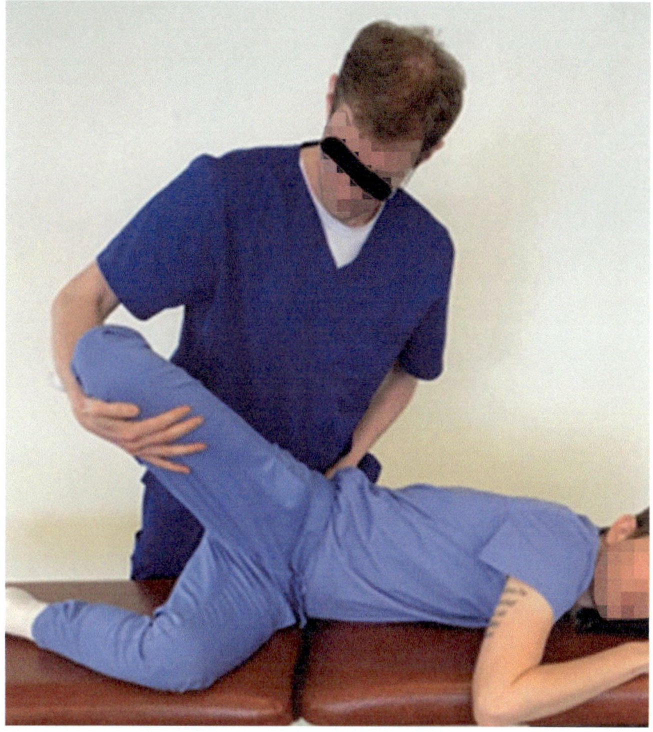

Fig. 59.4 Myofascial release (MFR) technique

59.3.4 Soft Tissue Techniques

These are a diverse group of techniques that may use longitudinal and/or perpendicular stretching of the muscles, as well as kneading and deep pressure (Fig. 59.5). These are used by themselves to treat hypertonicity of the muscles and fascial restrictions or may be employed prior to other treatments when the tissues are too restricted to comfortably engage the restrictive barrier.

59.3.5 Counter Strain

Also called strain/counterstrain (Fig. 59.6), it is a passive indirect technique that reduces pain from a specific tender point. Tender points are often referred to in the literature as tender points or Jones points, after the physician who developed the theory of counterstrain. They are believed to be a manifestation of somatic dysfunction of muscles and joints and are found in consistent locations associated with those

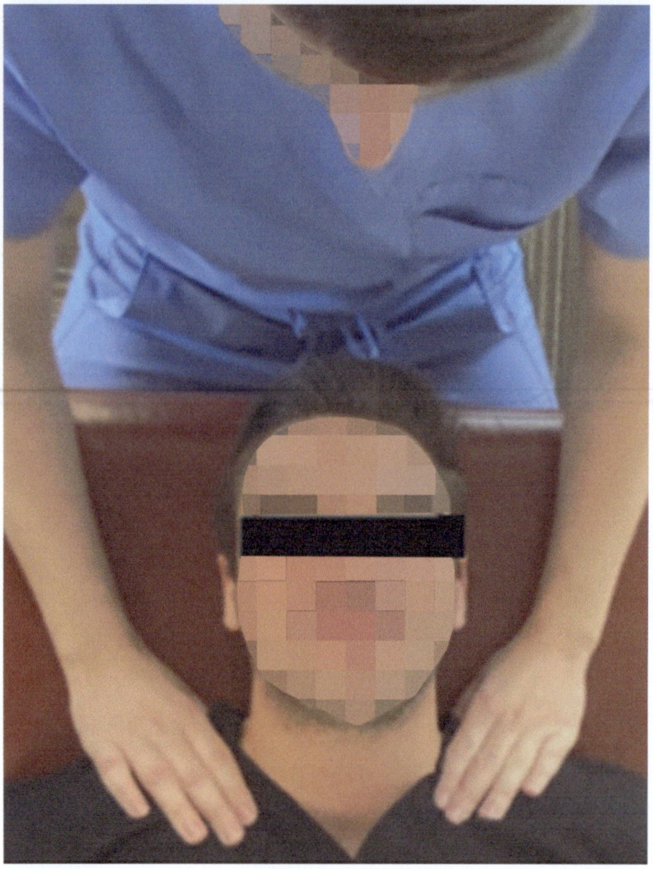

Fig. 59.5 Soft tissue technique

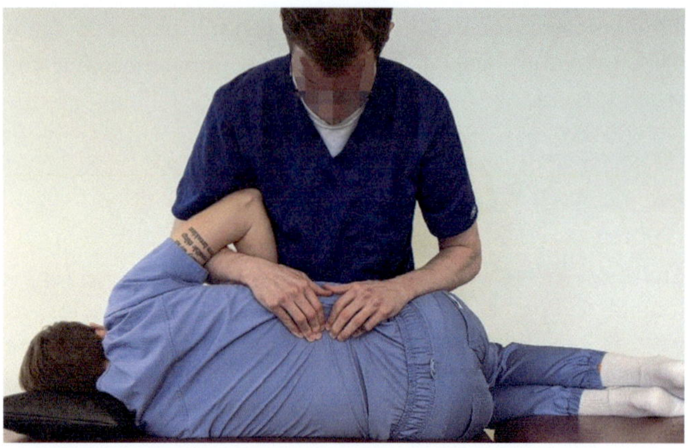

Fig. 59.6 Counterstrain technique

dysfunctions. Unlike myofascial trigger points, tender points do not radiate. The patient is positioned such that the tenderness in the point is nearly or completely relieved and that position is maintained for 90 s or until the tissues have completely relaxed. The patient is then passively returned to a neutral position, and the patient is re-examined for residual tenderness and somatic dysfunction. The indirect positioning of the patient is believed to reduce gamma efferent firing in

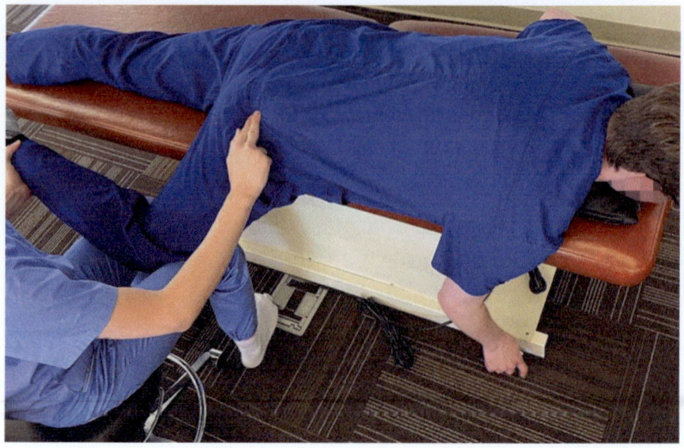

Fig. 59.7 Indirect technique

the involved muscles that are hypertonic due to the abnormal function of proprioceptive reflexes.

59.3.6 Indirect Techniques

Indirect techniques (Fig. 59.7) such as balanced ligamentous tension, facilitated positional release, and functional technique, among others, are presumed to function on the same physiologic mechanisms as counterstrain but are not based on locating particular tender points. Most commonly, a particular segmental or articular dysfunction is identified and positioned indirectly to affect the reflex hypertonicity that is maintaining the dysfunction. Often, they are differentiated by small features such as the addition of a compressive or decompressive force and whether the tissues are moved back through the restrictive barrier after initial treatment in the indirect position. One advantage to counterstrain and other indirect techniques is that they are well tolerated in cases of acute injury or severe pain and spasm.

59.4 Indications, Contraindication, and Complications of OMT

59.4.1 Indication for OMT

The indication for the application of osteopathic manipulative treatment techniques is the presence of somatic dysfunction diagnosed by palpation during an osteopathic structural exam. There are times in the setting of systemic illness that OMT such as a lymphatic pump or rib raising may be done to maximize a patient's physiologic function to aid in recovery without the diagnosis of somatic dysfunction. Those techniques can also help with the edema from an acute joint injury when performed proximal to that joint, where local techniques are likely contraindicated. Once a decision is made to do OMT, the type of technique selected is usually based on a combination of physician skill and experience together with patient condition and preference.

59.4.2 Contraindications for OMT

Contraindications can be either absolute or relative and are determined by many factors that are related to the patient's diagnosis, the type of technique, and the region being treated. For example, while any technique would be contraindicated at the site of an acute fracture or ligament rupture, once that is stabilized, gentle treatment of hypertonic muscles in adjacent regions may relieve the tension on the injured tissues. Most technique-related contraindications are for direct action techniques like HVLA, MET, or articulatory techniques, all of which are contraindicated in any type of acute tissue injury, severe osteoporosis, joint infection or inflammation, osteomyelitis, coagulation disorder, hypermobility, and severe arthritis or tumor, to name a few. Diagnosis-specific contraindications include things like rheumatoid arthritis, in which the upper cervical spine can become unstable in severe disease. Gentle indirect techniques in joints of the extremities that are not acutely inflamed may be safe and well tolerated, however. As long as the physician takes a thorough history, performs a detailed physical examination, and uses appropriate caution and common sense, it is easy to avoid using OMT in contraindicated situations.

59.4.3 Potential Complications with OMT

The most feared complication is vascular injury and CVA after cervical spine high-velocity manipulation. While statistically rare, the results can be devastating. Unfortunately, provocative tests have not been shown to predict who is vulnerable to vertebral artery insufficiency or injury and, in fact, creates the risk of causing the problem they are attempting to prevent. The position of extreme rotation combined with extension in the upper cervical spine should be avoided in both examination and treatment. Other possible complications can arise when too much force is used or force is applied too close to the endpoint of the range of motion, thus disrupting the anatomic barrier and causing tissue damage. Appropriate and judicious use of force should never put the patient at risk of tissue injury.

59.5 Complementary Effect of Osteopathic Care and Physical Therapy

Osteopathic physicians who do OMT have long recognized the benefit of adding physical therapy (PT) to their treatment plans. There are multiple ways these approaches can be synergistic. When patients presenting in such severe pain cannot tolerate structural examination and treatment in any meaningful fashion, starting with physical therapy modalities like heat, ultrasound, TENS, and gentle movement can reduce the patient's overall hyperalgesia and kinesiophobia prior to starting OMT. Patients who have been in chronic pain often become deconditioned which can impede their recovery process. Physical therapists can design a targeted exercise program to improve posture and core strength and stability, allowing the osteopathic treatments to be more effective and last longer. Chronic postural decompensation can create somatic dysfunction and pain that may be relieved by OMT but will return if those imbalances are not addressed.

59.6 Differentiating Osteopathic Manipulation from Chiropractic Manipulation

While both osteopathic and chiropractic manipulation were initially introduced around the same time in the late nineteenth century, they have evolved differently as evidenced by their treatment approaches and scope of practice. Of course, there are always exceptions to any generalization; however, some basic distinctions in these manipulative approaches can be made. Traditionally, chiropractors are thought to focus on spinal dysfunction in order to affect the neurologic function of the rest of the body via the spinal cord. Osteopathic physicians take a broader approach, also considering the osseous and soft tissue dysfunctions of the entire body to diagnose the cause of the patient complaint. Chiropractic manipulation is most commonly associated with primarily HVLA/thrust-type maneuvers, while OMT takes many different approaches as discussed in the beginning of this chapter. Osteopathic physicians rely on palpation to diagnose somatic dysfunction, while chiropractors typically diagnose subluxations on X-ray and may use other technology such as thermal scans to diagnose the paraspinal tissues. Lastly, chiropractors tend to see patients for shorter visits but with greater frequency than osteopathic physicians.

59.7 Osteopathic Applications to Common MSK Conditions

Manipulative treatment has been shown to be efficacious in many types of musculoskeletal conditions, but when looking for this evidence in the literature, it is important to remember to search broadly across all professions that provide manipulative treatment. These include osteopathic medicine, osteopathy performed by nonphysician osteopaths, chiropractic, and physical therapy. While these professions are by no means equivalent in their methods and scope of practice, the architecture and physiology of the joints and tissues do not change based on who is trying to affect them and, therefore, any studies showing the efficacy of manipulative treatment should be considered when evaluating the evidence. Some examples of manual treatment providing clinical benefit in common musculoskeletal conditions are provided here, but the body of literature is much greater than the scope of this chapter can detail.

59.7.1 Osteopathic Care in Shoulder Disorders

Shoulder pain is a common complaint and can have many different etiologies. Shwerla et al. performed a randomized controlled trial with a total of 70 patients utilizing five OMT treatments which demonstrated improvement in both the VAS and pain intensity measurements as well as improved frequency of pain episodes [4]. Atkinson et al. showed that chiropractic manipulation improved pain and range of motion in patients with rotator cuff tendinopathy [5]. Adhesive capsulitis has also been shown to respond well to manipulative treatment, including scapular mobilization and Spencer muscle energy technique [6, 7]. Because the shoulder girdle is a complex anatomical structure, it seems logical that ensuring free motion of all the associated articulations and soft tissues would be beneficial. In particular, many osteopathic physicians contend that since the scapula is almost entirely embedded within the muscle that attaches to the cervical and thoracic spine and ribcage as well as the clavicle and humerus, restoring optimal mechanics to all of those structures should be a prerequisite to addressing the actual shoulder dysfunction.

59.7.2 Osteopathic Care in Elbow Disorders

While elbow disorders such as medial and lateral epicondylitis are common, they have been less studied with regard to manipulation or other manual treatment as compared to other musculoskeletal diagnoses. However, a systematic review on the use of joint mobilization in the elbow, wrist, and hand did support the use of joint mobilization in lateral epicondylalgia [8]. Manipulation of the wrist has also been shown to be beneficial in lateral epicondylitis as compared to other physical therapy treatments [9].

59.7.3 Osteopathic Care in Wrist and Hand Disorders

With the almost constant use of computers, video game systems, and mobile devices, hand and wrist disorders like carpal tunnel syndrome (CTS) and de Quervain's tenosynovitis have become more prevalent. CTS has been shown to improve symptomatically with myofascial release and other manipulative techniques [10]. Additionally, an increase in the length of the transverse carpal ligament and improvement in nerve conduction studies have been demonstrated, although the number of patients in these studies has been small [11, 12]. Another small pilot study showed improvement in CTS symptomatology with multiple osteopathic treatments but no change in nerve conduction or functional morphology of the carpal tunnel to account for the symptomatic change [13]. Multiple case reports have shown the benefit of manual treatment in de Quervain's tenosynovitis, but no larger studies could be located.

59.7.4 Osteopathic Care in Pelvic Disorders

Sacroiliac (SI) joint pain and dysfunction can be a common component of mechanical low back pain [14, 15]. MET directed at the SI joint, along with moist heat, has been shown to improve pain and spinal ROM [16]. Dysfunction of the sacrum, innominates, and lumbar spine can affect leg length and weight-bearing [17], potentially leading to long-term articular and soft tissue changes. One study intended to compare thrust-type techniques, MET and a simulated technique applied to SI joint dysfunction in athletes, demonstrated improvement from both types of manipulation as compared to the sham technique [18, 13]. The SI joint also plays a role in intrapelvic complaints such as dysmenorrhea and chronic pelvic pain. Manipulation has been shown to improve the low back pain as well as serotonin levels in primary dysmenorrhea [19].

59.7.5 Osteopathic Care in Hip Disorders

Hip pain is a common complaint in athletes as well as the aging population experiencing degenerative changes to the femur and acetabulum. Interestingly, multiple studies regarding hip pain in athletes demonstrate that treatment of the SI joint actually affects hip pain, ROM, and performance, rather than the hip joint itself [20, 21]. This illustrates the osteopathic concepts of body unity and structure and function, specifically that the location of the pain is not always the location of the associated dysfunctions and a thorough structural exam is required rather than simply examining the area of the presenting complaint. With respect to osteoarthritis (OA) of the hip, one study from the Netherlands examined the impact of manual therapy versus exercise therapy on the pain and loss of function in 109 patients with hip OA. While both methods showed improvement, 81% of patients receiving manual therapy showed a decrease in pain and an increase in function as compared to 50% of the exercise therapy group [22].

59.7.6 Osteopathic Care in Knee Disorders

Patellofemoral pain syndrome (PFPS) is a common and well-studied diagnosis, and treatment is multifaceted, including different types of targeted exercise and manipulation of the knee as well as the rest of the body. One study that provided full-body osteopathic treatment showed statistically significant improvement in the Visual Analog Scale (VAS) for multiple measures of pain and function [23]. Zago et al. compared OMT applied to the lumbar spine, SI joint, hip, knee, and ankle to both exercise and no intervention in the treatment of PFPS. Both groups showed improvement in pain compared to the control group, but OMT also showed increased function and improvement in some individually measured lower extremity mechanics [24]. Osteoarthritis of the knee has been shown to respond well to OMT. In one study, OMT and exercise showed significantly higher functional improvement and pain relief when compared to exercise alone [25]. Another interesting study showed that full-body OMT performed preoperatively twice prior to total knee arthroplasty resulted in decreased postoperative pain and opioid consumption as compared to typical preoperative care [26].

59.7.7 Osteopathic Care in Ankle and Foot Disorders

Ankle sprains are a commonly seen injury in the emergency department and outpatient settings. Eisenhart et al. studied OMT in the emergency department for ankle injuries and demonstrated immediate improvement in pain and swelling and improvement in ROM when re-examined 5–7 days later [27]. A systematic review of manipulation in lateral ankle sprains showed improvement in multiple outcomes immediately after performing the treatments with no detrimental effects [28]. Plantar fasciitis is another common diagnosis that may be improved by the addition of manual therapy. Specifically, a systematic review by Fraser et al. showed a definite improvement in function and pain with the use of manual therapy as compared to more typical physical therapy treatments of stretching and strengthening, as well as other modalities [29]. As plantar fasciitis often has a prolonged course and significantly impacts patient quality of life, it is worth considering adding anything that will hasten full recovery.

59.7.8 Osteopathic Care in Spine Disorders

Most of the research on osteopathic treatment centers around spine disorders. One of the most influential articles has been the meta-analysis of studies on the treatment of low back pain [30] in which OMT was associated with highly significant reduction in pain ($p = 0.001$), significant reduction in pain associated with OMT for short-term, intermediate-term, and long-term follow-ups. Not many studies differentiate between types of OMT given the amount of clinical decision-making involved in each patient case; however, one study showed no difference between HVLA and MET which were both effective in reducing pain after the first session and after 15 days [31]. OMT has also been shown to be effective in neck pain and cervicogenic headache [32, 33]. Osteopathic treatment is commonly used in other frequently seen spine disorders including scoliosis, arthritis, and disc problems. There are a wide variety of studies showing a range of efficacy from positive long-term response to no statistical difference from standard care, but no major studies have shown negative outcomes [34]. Given that back pain is in the top five most common reasons for visits to a physician, there are many opportunities for integration of osteopathic treatment in the overall care plan for patients. Considering that back pain is a major cause of absenteeism from work, getting patients back to work more quickly using OMT as part of the treatment could have a positive effect on economic outcomes in terms of productivity and reduced health care and disability costs.

59.7.9 Osteopathic Care in Chest Wall Pain

Chest wall pain, also known as chest wall syndrome, is a nonspecific term that encompasses multiple diagnoses and etiologies including trauma, costochondritis, Tietze's syndrome, lower rib pain syndrome, and others. It is essentially used to account for chest wall symptoms after more serious visceral problems or rheumatic diseases that could be perceived as chest pain are ruled out. Hussain et al. detail the osteopathic approach to all types of chest pain [35]. Flodine and Thomas provide an excellent summary and treatment approach for inhaled rib somatic dysfunctions which are commonly seen in anterior chest wall pain [36], and the principles of evaluation and treatment described there represent a comprehensive approach to any chest wall complaints that are not due to any other diagnosis.

References

1. Trends in the use of complementary health in the United States: 2002–2012 [Internet]. Nih.gov. [cited 2021 Aug 6]. Available from: https://www.nccih.nih.gov/research/trends-in-the-use-of-complementary-health-in-the-united-states-20022012
2. Rebecca Giusti DO. Glossary of osteopathic terminology. Bethesda: American Association of Colleges of Osteopathic Medicine; 2017.
3. Kawchuk GN, Fryer J, Jaremko JL, Zeng H, Rowe L, Thompson R. Real-time visualization of joint cavitation. PLoS One. 2015;10(4):e0119470.
4. Schwerla F, Hinse T, Klosterkamp M, Schmitt T, Rütz M, Resch K-L. Osteopathic treatment of patients with shoulder pain. A pragmatic randomized controlled trial. J Bodyw Mov Ther. 2020;24(3):21–8.

5. Atkinson M, Mathews R, Brantingham JW, Globe G, Cassa T, Bonnefin D, Korporaal C. A randomized controlled trial to assess the efficacy of shoulder manipulation vs. placebo in the treatment of shoulder pain due to rotator cuff tendinopathy. J Am Chiropr Assoc. 2008;45(9):11–26.
6. Iqbal M, Riaz H, Ghous M, Masood K. Comparison of Spencer muscle energy technique and passive stretching in adhesive capsulitis: a single blind randomized control trial. J Pak Med Assoc. 2020;70(12(A)):2113–8.
7. Knebl JA, Shores JH, Gamber RG, Gray WT, Herron KM. Improving functional ability in the elderly via the Spencer technique, an osteopathic manipulative treatment: a randomized, controlled trial. J Am Osteopath Assoc. 2002;102(7):387–96.
8. Heiser R, O'Brien VH, Schwartz DA. The use of joint mobilization to improve clinical outcomes in hand therapy: a systematic review of the literature. J Hand Ther. 2013;26(4):297–311; quiz 311
9. Struijs PAA, Damen P-J, Bakker EWP, Blankevoort L, Assendelft WJJ, van Dijk CN. Manipulation of the wrist for management of lateral epicondylitis: a randomized pilot study. Phys Ther. 2003;83(7):608–16.
10. Sucher BM. Myofascial manipulative release of carpal tunnel syndrome: documentation with magnetic resonance imaging. J Am Osteopath Assoc. 1993;93(12):1273–8.
11. Sucher BM, Hinrichs RN. Manipulative treatment of carpal tunnel syndrome: biomechanical and osteopathic intervention to increase the length of the transverse carpal ligament. J Am Osteopath Assoc. 1998;98(12):679–86.
12. Sucher BM. Palpatory diagnosis and manipulative management of carpal tunnel syndrome. J Am Osteopath Assoc. 1994;94(8):647–63.
13. Burnham T, Higgins DC, Burnham RS, Heath DM. Effectiveness of osteopathic manipulative treatment for carpal tunnel syndrome: a pilot project. J Am Osteopath Assoc. 2015;115(3):138–48.
14. Sembrano JN, Polly DW Jr. How often is low back pain not coming from the back? Spine (Phila Pa 1976). 2009;34(1):E27–32.
15. Cohen SP. Sacroiliac joint pain: a comprehensive review of anatomy, diagnosis, and treatment. Anesth Analg. 2005;101(5):1440–53.
16. Rajesh Sewani SS. Effect of hot moist pack and muscle energy technique in subjects with Sacroilitis-iliac joint dysfunction. Int J Sci Res. 2017;6(2):669–72.
17. Qureshi Y, Kusienski A, Bemski JL, Luksch JR, Knowles LG. Effects of somatic dysfunction on leg length and weight bearing. J Am Osteopath Assoc. 2014;114(8):620–30.
18. García-Peñalver UJ, Palop-Montoro MV, Manzano-Sánchez D. Effectiveness of the muscle energy technique versus osteopathic manipulation in the treatment of sacroiliac joint dysfunction in athletes. Int J Environ Res Public Health. 2020;17(12):4490.
19. Molins-Cubero S, Rodríguez-Blanco C, Oliva-Pascual-Vaca A, Heredia-Rizo AM, Boscá-Gandía JJ, Ricard F. Changes in pain perception after pelvis manipulation in women with primary dysmenorrhea: a randomized controlled trial. Pain Med. 2014;15(9):1455–63.
20. Sandell J, Palmgren PJ, Björndahl L. Effect of chiropractic treatment on hip extension ability and running velocity among young male running athletes. J Chiropr Med. 2008;7(2):39–47.
21. Cibulka MT, Delitto A. A comparison of two different methods to treat hip pain in runners. J Orthop Sports Phys Ther. 1993;17(4):172–6.
22. Hoeksma HL, Dekker J, Ronday HK, Heering A, van der Lubbe N, Vel C, et al. Comparison of manual therapy and exercise therapy in osteoarthritis of the hip: a randomized clinical trial. Arthritis Rheum. 2004;51(5):722–9.
23. Tramontano M, Pagnotta S, Lunghi C, Manzo C, Manzo F, Consolo S, et al. Assessment and management of somatic dysfunctions in patients with patellofemoral pain syndrome. J Am Osteopath Assoc. 2020;120(3):165–73.
24. Zago J, Amatuzzi F, Rondinel T, Matheus JP. Osteopathic manipulative treatment versus exercise program in runners with patellofemoral pain syndrome: a randomized controlled trial. J Sport Rehabil. 2020;30(4):609–18.
25. Altınbilek T, Murat S, Yumuşakhuylu Y, İçağasıoğlu A. Osteopathic manipulative treatment improves function and relieves pain in knee osteoarthritis: a single-blind, randomized-controlled trial. Turk J Phys Med Rehabil. 2018;64(2):114–20.
26. Barral P, Klouche S, Barral N, Lemoulec Y-P, Thés A, Bauer T. Preoperative osteopathic manipulative therapy improves postoperative pain and reduces opioid consumption after total knee arthroplasty: a prospective comparative study. J Am Osteopath Assoc. 2020;120(7):436–45.
27. Eisenhart AW, Gaeta TJ, Yens DP. Osteopathic manipulative treatment in the emergency department for patients with acute ankle injuries. J Am Osteopath Assoc. 2003;103(9):417–21.
28. Loudon JK, Reiman MP, Sylvain J. The efficacy of manual joint mobilisation/manipulation in treatment of lateral ankle sprains: a systematic review. Br J Sports Med. 2014;48(5):365–70.
29. Fraser JJ, Corbett R, Donner C, Hertel J. Does manual therapy improve pain and function in patients with plantar fasciitis? A systematic review. J Man Manip Ther. 2018;26(2):55–65.
30. Licciardone JC, Brimhall AK, King LN. Osteopathic manipulative treatment for low back pain: a systematic review and meta-analysis of randomized controlled trials. BMC Musculoskelet Disord. 2005;6(1):43.
31. Sturion LA, Nowotny AH, Barillec F, Barette G, Santos GK, Teixeira FA, et al. Comparison between high-velocity low-amplitude manipulation and muscle energy technique on pain and trunk neuromuscular postural control in male workers with chronic low back pain: a randomised crossover trial. S Afr J Physiother. 2020;76(1):1420.
32. Fryer G, Alvizatos J, Lamaro J. The effect of osteopathic treatment on people with chronic and sub-chronic neck pain: a pilot study. Int J Osteopath Med. 2005;8(2):41–8.
33. Nilsson N, Christensen HW, Hartvigsen J. The effect of spinal manipulation in the treatment of cervicogenic headache. J Manip Physiol Ther. 1997;20(5):326–30.
34. Snelling NJ. Spinal manipulation in patients with disc herniation: a critical review of risk and benefit. Int J Osteopath Med. 2006;9(3):77–84.
35. Hussain MS, Kristen de Vries III OMS, Terzella MJ, Yao SC. Osteopathic considerations in the management of chest pain. Osteopat Fam Phys [Internet]. 2016 [cited 2021 Aug 6];8(3):20–26.
36. Flodine TE, Thomas M. Osteopathic manipulative treatment: inhaled rib dysfunction. In: StatPearls. Treasure Island: StatPearls Publishing; 2020.

Regenerative Medicine: Musculoskeletal Applications

60

Joshua Martin and Gerard Malanga

60.1 Prolotherapy

Prolotherapy is the use of an irritant to achieve tissue healing, typically at painful tendon and ligament insertions (enthesis) or joints. The term prolotherapy (from proliferant therapy) was coined based on the observation that a larger cross-sectional area (i.e., "proliferation") of ligamentous tissue was seen after prolotherapy injection in animal models [1]. Prolotherapy also has emerging evidence for its benefit in painful joints such as the knee OA, where the mechanism for improvements in pain and function is not yet fully understood. In practice, prolotherapy has been studied and offered as a series of 4–6 injections, which may be week(s) apart. Prolotherapy is very inexpensive, and the injectate is easy to mix in an office setting. Research on prolotherapy may be limited by the fact that it is not covered by CMS or other health insurance (Table 60.1). Prolotherapy does not involve the injection of any human blood or tissue product, so the above FDA regulation does not apply.

Mechanism Chemotactic agents are thought to elicit the inflammatory cascade in tendons and ligaments as some cells lyse with the net effect of an increase of growth factors, resulting in fibroblast proliferation and collagen formation. The ideal outcome of this treatment is stronger connective tissue, with improved soft tissue recovery.

Material The most common *irritant* used is hyperosmolar dextrose, but other irritants include zinc sulfate, glycerin, phenol, and guaiacol. Dextrose is felt to be an ideal proliferant because it is water-soluble and a normal constituent within blood, which can be injected safely. Dextrose is typically injected with a concentration above 10% (studies have ranged from 10% to 20%) as it can create an osmotic effect on local cells at this level. *Chemotactic agents* used include sodium morrhuate.

Table 60.1 Highest level of evidence for prolotherapy

Rotator cuff tendinopathy	Randomized prospective comparative trial, prolotherapy vs exercise, 1-year follow-up; improved VAS, SPADI, and WORC [2] Randomized controlled, blinded prospective comparative trial vs saline, 9-month follow-up, improved pain and satisfaction [3]
Plantar fasciitis	Randomized prospective comparative trial, prolotherapy vs stretching, 1-year follow-up improved VAS, FAOS [4]
Osgood-Schlatter disease	Randomized prospective comparative trial, prolotherapy vs lidocaine injection vs physical therapy. 1-year follow-up, improved pain scales in prolotherapy compared to either group [5]
Knee OA	Randomized controlled, blinded prospective comparative trial. Prolotherapy vs lidocaine vs home exercises. 1-year follow-up showed improved pain, function, and stiffness WOMAC scores [6] Randomized controlled, blinded prospective comparative trial. Prolotherapy vs lidocaine. 1-year follow-up, improved pain and swelling [7]
Lateral epicondylalgia	Randomized controlled, blinded prospective comparative trial prolotherapy vs steroids, 3-month follow-up. Improved VAS and quick DASH at 3 months [8]
Finger osteoarthritis	Prospective randomized double-blind placebo-controlled trial. Prolotherapy vs xylocaine, 6-month follow-up. Improved pain with motion [9]

60.2 Platelet-Rich Plasma (PRP)

Platelet-rich plasma (PRP) generally describes plasma consisting of platelet density above baseline. Platelets have alpha-granules containing cytokines, anabolic and anti-inflammatory

J. Martin
New Jersey Regenerative Institute, Hanover, NJ, USA

Regenerative Orthopedics and Sports Medicine (ROSM), Reston, VA, USA

G. Malanga (✉)
New Jersey Orthopaedic and Sports Medicine, New Jersey Regenerative Institute, Hanover, NJ, USA

Department of Physical Medicine & Rehabilitation, Rutgers School of Medicine, Newark, NJ, USA

© The Author(s), under exclusive license to Springer Nature Switzerland AG 2022

S. A. Mostoufi et al. (eds.), *Clinical Guide to Musculoskeletal Medicine*, https://doi.org/10.1007/978-3-030-92042-5_60

growth factors, as well as dense granules containing serotonin, adenosine diphosphate, dopamine, and adenosine triphosphate. Alpha-granules more specifically contain multiple key growth factors including insulin-like growth factor (IGF-I/III), transforming growth factor beta (TGF-β), platelet-derived growth factor (PDGF), vascular endothelial growth factor (VEGF), and basic fibroblast growth factor (bFGF). IGF-I stimulates fibroblast chemotaxis and proliferation, mostly during inflammatory and proliferative phases of healing. TGF-β has multiple functions including mesenchymal stem cell (MSC) stimulation and specialization, collagen synthesis, neovascularization, chemotaxis of endothelial cells, and regulation of mitosis. TGF-β also plays a role in fibrosis of skeletal muscle, ultimately leading to scar formation. PDGF stimulates other growth factors and modifies tissue during the process of healing. Taken together, these cytokines support anabolism, and there are also immunomodulatory properties of PRP that may counteract the effects of catabolic cytokines and interleukins.

There are additional components to consider in PRP, and not all PRP is created the same. PRP may be categorized by platelet concentration, concentration of total leukocytes, composition of leukocytes (neutrophils vs. monocytes), and concentration of RBCs. PRP may also be activated prior to injection. Various classification systems have been introduced, such as the PLRA classification (platelet count, leukocyte presence, RBC presence, and activation) without any particular classification system becoming standard for the field. Generally, RBCs are toxic to the cartilage and bone, do not provide helpful cell signaling, and should be removed from PRP products. The presence of leukocytes, especially neutrophils, is a current topic of research, and unfortunately, many studies on PRP do not fully quantify the cell counts of this component. The lack of PRP preparation protocols and injectate characterization, as well as heterogeneity in PRP preparation injection protocols, makes it difficult to compare studies and contributes to some mixed outcomes reported with PRP treatments. At this time, neutrophils are thought to be counterproductive in joints as they release free radicals and dominate the early stages of inflammation. Neutrophils have a catabolic profile with higher concentrations of tumor necrosis factor-α (TNF-α), interleukin 6 (IL-6), interferon-ϒ (IFN-ϒ), and interleukin-1 (IL-1), which may contribute to synoviocyte death and are counterproductive to the desired effect on joints. Yet, there is debate in the role of neutrophils in tendon pathologies as some postulate neutrophils may break down tendinopathic architecture for remodeling. Although, this theory has never been validated.

Monocytes and macrophages are other key leukocytes that play a critical role in injury repair. Monocytes and macrophages guide vascular remodeling, stimulation of local stem cells and progenitor cells, and structural repair in muscle and bone. These cells span a continuum of inflammatory (M1) macrophages to anti-inflammatory or pro-regenerative macrophages (M2), and their function depends on their microenvironment.

Table 60.2 Evidence for PRP use in orthopedics

Knee OA	The most heavily studied application for PRP. Best outcomes are for leukocyte poor PRP for mild knee osteoarthritis (KL 1–2). PRP lasts longer than HA injections (1 year vs 6 months)
Hip OA	Multiple studies found benefit with both PRP and HA [10]. More mild, higher platelet concentration, lower leukocytes tended to respond better [11]
SI joint dysfunction	Study with superiority to steroids [12]
Lateral epicondylosis	Multiple level 1 evidence supporting leukocyte-rich PRP over steroids [13, 14]
Greater trochanteric insertional tendinopathy	Multiple studies with superiority over steroids [15, 16]
Plantar fasciopathy	Supported by studies with US guidance +PRP characterization [17], not supported by studies without guidance or PRP characterization [18]
Patellar tendinopathy	Superior to dry needling for short-term outcomes [19], at 6 and 12 months superior to shockwave therapy [20]
Rotator cuff tendinopathies	Mixed results in the literature, although results supported PRP when ultrasound-guided and injectate described [21–23]
Achilles tendinopathy	Mixed results, without strong evidence to support PRP use

It is good practice to perform cell counts to determine the actual content of the PRP injected into an individual. These counts should include baseline as well as post-processing numbers. It is helpful to dose the number of the platelets given, as this is the intervention provided by the practitioner. It is also important to instruct patients to avoid NSAIDs and aspirin for 2 weeks before and after PRP injections to get the maximal effect from PRP. This is because NSAIDs interfere with platelet degranulation, and the lifespan of platelets is on average just over 10 days.

There are numerous studies regarding the use of PRP, in the treatment of various orthopedic conditions including tendinopathies and joint osteoarthritis (Table 60.2). There is additionally new emerging evidence regarding PRP use in the spine (epidural, facet, and sacroiliac joint injections) as well as around nerve sheaths, but there is currently a lack of high-quality studies.

60.3 Platelet-Poor Plasma (PPP)

Platelet-poor plasma (PPP) has been previously regarded as a waste product from the production of PRP, but there is laboratory evidence to suggest PPP has beneficial effects on myogenesis, the formation of skeletal muscle tissue. PPP contains fibrinogen and fibronectin, which mediate fibroblast proliferation, capillary tube proliferation, and angiogenesis, thereby promoting revascularization and wound healing. PPP also contains bioactive molecules such as PDGF and IGF-1, which may mediate the pro-myogenic effect on myoblasts. In laboratory studies, PPP induces myoblasts to differentiate and create myotubes, the multinucleated cells that result from the fusion of myoblasts which become muscle fibers. PRP does contain a greater quantity of platelet-derived factors such as TGFβ-1 that are detrimental for this differentiation and are pro-fibrotic, so PPP is thought to hold promise for skeletal muscle injuries [24]. More clinical studies are needed to determine whether PPP does improve muscle pain and function. Of note, PPP is in compliance with FDA guidelines for regenerative products.

60.4 Bone Marrow-Based Injections

Bone marrow is found in many areas of the body and is felt to contain various cells including cells often referred to as mesenchymal stem cells that may further differentiate or participate in cell signaling during the healing process. Mesenchymal stem cells, or MSCs, may be best referred to as "medicinal signaling cells," for their paracrine/immunomodulatory/trophic effects on nearby cells in the healing process as recommended by Arnold Caplan [25]. MSCs are also seen in umbilical cords, skeletal muscle, and synovial tissue but are particularly rich in the bone marrow and adipose [26]. MSCs can direct differentiation, replacing expired cells, although they may have even greater local effects through the secretion of growth factors, chemokines, cytokines, and exosomes known to promote tissue repair. MSCs have been shown to have paracrine effects through transforming growth factor beta (TGF-ß), fibroblast growth factor (FGF), and vascular endothelial growth factor (VEGF), which aid in the repair of tissue and modulation of inflammation. MSCs also have an immunomodulatory role through polarizing monocytes from inflammatory (M1) to anti-inflammatory or pro-regenerative cells (M2).

MSCs in bone are present in highest concentrations in central bone sites such as the sternum, vertebral bodies, and iliac crest. The iliac crest has been found to have the greatest concentration of MSCs, is in a convenient location for aspiration, and can be aspirated without significant discomfort, so it has become the most common source for aspirating MSCs in humans. Several studies have noted that to maximize yields of total nucleated cells, it is best to use small-volume aspirations from multiple sites or multiple depths [27]. After the first 10-15 cc of aspirate at each site, there is an increased amount of whole blood compared to the desired nucleated cells, and typically 60–120 mL of bone marrow aspirate is desirable between the multiple sites. Following aspiration, a concentration of the bone marrow aspirate is felt to be necessary to reduce the volume of the injectate and produce the greatest concentrations of cells per milliliter.

Table 60.3 Bone marrow aspirate-based injections and evidence

Knee OA	The most heavily studied, generally beneficial. It has been suggested 400 million cells are required [28]. Studies with less effect often have procedural mistakes (e.g., many RBCs injected rather than concentrated nucleated cells)
Elbow tendinopathy	Prospective case series with intra-tendinous injection of bone marrow concentrate beneficial through 12-week follow-up [29]
Rotator cuff Glenohumeral OA	Registry of 115 shoulders with generally good outcomes [30]
Hip OA	Improved numeric pain score, and Oxford Hip Scale, persisting with multiple-year follow-up [31]
Discogenic pain	Multiple publications for discogenic back pain, with dose-dependent improvement [32]

The following conditions listed in Table 60.3 have the most data regarding bone marrow aspirate efficacy. Some surgical applications such as treating cartilage defects, avascular necrosis, and hip osteonecrosis with procedures or injections below the cartilage are out of scope of this chapter.

60.5 Adipose-Based Injections

Adipose tissue also contains a heterogenous population of stromal cells which are involved in cell signaling, providing a supply of MSCs. Adipose tissue may be processed into several different products, including microfragmented adipose tissue (MFAT), enzyme-digested stromal vascular fraction (SVF), and cultured adipose stem cells (ASC). All of these products have different concentrations of their relative cellular components and may be different in their biological effects. At this time, certain devices that can create MFAT have 510(k) clearance to provide MFAT, which providers have been using for various orthopedic conditions. SVF and ASCs are not minimally manipulated, so they cannot yet be used in practice outside of an FDA-approved study.

Previously bone marrow was felt to be the preferred source for MSCs; however, bone marrow-derived MSCs have not been shown to have superiority over adipose-derived MSCs, and many providers prefer adipose due to ease of aspiration. In fact, mature adipocytes have been shown to be able to de-differentiate in vitro, expressing mesenchymal morphology and immunophenotype, with a similar DNA methylation condition to bone marrow-derived MSCs [33]. Studies comparing MFAT and bone marrow concentrate for knee osteoarthritis have not shown a significant difference between the two sources [34]. Bone marrow cellarity may decline as we age, while the content of fatty tissues does not change significantly, so clinicians may prefer to use adipose-derived products over bone marrow in the elderly for this reason as well.

60.5.1 Adipose Tissue Preparations

(a) *Microfragmented adipose tissue (MFAT)* contains many of the same heterogenous stromal cells as regular adipose, but with oils and debris removed. MFAT is obtained using tumescent anesthesia and lipoaspirating the adipose with a low-pressure syringe. Tumescent anesthesia refers to subcutaneous infiltration of large volumes of tumescent fluid containing lidocaine, saline, and epinephrine (1:1,000,000) to produce anesthesia and reduce bleeding of the targeted areas. Once harvested, MFAT is obtained by resizing the lipoaspirate tissue by mechanical processing. The adipose is washed with normal saline to remove oils, RBCs, and debris. The final product contains a variety of cells including mature adipocytes, endothelial cells, and adipose-derived stem cells. The processing meets the FDA's requirement of minimal manipulation. MFAT can be injected under ultrasound guidance to the location of interest.

There are also technical considerations for lipoaspirating the adipose that may make the procedure go smoothly. It is helpful to spend time to find areas that have sufficient fat reserves, often at the upper buttocks, or at the posterolateral thighs. Ultrasound can be considered to identify locations that contain sufficient adipose tissue. After injecting tumescent anesthesia, it is helpful to wait 15 minutes for the epinephrine to take effect. This will reduce bleeding and the number of RBCs in the product. Pre-tunneling (going back and forth with the cannula to create tracks) during the stage injecting tumescent anesthesia may make harvesting easier, faster, and with less trauma to other subcutaneous tissues.

(b) *Stromal vascular fraction (SVF)* is a heterogeneous population of various immune, precursor, progenitor, stromal, and stem cells, without the mature adipose cells as seen in MFAT. Obtaining SVF requires enzymatic dissociation, centrifugation, and filtration, which is more than minimal manipulation, as the properties of the adipose tissue are altered with disruption of the collagen-based extracellular matrix. After processing the product contains adipose-derived stem cells, pericytes, hematopoietic stem cells, endothelial progenitors, fibroblasts, smooth muscle cells, T regulatory cells, monocytes, macrophages, lymphocytes, and pre-adipocytes. FDA-approved studies are currently ongoing for specific indications, such as knee osteoarthritis, regarding the use of SVF.

Table 60.4 Applications and evidence of adipose-based injections

Knee OA	The most heavily studied, 80+ peer-reviewed publications with MFAT. Positive results for more advanced osteoarthritis compared to PRP (KL 2–3), many with 3-year follow-up
Meniscus injury	Cohort and case studies with favorable outcomes
Rotator cuff tears	Numerous cases of reduced shoulder pain, reduced defect size, studies have included MFAT and SVF [35]
Achilles tendinopathy	Randomized prospective clinical trial, SVF superior to PRP [36]
Lateral epicondylosis	SVF in 12 cases, improvement in pain scores, and tendon defect healing on ultrasound [37]
Osteonecrosis of the femoral head	SVF case reports with improvements in symptoms and bone regeneration on MRI [38–40]

(c) *Adipose stem cells (ASCs)* may also be culture expanded when seeking to obtain larger quantities of a purer stem cell product. Cells may be cultured in a medium such as fetal bovine serum or human serum. Adipose stem cell expansion can take weeks to obtain a large number of true stem cells, so this product is more than manipulated and not same-day use. These techniques are clearly not in accordance with FDA guidelines for regenerative procedures.

Clinical studies have included MFAT and SVF, with MFAT the most commonly used adipose product. Most common applications are given in Table 60.4. There have been additional studies with adipose-based products combined with various surgical procedures, but that is beyond the scope of ultrasound-guided injections.

60.6 Alpha-2 Macroglobulin (A2M)

Alpha-2 macroglobulin (A2M) is a plasma protein mostly found in blood and bone marrow. It is mainly produced in the liver but is also produced locally by macrophages and fibroblasts. A2M can block matrix metalloproteases (MMPs), such as collagenase and trypsin. Considering some of these MMPs are thought to break down cartilage in rheumatoid and osteoarthritis, there has been interest in using A2M to treat these conditions. There have been intra-articular animal models with A2M exerting an anti-inflammatory effect, attenuating cartilage and bone loss in a collagen II-induced arthritis model, the most common rheumatoid arthritis model [41]. There have also been animal models of osteoarthritis demonstrating chondroprotective effects of A2M in rats [42]. At this time, there have been no studies with long-term outcomes regarding the efficacy of using A2M to treat arthritis in humans.

60.7 Interleukin Receptor Antagonist Protein (IRAP)

IRAP is a member of the interleukin cytokine family, where IL-1RA protein is a natural inhibitor of the pro-inflammatory effect of IL1β, decreasing inflammation and modulating the immune response. IRAP is secreted by various types of cells including immune cells, epithelial cells, and adipocytes. IRAP has not been well studied for injections in humans, although it has been used in veterinary medicine to inject the joints of horses and other animals. Anakinra is a pharmaceutical recombinant and slightly modified version of the human interleukin 1 receptor antagonist protein, a subcutaneous injection, used for the treatment of rheumatoid arthritis in humans. Researchers in Germany have also published an IRAP product called Regenokine (US product name) and Orthokine (German product name). Obtaining this product from whole blood requires heating before centrifugation and is not FDA compliant.

60.8 Birth Tissues

Amniotic membrane and amniotic fluid products are obtained from donors from uncomplicated, elective C-sections, as this is relatively aseptic compared to vaginal delivery. After collection, the products are washed in antibiotic and anti-fungal agents, then stored as cryopreserved human amniotic membrane or dehydrated human amniotic membrane products. To date, birth tissues containing live cells such as umbilical cord blood and placental tissues cannot be used for orthopedic conditions (not FDA compliance for homologous use). There have additionally been issues with bacterially contaminated products in patients who have received non-FDA-approved umbilical cord blood-derived stem cell products. Cultures of unopened products have been identified with *E. coli* and *E. faecalis*, and patients with joint injections or infusions have suffered from bloodstream infections, joint infections, and epidural abscesses [43].

In 2018, a single product containing allogeneic micronized dehydrated human amnion/chorion membrane was given regenerative medicine advanced therapy (RMAT) designation by FDA for treatment of knee OA. Instead of cells, these products are thought to contain growth factors that may help in the healing response. Human clinical trials of these products are still lacking.

60.9 Exosomes

Exosomes are membrane-bound extracellular vesicles that contain and transfer not only protein and lipids but also mRNA and microRNA into acceptor cells. Exosomes were once thought to be a system to dispose of debris, but there is now evidence that the cargo has functional effects in recipient cells. Exosomes are thought to play roles in cell-cell communication and transmission of macromolecules between cells. It is not well understood how to specifically obtain and inject regenerative exosomes. Exosomes may play roles in tissue healing, but their exact functions are poorly understood, and under FDA regulations, there are currently no approved uses of exosomes.

60.10 Posttreatment Rehabilitation

There has been very little research regarding post-regenerative procedure rehabilitation.

Some procedures such as needle tenotomy of the Achilles may merit a few weeks of relative rest prior to starting aggressive physical therapy, and other applications may not require delay in rehab. Mautner et al. published a suggested rehabilitation protocol based on basic scientific understanding of tissue healing [44]. Regenerative procedures themselves also have some theoretical considerations that may guide current practice.

Physical therapy generally begins at 4 weeks following the procedure depending on the injection, and eccentric exercises with greater tendon loads may be introduced at 6 weeks for tendon procedures. Recovery after regenerative procedures can be considered in light of the stages of the healing response:

(a) *Initial Phase:* For the first few days, there is growth factor and cytokine release, chemotaxis, and synthesis of type III collagen. This initial phase with regenerative treatments may have differences compared to the typically described "inflammatory phase" of tissue healing as the tissue products have a different composition compared to whole blood.
(b) *Inflammatory Phase:* By preferentially selecting the appropriate blood or tissue products (like PRP or adipose), the local environment of the injection may have more of an anti-inflammatory cytokine profile in regard to mediators of pain and swelling. NSAIDs should be avoided for approximately 2 weeks before and after injection. NSAIDs have antiplatelet effects in regard to PRP, and depending on the dose and duration may impair soft tissue healing. After injection immobilization is not necessary in most cases, as this may be detrimental to the recovery of tendons, ligaments, and muscle. Tissues best respond to motion and load for healing, via mechanotranduction. Topical heat rather than ice may be considered, as ice may impair platelet function and degranulation after these procedures.
(c) *Proliferation phase:* Generally, it is few weeks after PRP injection where type II collagen is laid down with proteoglycan production. Activity as tolerated may be con-

sidered to preserve a range of motion, but the patient may not be ready for formal therapy that more aggressively loads the area. Rather, a gradual loading of tissue would be recommended. Finally, the remodeling phase takes place during the first 6 weeks to 1 year, where type 1 collagen is laid down. Physical therapy generally begins at 4 weeks following the procedure depending on the injection, and eccentric exercises with greater tendon loads may be introduced at 6 weeks for tendon procedures.

60.11 FDA Guidance for "Regenerative Treatments"

If a provider is to offer regenerative treatments, he or she must be aware of FDA guidelines regarding the use of these products in order to maintain compliance (Table 60.1). Products derived from human blood and tissues are regulated by the FDA's Center for Biologics Evaluation and Research (CBER). The regulatory process for these products is described in the FDA's 21 CFR 1271 of the Code of Regulations. Under these regulations, certain products, including blood products such as PRP, are exempt and therefore do not follow the FDA's traditional regulatory pathway that includes animal studies and clinical trials. There are numerous PRP preparation systems on the market today with FDA 510(k) clearance, although musculoskeletal injections with many of these systems are often technically considered "off-label." Clinicians are free to use a product off-label as long as certain responsibilities are met. Per CBER, when the intent is the practice of medicine, clinicians "have the responsibility to be well informed about the product, to base its use on firm scientific rationale and on sound medical evidence, and to maintain records of the product's use and effects."

Cellular products, including adipose- and bone marrow-based injections are currently looked at with more scrutiny compared to PRP. Human cells or tissue intended for implantation, transplantation, infusion, or transfer into a human recipient are regulated as a human cell, tissue, and cellular and tissue-based product or HCT/P. The Center for Biologics Evaluation and Research (CBER) regulates HCT/Ps under 21 CFR Parts 1270 and 1271. Examples of such tissues are bone, adipose, ligaments, tendons, and hematopoietic stem/progenitor cells derived from peripheral and cord blood. In order for these cellular products to be in FDA compliance for use in orthopedics, products should be homologues, minimally manipulated, and not combined with other products and have no systemic effect or dependency on the metabolic effect of living cells for its function. This is summarized in Table 60.5. In practice to be compliant with current regulation, providers should consider limiting orthobiologic injections to oneself for a same-day procedure from when the HCT/Ps were harvested.

Table 60.5 2021 FDA guidelines for orthobiologic injections

Minimal manipulation	Processing does not alter the original relevant characteristics of the tissue relating to the tissue's utility for reconstruction, repair, or replacement. The only processing steps that are considered minimal manipulation include rinsing, cleansing, sizing, and shaping
Homologous use	Product performs the same basic functions in the recipient as in the donor
Not combined with other products	Exception for water, crystalloids, or sterilizing, preserving, or storage agents drugs and other products may alter the function of cells
No systemic effects and is not dependent upon the metabolic activity of living cells for its primary function*	*Exceptions are made for autologous use (product goes back into the same person), allogeneic use in a first-degree or second-degree blood relative, or for reproductive use For surgical procedures, there is also an exemption from these criteria "if you are in an establishment that removes HCT/Ps from an individual and implants such HCT/Ps into the same individual during the same surgical procedure"

Certain biologic products would not be compliant with this FDA guidance including stromal vascular fraction, typically involving an enzymatic processing step which is more than minimal manipulation. There are FDA-approved studies (results pending) that may allow for the use of SVF for musculoskeletal conditions (knee osteoarthritis) in the near future. Umbilical cord products with live cells for musculoskeletal conditions are not compliant. Additionally, as of this writing, there are no FDA-approved exosome products. Furthermore, clinicians should be careful with how they describe adipose or bone marrow-based injections to the patient. For example, when considering adipose for the treatment of osteoarthritis pain, it may be discussed that adipose helps with local cell signaling. Marketing adipose injectate as a "stem cell" procedure that regenerates cartilage and bone would not be appropriate according to current guidelines.

References

1. Hackett GS, Hemwall GA, Montgomery GA. Ligament and tendon relaxation treated by prolotherapy. 5th ed. Oak Park: Gustav A. Hemwall; 1993.
2. Seven MM, Ersen O, Akpancar S, Ozkan H, Turkkan S, Yıldız Y, et al. Effectiveness of prolotherapy in the treatment of chronic rotator cuff lesions. Orthop Traumatol Surg Res. 2017;103:427–33.
3. Bertrand H, Reeves KD, Bennett CJ, Bicknell S, Cheng AL. Dextrose prolotherapy versus control injections in painful rotator cuff tendinopathy. Arch Phys Med Rehabil. 2016;97:17–25.

4. Ersen Ö, Koca K, Akpancar S, Seven MM, Akyıldız F, Yıldız Y, et al. A randomized-controlled trial of prolotherapy injections in the treatment of plantar fasciitis. Turk J Phys Med Rehabil. 2017;64:59–65.
5. Topol GA, Podesta LA, Reeves KD, Raya MF, Fullerton BD, Yeh HW. Hyperosmolar dextrose injection for recalcitrant Osgood-Schlatter disease. Pediatrics. 2011;128(5):e1121–8.
6. Rabago D, Patterson JJ, Mundt M, Kijowski R, Grettie J, Segal NA, et al. Dextrose prolotherapy for knee osteoarthritis: a randomized controlled trial. Ann Fam Med. 2013;11:229–37.
7. Reeves KD, Hassanein K. Randomized prospective double-blind placebo-controlled study of dextrose prolotherapy for knee osteoarthritis with or without ACL laxity. Altern Ther Health Med. 2000;6:68–74. 77-80
8. Bayat M, Raeissadat SA, Mortazavian Babaki M, Rahimi-Dehgolan S. Is dextrose prolotherapy superior to corticosteroid injection in patients with chronic lateral epicondylitis?: a randomized clinical trial. Orthop Res Rev. 2019;11:167–75.
9. Reeves KD, Hassanein K. Randomized, prospective, placebo-controlled double-blind study of dextrose prolotherapy for osteoarthritic thumb and finger (DIP, PIP, and trapeziometacarpal) joints: evidence of clinical efficacy. J Altern Complement Med. 2000;6:311–20.
10. Battaglia M, et al. Efficacy of ultrasound-guided intra-articular injections of platelet-rich plasma versus hyaluronic acid for hip osteoarthritis. Orthopedics. 2013;36(12):e1501–8.
11. Villanova-López MM, et al. Randomized, double-blind, controlled trial, phase III, to evaluate the use of platelet-rich plasma versus hyaluronic acid in hip coxarthrosis. Ensayo clínico fase III para evaluar la eficacia y seguridad del uso de plasma Rico en plaquetas frente a ácido hialurónico en coxartrosis. Rev Esp Cir Ortop Traumatol (Engl Ed). 2020;64(2):134–42.
12. Wallace P, Bezjian Wallace L, Tamura S, Prochnio K, Morgan K, Hemler D. Effectiveness of ultrasound-guided platelet-rich plasma injections in relieving sacroiliac joint dysfunction. Am J Phys Med Rehabil. 2020;99(8):689–93. https://doi.org/10.1097/PHM.0000000000001389.PMID: 31972616.
13. Mishra AK, et al. Efficacy of platelet-rich plasma for chronic tennis elbow: a double-blind, prospective, multicenter, randomized controlled trial of 230 patients. Am J Sports Med. 2014;42(2):463–71.
14. Gosens T, et al. Ongoing positive effect of platelet-rich plasma versus corticosteroid injection in lateral epicondylitis: a double-blind randomized controlled trial with 2-year follow-up. Am J Sports Med. 2011;39(6):1200–8.
15. Begkas D, Chatzopoulos ST, Touzopoulos P, Balanika A, Pastroudis A. Ultrasound-guided platelet-rich plasma application versus corticosteroid injections for the treatment of greater trochanteric pain syndrome: a prospective controlled randomized comparative clinical study. Cureus. 2020;12(1):e6583.
16. Fitzpatrick J, et al. The effectiveness of platelet-rich plasma injections in gluteal tendinopathy: a randomized, double-blind controlled trial comparing a single platelet-rich plasma injection with a single corticosteroid injection. Am J Sports Med. 2018;46(4):933–9.
17. Monto RR. Platelet-rich plasma efficacy versus corticosteroid injection treatment for chronic severe plantar fasciitis. Foot Ankle Int. 2014;35(4):313–8.
18. Tiwari M, Bhargava R. Platelet rich plasma therapy: a comparative effective therapy with promising results in plantar fasciitis. J Clin Orthop Trauma. 2013;4(1):31–5.
19. Dragoo JL, et al. Platelet-rich plasma as a treatment for patellar tendinopathy: a double-blind, randomized controlled trial. Am J Sports Med. 2014;42(3):610–8.
20. Vetrano M, et al. Platelet-rich plasma versus focused shock waves in the treatment of jumper's knee in athletes. Am J Sports Med. 2013;41(4):795–803.
21. Miller LE, et al. Efficacy of platelet-rich plasma injections for symptomatic tendinopathy: systematic review and meta-analysis of randomised injection-controlled trials. BMJ Open Sport Exerc Med. 2017;3(1):e000237.
22. Shams A, et al. Subacromial injection of autologous platelet-rich plasma versus corticosteroid for the treatment of symptomatic partial rotator cuff tears. Eur J Orthop Surg Traumatol. 2016;26(8):837–42.
23. Rha DW, et al. Comparison of the therapeutic effects of ultrasound-guided platelet-rich plasma injection and dry needling in rotator cuff disease: a randomized controlled trial. Clin Rehabil. 2013;27(2):113–22.
24. Chellini F, Tani A, Zecchi-Orlandini S, Sassoli C. Influence of platelet-rich and platelet-poor plasma on endogenous mechanisms of skeletal muscle repair/regeneration. Int J Mol Sci. 2019;20(3):683.
25. Caplan AI. Medicinal signaling cells: they work, so use them. Nature. 2019;566(7742):39.
26. Bora P, Majumdar AS. Adipose tissue-derived stromal vascular fraction in regenerative medicine: a brief review on biology and translation. Stem Cell Res Ther. 2017;8(1):145–54.
27. Hernigou P, et al. Benefits of small volume and small syringe for bone marrow aspirations of mesenchymal stem cells. Int Orthop. 2013;37(11):2279–87.
28. Centeno CJ, et al. A dose response analysis of a specific bone marrow concentrate treatment protocol for knee osteoarthritis. BMC Musculoskelet Disord. 2015;16:258.
29. Singh A, Gangwar DS, Singh S. Bone marrow injection: a novel treatment for tennis elbow. J Nat Sci Biol Med. 2014;5(2):389–91.
30. Centeno CJ, et al. A prospective multi-site registry study of a specific protocol of autologous bone marrow concentrate for the treatment of shoulder rotator cuff tears and osteoarthritis. J Pain Res. 2015;8:269–76.
31. Centeno CJP, Pitts JA, Al-Sayegh H, Freeman MD. Efficacy and safety of bone marrow concentrate for osteoarthritis of the hip; treatment registry results for 196 patients. J Stem Cell Res Ther. 2014;4(10):1–7.
32. Pettine KA, et al. Autologous bone marrow concentrate intradiscal injection for the treatment of degenerative disc disease with three-year follow-up. Int Orthop. 2017;41(10):2097–103.
33. Poloni A, Maurizi G, Leoni P, Serrani F, Mancini S, Frontini A, Zingaretti MC, Siquini W, Sarzani R, Cinti S. Human dedifferentiated adipocytes show similar properties to bone marrow-derived mesenchymal stem cells. Stem Cells. 2012;30:965–74. https://doi.org/10.1002/stem.1067.
34. Mautner K, Bowers R, Easley K, Fausel Z, Robinson R. Functional outcomes following microfragmented adipose tissue versus bone marrow aspirate concentrate injections for symptomatic knee osteoarthritis. Stem Cells Transl Med. 2019;8:1149–56. https://doi.org/10.1002/sctm.18-0285.
35. Cherian C, Malanga GA, Hogaboom N, Pollack MA, Dyson-Hudson TA. Autologous, micro-fragmented adipose tissue as a treatment for chronic shoulder pain in a wheelchair using individual with spinal cord injury: a case report. Spinal Cord Ser Cases. 2019;5:46.
36. de Girolamo L, Grassi M, Viganò M, Orfei CP, Montrasio UA, Usuelli F. Treatment of achilles tendinopathy with autologous adipose-derived stromal vascular fraction. Orthop J Sports Med [Internet]. 2016 [cited 2020 Jan 9];4(7):1.
37. Lee SY, Kim W, Lim C, Chung SG. Treatment of lateral epicondylosis by using allogeneic adipose-derived mesenchymal stem cells: a pilot study. Stem Cells. 2015;33(10):2995–3005.
38. Pak J. Regeneration of human bones in hip osteonecrosis and human cartilage in knee osteoarthritis with autologous adipose-tissue-derived stem cells: a case series. J Med Case Rep. 2011;5:296.

39. Pak J. Autologous adipose tissue-derived stem cells induce persistent bone-like tissue in osteonecrotic femoral heads. Pain Physician. 2012;15(1):75–85.
40. Pak J, Lee JH, Jeon JH, Lee SH. Complete resolution of avascular necrosis of the human femoral head treated with adipose tissue-derived stem cells and platelet-rich plasma. J Int Med Res. 2014;42(6):1353–62.
41. Li S, Xiang C, Wei X, et al. Early supplemental α2-macroglobulin attenuates cartilage and bone damage by inhibiting inflammation in collagen II-induced arthritis model. Int J Rheum Dis. 2019;22:654–65. https://doi.org/10.1111/1756-185X.13457.
42. Zhang Y, Wei X, Browning S, et al. Targeted designed variants of alpha-2-macroglobulin (A2M) attenuate cartilage degeneration in a rat model of osteoarthritis induced by anterior cruciate ligament transection. Arthritis Res Ther. 2017;19:175. https://doi.org/10.1186/s13075-017-1363-4.
43. Perkins KM, Spoto S, Rankin DA, et al. Notes from the field: infections after receipt of bacterially contaminated umbilical cord blood–derived stem cell products for other than hematopoietic or immunologic reconstitution — United States, 2018. MMWR Morb Mortal Wkly Rep. 2018;67:1397–9. https://doi.org/10.15585/mmwr.mm6750a5.
44. Mautner K, Malanga G, Colberg R. Optimization of ingredients, procedures and rehabilitation for platelet-rich plasma injections for chronic tendinopathy. Pain Manag. 2011;1(6):523–32. https://doi.org/10.2217/pmt.11.56. PMID: 24645763.

Tendinopathy

61

Richard Fontanez, Kevin De Jesus, Fernando Sepulveda, and William Micheo

61.1 Synonyms

- Tendinitis
- Tendonitis
- Tendinosis
- Paratenonitis
- Paratendinitis
- Enthesopathy/enthesitis
- Tendon ruptur

61.2 ICD-10

- *M67.90* – Soft tissue disorder related to use, overuse, and pressure of tendon
- *M65.2* – Calcific tendonitis
- *M75.1* – Rotator cuff syndrome
- *M75.2* – Bicipital tendonitis
- *M75.3* – Calcific tendonitis of shoulder
- *M76.0* – Gluteal tendonitis
- *M76.1* – Psoas tendonitis
- *M76.5* – Patellar tendonitis
- *M76.6* – Achilles tendonitis
- *M76.7* – Peroneal tendonitis
- *M77* – Other enthesopathies
- *M66.2* – Spontaneous rupture of extensor tendons
- *M66.3* – Spontaneous rupture of flexor tendons
- *M66.8* – Spontaneous rupture of other tendons

R. Fontanez · F. Sepulveda
Department PM&R and Sports Medicine, University of Puerto Rico, San Juan, PR, USA

Physical Medicine, Rehabilitation and Sports Medicine Department, University of Puerto Rico, School of Medicine, San Juan, PR, USA
e-mail: richard.fontanez1@upr.edu

K. De Jesus · W. Micheo (✉)
Department PM&R and Sports Medicine, University of Puerto Rico School of Medicine, San Juan, PR, USA
e-mail: kevin.dejesus1@upr.edu; william.micheo@upr.edu

61.3 Description

Tendon disease is a common cause of musculoskeletal complaints and presents in a wide variety of patients. Tendinopathy can be a descriptor of tendon disease and can be specifically categorized based on the pathophysiology of the disease, ranging from inflammation to degeneration. Tendinopathy can be associated with a clinical syndrome characterized by pain, swelling, and impaired performance [1]. The most frequently involved anatomical sites for the development of tendinopathy are the rotator cuff, the long head of the brachial biceps, the extensor and flexor tendons of the wrist, the thigh adductors, the posterior tibial tendon, the patellar tendon, and the Achilles tendon [2]. The type of sport and occupational activity in which the patient participates may influence the development of tendinopathy at specific anatomical locations. Despite being widely studied, its etiology is still uncertain and is now subclassified into different tendon lesions described in Fig. 61.1. As reviewed extensively in the medical literature [4–7], tendon dysfunction is caused by a failed healing response secondary to multiple factors like continuous inappropriate mechanical stimuli, repetitive movements, and poorly vascularized tissue [1]. Despite being described primarily as a degenerative condition, tendinopathy can present with inflammatory features in its early stages. There is an imbalance between tissue recovery and healing accompanied by a release of pro-inflammatory substances that contribute to the onset of pain, even if no clinical evidence of inflammation is found. Following the initial inflammatory phase, the healing process can still be impaired and subsequent changes that characterize tendinopathy as a degenerative condition occur [8]. Chronic changes (e.g., thickening of the tendon, collagen remodeling, neovascularization) disrupt tendinous fibers and promote the release of pro-inflammatory cytokines. This cellular response may lead to an increase in type 3 collagen deposition that hinders the original tendon composition and structure, making the tendon susceptible to damage. Both intrinsic and extrinsic factors play a critical role in the development of tendinopathy (Fig. 61.2).

© The Author(s), under exclusive license to Springer Nature Switzerland AG 2022
S. A. Mostoufi et al. (eds.), *Clinical Guide to Musculoskeletal Medicine*, https://doi.org/10.1007/978-3-030-92042-5_61

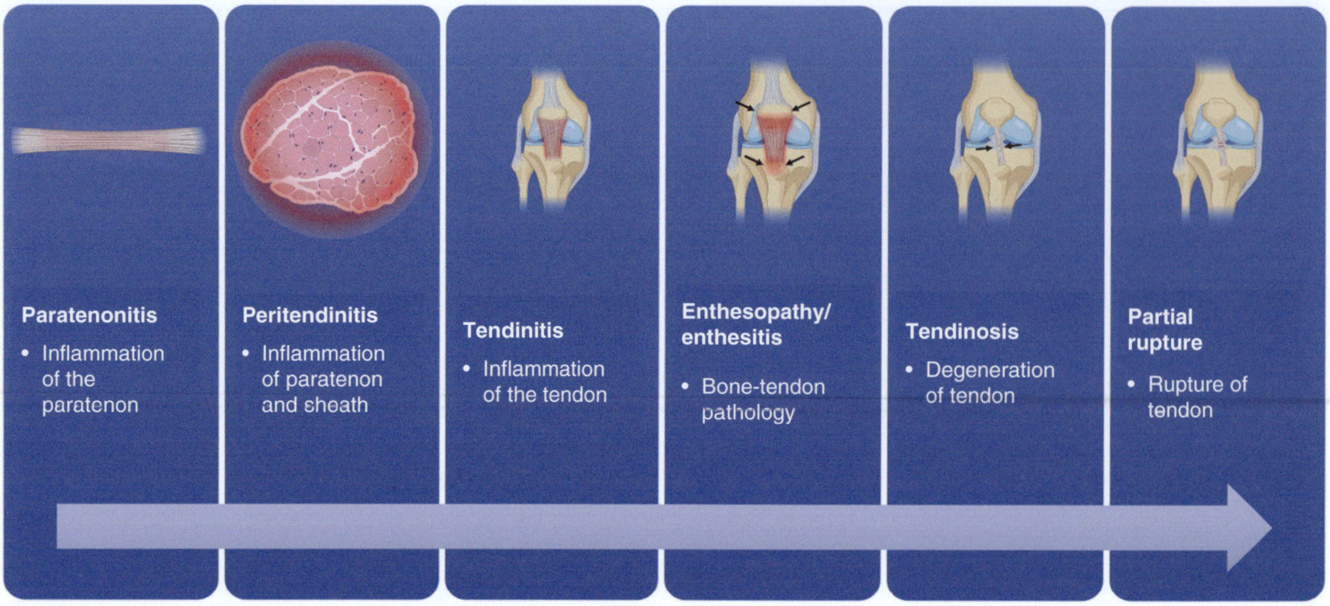

Fig. 61.1 Spectrum of tendon damage [3]. (Created with BioRender.com)

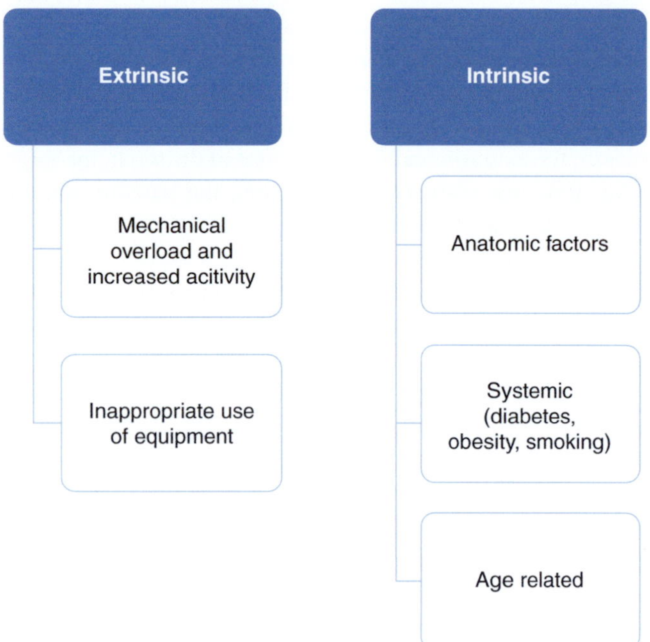

Fig. 61.2 Tendinopathy risk factors. (Modified from Federer et al. [3])

Additional key factors that trigger tendon degeneration include high temperature secondary to strenuous exercise, hypoxia, and loss of repair mechanisms [9, 10]. Degenerated fibers are infiltrated and replaced by lipid and mucoid materials that alter their parallel arrangement and the mechanical properties of the tendon. As a result, there is an alteration in the glycogen composition and tenocytes, creating a fragile and painful tendon [10].

61.3.1 Anatomy

Tendons are formed by different types of collagen molecules of which type I is the most abundant. These molecules are arranged in helical structures, which are grouped to form fascicles. These fascicles are bound by the endotenon to make the tendon unit. The tendon surface is wrapped by the epitenon, a connective tissue sheath continuous with the endotenon, which facilitates the sliding of the tendon in distal areas of joints. The paratenon surrounds the tendons and facilitates the movement of tendons below the skin [11]. All tendon cells are covered by the extracellular matrix where cell signaling, exchange of nutrients, and cell proliferation occur. Tendons' primary function is to transfer force produced by muscle contraction and create body movement [8]. Other functions are kinetic energy absorption and storage and participation in proprioception mechanisms.

61.4 Clinical Presentation

Symptoms may vary depending on the anatomical location, but all sites share some presenting features. Pain is often described as dull, insidious, and, on some occasions, sharp. Occupational activities, exercise, and sports may exacerbate and worsen the pain when using specific movements (e.g., rotator cuff tendinopathy in an overhead athlete may worsen with activity above the shoulder). Patient history evaluation should include the identification of modifiable (intrinsic) and activity-related (extrinsic) factors. Besides the classic musculoskeletal survey, it is also important to assess if the patient is engaging in any repetitive stress or increase in load of any particular joint (e.g., increasing time, intensity, or volume of practices). Ultimately, a thorough evaluation is warranted as tendinopathy may be confused with other etiologies. For example, radial tunnel syndrome and C7 radiculopathy can be confused with lateral epicondylitis, calcaneal apophysitis can be confused with Achilles tendinopathy, a stress fracture can be confused with posterior tibial tendinopathy, and an inflammatory arthropathy can be confused with patellar tendonitis.

61.5 Physical Examination

The clinical examination should be performed in an orderly manner, addressing specific complaints of the patient and possible causative or contributing factors. Physical examination begins with inspection, which may reveal local swelling, erythema, muscle atrophy, or tendon gap. In addition, observation for anatomical alignment or abnormal posture and biomechanics are important for identifying predisposing factors. Palpation of the tendon origin, insertion, or tendon substance can elicit tenderness or discomfort. Adjacent soft tissues, such as muscle or bursae, may also be tender. Range of motion (ROM) must be evaluated during active and passive movement. Loss of active motion may be associated with pain inhibition, muscle weakness, nerve injury, or tendon tear. Loss of passive motion may be seen in patients with tendon contracture. Muscle strength can be affected by muscle inhibition, immobilization, contracture, and tendon rupture. Clinical weakness in some cases can be attributed to the altered biomechanics and anatomic misalignment. Neurologic evaluation should reveal normal sensation and muscle stretch reflexes. Special tests directed at specific tendons to reproduce common mechanisms of injury should be included in the examination [12].

61.6 Diagnostic Workup

Ultrasound (US) and magnetic resonance imaging (MRI) are the most commonly used imaging approaches to evaluate tendon pathologies [13], as structural alterations of tendinopathies show in these imaging techniques. Various studies have assessed the accuracy and sensitivity of these two modalities, with no clear advantage on one being the gold standard [14, 15]. As both show non-inferior value compared to the other, each provides distinct benefits, and selection must be based on patient presentation.

Ultrasound With US, normal tendon texture appears homogeneous with parallel echogenic lines reflecting the internal fibrillar structure of the tendon. In tendinopathy, the fibrillary disorganization and the lack of parallel alignment of fibers generate multiple reflections and shadowing that are represented by an area of hypoechogenicity [8].

MRI Overall, *MR* has a higher diagnostic accuracy [15] with visualization of adjacent areas and the articulation, making it useful on instances where a distinction between diagnoses must be established [14]. The downsides of MRI are its high costs and it is less available than the ultrasound. In contrast, the US is highly sensitive and provides a practical tool that captures a dynamic image that makes it possible to evaluate passive and active movements in real time, while visualizing the intratendinous condition [14]. Potential disadvantages are that the quality of imaging is user-dependent and there is difficulty evaluating deep tendons. The diagnostic value of both imaging modalities may be limited in patients in which abnormal imaging findings do not correlate with the patient's clinical presentation or that are asymptomatic [14].

61.7 Treatment

61.7.1 Medical Management

Nonsteroidal Anti-Inflammatory Medications (NSAIDs) Oral NSAIDs are a drug class commonly used to alleviate pain and decrease inflammation and, consequently, used as a therapeutic intervention in the management of tendinopathy. In the acute setting, they help to reduce symptoms and allow participation in rehabilitation programs. In particular, ibuprofen has shown a lower risk profile compared with other NSAIDs [9]. However, long-term use is not recommended since the pathology of the disease is primarily degenerative, there is lack of sustained inflammation, and the possibility of delay in healing of tendinous tissue has been reported [16]. NSAIDs' potential downsides include the risk of reinjury and the common side effects associated with their mechanism of action (e.g., gastric ulcers, cardiovascular events, renal injury), particularly in older patients [16]. For patients at risk for gastrointestinal bleeding, selective COX-2 inhibitors (e.g., Celebrex) are associated with a safer profile. Topical NSAIDs like diclofenac have shown no significant differences in the efficacy of symptom management in comparison to oral NSAIDs [17]. In both modalities, effects may be short-lived and may inhibit the healing process, thus weakening the tendon.

Nitric Oxide Nitric oxide appears to have a role in the synthesis of new tissue during tendon healing [18]. Clinically, it has been used in the form of transdermal patches showing a positive effect in tendon healing response and pain control with short-term use. Headaches have been reported as a common secondary effect [18].

61.7.2 Rehabilitation

Exercise-Based Rehabilitation Rehabilitation of tendon injury should be individualized to the patient, requires activity modification to allow the tendon to heal, and combines therapeutic modalities and exercise. A progressive exercise program is the foundation for the treatment and rehabilitation of tendinopathies [8]. Different protocols have been established, including eccentric exercises, combined eccentric and concentric exercises, and heavy-slow resistance (HSR) training, with no protocol demonstrating an advantage over the others. Both eccentric and HSR exercises have shown long-term pain relief, principally in patients with patellar tendinopathy. Isotonic and isometric exercises provide immediate pain relief, with isometric exercises showing analgesic effects for longer than 45 min after a single exercise session. Isometric exercises also showed superior pain improvement scores up to 4 weeks later when compared in reevaluations with isotonic exercises [13].

In general, tendons respond more favorably to cyclic loading rather than large magnitudes of load [19]. Regular and well-structured exercise positively affects the tendon tissue by strengthening it through the production of new collagen fibers [20]. An ideal training plan will possibly combine more than one protocol to implement adequate load-bearing exercises, varying from patient to patient based on a comprehensive assessment of the patient's needs and conditioning. A sample rehabilitation program (Fig. 61.3) was proposed by Cardoso et al. for lower extremity tendinopathies consisting of progressive loading and unloading of the tendon promoting pain reduction [9]. This proposed routine can be customized for the patient's current and expected function. A recent systematic review by Burton et al. outlines the importance of resistance training exercise in different lower extremities tendinopathies and the need for implementation of a better methodology especially on the progression of exercises and individualization of the training program [21].

Extracorporeal Shock Wave Therapy (ESWT) ESWT, which releases growth factors that activate tenocytes, has shown effectiveness, mostly in insertional Achilles tendinopathy [22], gluteal [23] and proximal hamstring [24] tendinopathy, as well as calcific tendonitis [16]. The use of radial vs. focal ESWT and specific treatment parameters are yet to be described for accurate prescriptions in different types of tendinopathy, and further investigation is warranted.

Thermal Modalities Cold and hot treatments are simple approaches that have been widely used; cold treatment aims to decrease inflammation and cell metabolism, while therapeutic heat stimulates cell activity and increases blood flow

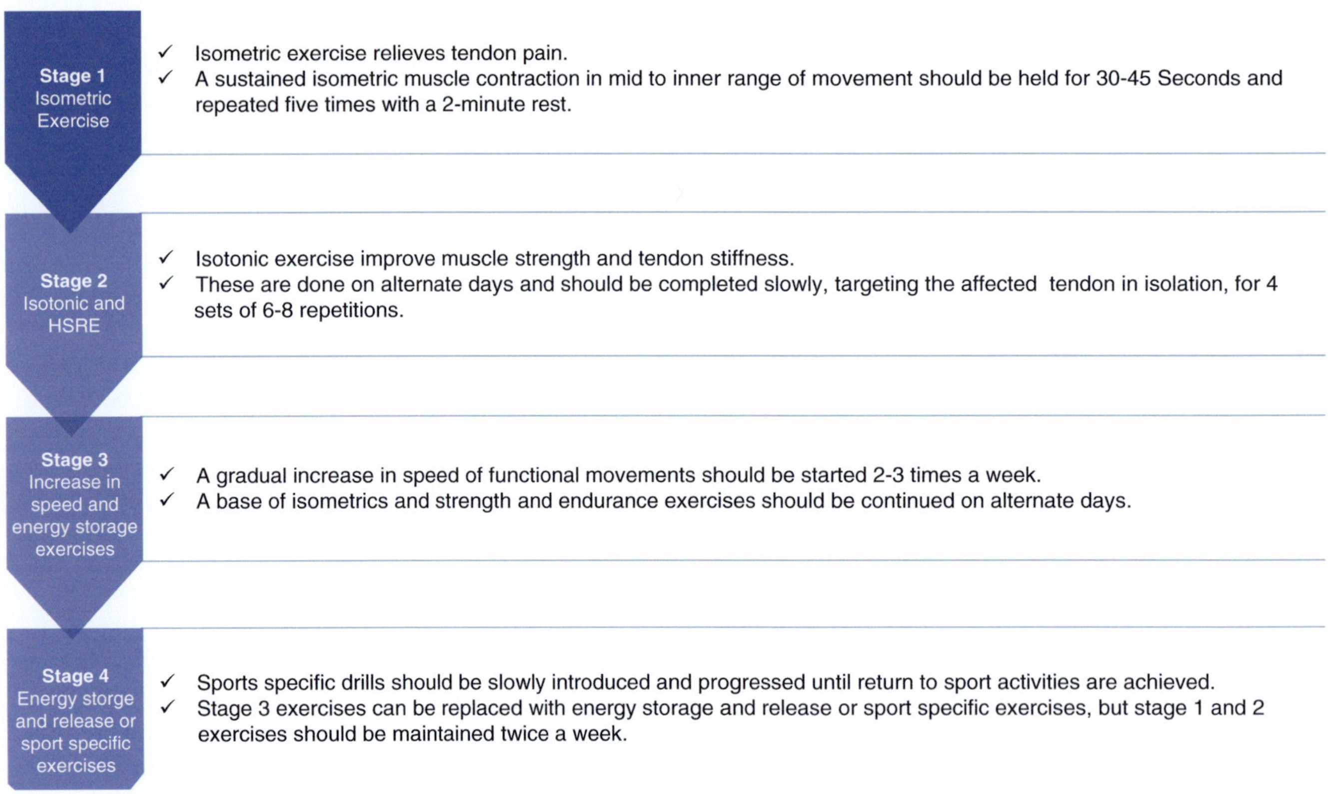

Fig. 61.3 Lower extremity tendinopathies sample exercise-based rehabilitation program. (Modified from Cardoso et al. [13])

[9]. Both may be helpful at different time periods across the development of the condition and used depending on the patient's symptoms. Cold may be used in initial stages with acute presentation of pain and swelling. Heat may be used after the initial inflammatory response to aid in analgesia and soft tissue distensibility and combined with exercise. In patients with recurring symptoms, both modalities can be combined to prevent exacerbation. They may be combined in exercise sessions, using heat before exercises and cold after exertion.

Low-Level Laser Therapy Laser therapy appears to have an effect on cellular activity promoting tissue regeneration, angiogenesis, fibroblast proliferation, and collagen synthesis while also having an analgesic effect [25]. Currently, this modality has low to very low evidence of efficacy, especially on Achilles tendinopathy, mainly due to poor research methodology.

61.7.3 Procedures

Corticosteroids Injections Similar to NSAIDs, corticosteroid injections are commonly used for the treatment of tendinopathies. In patients who present with acute symptoms that persist at rest despite medication and therapeutic modalities, a single peritendon injection using the lowest effective dose may be useful. The improvement in these cases in many instances is short-lived and lasts approximately 6 weeks in a study specifically focusing on lateral epicondylosis [26]. In addition, they are associated with detrimental structural and functional outcomes to the tendon [16]. Ultrasound-guided medication delivery in the peritendinous space, instead of direct tendon injection, may have a lower risk of complications [9, 16].

Platelet-Rich Plasma (PRP) Available data suggests the effectiveness of PRP as a good treatment alternative in early tendinopathy [16]. One study by Gosens et al. showed the usefulness of PRP in tendinopathy with long-term improvement for up to 2 years [27]. Also, a recent systematic review and meta-analysis by Hamid et al. concludes that PRP is safe and effective in alleviating long-term shoulder pain symptoms and shoulder function associated with injury to the rotator cuff [28]. Nonetheless, more randomized, controlled trials are needed to analyze this modality in-depth [16]. Initial studies show structural recovery and symptomatic improvement, which provides reasonable indications for use in selected patients before resorting to surgery [16].

Prolotherapy This method, in which usually hyperosmolar dextrose is injected into the affected tendon to elicit a targeted inflammatory response to promote healing and neovascularization, has shown promising results in early trial phases [9, 16]. However, further investigation and evaluation are needed.

Stem Cell Therapy Cellular [29, 30] and animal studies [31, 32] have assessed the potential of differentiating stem cells and potentially repairing tendinous tissue, principally for age-related tendinopathy. Small, early studies have showed promising results, especially in refractory cases, but the strength of the evidence is poor [33].

61.7.4 Surgery

Surgical intervention is a last resort in tendinopathies, providing variable results in these cases [9, 34]. Operative approach consists of debridement and decompression or repair of the tendon, when needed, being successful particularly in Achilles tendinopathy and calcific tendonitis [9]. Surgery may also be an alternative for cases of chronic tendinopathy when combined with strength training, with pre- and postoperative mechanical loading [34]. Nevertheless, studies evaluating surgical interventions fall short from supporting surgery as a treatment for tendinopathy, reporting conflicting data and needing further prospective, well-designed trials [13].

References

1. van Dijk CN, van Sterkenburg MN, Wiegerinck JI, Karlsson J, Maffulli N. Terminology for Achilles tendon related disorders. Knee Surg Sports Traumatol Arthrosc. 2011;19(5):835–41.
2. Frizziero A, Oliva (medico.) F, Maffulli N. Tendinopatie: stato dell'arte e prospettive. Italian medical publisher: Pacini Editore Medicina; 2011.
3. Wang JH-C, Iosifidis MI, Fu FH. Biomechanical basis for tendinopathy. Clin Orthop Relat Res. 2006;443:320–32.
4. Federer AE, Steele JR, Dekker TJ, Liles JL, Adams SB. Tendonitis and Tendinopathy. Foot Ankle Clin. 2017;22(4):665–76.
5. Loiacono C, Palermi S, Massa B, Belviso I, Romano V, Di Gregorio A, et al. Tendinopathy: pathophysiology, therapeutic options, and role of nutraceutics. A narrative literature review. Medicina. 2019;55(8):447.
6. Andarawis-Puri N, Flatow EL, Soslowsky LJ. Tendon basic science: development, repair, regeneration, and healing. J Orthop Res. 2015;33(6):780–4.
7. Järvinen TA. Neovascularisation in tendinopathy: from eradication to stabilisation? Br J Sports Med. 2019;54(1):1–2.
8. Ackermann PW, Domeij-Arverud E, Leclerc P, Amoudrouz P, Nader GA. Anti-inflammatory cytokine profile in early human tendon repair. Knee Surg Sports Traumatol Arthrosc. 2012;21(8):1801–6.
9. Ahmad Z, Parkar A, Shepherd J, Rushton N. Revolving doors of tendinopathy: definition, pathogenesis and treatment. Postgrad Med J. 2019;96(1132):94–101.
10. Magnusson SP, Langberg H, Kjaer M. The pathogenesis of tendinopathy: balancing the response to loading. Nat Rev Rheumatol. 2010;6(5):262–8.

11. Thorpe CT, Screen HRC. Tendon structure and composition. Metabolic influences on risk for tendon disorders [Internet]. 2016 [cited 2021 May 14];3–10. Available from: https://doi.org/10.1007/978-3-319-33943-6_1.
12. Martinez-Silvestrini J, Nava A, Elmore C. Tendinopathy [Internet]. PM&R knowledge now. 2021 [cited 2021 Apr 23]. Available from: https://now.aapmr.org/tendinopathy/.
13. Cardoso TB, Pizzari T, Kinsella R, Hope D, Cook JL. Current trends in tendinopathy management. Best Pract Res Clin Rheumatol. 2019;33(1):122–40.
14. Docking SI, Ooi CC, Connell D. Tendinopathy: is imaging telling us the entire story? J Orthop Sports Phys Ther. 2015;45(11):842–52.
15. Gatz M, Bode D, Betsch M, Quack V, Tingart M, Kuhl C, et al. Multimodal ultrasound versus MRI for the diagnosis and monitoring of achilles tendinopathy: a prospective longitudinal study. Orthop J Sports Med. 2021;9(4):232596712110068.
16. Aicale R, Bisaccia RD, Oliviero A, Oliva F, Maffulli N. Current pharmacological approaches to the treatment of tendinopathy. Expert Opin Pharmacother. 2020;21(12):1467–77.
17. Pattanittum P, Turner T, Green S, Buchbinder R. Non-steroidal anti-inflammatory drugs (NSAIDs) for treating lateral elbow pain in adults. Cochrane Database Syst Rev. 2013;5:CD003686.
18. Vasta S, Di Martino A, Zampogna B, Torre G, Papalia R, Denaro V. Role of VEGF, nitric oxide, and sympathetic neurotransmitters in the pathogenesis of tendinopathy: a review of the current evidences. Front Aging Neurosci. 2016;8:186.
19. Simonsen EB, Klitgaard H, Bojsen-MØller F. The influence of strength training, swim training and ageing on the Achilles tendon and m. soleus of the rat. J Sports Sci. 1995;13(4):291–5.
20. Killian ML, Cavinatto L, Galatz LM, Thomopoulos S. The role of mechanobiology in tendon healing. J Shoulder Elb Surg. 2012;21(2):228–37.
21. Burton I, McCormack A. The implementation of resistance training principles in exercise interventions for lower limb tendinopathy: a systematic review. Phys Ther Sport. 2021;50:97–113.
22. Jarin IJ, Bäcker HC, Vosseller JT. Functional outcomes of insertional Achilles tendinopathy treatment. JBJS Rev. 2021;9(6)1–11.
23. Mani-Babu S, Morrissey D, Waugh C, Screen H, Barton C. The effectiveness of extracorporeal shock wave therapy in lower limb tendinopathy. Am J Sports Med. 2014;43(3):752–61.
24. Cacchio A, Rompe JD, Furia JP, Susi P, Santilli V, De Paulis F. Shockwave therapy for the treatment of chronic proximal hamstring tendinopathy in professional athletes. Am J Sports Med. 2010;39(1):146–53.
25. Martimbianco ALC, Ferreira RES, Latorraca CDOC, Bussadori SK, Pacheco RL, Riera R. Photobiomodulation with low-level laser therapy for treating Achilles tendinopathy: a systematic review and meta-analysis. Clin Rehabil. 2020;34(6):713–22.
26. Lai WC, Erickson BJ, Mlynarek RA, Wang D. Chronic lateral epicondylitis: challenges and solutions. Open Access J Sports Med. 2018;9:243–51.
27. Gosens T, Peerbooms JC, van Laar W, den Oudsten BL. Ongoing positive effect of platelet-rich plasma versus corticosteroid injection in lateral epicondylitis. Am J Sports Med. 2011;39(6):1200–8.
28. Hamid MSA, Sazlina SG. Platelet-rich plasma for rotator cuff tendinopathy: a systematic review and meta-analysis. PLoS One. 2021;16(5):e0251111.
29. Migliorini F, Tingart M, Maffulli N. Progress with stem cell therapies for tendon tissue regeneration. Expert Opin Biol Ther. 2020;20(11):1373–9.
30. Kunze KN, Burnett RA, Wright-Chisem J, Frank RM, Chahla J. Adipose-derived mesenchymal stem cell treatments and available formulations. Curr Rev Musculoskelet Med. 2020;13(3):264–80.
31. Fedato RA, Francisco JC, Sliva G, de Noronha L, Olandoski M, Faria Neto JR, et al. Stem cells and platelet-rich plasma enhance the healing process of tendinitis in mice. Stem Cells Int. 2019;2019:1–9.
32. Oshita T, Tobita M, Tajima S, Mizuno H. Adipose-derived stem cells improve collagenase-induced tendinopathy in a rat model. Am J Sports Med. 2016;44(8):1983–9.
33. Dakkak A, Krill ML, Fogarty A, Krill MK. Stem cell therapy for the management of lateral elbow tendinopathy: a systematic literature review. Sci Sports. 2021;36(3):181–92.
34. Zhou B, Zhou Y, Tang K. An overview of structure, mechanical properties, and treatment for age-related tendinopathy. J Nutr Health Aging. 2014;18(4):441–8.

Autologous Orthobiologics

62

Peter A. Everts, Glenn Flanagan II, and Luga Podesta

62.1 Introduction

The human body has an endogenous system of regeneration through stem cells and progenitor cells, signaling cells, and other cell types, as they are found in almost every type of tissue. It is important to understand the terminology used in relation to tissue regeneration.

62.1.1 Regenerative Medicine

Regenerative medicine treatments using autologous PRP, bone marrow preparations, and adipose stem cells can be safely executed by well-trained physicians at the point of care (POC). The objectives of regenerative medicine applications are to support the body to form new functional tissues to replace degenerative or defective ones and to provide therapeutic treatment for conditions where conventional therapies are inadequate.

62.1.2 Orthobiologics

The term orthobiologics has recently been introduced for the treatment of a variety of musculoskeletal (MSK) disorders with autologous orthobiologic preparations such as PRP, bone marrow preparations, and adipose tissue concentrate. Such autologous products are showing promising results for the regenerative capacity of these heterogeneous biological active cellular cocktails. This chapter is not meant to be exhaustive, but our aims are to shed light on cell mechanisms following interventional procedures with orthobiologics. A solid understanding of employing interventional procedures using orthobiological preparations and their cellular responses to MSK disorders and tissue conditions is mandatory. FDA and other regulatory limitations of such products (local or federal) need to be understood by clinicians who have incorporated such treatments in their practice.

62.1.3 Regenerative Rehabilitation

The American Physical Therapy Association has defined regenerative rehabilitation as the combination of interventional orthobiological techniques and appropriate rehabilitation protocols that harness the bodies' intrinsic healing mechanisms through movement to augment orthobiologic injections [1].

62.2 Description

The purpose of this chapter is to provide detailed information on three autologous orthobiologic preparations: PRP, bone marrow–derived preparations, and adipose tissue concentrate.

62.2.1 Platelet-Rich Plasma

PRP therapies have been used for various indications for more than 30 years, resulting in considerable interest in the potential of PRP in regenerative medicine. Autologous PRP is the processed liquid fraction of autologous peripheral blood with a platelet concentration above the baseline [2]. Currently, PRP therapies are suitable treatment options with clinical benefits and encouraging patient outcomes reported [3–5]. However, new therapeutic insights and needs have

P. A. Everts (✉)
Research and Science Division, Gulf Coast Biologics, Fort Myers, FL, USA
e-mail: peter@gulfcoastbiologics.com

G. Flanagan II
Naples Regenerative Institute, Naples, FL, USA

L. Podesta
Regenerative Orthopedics & Sports Medicine, Naples, FL, USA

Physical Medicine and Rehabilitation and Sports Medicine at Western University of Health Sciences, Pomona, CA, USA

© The Author(s), under exclusive license to Springer Nature Switzerland AG 2022
S. A. Mostoufi et al. (eds.), *Clinical Guide to Musculoskeletal Medicine*, https://doi.org/10.1007/978-3-030-92042-5_62

challenged the practicality and effectiveness of PRP clinical applications as many different commercially available PRP and PRP-like systems are being used [6]. A profuse variability in final PRP cellular contents has been reported. Not surprising, different PRP devices contribute to distinctive PRP properties and bioformulations, which may explain inconsistencies in patient outcomes.

One of the authors (PE) published in 2006 a review on PRP technology, focusing on platelet function, PRP mode of action, platelet growth factor and effects during the various stages of the healing cascade, and the central role of platelet-derived growth factors in various PRP indications. Notably, in this period, PRP-gel research, was directed only toward the ability of PRP to release several platelet growth factors (PGFs) with their specific functions toward only bone growth and bone healing, during orthopedic and spine surgical procedures [7]. Later in this chapter, we will discuss the roles of individual cells that can be present in PRP preparation along with detailed information on their effects on tissue regenerative processes. Furthermore, recent advances in understanding PRP bioformulations, platelet dosing, the specific roles of particular leukocytes, and the effects of PGF concentrations and cytokines on mesenchymal stem cell (MSC) trophic effects [8] will be described, including the pivotal roles of PRP in targeting different cells and tissue environments following cell signaling and paracrine effects [9]. Likewise, we will discuss PRP mechanisms related to inflammation and angiogenesis in tissue repair and regenerative processes. Lastly, we will review the analgesic effects of PRP [10] and the effect of certain drugs on PRP activity.

62.2.2 Bone Marrow Aspirate/Concentrate

Bone marrow concentrates are commonly used autologous regenerative orthobiological therapies. In 1989, Wientroub et al. were the first to describe bone marrow aspiration procedures performed for musculoskeletal applications as a method to improve osteogenic potential of bone grafts in pediatric patients [11]. To produce a BMC, bone marrow aspirate (BMA) must be extracted via an aspiration device, which is inserted through the bony cortex. Bone marrow stroma is collected in syringes. A specific BMA volume is then processed by centrifugation to create a BMC buffy coat that should include mesenchymal and hematopoietic stem cells, myelopoietic and erythropoietic cells, mature leukocytes, platelets, and some megakaryocytes [12]. Later in this chapter, scientific information is provided on the bone marrow aspirate cellular content, their specific biological functions, and intercellular interactions, as these, among others, contribute to tissue regeneration following clinical regenerative medicine applications. Furthermore, we underline the differences between BMA and BMC specimen, both prepared at point of care from freshly aspirated bone marrow.

62.2.3 Adipose Tissue Concentrate

Another source for autologous mesenchymal stem cells is adipose (fat) grafts. Adipose tissue can be harvested via lipoaspiration of subcutaneous fat from various areas of the body like the abdomen, thighs, flank, and perigluteal region [13]. Later in the chapter, we will discuss recent developments in the three autologous orthobiological preparations regarding dosing, cellular structures, cell membrane receptors, and their effects on the innate and adaptive immunomodulatory actions, angiogenesis, and analgesic effects.

62.3 Platelet-Rich Plasma (PRP)

62.3.1 Description

The most well-known physiological role of platelets is the control of hemorrhage, where they accumulate at tissue injury sites and damaged blood vessels. These events are instigated by the expression of integrins and selectins that stimulate platelet adhesion and aggregation, leading to the formation of the platelet plug. However, during PRP preparation procedures, clothing should be always avoided as this will jeopardize the preparation of an adequate and viable e orthobiological injectate.

PRP can be characterized as a complex composition of autologous multicellular components in a small volume of plasma that is acquired from a fraction of peripheral blood after centrifugation. The essentials of a phlebotomy procedure are summarized in Table 62.1. After centrifugation, according to the different cellular densities (where platelets have the lowest density), PRP and their non-platelet cellular constituents can be retrieved from the concentration device.

Table 62.1 Essentials and considerations of a phlebotomy procedure for PRP preparation

Properly labeling relevant syringes with patient information
Sufficient anticoagulant in blood collection syringe
PPE and aseptic techniques
Harvesting site choice and preparation
Proper blood draw and draw time
Agitation of blood with anticoagulant during collection
Controlled transfer to PRP device
Following instructions for use to prepare PRP vial

62.3.1.1 PRP: Preparation

A clear consensus across treatment indications is nonexistent, making it difficult to compare PRP products with their related therapy outcomes. In the majority of reported cases, platelet concentrate therapies are all grouped under the term "PRP," even for the same clinical indication [14]. Therefore, this lack of a consensus in PRP preparation methods and validation continues to contribute to inconsistent PRP patient outcomes, based on enormous differences in PRP formulation, specimen quality, including platelet dosing. Nonetheless, for some medical fields (e.g., OA and tendinopathies), progress has been made in understanding the variations in the PRP formulations, delivery routes, platelet function, and other PRP constituents influencing tissue repair and tissue regeneration.

There are many methods and devices on the market for PRP preparation and this chapter is not promoting any specific device. In Fig. 62.1 (EmCyte Corporation, Fort Myers, FL, USA), cellular density separation of whole blood follows a two-spin centrifugation procedure using the proprietary device. After the first centrifugation procedure, the whole blood components are separated into two basic layers: the platelet (poor) plasma suspension and the RBC layer. After a second centrifugation step, the needed PRP volume can be extracted for patient application. The magnification in Fig. 62.1 shows at the bottom of the device the organized multicomponent buffy coat layer (indicated by the blue lines), containing high concentrations of platelets, monocytes, and lymphocytes, based on density gradients. In this example, a minimal percentage of neutrophils (< 0.3%) and RBCs (< 0.1%) will be extracted, following a neutrophil-poor PRP preparation protocol (modified from Everts et al. (IJMS) [15]).

62.3.1.2 PRP: Platelet Granules and Their Content

PRP should meet the prerequisites (platelet dosage, minimal RBC contamination, and addition or removal of particular leukocytes) to produce significant clinical outcomes. These PRP qualifications, combined with elucidating the activities of different PGFs, platelet proteins, cytokines, and chemokines, contribute to the understanding of the fundamental tissue repair mechanisms involving mitogenesis, angiogenesis, chemotaxis, and extracellular matrix formation.

In early PRP applications, α-granules were the most cited intra-platelet structures because of the presence of many PGFs [16]. To a lesser degree, coagulation factors and regulators of angiogenesis were referenced with PRP applications. Additional factors included less-famous chemokine and cytokine constituents, such as platelet factor 4 (PF4), pro-platelet basic protein, P-selectin (activator of integrin), and the chemokine RANTES (regulated upon activation of normal T cell, expressed and presumably secreted). The overall functions of these specific platelet granule constituents are to recruit and activate other immune cells or induce endothelial cell inflammation (Fig. 62.2) [17].

The number of potential interactions, both direct and indirect, between platelets and other (receptor) cells is wide-ranging. As a result, numerous inflammatory effects can be induced by PRP when applied in a local, pathological, tissue environment. The dense granule constituents like ADP, serotonin, polyphosphates, histamine, and epinephrine are more implicit as modifiers of platelet activation and thrombus formation [18]. Most importantly, many of these elements have immune cell-modifying effects. Platelet ADP is recognized by dendritic cells (DCs), increasing antigen endocytosis. DCs (antigen-presenting cells) are critical for initiating

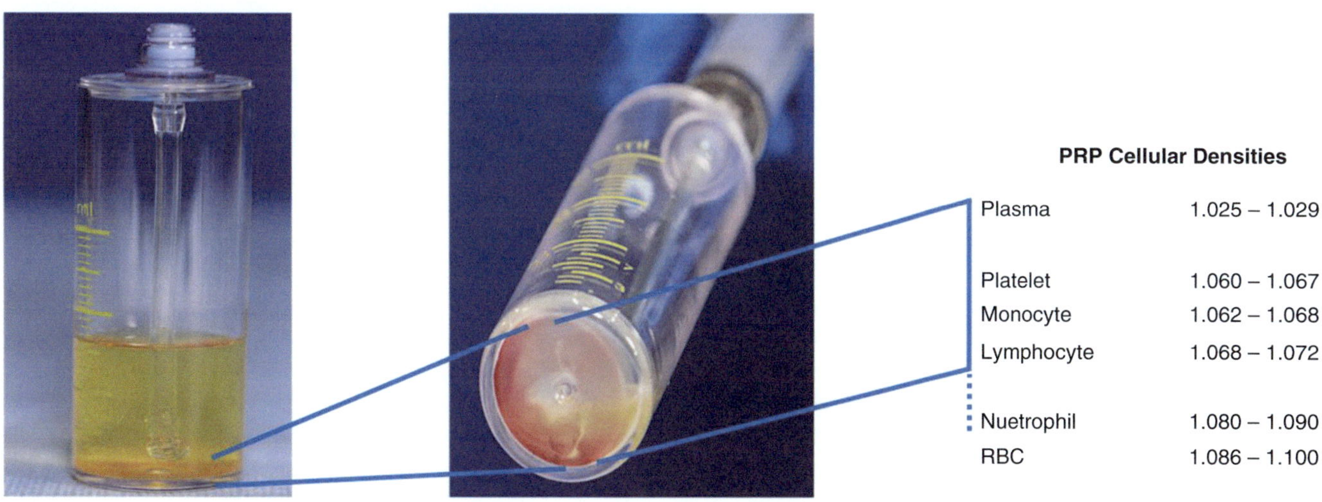

Fig. 62.1 Two-spin PRP preparation procedures result in cellular density gravitational separation. Cells are organized according to their specific densities. (Used with permission from EmCyte Corporation, Fort Myers, FL, USA, PurePRPI® device)

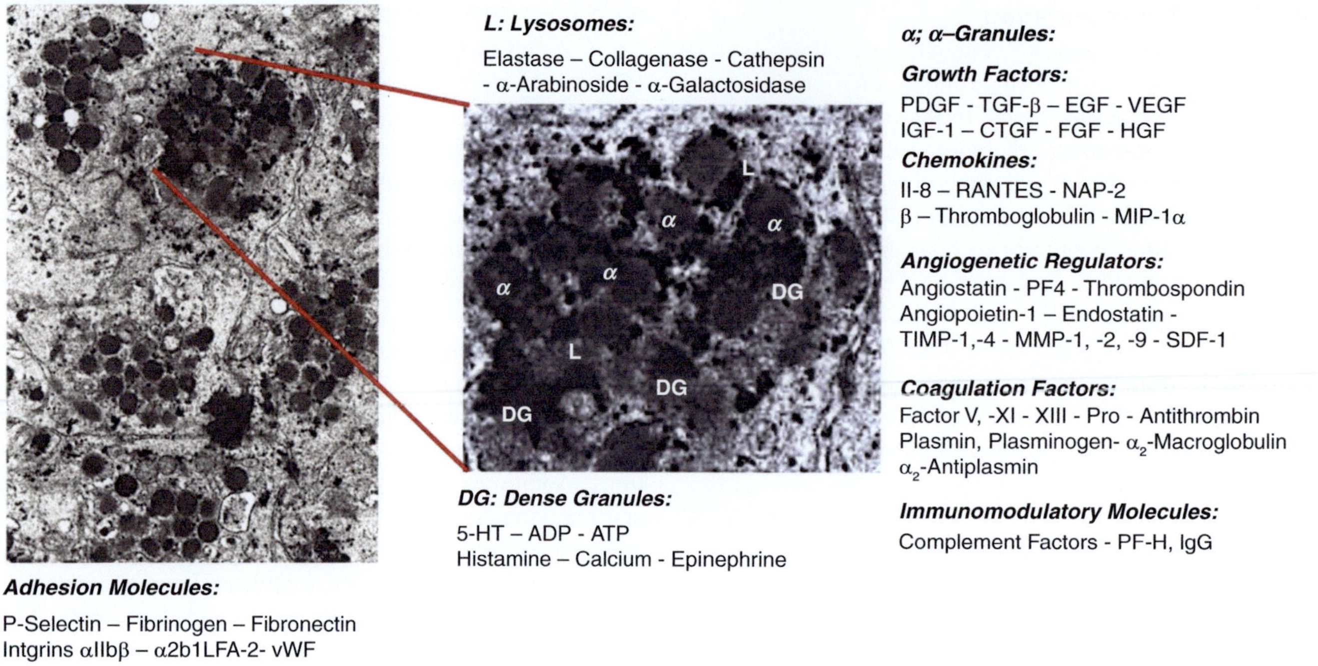

Fig. 62.2 Electron microscopic picture of a cluster of platelets after a PRP preparation showing the various intra-platelet structures at magnification X 10,000. The three platelet cellular constituents α-granules, dense granules (DG), and lysosomes (L) are clearly visible, including some platelet surface adhesion molecules. (Adapted and modified from Everts et al. [15])

T-cell immune responses and govern the protective immune response [18], linking the innate and adaptive immune systems. Moreover, platelet adenosine triphosphate (ATP) signals through the T-cell receptors, which results in an increase in the differentiation of CD4 T-helper cells to pro-inflammatory T helper 17 (Th17) cells [19]. Other platelet-dense granule constituents (e.g., glutamate and serotonin) induce T-cell migration and increase the differentiation of monocyte into DCs, respectively [20]. In PRP, these dense granule–derived immune modifiers are highly enriched and have substantial immune functions.

62.3.1.3 PRP: An Orthobiologic Treatment

PRP preparations have gained increasing popularity with widespread use in diverse medical fields. The underlying scientific rationale for PRP therapy is that an injection of concentrated platelets at sites of injury may initiate tissue repair via the release of many biologically active factors (growth factors, cytokines, lysosomes) and adhesion proteins that are responsible for initiating the hemostatic cascade, synthesis of new connective tissue, and revascularization. PRP is as complex as blood itself and likely more complex than traditional pharmaceutical drugs. PRP products are living biomaterials, and the outcomes of clinical PRP applications are dependent on the intrinsic, versatile, and adaptive characteristics of the patient's blood, including various other cell constituents that may be present in the PRP specimen [21] and the interaction with the recipient local microenvironment, which can be in an acute or chronic state.

PRP concentrates can stimulate the supraphysiological release of growth factors to jump-start healing in chronic injuries and accelerate the acute injury repair process [22]. At all stages of the tissue repair process, a wide variety of growth factors, cytokines, and locally acting regulators contribute to most basic cell functions via endocrine, paracrine, autocrine, and intracrine mechanisms (Table 62.2).

The main advantages of PRP include its safety and the ingenious preparation techniques of current commercial devices to prepare a biologic that can be used in a broad application profile [23]. Most importantly, PRP is an autologous product with no known adverse effects, in contrast to the commonly used corticosteroids and other non-autologous biological products [24, 25]. The enthusiasm to use PRP is often overshadowed as there are no clear regulations regarding the bioformulation and composition of an injectable PRP composition, and PRP compositions vary greatly regarding cellular content and PDGF concentrations [26, 27]. Furthermore, the vital roles of other cellular constituents present in these blood-derived products are partially understood, which was further aggravated by a lack of scientific data, mystical belief, commercial interests, and lack of standardization and classification [14]. In Table 62.3, an overview of the differences between some commercially available PRP and PRP-like devices is displayed, regarding platelet,

Table 62.2 PRP-based growth factors, angiogenetic factors, and platelet cytokines (Partial List)

Growth factors	Function and effects	
	PDGF (AA-BB-AB)	Mitogenic for mesenchymal cells and osteoblasts; stimulates chemotaxis and mitogenesis in fibroblast/glial/smooth muscle cells; regulates collagenase secretion and collagen synthesis; stimulates macrophage and neutrophil chemotaxis
	TGF (α – β)	Stimulates undifferentiated mesenchymal cell proliferation; regulates endothelial, fibroblastic, and osteoblastic mitogenesis; regulates collagen synthesis and collagenase secretion; regulates mitogenic effects of other growth factors; stimulates endothelial chemotaxis and angiogenesis; inhibits macrophage and lymphocyte proliferation
	HGF	Regulates cell growth and motility in epithelial/endothelial cells, supporting epithelial repair and neovascularization during wound healing
	EGF	Proliferation of keratinocytes, fibroblasts, stimulates mitogenesis for endothelial cells
	FGF (a-b)	Promotes growth and differentiation of chondrocytes and osteoblasts; mitogenic for mesenchymal cells, chondrocytes, and osteoblasts
	CTGF	Promotes angiogenesis, cartilage regeneration, fibrosis, and platelet adhesion
	IGF-1	Chemotactic for fibroblasts and stimulates protein synthesis; enhances bone formation by proliferation and differentiation of osteoblasts
	KGF	Regulates epithelial migration and proliferation
Angiogenetic factors	VEGF	Increases angiogenesis and vessel permeability; stimulates mitogenesis for endothelial cells
	IL-8	Pro-angiogenetic to stimulate angiogenesis
	5-HT	Pro-angiogenetic contributions
	Ang-1	Induces angiogenesis stimulating migration and proliferation of endothelial cells; supports and stabilizes blood vessel development via the recruitment of pericyte
	Endo	Endostatin
Cytokines	IL-1	Promotes systemic inflammation
	IL-6	Pro inflammation – anti-inflammation
	PF-4	Calls leucocytes and regulates their activation; has anti-angiogenetic properties
	SDF-1α	Calls CD34+ cells, induces their homing, proliferation, and differentiation into endothelial progenitor cells stimulating angiogenesis; calls mesenchymal stem cells and leukocytes
	TNF	Regulates monocyte migration, fibroblast proliferation, macrophage activation, angiogenesis

Modified from Everts et al. [32]

Abbreviations: *PDGF* platelet-derived growth factors, *TGF* transforming growth factor, *VEGF* vascular endothelial growth factor, *EGF* epidermal growth factor, *FGF* fibroblast growth factor, *CTCG* connective tissue growth factor, *IGF* insulin-like growth factor, *HGF* hepatocyte growth factor, *KGF* keratinocyte growth factor, *5-HT* serotonin, *Ang-1* angiopoietin-1, *Endo* endostatin, *IL-1* interleukin 1, *IL-6* interleukin 6, *IL-8* interleukin 8, *PF4* platelet factor 4, *SDF* stromal cell–derived factor, *TNF* tumor necrosis factor

Table 62.3 Variances in PRP commercial products and specimen differences

	Angel®	GPSIII®	PurePRP-A®	SmartPrep®	Regenkit®-A-PRP
PLT increase from BL	4.8	4.2	6.6	4.9	0.6
Platelets (× 10^6/mL)	856	754	1175	882	107
WBC (× 10^6/mL)	7.1	19.8	10.7	21.4	0.3
Monocyte %	33	15	72	27	0
RBC (× 10^9/mL) /HCT	0.3/2.8	1.1/8.1	0.1/1.1	0.9/7.9	0/0
PRP volume (mL)	3	6	7	7	5
T.D. PLTs (× 10^6/mL)	2568	4524	8225	6174	535

Same donor laboratory study ($N = 12$, only male donors), with average baseline platelet count of 178 × 10^6/mL, unpublished data

Abbreviations: *PLT* platelet, *BL* baseline, *WBC* white blood cell, *RBC* red blood cell, *PRP* platelet-rich plasma, *TD PLT* total deliverable platelets

Angel: Arthrex, Naples, FL, USA; GPS III: Zimmer Biomet, Warsaw, IN, USA; PurePRP: EmCyte Corporation, Fort Myers, FL, USA; SmartPrep: Terumo, Lakewood, CO, USA; Regenkit-A-PRP: Mont-sur-Lausanne, Switzerland

leukocyte cell (WBC) content, red blood cell (RBC) contamination, preparation volumes, and platelet dosing capabilities.

62.3.1.4 PRP Classification

Currently, orthobiological applications classify PRP into three groups: pure platelet-rich fibrin (P-PRF), leukocyte-rich PRP (LR-PRP), and leukocyte-poor PRP (LP-PRP) [28]. Although more specific than a generic PRP product definition, the LR-PRP and LP-PRP categories are significantly lacking any specificity regarding the leukocyte content. Regrettably, there is no consensus on a comprehensive classification system for PRP or any other autologous blood and blood-derived preparations. Ideally, a classification system should focus on the various PRP characteristics, definitions, and appropriate nomenclature that are relevant for therapeutic decision-making to treat patient-specific conditions.

62.3.2 PRP Component: Platelet

62.3.2.1 Platelet Activation and Tissue Repair Mechanisms

After the application of PRP on diseased tissues to initiate repair mechanism, PRP platelets interact with a broad range of cells to induce regenerative tissue remodeling mechanisms, following the classic functions of platelets. Underestimated are platelet functions where they interrelate with a variety of immune cells to regulate the immune responses following tissue injury and inflammation [29, 30]. During traumatic MSK disorders, platelets are among the first cells arriving at the site of vascular lesions and tissue breaches, where they interact with leukocytes, endothelial cells, and resident or circulating cells that are involved in tissue reorganization, following the induction and regulation of hemostasis [31].

After a controlled delivery of non-activated PRP, the platelets will be activated by interacting with platelet tissue factor (factor III), present in subendothelial tissues and leukocytes. Other activation pathways can be activiated by the addition of $CaCl_2$ and/or thrombin preparations.

Following platelet activation, the platelet α-, dense, lysosomal, and T granules undergo regulated exocytosis and release their contents into the extracellular environment (Fig. 62.3) [33, 34]. As a result, a platelet plug will develop in the injected microenvironment, as the first step of the healing cascade with the release of signaling molecules that trigger the recruitment and activation of inflammatory cells through a broad range of cell membrane receptors and soluble mediators, which are released upon PRP platelet activation [35].

62.3.2.2 PRP: Critical Platelet Count

PRP treatment protocols have evolved immensely over the past 10 years. Through experimental and clinical research, we now have a better understanding of platelet and other cellular physiology. Systematic reviews, meta-analyses, and randomized controlled trials denote the effectiveness of PRP biological technologies in many medical fields, including orthobiology and sports medicine [36, 37], spinal disorders [38], dermatology [39], cardiac surgery [40], plastic surgery [41], orthopedic surgery [42], and pain management [43].

The therapeutic actions of PRP and other platelet concentrates stem from the release of a multitude of factors involved in tissue repair and regeneration. Following platelet activation, a platelet plug is formed, which acts as a temporary extracellular matrix, allowing cells to proliferate and differentiate [2]. Therefore, it is fair to assume that higher platelet dosages will generate an elevated local concentration of released platelet bioactive factors. However, the correlation between platelet dose, concentration, and the concentration of released platelet bioactive growth factors and agents may not be precise because there are marked differences in baseline platelet counts between individual patients [44], and differences exist between PRP preparation methods [45, 46]. Likewise, several platelet growth factors involved in tissue repair mechanisms reside in the plasma fraction of PRP (e.g., hepatic growth factor and insulin-like growth factor 1). Therefore, higher platelet concentrations do not affect the repair potential of PGF [47].

In in vitro PRP research, study results are quickly obtained because the different parameters can be precisely controlled. Several studies have demonstrated that cells respond to PRP in a dose-dependent manner. Nguyen and Pham [48] showed

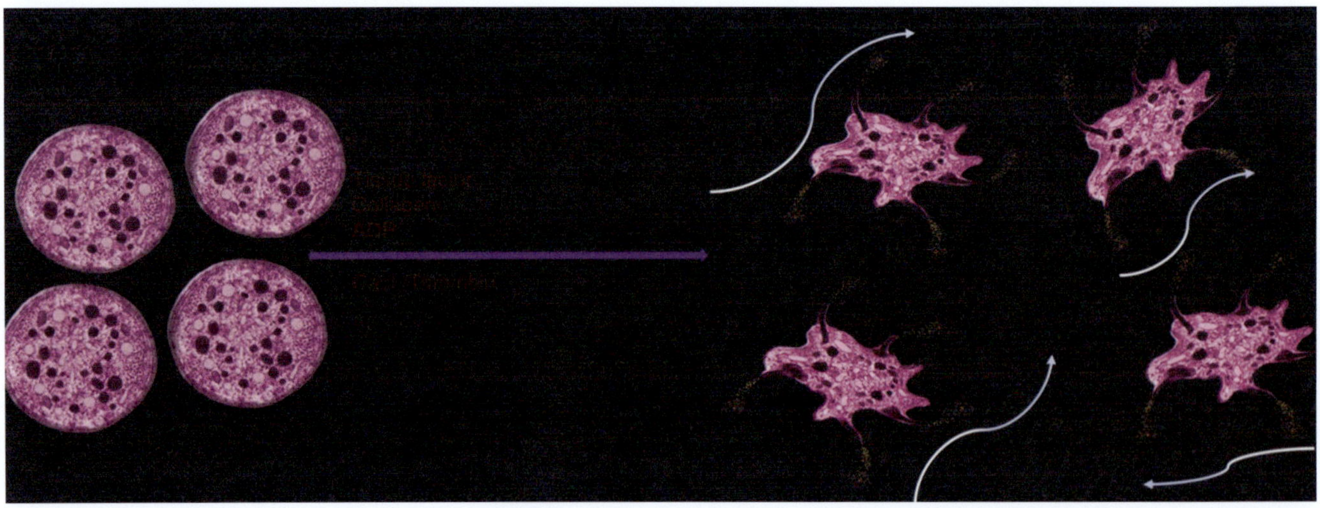

Fig. 62.3 Activated platelets change their shape with the development of pseudopods to promote platelet aggregation. Passive platelet activation is induced by platelet tissue factor and collagen, while active platelet activation can be accomplished by adding $CaCl_2$ and/or thrombin to the PRP specimen. Platelet activation will release the platelet content and all cellular components will invade the tissues

that very high concentrations of PGF are not necessarily advantageous for cell stimulatory processes and may be counterproductive. Some in vitro studies have indicated that high PGF concentrations may have detrimental effects [49]. One reason could be that the quantity of cell membrane receptors is limited. Thus, once the PGF levels are too high compared to the available receptors, they negatively affect cell function [50]. Although in vitro studies have many advantages, they also have some weaknesses.

62.3.2.3 PRP: Platelet Function: In Vitro vs. In Vivo

Due to tissue architecture and cell organization, there is a continuous interplay between many different cell types within any tissue, making it difficult to replicate in vitro in a two-dimensional monoculture setting. Cell density, which can affect cell signaling pathways, is usually less than 1% of the tissue situation. The two-dimensional in vitro culture dish organization precludes cells from being exposed to an extracellular matrix (ECM). Furthermore, typical culturing techniques lead to the accumulation of cellular waste products and continuous nutrient consumption. Thus, in vitro culturing does not resemble any homeostatic conditions, the tissue oxygen supply, or the sudden exchange of media, making it difficult to translate in vitro PRP dosing results into clinical practice. Conflicting results have been published comparing the clinical effects of PRP to in vitro studies for specific cells, tissue types, and platelet concentrations. Graziani et al. [51] found that in vitro, the maximum effect on the proliferation of osteoblasts and fibroblasts was achieved at a PRP platelet concentration that was 2.5-fold times higher than the baseline value. In contrast, clinical data presented by Park and associates [52] indicated that more than a fivefold increase in PRP platelet levels above baseline was required to induce a positive outcome after spinal fusion. Similar contradictory outcomes have been reported between in vitro tendon proliferation data and clinical outcome studies [36, 37]. It is apparent that in vitro and animal methodologies are not ideal study settings for successful translation into clinical practice.

62.3.2.4 PRP: Variation in Preparation

In general, PRP device comparison studies should not support decision-making, as they indicate a large variation in platelet concentrations among the large variety of available PRP devices [14], as demonstrated in an extensive review by Fadadu et al. [6]. In their study, 33 PRP systems and protocols were evaluated. Some of these systems produced final PRP preparations with a platelet count less than that of whole blood. They reported a PRP platelet factor increase as low as 0.52 with a single spin kit [53]. In contrast, the dual-spin device produced the highest platelet concentration ($1.6 \times 10^6/\mu L$) [6].

62.3.2.5 PRP: Clinically Required Platelet Concentration

It is important to understand the minimally required platelet concentration to induce an angiogenic response and stimulate cell proliferation and cell migration. Currently, PRP is characterized by its absolute platelet concentration, thereby shifting from the initial definition of PRP consisting of a platelet concentration above baseline values [2] to a minimum platelet concentration of more than $1 \times 10^6/\mu L$ or an approximately fivefold increase in platelets from baseline [54]. "Clinical PRP" should contain a critical dose of concentrated platelets to produce beneficial therapeutic effects. The platelets in clinical PRP should stimulate cell proliferation, synthesize mesenchymal and neurotrophic factors, contribute to chemotactic cell migration, and stimulate immunomodulatory activities [55, 56]. Marx was the first to demonstrate the enhancement of bone and soft tissue healing with a minimum platelet count of $1 \times 10^6/\mu L$ [2]. These results were confirmed in a transforaminal lumbar fusion study that demonstrated significantly more fusion when the platelet dose was greater than 1.3×10^6 platelets /μL [57]. Moreover, Giusti et al. [58] revealed that a dose of 1.5×10^9 platelets/mL is needed for tissue repair mechanisms to induce a functional angiogenic response through endothelial cell activity. In Giusti's study, higher concentrations reduced the angiogenic potential of platelets in follicular and perifollicular angiogenesis. Furthermore, earlier data indicate that the PRP dose also affects the magnitude of the therapy outcome [59]. Therefore, to significantly induce an angiogenic response and stimulate cell proliferation and cell migration, clinical PRP should contain at least 7.5×10^9 deliverable platelets in a 5-mL PRP treatment vial.

62.3.2.6 PRP: Dose Dependency

Apart from dose dependency, the effects of PRP on cell activity appear to be highly time-dependent. Soffer et al. [60] indicated that short-term exposure to human platelet lysate stimulates bone cell proliferation and chemotaxis. In contrast, long-term PRP exposure results in decreased levels of alkaline phosphatase and mineral formation. In a prospective, double-blinded, randomized controlled study from Bansal and associates, the effect of platelet dosing was unambiguously presented in patients with knee OA [61] This is the first study addressing the effect of leukocyte-poor PRP-platelet dosing. In their study, a single injection of 10 billion platelets, in a volume of 8 ml, improved functional and pain outcomes and preserved the articular cartilage for 12 months. Furthermore, decreased inflammatory markers were noted. From this study, one might conclude a sustained therapeutic effect with this high dose of platelets. Further studies need to elaborate whether higher doses are more beneficial or less effective.

62.3.3 PRP Component: Leukocytes

62.3.3.1 PRP: Leukocyte Fraction

The presence of leukocytes in PRP treatment is variable and dependent on the PRP preparation device. The presence of leukocytes in PRP preparations is dependent on the manufacturer's instruction and preparation protocol. The so-called plasma-based PRP devices do not contain any leukocytes. In buffy coat layer of PRP preparations, leukocytes are significantly concentrated [62], except for the eosinophils and basophils, as their cell membranes are too fragile to withstand the centrifugal processing forces.

Systematic reviews identified LP-PRP as the preferred PRP formulation to achieve effective treatment outcomes for joint OA [63]. However, Lana et al. [64] disagreed with this theory, suggesting that particular leukocytes play an important role in the inflammatory process preceding tissue regeneration due to their release of both pro- and anti-inflammatory molecules. They found that the combination of neutrophils and activated platelets could have a more positive than detrimental effect on tissue repair. They also indicated that the plasticity of monocytes is important for the non-inflammatory and reparative roles in tissue repair [64].

It is generally accepted that leukocytes greatly impact the intrinsic biology of chronic tissue lesions due to their immune and host-defense mechanisms. Much has been debated about the presence or absence of leukocytes and their contributions to different sub-PRP products, as reflected in Table 62.4 [64, 65]. In a recent review, six randomized controlled trials (level 1 evidence) and three prospective comparative studies (level 2 evidence) with a total of 1055 patients showed that LR-PRP and LP-PRP had similar safety profiles [66]. The authors concluded that the adverse reactions from PRP might not be directly related to the leukocyte concentration. In another study, LR-PRP did not modify systemic or local levels of the pro-inflammatory interleukins (IL-1β, IL-6, IL-8, and IL-17) in OA knees [67]. Those results support the idea that the in vivo role of leukocytes in the bioactivity of PRP might come from the crosstalk between the platelets and leukocytes. This interaction could promote the biosynthesis of other factors (e.g., lipoxins) that counteract or facilitate the resolution of inflammation [68].

After the initial release of inflammatory molecules (arachidonic acid, leukotrienes, and prostaglandins), lipoxin A4 is released from activated platelets to prevent neutrophil activation [64]. It is in this milieu that switches the MΦ phenotypes, from MΦ1 to MΦ2 [68]. Moreover, there has been accumulating evidence indicating that circulating monocytes can differentiate into a variety of non-phagocytic cell types due to their multipotential nature [69].

The type of PRP can influence MSC cultures. LR-PRP can induce significantly higher bone marrow–derived MSC (BM-MSC) proliferation than pure PRP or PPP samples, with faster release and better biological activity of PGFs [70].

Table 62.4 PRP and sub-PRP classifications

Platelet-rich plasma (PRP)
Pure-PRP (P-PRP)
Leukocyte-rich PRP (LR-PRP)
Leukocyte-poor PRP (LP-PRP)
Platelet-rich fibrin (PRF)
Platelet-rich fibrin matrix (PRFM)
Preparation rich in growth factors (PRGF)

62.3.3.2 PRP: Function of Specific Leukocyte

Leukocytes greatly influence the intrinsic biology of acute and chronic tissue conditions because of their immune and host-defense mechanisms. Therefore, the presence of specific leukocytes in PRP preparations can cause significant cellular and tissue effects. More specifically, different PRP buffy coat systems utilize different preparation protocols, thereby producing different neutrophil, lymphocyte, and monocyte cell ratios in PRP [71]. Further research is needed to develop a consensus regarding the role and magnitude of leukocytes in PRP bioformulations to treat certain pathologies and conditions adequately and safely.

- *Neutrophils*

Neutrophils are essential leukocytes in numerous healing pathways that create dense barriers against invading pathogens [72] in conjunction with antimicrobial proteins present in platelets [73]. The presence of neutrophils in PRP preparations is mostly based on the treatment objectives. Exacerbated tissue inflammatory levels can be necessary in chronic wound care PRP biological treatments [32] or applications directed toward bone growth or healing [74]. The use of a full buffy coat PRP treatment vial is also frequently mentioned in chronic tendinopathy treatments [75, 76]. Importantly, additional neutrophil functions have been uncovered in several models, emphasizing their roles in angiogenesis and tissue restoration [77]. However, neutrophils can also cause harmful effects and, thus, are not indicated for some applications. Zhou and Wang demonstrated that the use of PRP rich in neutrophils could result in a higher collagen type III to collagen type I ratio, adding to fibrosis and decreased tendon strength [78]. Other neutrophil-mediated deleterious properties are the release of inflammatory cytokines and metalloproteinases (MMPs) that promote pro-inflammatory and catabolic effects when applied to tissues [79].

- *Lymphocytes*

In the buffy coat of PRP preparations, mononuclear T and B lymphocytes are more concentrated than any other leukocytes. They are critically involved in cell-mediated cytotoxic adaptive immunity. Lymphocytes can elicit a cell response to fight infection and adapt to intruders [80]. Furthermore, T lymphocyte–derived cytokines (interferon-γ [IFN-γ] and interleukin-4 [IL-4]) strengthen macrophage polarization [81]. Weirather et al. demonstrated that regular T lymphocytes indirectly contribute to tissue healing in a mouse model by modulating monocyte and macrophage differentiation [82].

- *Monocytes and Macrophages*

Depending on the PRP preparation devices used, monocytes may be prominent or absent in prepared PRP. Unfortunately, their manifestation and regenerative capabilities are rarely discussed in the literature. Therefore, little attention is given to monocytes in preparation methods or final formulations. In the orthobiological literature, leukocyte differentiation is rarely addressed and the reporting of PRP preparation protocols has been highly inconsistent. Furthermore, most published studies do not present the PRP preparation methods needed for protocol reproducibility, even though PRP biological preparations containing specific leukocytes can significantly contribute to pro-inflammation, immune modulation, tissue repair, and regeneration. However, monocytes and macrophages play key roles in immunomodulatory processes and tissue repair mechanisms [83].

Monocyte populations are heterogeneous and originate from progenitor cells in the bone marrow via hematopoietic stem cell pathways and traffic via the bloodstream to peripheral tissues depending on the microenvironmental stimuli. During homeostasis and inflammation, circulating monocytes leave the bloodstream and are recruited to injured or degenerated tissues. They can act either as effector cells or as progenitors of macrophages (MΦs). Monocytes, macrophages, and dendritic cells represent the mononuclear phagocyte system (MPS) [84]. A typical feature of the MPS is the plasticity in their gene expression patterns and functional overlap between these cell types. In degenerated tissues, resident macrophages, local-acting growth factors, pro-inflammatory cytokines, apoptotic or necrotic cells, and microbial products initiate the differentiation of monocytes into MPS cell populations [85]. Hypothetically, when C-PRP containing high yields of monocytes is injected in a diseased local microenvironment, monocytes most likely differentiate into MΦs to provoke major cellular changes.

During the monocyte-to-MΦ transition, particular MΦ phenotypes are produced [83]. MΦ phenotype 1 (MΦ1) is characterized by inflammatory cytokine secretion and the production of both VEGF and FGF. The MΦ2 phenotype consists of anti-inflammatory cells, producing mainly extracellular matrix components and angiogenic factors [84]. From these data, it is reasonable to assume that C-PRP preparations containing a high concentration of monocytes and MΦs are likely to contribute to better tissue repair because of their anti-inflammatory tissue repair and cell signaling capabilities.

62.3.4 PRP Component: RBC

The role of RBCs in tissue regeneration has never been established. RBCs are responsible for transporting oxygen to tissues and removing carbon dioxide from tissues to the lungs [86]. They have no nucleus and are made of protein-bound heme molecules. Iron and heme components inside RBCs facilitate the binding of oxygen and carbon dioxide. Normally, the RBC life cycle is approximately 120 days. They are removed from circulation by macrophages by a process termed RBC senescence. Under conditions of shear forces (e.g., whole blood phlebotomy procedures, immune-mediated processes, oxidative stress, or inadequate PRP concentration protocols), RBCs in the PRP specimens could become damaged. As a consequence, the RBC cell membrane disintegrates and releases toxic hemoglobin (Hb), measured as plasma-free hemoglobin (PFH), hemin, and iron [87]. PFH and its degradation products (heme and iron) collectively lead to detrimental and cytotoxic effects on tissues, causing oxidative stress, loss of nitric oxide, activation of inflammatory pathways, and immunosuppression. These effects ultimately lead to microcirculatory dysfunction, local vasoconstriction with vascular damage, and significant tissue injury.

Most importantly, when PRP containing RBCs is delivered to tissues, it causes a local response called eryptosis, which triggers the release of a potent cytokine, macrophage migration inhibitory factor [88]. This cytokine inhibits the migration of monocytes and macrophages. It exerts profound pro-inflammatory signals to surrounding tissues that inhibit the migration of stem cells and fibroblast proliferation and causes significant local cellular dysfunction. Based on above explanation, limiting RBC contamination in PRP preparations is important. Adequate C-PRP centrifugation and preparation processes typically reduce or even eliminate the presence of RBCs, thereby avoiding the detrimental consequences of hemolysis and eryptosis.

62.3.5 PRP: Immunomodulatory Effects

The body can identify foreign bodies and injured tissues in acute or chronic conditions to initiate the wound healing cascade and related inflammatory pathways. The innate and adaptive immune systems protect the host from infection, with essential roles for leukocytes overlapping between both systems, as displayed in Fig. 62.4. Specifically, monocytes,

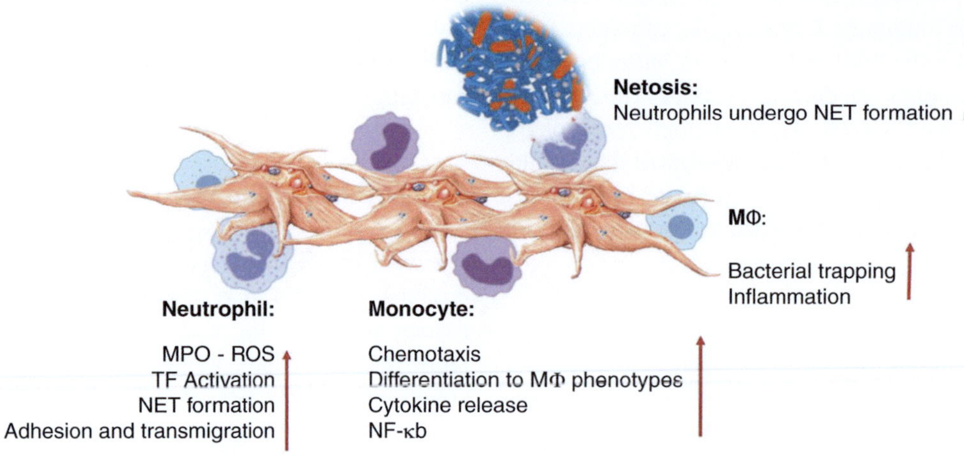

Fig. 62.4 Platelet and leukocyte interactions in innate immunity cell interactions. Platelets interact with neutrophils, monocytes, and ultimately with MΦs, modulating and increasing their effector functions. These platelet-leukocyte interactions result in inflammatory contributions through different mechanisms, including NETosis. Abbreviations: MPO myeloperoxidase, ROS reactive oxygen species, TF tissue factor, NETs neutrophil extracellular traps, NF-κB nuclear factor kappa B, MΦ macrophage

macrophages, neutrophils, and natural killer cells have pivotal roles in the innate system, whereas lymphocytes and their subsets play similar roles in the adaptive immune system [89].

- *Innate Immune System*

The role of the innate immune system is to identify intruding microbes or tissue fragments and stimulate their clearance. Activation of the innate immune system occurs when certain molecular structures, termed *surface-expressed pattern recognition receptors*, bind to *pathogen-associated molecular patterns* and *damage-associated molecular patterns*. Interestingly, platelets also express several immunomodulatory receptor molecules on their surface, such as P-selectin, transmembrane protein CD40 ligand (CD40L), cytokines (e.g., IL-1β), and platelet specific toll-like receptors (TLR), enabling them to interact with various immune cells [90].

Neutrophils, monocytes, and dendritic cells are the most common innate immune cells in the blood. Their recruitment is required for an adequate early-phase immune response. Platelet-leukocyte interactions regulate inflammation, wound healing, and tissue repair when PRP is used in regenerative medicine applications. More specifically, the platelet TLRs stimulate platelet-neutrophil interactions [91], which regulate the so-called leukocyte oxidative burst by modulating the release of reactive oxygen species (ROS) and myeloperoxidase (MPO) from neutrophils [92]. Furthermore, the platelet-neutrophil interaction with neutrophil degranulation results in the formation of neutrophil-extracellular traps (NETs). NETs comprise the neutrophil nucleus and other neutrophil intracellular contents that trap bacteria and kill them by NETosis. The formation of NETs is an essential killing mechanism for neutrophils [93]. As a result of PRP platelet activation, monocytes can migrate to diseased and degenerative tissues where they perform adhesion activities while secreting inflammatory molecules that may alter chemotaxis and modify proteolytic properties [94]. Additionally, platelets can modulate the effector functions of monocytes by inducing the activation of monocyte NF-κb [95], a critical mediator of the inflammatory response and the activation and differentiation of immune cells. Therefore, PRP preparation devices that can yield high concentrations of monocytes from whole blood have the advantage of this mechanism in tissue repair processes after PRP application.

- *Adaptive Immune System*

The adaptive immune system employs antigen-specific receptors and remembers previous pathogen encounters and destroys these pathogens during subsequent encounters with the host. However, these adaptive immune responses are slow to develop. Cognasse et al. [90] showed that platelet components contribute to danger sensing and tissue repair and suggested that the interaction of platelets with leukocytes facilitates the activation of the adaptive immune response.

During adaptive immune responses, platelets promote monocyte and macrophage responses. Thus, platelet granular constituents directly affect adaptive immunity by expressing CD40L [96], a molecule critical to the modulation of adaptive immune responses, as they promote T-cell responses to inflammatory stimuli for robust pro-and anti-inflammatory responses [97]. Moreover, platelets have an abundance of cell surface receptors that can prompt platelet activation, with the release of numerous inflammatory and bioactive molecules stored within different platelet granules, thus influencing both innate and adaptive immune responses [30].

Following the identification of microbes or tissue damage by the non-specific innate immune system, the specific adaptive immune system takes over. The adaptive system includes B lymphocytes (B cells), which bind antigens, and regular T lymphocytes (Treg), which coordinate the elimination of the pathogens. T cells can be broadly categorized into helper T cells (Th cells) and cytotoxic T cells (Tc cells, also known as T killer cells) [89]. The Th cells are further divided into Th1, Th2, and Th17 cells, with critical functions in inflammation. The Th cells can secrete pro-inflammatory cytokines (e.g., IFN-γ and TNF-β) and several interleukins. They are particularly effective in protecting against intracellular viral and bacterial infections. Th cells stimulate proliferation and differentiation of cells involved in the immunological response. Tc cells are effector cells that eliminate the targeted intracellular and extracellular microbes and cells [98].

Interestingly, the Th2 cells produce IL-4 and influence MΦ polarization, directing MΦs to the regenerative MΦ2 phenotype, while IFN-γ shifts MΦ toward the inflammatory MΦ1phenotype, depending on the dose and timing of the cytokines. Th cells guide MΦ phenotypes to pro-regenerative phenotypes in response to tissue-derived biologics in an IL-4-dependent manner [99]. This mechanism is based on the evidence that Th cells have a pronounced role in controlling both inflammation and tissue repair.

62.3.6 PRP: Nociceptive Effects

Activated platelets release many pro- and anti-inflammatory mediators that are proficient in inducing pain but can also reduce inflammation and pain. Once applied, the typical platelet dynamics of PRP alter the microenvironment prior to tissue repair and regeneration via multiple complex pathways related to anabolic and catabolic processes, cell proliferation, differentiation, and stem cell regulation. These PRP characteristics have led to the implementation of PRP applications in various clinical pathological conditions that are usually associated with chronic pain (e.g., sports injuries, orthopedic pathologies, spinal disorders, and complex chronic wounds), even though the exact mechanisms are not yet fully understood.

In 2008, Everts et al. [100] were the first to report a randomized controlled trial on the analgesic effects of a PRP formulation prepared from autologous buffy coat and activated with autologous thrombin following shoulder surgery. They noticed a significant reduction in visual analog scale scores, the use of opioid-based pain medication, and a more successful postsurgical rehabilitation. Of note, they reflected on the analgesic effects of activated platelets and postulated on the mechanism of platelet-released 5-HT. Briefly, platelets are dormant in freshly prepared PRP. After direct or indirect (tissue factor) platelet activation, platelets change shape and develop pseudopods to promote platelet aggregation. Subsequently, they release their intracellular α- and dense granules [22]. Tissues treated with activated PRP will be invaded by PGFs, cytokines, and other platelet lysosomes. More specifically, when the dense granules release their contents, an abundance of pain-modulating 5-HT will be discharged [101]. In PRP, the platelet concentration can be five- to sevenfold higher than in peripheral blood. Therefore, the release of 5-HT from the platelet is astronomical. Interestingly, Sprott et al. [102] reported observing substantial pain reduction following acupuncture and a significant decrease in platelet-derived 5-HT concentrations, with a subsequent increase in 5-HT plasma levels.

In the periphery, endogenous 5-HT is released from platelets, mast cells, and endothelial cells in response to tissue injury or surgical trauma [103]. Interestingly, multiple neuronal 5-HT receptors have been detected in the periphery, confirming that 5-HT can interfere with nociceptive transmission at peripheral sites. The 5-HT system represents a powerful system that can decrease and increase the magnitude of pain following noxious stimulation. Studies have indicated that 5-HT can affect nociceptive transmission at peripheral tissue sites through a variety of 5-HT receptors [104, 105].

In analgesic animal model trials, the potential of PRP analgesic effect was demonstrated by Yoshida et al. [106]. In several clinical studies, the nociceptive and analgesic effects of PRP were discussed. Several studies have indicated little to no pain relief in patients treated for tendinosis pathologies or rotator cuff tears [107, 108]. In contrast, several other studies indicated that PRP reduced or even eliminated pain in patients suffering from tendinosis, OA, plantar fasciitis, and other foot and ankle disorders [109, 110].

The final platelet concentration and the biocellular composition have been identified as key PRP characteristics that contributed to the consistent analgesic effects observed after PRP applications. Other variables included PRP delivery methods, platelet activation protocols, the bioactivity levels of the released PGFs and cytokines, the types of tissues to which PRP was applied, and the type of injury. Notably, Kuffler addressed the potential of PRP in pain relief in patients suffering from mild to severe chronic neuropathic pain, secondary to a damaged non-regenerated nerve. The objective of this study was to investigate whether neuropathic pain would decrease or resolve as a result of PRP's promotion of axonal regeneration and target reinnervation [111]. Strikingly, in treated patients, the neuropathic pain remained eliminated, or reduced, for a minimum of 6 years after the procedure and pain started to decrease within 3 weeks after the surgical PRP application, in all patients.

Recently, similar analgesic PRP effects were observed in the field of postsurgical wound and skincare [112]. Interestingly, the authors reported the physiological aspects of wound pain related to vascular injury and tissue hypoxia, addressing the importance of neoangiogenesis in optimizing oxygenation and nutrient delivery. More pain reduction was noted in PRP-treated patients compared to controls, with significantly higher angiogenetic development in post-PRP-treated patients.

Finally, Johal and co-workers performed a systematic review and meta-analysis and concluded that PRP leads to a reduction in pain following PRP administration in orthopedic indications, particularly in patients treated for lateral epicondylitis and knee OA [10]. Unfortunately, this study did not specify the effects of leukocytes, platelet concentration, or the use of exogenous platelet-activating agents, as these variables affect the overall PRP effectiveness. The optimal PRP platelet concentration that provokes maximal pain relief is yet unknown. In a rat tendinopathy model, complete pain relief was accomplished with a platelet concentration of 1.0 $x10^6/\mu L$, whereas PRP with half this platelet concentration induced significantly less pain relief [106]. Thus, more clinical studies to investigate the analgesic effects of different PRP formulations are needed.

62.3.7 PRP: Angiogenetic Effects

Ideally, the PRP preparations employed in precision regenerative orthobiological therapies allow for the delivery of biomolecules released by a high concentration of platelets, which are ultimately (passively) activated at the target tissue site. As a result, countless physiological cascades are initiated, resulting in on-site immunomodulatory and inflammatory processes, and angiogenesis stimulating healing and tissue repair activities [113].

Angiogenesis is a vibrant, multistep process involving the sprouting and organization of micro vessels from preexisting blood vessels. Angiogenesis progresses due to multiple biological mechanisms, including endothelial cell migration, proliferation, differentiation, and division. These cellular processes are prerequisites to the formation of new blood vessels. They are essential for the outgrowth of preexisting blood vessels to restore blood flow and support the high metabolic activity of tissue repair and tissue regeneration. These new vessels allow the delivery of oxygen and nutrients and the removal of by-products from the treated tissues [114].

Within a diseased and degenerative microenvironment (including a low oxygen tension, low pH, and high lactate levels), local angiogenic factors try to restore angiogenic activities. Following PRP treatment in these MSK pathologies, angiogenic activities are modulated by a balance between pro- and anti-angiogenetic factors. The most important factors are shown in Table 62.5.

Table 62.5 PRP – platelet pro- and anti-angiogenetic factors [15]

Platelet pro-angiogenetic factors	Platelet anti-angiogenetic factors
VEGF	PAI
PDGF-BB	TSP
TGF- β1	TGF- β1
Serotonin	PF-4
MMP-1,-2	Angiostatin
IL-8	TIMPS

Abbreviations: *VEGF* vascular endothelial growth factor, *PDGF-BB* platelet-derived growth factor BB, *TGF-β1* transforming growth factor, *MMP* matrix metalloprotenases, *IL* interleukin, *PAI* plasminogen activator inhibitor, *PF* platelet factor, *TIMPS* tissue inhibitors of metalloprotenases

It has been demonstrated that the overall PRP platelets effects on (neo)angiogenesis is pro-angiogenic and stimulatory [115]. Notably, Landsdown and Fortier [116] reported on the various outcome effects related to the PRP constituents, including intra-platelet sources of numerous angiogenic modulators. Furthermore, they concluded that an increase in angiogenesis contributes to the healing of MSK disorders in areas of poor vascularization, such as meniscal tears, tendon injuries, and other areas with poor vascularity. The administration of PRP, more specifically the delivery of high concentrations of PGFs and other platelet cytokines, can induce angiogenesis, vasculogenesis, and arteriogenesis because stromal cell-derived factor-1a binds to the specific cytokine receptors on endothelial progenitor cells. Another important and essential factor in restoring angiogenic pathways is synergy between multiple PGFs. Richardson et al. [117] demonstrated that the synergistic activities of the angiogenic factors platelet-derived growth factor BB (PDGF-BB) and VEGF result in the rapid formation of a mature vascular network compared to the individual growth factor activities. Most importantly, Giusti and co-workers concluded in a dose defining study that the optimal platelet dose to promote angiogenesis was 1.5×10^6 platelets/μL [64]. Therefore, it is fair to assume that PRP preparations with high concentrations of platelets contain high concentrations of the stimulatory pro-angiogenic PGF VEGF, contributing to significant angiogenetic effects, when compared to PRP preparations with less than 1.5×10^6 platelets/μL.

62.4 Bone Marrow Concentrate (BMC)

The human body has an endogenous system of tissue repair and tissue regeneration through stem cells, as they are found almost in every type of tissue. Clinicians utilizing regenerative medicine applications have a growing interest in using the concentrated bone marrow products, since it is well acknowledged that BM is a plentiful source of MSCs, progenitors, and other cells residing in the trabecular part of flat and long bones, acquired via appropriately performed BMA procedures [118, 119]. Orthobiological and regenerative medicine treatment options using autologous stem cells can be safely executed by well-trained physicians at point of care.

62.4.1 Bone Marrow Anatomy

The bone is an organ composed of cortical and trabecular bone, cartilage, and hematopoietic and connective tissues. The BM tissue is soft, similar to the peripheral blood, flexible connective tissue comprising the center and the epiphysis of bones, referred to as the BM cavity. In this place, a variety of new blood cells are produced and ultimately released to the peripheral circulation. The bone tissue has an essential role in the structure and protection of the human body. Spongy, or trabecular bone, is composed of a lattice of fine bone plates filled with hematopoietic marrow, fat-containing marrow, and arterial-venous sinusoidal blood vessels. Furthermore, it consists of bone cells at different developmental stages (including pre-osteoblasts, osteoblasts, and osteocytes), collagen fibrils, and calcium and phosphate deposits.

We recognize two categories of bone marrow tissue: the red and yellow marrow. Depending on age, the red marrow is replaced by the yellow marrow. In adults, the red bone marrow is a rich source of bone marrow-derived cells and present in most skeletal system bones of the iliac crest, tibia, spine vertebrae, humerus, calcaneus, ribs, and near point of attachment of long bones of legs and arms. In this well-shielded environment, an estimate of 500 billion cells per day can be produced, in particular erythrocytes, granulocytes, and platelets [120]. For orthobiological applications, the red bone marrow is the preferred type as it contains myeloid and lymphoid stem cells and MSCs.

62.4.2 Bone Marrow Regions

The trabecular bone cavity is subdivided into four region, Table 62.6 [121], according to the model of Lambertsen and Weis. In Fig. 62.5, we illustrate this model which we have adopted and modified for clarification purposes. In general, the bone marrow consists of a hematopoietic component

Table 62.6 Bone marrow regions

Subendosteal
Peri-sinusoidal region
Central region
Endosteal region

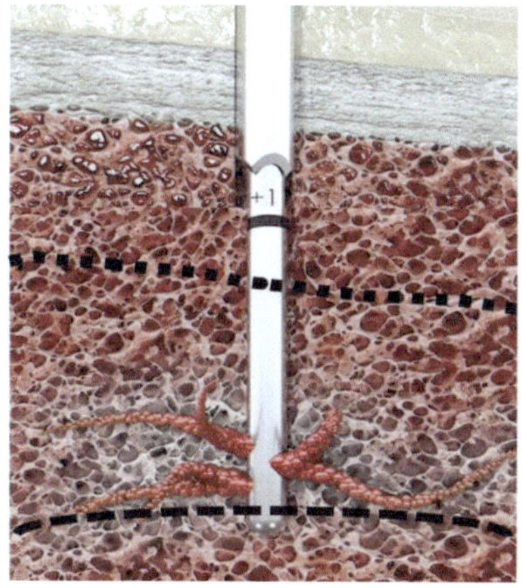

Fig. 62.5 Endosteal and subendosteal regions in a trabecular bone cavity

(parenchyma) and a vascular component (stroma). The parenchyma includes hematopoietic progenitor and hematopoietic stem cells (HSCs), which are localized close to the endosteum and around the blood vessels. BM stroma cells, including endothelial cells, are recognized as multipotential non-hematopoietic progenitor cells capable of differentiating into various tissues of mesenchymal origin, including osteoblasts, chondrocytes, tenocytes, endothelial cells, myocytes, fibroblasts, nerves, and adipocytes, as verified in in vitro and partially in in vivo research [122, 123]. The bone marrow's microvasculature includes single layers of endothelium arising in sinusoids, where they also contribute to rolling extravasations of leukocytic cells into and out of the BM tissue structures. The function of the vasculature and BM-derived endothelial cells is that they provide a barrier between the BM compartment as a functional and spatial entity from the extra-lymphoid BM section and the peripheral circulation [9]. The endothelial cells likewise contribute to tissue regeneration, as endothelial precursor cells are essential in improving vascularization of damaged and degenerative tissue cells by the secretion of pro-angiopoietic factors of invading cells [124].

62.4.3 Bone Marrow Niche

A niche is defined by anatomy and function. Stem cell niches are defined as specific cellular and molecular microenvironments regulating stem cell and progenitor functions. A niche consists of signaling molecules, intercellular contact, and the interaction between stem cells and their neighboring extracellular matrix (ECM). This three-dimensional microenvironment is thought to control genes and properties that define "stemness," including the control and balance between quiescence, self-renewal, proliferation, and differentiation of diverse cell types. Additionally, the microenvi-

Table 62.7 Bone marrow classical niches [26–28, 34]

Mesenchymal stem cell niche
Hematopoietic stem cell niche
Perivascular niche
Megakaryocyte niche

ronment provides stem cell autonomous signaling mechanisms [125, 126], and it engages in specific cascades to a stress response [127]. Acquired and prepared BM stem cells from one of the niches and subsequently injected into a totally different microenvironment can potentially differentiate into cell types of this new environment [128]. In Table 62.7, some of the bone marrow niches are given. Since autologously prepared MSCs originate from their specific and original BM niche but are used in other cellular tissue types to treat various pathologies, they can be successfully engaged in tissue repair and regeneration through regenerative medicine application techniques. This is a distinctly different approach in the physiological release of newly formed BM cells because they are retained in the BM cavity until they mature and thereafter released in the vascular peripheral circulation [123].

The role and function of the extracellular matrix (ECM) can be defined as key structural-functional components of cell niches, including soluble factors, cell-cell contacts, and cell-matrix adhesions present in these microenvironments. ECM components include fibrillar proteins, with, among others, collagen fibers, fibronectin, and other filamentous network components. The ECM's mechanical stability is provided by collagen [129]. Other significant ECM components supporting the BM niches are glycosaminoglycans and mainly hyaluronic acid via its receptor CD44. In general, no specific ECM components are identified that maintain MSCs in their immature state, as a niche matrix would do. However, it has become clear that the ECM can regulate MSC differentiation on a solitary basis, indicating potential applications for regenerative medicine applications and tissue engineering.

62.4.4 Stem Cells

Becker, McCulloch, and Till first conducted experiments that led to the discovery of stem cells in 1963 and they produced evidence that these cells were capable of endless self-renewal, which is a fundamental feature of stem cells [130]. A stem cell is a type of cell that is non-specific/specialized in its function. Generally, we recognize two types of stem cells, embryonic and non-embryonic, with two defining properties. Firstly, they have the capacity of self-renewal, therefore giving rise to more stem cells. Secondly, they can differentiate into different lineages under appropriate conditions.

Embryonic stem cells (ESCs) are obtained from 5- to 12-day-old embryos, and they are pluripotent and have a high plasticity as they can differentiate into ectoderm, mesoderm, and endoderm layers, whereas non-embryonic stem cells (non-ESCs) are multipotent, and it appears that they are able to form multiple cell lineages which form an entire tissue, usually specific to one germ layer, e.g., adult stem cells [131].

The capability of stem cell potency, in combination with the relative ease to prepare bone marrow stem cell injectates, is an invaluable property for regenerative medicine cell-based therapies in general and more specifically to treat, e.g., musculoskeletal disorders (MSK-D), chronic wounds, and critical limb ischemia. Friedenstein and colleagues reported first on the isolation of bone marrow–derived stem cells from BM stroma and their incubation in plastic culture dishes, and identified mesenchymal stem cells as colony-forming unit fibroblasts (CFU-Fs) [132]. The BM stroma is made up of a network of fibroblast-like cells and includes a subpopulation of multipotent cells which can generate the mesenchyme, known as the mass of tissue, that develops mainly from the mesoderm of the embryo subpopulation. The cells are referred to as mesenchymal stem cells (MSCs) [133]. The Friedenstein culture method revealed that MSCs can differentiate into several connective tissue cell types [134], described first by Pittenger and associates [135].

62.4.4.1 BMC: Bone Marrow–Specific Stem Cells

The literature articulates BMAs as a heterogeneous mix of cells, referring in most instances to HSCs, MSCs, and mononuclear cells. The roles of platelets, megakaryocytes, and RBCs are seldomly mentioned [136].

1. Hematopoietic Stem Cells

The major function of the bone marrow is to generate blood cells. In adults, marrow-derived HSCs are the principal cells of origin of all mature hematopoietic cell phenotypes, and the process is called hematopoiesis. HSCs are adult stem cells with extensive self-renewal capabilities and can differentiate into specialized blood cells with key roles in some biological activities: control homeostasis balance, immune functions, and response to microorganisms and inflammation. Most HSCs are in a quiescent state within the BM niches. They respond to the signals after the balance of blood cells, or HSC pool, is disturbed from either intrinsic or extrinsic stimuli and signaling processes [137]. Evolving evidence suggests that BM-derived endothelial cells and HSCs, including their progenitor cells, contribute to tissue vascularization. HSCs deliver specific angiogenetic factors, facilitating the incorporation of endothelial progenitor cells into newly sprouting vessels. Several clinical studies have shown that BM-derived cells contribute to neo-angiogenesis [138, 139]. This should contribute to the clinical discussion of the value of BM-derived HSC and vascular progenitor as they are able to contribute to tissue restoration by accelerating tissue vascularization and regeneration [140].

2. Mesenchymal Stem Cells

In recent decades, physicians performing orthobiological/regenerative medicine procedures have been more interested in the potential of BM-MSCs than of HSCs. Imaginable reasons for this particular interest in MSCs might be due to recently published expert opinions: the in vivo ability of MSCs to migrate into tissues, their sturdy regenerative and reparative properties, and MSC-mediated immunomodulatory actions. These typical characteristics and their particular mode of actions enable conceivable BM cell-based treatment options [141, 142]. MSCs do not express significant histocompatibility complexes and immune-stimulating molecules, leading to graft rejection. Likewise, a rapid development in clinical outcome reporting, with a better understanding of BM tissue molecular biology, improved bone marrow aspiration techniques and, and preparation methods, has increased the interest and indication for autologous BM stem and progenitor cell therapies.

MSC function: MSCs are multipotent stem cells which can be obtained from various adult tissues, like the BM stroma, adipose tissue, synovium, periosteum, and trabecular bone. Typical features are their ability for self-renewal, defined as sustaining biological pathways and mechanisms to preserve the undifferentiated stem state, and the regulation of lineage-specific differentiation [143]. Although the number of MSCs represents only a small fraction of non-hematopoietic, multipotent cells of the bone marrow (0.001–0.01%), understanding these unique cells has taken great strides forward. Under appropriate conditions and an optimal microenvironment, MSCs can differentiate into various mesodermal lineages like osteoblasts, chondrocytes, endothelial cells, adipose tissue, and smooth muscle cells [144]. These MSC proficiencies have led to the use of MSC as a potential strategy for treating various diseases, since they encourage biological processes, for example angiogenesis, cell proliferation, and cell differentiation [145]. Furthermore, they synthesize cytokines and trophic mediators which participate in tissue repair processes, immune modulation, and the regulation of inflammatory processes [146]. Based on the above characteristics, it can be assumed that MSCs are capable of instituting a regenerative microenvironment at the site of release and improving various cell recruitment, cell signaling, and differentiation of endogenous stem cells, with the potential to instigate tissue repair in a variety of disease states.

62.4.4.2 BMC: Harvesting and Preparation

Several groups have mentioned some considerations when performing BM harvesting procedures, addressing a variety of factors that have an impact on patient comfort and the quality of the harvested BM. Emphasis was given to procedural safety issues when using harvesting needle systems, level of experience of the operator, the choice for concentration technology and centrifugation devices, and pain management [147]. Autologous regenerative medicine BM-MSC applications may range from harvesting a low volume of BM and direct, unprocessed, tissue injection to the use of centrifugation protocols to concentrate and filter the BMA prior to injecting it in patients [148]. Various bone marrow harvesting systems are available on the market, each with their own proprietary design characteristics, and thus marrow cellular dynamics when extracting marrow. Potentially, different BM needle design features might affect the quality and cell viability of the harvested marrow tissue, as well as the cellular yields, before and after processing [149, 150]. Bone marrow aspiration anatomical sites: As MSCs represent a small population of BM cells [135], it is of critical importance to choose a BMA site that will yield the most MSCs. BM is relatively easy to harvest, largely available, and dispensable. Obviously, it is important that the BMA procedure is performed impeccably to obtain an optimal quality of viable BM tissue [133, 151]. In humans, the most common anatomical location to obtain BM is the iliac crest, but other BMA sites have been utilized [8]. Recently, McDaniel and co-workers, reported that all studied anatomical bone marrow harvesting locations contained MSCs, but the iliac crest was the most abundant source of MSCs [120], in particular posterior superior iliac spine (PSIS) [152].

62.4.4.3 Image Guidance for Bone Marrow Extraction

To perform BMC procedures, a certain volume and quality of bone marrow tissue are required. The aspiration volume is contingent on the processing volume of the BMC concentration system that is being used. It is imperative to precisely locate the BM donor site, as MSCs are mostly located in the endosteal and subendosteal marrow region and some are present around the blood vessels [127, 153, 154]. The precise delivery of local anesthetics and safe trocar placement before marrow extraction are accomplished by using image guidance [155]. In the following section, we focus on the posterior super iliac spine (PSIS) sites, as it is the most frequently reported anatomical site for BMA.

62.4.5 BMAC Harvesting: Ultrasound Guided

When the PSIS is targeted, patients are positioned in the prone position, while avoiding lumbar lordosis. The sonographic assessment uses a portable ultrasound system with a 5-2 low-frequency curvilinear transducer positioned in a transverse plane over the hyperechoic bilateral sacral cornual, with the patient lying prone and the monitor screen in the line of sight of the operator. The probe is then translated contralaterally from the physician, keeping the hyperechoic sacrum visualized. Next, the probe is translated proximally, with the hyperechoic ilium coming into view, while maintaining the hyperechoic sacrum, until the most superficial depth of the ilium is reached, known as the PSIS, contralateral to the examiner [156]. After identification of the PSIS, the most superficial depth is confirmed in both transverse and longitudinal orientation (Fig. 62.6). With the probe in the transverse plane at the PSIS, the slope of the iliac wing is noted for correct angulation of the BM trocar, and the most superficial depth of the PSIS is brought under the most medial aspect of the ultrasound probe. Using a sterile marker, a mark and directional line are made in both parallel and perpendicular orientations to form an intersection at the most superficial depth of the PSIS. This mark is maintained on the patient during skin preparation prior to the introduction of the BM trocar, and a superficial wheal of local anesthetic is placed at the point of planned trocar skin entry. Following the local antiseptic measures, sterile ultrasound gel is applied at the marked area, and a sterile probe cover is applied to the 5–2 MHz curvilinear array transducer. Typically, a mixture of local anesthetics is injected around the PSIS cortex and periosteal sleeve, under continued sonographic guidance, making sure to "walk off" the PSIS in four directions (superiorly, medially, laterally, and inferiorly), confirmed by sonographic guidance. The trocar is then introduced, using either a manual force that is perpendicular or slightly lateral to the patient, at 9–12 counterclockwise-clockwise rotations, or a mallet. The next step of the procedure is subject to the implementation of the instructions for use provided by the manufacturer of the aspiration harvesting system.

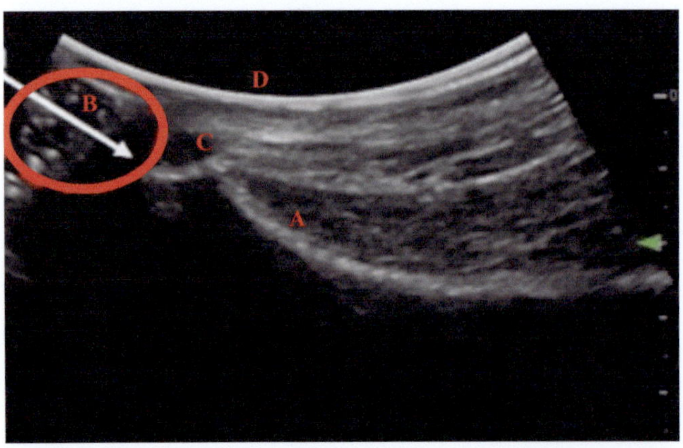

Fig. 62.6 Ultrasound image of the right PSIS, with the probe in transverse plane. A indicates the wing of the PSISI; B is the angulation of the trocar; C marks the superficial depth of the PSISI below the skin (D)

62.4.6 BMAC Harvesting: Fluoroscopic Guided

After proper patient positioning, the fluoroscopic equipment is installed to optimize the positioning for fluoroscopic imaging, using ipsilateral or contralateral oblique beam angulations for viewing the targeted PSIS site. The perpendicular fluoroscopic approach requires a beam angle around 15° ipsilateral to the PSIS entering laterally with angulation toward the sacroiliac joint. This angle will view the lateral ilium outer wall, and a needle is directed anteromedially. Fluoroscopic images support in positioning the tip of the trocar above the target area for entering the PSIS. The parallel fluoroscopic approach results in viewing down the PSIS table, at a 25° contralateral oblique beam position. This results in a classic view of the "teardrop" (Fig. 62.7).

Imaging can confirm the entry point into the PSIS table and visualize the angle through the cortex, allowing for safe trocar advancement in the BM cavity, at the tick part of the ilium bone [157]. Using proper fluoroscopic techniques, the parallel approach technique allows for a safe deeper marrow penetration. However, always, regardless of the approach,

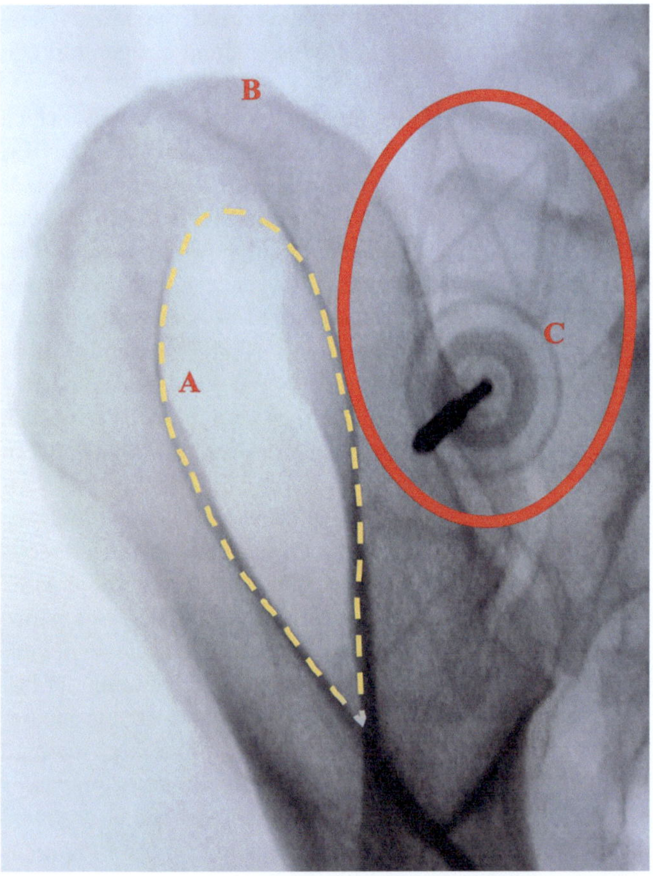

Fig. 62.7 The parallel fluoroscopic approach, viewing down the PSIS table (B), at a 25° contralateral oblique beam position. This results in a classic view of the "teardrop" (A). (Outline of the medial and lateral borders, in yellow). The tip of the BMA trocar and handle (C) marks the entry site in the marrow cavity

avoid increased manipulation and tissue trauma using the sharp trocar, as this will increase the risk for neurovascular injury, bleeding, tearing of lateral gluteal muscle origins, and post-procedural pain.

62.4.6.1 BMC: Immunomodulatory Effects

For MSCs to become "immunosuppressants," they need to be triggered by inflammatory cytokines, and the inflammatory environment is then a crucial factor for MSCs to exert their immunomodulatory effects. These are wielded by blocking apoptosis of native and activated neutrophils, aside from decreasing neutrophils from binding to vascular endothelial cells and mobilizing neutrophils to the area of damage [158]. However, the mechanisms by which MSCs are mobilized and recruited to damaged sites are not known. In addition, how they survive and differentiate into distinct cell types is still not clear. Once MSCs have been applied to the microenvironment of injured or degenerated tissues, many factors stimulate the release of many growth factors by MSCs. These growth factors stimulate the development of fibroblasts, endothelial cells, and tissue progenitor cells [159]. It is credible to state that the use of MSCs and their potential in immunomodulation in regenerative medicine applications hold great promise [160, 161].

62.4.6.2 BMC: Angiogenetic Effect

MSC paracrine trophic factors are potentially important in maintaining endothelial integrity and promoting angiogenesis through their ability to regulate endothelial cell proliferation and ECM production [162]. Furthermore, endothelial cell permeability is reduced, and MSCs inhibit interactions between leukocytes and endothelial cells [163]. Apart from MSC trophic factors, fibroblasts have fundamental functions in maintaining tissue integrity and promote tissue healing through their secretion of cytokines that support ECM building. These endothelial and angiogenetic capabilities have been demonstrated in clinical studies addressing chronic wound healing [164, 165] and recovery from post-myocardial infarction [166].

62.4.6.3 BMC: Tissue Repair Processes

BMACs are heterogeneous cell compositions that include BM-MSCs, making them endogenous cell sources for regenerative medicine repair treatments. They act by reducing cell apoptosis, fibrosis, and inflammation and activating cascades that lead to cell proliferation [167, 168]. In addition, BM-MSCs have the potential to differentiate into multiple cell lineages, including osteoblasts, adipocytes, myoblasts, epithelial, and neuronal cells [144]. They also contribute to angiogenesis via paracrine and autocrine pathways. Equally important, BM-MSCs are contributors to immunomodulatory actions independent of immune-specific cells, which participate in the inflammatory phase of wound repair [161, 169]. Moreover, BM-MSCs support the recruitment of cells to neoangiogenic treatment sites to accelerate local revascularization [170]. Kim et al. demonstrated that in the absence of an adequate scaffold, the survival rate of BM-MSCs and their reparative and differentiation capacity to enhance healing are jeopardized [171]. Although tissue harvesting, specimen preparation, and mechanism of action are different for PRP and BMCs, studies have shown that they can complement each other [172, 173].

62.4.7 BMC Trophic Effects Mediated by PGF

PRP platelet growth factors are crucial proteins that are involved in the BMC reparative processes and their role is to stimulate the various MSC capabilities, activities, and reparative functions, a phenomenon termed PRP trophic effects. The diversity of PDGFs and other cytokines involved in BMC trophic processes can initiate tissue repair by decreasing cell apoptosis and anabolic and anti-inflammatory effects, and by activating cell proliferation, differentiation, and angiogenesis via paracrine and autocrine pathways [174, 175]. Explicitly in OA treatments, PDGF plays a specific role in regenerating cartilage and maintaining homeostasis via MSC proliferation and inhibition of IL-1-induced chondrocyte apoptosis and inflammation [176]. Also, three TGF-β isoforms are active in stimulating chondrogenesis and inhibiting inflammation, and they express their ability to promote MSC-associated tissue healing via inter-molecular actions [174]. MSC trophic effects are associated with PGF activity and the secretion of reparative cytokines. Ideally, all of these cellular factors should be present in the BMA treatment vials and delivered to tissue injury sites to promote optimal MSC-associated therapeutic tissue healing [175].

Combining BMC and PRP: There is minimal information available on the presence or concentrations of PGFs in BMCs, or the ideal ratio needed to support BM-MSC trophic actions. Some clinicians combine high PRP concentrations with BMACs to have potentially more biologically active graft, projected to optimize regenerative medicine treatment outcomes [177]. However, there are minimal safety and efficacy data available that indicates that combining high PRP concentrations with BMAC is a more effective treatment option. Therefore, we believe that manipulating BMMSCs by priming them with high platelet concentrations may not be indicated at this stage.

62.5 Adipose Tissue Concentrate (ATC)

Aside from PRP and BMC preparations, adipose tissue (AT) has been used as a cell-based therapy in orthobiological and regenerative medicine procedures to create an adipose tissue concentrate (ATC), harvested and prepared at point-of-care in an office setting. Autologous AT is a heterogeneous biological source of various cellular tissue components. Furthermore, concentrated adipose tissue provides clinicians with a physiological 3D multicellular scaffold, including adipose stem cells (ASCs) and stromal cells. Both autologous and allogeneic ATCs have been employed in clinical trials to treat conditions such as lipoatrophy, muscular dystrophy, myocardial infarction, stroke, and spinal cord injury [178, 179]. ATCs have demonstrated to be effective in the treatment of MSK disorders and other regenerative applications, comparable to MSCs originating from BMCs. Like other MSCs, ASCs can differentiate into cells of mesodermal (osteoblasts, adipocytes, and chondrocytes), endodermal (hepatocytes, pancreatic cells), and ectodermal (neurons) primary layers [180]. These characteristics are of high interest when treating MSK disorders like osteoarthritis and chronic tendinopathies.

62.5.1 Adipose Tissue Structure

Adipose tissue is a highly vascularized connective tissue, abundantly present throughout the human body. White AT (WAT) is responsible for energy storage and plays a pivotal physiological role in maintaining metabolic homeostasis in the body by releasing several adipocytokines, growth factors, and cytokines that may act in an endocrine or paracrine fashion [181]. Brown AT (BAT) plays a significant role in thermogenesis via the actions of uncoupling protein 1. BAT cells present the ability to disperse energy by producing heat to ensure body temperature regulation, rather than storing it as triglycerides [182].

62.5.2 Adipose Tissue as a Source of Stem Cells

In 2002, Zuk et al. performed the first characterization of adult stem cells, isolated from lipoaspirates, demonstrating that ASC derived from WAT lipoaspirate exhibits MSC properties, like plastic-adherent, multipotency, and differential capacity [183–185]. AT MSCs have a high proliferation capacity and multilineage cell differentiation potential capable of differentiating into adipogenic, chondrogenic, myogenic, osteogenic, and neurogenic cells [186]. These AT-specific characteristics, combined with an abundance of MSCs when compared to MSCs derived from bone marrow [187, 188]. Therefore, ATs prepared form WAT have great potential in clinical orthobiological tissue repair applications [189, 190]. Furthermore, Yun et al. described the AT MSC-mediated effects on the reduction of proinflammatory cytokines, chemokines, cellular apoptosis, and collagenases [191]. Moreover, AD-MSCs have been shown to be immune-privileged [192]. AT has been one of the most studied tissues in the last decade [193–195] and they are increasingly popular. Practitioners value the high MSC content in ATC and they consider harvesting of subcutaneous WAT beneath the skin as a relatively easy procedure. Consequently, physicians might consider that MSCs from ATC have distinct advantages over "conventional" BMC preparations for orthobiological applications.

62.5.2.1 Stromal Vascular Fraction (SVF)

The use of AT in regenerative medicine is based on the separation of the vascular stroma contained in ATC, allowing for access to AD-MSCs [196, 197]. The isolation of AD-MSCs from WAT involves the separation of adipocytes from the remaining adipose cells of the SVF. SVF is a heterogeneous collection of cells contained within adipose tissue and can be isolated from fat using different disruption techniques, enzymatic digestion, or mechanical emulsification (ME).

Various techniques, including centrifugation (density gradient layer separation), are available for preparing a viable biological specimen to initiate SVF production. Centrifugation techniques have proven to be an effective means to safely wash, rinse, eliminate the infranatant-extracellular fluid, separate free lipids and residual oil, and prepare concentrated adipose tissue. In Fig. 62.8, the final processed adipose tissue is shown.

AD-MSCs and SVF cells, both contained in the SVF, meet the four criteria for MSCs as defined by the International Society for Cellular Therapy (ISCT) [198]. The presence of these cells can be measured by laboratory techniques, including flow cytometry techniques, as each cell has their own unique cell surface marker [199]. In Table 62.8, the heterogeneous SVF cellular distribution is shown.

62.5.3 Enzymatic Digestion vs. Mechanical Emulsification

Enzymatic digestion techniques use enzymes (collagenase) to isolate stromal and MSCs from adipose tissue by digesting the peptide bonds in the collagen of WAT with the destruction of extracellular structures. Centrifugation techniques are employed to separate the floating adipocytes from the pelleted SVF, following good manufacturing practices regarding closed, sterile, and safe isolation processes [200]. In these preparation protocols, a combination of enzymatic digestion and incubation/agitation has been identified, producing an adipose-derived cellular SVF (AD-cSVF). Freshly isolated SVF can directly be applied, without the need for further cell separation or in vitro expansion. AT-MSCs constitute as much as 1% of SVF cells compared with the 0.001–0.002% of BM-MSCs in bone marrow [201]. Furthermore,

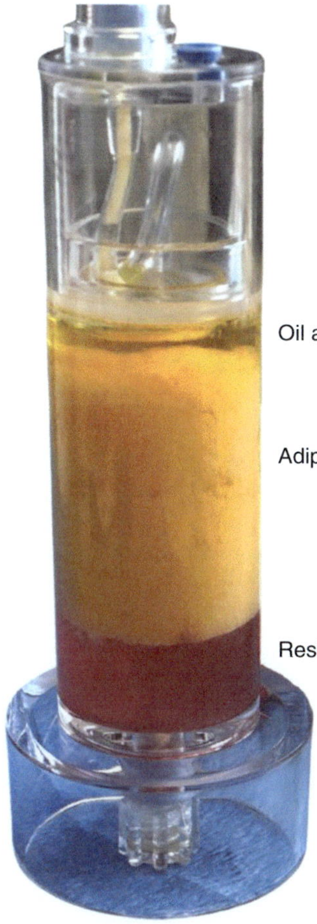

Fig. 62.8 Centrifugated density separation of adipose tissue, showing on top the oil and adipose fraction. The middle layer is the ATC, and at the bottom of the concentration device (Progenikine® Adipose Concentration System, EmCyte Corporation, Fort Myers, FL, USA, with permission) is the residual tumescent fluid

Table 62.8 SVF Cellular distribution

15–30% Stromal cells: AD-MSCs Pre-adipocytes Fibroblasts
35–45% Hematopoietic-lineage cells: Erythrocytes Platelets Neutrophils Lymphocytes Monocytes/macrophages
1–15% Hematopoietic stem and endothelial progenitor cells
3–5% Pericytes
10–20% Endothelial cells
5–15% Smooth muscle cells

Abbreviations: *AD-MSCs* adipose mesenchymal stem cells

detrimental erythrocytes are usually removed using a lysis buffer with a standard enzymatic processing protocol compared to a BMC product, which contains a significant number of erythrocytes [200]. In current FDA guidelines, enzymatic cellular prepared SVF products fall into the "more than manipulated" category and require specific clinical trials to examine and report the long-term safety and efficacy of such products in human clinical uses.

Another method to produce SVF refers to the definition of adipose-derived tissue SVF (AD-tSVF). This method addresses the adipose stromal population within a bioactive scaffold, or extra cellular matrix tissue, as described by Alexander. AT, acquired via lipoaspiration techniques, can be concentrated to an ATC by centrifugation and is thereafter subject to mechanical disruption by a process termed mechanical emulsification (ME) (Fig. 62.9). Hereafter, the final product is often termed microfat or nanofat, since it is composed of both cellular and native structural fragments [202, 203]. Therefore, emulsified AD-tSVF produces not a 100% concentrated cellular product when compared to AD-cSVF. Ultimately, after ME of ATC, the final AD-tSVF treatment specimen is injected into diseased tissue structures enabling the AD-MSCs to repair damaged and diseased tissues.

An advantage of this ME method is that prepared AD-tSVF offers the ability to provide a bioactive cellular tissue matrix after tissue application. Additionally, anti-inflammatory or immunosuppressive factors are secreted, capable of exerting immunomodulatory effects [204]. Noteworthy, AD-tSVF preparations and their subsequent applications are approved by the FDA.

62.5.3.1 Adipose Immunomodulatory Effects

Several studies have compared the immunomodulatory abilities of AD-MSCs and BM-MSCs and have shown that they exhibit similar effects when used in autoimmune diseases and chronic inflammatory conditions [205–207]. AD-MSCs can regulate the immune system directly via cell-cell communication and indirectly through the secretion of soluble mediators, growth factors, and extravascular vesicles [208, 209]. In adipose tissue, AD-MSC interact with numerous cell types, including immune cells, endothelial cells, pre-adipocytes, hematopoietic cells, nerve cells, endothelial cells, and pericytes surrounding the blood vessels. AD-MSCs and immune cells can interact because they can regulate and influence the activity of T cells, B cells, and macrophages in vitro and in vivo [210]. Indirect cell-cell communication is instigated by AD-MSCs when they secrete soluble mediators and extravascular vesicles (exosomes and micro vesicles) that are known to have therapeutic effects in regenerative medicine [211]. The most cited soluble mediators are pro-inflammatory and anti-inflammatory cytokines, adipokines, antioxidative, pro-angiogenic, anti-apoptotic, growth factors (like, VEGF, FGF, TGF), and specific interleukins (IL-6, IL-7). Currently, the clinical production of SVF to acquire AD-MSCs is subject to investigations addressing their

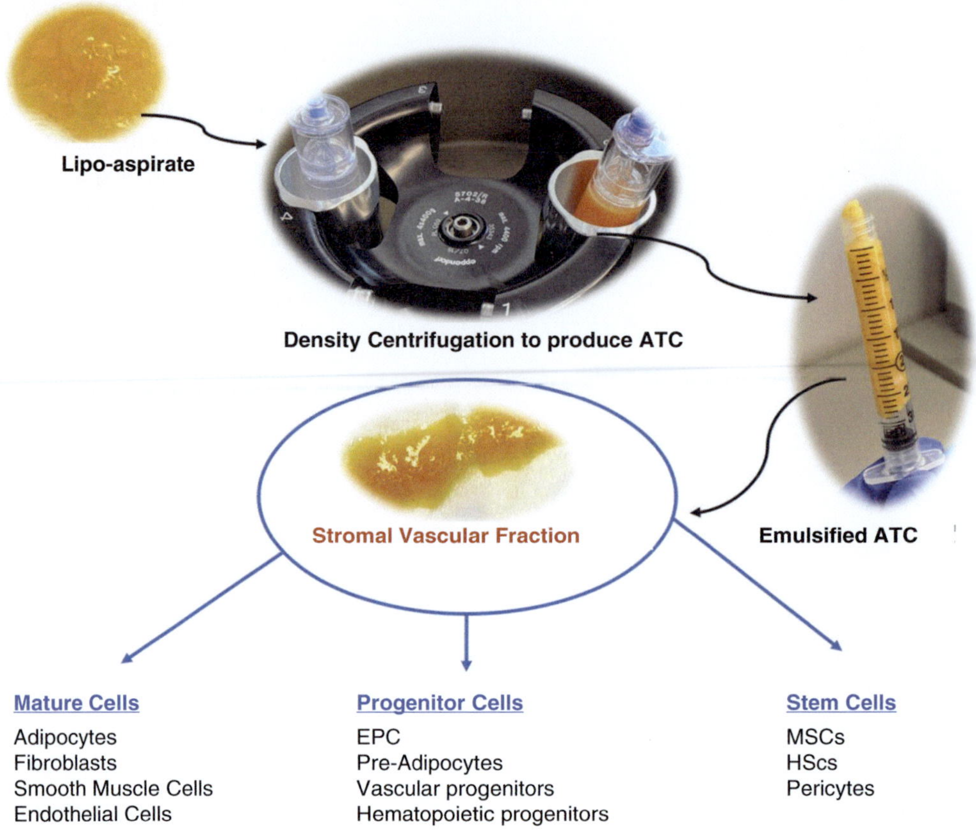

Fig. 62.9 SVF production steps. Adipose tissue is harvested following lipoaspiration and subsequently processed in a centrifuge for density cellular layering. After centrifugation, the ATC can be subject to ME before application as an orthobiological preparation. After EM, SVF cellular components will be liberated from the concentrated AT. This heterogeneous mixture is characterized as mature, progenitor stem cells

immunomodulatory potential in regenerative medicine. Critical aspects in these studies are the ability to develop standardized preparation protocols to ensure effective and safe use in orthobiological procedures.

62.5.3.2 ATC: Angiogenetic Effect

ATs have been intensely studied for the treatment of multiple conditions as they have great potential in orthobiological and regenerative medicine. AD-MSCs show paracrine activity and exhibit differentiation potential toward different cell lineages (adipogenic, osteogenic, chondrogenic, and myogenic lineages), while providing immunosuppressive properties and low immunogenicity [212]. AT produces and secretes various angiogenic factors such as angiopoietin-2 (Angpt2) and VEGF, as well as adipokines such as leptin and adiponectin, which influence and modulate angiogenesis and the vascular structure [213]. This suggests an autoregulatory function for angiogenesis in AT. Interestingly, precursor cells in blood vessel wall have been identified capable of differentiating into endothelial cells and/or adipocytes in WAT [214]. They concluded a high adipogenic potential, linking EC and adipocytes in terms of interchangeability based on cell-cell interactions, enabling them to participate in the formation of angiogenesis and neovascular structures. Therefore, AD-MSCs might affect the growth of capillary networks which are required in adipose tissue enlargement [215]. Furthermore, by enhancing angiogenesis and vasculogenesis, AD-MSCs promote neovascularization, which is fundamental in the treatment of tissue repair and post-(ischemic) injuries. These specialized characteristics of ATC were demonstrated by Miranville et al., revealing the expression of CD34 and CD133 of AD-MSCs which can differentiate into endothelial cells, contributing to revascularization [189]. Not only do AD-MSCs stimulate angiogenesis through differentiation into epithelial cells but also through paracrine activity, releasing angiogenic factors.

More specifically, the cellular components of SVF are rapidly restored to form new vessels in diseased tissue structures following orthobiological injections [216]. Neovascularization is further stimulated by stromal cells through the release of VEGF, TGF-b, and hepatocyte growth factor (HGF) [217]. Macrophages have demonstrated to be important cells in SVF for the proper structural organization of new blood vessels [216].

62.5.3.3 ATC: Tissue Repair Processes

Tissue repair processes following ATC and AD-tSVF preparations for orthobiological indications are based on their stromal, multipotent, and hematopoietic cell populations.

In addition, AD-tSVF can produce an assortment of angiogenic, hematopoietic, and anti-apoptotic factors that further expedite tissue repair (regeneration) via autocrine and paracrine actions [179].

SVF has the capacity to attain positive treatment outcomes through multiple cell components and tissue scaffold interactions with the extra cellular matrix (ECM).

The ECM is known as a potent scaffold in many tissues and accelerates the capability of regenerative functions by nearby cells [196]. The ECM encompasses structural proteins excreted by fibroblast, such as collagen, fibronectin, and elastin. A typical ECM characteristic is its ability to interact dynamically with integrin proteins on adhesive cells, triggering signaling pathways and changes in cell activity [218]. Furthermore, the ECM contributes to the growth of vascular infrastructure during angiogenesis [219]. Since the SVF comprises matrix-secreting fibroblasts and other stromal cells, the clinical application of ATC and SVF is possibly beneficial to various tissue types that benefit from a three-dimensional (3D) scaffold, like the ECM of tendons, which is composed of collagen and a smaller fraction of elastin embedded in a hydrated proteoglycan matrix [220].

ATC and AD-MSCs have been recognized as effective regenerative treatment modalities over the past decade. Aside from their capacity to differentiate into a variety of mature cell types, the stromal fraction within the SVF, including fibroblasts and stem cells, stimulates angiogenetic processes and the ECM secretes, among others, collagen proteins [221]. It has been suggested that fibroblast-derived ECM components are essential for the development of blood vessels and that angiogenesis necessitates synergy between stromal and endothelial populations [222]. Therefore, regenerative mechanisms demand synergy between angiogenesis and the synthesis of ECM proteins, founding a suitable milieu for tissue healing. Another tissue repair process is mediated by the presence of monocytes and macrophages in SVF. Approximately 5–15% of these cells are anti-inflammatory macrophage phenotype M2, an important component in controlling the environment for regeneration [223]. Additionally, 10–15% of the SVF comprises lymphocytes, including regulatory T cells contributing to tissue immune responses [223].

It appears that the heterogeneous composition of tissue SVF has distinct advantages. The interplay of controlled inflammation with immunomodulatory properties of AD-MSCs, as precursors to ECM formation and angiogenesis, provides the necessary constituents for cellular and musculotendinous repair processes and promotes the restoration of functional tissue.

62.5.3.4 Adipose Tissue Harvesting

Liposuction is the removal of subcutaneous fat by which it is possible to obtain the adipose tissue for autologous fat transplantations and for the preparation of ATC, for ASCs therapeutic treatments. The procedure is executed by means of aspiration cannulas, introduced through small skin incisions, assisted by suction. Its basic principles have been elaborated by Illouz, who was the first to introduce the modern, safe, and widespread method of liposuction with a blunt-tipped cannula as well as subcutaneous infiltration to facilitate adipose breakdown and aspiration [224, 225]. The procedure preserves neurovascular structures while maintaining fluid balance, with minimal patient discomfort [226]. In 1985, the tumescent liposuction technique was introduced by Klein [227]. Later, Coleman introduced a new three-step technique to decrease trauma to adipose tissue following liposuction: manual lipoaspiration under low pressure, centrifugation for 3 min at 3000 rpm, and 3D matrix reinjection [228]. In general, lipoaspiration techniques should not affect cell viability and consequently the yield of ASCs [198, 229]. Harvested WAT is transferred to a concentration device using minimal processing steps for autologous concentrated fat grafting preparations and ultimately ASC functionality (Fig. 62.10). An overview of adipose harvesting steps is given in Table 62.9.

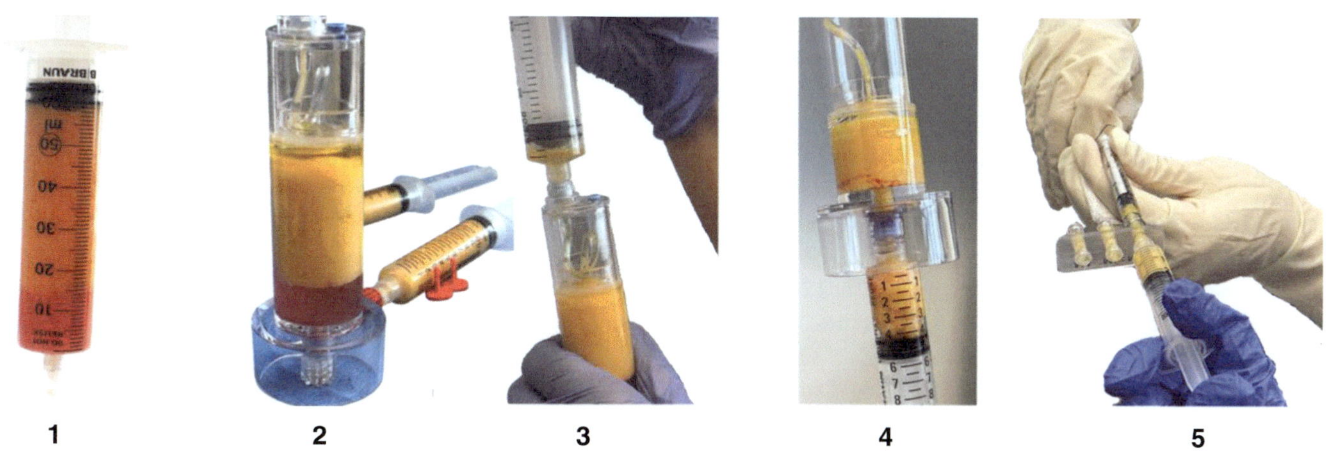

Fig. 62.10 ATC preparation techniques reviewed. After harvesting of AT, the extracted AT is racked and decanted from the syringe (1). After centrifugation (2), the oil (3) and tumescent fluid are removed, and subsequently the ATC is collected (4). Before injecting ATC, mechanical emulsification will size the ATC and break down the adipocytes (5)

Table 62.9 ATC preparation steps

A. Tumescent fluid preparation: a sterile NaCl solution consisting of anesthetics (lidocaine for pain relief and epinephrine for blood vessels to constrict to minimize RBC contamination in fat tissue during harvesting).
B. Tumescent injection: via small skin cuts, a thin blunt injector needle is injected in the target adipose harvesting area.
C. Waiting time: reports indicate to wait at least 20 minutes before starting the fat-harvesting procedure. This time is needed for the fluid to cause the injected area to swell and stiffen, supporting in easy fat removal.
D. Adipose harvesting: with a dedicated harvester cannula, fat tissue is harvested using liposuction; by applying manually negative pressure to a collection syringe, fat is removed from the area that was injected with tumescent fluid.
E. Racking and decanting: syringes filled with harvested fat are placed in a rack, with plunger in upward direction. After the adipose harvesting, leave all syringes in the rack for 10–15 minutes, with the luer connection of the syringe capped. Decant the supernatant (tumescent fluid) by removing the cap, until adipose tissue starts to block the luer.
F. Transfer the decanted fat into a disposable processing device and place it in a dedicated centrifuge to concentrate the AT specimen.
G. Centrifugation protocol: density layer separation by centrifugation, producing ATC. Follow the instruction for use of the preparation device to extract ATC.
H. Mechanical emulsification: a method to emulsify the ATC, by moving the two syringes back and forward through a restraining device to size the ATC, making it suitable for tissue injection.

62.5.3.5 Bone Marrow MSCs Versus Adipose MSCs

Adult MSCs are undifferentiated multipotent cells characterized by the capacity for self-renewal and the ability to differentiate into various cells of mesenchymal origin, including adipocytes, chondrocytes, myocytes, and osteoblasts, when exposed to specific growth signals [13], and the ISCT proposed clear criteria for the definition of both BM and AT MSCs [223].

Comparing AD-MSCs and BM-MSCs, the latter have been the most extensively used and investigated MSCs. However, some practitioners consider limitations with extracting BM-MSCs. Cited limitations are the possible pain and morbidity following harvesting and the limited number of MSCs that can be obtained, as only a relatively small amount (0.001–0.01%) of harvested BM cells are MSCs [135]. These issues have led for the search of alternative and comparable sources for MSCs. Abundant numbers of AD-MSCs have been reported to be easily isolated from adipose tissue by a minimally invasive procedure [190]. In addition, AT can be harvested from multiple sites [230–232]. Various studies indicate that BM-MSCs and AD-MSCs have comparable characteristics when it comes to CD markers and morphology [223], and like BM-MSCs, AD-MSCs can undergo multi-lineage differentiation, including osteogenic, chondrogenic, adipogenic, cardiomyocytic, hepatic, and neurogenic differentiation [233]. It has been postulated that the capability of proliferating and differentiating into different mesenchymal lineages make AD-MSCs a promising less-invasive alternative to BM-MSCs for cell-based therapeutic applications [234]. Klar et al., a cellular comparison was performed between BMC and SVF and a conclusion was made that the mononucleated fraction of the SVF is richer in stromal cells (15–30% of all cells) [235]. However, most of these studies compared AD-MSCs and BM-MSCs obtained from different individuals [236], lacking donor-matching MSCs from BM and AT tissues, and they were studied in MASC expansion studies. Furthermore, there is a lack of standardized methods and quality controls tests to translate scientific findings from basic science into the standard of orthobiological applications.

In an in vitro study, Mohamed-Ahmed and co-workers compared the properties of BM-MSCs and AD-MSCs, acquired from the same individuals [13]. They reported comparable multi-potencies, morphology, and immunophenotyping for both MSC types. Nevertheless, their tissue-specific differentiation capacity varied. BM-MSCs were superior to AD-MSCs in terms of osteogenic and chondrogenic differentiation, while AD-MSCs had higher proliferation and adipogenic potential. Furthermore, other reports have also concluded that MSCs preferentially differentiate into cells of their native microenvironment [237, 238].

62.6 Summary

Autologous PRP can be easily prepared from whole blood and can ultimately secrete multiple growth factors and other cytokines for regulating various physiological activities. These platelet constituents induce tissue repair and are capable of stimulating proliferation and differentiation of different stems cells in MSK injury models and have been used safely and effectively for decades. Current literature supports the use of PRP in early OA and other indications. Unfortunately, we are still in search for consensus of appropriate bioformulations and preparation standards to treat different maladies. PRP treatments require considerably less resources when compared to MSC cellular-based therapies.

Following PRP treatments, autologous progenitor and MSC stem cell-based therapy have emerged as an alternative strategy in MSK disorders to overcome the limitations and consequences of more invasive treatment procedures. These limitations include (post-surgical) treatment morbidity, risk of infection, wound healing disturbances, and hemorrhage [239]. Despite their safety, regulatory complexities have materialized to implement MSC cell-based therapies, with more restrictions to the use of adipose tissue, making these treatments less available for most patients. Although autologous orthobiological interventions demonstrate very promising results, some (competitive commercial) organizations consider them experimental, with unproven cost/efficacy data and treatment durability.

High expectations on the performance of all three discussed orthobiologics will be met after clarifying scientific barriers, through a clearer understanding of the underlying mechanisms of action. In addition, comprehending the various crucial clinical features of MSK pathologies, that potentially can be treated with orthobiologics, will allow for the improvement of orthobiological product definitions and application procedures. Combined with patient stratifications according to biological and clinical criteria, these aspects together will increase the efficacy of PRP, BMC, and ATC treatments and contribute to move the field of management of musculoskeletal and sports lesions forward, potentially increasing the utilization and acceptance of autologous orthobiological treatment modalities.

References

1. Centeno CJ, Pastoriza SM. Past, current and future interventional orthobiologics techniques and how they relate to regenerative rehabilitation: a clinical commentary. Int J Sports Phys Ther. 2020;15(2):301–25.
2. Marx RE. Platelet-rich plasma (PRP): what is PRP and what is not PRP? Implant Dent. 2001;10(4):225–8.
3. Filardo G, Di Matteo B, Kon E, Merli G, Marcacci M. Platelet-rich plasma in tendon-related disorders: results and indications. Knee Surg Sports Traumatol Arthrosc. 2018;26(7):1984–99.
4. Belk JW, Kraeutler MJ, Houck DA, Goodrich JA, Dragoo JL, McCarty EC. Platelet-rich plasma versus hyaluronic acid for knee osteoarthritis: a systematic review and meta-analysis of randomized controlled trials. Am J Sports Med. 2020;49(1):249–60. https://doi.org/10.1177/036354652090939.
5. Xuan Z, Yu W, Dou Y, Wang T. Efficacy of platelet-rich plasma for low back pain: a systematic review and meta-analysis. J Neurol Surg Part Cent Eur Neurosurg [Internet]. 2020 May; Available from: https://doi.org/10.1055/s-0040-1709170.
6. Fadadu PP, Mazzola AJ, Hunter CW, Davis TT. Review of concentration yields in commercially available platelet-rich plasma (PRP) systems: a call for PRP standardization. Reg Anesth Pain Med. 2019;44(6):652–9.
7. Everts PAM, Knape JTA, Weibrich G, Hoffmann J, Overdevest EP, Box HAM, et al. Platelet-rich plasma and platelet gel: a review. J Extra Corpor Technol. 2007;14
8. Everts P, Flanagan II G, Rothenberg J, Mautner K. The rationale of autologously prepared bone marrow aspirate concentrate for use in regenerative medicine applications. In: Regenerative medicine [Working Title] [Internet]. IntechOpen; 2020 [cited 2020 Jun 24]. Available from: https://www.intechopen.com/online-first/the-rationale-of-autologously-prepared-bone-marrow-aspirate-concentrate-for-use-in-regenerative-medi.
9. Hersant B, Sid-Ahmed M, Braud L, Jourdan M, Baba-Amer Y, Meningaud J-P, et al. Platelet-rich plasma improves the wound healing potential of mesenchymal stem cells through paracrine and metabolism alterations. Stem Cells Int. 2019;2019:1–14.
10. Johal H, Khan M, Yung SP, Dhillon MS, Fu FH, Bedi A, et al. Impact of platelet-rich plasma use on pain in orthopaedic surgery: a systematic review and meta-analysis. Sports Health Multidiscip Approach. 2019;11(4):355–66.
11. Wientroub S, Goodwin D, Khermosh O, Salama R. The clinical use of autologous marrow to improve osteogenic potential of bone grafts in pediatric orthopedics. J Pediatr Orthop. 1989;9(2):186–90.
12. Järvinen TAH, Järvinen TLN, Kääriäinen M, Kalimo H, Järvinen M. Muscle injuries: biology and treatment. Am J Sports Med. 2005;33(5):745–64.
13. Mohamed-Ahmed S, Fristad I, Lie SA, Suliman S, Mustafa K, Vindenes H, et al. Adipose-derived and bone marrow mesenchymal stem cells: a donor-matched comparison. Stem Cell Res Ther. 2018;9(1):168.
14. Chahla J, Cinque ME, Piuzzi NS, Mannava S, Geeslin AG, Murray IR, et al. A call for standardization in platelet-rich plasma preparation protocols and composition reporting: a systematic review of the clinical orthopaedic literature. J Bone Jt Surg. 2017;99(20):1769–79.
15. Everts P, Onishi K, Jayaram P, Lana JF, Mautner K. Platelet-rich plasma: new performance understandings and therapeutic considerations in 2020. Int J Mol Sci. 2020;21(20):7794.
16. Lubkowska A, Dołęgowska B, Banfi G. Growth factor content in PRP and their applicability in medicine. J Biol Regul Homeost Agents. 2012;26(2 Suppl 1):3S–22S.
17. Blair P, Flaumenhaft R. Platelet alpha-granules: basic biology and clinical correlates. Blood Rev. 2009;23(4):177–89.
18. Iberg CA, Hawiger D. Natural and induced tolerogenic dendritic cells. J Immunol. 2020;204(4):733–44.
19. Younas M, Hue S, Lacabaratz C, Guguin A, Wiedemann A, Surenaud M, et al. IL-7 modulates in vitro and in vivo human memory T regulatory cell functions through the CD39/ATP axis. J Immunol Baltim Md 1950. 2013;191(6):3161–3168.
20. Ganor Y, Besser M, Ben-Zakay N, Unger T, Levite M. Human T cells express a functional ionotropic glutamate receptor GluR3, and glutamate by itself triggers integrin-mediated adhesion to laminin and fibronectin and chemotactic migration. J Immunol Baltim Md 1950. 2003;170(8):4362–72.
21. Everts PAM, Hoffmann J, Weibrich G, Mahoney CB, Schönberger JPAM, van Zundert A, et al. Differences in platelet growth factor release and leucocyte kinetics during autologous platelet gel formation. Transfus Med. 2006;16(5):363–8.
22. Everts PAM, Knape JTA, Weibrich G, Hoffmann J, Overdevest EP, Box HAM, et al. Platelet-rich plasma and platelet gel: a review. J Extra Corpor Technol. 2006;38(2):174–87.
23. Andia I, Maffulli N. A contemporary view of platelet-rich plasma therapies: moving toward refined clinical protocols and precise indications. Regen Med. 2018;13(6):717–28.
24. Puzzitiello RN, Patel BH, Forlenza EM, Nwachukwu BU, Allen AA, Forsythe B, et al. Adverse impact of corticosteroids on rotator cuff tendon health and repair: a systematic review of basic science studies. Arthrosc Sports Med Rehabil. 2020;2(2):e161–9.
25. Kumar A, Kadamb AG, Kadamb KG. Hope, hype, hurdles and future perspective for PRP, PRP versus hyaluronic acid injection in osteoarthritis of the knee. Biol Orthop J. 2:12.
26. Beitzel K, Allen D, Apostolakos J, Russell R, McCarthy M, Gallo G, et al. US definitions, current use, and FDA stance on use of platelet-rich plasma in sports medicine. J Knee Surg. 2014;28(01):029–34.
27. Mazzucco L, Balbo V, Cattana E, Guaschino R, Borzini P. Not every PRP-gel is born equal evaluation of growth factor availability for tissues through four PRP-gel preparations: Fibrinet®, RegenPRP-Kit®, Plateltex® and one manual procedure. Vox Sang. 2009;97(2):110–8.
28. Dohan M, Ehrenfest D, Bielecki T, Mishra A, Borzini P, Inchingolo F, Sammartino G, et al. In search of a consensus terminology in the field of platelet concentrates for surgical use: platelet-rich plasma (PRP), platelet-rich fibrin (PRF), fibrin gel polymerization and leukocytes. Curr Pharm Biotechnol. 2012;13(7):1131–7.

29. Langer HF, Chavakis T. Platelets and neurovascular inflammation. Thromb Haemost. 2013;110(11):888–93.
30. Semple JW, Italiano JE, Freedman J. Platelets and the immune continuum. Nat Rev Immunol. 2011;11(4):264–74.
31. Koupenova M, Clancy L, Corkrey HA, Freedman JE. Circulating platelets as mediators of immunity, inflammation, and thrombosis. Circ Res. 2018;122(2):337–51.
32. Everts PA. Autologous platelet-rich plasma and mesenchymal stem cells for the treatment of chronic wounds. In: Hakan Dogan K, editor. Wound healing - current perspectives [Internet]. IntechOpen; 2019 [cited 2019 Oct 4]. Available from: https://www.intechopen.com/books/wound-healing-current-perspectives/autologous-platelet-rich-plasma-and-mesenchymal-stem-cells-for-the-treatment-of-chronic-wounds.
33. Morrell CN, Aggrey AA, Chapman LM, Modjeski KL. Emerging roles for platelets as immune and inflammatory cells. Blood. 2014;123(18):2759–67.
34. Thon JN, Peters CG, Machlus KR, Aslam R, Rowley J, Macleod H, et al. T granules in human platelets function in TLR9 organization and signaling. J Cell Biol. 2012;198(4):561–74.
35. Everts PA, Brown Mahoney C, Hoffmann JJ, Schönberger JP, Box HA, van Zundert A, et al. Platelet-rich plasma preparation using three devices: implications for platelet activation and platelet growth factor release. Growth Factors. 2006;24(3):165–71.
36. de Mos M, van der Windt AE, Jahr H, van Schie HTM, Weinans H, Verhaar JAN, et al. Can platelet-rich plasma enhance tendon repair?: a cell culture study. Am J Sports Med. 2008;36(6):1171–8.
37. Yuan T, Zhang C-Q, Wang H-C. Augmenting tendon and ligament repair with platelet-rich plasma (PRP). Muscle Ligaments Tendons J. 2019;03(03):139.
38. Tuakli-Wosornu YA, Terry A, Boachie-Adjei K, Harrison JR, Gribbin CK, LaSalle EE, et al. Lumbar intradiskal platelet-rich plasma (PRP) injections: a prospective, double-blind, randomized controlled study. PM&R. 2016;8(1):1–10.
39. Gupta AK, Cole J, Deutsch DP, Everts PA, Niedbalski RP, Panchaprateep R, et al. Platelet-rich plasma as a treatment for androgenetic alopecia. Dermatol Surg. 2019;45(10):1262–73.
40. Kirmani BH, Jones SG, Datta S, McLaughlin EK, Hoschtitzky AJ. A meta-analysis of platelet gel for prevention of sternal wound infections following cardiac surgery. Blood Transfus [Internet]. 2016 [cited 2020 Jul 7]; Available from: https://doi.org/10.2450/2016.0231-15.
41. Willemsen JCN, Van Dongen J, Spiekman M, Vermeulen KM, Harmsen MC, van der Lei B, et al. The addition of PRP to facial lipofilling: a double-blind placebo-controlled randomized trial. Plast Reconstr Surg. 2017;1
42. Muchedzi TA, Roberts SB. A systematic review of the effects of platelet rich plasma on outcomes for patients with knee osteoarthritis and following total knee arthroplasty. The Surgeon. 2018;16(4):250–8.
43. Cengiz IF, Pereira H, Espregueira-Mendes J, Reis RL, Oliveira JM. The clinical use of biologics in the knee lesions: does the patient benefit? Curr Rev Musculoskelet Med. 2019;12(3):406–14.
44. Amable P, Carias RB, Teixeira MV, da Cruz PÍ, Corrêa do Amaral RJ, Granjeiro J, et al. Platelet-rich plasma preparation for regenerative medicine: optimization and quantification of cytokines and growth factors. Stem Cell Res Ther. 2013;4(3):67.
45. Gentile P, Calabrese C, De Angelis B, Dionisi L, Pizzicannella J, Kothari A, et al. Impact of the different preparation methods to obtain autologous non-activated platelet-rich plasma (A-PRP) and activated platelet-rich plasma (AA-PRP) in plastic surgery: wound healing and hair regrowth evaluation. Int J Mol Sci. 2020;21(2):431.
46. Samadi P, Sheykhhasan M, Khoshinani HM. The use of platelet-rich plasma in aesthetic and regenerative medicine: a comprehensive review. Aesthet Plast Surg. 2019;43(3):803–14.
47. Gentile P, Garcovich S. Systematic review – the potential implications of different platelet-rich plasma (PRP) concentrations in regenerative medicine for tissue repair. Int J Mol Sci. 2020;21(16):5702.
48. Nguyen PA, Pham TAV. Effects of platelet-rich plasma on human gingival fibroblast proliferation and migration in vitro. J Appl Oral Sci [Internet]. 2018 Jul 10 [cited 2020 Jul 5];26(0). Available from: http://www.scielo.br/scielo.php?script=sci_arttext&pid=S1678-77572018000100480&lng=en&tlng=en.
49. Vahabi S, Yadegari Z, Mohammad-Rahimi H. Comparison of the effect of activated or non-activated PRP in various concentrations on osteoblast and fibroblast cell line proliferation. Cell Tissue Bank. 2017;18(3):347–53.
50. Miller EJ, Lappin SL. Physiology, cellular receptor [Internet]. Treasure Island: StatPearls Publishing; 2020. Available from: http://europepmc.org/books/NBK554403.
51. Graziani F, Ivanovski S, Cei S, Ducci F, Tonetti M, Gabriele M. The in vitro effect of different PRP concentrations on osteoblasts and fibroblasts. Clin Oral Implants Res. 2006;17(2):212–9.
52. Park MS, Moon S-H, Kim T-H, Oh JK, Yoon WY, Chang HG. Platelet-rich plasma for the spinal fusion. J Orthop Surg. 2018;26(1):230949901875577.
53. Kushida S, Kakudo N, Morimoto N, Hara T, Ogawa T, Mitsui T, et al. Platelet and growth factor concentrations in activated platelet-rich plasma: a comparison of seven commercial separation systems. J Artif Organs. 2014;17(2):186–92.
54. Haunschild ED, Huddleston HP, Chahla J, Gilat R, Cole BJ, Yanke AB. Platelet-rich plasma augmentation in meniscal repair surgery: a systematic review of comparative studies. Arthrosc J Arthrosc Relat Surg. 2020;36(6):1765–74.
55. Xu J, Gou L, Zhang P, Li H, Qiu S. Platelet-rich plasma and regenerative dentistry. Aust Dent J. 2020;65(2):131–42.
56. Zheng C, Zhu Q, Liu X, Huang X, He C, Jiang L, et al. Effect of platelet-rich plasma (PRP) concentration on proliferation, neurotrophic function and migration of Schwann cells *in vitro*: effect of platelet-rich plasma on Schwann cells. J Tissue Eng Regen Med. 2016;10(5):428–36.
57. Hee HT, Majd ME, Holt RT, Myers L. Do autologous growth factors enhance transforaminal lumbar interbody fusion? Eur Spine J. 2003;12(4):400–7.
58. Giusti I, Rughetti A, D'Ascenzo S, Millimaggi D, Pavan A, Dell'Orso L, et al. Identification of an optimal concentration of platelet gel for promoting angiogenesis in human endothelial cells. Transfusion (Paris). 2009;49(4):771–8.
59. Creeper F, Lichanska AM, Marshall RI, Seymour GJ, Ivanovski S. The effect of platelet-rich plasma on osteoblast and periodontal ligament cell migration, proliferation and differentiation. J Periodontal Res. 2009;44(2):258–65.
60. Soffer E, Ouhayoun J-P, Dosquet C, Meunier A, Anagnostou F. Effects of platelet lysates on select bone cell functions. Clin Oral Implants Res. 2004;15(5):581–8.
61. Bansal H, Leon J, Pont JL, Wilson DA, Bansal A, Agarwal D, et al. Platelet-rich plasma (PRP) in osteoarthritis (OA) knee: correct dose critical for long term clinical efficacy. Sci Rep. 2021;11(1):3971.
62. Fitzpatrick J, Bulsara MK, McCrory PR, Richardson MD, Zheng MH. Analysis of platelet-rich plasma extraction: variations in platelet and blood components between 4 common commercial kits. Orthop J Sports Med. 2017;5(1):232596711667527.
63. the GRIP (Groupe de Recherche sur les Injections de PRP, PRP Injection Research Group), Eymard F, Ornetti P, Maillet J, Noel É, Adam P, et al. Intra-articular injections of platelet-rich plasma in symptomatic knee osteoarthritis: a consensus statement from French-speaking experts. Knee Surg Sports Traumatol Arthrosc

[Internet]. 2020 Jun 24 [cited 2020 Jun 30]; Available from: http://link.springer.com/10.1007/s00167-020-06102-5.
64. Lana JF, Macedo A, Ingrao ILG, Huber SC, Santos GS, Santana MHA. Leukocyte-rich PRP for knee osteoarthritis: current concepts. J Clin Orthop Trauma. 2019;10:S179–82.
65. Lana JFSD, Purita J, Paulus C, Huber SC, Rodrigues BL, Rodrigues AA, et al. Contributions for classification of platelet rich plasma – proposal of a new classification: MARSPILL. Regen Med. 2017;12(5):565–74.
66. Riboh JC, Saltzman BM, Yanke AB, Fortier L, Cole BJ. Effect of leukocyte concentration on the efficacy of platelet-rich plasma in the treatment of knee osteoarthritis. Am J Sports Med. 2016;44(3):792–800.
67. Mariani E, Canella V, Cattini L, Kon E, Marcacci M, Di Matteo B, et al. Leukocyte-rich platelet-rich plasma injections do not up-modulate intra-articular pro-inflammatory cytokines in the osteoarthritic knee. De Rosa S, editor. PLoS One. 2016;11(6):e0156137.
68. Parrish WR. Physiology of blood components in wound healing: an appreciation of cellular co-operativity in platelet rich plasma action. J Exerc Sports Orthop. 2017;4(2):1–14.
69. Seta N, Kuwana M. Human circulating monocytes as multipotential progenitors. Keio J Med. 2007;56(2):41–7.
70. Perut F, Filardo G, Mariani E, Cenacchi A, Pratelli L, Devescovi V, et al. Preparation method and growth factor content of platelet concentrate influence the osteogenic differentiation of bone marrow stromal cells. Cytotherapy. 2013;15(7):830–9.
71. Melo L, Lana S. Centrifugation conditions in the L-PRP preparation affect soluble factors release and mesenchymal stem cell proliferation in fibrin nanofibers. Molecules. 2019;24(15):2729.
72. Moojen DJF, Schure R-M, Overdevest EP, van Zundert A, Knape JTA, Castelein RM, et al. Antimicrobial activity of platelet-leukocyte gel against Staphylococcus aureus. J Orthop Res. 2008;26(3):404–10.
73. Tang Y-Q, Yeaman MR, Selsted ME. Antimicrobial peptides from human platelets. Infect Immun. 2002;70(12):6524–33.
74. Institute of Orthopaedic Research and Biomechanics, University of Ulm, Helmholtzstr. 14, D-89081, Ulm, Germany, Kovtun A, Bergdolt S, Wiegner R, Radermacher P, Huber-Lang M, et al. The crucial role of neutrophil granulocytes in bone fracture healing. Eur Cell Mater. 2016;32:152–62.
75. Rossi LA, Piuzzi N, Giunta D, Tanoira I, Brandariz R, Pasqualini I, et al. Subacromial platelet-rich plasma injections decrease pain and improve functional outcomes in patients with refractory rotator cuff tendinopathy. Arthrosc J Arthrosc Relat Surg. 2021;37(9):2745–53.
76. Collins T, Alexander D, Barkatali B. Platelet-rich plasma: a narrative review. EFORT Open Rev. 2021;6(4):225–35.
77. Phillipson M, Kubes P. The healing power of neutrophils. Trends Immunol. 2019;40(7):635–47.
78. Zhou Y, Wang JH-C. PRP treatment efficacy for tendinopathy: a review of basic science studies. Biomed Res Int 2016;2016:1–8.
79. Fedorova NV, Ksenofontov AL, Serebryakova MV, Stadnichuk VI, Gaponova TV, Baratova LA, et al. Neutrophils release metalloproteinases during adhesion in the presence of insulin, but Cathepsin G in the presence of glucagon. Mediat Inflamm. 2018;2018:1–9.
80. Ubezio G, Ghio M. Bio-modulators in platelet-rich plasma: a comparison of the amounts in products from healthy donors and patients produced with three different techniques. Blood Transfus [Internet]. 2014 [cited 2020 Jul 8]; Available from: https://doi.org/10.2450/2012.0128-12.
81. Italiani P, Boraschi D. From monocytes to M1/M2 macrophages: phenotypical vs. functional differentiation. Front Immunol [Internet]. 2014 Oct 17 [cited 2020 Jul 8];5. Available from: http://journal.frontiersin.org/article/10.3389/fimmu.2014.00514/abstract.
82. Weirather J, Hofmann UDW, Beyersdorf N, Ramos GC, Vogel B, Frey A, et al. Foxp3 + CD4 + T cells improve healing after myocardial infarction by modulating monocyte/macrophage differentiation. Circ Res. 2014;115(1):55–67.
83. Ogle ME, Segar CE, Sridhar S, Botchwey EA. Monocytes and macrophages in tissue repair: implications for immunoregenerative biomaterial design. Exp Biol Med. 2016;241(10):1084–97.
84. Das A, Sinha M, Datta S, Abas M, Chaffee S, Sen CK, et al. Monocyte and macrophage plasticity in tissue repair and regeneration. Am J Pathol. 2015;185(10):2596–606.
85. Wynn TA, Vannella KM. Macrophages in tissue repair, regeneration, and fibrosis. Immunity. 2016;44(3):450–62.
86. Helms CC, Gladwin MT, Kim-Shapiro DB. Erythrocytes and vascular function: oxygen and nitric oxide. Front Physiol. 2018;9:125.
87. Schaer DJ, Buehler PW, Alayash AI, Belcher JD, Vercellotti GM. Hemolysis and free hemoglobin revisited: exploring hemoglobin and hemin scavengers as a novel class of therapeutic proteins. Blood. 2013;121(8):1276–84.
88. Repsold L, Joubert AM. Eryptosis: an erythrocyte's suicidal type of cell death. Biomed Res Int. 2018;2018:1–10.
89. Woodell-May JE, Sommerfeld SD. Role of inflammation and the immune system in the progression of osteoarthritis. J Orthop Res. 2020;38(2):253–7.
90. Cognasse F, Laradi S, Berthelot P, Bourlet T, Marotte H, Mismetti P, et al. Platelet inflammatory response to stress. Front Immunol. 2019;10:1478.
91. Vasina EM, Cauwenberghs S, Feijge MAH, Heemskerk JWM, Weber C, Koenen RR. Microparticles from apoptotic platelets promote resident macrophage differentiation. Cell Death Dis. 2011;2(9):e211.
92. Gros A, Syvannarath V, Lamrani L, Ollivier V, Loyau S, Goerge T, et al. Single platelets seal neutrophil-induced vascular breaches via GPVI during immune-complex-mediated inflammation in mice. Blood. 2015;126(8):1017–26.
93. Clark SR, Ma AC, Tavener SA, McDonald B, Goodarzi Z, Kelly MM, et al. Platelet TLR4 activates neutrophil extracellular traps to ensnare bacteria in septic blood. Nat Med. 2007;13(4):463–9.
94. Kapur R, Zufferey A, Boilard E, Semple JW. Nouvelle cuisine: platelets served with inflammation. J Immunol. 2015;194(12):5579–87.
95. Dale DC, Boxer L, Liles WC. The phagocytes: neutrophils and monocytes. Blood. 2008;112(4):935–45.
96. Henn V, Slupsky J, Gräfe M, Anagnostopoulos I, Förster R, Müller-Berghaus G, et al. CD40 ligand on activated platelets triggers an inflammatory reaction of endothelial cells. Nature. 1998;391(6667):591–4.
97. Yu Y, Ma X, Gong R, Zhu J, Wei L, Yao J. Recent advances in CD8+ regulatory Tï¿½cell research (Review). Oncol Lett [Internet]. 2018 Mar 29 [cited 2020 Sep 7]; Available from: http://www.spandidos-publications.com/10.3892/ol.2018.8378.
98. Gaudino SJ, Kumar P. Cross-talk between antigen presenting cells and T cells impacts intestinal homeostasis, bacterial infections, and tumorigenesis. Front Immunol. 2019;10:360.
99. Sadtler K, Estrellas K, Allen BW, Wolf MT, Fan H, Tam AJ, et al. Developing a pro-regenerative biomaterial scaffold microenvironment requires T helper 2 cells. Science. 2016;352(6283):366–70.
100. Everts PA, Devilee RJJ, Brown Mahoney C, van Erp A, Oosterbos CJM, Stellenboom M, et al. Exogenous application of platelet-leukocyte gel during open subacromial decompression contributes to improved patient outcome. Eur Surg Res. 2008;40(2):203–10.
101. Odem MA, Bavencoffe AG, Cassidy RM, Lopez ER, Tian J, Dessauer CW, et al. Isolated nociceptors reveal multiple specializations for generating irregular ongoing activity associated with ongoing pain. Pain. 2018;159(11):2347–62.
102. Sprott H, Franke S, Kluge H, Hein G. Pain treatment of fibromyalgia by acupuncture. Rheumatol Int. 1998;18(1):35–6.

103. Sommer C. Serotonin in pain and analgesia: actions in the periphery. Mol Neurobiol. 2004;30(2):117–25.
104. Nicholson R, Small J, Dixon A, Spanswick D, Lee K. Serotonin receptor mRNA expression in rat dorsal root ganglion neurons. Neurosci Lett. 2003;337(3):119–22.
105. Wu W-P, Hao J-X, Xu X-J, Wiesenfeld-Hallin Z, Koek W, Colpaert FC. The very-high-efficacy 5-HT1A receptor agonist, F 13640, preempts the development of allodynia-like behaviors in rats with spinal cord injury. Eur J Pharmacol. 2003;478(2–3):131–7.
106. Yoshida M, Funasaki H, Marumo K. Efficacy of autologous leukocyte-reduced platelet-rich plasma therapy for patellar tendinopathy in a rat treadmill model. Muscles Ligaments Tendons J. 2016;6(2):205–15.
107. Fu C-J, Sun J-B, Bi Z-G, Wang X-M, Yang C-L. Evaluation of platelet-rich plasma and fibrin matrix to assist in healing and repair of rotator cuff injuries: a systematic review and meta-analysis. Clin Rehabil. 2017;31(2):158–72.
108. Verhaegen F, Brys P, Debeer P. Rotator cuff healing after needling of a calcific deposit using platelet-rich plasma augmentation: a randomized, prospective clinical trial. J Shoulder Elb Surg. 2016;25(2):169–73.
109. Lin M-T, Wei K-C, Wu C-H. Effectiveness of platelet-rich plasma injection in rotator cuff tendinopathy: a systematic review and meta-analysis of randomized controlled trials. Diagnostics. 2020;10(4):189.
110. Urits I, Smoots D, Franscioni H, Patel A, Fackler N, Wiley S, et al. Injection techniques for common chronic pain conditions of the foot: a comprehensive review. Pain Ther. 2020;9(1):145–60.
111. Kuffler DP. Platelet-rich plasma promotes axon regeneration, wound healing, and pain reduction: fact or fiction. Mol Neurobiol. 2015;52(2):990–1014.
112. Mohammadi S, Nasiri S, Mohammadi MH, Malek Mohammadi A, Nikbakht M, Zahed Panah M, et al. Evaluation of platelet-rich plasma gel potential in acceleration of wound healing duration in patients underwent pilonidal sinus surgery: a randomized controlled parallel clinical trial. Transfus Apher Sci. 2017;56(2):226–32.
113. Deppermann C, Kubes P. Start a fire, kill the bug: the role of platelets in inflammation and infection. Innate Immun. 2018;24(6):335–48.
114. Hara GR, Basu T. Platelet-rich plasma in regenerative medicine. Biomedical Res Ther. 2014;1:5–6.
115. Brill A. Differential role of platelet granular mediators in angiogenesis. Cardiovasc Res. 2004;63(2):226–35.
116. Lansdown DA, Fortier LA. Platelet-rich plasma: formulations, preparations, constituents, and their effects. Oper Tech Sports Med. 2017;25(1):7–12.
117. Richardson TP, Peters MC, Ennett AB, Mooney DJ. Polymeric system for dual growth factor delivery. Nat Biotechnol. 2001;19(11):1029–34.
118. Hernigou P, Homma Y, Flouzat Lachaniette CH, Poignard A, Allain J, Chevallier N, et al. Benefits of small volume and small syringe for bone marrow aspirations of mesenchymal stem cells. Int Orthop. 2013;37(11):2279–87.
119. Oliver K, Awan T, Bayes M. Single- versus multiple-site harvesting techniques for bone marrow concentrate: evaluation of aspirate quality and pain. Orthop J Sports Med. 2017;5(8):232596711772439.
120. McDaniel JS, Antebi B, Pilia M, Hurtgen BJ, Belenkiy S, Necsoiu C, et al. Quantitative assessment of optimal bone marrow site for the isolation of porcine mesenchymal stem cells. Stem Cells Int. 2017;2017:1–10.
121. Bonomo A, Monteiro AC, Gonçalves-Silva T, Cordeiro-Spinetti E, Galvani RG, Balduino A. A T cell view of the bone marrow. Front Immunol [Internet]. 2016 May 17 [cited 2019 Nov 21];7. Available from: http://journal.frontiersin.org/Article/10.3389/fimmu.2016.00184/abstract.
122. Muguruma Y, Yahata T, Miyatake H, Sato T, Uno T, Itoh J, et al. Reconstitution of the functional human hematopoietic microenvironment derived from human mesenchymal stem cells in the murine bone marrow compartment. Blood. 2006;107(5):1878–87.
123. Fliedner TM, Graessle D, Paulsen C, Reimers K. Structure and function of bone marrow hemopoiesis: mechanisms of response to ionizing radiation exposure. Cancer Biother Radiopharm. 2002;17(4):405–26.
124. Rafii S, Lyden D. Therapeutic stem and progenitor cell transplantation for organ vascularization and regeneration. Nat Med. 2003;9(6):11.
125. Spradling A, Drummond-Barbosa D, Kai T. Stem cells find their niche. Nature. 2001;414(6859):98–104.
126. Li L, Xie T. Stem cell niche: structure and function. Annu Rev Cell Biol. 2005;21:605–31.
127. Ehninger A, Trumpp A. The bone marrow stem cell niche grows up: mesenchymal stem cells and macrophages move in. J Exp Med. 2011;208(3):421–8.
128. Wu P, Tarasenko YI, Gu Y, Huang L-YM, Coggeshall RE, Yu Y. Region-specific generation of cholinergic neurons from fetal human neural stem cells grafted in adult rat. Nat Neurosci. 2002;5(12):1271–8.
129. Discher DE, Mooney DJ, Zandstra PW. Growth factors, matrices, and forces combine and control stem cells. Science. 2009;324(5935):1673–7.
130. Becker AJ, McCULLOCH EA, Till JE. Cytological demonstration of the clonal nature of spleen colonies derived from transplanted mouse marrow cells. Nature. 1963;197(4866):452–4.
131. Lee EH, Hui JHP. The potential of stem cells in orthopaedic surgery. J Bone Jt Surg. 2006;88(7):11.
132. Charbord P. Bone marrow mesenchymal stem cells: historical overview and concepts. Hum Gene Ther. 2010;21(9):1045–56.
133. Caplan AI. Mesenchymal stem cells. J Orthop Res. 1991;9(5):641–50.
134. Samsonraj RM, Raghunath M, Nurcombe V, Hui JH, van Wijnen AJ, Cool SM. Concise review: multifaceted characterization of human mesenchymal stem cells for use in regenerative medicine: characterization of human mesenchymal stem cells. Stem Cells Transl Med. 2017;6(12):2173–85.
135. Pittenger MF. Multilineage potential of adult human mesenchymal stem cells. Science. 1999;284(5411):143–7.
136. Krebsbach PH, Kuznetsov SA, Bianco P, Gehron RP. Bone marrow stromal cells: characterization and clinical application. Crit Rev Oral Biol Med. 1999;10(2):165–81.
137. Chotinantakul K, Leeanansaksiri W. Hematopoietic stem cell development, niches, and signaling pathways. Bone Marrow Res. 2012;2012:1–16.
138. A. Everts P. Autologous platelet-rich plasma and mesenchymal stem cells for the treatment of chronic wounds. In: Hakan Dogan K, editor. Wound healing - current perspectives [Internet]. IntechOpen; 2019 [cited 2021 Mar 15]. Available from: https://www.intechopen.com/books/wound-healing-current-perspectives/autologous-platelet-rich-plasma-and-mesenchymal-stem-cells-for-the-treatment-of-chronic-wounds.
139. Pignon B, Sevestre M-A, Kanagaratnam L, Pernod G, Stephan D, Emmerich J, et al. Autologous bone marrow mononuclear cell implantation and its impact on the outcome of patients with critical limb ischemia – results of a randomized, double-blind, placebo-controlled trial. Circ J. 2017;81(11):1713–20.
140. Yancopoulos GD, Davis S, Gale NW, Rudge JS, Wiegand SJ, Holash J. Vascular-specific growth factors and blood vessel formation. Nature. 2000;407(6801):242–8.

141. Patel DM, Shah J, Srivastava AS. Therapeutic potential of mesenchymal stem cells in regenerative medicine. Stem Cells Int. 2013;2013:1–15.
142. Granero-Molto F, Weis JA, Longobardi L, Spagnoli A. Role of mesenchymal stem cells in regenerative medicine: application to bone and cartilage repair. Expert Opin Biol Ther. 2008;8(3):255–68.
143. Kolf CM, Cho E, Tuan RS. Mesenchymal stromal cells biology of adult mesenchymal stem cells: regulation of niche, self-renewal and differentiation. Arthritis Res Ther. 2007;9(1):204.
144. Badiavas EV. Treatment of chronic wounds with bone marrow–derived cells. Arch Dermatol. 2003;139(4):510.
145. da Silva ML, Fontes AM, Covas DT, Caplan AI. Mechanisms involved in the therapeutic properties of mesenchymal stem cells. Cytokine Growth Factor Rev. 2009;20(5–6):419–27.
146. Bashir J, Sherman A, Lee H, Kaplan L, Hare JM. Mesenchymal stem cell therapies in the treatment of musculoskeletal diseases. PM&R. 2014;6(1):61–9.
147. Lee S-H, Erber WN, Porwit A, Tomonaga M, Peterson LC, International Council for Standardization In Hematology. ICSH guidelines for the standardization of bone marrow specimens and reports. Int J Lab Hematol. 2008;30(5):349–64.
148. Scarpone M, Kuebler D, Chambers A, De Filippo CM, Amatuzio M, Ichim TE, et al. Isolation of clinically relevant concentrations of bone marrow mesenchymal stem cells without centrifugation. J Transl Med. 2019;17(1):10.
149. Everts PA, Ferrell J, Mahoney CB, Ii GF, Roman MI, Paul R, et al. A comparative quantification in cellularity of bone marrow aspirated with two new harvesting devices, and the non-equivalent difference between a centrifugated bone marrow concentrate and a bone marrow aspirate as biological injectates, using a bi-lateral patient model. J Stem Cell Res Therapy. 10(461):10.
150. Mautner K, Jerome MA, Easley K, Nanos K, Everts PA. Laboratory quantification of bone marrow concentrate components in unilateral versus bilateral posterior superior iliac spine aspiration. Cell Biol Res Therapy. (466):9.
151. Kunisaki Y, Bruns I, Scheiermann C, Ahmed J, Pinho S, Zhang D, et al. Arteriolar niches maintain haematopoietic stem cell quiescence. Nature. 2013;502(7473):637–43.
152. Marx RE, Tursun R. A qualitative and quantitative analysis of autologous human multipotent adult stem cells derived from three anatomic areas by marrow aspiration: tibia, anterior ilium, and posterior ilium. Int J Oral Maxillofac Implants. 2013;28(5):e290–4.
153. Siclari VA, Zhu J, Akiyama K, Liu F, Zhang X, Chandra A, et al. Mesenchymal progenitors residing close to the bone surface are functionally distinct from those in the central bone marrow. Bone. 2013;53(2):575–86.
154. Yusop N, Battersby P, Alraies A, Sloan AJ, Moseley R, Waddington RJ. Isolation and characterisation of mesenchymal stem cells from rat bone marrow and the endosteal niche: a comparative study. Stem Cells Int. 2018;2018:1–14.
155. Friedlis MF, Centeno CJ. Performing a better bone marrow aspiration. Phys Med Rehabil Clin N Am. 2016;27(4):919–39.
156. Hirahara AM, Panero A, Andersen WJ. An MRI analysis of the pelvis to determine the ideal method for ultrasound-guided bone marrow aspiration from the iliac crest. Am J Orthop Belle Mead NJ [Internet]. 2018;47(5) Available from: https://doi.org/10.12788/ajo.2018.0038.
157. Hernigou J, Alves A, Homma Y, Guissou I, Hernigou P. Anatomy of the ilium for bone marrow aspiration: map of sectors and implication for safe trocar placement. Int Orthop. 2014;38(12):2585–90.
158. Cassatella MA, Mosna F, Micheletti A, Lisi V, Tamassia N, Cont C, et al. Toll-like receptor-3-activated human mesenchymal stromal cells significantly prolong the survival and function of neutrophils. Stem Cells. 2011;29(6):1001–11.
159. Shi Y, Hu G, Su J, Li W, Chen Q, Shou P, et al. Mesenchymal stem cells: a new strategy for immunosuppression and tissue repair. Cell Res. 2010;20(5):510–8.
160. Li W, Ren G, Huang Y, Su J, Han Y, Li J, et al. Mesenchymal stem cells: a double-edged sword in regulating immune responses. Cell Death Differ. 2012;19(9):1505–13.
161. Regmi S, Pathak S, Kim JO, Yong CS, Jeong J-H. Mesenchymal stem cell therapy for the treatment of inflammatory diseases: challenges, opportunities, and future perspectives. Eur J Cell Biol. 2019;98(5–8):151041.
162. Lee JW, Fang X, Krasnodembskaya A, Howard JP, Matthay MA. Concise review: mesenchymal stem cells for acute lung injury: role of paracrine soluble factors. Stem Cells. 2011;29(6):913–9.
163. Giacca M, Zacchigna S. VEGF gene therapy: therapeutic angiogenesis in the clinic and beyond. Gene Ther. 2012;19(6):622–9.
164. Chen L, Tredget EE, Wu PYG, Wu Y. Paracrine factors of mesenchymal stem cells recruit macrophages and endothelial lineage cells and enhance wound healing. Bozza P, editor. PLoS One. 2008;3(4):e1886.
165. Herold J, Kalucka J. Angiogenesis in adipose tissue: the interplay between adipose and endothelial cells. Front Physiol. 2021;11:624903.
166. Timmers L, Lim SK, Hoefer IE, Arslan F, Lai RC, van Oorschot AAM, et al. Human mesenchymal stem cell-conditioned medium improves cardiac function following myocardial infarction. Stem Cell Res. 2011;6(3):206–14.
167. Morita Y, Ema H, Nakauchi H. Heterogeneity and hierarchy within the most primitive hematopoietic stem cell compartment. J Exp Med. 2010;207(6):1173–82.
168. Caplan AI, Dennis JE. Mesenchymal stem cells as trophic mediators. J Cell Biochem. 2006;98(5):1076–84.
169. Dabrowska S, Andrzejewska A, Janowski M, Lukomska B. Immunomodulatory and regenerative effects of mesenchymal stem cells and extracellular vesicles: therapeutic outlook for inflammatory and degenerative diseases. Front Immunol. 2021;11:591065.
170. King A, Balaji S, Keswani SG, Crombleholme TM. The role of stem cells in wound angiogenesis. Adv Wound Care. 2014;3(10):614–25.
171. Kim J-D, Lee GW, Jung GH, Kim CK, Kim T, Park JH, et al. Clinical outcome of autologous bone marrow aspirates concentrate (BMAC) injection in degenerative arthritis of the knee. Eur J Orthop Surg Traumatol. 2014;24(8):1505–11.
172. Hernigou P, Flouzat-Lachaniette C-H, Delambre J, Poignard A, Allain J, Chevallier N, et al. Osteonecrosis repair with bone marrow cell therapies: state of the clinical art. Bone. 2015;70:102–9.
173. Darrow M, Shaw B, Schmidt N, Boeger G, Budgett S. Treatment of shoulder osteoarthritis and rotator cuff tears with bone marrow concentrate and whole bone marrow injections. Schumacher U, editor. Cogent Med [Internet]. 2019 Jun 18 [cited 2019 Dec 11];6(1). Available from: https://www.cogentoa.com/article/10.1080/2331205X.2019.1628883.
174. Hernigou P, Daltro G, Hernigou J. Hip osteonecrosis: stem cells for life or behead and arthroplasty? Int Orthop. 2018;42(7):1425–8.
175. Tabatabaee RM, Saberi S, Parvizi J, Mortazavi SMJ, Farzan M. Combining concentrated autologous bone marrow stem cells injection with core decompression improves outcome for patients with early-stage osteonecrosis of the femoral head: a comparative study. J Arthroplast. 2015;30(9 Suppl):11–5.
176. Pepke W, Kasten P, Beckmann N, Janicki P, Egermann M. Core decompression and autologous bone marrow concentrate for treatment of femoral head osteonecrosis: a randomized prospective study. Orthop Rev [Internet]. 2016; Mar 21 [cited 2019 Dec 11];8(1). Available from: http://www.pagepress.org/journals/index.php/or/article/view/6162

177. Awad ME, Hussein KA, Helwa I, Abdelsamid MF, Aguilar-Perez A, Mohsen I, et al. Meta-analysis and evidence base for the efficacy of autologous bone marrow mesenchymal stem cells in knee cartilage repair: methodological guidelines and quality assessment. Stem Cells Int. 2019;2019:1–15.
178. Lim MH, Ong WK, Sugii S. The current landscape of adipose-derived stem cells in clinical applications. Expert Rev Mol Med. 2014;16. e8-undefined.
179. Argentati C, Morena F, Bazzucchi M, Armentano I, Emiliani C, Martino S. Adipose stem cell translational applications: from bench-to-bedside. Int J Mol Sci. 2018;19(11):3475.
180. Andrzejewska A, Lukomska B, Janowski M. Concise review: mesenchymal stem cells: from roots to boost: MSCs: from roots to boost. Stem Cells. 2019;37(7):855–64.
181. Karastergiou K, Mohamed-Ali V. The autocrine and paracrine roles of adipokines. Mol Cell Endocrinol. 2010;318(1–2):69–78.
182. Cinti S. Reversible physiological transdifferentiation in the adipose organ. Proc Nutr Soc. 2009;68(4):340–9.
183. Zuk PA, Zhu M, Ashjian P, Ugarte DAD, Huang JI, Mizuno H, et al. Human adipose tissue is a source of multipotent stem cells. Mol Biol Cell. 2002;13:17.
184. Zuk PA. The adipose-derived stem cell: looking back and looking ahead. Kellogg D, editor. Mol Biol Cell. 2010;21(11):1783–7.
185. Yang HJ, Kim K-J, Kim MK, Lee SJ, Ryu YH, Seo BF, et al. The stem cell potential and multipotency of human adipose tissue-derived stem cells vary by cell donor and are different from those of other types of stem cells. Cells Tissues Organs. 2014;199(5–6):373–83.
186. Wagner SJ, Leiby DA, Roback JD. Existing and emerging blood-borne pathogens: impact on the safety of blood transfusion for the hematology/oncology patient. Hematol Clin. 2019;33(5):739–48.
187. Baer PC. Adipose-derived mesenchymal stromal/stem cells: an update on their phenotype in vivo and in vitro. World J Stem Cells. 2014;6(3):256.
188. Dmitrieva RI, Minullina IR, Bilibina AA, Tarasova OV, Anisimov SV, Zaritskey AY. Bone marrow- and subcutaneous adipose tissue-derived mesenchymal stem cells: differences and similarities. Cell Cycle. 2012;11(2):377–83.
189. Miranville A, Heeschen C, Sengenès C, Curat CA, Busse R, Bouloumié A. Improvement of postnatal neovascularization by human adipose tissue-derived stem cells. Circulation. 2004;110(3):349–55.
190. Fraser JK, Wulur I, Alfonso Z, Hedrick MH. Fat tissue: an underappreciated source of stem cells for biotechnology. Trends Biotechnol. 2006;24(4):150–4.
191. Yun S, Ku S-K, Kwon Y-S. Adipose-derived mesenchymal stem cells and platelet-rich plasma synergistically ameliorate the surgical-induced osteoarthritis in Beagle dogs. J Orthop Surg. 2016;11(1):9.
192. Gonzalez-Rey E, Gonzalez MA, Varela N, O'Valle F, Hernandez-Cortes P, Rico L, et al. Human adipose-derived mesenchymal stem cells reduce inflammatory and T cell responses and induce regulatory T cells in vitro in rheumatoid arthritis. Ann Rheum Dis. 2010;69(01):241–8.
193. Kim E, Kim W, Oh K-J, Han B, Lee S, Bae K-H. Recent advances in proteomic studies of adipose tissues and adipocytes. Int J Mol Sci. 2015;16(3):4581–99.
194. Zimmerlin L, Park TS, Zambidis ET, Donnenberg VS, Donnenberg AD. Mesenchymal stem cell secretome and regenerative therapy after cancer. Biochimie. 2013;95(12):2235–45.
195. Coelho M, Oliveira T, Fernandes R. State of the art paper biochemistry of adipose tissue: an endocrine organ. Arch Med Sci. 2013;2:191–200.
196. Brown JC, Shang H, Li Y, Yang N, Patel N, Katz AJ. Isolation of adipose-derived stromal vascular fraction cells using a novel point-of-care device: cell characterization and review of the literature. Tissue Eng Part C Methods. 2017;23(3):125–35.
197. Gimble JM, Katz AJ, Bunnell BA. Adipose-derived stem cells for regenerative medicine. Circ Res. 2007;100(9):1249–60.
198. Gentile P, Calabrese C, De Angelis B, Pizzicannella J, Kothari A, Garcovich S. Impact of the different preparation methods to obtain human adipose-derived stromal vascular fraction cells (AD-SVFs) and human adipose-derived mesenchymal stem cells (AD-MSCs): enzymatic digestion versus mechanical centrifugation. Int J Mol Sci. 2019;20(21):5471.
199. Bora P, Majumdar AS. Adipose tissue-derived stromal vascular fraction in regenerative medicine: a brief review on biology and translation. Stem Cell Res Ther. 2017;8(1):145.
200. Sugii S, Kida Y, Berggren WT, Evans RM. Feeder-dependent and feeder-independent iPS cell derivation from human and mouse adipose stem cells. Nat Protoc. 2011;6(3):346–58.
201. Varma MJO, Breuls RGM, Schouten TE, Jurgens WJFM, Bontkes HJ, Schuurhuis GJ, et al. Phenotypical and functional characterization of freshly isolated adipose tissue-derived stem cells. Stem Cells Dev. 2007;16(1):91–104.
202. Tonnard P, Verpaele A, Peeters G, Hamdi M, Cornelissen M, Declercq H. Nanofat grafting: basic research and clinical applications. Plast Reconstr Surg. 2013;132(4):1017–26.
203. Bianchi F, Maioli M, Leonardi E, Olivi E, Pasquinelli G, Valente S, et al. A new nonenzymatic method and device to obtain a fat tissue derivative highly enriched in pericyte-like elements by mild mechanical forces from human lipoaspirates. Cell Transplant. 2013;22(11):2063–77.
204. Ong WK, Sugii S. Adipose-derived stem cells: fatty potentials for therapy. Int J Biochem Cell Biol. 2013;45(6):1083–6.
205. Hao T, Chen J, Zhi S, Zhang Q, Chen G, Yu F. Comparison of bone marrow-vs. adipose tissue-derived mesenchymal stem cells for attenuating liver fibrosis. Exp Ther Med [Internet]. 2017 Oct 18 [cited 2021 Nov 2]; Available from: http://www.spandidos--publications.com/10.3892/etm.2017.5333.
206. Pendleton C, Li Q, Chesler DA, Yuan K, Guerrero-Cazares H, Quinones-Hinojosa A. Mesenchymal stem cells derived from adipose tissue vs bone marrow: in vitro comparison of their tropism towards gliomas. Najbauer J, editor. PLoS One. 2013;8(3):e58198.
207. Puissant B, Barreau C, Bourin P, Clavel C, Corre J, Bousquet C, et al. Immunomodulatory effect of human adipose tissue-derived adult stem cells: comparison with bone marrow mesenchymal stem cells. Br J Haematol. 2005;129(1):118–29.
208. Fang Y, Zhang Y, Zhou J, Cao K. Adipose-derived mesenchymal stem cell exosomes: a novel pathway for tissues repair. Cell Tissue Bank. 2019;20(2):153–61.
209. Braga Osorio Gomes Salgado AJ, Goncalves Reis RL, Jorge Carvalho Sousa N, Gimble JM, Salgado AJ, Reis RL, et al. Adipose tissue derived stem cells secretome: soluble factors and their roles in regenerative medicine. Curr Stem Cell Res Ther. 2010;5(2):103–10.
210. Naik S, Larsen SB, Cowley CJ, Fuchs E. Two to tango: dialog between immunity and stem cells in health and disease. Cell. 2018;175(4):908–20.
211. Mitchell R, Mellows B, Sheard J, Antonioli M, Kretz O, Chambers D, et al. Secretome of adipose-derived mesenchymal stem cells promotes skeletal muscle regeneration through synergistic action of extracellular vesicle cargo and soluble proteins. Stem Cell Res Ther. 2019;10(1):116.
212. Wang K, Yu L-Y, Jiang L-Y, Wang H-B, Wang C-Y, Luo Y. The paracrine effects of adipose-derived stem cells on neovascularization and biocompatibility of a macroencapsulation device. Acta Biomater. 2015;15:65–76.
213. Sorop O, Olver TD, van de Wouw J, Heinonen I, van Duin RW, Duncker DJ, et al. The microcirculation: a key player in

obesity-associated cardiovascular disease. Cardiovasc Res. 2017;113(9):1035–45.
214. Tran K-V, Gealekman O, Frontini A, Zingaretti MC, Morroni M, Giordano A, et al. The vascular endothelium of the adipose tissue gives rise to both white and brown fat cells. Cell Metab. 2012;15(2):222–9.
215. Planat-Benard V, Silvestre J-S, Cousin B, André M, Nibbelink M, Tamarat R, et al. Plasticity of human adipose lineage cells toward endothelial cells: physiological and therapeutic perspectives. Circulation. 2004;109(5):656–63.
216. Koh YJ, Koh BI, Kim H, Joo HJ, Jin HK, Jeon J, et al. Stromal vascular fraction from adipose tissue forms profound vascular network through the dynamic reassembly of blood endothelial cells. Arterioscler Thromb Vasc Biol. 2011;31(5):1141–50.
217. Rehman J, Traktuev D, Li J, Merfeld-Clauss S, Temm-Grove CJ, Bovenkerk JE, et al. Secretion of angiogenic and anti-apoptotic factors by human adipose stromal cells. Circulation. 2004;109(10):1292–8.
218. Bosman FT, Stamenkovic I. Functional structure and composition of the extracellular matrix: structure and composition of the extracellular matrix. J Pathol. 2003;200(4):423–8.
219. Bauer AL, Jackson TL, Jiang Y. Topography of extracellular matrix mediates vascular morphogenesis and migration speeds in angiogenesis. Czirók A, editor. PLoS Comput Biol. 2009;5(7):e1000445.
220. Docheva D, Müller SA, Majewski M, Evans CH. Biologics for tendon repair. Adv Drug Deliv Rev. 2015;84:222–39.
221. Narayanan AS, Page RC, Swanson J. Collagen synthesis by human fibroblasts. Biochem J. 1989;260:7.
222. Newman AC, Nakatsu MN, Chou W, Gershon PD, Hughes CCW. The requirement for fibroblasts in angiogenesis: fibroblast-derived matrix proteins are essential for endothelial cell lumen formation. Adams JC, editor. Mol Biol Cell. 2011;22(20):3791–800.
223. Bourin P, Bunnell BA, Casteilla L, Dominici M, Katz AJ, March KL, et al. Stromal cells from the adipose tissue-derived stromal vascular fraction and culture expanded adipose tissue-derived stromal/stem cells: a joint statement of the International Federation for Adipose Therapeutics and Science (IFATS) and the International Society for Cellular Therapy (ISCT). Cytotherapy. 2013;15(6):641–8.
224. Simonacci F, Bertozzi N, Grieco MP, Raposio E. From liposuction to adipose-derived stem cells: indications and technique. Acta Bio Medica Atenei Parm. 2019;90(2):197–208.
225. Berry M, Davies D. Liposuction: a review of principles and techniques. J Plast Reconstr Amp Aesthetic Surg JPRAS. 2011;64(8):985–92.
226. Illouz Y. Body contouring by lipolysis: a 5-year experience with over 3000 cases. Plast Reconstr Surg. 1983;72(5):591–7.
227. Klein JA. The tumescent technique: anesthesia and modified liposuction technique. Dermatol Clin. 1990;8(3):425–37.
228. Coleman SR. Structural fat grafting: more than a permanent filler. Plast Reconstr Surg. 2006;118(Suppl):108S–20S.
229. Kurita M, Matsumoto D, Shigeura T, Sato K, Gonda K, Harii K, et al. Influences of centrifugation on cells and tissues in liposuction aspirates: optimized centrifugation for lipotransfer and cell isolation. Plast Reconstr Surg. 2008;121(3):1033–41.
230. Oedayrajsingh-Varma MJ, van Ham SM, Knippenberg M, Helder MN, Klein-Nulend J, Schouten TE, et al. Adipose tissue-derived mesenchymal stem cell yield and growth characteristics are affected by the tissue-harvesting procedure. Cytotherapy. 2006;8(2):166–77.
231. Farré-Guasch E, Martí-Pagès C, Hernández-Alfaro F, Klein-Nulend J, Casals N. Buccal fat pad, an oral access source of human adipose stem cells with potential for osteochondral tissue engineering: an *in vitro* study. Tissue Eng Part C Methods. 2010;16(5):1083–94.
232. Iyyanki T, Hubenak J, Liu J, Chang EI, Beahm EK, Zhang Q. Harvesting technique affects adipose-derived stem cell yield. Aesthet Surg J. 2015;35(4):467–76.
233. Huang S-J, Fu R-H, Shyu W-C, Liu S-P, Jong G-P, Chiu Y-W, et al. Adipose-derived stem cells: isolation, characterization, and differentiation potential. Cell Transplant. 2013;22(4):701–9.
234. De Ugarte DA, Morizono K, Elbarbary A, Alfonso Z, Zuk PA, Zhu M, et al. Comparison of multi-lineage cells from human adipose tissue and bone marrow. Cells Tissues Organs. 2003;174(3):101–9.
235. Klar AS, Zimoch J, Biedermann T. Skin tissue engineering: application of adipose-derived stem cells. BioMed Res Int. 2017;2017:1–12.
236. Phinney DG, Kopen G, Righter W, Webster S, Tremain N, Prockop DJ. Donor variation in the growth properties and osteogenic potential of human marrow stromal cells. J Cell Biochem. 1999;75(3):424–36.
237. Guneta V, Tan NS, Chan SKJ, Tanavde V, Lim TC, Wong TCM, et al. Comparative study of adipose-derived stem cells and bone marrow-derived stem cells in similar microenvironmental conditions. Exp Cell Res. 2016;348(2):155–64.
238. Woo D-H, Hwang HS, Shim JH. Comparison of adult stem cells derived from multiple stem cell niches. Biotechnol Lett. 2016;38(5):751–9.
239. Dimitriou R, Mataliotakis GI, Angoules AG, Kanakaris NK, Giannoudis PV. Complications following autologous bone graft harvesting from the iliac crest and using the RIA: a systematic review. Injury. 2011;42:S3–15.

Index

© The Editor(s) (if applicable) and The Author(s), under exclusive license to Springer Nature Switzerland AG 2022
S. A. Mostoufi et al. (eds.), *Clinical Guide to Musculoskeletal Medicine*, https://doi.org/10.1007/978-3-030-92042-5

D

M

N

O

Q

U

MIX
Papier aus verantwortungsvollen Quellen
Paper from responsible sources
FSC® C105338

If you have any concerns about our products,
you can contact us on
ProductSafety@springernature.com

In case Publisher is established outside the EU,
the EU authorized representative is:
Springer Nature Customer Service Center GmbH
Europaplatz 3, 69115 Heidelberg, Germany

Printed by Libri Plureos GmbH
in Hamburg, Germany